D0724716

ADA/PDR Guide to

DENTAL THERAPEUTICS

Fifth Edition

ADA American Dental Association®
America's leading advocate for oral health

ADA/PDR Guide to

DENTAL THERAPEUTICS

Fifth Edition

ADA American Dental Association®
America's leading advocate for oral health
211 East Chicago Avenue, Chicago, Illinois 60611
T 312.440.2500 F 312.440.7494 www.ada.org

PDR Publishing Staff

Senior Director, Editorial & Publishing: Bette Kennedy
Senior Director, Client Services: Stephanie Struble
Director, Clinical Services: Sylvia Nashed, PharmD
Manager, Editorial Services: Lori Murray
Manager, Clinical Services: Nermin Shenouda, PharmD
Clinical Editor: Christine Sunwoo, PharmD
Contributing Clinical Editor: Majid Kerolous, PharmD
Drug Information Specialist: Anila Patel, PharmD
Project Managers: Deana DiVizio, Gary Lew
Associate Editor: Jennifer Reed
Contributing Editor: Kathleen Engel
Index Editor: Caryn Sobel
Manager, Art Department: Livio Udina
Electronic Publishing Designer: Carrie Spinelli Faeth
Manager, Production Purchasing: Thomas Westburgh
Senior Print Production Manager: Dawn Dubovich
Senior Promotion Manager: Linda Levine

Physicians' Desk Reference

Executive Vice President: Thomas Rice
Vice President, Product Management: Cy Caine
Vice President, Publishing & Operations: Valerie Berger
Vice President, Clinical Relations: Mukesh Mehta, RPh
Vice President, Strategy & Business Development: Ray Zoeller
Vice President, Finance: Donna Santarpia
Senior Director, Copy Sales: Bill Gaffney
Senior Product Manager: Richard Buchwald

DISCLAIMER

The American Dental Association (ADA) and Physicians' Desk Reference Inc. (together the "Publishers") publish and present this book to you. The editor and authors of the *ADA/PDR Guide to Dental Therapeutics* have used care to confirm that the drugs and treatment schedules set forth in this book are in accordance with current recommendations and practice at the time of publication. This guide does not, however, constitute policy of the ADA, establish a standard of care or restrict a dentist's exercise of professional judgment. As the science of dental therapeutics evolves, changes in drug treatment and use become necessary. The ADA was not involved in the preparation of the drug information. The reader is advised to consult the package insert for each drug to consider and adopt all safety precautions before use, particularly with new and infrequently used drugs. The reader is responsible for ascertaining the U.S. Food and Drug Administration clearance of each drug and device used in his or her practice.

The treatment and pharmacotherapy discussed in this book should be undertaken only within the bounds of applicable federal and state laws, including those pertaining to privacy and confidentiality, such as the Health Insurance Portability and Accountability Act and similar state laws. This book does not provide legal advice, and readers must consult with their own attorneys for such advice.

The Publishers, editor, and authors disclaim all responsibility for any liability, loss, injury or damage resulting directly or indirectly from the reader's use and application of the information in this book and make no representations or warranties with respect to such information, including the products described herein.

The Publishers, editor, and authors have produced this book in their individual capacities and not on behalf or in the interest of any pharmaceutical companies or state or federal agencies. Many of the proprietary names of the products listed in this book are trademarked and registered in the U.S. Patent Office. It should be understood that by making this material available, the Publishers are not advocating the use of any product described herein, nor are the Publishers responsible for misuse of a product due to typographical error. Additional information on any product may be obtained from the manufacturer.

Copyright © 2009 American Dental Association and Physicians' Desk Reference Inc. Published by Physicians' Desk Reference Inc., Montvale, NJ. All rights reserved. No part of this publication may be reproduced or transmitted, in any form or by any means, electronic or mechanical, including photocopying, recording, information storage and retrieval system, or otherwise, without the prior written permission of Physicians' Desk Reference Inc. American Dental Association®, Physicians' Desk Reference®, and PDR® are registered trademarks used herein under license of their respective owners.

ISBN: 978-1-56363-769-8 P064

EDITORIAL BOARD

EDITOR

Sebastian G. Ciancio, D.D.S.
Distinguished Service Professor and Chair
Department of Periodontics and Endodontics
Adjunct Professor of Pharmacology
Director, Center for Dental Studies
University at Buffalo
State University of New York
Buffalo, New York

AUTHORS

Jennifer P. Bassiur, D.D.S.
Director, The Center for Oral, Facial and Head Pain
Assistant Professor of Clinical Dentistry
Division of Oral and Maxillofacial Surgery
College of Dental Medicine
Columbia University
New York, New York

Barry C. Boyd, D.M.D., M.D.
Clinical Associate Professor
Department of Oral and Maxillofacial Surgery
University at Buffalo
State University of New York
Buffalo, New York

Kenneth H. Burrell, D.D.S., S.M.
President
Burrell Consulting, Inc.
Lisle, Illinois
Former Senior Director
Council on Scientific Affairs
American Dental Association
Chicago, Illinois

B. Ellen Byrne, D.D.S., Ph.D.
Associate Professor
Department of Endodontics
School of Dentistry
Medical College of Virginia
Virginia Commonwealth University
Richmond, Virginia

James Fricton, D.D.S., M.S.
Professor
Division of TMD and Orofacial Pain
Department of Diagnostic and Biological Sciences
School of Dentistry
Fellow, Institute for Health Informatics
University of Minnesota
Minneapolis, Minnesota

Adriane Fugh-Berman, M.D.
Associate Professor
Complementary and Alternative Medicine Masters Program
Department of Physiology and Biophysics
Georgetown University Medical Center
Washington, D.C.

Steven Ganzberg, D.M.D., M.S.
Professor of Clinical Anesthesiology
College of Dentistry
College of Medicine & Public Health
Dental Anesthesiology Residency Program Director
The Ohio State University
Columbus, Ohio

Martin S. Greenberg, D.D.S.
Professor and Chair, Oral Medicine
Associate Dean, Hospital Affairs
University of Pennsylvania School of Dental Medicine
Philadelphia, Pennsylvania

Richard E. Hall, D.D.S., M.D., Ph.D., F.A.C.S.
Professor and Chairman
Department of Oral and Maxillofacial Surgery
University at Buffalo
State University of New York
Buffalo, New York

Alan M. Kramer, M.D.
Clinical Associate Professor of Medicine
University of California, San Francisco
San Francisco, California

Angelo J. Mariotti, D.D.S., Ph.D.
Professor and Chair
Section of Periodontology
College of Dentistry
The Ohio State University
Columbus, Ohio

Frederick McIntyre, D.D.S., M.S.
Clinical Professor Emeritus of Restorative Dentistry
University at Buffalo
State University of New York
Staff prosthodontist
VA Medical Center
Buffalo, New York

Robert L. Merrill, D.D.S., M.S.
Adjunct Professor
Section of Oral Medicine and Orofacial Pain
Director, Orofacial Pain and Dental Sleep Medicine
Graduate Program
UCLA School of Dentistry
Los Angeles, California

Brian C. Muzyka, D.M.D., M.S., M.B.A.
Associate Professor of Family Medicine
Brody School of Medicine
East Carolina University
Greenville, North Carolina

Lida Radfar, D.D.S., M.S.
Diplomate, American Board of Oral Medicine
Associate Professor of Oral Medicine
Oral Diagnosis and Radiology Department
University of Oklahoma College of Dentistry
Oklahoma City, Oklahoma

Maria Salnik, M.S., D.D.S. candidate
D.D.S. Candidate Research Assistant
Complementary and Alternative Medicine Masters Program
Department of Physiology and Biophysics
Georgetown University
Washington, D.C.

Luciana M. Shaddox, D.D.S., Ph.D.
Assistant Professor
Department of Periodontology
College of Dentistry
University of Florida
Gainesville, Florida

Sol Silverman Jr., D.D.S., M.A
Professor of Oral Medicine
University of California, San Francisco
School of Dentistry
San Francisco, California

Martha Somerman, D.D.S., Ph.D.
Dean and Professor of Periodontics
University of Washington
School of Dentistry
Seattle, Washington

Eric T. Stoopler, D.M.D.
Assistant Professor of Oral Medicine
Director, Oral Medicine Residency Program
University of Pennsylvania School of Dental Medicine
Philadelphia, Pennsylvania

Lakshmanan Suresh, D.D.S., M.S.
Assistant Director of Oral Pathology and Immunopathology
IMMCO Diagnostics, Inc.
Buffalo, New York

Leonard S. Tibbetts, D.D.S., M.S.D.
Private Practitioner
Arlington, Texas
Visiting Assistant Professor of Periodontics
University of Washington
Seattle, Washington

Clay Walker, Ph.D.
Professor of Oral Biology
Department of Oral Biology and Periodontal
Disease Research Clinics
College of Dentistry
University of Florida
Gainesville, Florida

John A. Yagiela, D.D.S., Ph.D.
Professor and Chair
Division of Diagnostic and Surgical Sciences
School of Dentistry
Professor, Department of Anesthesiology
School of Medicine
University of California, Los Angeles
Los Angeles, California

TABLE OF CONTENTS

FOREWORD

Dentists are prescribing more medications today than ever before. In view of our aging and mobile population, patients seeking dental care are using a wide range of medications for medical problems. And both dentists and patients have choices to make about the variety of nonprescription products available for treating various disorders of the mouth.

Dentists have expressed their need for a quick and accurate drug reference that is more than a dictionary and yet not a textbook of pharmacology. In response, the ADA published the first edition of the *ADA Guide to Dental Therapeutics* in 1998. The guide was based on what dentists in focus groups told us they needed to make their practices complete: concise and accurate information about the medications they use, information based on the science of pharmacology and organized by drug category in an easy-to-use tabular format. This fifth edition continues the collaboration of the ADA and the *Physicians' Desk Reference®* (*PDR*), making it the most comprehensive dental drug reference of its kind—the only one complete enough to bear both the ADA and PDR names.

For this latest edition, every chapter and table containing pertinent chairside information has been updated.

As a practical chairside resource, the guide offers easy access to crucial information about the drugs prescribed for and taken by dental patients—nearly 1,000 generic drugs and 3,000 brand-name drugs in all. Every practicing dentist, dental educator, dental student, and member of the dental team can profit from using this book. In addition, it serves as a useful resource in preparing for various board examinations.

A major strength of this book is that it was written by both academicians and clinicians in a team approach. Writers were selected because of their expertise and reputations in dental therapeutics. The content is as up-to-the minute as possible and is scheduled to be updated every three years. Readers and reviewers of earlier editions gave us their comments, many of which were incorporated into this fifth edition. I encourage you to send us your comments so that the sixth edition can grow even more than the fifth.

This edition identifies nonprescription products that carry the ADA Seal of Acceptance. This Seal is designed to help the public and dental professionals make informed decisions about dental products. The Seal provides an assurance that all products have met the ADA's standards of efficacy, safety and truth in advertising. Knowing which products carry the ADA Seal will enable all members of the dental team to select professional products knowledgeably and to discuss various toothpastes, mouthrinses, and other nonprescription medications with their patients.

KEY FEATURES

The guide is unlike any other drug information reference available, offering a host of benefits to the practicing dentist:

- clear, well-organized tables that offer rapid access to information on more than 900 drugs used in dentistry, including therapeutic products that carry the ADA Seal of Acceptance;
- crucial data on dosage, interactions, precautions, and adverse effects at the reader's fingertips;
- brief but informative descriptions of drug categories that bridge the gap between drug handbooks and pharmacology texts;
- information on more than 3,000 drugs used in medicine, enabling dentists to communicate knowledgeably with other medical professionals about patients' medications and their dental side effects;
- an evidence-based overview of herbs and dietary supplements;
- a one-of-a-kind chapter on oral manifestations of systemic agents;
- an appendix on drugs that cause photosensitivity;
- other appendices covering drug-related issues that affect dental practice: substance abuse, tobacco-use cessation, infection control, and many others;
- suggested reading lists at the end of each chapter for practitioners who want additional information.

DRUGS USED IN DENTISTRY

This book is arranged in three sections. The first focuses on drugs prescribed primarily by dentists, so that the practitioner can readily prescribe them with a full understanding of their actions, adverse effects, and interactions. It contains drug information essential to solving patients' dental problems. Dentists will be able to quickly locate dosages and information of clinical significance (interactions, adverse effects, precautions, and contraindications). Drugs and products that have received the ADA Seal of Acceptance are identified with a star ★.

In Section I, each chapter is organized by:

- description of the general category of drugs and the accepted indications;
- special dental considerations—drug interactions, pertinent laboratory value alterations, drug cross-sensitivities, and effects on pregnant and nursing women, children, elderly patients, and other patients with special needs;
- adverse effects and precautions, arranged by drug class or body system;
- pharmacology;
- information for patient/family consultation.
- tables with specific drugs by generic and brand name—including adult and child dosages, forms, and strengths.

If any of these categories or subcategories does not appear (for instance, laboratory value alterations), it is because it did not pertain to the particular type of drug or because there was no such information available.

In each chapter in Section I, the prescribing information table (which appears at the end of the chapter text) is based on the assumption that the dentist has determined—through taking a health history and interviewing the patient—that the patient is in general good health and is not taking any medications that may interact with the drug in question. For quick reference, drug interactions are detailed in a separate table that also appears at the end of each chapter.

This book includes all ADA-accepted products in the various categories discussed. However, in some cases we have included only a representative sampling of products in a category—ADA-accepted or not. Inclusion of a particular product in no way indicates that it is superior to others.

DRUGS USED IN MEDICINE

Increasingly, dental patients are taking one or more prescription drugs. To assist the dentist, the second section of the book focuses on drugs prescribed primarily by physicians. It presents drug information in a more abbreviated form, emphasizing each drug's effect on dental diagnosis and treatment planning. The information here will help the dentist interact effectively with the patient's physician about the patient's medications, particularly when a modification of drug therapy is in question. Helpful dosage ranges enable dentists to anticipate potential side effects in patients at the upper end of the dosage range.

DRUG ISSUES IN DENTAL PRACTICE

The book's third section focuses on issues related to dental pharmacology that affect the dentist's practice, including legal considerations of using drugs in dentistry and information on herbs and dietary supplements. As part of the community of practitioners interested in patients as people and not just as "teeth and gums," dentists can use the information discussed here as building blocks for a successful and expanding practice. A highlight of this section is the chapter on oral manifestations of systemic medications. The topics presented in Section III are not addressed in most dental drug handbooks.

APPENDICES AND INDEX

The book features several appendices covering a broad range of topics, including a section on bisphosphonate-associated osteonecrosis of the jaw. The comprehensive index at the back of the book is designed to help you find information quickly and easily.

ACKNOWLEDGMENTS

I wish to acknowledge the pioneering efforts of contributors to the ADA's *Accepted Dental Therapeutics* (which ceased publication in 1984), who laid the foundation for this book. I also wish to thank the authors, who applied their time and their broad talents generously to this task. I am grateful to my dean, Richard N. Buchanan, D.M.D., and to my wife, Marilyn, both of whom gave me the time and support needed to serve as editor. The authors and I would also like to thank Dr. John S. Findley, president of the ADA, and Dr. William R. Calnon, ADA trustee for my district. Finally, a special thanks is due to Carolyn B. Tatar, Senior Manager of Product Development and Management at the ADA, and to my staff for helping me through the months of preparation; and especially to Lori Murray, Bette Kennedy, Bill Gaffney, and Mike Bennett of PDR for their patience, persistence, and devotion to excellence. The combined efforts of these people as well as our chapter authors helped make this a dental therapeutics book of true distinction.

Sebastian G. Ciancio, D.D.S.
University at Buffalo
State University of New York

August 2009

HOW TO USE THIS BOOK

The fifth edition of the *ADA/PDR Guide to Dental Therapeutics* features a table format designed to help you find the information you need as quickly and easily as possible. Book chapters are divided into three parts, allowing you to go directly to a particular therapeutic category:

I. **Drugs Used in Dentistry**
II. **Drugs Used in Medicine: Treatment and Pharmacological Considerations for Dental Patients Receiving Medical Care**
III. **Drug Issues in Dental Practice**

Chapter text is organized by drug or product class. Each section includes general pharmacological information and special dental considerations. References and suggested reading are given at the end of each section or chapter, where applicable.

Drug tables are organized by therapeutic drug class. Within each class, products are listed alphabetically. **For ease of use, all tables are located at the end of each chapter.** For definitions of the abbreviations used in these tables, see the key at the end of this discussion.

Tables with prescribing information appear first and give pertinent details on the following:

- **Generic name:** Listed in bold, with brand names appearing in parentheses. Controlled substances are marked with their corresponding classification (eg, CII) after the drug name. Appendix A gives definitions of these classifications. In addition, products bearing the ADA Seal of Acceptance are marked with a star (★) after the name.
- **Drug forms and strengths:** Indicates whether the drug comes as a tablet, capsule, injection, etc. Scored tablets are noted with an asterisk.
- **Dosage:** Highlights adult and pediatric dosages in bold italics. Dosages are arranged according to each drug's indication, shown in bold type. Special dosing considerations—maximum dose, titration, dosage reductions for special patient groups—are also highlighted in bold.
- **Warnings/precautions and contraindications:** Lists crucial warnings and precautions (denoted with **W/P**), followed by contraindications (denoted with **Contra**) and pregnancy/nursing information (denoted with **P/N**). Pregnancy categories (eg, Category C) are defined in Appendix B. Where applicable, "black box" warnings—that is, those that require special vigilance—are listed first and denoted with **BB**.
- **Adverse effects:** Lists the most common side effects occurring in ≥3% of patients as noted in the manufacturer's package insert. Dental-related side effects are noted in bold.

Tables with drug interactions appear after the prescribing information. These are also organized alphabetically by therapeutic class and generic name. Please keep in mind that the chance of an interaction varies among patients, and that previously undocumented drug interactions are always a possibility.

Other pharmacological tables are also included at the end of each chapter as necessary. These may include overall class definitions or special dental-related information.

Prescribing information for drug entries provided by *PDR* is drawn from FDA-approved product labeling as published in *Physicians' Desk Reference®* or supplied by the manufacturer. The entries are compiled and updated on a regular basis by a staff of experienced pharmacists. While diligent efforts have been made to ensure the accuracy of each entry, it is essential to bear in mind that the information presented here is merely a synopsis of key points in the official labeling, and that the complete labeling contains additional precautionary information that may be of significance in specific cases. Similarly, please remember that only common and dangerous adverse reactions and interactions are included here, and that numerous less-prevalent adverse effects may be reported in the complete labeling. If an entry leaves any question unanswered, be sure to consult *Physicians' Desk Reference* or the manufacturer for additional information.

APPENDICES AND INDEX

These appear at the end of the book. Appendix topics are outlined in the Table of Contents. The comprehensive alphabetical Index contains all brand and generic names as well as general subject and chapter entries. Information appearing in a table is denoted with a "t" after the page number. Products with the ADA Seal are denoted with a star (★).

KEY TO ABBREVIATIONS USED IN THIS BOOK

ac	before meals
ACEI	angiotensin-converting enzyme inhibitor
ACTH	adrenocorticotropan hormone
ADHD	attention deficit hyperactivity disorder
AED	anti-epileptic drug
ANC	absolute neutrophil count
ARB	angiotensin II receptor blocker
AS	ankylosing spondylitis
ASA	acetylsalicylic acid (aspirin)
AST	aspartate aminotransferase
AUC	area under the concentration-time curve
BB	black box warning
bid	twice a day
BMD	bone mineral density
BMT	bone marrow transplantation
BP	blood pressure
BPH	benign prostatic hyperplasia
BUN	blood urea nitrogen
BZD	benzodiazepine
CAD	coronary artery disease
cap	capsule
CAPD	continuous ambulatory peritoneal dialysis
CBC	complete blood count
CCB	calcium channel blocker
CHF	congestive heart failure
CINV	chemotherapy-induced nausea and vomiting
CML	chronic myeloid leukemia
CMV	cytomegalovirus
CNS	central nervous system
Contra	contraindications
COPD	chronic obstructive pulmonary disease
CPK	creatine phosphokinase
CrCl	creatinine clearance
cre	cream
CSF	cerebrospinal fluid
CV	cardiovascular
CVD	cardiovascular disease
D/C	discontinued
DM	diabetes mellitus
DSST	Digital Symbol Substitution Test
DVT	deep vein thrombosis
ECG	electrocardiogram/electrocardiograph
EEG	electroencephalogram
EIAED	enzyme-inducing anti-epileptic drug
EIB	exercise-induced bronchospasm
EPS	extrapyramidal syndrome
ESRD	end-stage renal disease
ETFN	empiric therapy in febrile neutropenia
FBG	fasting blood glucose
FBS	fasting blood sugar
FSH	follicle-stimulating hormone
GH	growth hormone
GHD	growth hormone deficiency
GI	gastrointestinal
HBV	hepatitis B virus
hCG	human chorionic gonadotropin
Hct	hematocrit
HCV	hepatitis C virus
HDL	high-density lipoprotein
HFA	hydrofluoroalkane
hFSH	human follicle-stimulating hormone
hgb	hemoglobin
HIV	human immunodeficiency virus
HPA	hypothalamic-pituitary-adrenal
HR	heart rate
hs	at bedtime
HSCT	hematopoietic stem cell transplantation
HSV	herpes simplex virus
HTN	hypertension
ICU	intensive care unit
IgE	immunoglobulin type E
IM	intramuscular
inh	inhaler
inj	injection
INR	international normalized ratio
IOP	intraocular pressure
IPPB	intermittent positive pressure breathing
IU	international unit
IV	intravenous
JRA	juvenile rheumatoid arthritis
KOH	potassium hydroxide
LFT	liver function test
lot	lotion
loz	lozenge
maint	maintenance dose
MAOI	monoamine oxidase inhibitor
MDI	metered dose inhaler
MI	myocardial infarction
MIU	million international units
MDD	minimum daily dose
MMD	major mood disorder
NG	nasogastric
NMS	neuroleptic malignant syndrome
NNRTI	non-nucleoside reverse transcriptase inhibitor
NRTI	nucleoside reverse transcriptase inhibitor
NSAID	nonsteroidal anti-inflammatory drug
N/V	nausea and vomiting
NYHA	New York Heart Association
OA	osteoarthritis
OCD	obsessive-compulsive disorder
oint	ointment
OSAHS	obstructive sleep apnea/hypopnea syndrome
OTC	over the counter
P/N	pregnancy category rating and nursing considerations
pc	after meals
PE	pulmonary embolism
PKU	phenylketonuria
PO	by mouth
PONV	post-operative nausea and vomiting

PT	prothrombin time
PTT	partial thromboplastin time
q4-6h	every 4 to 6 hours
q6h	every 6 hours
q8h	every 8 hours
q12h	every 12 hours
qam	every morning
qd	every day
qhs	every night at bedtime
qid	four times daily
qod	every other day
qow	every other week
qpm	every evening
RA	rheumatoid arthritis
SC/SQ	subcutaneous
SCr	serum creatinine
SIADH	syndrome of inappropriate antidiuretic hormone
SLE	systemic lupus erythematosus
sol	solution
SNRI	serotonin and norepinephrine reuptake inhibitor
SSRI	selective serotonin reuptake inhibitor
sup	suppository
sus	suspension
SWSD	shift work sleep disorder
syr	syrup
tab	tablet, caplet
TB	tuberculosis
tbs	tablespoon
TCA	tricyclic antidepressants
TIA	transient ischemic attack
tid	three times per day
tiw	three times per week
ULN	upper limit of normal
UTI	urinary tract infection
W/P	warnings/precautions
WBC	white blood cell count

Section I.

Drugs Used in Dentistry

Chapter 1

Injectable and Topical Local Anesthetics

John A. Yagiela, D.D.S., Ph.D.

INJECTABLE LOCAL ANESTHETICS

Local anesthetics reversibly block neural transmission when applied to a circumscribed area of the body. Cocaine, the first local anesthetic (introduced in 1884), remains an effective topical agent, but it proved too toxic for parenteral use. Procaine, introduced in 1904, was the first practical local anesthetic for injection and contributed greatly to breaking the historic connection between dentistry and pain.

Vasoconstrictors are agents used in local anesthetic solutions to retard systemic absorption of the local anesthetic from the injection site. Although not active themselves in preventing neural transmission, vasoconstrictors such as epinephrine and related adrenergic amines can significantly increase the duration and even the depth of anesthesia. The vasoconstriction they produce also may be useful in reducing bleeding during intraoral procedures.

Chemistry and classification

Injectable local anesthetics consist of amphiphilic molecules; that is, they can dissolve in both aqueous and lipid environments. A lipophilic ring structure on one end of the molecule confers fat solubility, and a secondary or tertiary amino group on the other end permits water solubility. Local anesthetics intended for injection are prepared commercially as the hydrochloride salt.

Two major classes of injectable local anesthetics are recognized: esters and amides. They are distinguished by the type of chemical bond joining the two ends of the drug molecules. Early local anesthetics, such as cocaine and procaine, were esters. Most local anesthetics introduced since 1940 have been amides.

The use of injectable local anesthetics in dentistry is almost exclusively limited to amide-type drugs. In fact, no ester agent is currently being marketed in dental cartridge form in the United States. Given the number of local anesthetic injections administered in dentistry (conservatively estimated at more than 300 million in the United States annually), a drug with a minimal risk of allergy is desirable. Amide anesthetics offer a significantly lower risk of allergy than ester anesthetics. Conversely, amides also have a somewhat greater risk of systemic toxicity than do esters. However, as toxic reactions usually are dose-related, adherence to proper injection techniques—including the use of minimal volumes of anesthetic—minimizes this risk. Amide formulations have also proved more effective than esters for achieving intraoral anesthesia. Thus, amide local anesthetics, as used in dentistry, offer the fewest overall risks and the greatest clinical benefits.

Selecting a local anesthetic

The selection of a local anesthetic for use in a dental procedure is based on four criteria:

- duration of the dental procedure
- requirement for hemostasis
- requirement for postsurgical pain control
- contraindication(s) to specific anesthetic drugs or vasoconstrictors

Duration

Local anesthetic formulations intended for use in dentistry are categorized by their expected duration of pulpal anesthesia as short-, intermediate-, and long-acting drugs.

- **Short-acting drugs**, which typically provide pulpal and hard tissue anesthesia for up to 30 minutes after submucosal infiltration: 2% lidocaine, 3% mepivacaine, and 4% prilocaine.
- **Intermediate-acting agents**, which typically provide up to 60 minutes of pulpal anesthesia after submucosal infiltration and 90 minutes after inferior alveolar nerve block: 4% articaine with 1:100,000 or 1:200,000 epinephrine, 2% lidocaine with 1:50,000 or 1:100,000 epinephrine, 2% mepivacaine with 1:20,000 levonordefrin, and 4% prilocaine with 1:200,000 epinephrine.
- **Long-acting drugs**, which last up to 8 hours after nerve block anesthesia: 0.5% bupivacaine with 1:200,000 epinephrine.

For most clinical situations, an intermediate-acting formulation is appropriate. These agents are highly effective and have durations of action that can accommodate most intraoral procedures. The 4% prilocaine and 3% mepivacaine solutions, however, may be preferred for maxillary supraperiosteal injections when there is a need for pulpal anesthesia of only short duration. (The 2% lidocaine plain formulation cannot be recommended because pulpal anesthesia is not consistently achieved.) Long-acting local anesthetics are helpful for providing anesthesia of extended duration. Unfortunately, pulpal anesthesia after supraperiosteal injection is less reliable than with the intermediate-acting drugs, because the highly lipophilic long-acting drugs do not readily reach the superior dental nerve plexus.

Hemostasis

Lidocaine with epinephrine is the formulation usually administered to achieve temporary hemostasis in tissues undergoing treatment. Although the 1:50,000 strength of epinephrine provides little benefit over the 1:100,000 concentration with regard to the duration of local anesthesia, it can significantly decrease bleeding associated with periodontal tissue when given by local infiltration.

Postsurgical pain control

The bupivacaine formulation can help the surgical patient remain pain-free for up to 8 hours after treatment. This agent may be administered before the procedure to provide local anesthesia intraoperatively or afterward to maximize the duration of postsurgical pain relief.

Contraindications

True allergy is the only absolute contraindication to the use of any local anesthetic formulation. Although there is little evidence of cross-allergenicity among the amides, it is probably prudent to avoid amides with the greatest molecular similarity to the putative allergen. Lidocaine is most similar to prilocaine in structure, whereas mepivacaine is most similar to bupivacaine. Articaine is identical in structure to prilocaine except that it contains a thiophene group instead of the typically substituted benzene ring. If a sulfite preservative is the allergen, then the 3% mepivacaine and 4% prilocaine solutions without vasoconstrictor are the formulations of choice because they are free of sulfites.

These plain solutions also are indicated when the use of epinephrine and levonordefrin is not recommended. However, formulations containing 1:200,000 epinephrine may be considered when modest doses of vasoconstrictor are permissible and when the plain solutions might not provide anesthesia of sufficient depth or duration. (Specific contraindications and restrictions to vasoconstrictors are reviewed later in this chapter.)

Accepted Indications

Injectable local anesthetics are used to provide local or regional analgesia for surgical and other dental procedures. They are also used for diagnostic or other therapeutic purposes via routes of administration specified in product labeling.

General Dosing Information

General dosing information is provided in **Table 1.1**. In addition, standard textbooks provide information on the appropriate dosage (both concentration and injection volume) of local anesthetic to be used for specific injection techniques and dental procedures. The dosage depends on:

- the specific anesthetic technique and operative procedure
- tissue vascularity in the area of injection
- individual patient response

In general, the dentist should administer the lowest concentration and volume of anesthetic solution that provide adequate anesthesia.

Maximum Recommended Doses

Table 1.1 lists the maximum recommended doses for local anesthetic formulations per procedure or appointment, as approved by the U.S. Food and Drug Administration (FDA). Additional anesthetic may be administered only after sufficient time is allowed for elimination of the initial dose.

Dosage Adjustments

The actual maximum dose for each patient must be individualized depending on his or her size, age, and physical status; other drugs he or she may be taking; and the anticipated rate of absorption of the local anesthetic from the injected tissues. Reduced maximum doses are often indicated for pediatric and geriatric patients, patients who have serious illness or disability, and patients who have medical conditions or are taking drugs that alter responses to local anesthetics or vasoconstrictors.

Table 1.1 presents specific limits for local anesthetic doses in pediatric patients.

VASOCONSTRICTORS

A vasoconstrictor added to a local anesthetic may significantly prolong the anesthetic's duration of action by reducing blood flow around the injection site. This, in turn, may reduce the local anesthetic's peak plasma concentration and the risk of adverse systemic reactions.

Repeated injection of vasoconstrictors in local anesthetics also may decrease blood flow sufficiently to cause anoxic injury in the local tissue, leading to delayed wound healing, edema, or necrosis. The use of local anesthetic solutions containing vasoconstrictors may be restricted or contraindicated in patients who have advanced cardiovascular disease or who are taking medications that increase the activity of the vasoconstrictor.

Although there are no officially recognized maximum doses for vasoconstrictors when administered with local anesthesia, it is widely accepted that vasoconstrictor usage be minimized in patients with increased risk of vasoconstrictor toxicity. Because plasma concentrations of epinephrine measured in subjects performing normal activities of daily living are comparable to those achieved by the intraoral injection of two cartridges of lidocaine with 1:100,000 epinephrine (about 0.04 mg epinephrine) in reclining subjects, it is assumed that this dosage should be safe in the ambulatory patient with cardiovascular disease. Slow, careful injection with frequent aspiration attempts and avoidance of the 1:50,000 epinephrine formulation are additional precautions to take for the patient with reduced vasoconstrictor tolerance.

Special Dental Considerations

Drug Interactions of Dental Interest

Drug interactions and related problems involving local anesthetics and vasoconstrictors (**Table 1.2**) are potentially of clinical significance in dentistry.

Laboratory Value Alterations

Pancreatic function tests using bentiromide are altered by ester local anesthetics or lidocaine.

Cross-Sensitivity

Table 1.3 describes potential cross-sensitivity considerations.

Special Patients

Pregnant and nursing women

Local anesthetics readily cross the placenta and enter the fetal circulation. Although retrospective investigations of pregnant women receiving local anesthesia during the first trimester of pregnancy have found no evidence of fetal toxicity, animal investigations indicate a potential for birth defects—albeit at enormous doses—with some local anesthetics.

Considerations of risk/benefit suggest that purely elective treatment be delayed until after delivery and that other dental care be performed, if possible, during the second trimester. Lidocaine and, most likely, other local anesthetics are distributed into breast milk; again, however, no problems with injected local anesthetics have been documented in humans.

Table 1.1 lists the FDA pregnancy risk category classifications for injectable local anesthetics used in dentistry.

Pediatric, geriatric, and other special patients

Although there are some data to suggest that adverse reactions to local anesthetics may be more prevalent in pediatric and geriatric populations, studies involving mepivacaine and other local anesthetics have found no age-specific problem that would limit their use. However, overdosage is more likely to occur in young children because of their small size and the commensurately low margin for error. Increased variability of response to the local anesthetic or vasoconstrictor is likely to be encountered in elderly patients and in those with significant medical problems. Lower maximum doses in these patients provide an extra margin of safety.

Local anesthetics are less effective than normal in the presence of inflammation or infection. Strategies that may assist the clinician in achieving pain control include the use of nerve blocks proximal to the affected tissue and intraosseous anesthesia.

Patient Monitoring: Aspects to Watch

- State of consciousness
- Respiratory status
- Cardiovascular status

Adverse Effects and Precautions

The incidence of adverse reactions to local anesthetic agents is low. Many reactions (eg, headache, palpitation, tremor, nausea, dyspnea, hyperventilation syndrome, syncope) result from the perceived stress of injection and are not caused by the agents themselves. Toxic systemic reactions generally are associated with high plasma concentrations of the local anesthetic or vasoconstrictor, or both, after an accidental intravascular injection, administration of a drug in a manner that causes rapid absorption, administration of a true overdosage, or selection of a drug formulation inappropriate for the specific patient. Idiosyncratic and allergic reactions account for a small minority of adverse responses. In addition, a small subset of asthmatic patients intolerant of inhaled or dietary sulfites may develop bronchospasm after injection of local anesthetic solutions containing sulfite antioxidants.

Systemic reactions to local anesthetics may occur immediately on administration or may be delayed for up to 30 minutes or more. Oxygen, resuscitative equipment, and drugs necessary to treat systemic emergencies must be immediately available whenever a local anesthetic is administered. **Table 1.1** lists adverse effects for injectable local anesthetics and vasoconstrictors.

Local anesthetics can produce tissue damage in the area of injection. Muscle tissue appears to be highly sensitive to local anesthetics; mucosal lesions most commonly occur when relatively large amounts of local anesthetic are injected under high pressure into attached gingiva or palatal mucosa. Vasoconstrictors enhance the likelihood and extent of damage. Generally, complete healing progresses uneventfully.

Rarely, local anesthetics may cause neuronal damage resulting in permanent alteration of sensation. The inferior alveolar nerve block is usually involved, leading to damage of the lingual nerve (most frequently), inferior alveolar nerve, or both nerves (least frequently). The neurotoxic response is not caused by the physical trauma of needle insertion but appears to be a direct toxic effect of the local anesthetic. High-concentration local anesthetics with vasoconstrictors (ie, 4% articaine or 4% prilocaine, both with epinephrine) are more likely to result in permanent paresthesia or anesthesia.

Pharmacology

Local Anesthetics

Local anesthetics bind to sodium channels in the nerve membrane and prevent the entry of sodium ions in response to the membrane's depolarization. Propagation of the action potential is inhibited in the area of injection, and nerve conduction fails when an adequate length of nerve is exposed to a sufficient concentration of local anesthetic. Nerve conduction is restored as the anesthetic diffuses away from the injection site and is absorbed into the systemic circulation. Systemic effects, should they occur, are largely the result of the local anesthetic inhibiting other excitable tissues. Systemic reactions are minimized when metabolism of the local anesthetic is able to inactivate the drug as it is absorbed into the bloodstream.

The rate of absorption of a local anesthetic is governed by several factors, including the drug, its concentration and dose, the vascularity of the injection site, and the presence of a vasoconstrictor. Generally, peak concentrations are achieved in 10 to 30 minutes.

Most amide anesthetics are metabolized in the liver. Prilocaine is unusual in that it is metabolized in the kidneys to some extent.

Most esters are hydrolyzed by plasma esterase to inactive products; some metabolism also occurs in the liver. Although classified as an amide local anesthetic, articaine is largely inactivated by blood and tissue esterases, which cleave a vital ester side chain from the drug.

Small amounts of local anesthetics (2% to 20%) and the various metabolites eventually are excreted into the urine.

Vasoconstrictors

Epinephrine, levonordefrin, and other adrenergic amine vasoconstrictors help retard absorption of the local anesthetic by stimulating α-adrenergic receptors in the local vasculature. The resultant reduction in tissue blood flow gives the local anesthetic more time to reach its site of action in the nerve membrane.

Systemic effects of vasoconstrictors are associated with stimulation of both α- and β-adrenergic receptors. The intensity and duration of these effects parallel the rate of absorption of the vasoconstrictor from the injection site. Stimulation of β receptors results in cardiac stimulation and vasodilation in skeletal muscle (β_2 receptors only). Stimulation of α receptors causes constriction of resistance arterioles throughout the body as well as capacitance veins in the legs and abdomen, which increases peripheral vascular resistance and venous return to the heart. Both α- and β-receptor effects contribute to the potential for cardiac dysrhythmias.

The adrenergic vasoconstrictors used in dentistry are quickly inactivated (plasma half-life of 1 to 2 minutes) by the enzyme catechol-O-methyltransferase. Additional metabolism of epinephrine by monoamine oxidase may occur, and the products are then excreted in the urine.

Patient Advice

- Injury to the anesthetized tissues may occur without any resulting sensation.
- To prevent injury, patients should not test for anesthesia by biting the lip or tongue, nor should they eat or chew anything until the anesthetic effect has dissipated.
- Children should be warned not to bite their lip or tongue and be monitored by their parents to prevent injury.

Reversal of Soft-Tissue Anesthesia

Phentolamine mesylate (OraVerse) has recently been approved by the FDA for the "reversal of soft-tissue anesthesia, ie, anesthesia of the lip and tongue, and the associated functional deficits resulting from an intraoral submucosal injection of a local anesthetic containing a vasoconstrictor." Marketed in dental cartridges containing 0.4 mg/1.7 mL, the drug is injected in the same manner and volume as the local anesthetic (up to a total of two cartridges in adults, one cartridge in children 6 years of age and older) once the need for pain control has passed. The agent is not recommended for use after surgical procedures when maintenance of local anesthesia is desired. Clinical trials indicate that phentolamine reduces the median duration of soft-tissue anesthesia by 70 (tongue) to 85 (lips) minutes in adults, and by 50 (upper lip) to 120 (lower lip) minutes in children. Patients regain the ability to drink, speak, and smile normally as sensation returns to normal. Although toxic reactions or adverse drug interactions with the small doses of phentolamine used for local anesthesia reversal have not been observed, larger doses (eg, 5 to 10 mg) injected intravenously may cause marked hypotension and reactive tachycardia and lead to cardiac dysrhythmias, myocardial infarction, and cerebrovascular accidents.

SUGGESTED READING

Haas DA. Articaine and paresthesia: epidemiological studies. *J Am Coll Dent*. 2006;73(3):5-10.

Hersh EV, Moore PA, Papas AS, et al. Reversal of soft-tissue local anesthesia with phentolamine mesylate in adolescents and adults. *JADA*. 2008;139(8):1080-1093.

Malamed SF. *Handbook of Local Anesthesia*. 5th ed. St. Louis: Mosby; 2004.

Moore PA. Adverse drug interactions associated with local anesthetics, sedatives and anxiolytics. *JADA*. 1999;130(4):541–554.

Yagiela JA. Adverse drug interactions in dental practice: interactions associated with vasoconstrictors. *JADA*. 1999;130(5):701–709.

Yagiela JA. Local anesthetics. In Yagiela JA, Dowd FJ, Neidle EA, eds. *Pharmacology and Therapeutics for Dentistry*. 5th ed. St. Louis: Mosby; 2004.

TOPICAL LOCAL ANESTHETICS

Topical local anesthetic preparations used on oral mucosa differ in several respects from injectable preparations. Topical agents are selected for their ability to penetrate the oral mucosa and depend on diffusion to reach their site of action. Many of the anesthetics effective for nerve block or infiltration do not cross the mucosa adequately and, therefore, are not used for topical anesthesia.

In contrast to their injectable counterparts, topical ester-type agents are important for producing anesthesia, and some drugs used for mucosal anesthesia are neither esters nor amides. Life-threatening allergic reactions are extremely unlikely with topical anesthetics, regardless of type, and the inclusion of paraben preservatives in some topical amide formulations reduces the disparity in risk of allergy among these preparations.

Topical anesthetics are manufactured in a variety of forms. Gels, viscous gels, and ointments are best used to limit the area of coverage of the topical anesthetic; aerosol sprays and solution rinses are best used for widespread application; lozenges, pastes, and film-forming gels are specifically formulated to provide prolonged pain relief.

Several drugs used as topical anesthetics are so insoluble in water that they cannot be prepared in aqueous solutions. They are soluble in alcohol, propylene glycol, polyethylene glycol, volatile oils, and other vehicles suitable for surface application. Included in this group of anesthetics are benzocaine and lidocaine bases. The poor water solubility of benzocaine in particular makes it safe for topical use on abraded or lacerated tissue.

To facilitate diffusion, the concentration of anesthetic used for surface application usually is much higher than that of injectable preparations. As a consequence, the potential toxicity of these preparations can be significant if large quantities are absorbed or even ingested. Systemic absorption of some topical anesthetics applied to the mucosa can be rapid, and blood concentrations approaching those with intravenous infusion may be achieved with tetracaine, depending on the area of coverage and method of application.

The rate of onset for topical anesthesia varies from 30 seconds to 5 minutes, depending on the anesthetic agent. Optimum effectiveness may be delayed, depending on the preparation. The mucosa should be dried before application to improve local uptake. The duration of topical anesthesia is generally shorter than with injected anesthesia. **Table 1.4** indicates the approximate durations of action of the various topical anesthetics for mucosal anesthesia.

An occlusive dressing preventing the loss of agent can extend the duration; removing the residual agent and rinsing the mouth can shorten it. Topical preparations do not contain adrenergic vasoconstrictors.

Generally, mucosal anesthesia is only about 2 mm deep and is poor or nonexistent in the hard palate. Lidocaine and prilocaine prepared together in a eutectic mixture have been shown to improve anesthetic depth; however, the only preparation currently available for intraoral use is approved only for anesthesia of periodontal pockets. Given the trade name Oraqix, this lidocaine and prilocaine periodontal gel is marketed in special cartridge form and is applied into the pocket. Anesthesia begins in 30 seconds and lasts for about 20 minutes. A mucoadhesive patch containing lidocaine—DentiPatch Lidocaine Transoral Delivery System—also has shown increased efficacy as a topical anesthetic agent. The patch is applied directly to the mucosa in the area where anesthesia is desired so that the lidocaine's effect is maximized and the flow and dilution of the medication are limited. Anesthesia begins in 2.5 minutes, but the patch can be left in place for up to 15 minutes to increase the effect. Site-specific topical anesthesia additionally can be obtained with the use of a solid gel patch containing

18% benzocaine (Topicale GelPatch). The patch can be trimmed and shaped to fit the intended target. Anesthesia begins in about 30 seconds and is maintained as the patch dissolves during the next 20 minutes.

Accepted Indications

Topical local anesthetics are used to provide mucosal analgesia before local anesthetic injection; to facilitate dental examination, including pocket probing, the taking of radiographs, periodontal pocket scaling and other relatively noninvasive dental procedures by minimizing pain and the gag reflex; and to provide temporary symptomatic relief of toothache, oral lesions and wounds, as well as irritation caused by dentures and other appliances.

Additional uses for diagnostic and therapeutic purposes are described in product labeling.

General Dosing Information

The dosage of topical anesthetics depends on the anesthetic preparation selected, the area to be anesthetized, the ability to maintain the anesthetic agent on the area of application, the vascularity of the administration site and the patient's age, size, and health status. Physical removal of the anesthetic and rinsing of the mouth once the need for topical anesthesia has passed preclude further absorption of the drug.

Maximum Recommended Doses

Table 1.5 lists the usual dose and the maximum recommended dose for topical anesthetic formulations per application and, where appropriate or available, the application interval.

Dosage Adjustments

The actual maximum dose for each patient must be individualized depending on his or her size, age, and physical status; other drugs he or she may be taking; and the anticipated rate of absorption of the topical anesthetic from the application site. Reduced maximum doses are often indicated for pediatric and geriatric patients, people who have serious illness or disability, and patients who have medical conditions or are taking drugs that alter responses to topical anesthetics.

Specific limits for topical anesthetic use in pediatric patients appear in **Table 1.5**.

Special Dental Considerations

Drug Interactions of Dental Interest

Drug interactions and related problems involving topical anesthetics are in general the same as those listed in **Table 1.2**. Interactions specific to cocaine are not included, since this drug is rarely used in dentistry.

Cross-Sensitivity

The potential for cross-sensitivity of topical local anesthetics is addressed in **Table 1.3**.

Special Patients

Pregnant and nursing women

Once absorbed into the systemic circulation, topical anesthetics can cross the placenta to enter the fetal circulation. **Table 1.5** includes the FDA pregnancy category classifications for topical anesthetics used in dentistry. Considerations of risk/benefit suggest that purely elective treatment should be delayed until after delivery and that other dental care should be performed, if possible, during the second trimester. Lidocaine and probably other topical anesthetics are distributed into breast milk, but no problems have been documented in humans, except with cocaine. Cocaine intake by infants during nursing has led to overt toxicity, including convulsions and cardiovascular derangements.

Pediatric, geriatric, and other special patients

Adverse reactions to topical anesthetics are rare in dentistry but may be more prevalent in pediatric and geriatric populations. Overdosage is more likely to occur in young children because of their small size and the commensurately low margin for error. Methemoglobinemia with use of benzocaine is largely limited to young children. Increased variability of response to local anesthetics is likely to be encountered in elderly patients and in those with significant medical problems. Lower maximum doses in these patients provide an extra margin of safety.

Patient Monitoring: Aspects to Watch

- State of consciousness
- Respiratory status
- Cardiovascular status

Adverse Effects and Precautions

Systemic reactions may occur when local anesthetics are applied topically. Systemic absorption of these agents should be minimized by limiting the concentration of the drug, the area of application, the total amount of agent applied, and the time of exposure for drugs that can be removed once the effect has been achieved. To minimize absorption, special caution is needed when applying topical agents to severely traumatized mucosa or to areas of sepsis.

Several topical anesthetic preparations are marketed in pressurized spray containers. It is difficult to control the amount of drug expelled with unmetered spray devices and to confine the agent to the desired site. Thus, a patient inadvertently may inhale sufficient quantities of the aerosol spray to provoke an adverse reaction. Therefore, caution is advised when using any spray device, and metered spray devices are preferred because they dispense a measured amount of drug.

In recent years, certain compounding pharmaceutical companies have marketed topical anesthetic formulations containing multiple anesthetic and vasoconstrictor agents in high concentrations. These agents have been used by dentists seeking therapeutic efficacies not available with existing products. Several deaths attributed to the unregulated use of these products have prompted the FDA to move against their distribution. Although compounding of drugs for individual patient use is an accepted practice, sale of such preparations for general use is illegal. Dentists are advised to avoid such preparations and rely instead on FDA-approved agents for their anesthetic needs.

Adverse effects and precautions for topical anesthetics are included in **Table 1.5**.

Pharmacology

Topical local anesthetics provide anesthesia by anesthetizing the free nerve endings in the mucosa. The mechanism of action is identical to that described in the previous section for injectable local anesthetics. Cocaine, however, has a distinct pharmacology. In addition to its local anesthetic action, cocaine blocks the reuptake of released adrenergic neurotransmitters (norepinephrine, dopamine) back into the nerve terminal. This action gives cocaine its vasoconstrictor and CNS-stimulant properties, as well as its addictive potential and increased risk of cardiovascular toxicity.

The rate of absorption of a topical anesthetic depends on the dose administered, the duration of exposure, the area of coverage, the mucosa's permeability, the mucosa's intactness, and the vascularity of the tissue. Benzocaine is unique in its poor solubility in water and is the least absorbed into the bloodstream.

A considerable portion of topical anesthetics administered intraorally is swallowed. Although absorption from the gastrointestinal tract occurs, extensive metabolism of the drug in the hepatic-portal system prevents toxic blood concentrations except with excessive doses. The metabolic fate and excretion of these drugs is covered in the first part of this chapter, in the section on injectable local anesthetics.

Patient Advice

- Injury to the anesthetized tissues may occur without any resulting sensation.
- To prevent pulmonary aspiration, patients who have undergone topical anesthesia of the pharynx should use caution when eating or drinking until normal sensation has returned.
- To prevent injury, patients should not test for anesthesia by biting the lip or tongue, nor should they eat or chew anything until the anesthetic effect has dissipated.
- Children should be warned not to bite their lips or tongue and be monitored by their parents to prevent injury.
- Patients using topical anesthetics to manage toothache, intraoral conditions, or ill-fitting dental appliances should seek professional dental care for definitive treatment.

SUGGESTED READING

Kravitz ND. The use of compound topical anesthetics. *JADA*. 2007;138(10):1333-1339.

Magnusson I, Jeffcoat MK, Donaldson D, et al. Quantification and analysis of pain in nonsurgical scaling and/or root planing. *JADA*. 2004;135(12):1747-1754.

Malamed SF. *Handbook of Local Anesthesia*. 5th ed. St. Louis: Mosby; 2004.

Meechan JG. Intra-oral topical anaesthetics: a review. *J Dent*. 2000;28(1):3-14.

Table 1.1. PRESCRIBING INFORMATION FOR INJECTABLE LOCAL ANESTHETICS

NAME	FORM/ STRENGTH	DOSAGE	WARNINGS/PRECAUTIONS & CONTRAINDICATIONS	ADVERSE EFFECTS
Articaine HCl w/ Epinephrine (Septocaine w/ Epinephrine, Zorcaine)	**Sol, Inj:** (Articaine-Epinephrine) 4%-1:100,000/1.7mL; 2%-1:200,000/ 1.7mL	***Adults:* Submucosal Infiltration:** 0.5-2.5mL. **Nerve Block:** 0.5-3.4mL. **Oral Surgery:** 1-5.1mL. **Max:** 7mg/kg (0.175mL/kg) or 3.2mg/lb (0.0795mL/lb). ***Pediatrics:* ≥4 yrs: Submucosal Infiltration/Nerve Block/Oral Surgery:** Up to 7mg/kg (0.175mL/kg) or 3.2mg/lb (0.0795mL/lb).	**W/P:** Avoid intravascular injection; aspirate needle before use. Intravascular injection is associated with convulsions, followed by CNS or cardiorespiratory depression and coma progressing to respiratory arrest. CNS or cardiovascular effects may also occur with systemic absorption. Epinephrine can cause local tissue necrosis or systemic toxicity. Multiple injections at same tissue site increase likelihood of local tissue damage. Cardiovascular toxicity is more likely in patients with pre-existing cardiac defects, disease or dysrhythmias; peripheral vascular disease; hypokalemia; or uncontrolled hypertension, pheochromocytoma or thyroid disease. **Contra:** Known hypersensitivity to amide local anesthetics or sulfite preservatives. **P/N:** Category C, caution in nursing.	Confusion, restlessness, anxiety, dizziness, tinnitus, blurred vision, tremors, convulsions, nausea, vomiting, chills, unconsciousness, respiratory depression and arrest, hypotension, bradycardia, tachycardia, ventricular dysrhythmias, palpitation, angina pectoris, cardiac arrest, urticaria, pruritus, erythema, bronchospasm, anaphylaxis, facial edema, trismus, headache, infection, pain, local tissue damage, long-lasting paresthesia.
Bupivacaine HCl w/ Epinephrine (Marcaine w/ Epinephrine, Vivacaine)	**Sol, Inj:** (Bupivacaine-Epinephrine) 0.5%-1:200,000/ 1.8mL	***Adults:*** Individualize dose. Dosage varies depending on procedure, area to be anesthetized, vascularity of tissues, and patient tolerance and physical condition. **Single Dose Max:** 90mg (225mg for nondental uses). **Elderly/Debilitated/Cardiac or Liver Disease:** Reduce dose. ***Pediatrics:* ≥12 yrs:** Individualize dose. Dosage varies depending on procedure, area to be anesthetized, ascularity of tissues, and patient tolerance and physical condition.	**W/P:** Avoid intravascular injection; aspirate needle before use. Acidosis, cardiac arrest, and death reported from delay in toxicity management. Monitor cardiovascular and respiratory vital signs and state of consciousness after each injection. Caution with hepatic disease and impaired cardiovascular function. Epinephrine can cause local tissue necrosis or systemic toxicity. Multiple injections at same tissue site increase likelihood of local tissue damage. Cardiovascular toxicity is more likely in patients with pre-existing cardiac defects, disease or dysrhythmias; peripheral vascular disease; hypokalemia; or uncontrolled hypertension, pheochromocytoma or thyroid disease. Patients should be warned about inadvertent trauma to oral tissues and advised not to chew solid food while anesthetized. **Contra:** Known hypersensitivity to amide local anesthetics or sulfite preservatives. **P/N:** Category C, not for use in nursing.	Confusion, restlessness, anxiety, dizziness, tinnitus, blurred vision, tremors, convulsions, nausea, vomiting, chills, unconsciousness, respiratory depression and arrest, hypotension, bradycardia, tachycardia, ventricular dysrhythmias, palpitation, angina pectoris, myocardial depression, cardiac arrest, urticaria, pruritus, erythema, bronchospasm, anaphylaxis, facial edema, trismus, local tissue damage.
Lidocaine HCl (Xylocaine)	**Sol, Inj:** 2%/1.8mL	***Adults:*** Dosage varies depending on procedure, area to be anesthetized, vascularity of tissues, and patient tolerance and physical condition. **Max:** 4.5mg/kg (2mg/lb) or total dose of 300mg. **Children/Elderly/Debilitated/Cardiac or Liver Disease:** Reduce dose. ***Pediatrics:* >3 yrs: Max:** 4.5mg/kg (2mg/lb).	**W/P:** Avoid intravascular injection; aspirate needle before use. Acidosis, cardiac arrest, and death reported from delay in toxicity management. Use lowest effective dose. Reduce dose with debilitated, elderly, acutely ill, and children. Monitor cardiovascular and respiratory vital signs and state of consciousness after each injection. Caution with hepatic disease and cardiovascular disorders. **Contra:** Known hypersensitivity to amide local anesthetics. **P/N:** Category B, caution in nursing.	Confusion, restlessness, anxiety, dizziness, tinnitus, blurred vision, tremors, convulsions, nausea, vomiting, chills, unconsciousness, respiratory depression and arrest, hypotension, bradycardia, ventricular dysrhythmias, cardiac arrest, urticaria, pruritus, erythema, anaphylaxis, facial edema, trismus.

W/P = warnings/precautions; **Contra** = contraindications; **P/N** = pregnancy category rating and nursing considerations.

Table 1.1. PRESCRIBING INFORMATION FOR INJECTABLE LOCAL ANESTHETICS *(cont.)*

NAME	FORM/ STRENGTH	DOSAGE	WARNINGS/PRECAUTIONS & CONTRAINDICATIONS	ADVERSE EFFECTS
Lidocaine HCl w/ Epinephrine (Lignospan Standard, Lignospan Forte, Octocaine 50, Octocaine 100, Xylocaine w/ Epinephrine)	**Sol, Inj:** (Lidocaine-Epinephrine) 2%-1:50,000/1.7-1.8mL; 2%-1:100,000/1.7-1.8mL	***Adults:*** Dosage varies depending on procedure, area to be anesthetized, vascularity of tissues, and patient tolerance and physical condition. **Max:** 7mg/kg (3.2 mg/lb) or total dose of 500mg. **Children/Elderly/ Debilitated/ Cardiac or Liver Disease:** Reduce dose. ***Pediatrics:*** **>3 yrs: Max:** 7mg/kg (3.2 mg/lb).	**W/P:** Avoid intravascular injection; aspirate needle before use. Acidosis, cardiac arrest, and death reported from delay in toxicity management. Use lowest effective dose. Reduce dose with debilitated, elderly, acutely ill, and children. Multiple injections at same tissue site increase likelihood of local tissue damage. Epinephrine can cause local tissue necrosis or systemic toxicity. Multiple injections at same tissue site increase likelihood of local tissue damage. Cardiovascular toxicity is more likely in patients with pre-existing cardiac defects, disease or dysrhythmias; peripheral vascular disease; hypokalemia; or uncontrolled hypertension, pheochromocytoma or thyroid disease. Monitor cardiovascular and respiratory vital signs and state of consciousness after each injection. Caution with hepatic disease and cardiovascular disorders. **Contra:** Known hypersensitivity to amide local anesthetics or sulfite preservatives. **P/N:** Category B, caution in nursing.	Confusion, restlessness, anxiety, dizziness, tinnitus, blurred vision, tremors, convulsions, nausea, vomiting, chills, unconsciousness, respiratory depression and arrest, hypotension, bradycardia, tachycardia, ventricular dysrhythmias, palpitation, angina pectoris, cardiac arrest, urticaria, pruritus, erythema, bronchospasm, anaphylaxis, facial edema, trismus, local tissue damage.
Mepivacaine HCl (Carbocaine, Isocaine, Polocaine, Scandonest 3% Plain)	**Sol, Inj:** 3%/1.7-1.8mL	***Adults:*** Dose varies with anesthetic procedure, area to be anesthetized, vascularity of tissues, number of neuronal segments to be blocked, depth of anesthesia and degree of muscle relaxation required, and duration of anesthesia required. **Max:** 6.6mg/kg or total dose of 400mg. ***Pediatrics:*** Dose not to exceed 5-6mg/kg.	**W/P:** Aspiration for blood should be done prior to injection of initial and all subsequent doses to avoid intravascular injection. Use with caution if inflammation and/or sepsis in region of proposed injection. Avoid injecting mepivacaine too rapidly or into intravascular spaces (systemic toxicity could result). Use with caution in patients with hepatic disease. **Contra:** Hypersensitivity to amide-type anesthetics. **P/N:** Category C, caution in nursing.	Lightheadedness, nervousness, euphoria, confusion, dizziness, drowsiness, tinnitus, blurred vision, vomiting, heat/cold sensations, twitching, tremors, convulsions, respiratory depression, bradycardia, ventricular dysrhythmias, hypotension, urticaria, edema, anaphylaxis, trismus.
Mepivacaine HCl w/ Levonordefrin (Carbocaine w/ NeoCobefrin, Isocaine w/ Levonordefrin, Scandonest 2% L)	**Sol, Inj:** (Mepivacaine-Levonordefrin) 2%-1:20,000/ 1.8mL	***Adults:*** Dose varies with anesthetic procedure, area to be anesthetized, vascularity of tissues, number of neuronal segments to be blocked, depth of anesthesia and degree of muscle relaxation required, and duration of anesthesia required. **Max:** 6.6mg/kg or total dose of 400mg. ***Pediatrics:*** Dose not to exceed 5-6mg/kg.	**W/P:** Aspiration for blood should be done prior to injection of initial and all subsequent doses to avoid intravascular injection. Use with caution if inflammation and/or sepsis in region of proposed injection. Levonordefrin can cause local tissue necrosis or systemic toxicity. Multiple injections at same tissue site increase likelihood of local tissue damage. Cardiovascular toxicity is more likely in patients with pre-existing cardiac defects, disease or dysrhythmias; peripheral vascular disease; hypokalemia; or uncontrolled hypertension, pheochromocytoma or thyroid disease. Use with caution in patients with hepatic disease. **Contra:** Hypersensitivity to amide-type anesthetics and sulfite preservatives. **P/N:** Category C, caution in nursing.	Lightheadedness, nervousness, euphoria, confusion, dizziness, drowsiness, tinnitus, blurred vision, vomiting, heat/cold sensations, twitching, tremors, convulsions, respiratory depression, bradycardia, ventricular dysrhythmias, palpitation, angina pectoris, hypotension, hypertension, urticaria, edema, bronchospasm, anaphylaxis, trismus, local tissue damage.

W/P = warnings/precautions; **Contra** = contraindications; **P/N** = pregnancy category rating and nursing considerations.

NAME	FORM/ STRENGTH	DOSAGE	WARNINGS/PRECAUTIONS & CONTRAINDICATIONS	ADVERSE EFFECTS
Prilocaine HCl (Citanest Plain)	**Sol, Inj:** 4%/1.8mL	***Adults:*** **Maxillary Infiltration: Initial:** 1-2mL. **<70kg: Max:** 8mg/kg per injection. **≥70kg: Max:** 600mg (15mL) per injection. The dosage varies and depends on the physical status of the patient. Aspiration prior to injection is recommended. ***Pediatrics:*** **<10 yrs:** 40mg per procedure. **Max:** 8mg/kg.	**W/P:** Avoid intravascular injection; aspiration should be performed. Caution in patients with congenital or idiopathic methemoglobinemia, or patients with glucose-6-phosphate deficiencies, and very young patients. Use with caution in patients with severe shock or heart block. Use with caution in patients with hepatic disease. **Contra:** Congenital methemoglobinemia; hypersensitivity to amide containing anesthetics. **P/N:** Category B, caution in nursing.	Lightheadedness, nervousness, euphoria, confusion, dizziness, drowsiness, tinnitus, blurred vision, vomiting, heat/cold sensations, twitching, tremors, convulsions, respiratory depression, or idiopathic tachypnea and hypoxemia, bradycardia, ventricular dysrhythmias, hypotension, urticaria, edema, anaphylaxis, cardiac arrest, long-lasting paresthesia.
Prilocaine HCl w/ Epinephrine (Citanest Forte)	**Sol, Inj:** (Prilocaine-Epinephrine) 4%-1:200,000/1.8mL	***Adults:*** **Maxillary Infiltration: Initial:** 1-2mL. **<70kg: Max:** 8mg/kg per injection. **≥70kg: Max:** 600mg (15mL) per injection. The dosage varies and depends on the physical status of the patient. Aspiration prior to injection is recommended. ***Pediatrics:*** **<10 yrs:** 40mg per procedure. **Max:** 8mg/kg.	**W/P:** Avoid intravascular injection; aspiration should be performed. Caution in patients with congenital or idiopathic methemoglobinemia, or patients with glucose-6-phosphate deficiencies, and very young patients. Use with caution in patients with severe shock or heart block. Epinephrine can cause local tissue necrosis or systemic toxicity. Multiple injections at same tissue site increase likelihood of local tissue damage. Cardiovascular toxicity is more likely in patients with pre-existing cardiac defects, disease or dysrhythmias; peripheral vascular disease; hypokalemia; or uncontrolled hypertension, pheochromocytoma or thyroid disease. Use with caution in patients with hepatic disease. **Contra:** Congenital or idiopathic methemoglobinemia; hypersensitivity to amide-type anesthetics and sulfite preservatives. **P/N:** Category B, caution in nursing.	Lightheadedness, nervousness, euphoria, confusion, dizziness, drowsiness, tinnitus, blurred vision, vomiting, heat/cold sensations, twitching, tremors, convulsions, respiratory depression, tachypnea and hypoxemia, bradycardia, tachycardia, ventricular dysrhythmias, palpitation, angina pectoris, hypotension, urticaria, edema, bronchospasm, anaphylaxis, ventricular dysrhythmias, cardiac arrest, trismus, local tissue damage, long-lasting paresthesia.

Table 1.2. DRUG INTERACTIONS FOR INJECTABLE LOCAL ANESTHETICS

Articaine HCl w/ Epinephrine (Septocaine w/ Epinephrine, Zorcaine)	
α-Adrenergic blockers (prazosin), butyrophenones (haloperidol) and phenothiazines (thioridazine)	May reduce or reverse pressor effect of epinephrine (large doses only); use vasoconstrictor cautiously.
Antidysrhythmic agents (class I)	Additive CNS and cardiac toxicity; use local anesthetic cautiously and in reduced maximum doses.
β-Adrenergic blockers (nonselective)	May cause hypertension and bradycardia with vasoconstrictor; monitor patient and use vasoconstrictor cautiously.
CNS depressants (including alcohol, opioids, antidepressants, and other local anesthetics)	Additive or supra-additive CNS and respiratory depression; use local anesthetic cautiously and in reduced maximum doses.
CNS stimulants (amphetamine) and ergot derivatives (dihydroergotamine)	May cause hypertension with vasoconstrictor; monitor patient and use vasoconstrictor cautiously.
Cocaine	May increase cardiovascular responses to vasoconstrictor; avoid vasoconstrictor use in patient under influence of cocaine.
COMT inhibitors (entacapone)	Inhibition of metabolism may enhance systemic effects of vasoconstrictor; monitor patient and use vasoconstrictor cautiously.
Digoxin	May increase risk of cardiac dysrhythmias; use vasoconstrictor in consultation with physician.
Hydrocarbon inhalation anesthetics (halothane)	May cause cardiac dysrhythmias with vasoconstrictors; consult anesthesiologist about vasoconstrictor use.
Levodopa and thyroid hormones (levothyroxine)	Large doses (beyond replacement doses of thyroid hormone) may increase risk of cardiac toxicity; use vasoconstrictor cautiously.
Methyldopa and adrenergic neuron blockers (guanadrel)	May enhance systemic effects of vasoconstrictor; use vasoconstrictor cautiously.
Tricyclic (imipramine) and heterocyclic (amoxapine) antidepressants	May enhance systemic effects of epinephrine; use vasoconstrictor cautiously.
Bupivacaine HCl w/ Epinephrine (Marcaine w/ Epinephrine, Vivacaine)	
α-Adrenergic blockers (prazosin), butyrophenones (haloperidol) and phenothiazines (thioridazine)	May reduce or reverse pressor effect of epinephrine (large doses only); use vasoconstrictor cautiously.
Antidysrhythmic agents (class I)	Additive CNS and cardiac toxicity; use local anesthetic cautiously and in reduced maximum doses.
β-Adrenergic blockers (nonselective)	May cause hypertension and bradycardia with vasoconstrictor; monitor patient and use vasoconstrictor cautiously.

Table 1.2. DRUG INTERACTIONS FOR INJECTABLE LOCAL ANESTHETICS *(cont.)*

Bupivacaine HCl w/ Epinephrine *(cont.)*	
CNS depressants (including alcohol, opioids, antidepressants, and other local anesthetics)	Additive or supra-additive CNS and respiratory depression; use local anesthetic cautiously and in reduced maximum doses.
CNS stimulants (amphetamine) and ergot derivatives (dihydroergotamine)	May cause hypertension with vasoconstrictor; monitor patient and use vasoconstrictor cautiously.
Cocaine	May increase cardiovascular responses to vasoconstrictor; avoid vasoconstrictor use in patient under influence of cocaine.
COMT inhibitors (entacapone)	Inhibition of metabolism may enhance systemic effects of vasoconstrictor; monitor patient and use vasoconstrictor cautiously.
Digoxin	May increase risk of cardiac dysrhythmias; use vasoconstrictor in consultation with physician.
Hydrocarbon inhalation anesthetics (halothane)	May cause cardiac dysrhythmias with vasoconstrictors; consult anesthesiologist about vasoconstrictor use.
Levodopa and thyroid hormones (levothyroxine)	Large doses (beyond replacement doses of thyroid hormone) may increase risk of cardiac toxicity; use vasoconstrictor cautiously.
Methyldopa and adrenergic neuron blockers (guanadrel)	May enhance systemic effects of vasoconstrictor; use vasoconstrictor cautiously.
Tricyclic (imipramine) and heterocyclic (amoxapine) antidepressants	May enhance systemic effects of epinephrine; use vasoconstrictor cautiously.
Lidocaine HCl (Xylocaine)	
Amiodarone, β-adrenergic blockers (propranolol), cimetidine	Hepatic metabolism may be decreased; use local anesthetic cautiously, especially regarding repeat dosing.
Antidysrhythmic agents (class I)	Additive CNS and cardiac toxicity; use local anesthetic cautiously and in reduced maximum doses.
CNS depressants (including alcohol, opioids, antidepressants, and other local anesthetics)	Additive or supra-additive CNS and respiratory depression; use local anesthetic cautiously and in reduced maximum doses.
Lidocaine HCl w/ Epinephrine (Lignospan Standard, Lignospan Forte, Octocaine 50, Octocaine 100, Xylocaine w/ Epinephrine)	
α-Adrenergic blockers (prazosin), butyrophenones (haloperidol) and phenothiazines (thioridazine)	May reduce or reverse pressor effect of epinephrine (large doses only); use vasoconstrictor cautiously.
Amiodarone, β-adrenergic blockers, cimetidine	Hepatic metabolism may be decreased; use local anesthetic cautiously, especially regarding repeat dosing.

Lidocaine HCl w/ Epinephrine *(cont.)*	
Antidysrhythmic agents (class I)	Additive CNS and cardiac toxicity; use local anesthetic cautiously and in reduced maximum doses.
β-Adrenergic blockers (nonselective)	May cause hypertension and bradycardia with vasoconstrictor; monitor patient and use vasoconstrictor cautiously.
CNS depressants (including alcohol, opioids, antidepressants, and other local anesthetics)	Additive or supra-additive CNS and respiratory depression; use local anesthetic cautiously and in reduced maximum doses.
CNS stimulants (amphetamine) and ergot derivatives (dihydroergotamine)	May cause hypertension with vasoconstrictor; monitor patient and use vasoconstrictor cautiously.
Cocaine	May increase cardiovascular responses to vasoconstrictor; avoid vasoconstrictor use in patient under influence of cocaine.
COMT inhibitors (entacapone)	Inhibition of metabolism may enhance systemic effects of vasoconstrictor; monitor patient and use vasoconstrictor cautiously.
Digoxin	May increase risk of cardiac dysrhythmias; use vasoconstrictor in consultation with physician.
Hydrocarbon inhalation anesthetics (halothane)	May cause cardiac dysrhythmias with vasoconstrictors; consult anesthesiologist about vasoconstrictor use.
Levodopa and thyroid hormones (levothyroxine)	Large doses (beyond replacement doses of thyroid hormone) may increase risk of cardiac toxicity; use vasoconstrictor cautiously.
Methyldopa and adrenergic neuron blockers (guanadrel)	May enhance systemic effects of vasoconstrictor; use vasoconstrictor cautiously.
Tricyclic (imipramine) and heterocyclic (amoxapine) antidepressants	May enhance systemic effects of epinephrine; use vasoconstrictor cautiously.
Mepivacaine HCl (Carbocaine, Isocaine, Polocaine, Scandonest 3% Plain)	
Amiodarone, β-adrenergic blockers, cimetidine	Hepatic metabolism may be decreased; use local anesthetic cautiously, especially regarding repeat dosing.
Antidysrhythmic agents (class I)	Additive CNS and cardiac toxicity; use local anesthetic cautiously and in reduced maximum doses.
CNS depressants (including alcohol, opioids, antidepressants, and other local anesthetics)	Additive or supra-additive CNS and respiratory depression; use local anesthetic cautiously and in reduced maximum doses.
Mepivacaine HCl w/ Levonordefrin (Carbocaine w/ NeoCobefrin, Isocaine w/ Levonordefrin, Scandonest 2% L)	
Amiodarone, β-adrenergic blockers, cimetidine	Hepatic metabolism may be decreased; use local anesthetic cautiously, especially regarding repeat dosing.
Antidysrhythmic agents (class I)	Additive CNS and cardiac toxicity; use local anesthetic cautiously and in reduced maximum doses.

Table 1.2. DRUG INTERACTIONS FOR INJECTABLE LOCAL ANESTHETICS *(cont.)*

Mepivacaine HCl w/ Levonordefrin *(cont.)*	
β-Adrenergic blockers (nonselective)	May cause hypertension and bradycardia with vasoconstrictor; monitor patient and use vasoconstrictor cautiously.
CNS depressants (including alcohol, opioids, antidepressants, and other local anesthetics)	Additive or supra-additive CNS and respiratory depression; use local anesthetic cautiously and in reduced maximum doses.
CNS stimulants (amphetamine) and ergot derivatives (dihydroergotamine)	May cause hypertension with vasoconstrictor; monitor patient and use vasoconstrictor cautiously.
Cocaine	May increase cardiovascular responses to vasoconstrictor; avoid vasoconstrictor use in patient under influence of cocaine.
COMT inhibitors (entacapone)	Inhibition of metabolism may enhance systemic effects of vasoconstrictor; monitor patient and use vasoconstrictor cautiously.
Digoxin	May increase risk of cardiac dysrhythmias; use vasoconstrictor in consultation with physician.
Hydrocarbon inhalation anesthetics (halothane)	May cause cardiac dysrhythmias with vasoconstrictors; consult anesthesiologist about vasoconstrictor use.
Levodopa and thyroid hormones (levothyroxine)	Large doses (beyond replacement doses of thyroid hormone) may increase risk of cardiac toxicity; use vasoconstrictor cautiously.
Methyldopa and adrenergic neuron blockers (guanadrel)	May enhance systemic effects of vasoconstrictor; use vasoconstrictor cautiously.
Tricyclic (imipramine) and heterocyclic (amoxapine) antidepressants	May strongly enhance systemic effects of levonordefrin; avoid concurrent use.
Prilocaine HCl (Citanest Plain)	
Acetaminophen, acetanilid, aniline dyes, benzocaine, chloroquine, dapsone, naphthalene, nitrates and nitrites, nitrofurantoin, nitroglycerin, nitroprusside, pamaquine, para-aminosalicylic acid, phenacetin, phenobarbital, phenytoin, primaquine, quinine, and sulfonamides	Increased risk for developing methemoglobinemia; use prilocaine in reduced maximum doses.
Amiodarone, β-adrenergic blockers, cimetidine	Hepatic metabolism may be decreased; use local anesthetic cautiously, especially regarding repeat dosing.
Antidysrhythmic agents (class I)	Additive CNS and cardiac toxicity; use local anesthetic cautiously and in reduced maximum doses.
CNS depressants (including alcohol, opioids, antidepressants, and other local anesthetics)	Additive or supra-additive CNS and respiratory depression; use local anesthetic cautiously and in reduced maximum doses.

able 1.3. LOCAL ANESTHETICS: POTENTIAL CROSS-SENSITIVITY WITH OTHER DRUGS

ERSON WITH A SENSITIVITY TO	MAY ALSO HAVE A SENSITIVITY TO
a-aminobenzoic acid (PABA) or aben preservative	Procaine, chloroprocaine, benzocaine, butamben, tetracaine, other local anesthetic solutions containing paraben preservatives (as in multidose vials)
y ester local anesthetic	Other ester local anesthetics
y amide local anesthetic	Other amide local anesthetics (rarely)
lfites	Any local anesthetic with an adrenergic vasoconstrictor (sulfites are included with vasoconstrictors as antioxidants)

Table 1.4. TOPICAL ANESTHETICS: DURATION OF ACTION

DRUG	DURATION OF ANESTHETIC ACTION
Benzocaine	10-20 min
Cocaine	20-40 min
Dyclonine	20-40 min
Lidocaine	10-20 min*
Tetracaine	20-60 min

*Duration can be extended up to 45 min if lidocaine transoral delivery patch is applied for 15 min.

Prilocaine HCl w/ Epinephrine (Citanest Forte)	
Acetaminophen, acetanilid, aniline dyes, benzocaine, chloroquine, dapsone, naphthalene, nitrates and nitrites, nitrofurantoin, nitroglycerin, nitroprusside, pamaquine, para-aminosalicylic acid, phenacetin, phenobarbital, phenytoin, primaquine, quinine, and sulfonamides	Increased risk for developing methemoglobinemia; use prilocaine maximum doses.
α-Adrenergic blockers (prazosin), butyrophenones (haloperidol) and phenothiazines (thioridazine)	May reduce or reverse pressor effect of epinephrine (large doses only); vasoconstrictor cautiously.
Amiodarone, β-adrenergic blockers, cimetidine	Hepatic metabolism may be decreased; use local anesthetic cautiously, especially regarding repeat dosing.
Antidysrhythmic agents (class I)	Additive CNS and cardiac toxicity; use local anesthetic cautiously and in reduced maximum doses.
β-Adrenergic blockers (nonselective)	May cause hypertension and bradycardia with vasoconstrictor; monitor patie and use vasoconstrictor cautiously.
CNS depressants (including alcohol, opioids, antidepressants, and other local anesthetics)	Additive or supra-additive CNS and respiratory depression; use cautiously and in reduced maximum doses.
CNS stimulants (amphetamine) and ergot derivatives (dihydroergotamine)	May cause hypertension with vasoconstrictor; monitor patient and use vasoconstrictor cautiously.
Cocaine	May increase cardiovascular responses to vasoconstrictor; avoid vasoconstrictor use in patient under influence of cocaine.
COMT inhibitors (entacapone)	Inhibition of metabolism may enhance systemic effects of vasoconstrictor; monitor patient and use vasoconstrictor cautiously.
Digoxin	May increase risk of cardiac dysrhythmias; use vasoconstrictor in consultation with physician.
Hydrocarbon inhalation anesthetics (halothane)	May cause cardiac dysrhythmias with vasoconstrictors; consult anesthesiologist about vasoconstrictor use.
Levodopa and thyroid hormones (levothyroxine)	Large doses (beyond replacement doses of thyroid hormone) may increase risk of cardiac toxicity; use vasoconstrictor cautiously.
Methyldopa and adrenergic neuron blockers (guanadrel)	May enhance systemic effects of vasoconstrictor; use vasoconstrictor cautiously.
Tricyclic (imipramine) and heterocyclic (amoxapine) antidepressants	May enhance systemic effects of epinephrine; use vasoconstrictor cautiously.

Table 1.5. PRESCRIBING INFORMATION FOR TOPICAL LOCAL ANESTHETICS

NAME	FORM/ STRENGTH	DOSAGE	WARNINGS/PRECAUTIONS & CONTRAINDICATIONS	ADVERSE EFFECTS†
Benzocaine	**Cre:** Banadyne-3 5%, Benzodent 20%, Orajel PM Maximum Strength 20%; **Gel:** HDA Toothache 6.5%, Baby Anbesol 7.5%, Baby Orajel Teething Pain Medicine 7.5%, Anbesol Jr. 10%, Anbesol Regular Strength 10%, Baby Orajel Teething Nighttime Formula 10%, Orajel Regular Strength 10%, Zilactin-B 10%, Orajel Denture Plus 15%, Orajel Ultra Mouth Sore Medicine 15%, Anbesol Maximum Strength 20%, ComfortCaine 20%, Darby Super-Dent Benzocaine Topical Anesthetic 20%, Dentapaine 20%, Dentsply Oral Anesthetic 20%, Gingicaine 20%, HurriCaine 20%, Kank-A Soft Brush 20%, Orabase with Benzocaine 20%, Orabase-B 20%, Orajel Maximum Strength 20%, Orajel Mouth Sore Medicine 20%, Orajel Ultra Mouth Sore Medicine 20%, ProJel-20 20%, Topex 20%, Topicale 18%, Topicale Xtra 20%; **Disc:** Orajel Protective Mouth Sore Discs 20mg/disc; **Gel patch:** Topicale GelPatch 36mg/patch; **Gum:** Dent's Extra Strength Toothache 20%; **Liquid:** Rid-A-Pain Dental Drops 6.3%, Baby Orajel Teething Pain Medicine 7.5%, Anbesol Regular Strength 10%, Orajel Regular Strength 10%, Tanac Liquid 10%, Anbesol Maximum Strength 20%, Gingicaine 20%, HurriCaine 20%, Kank-A 20%, Orajel Maximum Strength 20%, Topex 20%; **Loz:** Chloraseptic Sore Throat 6 mg, Cepacol 15 mg, Chloraseptic Max Sore Throat Relief 15 mg; **Oint:** Cora-Caine 16%, Anbesol Cold Sore Therapy 20%, Red Cross Canker Sore Medication 20%, Topicale 20%; **Paste:** Orabase with Ben-zocaine 20%; **Spray:** Americaine 20%, HurriCaine 20%, Topex 20%; **Swab:** Baby Orajel Teething Swabs 7.5%, CaineTips 20%, Dentemp's Oral Pain Relief 20%, HurriCaine 20%, Orajel Medicated Mouth Sore Swabs 20%, Orajel Medicated Toothache Swabs 20%, Topex HandiCaine Stix 20%, Zilactin Toothache Maximum Strength 20%	**(Cre)** ***Adults:*** Apply to affected area up to 4 times daily or as directed. ***Pediatrics:*** **<2 yrs:** Dose must be individualized by dentist or physician. **(Disc)** ***Adults:*** Apply disc to affected area, hold for 5-10 sec and allow product to dissolve slowly in the mouth. May be repeated every 2 hrs as needed. ***Pediatrics:*** **<2 yrs:** Dose must be individualized by dentist or physician. **(Gel)** ***Adults:*** Apply to affected area up to 4 times daily or as directed. ***Pediatrics:*** **<4 months:** Nonprescription teeth-ing products should not be used. **<2 yrs:** Dosages of all benzocaine products for children under 2 yrs should be individualized based on child's age, weight, and physical status. **(Gel Patch)** Apply to affected area up to 4 times daily or as directed. **(Gum)** Clean tooth cavity by rinsing with warm water; then cut gum to fit and press into cavity. **(Liq)** ***Adults:*** Apply to affected area up to 4 times daily or as directed. ***Pediatrics:*** **<2 yrs:** Dosages for children should be in-dividualized based on child's age, weight, and physical status. **(Loz)** ***Adults:*** Dissolve 1 lozenge no more frequently than every 2 hrs. ***Pediatrics:*** **2-12 yrs:** Varies by individual product. **(Oint)** ***Adults:*** Apply to affected area up to 4 times daily or as directed. **(Paste)** ***Adults:*** Apply to affected area up to 4 times daily or as directed. ***Pediatrics:*** **<6 yrs:** Dose must be individualized by dentist or physician. **(Spray)** ***Adults:*** Spray should be applied for 1 sec or less for normal anesthesia. Spray in excess of 2 sec is contraindicated. **(Swab)** Apply to affected area up to 4 times daily or as directed.	**W/P:** Patients with a history of allergy to local anesthetics such as procaine, butacaine, benzocaine, or other "caine" anesthetics should be instructed not to use these products. Methemoglobinemia (rare) has been reported with benzocaine-containing products, especially with unmetered spray formulations. Benzocaine sprays should not exceed 2 sec in total. Avoid contact with eyes. Patients should be instructed that fever and nasal congestion are not symptoms of teething and may indicate the presence of infection. Patient should not use for more than 7 days unless directed to. Patients should be instructed to alert dentist or physician if sore mouth symp-toms do not get better in 7 days; irritation, pain, or redness does not go away; or swelling, rash, or fever develops. Keep out of reach of children. **Contra:** Hypersensitivity to benzocaine/ester-type local anes-thetics. **P/N:** Category C, caution in nursing.	**Burning, stinging, swelling, skin rash, redness, itching, or hives in or around the mouth;** methe-moglobinemia, dizziness, tired-ness, headache, weakness.

†Bold entries denote special dental considerations.
W/P = warnings/precautions; **Contra** = contraindications; **P/N** = pregnancy category rating and nursing considerations.

Table 1.5. PRESCRIBING INFORMATION FOR TOPICAL LOCAL ANESTHETICS *(cont.)*

NAME	FORM/ STRENGTH	DOSAGE	WARNINGS/PRECAUTIONS & CONTRAINDICATIONS	ADVERSE EFFECTS†
Benzocaine, Butambin, and Tetracaine HCl	**Gel:** Cetacaine Hospital 14%/2%/2%; **Sol:** Cetacaine 14%/2%/2%; **Spray:** Cetacaine 14%/2%/2%	**(Gel)** ***Adults:*** Apply up to 1mL to affected area. **(Sol)** ***Adults:*** Apply up to 1mL to affected area. **(Spray)** ***Adults:*** Spray up to 1mL (or 2 sec) on affected area.	**W/P:** Patients with a history of allergy to ester local anesthetics such as procaine, butacaine, benzocaine, or tetracaine should be instructed not to use these products. Methemoglobinemia (rare) has been reported with benzocaine-containing products, especially with unmetered spray formulations. Sprays should not exceed 2 sec in total. Avoid inhalation, which could result in rapid absorption and systemic toxicity. Do not exceed recommended dose. Keep out of the reach of children. Avoid contact with eyes. **Contra:** Hypersensitivity to ester-type local anesthetics. **P/N:** Category C, caution in nursing.	Burning, stinging, swelling, or tenderness not present before treatment; **skin rash, redness, itching, or hives in or around the mouth;** methemoglobinemia, dizziness, tiredness, headache, weakness, lightheadedness, nervousness, confusion, euphoria, dizziness, drowsiness, blurred vision, tremors, convulsions, respiratory depression, bradycardia, hypotension.
Dyclonine HCl	**Loz:** Sucrets Children's 1.2mg, Sucrets Regular Strength 2mg, Sucrets Maximum Strength 3mg; **Sol:** Dyclone 1%	**(Loz)** ***Adults:*** Dissolve 1 lozenge slowly no more than once every 2 hrs up to a maximum of 10 lozenges per day. ***Pediatrics:*** **2-12 yrs:** Limit dose to 1.2 mg/lozenge. **(Sol)** ***Adults:*** Apply up to 300mg (30mL) to affected area per examination. May be used after dilution to a 0.5% concentration as a mouthwash or gargle and the excess expelled.	**W/P:** Reduce dose in elderly, debilitated, acutely ill. Increased likelihood for local or systemic reactions when applied to traumatized mucosa or areas with sepsis Caution with heart block and severe shock. Excessive dose or too-frequent administration may result in high plasma levels and serious adverse effects requiring resuscitative measures. Dosing not established in children under 12 yrs. **P/N:** Category C, caution in nursing.	Lightheadedness, nervousness, confusion, euphoria, dizziness, drowsiness, blurred vision, tremors, convulsions, respiratory depression, bradycardia, hypotension, edema, irritation, stinging, swelling, urticaria.
Lidocaine	**Oint:** Octocaine 5%, Xylocaine 5%; **Patch:** DentiPatch 46.1mg	**(Oint)** ***Adults:*** Apply to affected area or denture up to a maximum of 5g (250mg lidocaine) in 6 hrs. ***Pediatrics:*** Limit dose to 4.5mg/kg body weight (lidocaine) or 2.5g in 6 hrs. **(Patch)** ***Adults:*** Apply single patch.	**W/P:** Reduce dose in elderly, debilitated, acutely ill, and pediatrics. Caution with heart block and severe shock. Excessive dose or too-frequent administration may result in high plasma levels and serious adverse effects requiring resuscitative measures. Extreme caution if mucosa traumatized; risk of rapid systemic absorption. Overdose reported in pediatrics due to inappropriate dosing. **Contra:** Hypersensitivity to amide-type local anesthetics. **P/N:** Category B, caution in nursing.	Lightheadedness, nervousness, confusion, euphoria, dizziness, drowsiness, blurred vision, tremors, convulsions, respiratory depression, bradycardia, hypotension, urticaria, edema, anaphylactoid reactions.
Lidocaine HCl	**Gel:** Xylocaine Jelly 2%; **Oral Topical Sol:** Xylocaine Viscous 2%; **Sol:** Xylocaine 4%	**(Gel)** Apply to affected area up to a maximum of 4.5mg/kg or 300mg lidocaine. **(Oral Topical Sol)** ***Adults:*** Apply to affected area or swish or gargle and then expectorate, using up to a maximum dose of 4.5mg/kg or 300mg lidocaine every 3 hrs. ***Pediatrics:*** **≤ 3 yrs:** Apply up to 1.25mL solution (25mg lidocaine) every 3 hrs. **(Sol)** Apply to affected area up to a maximum of 4.5mg/kg or 300mg lidocaine.	**W/P:** Reduce dose in elderly, debilitated, acutely ill, and pediatrics. Caution with heart block and severe shock. Excessive dose or too-frequent administration may result in high plasma levels and serious adverse effects requiring resuscitative measures. Extreme caution if mucosa traumatized; risk of rapid systemic absorption. Overdose reported in pediatrics due to inappropriate dosing. **Contra:** Hypersensitivity to amide-type local anesthetics. **P/N:** Category B, caution in nursing.	Lightheadedness, nervousness, confusion, euphoria, dizziness, drowsiness, blurred vision, tremors, convulsions, respiratory depression, bradycardia, hypotension, urticaria, edema, anaphylactoid reactions.

†Bold entries denote special dental considerations.
W/P = warnings/precautions; **Contra** = contraindications; **P/N** = pregnancy category rating and nursing considerations.

NAME	FORM/ STRENGTH	DOSAGE	WARNINGS/PRECAUTIONS & CONTRAINDICATIONS	ADVERSE EFFECTS†
Lidocaine and Prilocaine Periodontal Gel (Oraqix)	**Gel:** 2.5%/2.5%	***Adults:*** Apply Oraqix on the gingival margin around selected teeth using blunt-tipped applicator included with package. Wait 30 sec, then fill periodontal pockets with Oraqix using blunt-tipped applicator until gel becomes visible at the gingival margin. Wait another 30 sec before starting treatment. Maximum 8.5g gel per treatment session.	**W/P:** Allergic reactions, including anaphylaxis, can occur. Elevated methemoglobin levels. Patients with elevated methemoglobin levels, glucose-6-phosphate dehydrogenase deficiency, or congenital or idiopathic methemoglobinemia should not use Oraqix. Oraqix should not be used with standard dental syringes. Only use this product with the Oraqix Dispenser. **Contra:** Hypersensitivity to amide-type local anesthetics. **P/N:** Category B, caution in nursing women.	**Pain, soreness, irritation, numbness, vesicles, ulcerations, edema and/or redness in the treated area,** headache, nausea, **taste alteration,** fatigue, flu, respiratory infection, musculoskeletal pain, accidental injury.
Tetracaine HCl (Pontocaine)	**Sol:** 2%	***Adults:*** Apply as a 0.25% or 0.5% topical solution or as a 0.5% nebulized spray; total dosage not to exceed 20mg.	**W/P:** Patients should be instructed not to use tetracaine if they have a history of allergy to ester local anesthetics such as procaine, butacaine, or benzocaine. Avoid contact with eyes. Do not exceed recommended dose. Caution with heart block and severe shock. Excessive dose or too-frequent administration may result in high plasma levels and serious adverse effects requiring resuscitative measures. Keep out of reach of children. **Contra:** Hypersensitivity to tetracaine/ester-type local anesthetics. **P/N:** Category C, caution in nursing.	Burning, stinging, swelling, or tenderness not present before treatment; skin rash, redness, itching, or hives; lightheadedness, nervousness, confusion, euphoria, dizziness, drowsiness, blurred vision, tremors, convulsions, respiratory depression, bradycardia, hypotension.

Chapter 2

Conscious Sedation and Agents for the Control of Anxiety

B. Ellen Byrne, D.D.S., Ph.D.; Leonard S. Tibbetts, D.D.S., M.S.D.

All types of dental care—from that rendered with no anesthesia to treatment rendered under general anesthesia—require accurate diagnosis, proper treatment, and effective patient monitoring. This involves obtaining a current complete medical history, performing a comprehensive examination, and a thorough pretreatment evaluation.

The administration of local anesthesia, sedation, and general anesthesia is an integral part of dental practice. The American Dental Association is committed to the safe and effective use of these modalities by appropriately educated and trained dentists. To assist practitioners, the ADA has issued "Guidelines for the Use of Sedation and General Anesthesia by Dentists" (see "Suggested Reading" at the end of this section for more information). Dentists providing sedation and anesthesia in compliance with their state rules and/or regulations prior to the adoption of these guidelines are not subject to the educational requirements outlined in Section III of the document.

Providing care and ensuring the well-being of patients in the dental office is based on a continuum of techniques that are available for the management of anxiety and pain. This chapter focuses on the calming of apprehensive and/or nervous patients through the use of drugs, without causing the loss of consciousness.

Using various techniques to control anxiety and pain has been an integral part of the practice of dentistry since the profession's early years. Today, the term "conscious sedation" is used to describe the amelioration of patient anxiety, the blunting of the stress response, and often some degree of amnesia produced by a combination of psychological techniques and drugs. Unfortunately, the term "intravenous sedation" means general anesthesia to much of the public and to many medical and dental professionals. When properly understood, the term "conscious sedation," coined by dentist/anesthesiologist Richard Bennett in the 1970s, does much to alleviate this misconception. Conscious sedation is a minimally depressed level of consciousness in which the patient retains the ability to independently and continuously maintain an airway—as well as to respond appropriately to physical stimulation or verbal command—that can be produced by a pharmacological or nonpharmacological method or both. Examples of nonpharmacological methods used for anxiety and pain management are hypnosis, acupuncture, acupressure, audio-analgesia, biofeedback, electroanesthesia (transcutaneous electrical nerve stimulation), and electrosedation.

Appropriately trained dentists may use any of a number of preoperative and operative pharmacological conscious sedation techniques to achieve the goals of anxiety reduction and pain control. Such techniques may include sedation by enteral (absorption by way of the alimentary canal), inhalation (absorption into the lungs), and parenteral (introduction via subcutaneous, intramuscular, intraorbital, or intravenous routes) means.

Each category of pharmacological conscious sedation has specific educational and monitoring requirements for safe, effective, and efficacious patient usage, as well as specific licensing requirements mandated by regulatory agencies. The use of conscious sedation techniques in the various categories by appropriately trained dentists has a remarkable safety record. (See "Suggested Reading" at the end of this section for information on these ADA statements: "Policy Statement: The Use of Sedation and General Anesthesia by Dentists," and "Guidelines for Teaching Pain Control and Sedation to Dentists and Dental Students.")

Whatever the methods of conscious sedation in which dentists strive to be educationally and professionally competent, the use of a wide array of drugs for various types of conscious sedation is contraindicated without an adequately detailed working knowledge about them. In fact, using as few drugs as possible to appropriately and adequately sedate patients is advised as the dentist can become intimately familiar with a limited number of drugs, their pharmacological actions, indications, contraindications, precautions, and drug interactions.

Intravenous conscious sedation induced in the dental office, for example, can be handled almost entirely by a combination of the following seven drugs, which fall into these three classes:

- benzodiazepines—diazepam, midazolam
- sedatives—pentobarbital
- narcotic analgesics—morphine, meperidine, fentanyl, nalbuphine

Today, the most common pharmacological method of controlling anxiety with intravenous sedation is through the use of one of the benzodiazepines in combination with a narcotic analgesic. The benzodiazepines are used to reduce the apprehension and fear, as well as to provide an amnesia effect, while the narcotics produce analgesia and euphoria. The sedative pentobarbital, in combination with meperidine, can be used when there are contraindications to the use of the benzodiazepines.

Administration Routes

Of the various administration routes for conscious sedation drugs, each has advantages and disadvantages.

The oral route is most commonly used, and it has the advantages of almost universal acceptance by patients, ease of administration, and relative safety. Its disadvantages include its requirement of a bolus dosage of medication, based on the patient's weight and age; its long latent period; its unreliable absorption; its inability to be titrated due to the long latency period; and its prolonged duration of action.

Titration of oral medication for the purpose of sedation, therefore, is unpredictable. Repeated dosing of orally administered sedative agents may result in an alteration in the state of consciousness beyond the practitioner's intent. Except in unusual circumstances, the maximum recommended dose of an oral medication should not be exceeded.

The rectal route of administration is used in dentistry only occasionally, when patients are either unwilling or unable to take the drugs by mouth. This route's advantages and disadvantages are similar to those of oral administration.

Another option is the combined inhalation-enteral route of conscious sedation. The advantages of using this combination include greater patient acceptance and a higher degree of effectiveness than either technique offers individually. The disadvantage is that the dentist must be proficient in the pharmacology of agents used in the management of both inhalation and enteral sedation—drug interactions and incompatibilities, problems and complications—as well as in making the distinction between the conscious and unconscious state and in clinical airway management.

All other routes of drug administration bypass the gastrointestinal system. In these routes, the drugs are absorbed directly by the body from the site of administration into the cardiovascular system. This includes inhalation and parenteral routes of administration. In dentistry, nitrous oxide and oxygen sedation are synonymous with inhalation sedation. The advantages of inhalation conscious sedation with nitrous oxide and oxygen are that the observed latent period is short, the administrator can titrate the agent appropriately, actions of the agent can be quickly adjusted to decrease or increase the depth of sedation, and recovery is rapid. The disadvantage is that the nitrous oxide–oxygen combination, with no less than a 70:30 ratio, is not a very potent agent, and a certain proportion of patients will not experience the desired effect.

The subcutaneous (SQ) route of administration is used primarily in pediatric dentistry. It offers advantages and disadvantages similar to those of intramuscular (IM) administration as compared with enteral administration. Compared with enteral administration, both SQ and IM administrations offer more rapid onset of action, as well as a more pronounced clinical effect with the same dosage. The SQ route is useful for injecting nonvolatile, water- and fat-soluble hypnotic and narcotic drugs. The relatively poor blood supply of subcutaneous tissues, however, limits the effectiveness of this technique. For the uncooperative pediatric patient, both SQ and IM techniques require a short period of restraint during administration. The major disadvantage of both techniques is the inability to titrate the medications accurately, so typically a bolus dosage is administered based on the patient's age and size. It is also impossible to retrieve the dosage should overdosage occur. For this reason, proper patient monitoring is extremely important, so complications can be intercepted early.

Intravenous (IV) conscious sedation represents the most effective method of acquiring adequate and predictable sedation in virtually all patients, with the exception of disruptive patients, whose cooperation is needed for successful venipuncture. IV conscious sedation allows effective blood levels of drugs to be achieved rapidly with titration (the incremental administration of small drug dosages over appropriate time intervals until the desired level of sedation is achieved) and rapidly enhances the action of a drug. For many IV-administered drugs, the desired and maximum clinical sedative effects are reached within 2 to 8 minutes. Some of the currently available drugs for anxiety reduction are capable of producing an amnesia effect in 80% to 90% of patients for 20 to 40 minutes after administration.

While it is possible with the use of specific antagonists to reverse the actions of some medications in conscious sedation, it is not possible to reverse the action of all drugs after they have been injected. The rapid onset of action and the pronounced clinical actions of intravenously injected drugs will result in exaggerated problems with overdosage. This means the entire dental office staff must be well-trained in the recognition and management of adverse reactions and emergencies that may accompany the drugs used so that patient safety and quality dental care are never compromised.

Records and Monitoring

Written, advised, informed consent for all forms of conscious sedation is essential. The standard of care for physiological and vital-sign monitoring for the various types of conscious sedation is well-established, as is that for documentation of drugs used, dosage, adverse reactions to medications and recovery from the anesthetic.

State-of-the-art monitoring of patients'

vital signs has improved dramatically in the past several years. Pulse rate, blood pressure, and respiration now can be monitored either physically or electronically. Today, pulse oximetry offers a rapid and effective means of monitoring the blood oxygen saturation and pulse rate and should be used for all methods of conscious sedation, including oral conscious sedation. These methods, in combination with the old standbys of close patient observation and conversation, are the current standards of monitoring care for patients in ASA Class I and II (healthy or with mild-to-moderate systemic disease) who are undergoing any type of parenteral conscious sedation or inhalation-enteral conscious sedation. In the treatment of patients of ASA Class III (with severe systemic disease that limits activity) or higher (ranging from IV: with severe life-threatening systemic disease, to VI: clinically dead but being maintained for harvesting of organs), electrocardiogram monitoring also becomes the standard of care, in addition to the other means of monitoring.

This chapter covers the drugs most frequently used in dental conscious sedation (benzodiazepines and their antagonist flumazenil; barbiturates, opioids and their antagonist naloxone). It also addresses older, less frequently used drugs: chloral hydrate, ethchlorvynol, and meprobamate.

BENZODIAZEPINES

The benzodiazepines are among the most popular classes of drugs available today, having been used since the late 1950s for effective and safe treatment of a variety of anxiety states, as well as for epilepsy (diazepam, clonazepam) and sleep disorders (flurazepam, temazepam, triazolam).

Along with their use for anxiety, the benzodiazepines have extensive clinical applications in anesthesia procedures (diazepam, midazolam) and as muscle relaxants (diazepam). In addition, triazolam is increasing in popularity as oral/sublingual premedication prescribed by dentists for anxious patients. Recent anecdotal reports suggest that incremental dosing of triazolam may be an effective technique for producing conscious sedation in the dental setting. While showing promise, no laboratory or clinical data are available to evaluate the efficacy or safety of this approach.

Although the benzodiazepines have a wide margin of safety, they are not without adverse effects. Their time course of action is variable among patients as well as among various agents. Although all benzodiazepines are effective, there are significant differences among them. When used enterally, diazepam and flurazepam are among the most rapidly absorbed, whereas oxazepam is one of the most slowly absorbed. Use of IM routes of administration for benzodiazepines often results in erratic and poor absorption. Most of the benzodiazepines are poorly soluble in water and are not available for IV use. Diazepam and midazolam, however, are the two agents most commonly used for IV conscious sedation, and an anterograde amnesia is strongly associated with this class of drugs. The level of amnesia varies with agent and route of administration.

All benzodiazepines in use are bound 50% or more to plasma proteins. Their distribution to tissue depends on their lipid solubility.

The metabolism and excretion of the benzodiazepines are complex. Clorazepate is a prodrug converted by metabolism to the active form; others are inactivated by metabolism; still others are biotransferred to metabolites that retain activity. Many of the metabolites of benzodiazepines have longer half-lives than the parent compound and so accumulate to a greater extent. It is important to recognize that some of these compounds have the potential for extremely long durations of action. Thus, benzodiazepine half-lives vary from a few hours to as long as a week.

The imidazopyridine sedative hypnotic zolpidem is included in this section of the chapter because, although it is structurally dissimilar to the benzodiazepines, many of its actions are explained by its action on the benzodiazepine receptor.

Antagonist. The benzodiazepines have a specific antagonist, flumazenil, which is administered intravenously. It reverses the CNS effects of benzodiazepines, including respiratory depression. Its duration of action may be as brief as 30 minutes, so treatment with it requires continuous monitoring of the patient and possibly repeated administration.

Accepted Indications

Benzodiazepines are used for the treatment of anxiety, insomnia, epilepsy, panic disorders, and alcohol withdrawal. As adjuncts in anesthesia, they are used as a preanesthetic medication to produce sedation, relieve anxiety, and produce anterograde amnesia.

General Dosing Information

All benzodiazepines have similar pharmacologic actions. Their different clinical uses are often based on pharmacokinetic differences and availability of clinical use data. Optimal dosage of benzodiazepines varies with diagnosis, method of administration, and patient response. The minimum effective dose should be used for the shortest period of time. Prolonged enteral use (for weeks or months) may result in psychological or physical dependence. After prolonged administration, benzodiazepines should be withdrawn gradually to prevent withdrawal symptoms.

For parenteral dosing, after administration of the drug, patients should be kept under observation until they have recovered sufficiently to return home. Bolus doses and rapidly administered IV doses may result in respiratory depression, apnea, hypotension, bradycardia, and cardiac arrest. When parenteral benzodiazepines are administered intravenously, equipment necessary to secure and maintain an airway should be immediately available.

Table 2.1 provides benzodiazepine dosing information.

Dosage Adjustments

Geriatric or debilitated patients, children, and patients with hepatic or renal function impairment should receive a lower initial dosage, as elimination of benzodiazepines may be slower in these patients, resulting in impaired coordination, dizziness, and excessive sedation.

Special Dental Considerations

Drug Interactions of Dental Interest

Table 2.2 lists possible interactions of the benzodiazepines and zolpidem with other drugs.

Cross-Sensitivity

There may be cross-sensitivity between benzodiazepines.

Special Patients

Pregnant and nursing women

See **Table 2.1** for pregnancy risk categories.

Benzodiazepines are reported to increase the risk of congenital malformations when used during the first trimester; chronic use may cause physical dependence in the neonate, resulting in withdrawal symptoms and CNS depression.

Benzodiazepines and their metabolites may distribute into breast milk, thus creating feeding difficulties and weight loss in the infant.

Pediatric, geriatric, and other special patients

Children (especially the very young) and geriatric patients are usually more sensitive to the CNS effects of benzodiazepines. In the neonate, prolonged CNS depression may be produced because of the newborn's inability to metabolize the benzodiazepine into inactive products. In the geriatric patient, the dosage should be limited to the smallest effective dose and increased gradually to minimize ataxia, dizziness, and oversedation.

Patient Monitoring: Aspects to Watch

- Respiratory status
- Patient requests for benzodiazepines (all of which are Schedule IV controlled substances in the United States)
- Possible abuse and dependence

Adverse Effects and Precautions

Table 2.1 lists adverse effects, precautions, and contraindications for benzodiazepines.

Pharmacology

Benzodiazepines depress all levels of the CNS, resulting in mild sedation, hypnosis, or coma, depending on the dose. It is believed that benzodiazepines enhance or facilitate the inhibitory neurotransmitter action of γ-aminobutyric acid (GABA). After oral administration, benzodiazepines are absorbed well from the gastrointestinal tract. After IM injection, absorption of lorazepam and midazolam is rapid and complete, whereas that of chlordiazepoxide and diazepam may be slow and erratic. Rectal absorption of diazepam is rapid. The benzodiazepines are metabolized by the liver to inactive or other active metabolites. During repeated dosing with long half-life benzodiazepines, there is accumulation of the parent compound and/or active metabolites. During repeated dosing with short to intermediate half-life benzodiazepines, accumulation is minimal.

Patient Advice

- Avoid concurrent use of alcohol and other CNS depressants.
- Until CNS effects are known, avoid activities needing good psychomotor skills.
- A responsible adult should drive the patient to and from dental appointments.
- Recurrent use of these drugs may cause physical or psychological dependence.
- Benzodiazepines may cause xerostomia, which can be countered using sugarless candy, sugarless gum, or a commercially available saliva substitute.

BENZODIAZEPINE ANTAGONIST: FLUMAZENIL

Accepted Indications

Flumazenil is used to reverse the pharmacological effects of benzodiazepines used in anesthesia and to manage benzodiazepine overdose.

General Dosing Information

Flumazenil selectively reverses the pharmacologic effects of benzodiazepines used in anesthesia and is used to manage benzodiazepine overdose. Flumazenil does not antagonize other CNS depressants except for zolpidem. See **Table 2.1**.

Special Dental Considerations

Drug Interactions of Dental Interest

Table 2.2 lists the possible interactions of flumazenil with other drugs.

Cross-Sensitivity

There may be cross-sensitivity to benzodiazepines.

Special Patients

Pregnant and nursing women

Caution should be used in administering flumazenil to a nursing woman because it is not known whether flumazenil is excreted in breast milk.

Pediatric, geriatric, and other special patients

Flumazenil is not recommended for use in children, either for the reversal of sedation, the management of overdose, or resuscitation of newborns. Pulmonary management is advised as the treatment of choice.

The pharmacokinectics of flumazenil have been studied in elderly people and are not significantly different from those in younger patients.

Patient Monitoring: Aspects to Watch

- Respiratory status
- Alertness
- Possible resedation
- Possible seizure activity

Adverse Effects and Precautions

Table 2.1 lists adverse effects, precautions, and contraindications related to flumazenil.

Pharmacology

Flumazenil, an imidazobenzodiazepine derivative, antagonizes the actions of benzodiazepines on the CNS. Flumazenil competitively inhibits the activity at the benzodiazepine recognition site on the benzodiazepine-GABA receptor-chloride ionophore complex. Flumazenil is a weak partial agonist in some animal models of activity, but has little or no agonist activity in humans.

The onset of reversal is usually evident 1 to 2 minutes after the injection is completed. Eighty percent response will be reached within 3 minutes, with peak effect occurring at 6 to 10 minutes. The duration and degree of reversal are related to the plasma concentration of the sedating benzodiazepine as well as the dose of flumazenil given. Resedation is possible if a large single or cumulative dose of benzodiazepine has been given in the course of a long procedure and is least likely in cases where flumazenil is administered to reverse a low dose of a short-acting benzodiazepine.

SUGGESTED READING

American Dental Association. Guidelines for Teaching Pain Control and Sedation to Dentists and Dental Students. Adopted by the ADA House of Delegates, October 2007. Available at: www.ada.org/prof/resources/positions/statements/anxiety_guidelines.pdf.

American Dental Association. Guidelines for the Use of Sedation and General Anesthesia by Dentists. Adopted by the ADA House of Delegates, October 2007. Available at: www.ada.org/prof/resources/positions/statements/anesthesia_guidelines.pdf.

American Dental Association. Policy Statement: The Use of Sedation and General Anesthesia by Dentists. Adopted by the ADA House of Delegates, October 2007. Available at: www.ada.org/prof/resources/positions/statements/statements_anesthesia.pdf.

Giangrego E. Conscious sedation: benefits and risks. *JADA*. 1984;109:546-557.

Jackson DL, Milgrom P, Heacox GA, et al. Pharmacokinetics and clinical effects of multidose sublingual triazolam in healthy volunteers. *J Clin Psychopharmacol*. 2006;26(1):4-8.

Kallar SK, Dunwiddie WC. In: Wetchler BV, ed. *Problems in Anesthesia*. Philadelphia: JB Lippincott Co.; 1988:93-100.

Malamed SF. *Sedation: A Guide to Patient Management*. 4th ed. St. Louis: Mosby; 2003.

Miller RD. *Clinical Therapeutics*. 1992;14(suppl):861-995.

BARBITURATES

The barbiturates were the first drugs truly effective for the management of anxiety. The barbiturates are generalized CNS depressants, depressing the cerebral cortex, the limbic system, and the reticular activating system. These actions produce reduction in anxiety level, decreased mental acuity, and a state of drowsiness. Barbiturates are capable of producing any level of CNS depression, ranging from light sedation through hypnosis, general anesthesia, coma, and death. IV barbiturate compounds can be infused in subhypnotic doses to produce sedation. The barbiturates used for conscious sedation are classified as sedative hypnotics and are categorized by their duration of clinical action following an average oral dose.

Short-acting barbiturates (with 3- to 4-hour duration of action), most notably pentobarbital and secobarbital, are the barbiturates best suited for dental situations. The ultrashort-acting barbiturates (described in Chapter 3) are classified as general anesthetics and are contraindicated for conscious sedation. The long-acting (16- to 24-hour duration of action) and the intermediate-acting (6- to 8-hour duration of action) barbiturates produce clinical levels of sedation for a period exceeding that required for the usual dental or surgical appointment. The long-acting barbiturates, such as phenobarbital, are commonly used as anticonvulsants or when long-term sedation is necessary. The intermediate-acting barbiturates occasionally are used as "sleeping pills" for some types of insomnia.

Accepted Indications

Barbiturates have been used in routine cases requiring conscious sedation to relieve anxiety, tension, and apprehension; however, these agents have generally been replaced with the benzodiazepines for these uses. Barbiturates are used as adjuncts in anesthesia to reduce anxiety and facilitate induction of anesthesia. They are also used in the treatment of epilepsy and insomnia.

General Dosing Information

IV dosage of the barbiturates must be titrated individually in all patients, particularly for patients with impaired hepatic function; a low dose should be used initially. Tolerance and physical dependence occurs with repeated administration. These agents are controlled substances in the United States and Canada. See **Table 2.1**.

Special Dental Considerations

Drug Interactions of Dental Interest

Possible drug interactions and/or related problems of clinical significance in dentistry are shown in **Table 2.2**.

Special Patients

Pregnant and nursing women

Barbiturates readily cross the placenta and increase the risk of fetal abnormalities. Use during the third trimester may result in physical dependence and respiratory depression in newborns.

Barbiturates are excreted in breast milk and may cause CNS depression in the infant.

Patient Monitoring: Aspects to Watch

- Respiratory status

Adverse Effects and Precautions

Adverse effects and precautions related to barbiturates are listed in **Table 2.2**.

Pharmacology

Barbiturates can produce all levels of CNS mood alteration, from excitation to sedation, hypnosis and coma. In sufficient therapeutic doses, barbiturates induce anesthesia, and overdose can produce death. These agents depress the sensory cortex, decrease motor activity, alter cerebellar function, and produce drowsiness, sedation, and hypnosis.

Barbiturates are respiratory depressants and the degree of respiratory depression is dose-dependent. All barbiturates exhibit anticonvulsant activity.

Barbiturates are enzyme-inducing drugs. This class of drugs can enhance the metabolism of other agents. The onset of this enzyme induction is gradual and depends on the accumulation of the barbiturate and the synthesis of the new enzyme, while offset depends on elimination of the barbiturate and decay of the increased enzyme stores.

Absorption varies depending on the route of administration: oral or rectal, 20 to 60 minutes; IM, slightly faster than oral or rectal routes; IV, immediate to 5 minutes. The sodium salts of the barbiturates are more rapidly absorbed than the free acids because they dissolve rapidly. The rate of absorption is increased if the agents are taken on an empty stomach. The barbiturates are weak acids and distribute rapidly to all tissues, with high concentrations initially in the brain, liver, lungs, heart, and kidneys. The more lipid-soluble the drug, the more rapidly it penetrates all tissues of the body. The barbiturates are metabolized by the liver; phenobarbital is partially excreted unchanged in the urine.

OPIOIDS

The term "opioid" is used in a broad sense to include both opioid agonists and opioid agonists/antagonists. The opioids are administered for their analgesic properties and are considered excellent drugs for the relief of moderate to severe pain. The parenteral dosage forms of this class of drugs are also used as general anesthesia adjuncts in conjunction with other drugs, such as the benzodiazepines, neuromuscular blocking agents, and nitrous oxide for the maintenance of "balanced" anesthesia. Sufentanil, alfentanil, and remifentanil are discussed in Chapter 3, as they are used most often in dentistry for deep sedation and general anesthesia. Most opioids are classified as controlled substances in the U.S. and Canada. Opioids are grouped into three types: agonists, antagonists, and mixed agents. Agonists include codeine, fentanyl, hydrocodone, hydromorphone, levorphanol, meperidine, methadone, morphine, oxycodone, and oxymorphone. Antagonists are naloxone and naltrexone. Mixed agents are buprenorphine, butorphanol, nalbuphine, and pentazocine.

General Dosing Information

Narcotic drugs are used to produce mood changes, provide analgesia, and elevate the pain threshold. Opioid analgesics may not provide sufficient analgesia when used with nitrous oxide for the maintenance of balance anesthesia. Narcotic agents can be used in combination with other agents such as benzodiazepines, antihistamines, ultrashort-acting barbiturates, and a potent hydrocarbon inhalation anesthetic. Dosage and dosing intervals should be individualized for the patient based on duration of action of the specific drug, other medications the patient is currently taking, the patient's condition, and the patient's response. See **Chapter 3, Table 3.1**.

Special Dental Considerations

Drug Interactions of Dental Interest

Possible drug interactions of clinical significance in dentistry are shown in **Chapter 3, Table 3.2**.

Laboratory Value Alterations

- Opioids delay gastric emptying, thereby invalidating gastric emptying studies.
- In hepatobiliary imaging, delivery of technetium Tc99m disofenin to the small bowel may be prevented because opioids may constrict sphincter of Oddi; this results in delayed visualization and resembles an obstruction in the common bile duct.

- Cerebrospinal fluid may be increased secondary to respiratory depression–induced carbon dioxide retention.
- Plasma amylase activity may be increased.
- Plasma lipase activity may be increased.
- Serum alanine aminotransferase may be increased.
- Serum alkaline phosphatase may be increased.
- Serum aspartate aminotransferase may be increased.
- Serum bilirubin may be increased.
- Serum lactate dehydrogenase may be increased.

Cross-Sensitivity

Patients hypersensitive to fentanyl may be hypersensitive to the chemically related alfentanil or sufentanil.

Special Patients

Pregnant and nursing women

Risk-benefit must be considered because opioid analgesics cross the placenta.

Pediatric, geriatric, and other special patients

Geriatric patients are more susceptible to the effects of opioids, especially respiratory depression. Clearance of opioid analgesics can be reduced in the geriatric patient, which leads to a delayed postoperative recovery. Children aged up to 2 years may be more susceptible to opioids' effects, especially respiratory depression. Paradoxical excitation is especially likely to occur in the pediatric population.

Patient Monitoring: Aspects to Watch

- Respiratory status
- State of consciousness
- Heart rate
- Blood pressure

Opioids: Effect on Types of Nerve Receptors

Receptor	Effect
mu$_1$ (μ_1)	Supraspinal analgesia.
mu$_2$ (μ_2)	Respiratory depression, bradycardia, hypothermia, euphoria, moderate sedation, physical dependence, miosis.
kappa (K)	Spinal analgesia, heavy sedation, miosis.
sigma (σ)	Dysphoria, tachycardia, tachypnea, mydriasis.
delta (Δ)	Modulation of μ receptor.
epsilon (ε)	Altered neurohumoral functions.

Adverse Effects and Precautions

Table 2.1 lists adverse effects, precautions, and contraindications related to opioids.

Pharmacology

Opioid analgesics bind to receptors within the central nervous system and peripheral nervous system. This interaction affects both the perception of pain and the emotional response to pain. There are at least five types of opioid receptors—mu (μ), kappa (K), sigma (σ), delta (Δ) and epsilon (ε)—located throughout the body that may be activated by exogenous or endogenous opioid-like substances (endorphins). The action of various opioids at the various receptors determines the agents' specific actions and side effects (see box above).

Based on their actions at these receptors, the commercially available opioids may be divided into three groups: pure agonists, pure antagonists, and mixed agents (agonists/antagonists or partial agonists).

All opioids are respiratory depressants. By exerting a depressant action on respiratory center neurons in the medulla, they decrease respiratory rate, tidal volume, and minute ventilation. They may increase arterial CO_2 tensions. All opioids affect the cardiovascular system by their actions on the autonomic nervous system. Hypotension may result from arteriolar and venous dilation as a result of either histamine release or decreased sympathetic nervous system tone. Bradycardia results from vagal stimulation. Finally, all opioids disorganize GI function, causing increased tone and muscle spasm but delayed emptying and decreased motility and secretions.

OPIOID (NARCOTIC) ANTAGONISTS: NALOXONE, NALTREXONE

Like the benzodiazepines, the opioids have specific antagonists that reverse the pharmacologic effects caused by the opioid drugs.

Accepted Indications

Naloxone and naltrexone are competitive antagonists at the mu, kappa, and sigma receptors with a higher affinity for the mu receptor. Both drugs act centrally and peripherally, but have differing pharmacokinetic profiles favoring different therapeutic uses. Naloxone has low oral bioavailability, but a fast onset of action following parenteral administration and is used for the complete or partial reversal of narcotic depression, such as respiratory depression induced by opioids (including both natural and synthetic narcotics). Its short duration of action risks the potential for "re-narcotization," thus not providing adequate duration of effect for opioid maintenance or deterrent therapy. Naloxone is also used for the diagnosis of suspected acute opioid overdose.

Naltrexone is orally active with a longer duration of action, making it useful in abuse deterrent, detoxification, and maintenance treatment. Nalmefene, a mu opioid receptor antagonist, is a water-soluble naltrexone derivative with a longer duration of action than naloxone.

Naloxone and naltrexone can be combined with mu agonists or partial antagonists to prevent the intravenous abuse of the agonist.

General Dosing Information

Varying amounts of naloxone may be needed to antagonize the effects of different agents. Lack of significant improvement of CNS depression and/or respiration after administration of an adequate dose (10 mg) of naloxone may indicate that the condition is due to a nonopioid CNS depressant. Naloxone reverses the analgesic effects of the opioid and may precipitate withdrawal symptoms in physically dependent patients. See **Table 2.1** for dosage and prescribing information for naloxone.

Dosage Adjustments

Repeat dosing may be required within 1- or 2-hour intervals depending on the amount and type (short- or long-acting) of narcotic and the interval since its last administration. Supplemental IM doses can produce a long-lasting effect.

Special Dental Considerations

Drug Interactions of Dental Interest

Possible drug interactions of clinical significance in dentistry are shown in **Table 2.2**.

Special Patients

Pregnant and nursing women

Naloxone crosses the placenta and may precipitate withdrawal in the fetus as well as the mother. Breastfeeding problems in humans have not been documented.

Pediatric, geriatric, and other special patients

Studies performed in pediatrics have not shown problems that would limit the usefulness of naloxone in children. Geriatric-specific problems do not seem to limit the usefulness of this medication in elderly patients.

Patient Monitoring: Aspects to Watch

- Cardiac status
- State of consciousness
- Respiratory status, oxygen saturation

Adverse Effects and Precautions

Adverse effects, precautions, and contraindications related to naloxone are listed in **Table 2.1**.

Pharmacology

Naloxone reverses the CNS and respiratory depression associated with narcotic overdose. It also reverses postoperative opioid depression. Naloxone competes with and displaces narcotics at narcotic receptor sites.

Because of naloxone's short half-life, a continuous infusion may be required to maintain alertness. A patient should never be released soon after receiving naloxone because the ingested narcotic may have a longer half-life than naloxone, and its toxic effects—such as respiratory depression—may break through.

CHLORAL HYDRATE

Chloral hydrate is an oral sedative-hypnotic that is used when providing dental treatment to the uncooperative preschool child.

Accepted Indications

Accepted indications for chloral hydrate are nocturnal sedation; preoperative sedation to lessen anxiety; in postoperative care, and control of pain as an adjunct to opiates and analgesics.

General Dosing Information

Deaths have been associated with the use of chloral hydrate, especially in children. Repetitive dosing of chloral hydrate is not recommended owing to the accumulation of the active metabolite trichloroethylene. As with any sedation procedure, this sedative should be administered where there can be proper monitoring. Practitioners must know how to properly calculate and administer the appropriate dose. See **Table 2.1**.

Special Dental Considerations

Drug Interactions of Dental Interest

Drug interactions between chloral hydrate and other drugs are listed in **Table 2.2**.

Laboratory Value Alterations

- Chloral hydrate may interfere with the copper sulfate test for glucosuria (confirm suspected glucosuria by glucose oxidase test) and with fluorometric tests for urine catecholamines (do not administer chloral hydrate for 48 hours preceding the test).

Special Patients

Pregnant and nursing women

Chloral hydrate crosses the placenta, and chronic use of chloral hydrate during pregnancy may cause withdrawal symptoms in the neonate. In addition, since chloral hydrate is excreted in breast milk, its use by nursing mothers may cause sedation in the infant.

Pediatric, geriatric, and other special patients

Chloral hydrate is not recommended for use in infants and children in cases in which repeated dosing would be necessary. With repeated dosing, accumulation of trichloroethanol and trichloroacetic acid metabolites may increase the potential for excessive CNS depression.

No information is available on the relationship of age to the effects of chloral hydrate in geriatric patients. Elderly patients are more likely to have age-related hepatic function impairment and renal function impairment. Dose reduction may be required.

Patient Monitoring: Aspects to Watch

- Respiratory status
- Possible abuse and dependence
- Blood pressure

Adverse Effects and Precautions

Table 2.1 lists adverse effects, precautions, and contraindications related to chloral hydrate.

Pharmacology

The mechanism of action of chloral hydrate is unknown; however, it is believed that the CNS depressant effects are due to its active metabolite, trichloroethanol. It is rapidly absorbed from the gastrointestinal tract after oral administration and is metabolized in red blood cells in the liver to the active metabolite. Its onset of action is usually within 30 minutes and its duration of action is 4-8 hours.

Patient Advice

- Swallow the capsule whole; do not chew because of unpleasant taste.
- Take with a full glass of water or juice to reduce gastric irritation.
- For syrup dose: Mix with glassful of juice or water to improve flavor and reduce gastric irritation.
- For suppository form: If too soft for insertion, chill suppository in refrigerator for 30 minutes before removing foil wrapper.

MEPROBAMATE

Meprobamate is an antianxiety agent used for the management of anxiety disorders. It is not indicated for the treatment of anxiety or tension associated with everyday life. Prolonged use of meprobamate may decrease or inhibit salivary flow, thus contributing to the development of caries, periodontal disease, oral candidiasis, and oral discomfort.

Accepted Indications

Meprobamate is used for management of anxiety disorders.

General Dosing Information

Dosing information for meprobamate is listed in **Table 2.1**.

Special Dental Considerations

Drug Interactions of Dental Interest

Drug interactions with meprobamate are listed in **Table 2.2**.

Cross-Sensitivity

Patients sensitive to other carbamate derivatives (carbromal, carisoprodol, mebutamate, or tybamate) may be sensitive to this medication.

Special Patients

Pregnant and nursing women

Meprobamate crosses the placenta and has been associated with congenital malformations. It is excreted in the breast milk in a concentration 2 to 4 times that of maternal plasma concentration and may cause sedation in the infant.

Pediatric, geriatric, and other special patients

No pediatric-specific problems have been documented. Elderly patients are more sensitive to the effects of meprobamate.

Adverse Effects and Precautions

Adverse effects and precautions related to meprobamate are listed in **Table 2.1**.

Pharmacology

Mechanism of action of meprobamate is unknown. It is well absorbed from the gastrointestinal tract, with an onset of action within 1 hour.

SUGGESTED READING

Briggs GG, Freeman RK, Vaffe SJ. *Drugs in Pregnancy and Lactation*. 4th ed. Baltimore: Williams & Wilkins; 1994.

Helm S, Trescot AM, Colson J, Sehgla N, Silverman S. Opioid anatgonists, partial agonists, and agonists/antagonists: The role of office-based detoxification. *Pain Physician*. 2008;11:225-235.

Jastak JT, Donaldson D. Nitrous oxide. *Anesth Prog*. 1991;38:142-153.

Kallar SK, Dunwiddie WC. *Problems in Anesthesia: Outpatient Anesthesia*. In: Wetchler BV, ed. Conscious sedation. Philadelphia: JB Lippincott Co.; 1988:93-100.

Malamed SF. *Sedation: A Guide to Patient Management*. 4th ed. St. Louis: Mosby; 2003.

Table 2.1. PRESCRIBING INFORMATION FOR CONSCIOUS SEDATION/ANTIANXIETY AGENTS

NAME	FORM/ STRENGTH	DOSAGE	WARNINGS/PRECAUTIONS & CONTRAINDICATIONS	ADVERSE EFFECTS†
ANTIANXIETY/HYPNOTIC AGENTS				
Amitriptyline HCl/ Chlordiazepoxide (Limbitrol, Limbitrol DS) CIV	**Tab (Chlordiazepoxide-Amitriptyline):** (Limbitrol) 5mg-12.5mg, (Limbitrol DS) 10mg-25mg	***Adults:*** **Initial:** 3-4 tabs/day in divided doses. **Max:** (Limbitrol DS) 6 tabs/ day. **Elderly:** Start at low end of dosing range.	**BB:** Antidepressants increased the risk of suicidal thinking and behavior (suicidality) in short-term studies in children, adolescents, and young adults with major depressive disorder and other psychiatric disorders. Limbitrol is not approved for use in pediatric patients. **W/P:** Caution with urinary retention, angle-closure glaucoma, cardiovascular disorder, history of seizures, hyperthyroidism, renal or hepatic dysfunction. May produce arrhythmia, sinus tachycardia, and conduction time prolongation. May impair mental alertness. Caution in elderly. Avoid abrupt withdrawal. Monitor blood and LFTs periodically with long-term therapy. **Contra:** MAOI use during or within 14 days, acute recovery period following MI. **P/N:** Not for use in pregnancy or nursing.	Drowsiness, **dry mouth**, constipation, blurred vision, dizziness, bloating, anorexia, fatigue, weakness, restlessness, lethargy.
Amitriptyline HCl/ Perphenazine	**Tab (Amitriptyline-Perphenazine):** 10mg-2mg, 10mg-4mg, 25mg-2mg, 25mg-4mg, 50mg-4mg	***Adults:*** **Initial:** 25mg-2mg tab or 25mg-4mg tab tid-qid, or 50mg-4mg bid. **Maint:** 25mg-2mg tab or 25mg-4mg tab bid-qid, or 50mg-4mg bid. **Max:** 4 tabs/day of 50mg-4mg or 8 tabs/day any other strength. **Severe Illness with Schizophrenia: Initial:** 2 tabs of 25mg-4mg tid and hs prn. **Elderly/Adolescents: Initial:** 10mg-4mg tab tid-qid.	**BB:** Antidepressants increased the risk of suicidal thinking and behavior (suicidality) in short-term studies in children and adolescents with major depressive disorder and other psychiatric disorders. **W/P:** Tardive dyskinesia may develop. NMS reported. May alter blood glucose levels. D/C before elective surgery. Caution with urinary retention, angle-closure glaucoma, increased IOP, hyperthyroidism, convulsive disorders, hepatic dysfunction, and cardiovascular disorders. May increase prolactin levels. May obscure diagnosis of brain tumor or intestinal obstruction due to antiemetic effects. D/C if significant increase in body temperature develops. May impair mental/physical abilities. **Contra:** CNS depression from drugs, bone marrow depression, MAOI use within 14 days, acute recovery phase following MI. **P/N:** Not for use in pregnancy or nursing.	Sedation, hypotension, HTN, neurological impairment, **dry mouth**.
Buspirone HCl (BuSpar)	**Tab:** 5mg*, 10mg*, 15mg*, 30mg*	***Adults:*** **Usual:** 7.5mg bid. **Titrate:** May increase by 5mg/day every 2-3 days. **Usual:** 20-30mg/day. **Max:** 60mg/day. Use low dose with potent CYP450 3A4 inhibitors (eg, 2.5mg qd with nefazodone). Take consistently with or without food; bioavailability increased with food.	**W/P:** Avoid with hepatic or renal impairment. **P/N:** Category B, not for use in nursing.	Dizziness, nausea, headache, nervousness, lightheadedness, excitement, dystonia, fatigue, parkinsonism, akathisia, restless leg syndrome, restlessness.
Chloral Hydrate CIV	**Syrup:** 500mg/5mL	***Adults:*** Dilute in half glass of water, fruit juice, or ginger ale. **Hypnotic: Usual:** 500mg-1g 15-30 min before bedtime. **Sedative: Usual:** 250mg tid pc. **Alcohol Withdrawal: Usual:** 500mg-1g q6h prn. **Max:** 2g/day. ***Pediatrics:*** **Hypnotic:** 50mg/kg. **Max:** 1g/dose. **Sedative:** 8mg/kg tid. **Max:** 500mg tid. **Prior to EEG:** 20-25mg/kg.	**W/P:** May be habit forming. Caution with depression, suicidal tendencies, history of drug abuse. Avoid with esophagitis, gastritis or gastric or duodenal ulcers, large doses with severe cardiac disease. May impair mental/physical abilities. Risk of gastritis, skin eruptions, parenchymatous renal damage with prolonged use. Withdraw gradually with chronic use. **Contra:** Marked hepatic or renal impairment. **P/N:** Category C, caution in nursing.	N/V, diarrhea, ataxia, dizziness.

*Scored. †Bold entries denote special dental considerations.

BB = black box warning; **W/P** = warnings/precautions; **Contra** = contraindications; **P/N** = pregnancy category rating and nursing considerations.

CII = high potential for abuse; CIII = some potential for abuse; CIV = low potential for abuse. For more information on controlled substances categories, see Appendix A.

Table 2.1. PRESCRIBING INFORMATION FOR CONSCIOUS SEDATION/ANTIANXIETY AGENTS *(cont.)*

NAME	FORM/ STRENGTH	DOSAGE	WARNINGS/PRECAUTIONS & CONTRAINDICATIONS	ADVERSE EFFECTS†
ANTIANXIETY/HYPNOTIC AGENTS *(cont.)*				
Doxylamine Succinate (Unisom) OTC	**Tab:** 25mg	***Adults/Pediatrics:* >12 yrs:** 1 tab 30 min prior to going to bed. **Max:** 1 tab qhs.	**W/P:** Caution in emphysema, chronic bronchitis, glaucoma, and difficulty in urination due to BPH. Caution with alcohol. Re-evaluate therapy if sleeplessness persists >2 weeks. **Contra:** Pregnancy, nursing, asthma, glaucoma, prostate enlargement. **P/N:** Not for use in pregnancy or nursing.	Anticholinergic effects.
Eszopiclone (Lunesta) CIV	**Tab:** 1mg, 2mg, 3mg	***Adults:* Initial:** 2mg qhs. **Max:** 3mg qhs. **Elderly: Difficulty Falling Asleep: Initial:** 1mg qhs. **Max:** 2mg qhs. **Difficulty Staying Asleep: Initial/Max:** 2mg qhs. Avoid high-fat meal.	**W/P:** Abnormal thinking and behavioral changes reported. Amnesia and other neuropsychiatric symptoms may occur. Worsening of depression, including suicidal thinking, reported in primarily depressed patients. Avoid rapid dose decrease or abrupt discontinuation. Should only be taken immediately prior to bed or after going to bed and experiencing difficulty falling asleep. Avoid hazardous occupations. Caution in elderly, debilitated, or conditions affecting metabolism or hemodynamic responses. Reduce dose with severe hepatic impairment or concurrent use of potent CYP3A4 inhibitors. Caution with signs and symptoms of depression or suicidal tendencies. **P/N:** Category C, caution in nursing.	Headache, **unpleasant taste**, somnolence, **dry mouth**, dizziness, infection, rash, chest pain, peripheral edema, migraine.
Meprobamate CIV	**Tab:** 200mg, 400mg	***Adults:* Usual:** 1200-1600mg/day given tid-qid. **Max:** 2400mg/day. **Elderly: >65 yrs:** Start at low end of dosing range. ***Pediatrics:* 6-12 yrs:** 200-600mg/day, given bid-tid.	**W/P:** Physical and psychological dependence reported. Avoid abrupt withdrawal after prolonged or excessive use. Increased risk of congenital malformations with use during 1st trimester of pregnancy. Caution with liver or renal dysfunction, and in elderly. May precipitate seizures in epileptic patients. Prescribe small quantities in suicidal patients. **Contra:** Porphyria, allergic or idiosyncratic reactions to carisoprodol, mebutamate, tybamate, carbromal. **P/N:** Safety in pregnancy and nursing not known.	Drowsiness, ataxia, slurred speech, vertigo, weakness, N/V, diarrhea, tachycardia, transient ECG changes, rash, leukopenia, petechiae.
Ramelteon (Rozerem)	**Tab:** 8mg	***Adults:*** 8mg within 30 min of bedtime. Do not take with or after high-fat meal.	**W/P:** Severe anaphylactic and anaphylactoid reactions reported. Sleep disturbances may manifest as a physical and/or psychiatric disorder; symptomatic treatment of insomnia should be initiated after evaluation. Abnormal thinking, behavioral changes, hallucinations, complex behaviors (eg, sleep driving), worsening depression, suicidal ideation reported. D/C therapy if complex sleep behavior occurs. May impair physical/mental abilities. May affect reproductive hormones. Avoid with severe hepatic impairment, severe sleep apnea, and severe COPD. Caution in moderate hepatic impairment. **Contra:** Avoid with fluvoxamine. **P/N:** Category C, caution in nursing.	Headache, somnolence, fatigue, dizziness, nausea, exacerbated insomnia, upper respiratory tract infection.

*Scored. †Bold entries denote special dental considerations.
BB = black box warning; **W/P** = warnings/precautions; **Contra** = contraindications; **P/N** = pregnancy category rating and nursing considerations.
CII = high potential for abuse; CIII = some potential for abuse; CIV = low potential for abuse. For more information on controlled substances categories, see "How to Use This Book" on page iv.

NAME	FORM/ STRENGTH	DOSAGE	WARNINGS/PRECAUTIONS & CONTRAINDICATIONS	ADVERSE EFFECTS†
Zaleplon (Sonata) CIV	**Cap:** 5mg, 10mg	***Adults:*** **Insomnia:** 10mg qhs. **Low-Weight Patients:** Start with 5mg hs. **Max:** 20mg/day. **Elderly/Debilitated/ Concomitant Cimetidine:** 5mg qhs. **Max:** 10mg/day. **Mild to Moderate Hepatic Dysfunction:** 5mg qhs. Take immediately prior to bedtime.	**W/P:** Monitor elderly/debilitated closely. Abnormal thinking and behavioral changes reported. Avoid abrupt withdrawal. Abuse potential exists. Caution in respiratory disorders, depression, conditions affecting metabolism or hemodynamic responses, and mild-to-moderate hepatic insufficiency. Not for use in severe hepatic impairment. May cause impaired coordination even the following day. Re-evaluate if no improvement of insomnia after 7-10 days of therapy. Contains tartrazine. **P/N:** Category C, not for use in nursing.	Headache, asthenia, nausea, dizziness, amnesia, somnolence, eye pain, dysmenorrhea, abdominal pain.
Zolpidem Tartrate (Ambien CR) CIV	**Tab, Extended-Release:** 6.25mg, 12.5mg	***Adults:*** 12.5mg qhs. **Elderly/Debilitated/Hepatic Insufficiency:** 6.25mg qhs. Swallow whole; do not divide, crush, or chew.	**W/P:** Use smallest possible effective dose, especially in elderly. Abnormal thinking and behavior changes reported with use of sedative/hypnotics. Caution with depression and conditions that could affect metabolism or hemodynamic responses. Signs and symptoms of withdrawal reported with abrupt discontinuation of sedative/hypnotics. Monitor elderly and debilitated patients for impaired motor and/or cognitive performance. **P/N:** Category C, not for use in nursing.	Headache, somnolence, dizziness, nausea, hallucinations, back pain, myalgia, fatigue.
Zolpidem Tartrate (Ambien) CIV	**Tab:** 5mg, 10mg	***Adults:*** **Usual:** 10mg qhs. **Elderly/ Debilitated/Hepatic Insufficiency: Initial:** 5mg. Decrease dose with other CNS depressants. **Max:** 10mg qd. Re-evaluate if insomnia persists after 7-10 days.	**W/P:** Severe anaphylactic/anaphylactoid reactions reported. Abnormal thinking, behavior changes, and complex behaviors (eg, sleep driving) reported. Worsening of depression or suicidal thinking may occur; use lowest feasible amount to avoid intentional overdose. Withdrawal symptoms may occur with rapid dose reduction or discontinuation. Potential impairment of activities requiring complete mental alertness (eg, operating machinery) after ingestion and on following day. Avoid with alcohol. Monitor elderly and debilitated patients for impaired motor performance. Caution with hepatic impairment, mild to moderate COPD or sleep apnea, impaired drug metabolism or hemodynamic responses. Avoid if you cannot get a full night's sleep. **P/N:** Category B, not for use in nursing.	Drowsiness, dizziness, headache, nausea, diarrhea, drugged feeling, dyspepsia, myalgia, lethargy, memory loss, anxiety, abnormal thoughts and behavior, **tongue or throat swelling.**
BARBITURATES				
Mephobarbital (Mebaral) CIV	**Tab:** 32mg*, 50mg*, 100mg	***Adults:*** **Epilepsy:** 400-600mg/day. Start with small dose, gradually increase over 4-5 days until optimum dose. **Elderly/Debilitated/Renal or Hepatic Dysfunction:** Reduce dose. **Concomitant Phenobarbital:** Give 50% of each drug. **Concomitant Phenytoin:** Reduce phenytoin dose. **Sedation:** 32-100mg tid-qid. **Optimum Dose:** 50mg tid-qid. ***Pediatrics:*** **Epilepsy: >5 yrs:** 32-64mg tid-qid. **<5 yrs:** 16-32mg tid-qid. Start with small dose, gradually increase over 4-5 days until optimum dose. **Sedation:** 16-32mg tid-qid.	**W/P:** May be habit forming; tolerance and dependence may occur with continued use. Avoid abrupt withdrawal. Caution in acute/chronic pain; paradoxical excitement may occur or symptoms masked. Can cause fetal damage. May cause marked excitement, depression, and confusion in elderly or debilitated. Reduce initial dose with hepatic damage. Careful adjustment in impaired renal, cardiac, or respiratory function, myasthenia gravis, and myxedema. May increase vitamin D requirements. Caution with depression, suicidal tendencies, and history of drug abuse. **Contra:** Manifest or latent porphyria. **P/N:** Category D, caution with nursing.	Somnolence, agitation, confusion, hyperkinesia, ataxia, CNS depression, hypoventilation, apnea, bradycardia, hypotension, syncope, N/V, headache.

Table 2.1. PRESCRIBING INFORMATION FOR CONSCIOUS SEDATION/ANTIANXIETY AGENTS *(cont.)*

NAME	FORM/ STRENGTH	DOSAGE	WARNINGS/PRECAUTIONS & CONTRAINDICATIONS	ADVERSE EFFECTS†
BARBITURATES *(cont.)*				
Pentobarbital Sodium (Nembutal Sodium Solution) CII	**Inj:** 50mg/mL	***Adults:* Usual:** 150-200mg as a single IM injection. (IV) 100mg (commonly used initial dose for 70kg adult); if needed, additional small increments may be given up to 200-500mg total dose. Rate of IV injection should not exceed 50mg/min. **Elderly/Debilitated/ Renal or Hepatic Impairment:** Reduce dose. ***Pediatrics:*** (IM) 2-6mg/kg as a single IM injection. **Max:** 100mg. (IV) Proportional reduction in dosage. Slow IV injection is essential.	**W/P:** May be habit-forming; avoid abrupt cessation after prolonged use. Avoid rapid administration. Tolerance to hypnotic effect can occur. Prehepatic coma use not recommended. Use with caution in patients with chronic or acute pain, mental depression, suicidal tendencies, history of drug abuse, or hepatic impairment. Monitor blood, liver, and renal function. May impair mental/ physical abilities. Avoid alcohol. **Contra:** History of manifest or latent porphyria. **P/N:** Category D, caution with nursing.	Agitation, confusion, hyperkinesia, ataxia, CNS depression, somnolence, brady-cardia, hypotension, N/V, constipation, headache, hyper-sensitivity reactions, liver damage.
Phenobarbital CIV	**Elixir:** 20mg/ 5mL; **Tab:** 15mg, 30mg, 32.4mg, 60mg, 64.8mg, 100mg	***Adults:* Sedation:** 30-120mg/day given bid-tid. **Max:** 400mg/24h. **Hypnotic:** 100-200mg. **Seizures:** 60-200mg/day. **Elderly/Debilitated/Renal or Hepatic Dysfunction:** Reduce dosage. ***Pediatrics:* Seizures:** 3-6mg/kg/day.	**W/P:** May be habit-forming. Avoid abrupt withdrawal. Caution with acute or chronic pain; may mask symptoms or paradoxical excitement may occur. Cog-nitive deficits reported in children with febrile seizures. May cause excitement in children and excitement, depression, or confusion in elderly, debilitated. Caution with hepatic dysfunction, borderline hypoadrenal function, depression. **Contra:** Respiratory disease with dyspnea or obstruction, porphyria, severe liver dysfunction. Large doses with nephritic patients. **P/N:** Category D, caution in nursing.	Drowsiness, residual sedation, lethargy, vertigo, somnolence, respi-ratory depression, hypersensitivity reactions, N/V, headache.
Secobarbital Sodium (Seconal Sodium) CII	**Cap:** 100mg	***Adults:* Hypnotic:** 100mg hs; **Preop-eratively:** 200-300mg, 1-2 hrs before surgery; **Elderly/Debilitated/Renal or Hepatic Dysfunction:** Reduce dose. ***Pediatrics:* Preoperatively:** 2-6mg/kg. **Max:** 100mg.	**W/P:** May be habit-forming; avoid abrupt cessation after prolonged use. Tolerance, psychological and physical dependence may occur with continued use. Use with caution, if at all, in patients who are mentally depressed, have suicidal tendencies, or have a history of drug abuse. In patients with hepatic damage, use with caution and initially reduce dose. Caution when administering to patients with acute or chronic pain. May impair mental and/or physical abilities. Avoid alcohol. **Contra:** History of manifest or latent porphyria, marked impairment of liver function, or respiratory disease in which dyspnea or obstruction is evident. **P/N:** Category D, caution in nursing.	Agitation, confusion, hyperkinesia, ataxia, CNS depression, somnolence, brady-cardia, hypotension, N/V, constipation, headache, hyper-sensitivity reactions, liver damage.
BENZODIAZEPINES				
Alprazolam (Niravam) CIV	**Tab, Orally Disintegrating:** 0.25mg*, 0.5mg*, 1mg*, 2mg*	***Adults:* Anxiety: Initial:** 0.25-0.5mg tid. **Titrate:** May increase every 3-4 days. **Max:** 4mg/day. **Panic Disorder: Initial:** 0.5mg tid. **Titrate:** Increase by no more than 1mg/day every 3-4 days; slower titration if ≥4mg/day. **Usual:** 1-10mg/ day. Decrease dose slowly (no more than 0.5mg every 3 days). **Elderly/ Advanced Liver Disease/Debilitated: Initial:** 0.25mg bid-tid. **Titrate:** Increase gradually as tolerated.	**W/P:** Risk of dependence. Withdrawal symptoms, including seizure, reported with dose reduction or abrupt discon-tinuation; avoid abrupt withdrawal. Risk of CNS depression and impaired performance. May cause fetal harm. Caution with impaired renal, hepatic, or pulmonary function, severe depression, obesity, elderly, and debilitated. Hypomania/mania reported with depression. Weak uricosuric effect. **Contra:** Acute narrow-angle glaucoma, untreated open-angle glaucoma, con-comitant ketoconazole or itraconazole. **P/N:** Category D, not for use in nursing.	Drowsiness, fatigue/ tiredness, impaired coordination, irrita-bility, memory im-pairment, cognitive disorder, dysarthria, decreased libido, confusional state, light-headedness, **dry mouth**, hypoten-sion, **increased salivation**.

*Scored. †Bold entries denote special dental considerations.
BB = black box warning; **W/P** = warnings/precautions; **Contra** = contraindications; **P/N** = pregnancy category rating and nursing considerations.
CII = high potential for abuse; CIII = some potential for abuse; CIV = low potential for abuse. For more information on controlled substances categories, see "How to Use This Book" on page iv.

NAME	FORM/ STRENGTH	DOSAGE	WARNINGS/PRECAUTIONS & CONTRAINDICATIONS	ADVERSE EFFECTS†
Alprazolam (Xanax XR) CIV	**Tab, Extended-Release:** 0.5mg, 1mg, 2mg, 3mg	***Adults:* ≥18 yrs: Initial:** 0.5-1mg qd, preferably in the am. **Titrate:** Increase by no more than 1mg/day every 3-4 days. **Maint:** 1-10mg/day. **Usual:** 3-6mg/day. Decrease dose slowly (no more than 0.5mg every 3 days). **Elderly/Advanced Liver Disease/ Debilitated: Initial:** 0.5mg qd.	**W/P:** Risk of dependence. Withdrawal symptoms, including seizures, reported with dose reduction or abrupt discontinuation; avoid abrupt withdrawal. Caution with impaired renal, hepatic, or pulmonary function, severe depression, obesity, elderly, and debilitated. May cause fetal harm. Hypomania/ mania reported with depression. Weak uricosuric effect. Periodically reassess usefulness. **Contra:** Acute narrow-angle glaucoma, untreated open-angle glaucoma, concomitant ketoconazole or itraconazole. **P/N:** Category D, not for use in nursing.	Sedation, somnolence, memory impairment, dysarthria, abnormal coordination, fatigue, depression, constipation, mental impairment, ataxia, **dry mouth**, decreased libido, increased/decreased appetite.
Alprazolam (Xanax) CIV	**Tab:** 0.25mg*, 0.5mg*, 1mg*, 2mg*	***Adults:* Anxiety: Initial:** 0.25-0.5mg tid. **Titrate:** May increase every 3-4 days. **Max:** 4mg/day. **Elderly/Advanced Liver Disease/Debilitated: Initial:** 0.25mg bid-tid. **Titrate:** Increase gradually as tolerated. **Panic Disorder: Initial:** 0.5mg tid. **Titrate:** Increase by no more than 1mg/day every 3-4 days; slower titration if ≥4mg/day. **Usual:** 1-10mg/ day. Decrease dose slowly (no more than 0.5mg every 3 days).	**W/P:** Risk of dependence. Withdrawal symptoms, including seizures, reported with dose reduction or abrupt discontinuation; avoid abrupt withdrawal. Caution with impaired renal, hepatic, or pulmonary function, severe depression, obesity, elderly, and debilitated. May cause fetal harm. Hypomania/ mania reported with depression. Weak uricosuric effect. Periodically reassess usefulness. **Contra:** Acute narrow-angle glaucoma, untreated open-angle glaucoma, concomitant ketoconazole or itraconazole. **P/N:** Category D, not for use in nursing.	Drowsiness, light-headedness, depression, headache, confusion, insomnia, **dry mouth**, constipation, diarrhea, N/V, tachycardia/palpitations, blurred vision, nasal congestion.
Chlordiazepoxide HCl (Librium) CIV	**Cap:** 5mg, 10mg, 25mg	***Adults:* Mild-Moderate Anxiety:** 5-10mg tid-qid. **Severe Anxiety:** 20-25mg tid-qid. **Alcohol Withdrawal:** 50-100mg; repeat until agitation controlled. **Max:** 300mg/day. **Preoperative Anxiety:** 5-10mg PO tid-qid on days prior to surgery. **Elderly/Debilitated:** 5mg bid-qid. ***Pediatrics:* ≥6 yrs:** 5mg bid-qid. May increase to 10mg bid-tid.	**W/P:** Avoid in pregnancy. Paradoxical reactions reported in psychiatric patients and in hyperactive aggressive pediatrics. Caution with porphyria, renal or hepatic dysfunction. Reduce dose in elderly, debilitated. Avoid abrupt withdrawal after extended therapy. May impair mental/ physical abilities. **P/N:** Not for use in pregnancy, safety in nursing not known.	Drowsiness, ataxia, confusion, skin eruptions, edema, nausea, constipation, extrapyramidal symptoms, libido changes, EEG changes.
Clonazepam (Klonopin, Klonopin Wafers) CIV	**Tab:** 0.5mg*, 1mg, 2mg; **Tab, Disintegrating (Wafer):** 0.125mg, 0.25mg, 0.5mg, 1mg, 2mg	***Adults:* Seizure Disorders: Initial:** Not to exceed 1.5mg/day given tid. **Titrate:** May increase by 0.5-1mg every 3 days. **Max:** 20mg qd. **Panic Disorder: Initial:** 0.25mg bid. **Titrate:** Increase to 1mg/ day after 3 days, then may increase by 0.125-0.25mg bid every 3 days. **Max:** 4mg/day. (Wafer) Dissolve in mouth with or without water. ***Pediatrics:* <10 yrs or 30kg: Seizure Disorders: Initial:** 0.01-0.03mg/kg/day up to 0.05mg/ kg/day given bid-tid. **Titrate:** Increase by no more than 0.25-0.5mg every 3 days. **Maint:** 0.1-0.2mg/kg/day given tid. (Wafer) Dissolve in mouth with or without water.	**W/P:** May increase incidence of generalized tonic-clonic seizures. Monitor blood counts and LFTs periodically with long-term therapy. Caution with renal dysfunction, chronic respiratory depression. Increased fetal risks during pregnancy. Avoid abrupt withdrawal. Hypersalivation reported. Caution may alter mental alertness. **Contra:** Significant liver disease, acute narrow-angle glaucoma, untreated open-angle glaucoma. **P/N:** Category D, not for use in nursing.	Somnolence, depression, ataxia, CNS depression, upper respiratory tract infection, fatigue, dizziness, sinusitis, colpitis.

Table 2.1. PRESCRIBING INFORMATION FOR CONSCIOUS SEDATION/ANTIANXIETY AGENTS *(cont.)*

NAME	FORM/ STRENGTH	DOSAGE	WARNINGS/PRECAUTIONS & CONTRAINDICATIONS	ADVERSE EFFECTS†
BENZODIAZEPINES *(cont.)*				
Clorazepate Dipotassium (Tranxene T-Tab) CIV	**Tab:** (Tranxene T-Tab) 3.75mg*, 7.5mg*, 15mg*	***Adults:* Anxiety: Usual:** 30mg/day in divided doses or as a single dose qhs, starting at 15mg qhs. Adjust dosage based on individual patient responses. **Max:** 60mg/day. **Elderly/ Debilitated: Initial:** 7.5-15mg/day. **Alcohol Withdrawal: Day 1:** 30mg initially, then 30-60mg in divided doses. **Day 2:** 45-90mg in divided doses. **Day 3:** 22.5-45mg in divided doses. **Day 4:** 15-30mg in divided doses. After, gradually reduce dose to 7.5-15mg/ day; discontinue when stable. **Max:** 90mg/day. ***Adults/Pediatrics:* >12yrs: Antiepileptic Adjunct: Initial:** 7.5mg tid. **Titrate:** Increase by no more than 7.5mg/week. **Max:** 90mg/day. **9-12 yrs: Initial:** 7.5mg bid. **Titrate:** Increase by no more than 7.5mg/week. **Max:** 60mg/day.	**W/P:** Avoid with depressive neuroses or psychotic reactions. Withdrawal symptoms with abrupt withdrawal; taper gradually. Caution with known drug dependency, renal/hepatic impairment. Suicidal tendencies reported; give lowest effective dose. Monitor LFTs and blood counts periodically with long-term therapy. Use lowest effective dose in elderly. **Contra:** Acute narrow-angle glaucoma. **P/N:** Safety in pregnancy not known, not for use in nursing.	Drowsiness, dizziness, GI complaints, nervousness, blurred vision, **dry mouth**, headache, mental confusion.
Diazepam (Diastat) CIV	**Kit:** 2.5mg, 5mg, 10mg, 15mg, 20mg	***Adults/Pediatrics:* ≥12 yrs:** 0.2mg/kg rectally. **6-11 yrs:** 0.3mg/kg. **2-5 yrs:** 0.5mg/kg. Calculate amount and round upwards to next available dose. May give 2nd dose 4-12 hrs later. For rectal administration. **Max:** 5 episodes/month and 1 episode every 5 days.	**W/P:** Produces CNS depression. Avoid abrupt withdrawal. Caution with elderly, hepatic/renal dysfunction, compromised respiratory function, neurologic damage. Not for daily chronic use. Withdrawal symptoms reported with discontinuation. **Contra:** Acute narrow-angle glaucoma, untreated open-angle glaucoma. **P/N:** Category D, not for use in nursing.	Somnolence, dizziness, headache, pain, abdominal pain, nervousness, vasodilation, diarrhea, ataxia, euphoria, incoordination, asthma, rhinitis, rash.
Diazepam Injection CIV	**Inj:** 5mg/mL	***Adults:* Anxiety (moderate):** 2-5mg IM/IV, may repeat in 3-4 hrs. **Anxiety (severe):** 5-10mg IM/IV, may repeat in 3-4 hrs. **Alcohol Withdrawal (acute):** 10mg IM/IV, then 5-10mg in 3-4 hrs if needed. **Endoscopic Procedures: Usual:** ≤10mg IV (up to 20mg) or 5-10mg IM 30 min prior to procedure. **Muscle Spasm:** 5-10mg IM/IV, then 5-10mg in 3-4 hrs if needed. **Status Epilepticus/Severe Seizures: Initial:** 5-10mg IV. **Maint:** May repeat at 10-15 min intervals. **Max:** 30mg. **Preoperative:** 10mg IM. **Cardioversion:** 5-15mg IV, 5-10 min prior to procedure. **Elderly/Debilitated: Usual:** 2-5mg. ***Pediatrics:* Tetanus: 30 days-5 yrs:** 1-2mg IM/IV (slowly), may repeat every 3-4 hrs prn. **≥5 yrs**: 5-10mg IM/IV, may repeat every 3-4 hrs. **Status Epilepticus/Severe Seizures: 30 days-5 yrs:** 0.2-0.5mg IV (slowly) every 2-5 min up to 5mg. **≥5 yrs:** 1mg IV (slowly) every 2-5 min up to 10mg, may repeat in 2-4 hrs.	**W/P:** Inject slowly and avoid small veins with IV. Do not mix or dilute with other products in syringe or infusion flask. Extreme caution in elderly, severely ill, and those with limited pulmonary reserve. Avoid if in shock, coma, or acute alcohol intoxication with depressed vital signs. May impair mental/physical abilities. Increase in grand mal seizures reported. Caution with kidney or hepatic dysfunction. Not for obstetrical use. Withdrawal symptoms may occur. Hypotension and muscular weakness reported. Monitor blood counts and LFTs. Not for maintenance of seizures once controlled. **Contra:** Acute narrow-angle glaucoma, untreated open-angle glaucoma. **P/N:** Not for use during pregnancy, safety in nursing unknown.	Drowsiness, fatigue, ataxia, venous thrombosis and phlebitis (injection site).

*Scored. †Bold entries denote special dental considerations.

BB = black box warning; **W/P** = warnings/precautions; **Contra** = contraindications; **P/N** = pregnancy category rating and nursing considerations.

CII = high potential for abuse; CIII = some potential for abuse; CIV = low potential for abuse. For more information on controlled substances categories, see "How to Use This Book" on page iv.

NAME	FORM/ STRENGTH	DOSAGE	WARNINGS/PRECAUTIONS & CONTRAINDICATIONS	ADVERSE EFFECTS†
Diazepam (Valium) CIV	**Tab:** 2mg*, 5mg*, 10mg*	***Adults:*** **Anxiety:** 2-10mg bid-qid. **Alcohol Withdrawal:** 10mg tid-qid for 24 hours. **Maint:** 5mg tid-qid prn. **Skeletal Muscle Spasm:** 2-10mg tid-qid: **Seizure Disorders:** 2-10mg bid-qid. **Elderly/Debilitated:** 2-2.5mg qd-bid initially; may increase gradually as needed and tolerated. ***Pediatrics:*** **≥6 months:** 1-2.5mg tid-qid initially; may increase gradually as needed and tolerated.	**W/P:** Monitor blood counts and LFTs in long-term use. Neutropenia and jaundice reported. Increase in grand mal seizures reported. Avoid abrupt withdrawal. Caution with kidney or hepatic dysfunction. **Contra:** Acute narrow-angle glaucoma, untreated open-angle glaucoma, patients <6 months. **P/N:** Not for use during pregnancy, safety in nursing not known.	Drowsiness, fatigue, ataxia, paradoxical reactions, minor EEG changes.
Estazolam CIV	**Tab:** 1mg*, 2mg*	***Adults:*** **Initial:** 1mg qhs. May increase to 2mg qhs. **Small Stature/Debilitated/ Elderly: Initial:** 0.5mg qhs.	**W/P:** Avoid abrupt withdrawal after prolonged use. Caution with depression, elderly/debilitated, renal/hepatic impairment. May cause respiratory depression. May impair mental/physical abilities. **Contra:** Pregnancy. **P/N:** Category X, not for use in nursing.	Somnolence, hypokinesia, dizziness, abnormal coordination, headache, malaise, nervousness, cold symptoms, asthenia.
Flurazepam HCl (Dalmane) CIV	**Cap:** 15mg, 30mg	***Adults/Pediatrics:*** **≥15 yrs: Usual:** 30mg hs. May give 15mg hs. **Elderly/ Debilitated: Initial/Usual:** 15mg hs.	**W/P:** Caution in elderly, debilitated, severely depressed, those with suicidal tendencies, hepatic/renal impairment, respiratory disease. Ataxia and falls reported in elderly and debilitated. Withdrawal symptoms after discontinuation; avoid abrupt discontinuation. Rare cases of angioedema involving the tongue, glottis, or larynx reported. Complex behaviors such as sleep driving, and other complex behaviors (eg, preparing and eating food, making phone calls, and having sex) reported in patients who are not fully awake. **Contra:** Pregnancy. **P/N:** Not for use in pregnancy or nursing.	Confusion, dizziness, drowsiness, lightheadedness, ataxia.
Lorazepam (Ativan Injection) CIV	**Inj:** 2mg/mL, 4mg/mL	***Adults:*** **≥18 yrs: Status Epilepticus:** 4mg IV (given slowly at 2mg/min); may repeat 1 dose after 10-15 min if seizures recur or fail to cease. **Preanesthetic Sedation: Usual:** 0.05mg/kg IM; 2mg or 0.044mg/kg IV (whichever is smaller). **Max:** 4mg IM/IV.	**W/P:** Monitor all parameters to maintain vital function. Risk of respiratory depression or airway obstruction in heavily sedated patients. May cause fetal damage during pregnancy. Increased risk of CNS and respiratory depression in elderly. Avoid with hepatic/renal failure. Caution with mild to moderate hepatic/renal disease. Avoid outpatient endoscopic procedures. Possible propylene glycol toxicity in renal impairment. Extreme caution when administering injections to elderly, very ill, or to patients with limited pulmonary reserve, hypoventilation and/or hypoxic cardiac arrest may occur. Gasping syndrome, characterized by CNS depression, metabolic acidosis, gasping respirations, and high levels of benzyl alcohol, may occur. **Contra:** Acute narrow-angle glaucoma, sleep apnea syndrome, severe respiratory insufficiency. Not for intra-arterial injection. **P/N:** Category D, not for use in nursing.	Respiratory depression/failure, hypotension, somnolence, headache, hypoventilation.

Table 2.1. PRESCRIBING INFORMATION FOR CONSCIOUS SEDATION/ANTIANXIETY AGENTS *(cont.)*

NAME	FORM/ STRENGTH	DOSAGE	WARNINGS/PRECAUTIONS & CONTRAINDICATIONS	ADVERSE EFFECTS†
BENZODIAZEPINES *(cont.)*				
Lorazepam (Ativan) CIV	**Tab:** 0.5mg, 1mg*, 2mg*	***Adults/Pediatrics:*** **>12 yrs: Initial:** 2-3mg/day given bid-tid. **Usual:** 2-6mg/day in divided doses. **Insomnia:** 2-4mg qhs. **Elderly/Debilitated:** 1-2mg/day in divided doses.	**W/P:** Avoid with primary depression or psychosis. Withdrawal symptoms with abrupt discontinuation. Careful supervision if addiction-prone. Caution in patients with compromised respiratory function. Caution with elderly, and renal or hepatic dysfunction. Monitor for GI disease with prolonged therapy. Periodic blood counts and LFTs with long-term therapy. **Contra:** Acute narrow-angle glaucoma. **P/N:** Not for use in pregnancy or nursing.	Sedation, dizziness, weakness, unsteadiness, transient amnesia, memory impairment, visual disturbance, depression, respiratory depression, constipation, vertigo, change in appetite, headache.
Midazolam HCl Injection CIV	**Inj:** 1mg/mL, 5mg/mL	***Adults:*** **IV: Sedation/Anxiolysis/ Amnesia Induction: <60 yrs: Initial:** 1-2.5mg IV over 2 min. **Max:** 5mg. **Titrate:** In small increments at 2 min intervals if needed. **Concomitant Narcotics/Other CNS Depressants:** Reduce by 30%. **≥60 yrs/Debilitated/ Chronically Ill: Initial:** 1-1.5mg IV over 2 min. **Max:** 3.5mg. **Titrate:** In small increments at 2 min intervals if needed. **Concomitant Narcotics/Other CNS Depressants:** Reduce by 50%. **Maint:** 25% of sedation dose by slow titration. **IM: Preoperative Sedation/Anxiolysis/ Amnesia: <60 yrs:** 0.07-0.08mg/kg IM up to 1 hr before surgery. **≥60 yrs/ Debilitated:** 1-3mg IM. **Anesthesia Induction: Unpremedicated: <55 yrs: Initial:** 0.3-0.35mg/kg IV over 20-30 seconds. May give additional doses of 25% of initial dose to complete induction. **>55 yrs: Initial:** 0.3mg/kg IV. **Debilitated: Initial:** 0.15-0.25mg/ kg IV. **Premedicated: <55 yrs: Initial:** 0.25mg/kg IV over 20-30 seconds. **>55 yrs: Initial:** 0.2mg/kg IV. **Debilitated:** 0.15mg/kg IV. **Maintenance Sedation: LD:** 0.01-0.05mg/kg IV. May repeat dose at 10-15 min intervals until adequate sedation. **Maint:** 0.02-0.1mg/ kg/hr. Titrate to desired level of sedation using 25-50% adjustments. Infusion rate should be decreased 10-25% every few hrs to find minimum effective infusion rate. ***Pediatrics:*** **Sedation/ Anxiolysis/Amnesia Induction: IV: <6 months:** Limited information; titrate with small increments and monitor. **6 months-5 yrs: Initial:** 0.05-0.1mg/kg IV over 2-3 min, up to 0.6mg/kg if needed. **Max:** 6mg. **6-12 yrs: Initial:** 0.025-0.05mg/kg IV over 2-3 min, up to 0.4mg/kg if needed. **Max:** 10mg. **12-16 yrs:** 1-2.5mg IV over 2 min. **Titrate:** In small increments at 2 min intervals if needed. **Max:** 10mg. **IM:** 0.1-0.15mg/ kg IM, up to 0.5mg/kg if needed. **Max:** 10mg. **Sedation: LD:** 0.05-0.2mg/ kg IV infusion over 2-3 min. **Maint:** 0.06-0.12mg/kg/hr IV infusion. May adjust dose by 25%. **Sedation in Critical Care: Neonatal Dose: <32 weeks: Initial:** 0.03mg/kg/hr IV infusion. **>32 weeks: Initial:** 0.06mg/kg/hr IV infusion. Adjust to lowest effective dose.	**BB:** Associated with respiratory depression and respiratory arrest, especially when used for sedation in noncritical care settings. Do not administer by rapid injection to neonates. Continuous monitoring required. **W/P:** Agitation, involuntary movements, hyperactivity, and combativeness reported. Caution with CHF, chronic renal failure, pulmonary disease, uncompensated acute illnesses (eg, severe fluid or electrolyte disturbances), elderly, or debilitated. Avoid use with shock or coma, or in acute alcohol intoxication with depression of vital signs. Contains benzyl alcohol. Administer IM or IV only. **Contra:** Acute narrow-angle glaucoma, untreated open-angle glaucoma, intrathecal or epidural use. **P/N:** Category D, caution in nursing.	Decreased tidal volume and/or respiratory rate, BP/HR variations, apnea, hypotension, pain and local reactions at injection site, hiccoughs, nausea, vomiting.

*Scored. †Bold entries denote special dental considerations.

BB = black box warning; **W/P** = warnings/precautions; **Contra** = contraindications; **P/N** = pregnancy category rating and nursing considerations.

CII = high potential for abuse; CIII = some potential for abuse; CIV = low potential for abuse. For more information on controlled substances categories, see "How to Use This Book" on page iv.

NAME	FORM/ STRENGTH	DOSAGE	WARNINGS/PRECAUTIONS & CONTRAINDICATIONS	ADVERSE EFFECTS†
Midazolam HCl Syrup CIV	**Syrup:** 2mg/mL [118mL]	***Pediatrics:*** **Usual:** Single dose of 0.25-1mg/kg. **Max:** 20mg. **6 months-<6 yrs/Less Cooperative:** 1mg/kg. **6-<16 yrs/Cooperative:** 0.25mg/kg. **Cardiac or Respiratory Compromise/ High-Risk Surgery/Concomitant Narcotics or Other CNS Depressants:** 0.25mg/kg. **Obesity:** Calculate dosage based on ideal body wt.	**BB:** Associated with respiratory depression and respiratory arrest, especially when used for sedation in noncritical care settings. Reports of airway obstruction, desaturation, hypoxia, and apnea, especially with other CNS depressants. Continuous monitoring required. **W/P:** Monitor for respiratory adverse events and paradoxical reactions. Agitation, involuntary movements, hyperactivity, and combativeness reported. Caution with CHF, chronic renal failure, chronic hepatic disease, pulmonary disease, cardiac or respiratory compromised patients. Avoid use with shock or coma, or in acute alcohol intoxication with depression of vital signs. For use only in hospital or ambulatory settings equipped to provide continuous monitoring of respiratory and cardiac function. **Contra:** Acute narrow-angle glaucoma. **P/N:** Category D, caution in nursing.	Emesis, nausea, agitation, hypoxia, **laryngospasm**, agitation.
Oxazepam CIV	**Cap:** 10mg, 15mg, 30mg; **Tab:** 15mg	***Adults:*** **Anxiety: Mild-Moderate:** 10-15mg tid-qid. **Severe:** 15-30mg tid-qid. **Elderly: Initial:** 10mg tid. **Titrate:** Increase to 15mg tid-qid. **Alcohol Withdrawal:** 15-30mg tid-qid.	**W/P:** May impair mental/physical abilities. Withdrawal symptoms with abrupt discontinuation. Caution in sensitivity to hypotension, elderly. Caution with tablets in tartrazine or ASA allergy. Risk of congenital malformations; avoid in pregnancy. **Contra:** Psychoses. **P/N:** Not for use in pregnancy or nursing.	Drowsiness, dizziness, vertigo, headache, paradoxical excitement, transient amnesia, memory impairment.
Temazepam (Restoril) CIV	**Cap:** 7.5mg, 15mg, 22.5mg, 30mg	***Adults*:** **Usual:** 15mg qhs. **Range:** 7.5-30mg qhs. **Transient Insomnia:** 7.5mg qhs. **Elderly/Debilitated: Initial:** 7.5mg qhs.	**W/P:** Caution in elderly, debilitated, severely depressed, those with suicidal tendencies, hepatic/renal impairment, pulmonary insufficiency. Avoid abrupt discontinuation. If no improvement after 7-10 days, may indicate primary psychiatric and/or medical condition. **Contra:** Pregnancy. **P/N:** Category X, caution in nursing.	Headache, dizziness, drowsiness, fatigue, nervousness, nausea, lethargy, hangover.
Triazolam (Halcion) CIV	**Tab:** 0.125mg, 0.25mg*	***Adults:*** 0.25mg qhs. **Max:** 0.5mg. **Elderly/Debilitated: Initial:** 0.125mg. **Max:** 0.25mg.	**W/P:** Worsening or failure of response after 7-10 days may indicate other medical conditions. Increased daytime anxiety, abnormal thinking, and behavioral changes have occurred. May impair mental/physical abilities. Anterograde amnesia reported with therapeutic doses. Caution with baseline depression, suicidal tendencies, history of drug dependence, elderly/debilitated, renal/hepatic impairment, chronic pulmonary insufficiency, and sleep apnea. Withdrawal symptoms after discontinuation; avoid abrupt withdrawal. **Contra:** Pregnancy. With ketoconazole, itraconazole, nefazodone, medications that impair CYP3A. **P/N:** Category X, not for use in nursing.	Drowsiness, dizziness, lightheadedness, headache, NV, coordination disorders, ataxia.

Table 2.1. PRESCRIBING INFORMATION FOR CONSCIOUS SEDATION/ANTIANXIETY AGENTS *(cont.)*

NAME	FORM/ STRENGTH	DOSAGE	WARNINGS/PRECAUTIONS & CONTRAINDICATIONS	ADVERSE EFFECTS†
BENZODIAZEPINE ANTAGONIST				
Flumazenil (Romazicon)	**Inj:** 0.1mg/mL	***Adults:* Reversal of Conscious Sedation/General Anesthesia:** Give IV over 15 seconds. **Initial:** 0.2mg. May repeat dose after 45 seconds and again at 60-second intervals, up to a max of 4 additional times until desired level of consciousness is reached. **Max Total Dose:** 1mg. In event of resedation, repeated doses may be given at 20-min intervals. **Max:** 1mg/dose (0.2mg/min) and 3mg/hr. **Benzodiazepine (BZD) Overdose:** Give IV over 30 seconds. **Initial:** 0.2mg. May repeat with 0.3mg after 30 seconds and then 0.5mg at 1-min intervals until desired level of consciousness is reached. **Max Total Dose:** 3mg. In event of resedation, repeated doses may be given at 20-min intervals. **Max:** 1mg/dose (0.5mg/min); 3mg/hr. ***Pediatrics:* >1yr:** Give IV over 15 seconds. **Initial:** 0.01mg/kg (up to 0.2mg). May repeat dose after 45 seconds and again at 60-second intervals, up to a max of 4 additional times until desired level of consciousness is reached. **Max Total Dose:** 0.05mg/kg or 1mg, whichever is lower.	**W/P:** Caution in overdoses involving multiple drug combinations. Risk of seizures, especially with long-term BZD-induced sedation, cyclic antidepressant overdose, concurrent major sedative-hypnotic drug withdrawal, recent therapy with repeated doses of parenteral BZDs, myoclonic jerking or seizure prior to flumazenil administration. Monitor for resedation, respiratory depression, or other residual BZD effects (up to 2 hrs). Avoid use in the ICU; increased risk of unrecognized BZD dependence. Caution with head injury, alcoholism, and other drug dependencies. Does not reverse respiratory depression/hypoventilation or cardiac depression. May provoke panic attacks with history of panic disorder. Adjust subsequent doses in hepatic dysfunction. Not for use as treatment for BZD dependence or for management of protracted abstinence syndromes. May trigger dose-dependent withdrawal syndromes. Extravasation may occur; administer IV into a large vein. **Contra:** Patients given BZDs for life-threatening conditions (eg, control of ICP or status epilepticus), signs of serious cyclic antidepressant overdose. **P/N:** Category C, caution in nursing.	N/V, dizziness, injection-site pain, increased sweating, headache, abnormal or blurred vision, agitation.
OPIOID ANTAGONISTS				
Naloxone HCl (Narcan)	**Inj:** 0.4mg/mL, 1mg/mL	***Adults:* Opioid Overdose: Initial:** 0.4-2mg IV every 2-3 minutes, up to 10mg. IM/SQ if IV route not available. **Post-Op Opioid Depression:** 0.1-0.2mg IV every 2-3 min to desired response. May repeat in 1-2 hr intervals. Supplemental IM doses last longer. **Naloxone Challenge Test:** IV: 0.1-0.2mg, observe 30 seconds for signs of withdrawal, then 0.6mg, observe for 20 min. SQ: 0.8mg, observe for 20 min. ***Pediatrics:* Opioid Overdose: Initial:** 0.01mg/kg IV. **Inadequate Response:** repeat 0.1mg/kg once. IM/SQ in divided doses if IV route not available. **Post-Op Opioid Depression:** 0.005-0.01mg IV every 2-3 min to desired response. May repeat in 1-2 hr intervals. Supplemental IM doses last longer. **Neonates: Opioid-Induced Depression:** 0.01mg/kg IV/IM/SQ, may repeat every 2-3 min until desired response.	**W/P:** Caution in patients including newborns of mothers known or suspected of opioid physical dependence. May precipitate acute withdrawal syndrome. Have other resuscitative measures available. Caution with cardiac, renal, or hepatic disease. Monitor patients satisfactorily responding due to extended opioid duration of action. Abrupt postoperative opioid depression reversal may result in serious adverse effects leading to death. **P/N:** Category B, caution in nursing.	HTN, hypotension, ventricular tachycardia and fibrillation, dyspnea, pulmonary edema, cardiac arrest, N/V, sweating, seizures, body aches, fever, nervousness.

*Scored. †Bold entries denote special dental considerations.

BB = black box warning; **W/P** = warnings/precautions; **Contra** = contraindications; **P/N** = pregnancy category rating and nursing considerations.

CII = high potential for abuse; CIII = some potential for abuse; CIV = low potential for abuse. For more information on controlled substances categories, see "How to Use This Book" on page iv.

NAME	FORM/ STRENGTH	DOSAGE	WARNINGS/PRECAUTIONS & CONTRAINDICATIONS	ADVERSE EFFECTS†
Naltrexone (Vivitrol)	**Inj, Extended-Release:** 380mg	***Adults:*** Administer 380mg IM gluteal inj every 4 weeks or once a month using alternating buttocks.	**W/P:** Hepatotoxicity with excessive doses; does not appear to be hepatotoxic at recommended doses. May cause eosinophilic pneumonia. Only treat patients opioid-free for 7-10 days. Perform naloxone challenge test if risk of precipitating withdrawal. Attempting to overcome the opiate blockade using opioids is very dangerous. More sensitive to lower doses of opioids after naltrexone is discontinued. In emergency situation, suggested plan for pain management is regional analgesia, conscious sedation with a benzodiazepine, or use of non-opioid analgesics or general anesthesia. Monitor for development of depression or suicidal thinking. Caution in renal or hepatic impairment. Administration will not eliminate or diminish alcohol withdrawal symptoms. **Contra:** Acute hepatitis or liver failure, concomitant opioid analgesics, physiologic opioid dependence, acute opiate withdrawal, positive urine screen for opioids or failed naloxone challenge test. **P/N:** Category C, not for use in nursing.	N/V, diarrhea, abdominal pain, upper respiratory tract infection, pharyngitis, insomnia, anxiety, depression, injection site reactions, arthralgia, muscle cramps, dizziness, syncope, appetite disorder, retinal artery occlusion.
Naltrexone HCl (ReVia)	**Tab:** 50mg*	***Adults:*** **Alcoholism:** 50mg qd up to 12 weeks. **Opioid Dependence: Initial:** 25mg qd. **Maint:** 50mg qd. **Naloxone Challenge Test:** 0.2mg IV, observe for 30 seconds, then 0.6mg IV, observe for 20 min; or 0.8mg SQ, observe for 20 min.	**W/P:** Hepatotoxicity with excessive doses; does not appear to be hepatotoxic at recommended doses. Only treat patients opioid-free for 7-10 days. Attempting to overcome opiate blockade is very dangerous. More sensitive to lower doses of opioids after naltrexone is discontinued. Safety in ultra-rapid opiate detoxification is not known. Increased risk of suicide in substance abuse patients. Severe opioid withdrawal syndromes reported with accidental ingestion in opioid-dependent patients. Monitor closely during blockade reversal. Caution in renal or hepatic impairment. Perform naloxone challenge test if question of opioid dependence. **Contra:** Acute hepatitis or liver failure, patients failing naloxone challenge or opioid-dependent, concomitant opioid analgesics, acute opioid withdrawal, positive urine screen for opioids or failed naloxone challenge test, phenanthrene sensitivity. **P/N:** Category C, caution in nursing.	N/V, headache, dizziness, nervousness, fatigue, restlessness, insomnia, anxiety, somnolence.

Table 2.1. PRESCRIBING INFORMATION FOR CONSCIOUS SEDATION/ANTIANXIETY AGENTS *(cont.)*

NAME	FORM/ STRENGTH	DOSAGE	WARNINGS/PRECAUTIONS & CONTRAINDICATIONS	ADVERSE EFFECTS†
PARTIAL OPIOID AGONIST/OPIOID ANTAGONISTS				
Buprenorphine HCl (Subutex) CIII **Buprenorphine HCl/ Naloxone HCl** (Suboxone) CIII	**Tab, SL (Buprenorphine-Naloxone):** (Suboxone) 2mg-0.5mg, 8mg-2mg. **Tab, SL (Buprenorphine):** (Subutex) 2mg, 8mg	***Adults/Pediatrics:* ≥16 yrs:** Give either agent SL as a single daily dose in the range of 12-16mg. Hold tabs under tongue until dissolved; swallowing tabs reduces bioavailability. **Induction: Subutex:** Give at least 4 hrs after last short-acting opioid (eg, heroin) use or preferably when early signs of opioid withdrawal appear. **Maint: Suboxone: Range:** 4mg-24mg/day. **Target dose:** 16mg/day. **Titrate:** Adjust by 2mg or 4mg to a level that maintains treatment and suppresses opioid withdrawal effects. **Hepatic Impairment:** Adjust dose and observe for precipitated opioid withdrawal. **Concomitant CNS Depressants:** Consider dose reduction.	**W/P:** Significant respiratory depression reported with buprenorphine; caution with compromised respiratory function. Naloxone may not be effective in reversing any respiratory depression produced by buprenorphine. Cytolytic hepatitis and hepatitis with jaundice reported. Obtain LFTs prior to initiation and periodically thereafter. Acute and chronic hypersensitivity reactions reported. May increase CSF pressure; caution with head injury, intracranial lesions. May cause miosis, changes in level of consciousness, and orthostatic hypotension. Caution with elderly, debilitated, myxedema, hypothyroidism, acute alcoholism, Addison's disease, CNS depression or coma, toxic psychoses, prostatic hypertrophy, urethral stricture, delirium tremens, kyphoscoliosis, biliary tract dysfunction, or severe hepatic/ renal/pulmonary impairment. Suboxone may cause opioid withdrawal symptoms. May obscure diagnosis of acute abdominal conditions. May produce dependence. **P/N:** Category C, not for use in nursing.	Headache, infection, pain (general, abdomen, back), withdrawal syndrome, constipation, nausea, insomnia, sweating, asthenia, anxiety, depression, rhinitis.

*Scored. †Bold entries denote special dental considerations.
BB = black box warning; **W/P** = warnings/precautions; **Contra** = contraindications; **P/N** = pregnancy category rating and nursing considerations.
CII = high potential for abuse; CIII = some potential for abuse; CIV = low potential for abuse. For more information on controlled substances categories, see "How to Use This Book" on page iv.

Table 2.2. DRUG INTERACTIONS FOR CONSCIOUS SEDATION/ANTIANXIETY AGENTS

ANTIANXIETY/HYPNOTIC AGENTS	
Amitriptyline HCl/Chlordiazepoxide (Limbitrol, Limbitrol DS) CIV	
Alcohol	Additive CNS-depressant effects with alcohol.
Anticholinergics	Severe constipation may occur with anticholinergics.
CNS depressants	Additive CNS-depressant effects with other CNS depressants.
CYP2D6 inhibitors	May increase levels with CYP2D6 inhibitors (eg, quinidine, cimetidine, SSRIs).
CYP2D6 substrates	May increase levels with CYP2D6 substrates (eg, other antidepressants, phenothiazines, propafenone, flecainide).
Fluoxetine	May increase levels with SSRIs. Avoid within 5 weeks of fluoxetine use.
Guanethidine	May block the antihypertensive effects of guanethidine and other similarly acting antihypertensives. Concomitant use not recommended.
MAOIs	Concurrent use with MAOIs contraindicated. Avoid within 14 days of MAOI use.
Psychotropic agents	Possible additive sedative effects with psychotropics.
Thyroid agents	Caution with concurrent use of thyroid agents.
Amitriptyline HCl/Perphenazine	
Anticholinergics	Additive anticholinergic effects with concomitant use.
Anticonvulsants	May require increased dosage of anticonvulsants.
CNS depressants	Concurrent use with CNS depressants (eg, barbiturates, alcohol, narcotics, analgesics, antihistamines) contraindicated.
CYP2D6 inhibitors	May increase levels with CYP2D6 inhibitors (eg, quinidine, cimetidine, SSRIs).
CYP2D6 substrates	May increase levels with CYP2D6 substrates (other antidepressants, phenothiazines, propafenone, flecainide).
Disulfiram	Concomitant administration may cause delirium.
Ethchlorvynol	Concomitant administration may cause transient delirium.
Guanethidine	May block the antihypertensive effects of guanethidine and other similarly acting antihypertensives. Concomitant use not recommended.
MAOIs	Concurrent use with MAOIs contraindicated. Avoid within 14 days of MAOI use.
Fluoxetine	May increase levels with SSRIs. Avoid within 5 weeks of fluoxetine use.
Sympathomimetics	Caution with sympathomimetics; may require dose adjustment.
Thyroid agents	Caution with concurrent use of thyroid agents.
Buspirone HCl (BuSpar)	
Alcohol	Caution with concomitant alcohol use.
CCBs, non-dihydropyridine	May increase levels with non-dihydropridine CCBs; may require dose adjustment.
CYP3A4 inhibitors	May increase levels with CYP3A4 inhibitors; may require dose reduction.
CYP3A4 inducers	May decrease levels with CYP3A4 induces; may require dose adjustment.
Cimetidine	Concomitant administration may increase levels with cimetidine.

Table 2.2. DRUG INTERACTIONS FOR CONSCIOUS SEDATION/ANTIANXIETY AGENTS *(cont.)*

ANTIANXIETY/HYPNOTIC AGENTS *(cont.)*	
Buspirone HCl (BuSpar) *(cont.)*	
Diazepam	Possible additive effects of diazepam.
Haloperidol	Increases plasma levels of haloperidol.
MAOIs	Avoid with MAOIs; elevated blood pressure reported.
Psychotropic agents	Caution with other psychotropic agents.
Trazodone	Elevated liver transaminases reported with trazodone.
Warfarin	Caution with warfarin; prolonged PT reported.
Chloral Hydrate CIV	
Alcohol	May cause vasodilation reaction, including tachycardia and palpitations.
Anticoagulants, oral	Caution with oral anticoagulants. Coadministration increases anticoagulant levels and may cause excessive hypoprothrombinemia.
CNS depressants	Additive CNS-depressant effects with other CNS depressants, including alcohol.
Furosemide injection	May cause reaction characterized by diaphoresis, flushes, variable blood pressure, and uneasiness.
Eszopiclone (Lunesta) CIV	
Alcohol	Caution with alcohol; additive effect on psychomotor performance.
Anticonvulsants	Possible additive CNS-depressant effects with coadministration.
Antihistamines	Possible additive CNS-depressant effects with coadministration.
CNS depressants	Additive CNS-depressant effects with other CNS depressants.
CYP3A4 inducers	May decrease levels with CYP3A4 inducers.
CYP3A4 inhibitors	May increase levels with CYP3A4 inhibitors (eg, ketoconazole); may require dose reduction of eszopiclone.
Olanzapine	Coadministration may decrease DSST scores.
Psychotropic agents	Possible additive sedative effects with psychotropic agents.
Meprobamate CIV	
Alcohol	Additive CNS-depressant effects with alcohol.
CNS depressants	Additive CNS-depressant effects with other CNS depressants.
Psychotropic agents	Possible additive sedative effects with psychotropic agents.
Ramelteon (Rozerem)	
Alcohol	Additive CNS-depressant effects with alcohol.
CYP450 inducers	Strong CYP inducers (eg, rifampin) may reduce efficacy of ramelteon.
CYP1A2 inhibitors	Caution with less potent CYP1A2 inhibitors, may increase levels of ramelteon.
CYP2C9 inhibitors	May increase levels with strong CYP2C9 inhibitors (eg, fluconazole).
CYP3A4 inhibitors	May increase levels with strong CYP3A4 inhibitors (eg, ketoconazole).
Fluvoxamine	Contraindicated with fluvoxamine (strong CYP1A2 inhibitor); increases AUC and C_{max} of ramelteon.

ANTIANXIETY/HYPNOTIC AGENTS *(cont.)*

Zaleplon (Sonata) CIV	
Alcohol	Caution with alcohol; additive CNS-depressant effects.
Anticonvulsants	Additive CNS-depressant effects with anticonvulsants.
Antihistamines	Potentiation of CNS-depressant effects with antihistamines.
Cimetidine	May increase plasma levels with cimetidine; may reduce zaleplon dose.
CNS depressants	Additive CNS-depressant effects with other CNS depressants.
CYP3A4 inhibitors	May increase levels with strong CYP3A4 inhibitors (eg, erythromycin, ketoconazole).
CYP3A4 inducers	Strong or multiple-doses of CYP3A4 inducers (eg, rifampin) may decrease efficacy of zaleplon.
Imipramine	Coadministration may cause additive effects on decreased alertness and impaired psychomotor performance.
Opioids	Potentiation of CNS-depressant effects with opioids.
Promethazine	Coadministration may decrease plasma levels of zaleplon.
Psychotropic agents	Additive decreased alertness and impaired psychomotor performance with psychotropic agents.
Thioridazine	Additive decreased alertness and impaired psychomotor performance with thioridazine.
Zolpidem Tartrate (Ambien, Ambien CR) CIV	
Chlorpromazine	Additive effect of decreased alertness and impaired psychomotor performance with coadministration.
CNS depressants	Potentiation of CNS-depressant effect with other CNS depressants, including alcohol.
CYP3A4 inhibitors	CYP3A4 inhibitors (eg, ketoconazole) may increase plasma levels of zolpidem; may cause additive sedative effects.
Flumazenil	Coadministration may reverse the sedative/hypnotic effect of zolpidem.
Imipramine	Coadministration may potentiate decrease in alertness.
Rifampin	Decreases plasma levels of zolpidem; may reduce efficacy.

BARBITURATES

Mephobarbital (Mebaral) CIV	
Alcohol	Additive CNS-depressant effects with alcohol.
Antihistamines	Additive CNS-depressant effects with antihistamines.
CNS depressants	Additive CNS-depressant effects with other CNS depressants.

Table 2.2. DRUG INTERACTIONS FOR CONSCIOUS SEDATION/ANTIANXIETY AGENTS *(cont.)*

BARBITURATES *(cont.)*	
Mephobarbital (Mebaral) CIV *(cont.)*	
Corticosteroids	Increases corticosteroid metabolism; may require dose adjustment of corticosteroid.
Coumarins	Decreases anticoagulant effect; may require dose adjustment of anticoagulant.
Doxycycline	Shortens half-life of doxycyline for as long as 2 weeks after barbiturate therapy discontinued; monitor for clinical response to doxycyline treatment.
Griseofulvin	Avoid concomitant administration; decreases griseofulvin absorption.
MAOIs	Inhibits metabolism of mephobarbital; may prolong barbiturate effect.
Phenytoin	May alter phenytoin metabolism; monitor blood levels of both medications.
Steroidal hormones/ oral contraceptives	Decreases efficacy of steroidal hormones.
Valproic acid/sodium valproate	Decreases mephobarbital metabolism; monitor blood levels and adjust dose accordingly.
Pentobarbital Sodium (Nembutal Sodium Solution) CII	
Antihistamines	Additive CNS-depressant effects with antihistamines.
CNS depressants	Additive CNS-depressant effects with other CNS depressants.
Corticosteroids	Increases corticosteroid metabolism; may require dose adjustment of corticosteroid.
Coumarins	Decreases anticoagulant effect; may require dose adjustment of anticoagulant.
Doxycycline	Shortens half-life of doxycyline for as long as 2 weeks after barbiturate therapy discontinued; monitor for clinical response to doxycyline treatment.
Griseofulvin	Avoid concomitant administration; decreases griseofulvin absorption.
MAOIs	Inhibits metabolism of pentobarbital; may prolong barbiturate effect.
Phenytoin	May alter phenytoin metabolism; monitor blood levels of both medications.
Steroidal hormones/ oral contraceptives	Decreases efficacy of steroidal hormones.
Valproic acid/sodium valproate	Decreases pentobarbital metabolism; monitor blood levels and adjust dose accordingly.
Phenobarbital CIV	
Antihistamines	Additive CNS-depressant effects with antihistamines.
CNS depressants	Additive CNS-depressant effects with other CNS depressants.
Corticosteroids	Increases corticosteroid metabolism; may require dose adjustment of corticosteroid.
Coumarins	Decreases anticoagulant effect; may require dose adjustment of anticoagulant.
Doxycycline	Shortens half-life of doxycyline for as long as 2 weeks after barbiturate therapy discontinued; monitor for clinical response to doxycyline treatment.

BARBITURATES *(cont.)*

Phenobarbital CIV *(cont.)*	
Griseofulvin	Avoid concomitant administration; decreases griseofulvin absorption.
MAOIs	Inhibits metabolism of phenobarbital; may prolong barbiturate effect.
Phenytoin	May alter phenytoin metabolism; monitor blood levels of both medications.
Steroidal hormones/ oral contraceptives	Decreases efficacy of steroidal hormones.
Valproic acid/sodium valproate	Decreases phenobarbital metabolism; monitor blood levels and adjust dose accordingly.
Secobarbital Sodium (Seconal Sodium) CII	
Antihistamines	Additive CNS-depressant effects with antihistamines.
CNS depressants	Additive CNS-depressant effects with other CNS depressants.
Corticosteroids	Increases corticosteroid metabolism; may require dose adjustment of corticosteroid.
Coumarins	Decreases anticoagulant effect; may require dose adjustment of anticoagulant.
Doxycycline	Shortens half-life of doxycyline for as long as 2 weeks after barbiturate therapy discontinued; monitor for clinical response to doxycyline treatment.
Griseofulvin	Avoid concomitant administration; decreases griseofulvin absorption.
MAOIs	Inhibits metabolism of secobarbital; may prolong barbiturate effect.
Phenytoin	May alter phenytoin metabolism; monitor blood levels of both medications.
Steroidal hormones/ oral contraceptives	Decreases efficacy of steroidal hormones.
Valproic acid/sodium valproate	Decreases secobarbital metabolism; monitor blood levels and adjust dose accordingly.

BENZODIAZEPINES

Alprazolam (Niravam, Xanax, Xanax XR) CIV	
Amiodarone	Caution with amiodarone; may increase levels.
Anticonvulsants	Additive CNS depressant effects with anticonvulsants.
Antihistamines	Additive CNS depressant effects with antihistamines.
Carbamazepine	May decrease plasma levels with carbamazepine.
Cimetidine	Potentiated by cimetidine.
Contraceptives, oral	Potentiated by oral contraceptives
Cyclosporine	Caution with cyclosporine; may increase levels.
CYP3A inducers	May decrease levels with CYP3A inducers (eg, carbamazepine)
CYP3A inhibitors	Avoid with potent CYP3A inhibitors (eg, azole antifungals)
Desimipramine	May increases levels of desimipramine.
Diltiazem	Caution with diltiazem; may increase levels.
Ergotamine	Caution with ergotamine; may increase levels.

Table 2.2. DRUG INTERACTIONS FOR CONSCIOUS SEDATION/ANTIANXIETY AGENTS *(cont.)*

BENZODIAZEPINES *(cont.)*

Alprazolam (Niravam, Xanax, Xanax XR) CIV *(cont.)*	
Ethanol	Additive CNS depressant effects with ethanol.
Fluoxetine	Potentiated by fluoxetine.
Fluvoxamine	Potentiated by fluvoxamine.
Grapefruit juice	Caution with grapefruit juice; may increase levels.
Imipramine	May increase levels of imipramine.
Isoniazid	Caution with isoniazid; may increase levels.
Itraconazole	Contraindicated with itraconazole.
Ketoconazole	Contraindicated with ketoconazole.
Macrolides	Caution with macrolides; may increase levels.
Nefazodone	Potentiated by nefazodone.
Nicardipine	Caution with nicardipine; may increase levels.
Nifedipine	Caution with nifedipine; may increase levels.
Paroxetine	Caution with paroxetine; may increase levels.
Propxyphene	May decrease plasma levels with propoxyphene.
Psychotropic agents	Additive CNS depressant effects with psychotropic agents.
Saliva/stomach pH, drugs affecting	May slow or decrease alprazolam absorption (Niravam).
Sertraline	Caution with sertraline, may increase levels.
Chlordiazepoxide HCl (Librium) CIV	
Alcohol	Additive CNS-depressant effects with alcohol.
CNS depressants	Additive CNS-depressant effects with other CNS depressants.
Psychotropic agents	Avoid concomitant use of psychotropic agents (eg, MAOIs, phenothiazines) with chlordiazepoxide.
Clonazepam (Klonopin, Klonopin Wafers) CIV	
Alcohol	Additive CNS-depressant effects with alcohol.
Anticonvulsants	Potentiates CNS-depressant effects with anticonvulsants.
Barbiturates	Potentiates CNS-depressant effects with barbiturates.
CNS depressants	Additive CNS-depressant effects with other CNS depressants.
CYP450 inducers	May decrease levels with CYP450 inducers (eg, carbamazepine, phenobarbital, phenytoin).
CYP3A4 inhibitors	Caution with CYP3A inhibitors (eg, azole antifungals); may increase levels of clonazepam.
MAOIs	Potentiates CNS-depressant effects with MAOIs.
Narcotics	Potentiates CNS-depressant effects with narcotics.
Psychotropic agents	Potentiates CNS-depressant effects with psychotropic agents.

BENZODIAZEPINES *(cont.)*

Clorazepate Dipotassium (Tranxene T-Tab) CIV	
Alcohol	Additive CNS-depressant effects with alcohol.
Barbiturates	Potentiates CNS-depressant effects with barbiturates.
CNS depressants	Additive CNS-depressant effects with other CNS depressants.
Hypnotics	Increases sedation with hypnotics.
MAOIs	Potentiates CNS-depressant effects with MAOIs.
Narcotics	Potentiates CNS-depressant effects with narcotics.
Psychotropic agents	Potentiates CNS-depressant effects with psychotropic agents.
Diazepam (Diastat) CIV	
Alcohol	Additive CNS-depressant effects with alcohol.
Barbiturates	Potentiates CNS-depressant effects with barbiturates.
Cimetidine	Coadministration may delay clearance of diazepam.
CNS depressants	Additive CNS-depressant effects with other CNS depressants.
CYP2C19 inducers	CYP2C19 inducers (eg, rifampin) increase the rate of diazepam elimination.
CYP2C19 inhibitors	CYP2C19 inhibitors (eg, cimetidine, quinidine, tranylcypromine) decrease rate of diazepam elimination.
CYP3A4 inducers	CYP3A4 inducers (eg, carbamazepine, dexamethasone, phenobarbital, phenytoin) increase the rate of diazepam metabolism.
CYP3A4 inhibitors	CYP3A4 inhibitors (eg, clotrimazole, ketoconazole, troleandomycin) decrease the rate of diazepam elimination.
CYP2C19 substrates	May interfere with the metabolism of drugs which are substrates for CYP2C19 (eg, omeprazole, propranolol, imipramine).
CYP3A4 substrates	May interfere with the metabolism of drugs which are substrates for CYP3A4 (eg, cyclosporine, paclitaxel, terfenadine, theophylline, warfarin).
MAOIs	Potentiates CNS-depressant effects with MAOIs.
Narcotics	Potentiates CNS-depressant effects with narcotics.
Psychotropic agents	Potentiates CNS-depressant effects with psychotropic agents.
Valproate	May potentiate CNS-depressant effects of diazepam.
Diazepam (Diazepam Injection, Valium) CIV	
Alcohol	Increases CNS-depressant effect; avoid concomitant use.
Antacids	May slow rate of absorption; decreases peak diazepam concentration.
Anticonvulsants	Potentiates CNS-depressant effects with anticonvulsants.
Antihistamines	Additive CNS-depressant effects with antihistamines.
Barbiturates	Potentiates CNS-depressant effects with barbiturates.
Cimetidine	Coadministration may delay clearance of diazepam.
CNS depressants	Additive CNS-depressant effects with other CNS depressants.
CYP2C19 inhibitors	May increase plasma levels of diazepam and cause increased and prolonged sedation.

Table 2.2. DRUG INTERACTIONS FOR CONSCIOUS SEDATION/ANTIANXIETY AGENTS *(cont.)*

BENZODIAZEPINES *(cont.)*	
Diazepam (Valium) CIV *(cont.)*	
CYP3A4 inhibitors	May increase plasma levels of diazepam and cause increased and prolonged sedation.
MAOIs	Potentiates CNS-depressant effects with MAOIs.
Narcotics	Potentiates CNS-depressant effects with narcotics.
Phenytoin	May decrease elimination of phenytoin.
Psychotropic agents	Potentiates CNS-depressant effects with psychotropic agents.
Estazolam CIV	
Anticonvulsants	Potentiates CNS-depressant effects with anticonvulsants.
Antihistamines	Additive CNS-depressant effects with antihistamines.
Azole antifungals	Contraindicated with ketoconazole and itraconazole.
Barbiturates	Potentiates CNS-depressant effects with barbiturates.
CNS depressants	Additive CNS-depressant effects with other CNS depressants.
CYP3A inducers	Potent CYP3A inducers (eg, barbiturates, carbamazepine, phenytoin, rifampin) may decrease plasma levels of estazolam.
CYP3A inhibitors	CYP3A inhibitors (eg, diltiazem, nefazodone, fluvoxamine, cimetidine, some macrolides) increase levels of estazolam. Avoid with potent CYP3A inhibitors (eg, azole antifungals).
MAOIs	Potentiates CNS-depressant effects with MAOIs.
Narcotics	Potentiates CNS-depressant effects with narcotics.
Psychotropic agents	Potentiates CNS-depressant effects with psychotropic agents.
Flurazepam HCl (Dalmane) CIV	
Alcohol	Additive CNS-depressant effects with alcohol.
CNS depressants	Additive CNS-depressant effects with other CNS depressants.
Lorazepam (Ativan Injection) CIV	
Antidepressants	Additive CNS-depressant effects with antidepressants.
Barbiturates	Additive CNS-depressant effects with barbiturates.
Clozapine	Caution with clozapine; marked sedation, excessive salivation, ataxia, and death reported.
Haloperidol	Caution with haloperidol; apnea, coma, bradycardia, arrhythmia, and death reported.
Loxapine	Caution with loxapine; respiratory depression, stupor, and hypotension reported.
MAOIs	Additive CNS-depressant effects with MAOIs.
Narcotics	Additive CNS-depressant effects with narcotics.
Phenothiazines	Additive CNS-depressant effects with phenothiazines.
Probenecid	Decreases clearance and prolongs half-life of lorazepam; reduce lorazepam dose by 50%.

BENZODIAZEPINES *(cont.)*

Lorazepam (Ativan Injection) CIV *(cont.)*	
Scopolamine	Caution with scopolamine; sedation, hallucination, and irrational behavior reported.
Steroidal hormones/ oral contraceptives	Increases clearance and decreases half-life of lorazepam; may require increased dosage.
Valproate	Increases plasma levels of lorazepam; reduce lorazepam dose by 50%.
Lorazepam (Ativan) CIV	
Aminophylline	May reduce sedative effects of lorazepam.
Anticonvulsants	Potentiates CNS-depressant effects with anticonvulsants.
Antihistamines	Additive CNS-depressant effects with antihistamines.
Barbiturates	Additive CNS-depressant effects with barbiturates.
Clozapine	Caution with clozapine; marked sedation, excessive salivation, ataxia, delirium, and respiratory arrest reported.
CNS depressants	Additive CNS-depressant effects; may cause potentially fatal respiratory depression.
Narcotics	Potentiates CNS-depressant effects with narcotics.
Probenecid	Decreases clearance and increases half-life of lorazepam; may cause a more rapid onset or prolonged effect of lorazepam. Reduce lorazepam dose by 50% with probenecid.
Theophylline	May reduce sedative effects of lorazepam.
Valproate	Increases levels of lorazepam; reduce lorazepam dose by 50% with valproate.
Midazolam HCl (Midazolam Injection) CIV	
Barbiturates	Potentiates CNS-depressant effects with barbiturates; increased risk of hypoventilation and apnea.
CNS depressants	Additive CNS-depressant effects with other CNS depressants; increases risk of hypoventilation and apnea.
CYP3A4 inhibitors	CYP3A4 inhibitors (eg, cimetidine, erythromycin, diltiazem, verapamil, ketoconazole, itraconazole) decrease clearance of midazolam; may cause prolonged sedation.
Erythromycin	Caution with erythromycin; decreases plasma clearance of midazolam.
Fentanyl	May cause severe hypotension with concomitant use of fentanyl in neonates.
Halothane	May decrease the minimum alveolar concentration of halothane required for anesthesia.
Narcotics	Potentiates CNS-depressant effects with narcotics; may cause increased sedation.
Midazolam HCl (Midazolam Syrup) CIV	
Anesthetic agents	Caution with anesthetics; may cause increased sedation.
Barbiturates	Potentiates CNS-depressant effects with barbiturates.
CNS depressants	Additive CNS-depressant effects with other CNS depressants, including alcohol.

Table 2.2. DRUG INTERACTIONS FOR CONSCIOUS SEDATION/ANTIANXIETY AGENTS *(cont.)*

BENZODIAZEPINES *(cont.)*	
Midazolam HCl (Midazolam Syrup) CIV *(cont.)*	
CYP3A4 inducers	CYP3A4 inducers (eg, rifampin, carbamazepine, phenytoin) decrease plasma levels of midazolam; may require dose adjustment.
CYP3A4 inhibitors	CYP3A4 inhibitors (eg, diltiazem, erythromycin, ketoconazole, itraconazole, nelfinavir, ritonavir, saquinavir, verapamil) decrease clearance of midazolam; may cause prolonged sedation.
Narcotics	Potentiates CNS-depressant effects with narcotics; may cause increased sedation.
Oxazepam CIV	
Alcohol	Additive CNS-depressant effects with alcohol.
CNS depressants	Additive CNS-depressant effects with other CNS depressants.
Temazepam (Restoril) CIV	
Alcohol	Additive CNS-depressant effects with alcohol.
CNS depressants	Additive CNS-depressant effects with other CNS depressants.
Diphenhydramine	Caution with diphenhydramine; possible synergistic effect.
Triazolam (Halcion) CIV	
Alcohol	Additive CNS-depressant effects with alcohol.
Amiodarone	Caution with concomitant administration of amiodarone.
Anticonvulsants	Potentiates CNS-depressant effects with anticonvulsants.
Antihistamines	Additive CNS-depressant effects with antihistamines.
CCBs	Caution with concomitant use of CCBs (eg, diltiazem, verapamil, nicardipine, nifedipine).
CNS depressants	Additive CNS-depressant effects with other CNS depressants.
Contraceptives, oral	Increases plasma levels and half-life of triazolam.
CYP3A inhibitors	Contraindicated with potent CYP3A inhibitors: ketoconazole, itraconazole, and nefazodone. Caution with less potent CYP3A inhibitors (eg, cimetidine, macrolide antibiotics); may increase plasma levels and decrease clearance of midazolam.
Cyclosporine	Caution with concomitant administration of cyclosporine.
Ergotamine	Caution with concomitant administration of ergotamine.
Fluvoxamine	Caution with concomitant administration of fluvoxamine.
Isoniazid	Increases plasma levels and half-life of triazolam.
Paroxetine	Caution with concomitant administration of paroxetine.
Psychotropic agents	Additive CNS-depressant effects with psychotropic agents.
Ranitidine	Caution with ranitidine; increases plasma levels and half-life of triazolam.
Sertraline	Caution with concomitant administration of sertraline.

BENZODIAZEPINE ANTAGONISTS

Flumazenil (Romazicon)	
Cyclic antidepressants	Toxic effects including convulsions and cardiac dysrhythmias may occur with mixed drug overdose.
Neuromuscular blocking agents	Avoid use until effects of neuromuscular blockage has been fully reversed.
Non-benzodiazepine hypnotics	Blocks effects of non-benzodiazepine hypnotics (eg, zolpidem, eszopiclone).

OPIOID ANTAGONISTS

Naloxone HCl (Narcan)	
Buprenorphine	Reversal of buprenorphine-induced respiratory depression may be incomplete; may require higher doses of naloxone.
Cardiovascular effects, drugs causing	Caution with increased risk of cardiovascular events, including ventricular tachycardia/fibrillation, pulmonary edema, and cardiac arrest with coadministration.
Pentazocine	Reversal of pentazocine-induced respiratory depression may be incomplete; may require higher doses of naloxone.
Naltrexone (Vivitrol)	
Opioid analgesics	Contraindicated with opioid analgesics; antagonizes analgesic effect.
Naltrexone HCl (ReVia)	
Antidiarrheals, opioid-containing	Antagonizes the effect of opioid-containing antidiarrheals.
Cough and cold perparations, opioid-containing	Antagonizes the effect of opioid-containing cough and cold preparations.
Disulfiram	Avoid concomitant use; increases risk of hepatotoxicity.
Opioid analgesics	Contraindicated with opioid analgesics; antagonizes analgesic effect.
Thioridazine	Lethargy and somnolence reported with thioridazine.

PARTIAL OPIOID AGONISTS/OPIOID ANTAGONISTS

Buprenorphine/Naloxone (Suboxone, Subutex) CIII	
CNS depressants	Additive CNS-depressant effect; increases risk of respiratory depression and death with coadministration.
CYP3A4 inhibitors	CYP3A4 inhibitors (eg, azole antifungals, macrolide antibiotics, protease inhibitors) increase plasma levels of buprenorphine; may require dose adjustment.
CYP3A4 inducers	Caution with CYP3A4 inducers (eg, carbamazepine, phenobarbital, phenytoin); close monitoring recommended.
Narcotics	Increases CNS-depressant effect with narcotics.

Chapter 3

Analgesics: Opioids and Nonopioids

Steven Ganzberg, D.M.D., M.S.
James Fricton, D.D.S., M.S.

The use of systemically acting medications to reduce pain perception is an integral part of dental practice. Analgesic medications in dentistry are indicated for the relief of acute pain, postoperative pain, and chronic pain, as well as for adjunctive intraoperative pain control. In addition, these medications can be given preoperatively to decrease expected postoperative pain. There are two general categories of analgesic medications: opioid and nonopioid.

OPIOID ANALGESICS

Accepted Indications

Moderate-to-Severe Pain

Opioid medications are generally reserved for moderate-to-severe pain. Codeine, hydrocodone, dihydrocodeine, and oxycodone—in combination preparations that contain aspirin, acetaminophen, or ibuprofen—are commonly prescribed to manage acute orodental and postoperative pain in dental practice. Based on the amount of drug needed to produce a specific analgesic effect, oxycodone is a more potent analgesic than these other medications, but an equianalgesic dose can be found with any of the other agents. At an equianalgesic dose, the side effects of opioids, including sedation, nausea, vomiting, constipation, respiratory depression, and pupillary constriction, are relatively similar.

Table 3.1 lists the commonly prescribed combination opioids, along with oral dosages and schedule of dosing. For severe pain, opioids such as oxycodone, morphine, and hydromorphone are available without a nonsteroidal anti-inflammatory drug (NSAID) or acetaminophen. Other accepted indications for opioids include treatment of diarrhea, cough, and some types of acute pulmonary edema; as an adjunct to anesthesia and sedation; and detoxification from opioids. **Table 3.1** also lists commonly prescribed opioids not in combination with other analgesics, along with oral dosages and schedule of dosing.

Cancer and Chronic Nonmalignant Pain

Long-acting opioid analgesics, such as MS Contin, Opana, Oramorph, OxyContin, methadone, levorphanol, and fentanyl patches, are available for treating oral cancer pain and selected cases of chronic nonmalignant orofacial pain. These agents are not indicated for acute pain relief and should be prescribed only for people who can tolerate short-acting opioids. Only practitioners who are skilled in the management of chronic pain should prescribe these agents due to the potential for long-term adverse events (including depression, constipation, and bowel obstruction), sedation and cognitive deficits, escalation of dose, solicitation from multiple practitioners, and common polypharmaceutical overuse. Zitman et al

(1990) noted that chronic pain is a treatment-resistant condition, and that even modest improvement may be considered worthwhile.

Another potentially useful agent for chronic pain management is tramadol (Ultram), which acts as a mu (μ) agonist and weak serotonin/norepinehprine reuptake blocker. The latter effect, which would be expected to be helpful for chronic pain conditions, may also produce analgesia. The intravenous use of opioid medications for intraoperative sedation is discussed in **Chapter 2** and **Appendix L**.

General Dosing Information

Analgesic medications should be prescribed in a manner that affords the patient the greatest degree of comfort within a high margin of safety. If it is suspected that a patient will have pain for 24 to 48 hours after a dental or surgical procedure, it is prudent to prescribe either opioid or NSAID analgesics on a regularly scheduled basis for at least 24 to 36 hours rather than on an as-needed (prn) basis. The rationale for this approach is to provide as continuous a plasma level of medication as possible. If a patient waits until an analgesic medication loses effect and then takes another dose, he or she will be in pain for an additional 30 to 60 minutes. Furthermore, it requires more analgesic medication to overcome pain than to maintain pain relief once it has been established. Therefore, knowledge of a specific analgesic's duration of action is needed to prescribe appropriately. Likewise, it is well-established that if an NSAID or an opioid is given preoperatively or prior to loss of local anesthetic activity, pain relief can be more easily achieved with postoperative analgesics. Since oral surgery studies comparing the analgesic benefit of many of these pharmacological agents to nonopioid analgesic medications (such as NSAIDs) fail to show increased analgesic efficacy of opioid combination analgesics, it may be appropriate to consider the use of a nonopioid agent as the primary analgesic for postoperative oral pain.

All opioid medications can cause tolerance, a reduced drug effect that results from continued use and the need for higher doses to produce the same effect. These medications also can cause physical dependence, the physiological state associated with discontinuation of the drug after prolonged use (withdrawal), and psychological dependence, which is an intense craving for the drug and compulsive drug-seeking behavior. For these reasons, most opioids are classified as controlled substances in the U.S. and Canada. Because the pain commonly encountered in dental practice is of the acute type, tolerance of and physical and psychological dependence upon opioids are so rare as to be of little concern, because such drugs are used only over the short term. Opioid medications should be used in sufficiently large doses for high-quality management of acute pain without fear that patients will develop dependence. The one exception may be patients with a history of drug abuse. For these patients, nonopioid analgesics should be prescribed initially.

It should also be appreciated that a significant portion of the analgesic activity of codeine, hydrocodone, and, likely, oxycodone occurs following hepatic metabolism by CYP2D6, one of the cytochrome P450 group of hepatic microsomal enzymes. As many as 10% of patients may not have a functional form of CYP2D6, which may significantly decrease analgesic efficacy of the above agents. If adequate analgesia does not occur with one of the above agents, it may be of value to try another opioid. Agents such as morphine and hydromorphone do not require hepatic metabolism to achieve analgesia. The majority of important drug interactions involve the possibility of sedative and gastrointestinal side effects, among others. A complete listing of these is provided in **Table 3.1**.

Maximum Recommended Doses

The choice of a pharmacologic agent or agents is based on a balance between higher efficacy and lower side effects, since almost every medication has some adverse effects. It is important to be familiar with indications, precautions, adverse effects, and drug interactions of all medications used. The adverse effect profile of some medications will affect patient adherence, but the patient's understanding of the proper use and therapeutic purpose of the medications can mitigate this negative influence.

Adults

Recommended doses for the combination products are listed in **Table 3.1**. The combination opioid products are generally limited by the dosage of the nonopioid product (for example, 4,000 mg per day for acetaminophen or aspirin). In general, there is no maximum dose of an opioid alone if proper titration has occurred, other than the dose at which side effects are not tolerated. The use of opioids not formulated as a combination product is generally reserved for the management of severe acute pain and selected chronic pain.

Pediatric Patients

In pediatric patients, codeine with acetaminophen and hydrocodone with acetaminophen is approved for pediatric pain not responsive to acetaminophen or ibuprofen alone. The maximum dosages for codeine with acetaminophen are shown in **Table 3.1**. Other opioids can be considered.

Geriatric Patients

Geriatric patients may develop exaggerated sedative effects with opioid medications. Postural hypotension may occur. Consider starting at lower dose ranges.

Dosage Adjustments

Clinicians should adjust the dosage based on patient response. If duration of analgesia is insufficient, a shorter period between doses (for example, q3h vs q4h) or a higher dosage (for example, 7.5 mg vs 5 mg of hydrocodone) is appropriate. If analgesia itself is insufficient, a higher dosage of pain medication is appropriate. For short-term acute pain conditions, dependence on opioids is generally not of concern and efforts should be made to provide adequate postoperative analgesia.

Dosage Forms

Opioid medications are available for oral, intravenous, intramuscular, intranasal, transmucosal, or transdermal use. Oral forms will likely be used (eg, capsule, tablet or elixir—see **Table 3.1**) or perhaps butorphanol, which is available in a nasal spray form.

Special Dental Considerations

Opioids may decrease salivary flow. Consider long-term opioid use in the differential diagnosis of caries, periodontal disease, or oral candidiasis. Also evaluate patients using oral opioid drugs that dissolve in the mouth, since these products often contain citric acid, sugars, and/or starch and may increase the risk of caries.

Drug Interactions of Dental Interest

The most common drug interactions of concern for dentistry involve the potential sedative side effects, which are exaggerated in patients taking other CNS depressants (**see Table 3.2**).

Cross-Sensitivity

Cross-sensitivity is possible with opioids. It is important to distinguish whether a true allergic reaction occurred, as most opioids can produce nausea and/or vomiting and some cause histamine release. These reactions are typically referred to as "allergic" by patients. Clinicians should consider using a nonopioid analgesic in these patients. Switching to a different opioid may produce fewer side effects.

Special Patients

Opioids should be used with caution in patients with chronic obstructive pulmonary disease (COPD), such as emphysema or chronic bronchitis, owing to possible respiratory compromise. Opioids may precipitate an asthmatic episode because of their potential for histamine release. This is considerably more likely with parenteral vs oral administration of opioids. Asthmatic patients should be instructed to discontinue use of oral opioids if they experience asthmatic symptoms during therapy. Combination opioid products that contain aspirin should not be prescribed to asthmatic patients. Likewise, patients with severe cardiac disease, such as advanced congestive heart failure, may not tolerate hypotensive side effects. If mentally challenged patients are prescribed opioid medications, they should be closely monitored by an appropriate caregiver. Opioids should be prescribed cautiously for a patient with emotional instability, suicidal ideation or attempts, or a history of substance abuse.

Pregnant and nursing women

Opioids should not be prescribed for a pregnant or nursing patient without consultation with the patient's physician.

Pediatric, geriatric, and other special patients

Clinicians should consider lower opioid dosages for pediatric and geriatric patients.

Patient Monitoring: Aspects to Watch

- Respiratory depression and sedation: the patient should contact the dentist if these side effects are observed.
- Nausea, vomiting, or both.

Adverse Effects and Precautions

The majority of important drug interactions involve the possibility of sedative and gastrointestinal side effects; a more complete listing is provided in **Table 3.1**.

Pharmacology

Opioid medications produce analgesia by interaction at specific receptors in the central nervous system, mimicking the effect of endogenous pain-relieving peptides (eg, dynorphin, enkephalin, and β-endorphin). These receptors are present in higher brain centers such as the hypothalamus and periaqueductal gray regions, as well as in the spinal cord and trigeminal nucleus. The result of this interaction is a decrease in pain transmission to higher thalamocortical centers and a corresponding decrease in pain perception. Recent evidence suggests a possible peripheral effect of opioid analgesics.

Opioids undergo hepatic transformation generally to inactive metabolites, which are excreted in the urine and/or bile. These drugs are subdivided into agonist, agonist-antagonist, or antagonist compounds based on their receptor effects.

Agonists

The opioid medications typified by morphine act primarily in the CNS through varied activity on specific opioid receptor subgroups. Although there is activity at all opioid receptors, morphine and related agents—such as codeine, hydrocodone, dihydrocodeine, and oxycodone, as well as meperidine and the fentanyl derivatives—provide analgesia chiefly through agonist activity at the μ receptor.

Agonist-Antagonists

Another group of opioid analgesics, the agonist-antagonists—including pentazocine, nalbuphine and butorphanol—are agonists at the kappa (κ) receptor, and antagonists at the mu (μ) receptor.

Antagonists

Specific competitive opioid antagonist medications—namely, naloxone and naltrexone—have also been developed. Naloxone's main use in dentistry is reversal of excessive opioid

IV sedation (See page 48 for more information). Naltrexone is used to treat former opioid abusers and recently has been used for patients with certain CNS disorders.

Patient Advice

- Patients should avoid use of alcohol or other CNS depressant medications unless a physician or dentist gives approval.
- The patient should notify the dentist if nausea, vomiting, excessive dry mouth, dizziness or light-headedness, ataxia, itching, hives, or difficulty in breathing occurs.
- Instruct patients to exercise caution when getting up suddenly from a lying or sitting position.
- Also instruct patients to avoid driving a motor vehicle or operating heavy machinery, especially if sedative side effects are present.

SUGGESTED READING

Dionne RA, Snyder J, Hargreaves KM. Analgesic efficacy of flubriprofen in comparison with acetaminophen, acetaminophen plus codeine, and placebo after impacted third molar removal. *J Oral Maxillofac Surg*. 1994;52(9):919-924.

Forbes JA, Bates JA, Edquist IA, et al. Evaluation of two opioid-acetaminophen combinations and placebo in post-operative oral surgery pain. *Pharmacotherapy*. 1994;14(2):139-146.

Hargreaves KM, Troullos ES, Dionne RA. Pharmacologic rationale for the treatment of acute pain. *Dent Clin North Am*. 1987;31(4):675-694.

The United States Pharmacopeial Convention, Inc. *USP Dispensing Information: drug information for the health care professional*. Vol. I. 23rd ed. Greenwood Village, CO: Thomson Micromedex; 2003.

Zitman FG, Linssen ACG, Edelbroek PM, Stijnen T. Low dose amitriptyline in chronic pain: the gain is modest. *Pain*. 1990;42:35-42.

NONOPIOID ANALGESICS

This group of analgesics includes the nonsteroidal anti-inflammatory drugs and acetaminophen. The site of action of these drugs is both peripheral and in the CNS.

Nonsteroidal Anti-Inflammatory Drugs and Acetaminophen

Although NSAIDs influence a number of systems, the primary analgesic effect is the inhibition of the synthesis of prostaglandins, which are potent vasodilators and mediators of the inflammatory response at the site of injury. By decreasing the production of peripheral prostaglandins, NSAIDs depress the inflammatory response. This decrease in prostaglandin concentration also raises the threshold for pain-conducting nerves to discharge, thus providing an analgesic effect. In the CNS, NSAIDs reduce prostaglandin formation in critical pain processing regions, hence producing decreased pain transmission and perception. NSAIDs also reduce fever by decreasing the concentration of prostaglandins in the hypothalamus, a brain center regulating body temperature.

The NSAIDs consist of several groups of drugs, based on structure and enzyme selectivity, that have similar mechanisms of action. They are primarily indicated for relief of mild-to-moderate pain and for chronic inflammatory conditions. Although no individual NSAID has been shown to be significantly superior for pain relief in all patients, NSAIDs do differ in duration of action and particularly side-effect profile. In regard to side effects, NSAIDs can be divided into traditional cyclooxygenase 1 and 2 (COX-1 and COX-2) inhibitors and selective COX-2 inhibitors. COX-1 is responsible for the physiologic production of homeostatic and cytoprotective prostanoids in the gastric mucosa, endothelium, platelets, and kidneys. Its inhibition is linked to many of the adverse effects of NSAIDs. Common side effects associated with NSAIDs include epigastric pain, nausea, vomiting, constipation, and diarrhea. Evidence suggests that these agents can also be associated with significant toxicities and adverse effects, such as renal damage, especially in high-risk patients. These adverse effects of NSAIDs are especially severe in patients over the age of 60, and those with a history of peptic ulcer disease, gastrointestinal (GI) bleeding, or use of tobacco and alcohol. COX-2 inhibitors affect the production of mainly proinflammatory prostaglandins and have considerably fewer gastrointestinal and impaired platelet aggregation effects, but adverse renal effects are still present. The traditional agents affect both forms of cyclooxygenase (COX-1 and COX-2) in variable proportions, but generally with greater likelihood of those adverse effects mentioned above. Some traditional agents, however, have favorable COX-1/COX-2 activity ratios and have a decreased incidence of some adverse effects (eg, nabumetone, etodolac, and meloxicam). For patients at increased risk of adverse effects (for example, history of peptic ulcer disease, gastroesophageal reflux disease [GERD], and inflammatory bowel disease), a predominantly COX-2–active drug may be preferred. Celecoxib is the only selective COX-2 inhibitor currently available in the U.S. that is able to completely inhibit COX-2 and the proinflammatory prostaglandins at doses that cause fewer GI side effects. The efficacy of selective COX-2 inhibitors for acute dental pain and systemic arthritic conditions is well supported. However, the COX-2 inhibitors have been found to increase embolic phenomena (eg, myocardial infarction and stroke), in part due to alteration of nitric oxide and prostacyclin formation, leading to the removal of two COX-2 selective agents from the market. Long-term use of COX-2 inhibitors requires weighing the benefit/risk profile for an individual patient. There is also risk of embolic phenomena with long-term use of traditional NSAIDs, although this is variable among this group.

The mechanism of action of acetaminophen is still the subject of debate, but current research suggests a CNS mechanism of action that may be mediated by COX-3. While acetaminophen has analgesic and antipyretic properties comparable to those of aspirin, it fails to exert significant anti-inflammatory action due to its susceptibility to the high level of peroxides present in inflammatory lesions. Acetaminophen (Paracetamol in many other countries), is a common analgesic and antipyretic drug used for the relief of headaches, fever, and minor aches and pains, including toothache. Acetaminophen is also useful in the management of more severe pain, with fewer side effects, allowing for the use of lower dosages of additional NSAIDs or opioid analgesics. Acetaminophen is usually classified along with NSAIDs. It is considered safe for human use with minimal adverse events at the recommended doses; it is a major ingredient in cold and flu medications, as well as many prescription analgesics. However, because of its wide availability, deliberate or accidental overdoses are common and may result in liver damage. Some acetaminophen and aspirin compounds include the addition of caffeine, which has been shown to improve management of some pain, such as tension-type headaches.

Accepted Indications

NSAIDs are indicated for use as analgesics for mild to moderate pain, including pain of acute dental origin or for postoperative dental pain. These drugs are also indicated for pain of inflammatory origin, especially for rheumatic conditions and primary non-rheumatic inflammatory conditions. Some (ibuprofen and naproxen) may also be used as antipyretics and for treatment of primary dysmenorrhea.

NSAIDs may be indicated for longer-term use in patients with chronic orofacial pain, especially pain with an inflammatory component, such as temporomandibular joint synovitis. Seven placebo-controlled RCTs have been conducted to evaluate the treatment of tension-type headaches with NSAIDs. Seven RCTs have evaluated NSAIDS for temporomandibular joint pain, with one of them testing Celecoxib. No individual NSAID has been found to be superior in analgesic effect to others, but NSAIDs appear overall to be better than acetaminophen for temporomandibular disorders. Individual patient response is variable, and failure of one NSAID is not an indication to forgo the use of others.

If these medications are prescribed for a longer term, consider conducting appropriate laboratory studies—including CBC, renal function tests, and liver function tests. For long-term use, the COX-2 inhibitors have the advantage of fewer gastrointestinal and impaired platelet aggregation adverse effects, although renal complications and embolic phenomena must be considered. The long-term use of these agents should be undertaken only by those skilled in chronic pain management.

General Dosing Information

Many NSAIDs have a ceiling dose for analgesia and require a higher dose for the anti-inflammatory effect. For instance, ibuprofen, at 400 mg taken qid, provides close to a maximum analgesic effect, but a dose of 2,400 to 3,200 mg per day may be required for the anti-inflammatory effect. Depending on the condition being treated, consider higher or lower dosages. Some NSAIDs may be better analgesics while others are better anti-inflammatories.

In regard to pain control, one NSAID may be ineffective while another provides excellent pain relief. If one NSAID is ineffective for pain control, keep in mind that another NSAID from a different structural group may be effective and consider switching NSAIDs to obtain the desired results.

NSAIDs with an easier dosing schedule, such as bid or tid, may provide better patient compliance and result in a more pain-free patient. As a general rule, analgesic medications should be prescribed in a manner that affords the patient the greatest degree of comfort within a high margin of safety. See the section on General Dosing under "Opioid Analgesics" above for guidelines for both opioids and NSAIDs. Owing to the possible gastrointestinal side effects, NSAIDs should be prescribed with meals and/or taken with a full glass of water.

Table 3.1 lists acetaminophen and traditional NSAIDs as well as the COX-2 inhibitors. Dosing schedules and maximum daily doses are also provided.

Maximum Recommended Doses

Adults

See **Table 3.1**.

Pregnant women

NSAIDs are generally contraindicated during pregnancy. Some NSAIDs do carry Pregnancy Category B classification during the first trimester of pregnancy. Regardless, the use of NSAIDs should be considered contraindicated in dental practice for all pregnant patients, unless prescribed in consultation with the patient's obstetrician. Acetaminophen, although generally acceptable, should be prescribed in consultation with the patient's obstetrician if there are any questions about the appropriateness of its use in an individual case.

Pediatric patients

Dosages should be reduced for children. Owing to their possible gastrointestinal side effects, NSAIDs should be prescribed with meals. Ibuprofen is the only NSAID that has been approved for use as an analgesic in children >2 years, although naproxen has been approved for juvenile rheumatoid arthritis for children >2 years.

Geriatric Patients

Dosages should be reduced for elderly patients. Owing to their possible gastrointestinal side effects, NSAIDs should be prescribed with meals.

Dosage Forms

NSAIDs and acetaminophen are available for oral use except for ketorolac tromethamine, which is also available in an IV/IM preparation. Elixir, liquid, and rectal preparations are available for aspirin and acetaminophen. Liquid forms of ibuprofen are also available.

Special Dental Considerations

In the differential diagnosis of appropriate conditions, dentists should take into consideration that NSAIDs may cause soreness or irritation of the oral mucosa. Although very rare, some NSAIDs may cause leukopenia and/or thrombocytopenia.

Drug Interactions of Dental Interest

Major drug interactions with NSAIDs stem from the effect of these drugs on platelet, gastrointestinal, and renal function. A specific absolute contraindication is warfarin anticoagulants (eg, Coumadin) and NSAIDs. NSAIDS may decrease the effects of antihypertensive medications and, when used longer term in combination with ACE inhibitors or beta blockers, may compromise renal function. Others involve pharmacokinetic interactions. See **Table 3.2** for major drug interactions.

Laboratory Value Alterations

- There are no laboratory tests results specifically altered by NSAIDs and acetaminophen.
- The effect of these drugs on platelet function will likely increase bleeding times.
- There may also be changes in renal and hepatic function, especially with long-term NSAID use.

Cross-Sensitivity

All NSAIDs and aspirin may exhibit cross-sensitivity. Any of these drugs should be used with extreme caution, if at all, in patients who have developed signs and symptoms of allergic reaction to any NSAID, including aspirin. It should also be noted that patients with a history of nasal polyps and asthma have an increased risk of sensitivity, including allergic reactions, to aspirin, particularly, but also to other NSAIDs. Celecoxib has a sulfonamide structure and should not be prescribed to patients who report sulfonamide ("sulfa") allergy.

Special Patients

Pregnant and nursing women

NSAIDs should not be prescribed by dentists for pregnant or nursing women. Acetaminophen is generally prescribed in consultation with the patient's physician.

Pediatric, geriatric, and other special patients

Only acetaminophen, aspirin, ibuprofen, and naproxen are approved for pediatric pain relief. Aspirin may cause Reye's syndrome in children infected with influenza virus. Reye's syndrome is a serious medical condition that can lead to severe hepatic and CNS disease, as well as death. Because other drugs are available that do not manifest this concern, consider avoiding use of aspirin in all children with fever.

Geriatric patients may be more susceptible to the gastrointestinal and renal side effects of NSAIDs. Start at lower dosages and avoid longer-acting agents that may accumulate.

Patient Monitoring: Aspects to Watch

- Short-term NSAID therapy: Laboratory monitoring is generally not necessary, but the patient should notify the dentist of symptoms of dyspepsia, fluid retention, or worsening hypertension
- Long-term NSAID therapy: As with short-term therapy, hematologic parameters, and renal and hepatic function require periodic laboratory evaluation

Adverse Effects and Precautions

These drugs have numerous side effects (**Table 3.1**) and drug interactions (**Table 3.2**). For short-term use, gastrointestinal side effects such as dyspepsia, diarrhea, and abdominal pain are the most common. Longer-term use can lead to gastrointestinal ulceration, bleeding, or perforation. As a precaution, NSAIDs should be taken with meals and/or a full glass of water. Various drugs have been developed to counteract some of the gastrointestinal side effects of NSAIDs, and NSAIDs that have fewer gastrointestinal side effects are listed later in this section. NSAIDs are contraindicated in patients who have active peptic ulcer disease and should be prescribed with extreme caution to patients who have a history of peptic ulcer disease or a history of long-term corticosteroid use.

Renal complications can also occur as idiosyncratic reactions with short-term use or as renal failure with long-term use. These medications are metabolized by the liver and should be prescribed cautiously to people who have liver disease.

It is important to note that NSAIDs can increase bleeding through their reversible inhibition of platelet aggregation by their effect on a platelet-aggregating agent, thromboxane A_2. This is the case with all NSAIDs except aspirin, which irreversibly inhibits platelet aggregation for the entire life of the platelet (11 days). If major oral surgery is planned:

- discontinue aspirin use for 5 to 6 days before surgery
- for NSAIDs that require dosing of 4 to 6 times per day, stop NSAID use 1 to 2 days before surgery
- for NSAIDs that require bid-tid dosing, stop NSAID use 2 to 3 days before surgery
- for q day NSAIDs, stop NSAID use 3 to 4 days before surgery to avoid excessive bleeding.

Drug interactions are presented in **Table 3.2**. An important contraindication involves the use of aspirin in children, which can lead to Reye's syndrome. Hypersensitivity reactions, such as anaphylactoid reactions, also have occurred with NSAIDs, especially aspirin. Patients with a history of bronchospastic disease and/or nasal polyps have an increased risk of having hypersensitivity reactions, particularly to aspirin. If a patient's medical history indicates that this type of reaction could be encountered, it is prudent not to prescribe another NSAID. Some patients may exhibit minor hypersensitivity reactions to one NSAID but not another. If a patient tolerates a specific NSAID without difficulty, it seems reasonable to allow him or her to continue using that agent. Medical consultation may be appropriate. A history of anaphylactoid/anaphylactic reaction to any NSAID precludes use of another NSAID.

Some NSAIDs have potentially fewer gastrointestinal complications. The following drugs may cause less gastrointestinal irritation in a patient who, for instance, has a history of peptic ulcer disease and no longer requires ulcer medication but for whom an NSAID is indicated:

- celecoxib
- etodolac
- meloxicam
- salsalate (long-term use)

Pharmacology

Although NSAIDs influence a number of systems, a primary effect is the inhibition of the metabolism of arachidonic acid—a by-product of cell wall breakdown—by the enzyme cyclooxygenase. Prostaglandins are one of the derivatives of this breakdown and are potent vasodilators and mediators of the inflammatory response. By decreasing the production of peripheral prostaglandins, NSAIDs depress the inflammatory response. This decrease in prostaglandin concentration also raises the threshold for pain-conducting nerves to discharge, thus providing an analgesic effect. In the CNS, NSAIDs reduce prostaglandin formation in critical pain-processing regions producing decreased pain transmission and perception. NSAIDs also reduce fever, in part by decreasing the concentration of prostaglandins in the hypothalamus, a brain center regulating body temperature.

Three forms of cyclooxygenase have now been identified and are designated COX-1, COX-2, and COX-3. COX-1 is a constitutive form of the enzyme-producing "protective" prostaglandins that, for example, serves to promote renal blood flow and decrease gastric acid secretion. COX-2 is an inducible form of the enzyme whose concentration significantly increases during inflammation. Specific agents—COX-2 inhibitors—have been developed that take advantage of this distinction. Clinical trials have shown decreased gastrointestinal and clotting side effects but an increase in embolic phenomena. Celecoxib is the only COX-2 inhibitor currently available. COX-3 is a CNS form and may be inhibited by acetaminophen.

Short-term use of NSAIDs, such as for 3 or 4 days of acute pain management after dental surgery, is unlikely to lead to serious sequelae (including embolic phenomena) in most healthy patients. It should be noted that idiosyncratic reactions (primarily manifesting as renal complications) can occur, and gastric mucosal irritation has been reported even with very brief use of NSAIDs.

Cyclooxygenase metabolism of arachidonic acid also produces thromboxane A_2, which increases platelet aggregability. NSAIDs decrease the production of thromboxane A_2; which decreases platelet aggregation and causes an increased tendency toward bleeding. NSAID inactivation of cyclooxygenase, and thus increased bleeding tendency, is reversible for all drugs except aspirin, which binds cyclooxygenase irreversibly.

Patient Advice

- Patients should be cautioned regarding the gastrointestinal side effects of these medications.
- These medications preferably should be taken with or after meals with a full glass of water to prevent lodging of the capsule or tablet in the esophagus.
- The patient should notify the dentist of any side effects that occur after starting use of the medication.

SUGGESTED READING

Brandt KD. The mechanism of action of non-steroidal anti-inflammatory drugs. *J Rheumatol.* 1991;27(suppl):120-121.

Dionne RA, Berthold CW. Therapeutic uses of non-steroidal anti-inflammatory drugs in dentistry. *Crit Rev Oral Biol Med.* 2001;12(4):315-330.

Dionne RA, Gordon SM. Nonsteroidal anti-inflammatory drugs for acute pain control. *Dent Clin North Am.* 1994;38(4):645-667.

Hargreaves KM, Keiser K. Development of new pain management strategies. *J Dent Educ.* 2002;66(1):113-121.

Hofer I, Battig K. Cardiovascular, behavioral, and subjective effects of caffeine under field conditions. *Pharmacology, Biochemistry & Behavior.* 1994;48(4):899-908.

Joris J. Efficacy of nonsteroidal anti-inflammatory drugs in post-operative pain. *Acta Anaesthesiol Belg.* 1996; 47(3):115-123.

Khan AA, Dionne RA. The COX-2 inhibitors: new analgesic and anti-inflammatory drugs. *Dent Clin North Am.* 2002;46:679-690.

Lawton GM, Chapman PJ. Diflunisal—a long acting non-steroidal anti-inflammatory drug. A review of its pharmacology and effectiveness in management of dental pain. *Aust Dent J.* 1993;38(4):265-271.

Migliardi JR, Armellino JJ, Friedman M, Gillings DB, Beaver WT. Caffeine as an analgesic adjuvant in tension headache. *Clin Pharmacol Ther.* 1994;56(5):576-86.

Steiner TJ, Lange R. Ketoprofen (25 mg) in the symptomatic treatment of episodic tension- type headache: double-blind placebo-controlled comparison with acetaminophen (1000 mg). *Cephalalgia.* 1998;18(1):38-43.

Woolf CJ, Chong MS. Preemptive analgesia—treating postoperative pain by preventing the establishment of central sensitization. *Anesth Analg.* 1993;77(2):362-379.

Table 3.1. PRESCRIBING INFORMATION FOR ANALGESICS

NAME	FORM/ STRENGTH	DOSAGE	WARNINGS/PRECAUTIONS & CONTRAINDICATIONS	ADVERSE EFFECTS†
NONOPIOID ANALGESICS				
ACETAMINOPHEN				
Acetaminophen (Feverall) OTC	**Sup:** 80mg, 120mg, 325mg, 650mg	***Pediatrics:*** Insert sup rectally. **3-11 months:** 80mg q6h. **Max:** 480mg/24 hrs. **12-36 months:** 80mg q4h. **Max:** 480mg/24 hrs. **3-6 yrs:** 120mg q4-6h. **Max:** 720mg/24 hrs. **6-12 yrs:** 325mg q4-6h. **Max:** 2600mg/24 hrs.	**P/N:** Safety in pregnancy or nursing not known.	—
Acetaminophen (Tylenol 8 Hour, Tylenol Arthritis Pain, Children's Tylenol, Tylenol Extra Strength, Infants' Tylenol, Tylenol Junior, Tylenol Regular Strength) OTC	**Caplets:** (Arthritis Pain, 8 Hour) 650mg; **Drops:** (Infants') 80mg/0.8mL [15mL, 30mL]; **Geltabs:** (Arthritis Pain) 650mg; **Sol:** (Extra Strength) 500mg/15mL; **Sus:** (Children's) 160mg/5mL; **Tab:** (Regular Strength) 325mg; (Extra Strength EZ Tabs, GoTabs, Caplets, Cool Caplets, Rapid Release Gels) 500mg; **Tab, Chewable:** (Children's) 80mg, (Junior) 160mg	***Adults:*** **≥12 yrs:** (Regular Strength) 650mg q4-6h prn. **Max:** 3900mg/day. (Extra Strength GoTabs, EZ Tabs, Rapid Release Gels, Caplets, Cool Caplets) 1000mg q4-6h prn. **Max:** 4000mg/day. (Arthritis Pain, 8 Hour) 2 caplets or geltabs q8h with water. **Max:** 6 caplets or geltabs/day. ***Pediatrics:*** **Max:** 5 doses/day. **0-3 months (6-11 lbs):** 40mg q4h prn. **4-11 months (12-17 lbs):** 80mg q4h prn. **12-23 months (18-23 lbs):** 120mg q4h prn. **2-3 yrs (24-35 lbs):** 160mg q4h prn. **4-5 yrs (36-47 lbs):** 240mg q4h prn. **6-8 yrs (48-59 lbs):** 320mg q4h prn. **9-10 yrs (60-71 lbs):** 400mg q4h prn. **11 yrs (72-95 lbs):** 480mg q4h prn. **12 yrs (≥96 lbs):** 640mg q4h prn. **Older Children:** (Regular Strength) **6-11 yrs:** 325mg q4-6h prn. **Max:** 1625mg/day.	**W/P:** Taking more than the recommended dose (overdose) may cause liver damage. **P/N:** Safety in pregnancy or nursing not known.	—
NSAIDs				
Celecoxib (Celebrex)	**Cap:** 50mg, 100mg, 200mg, 400mg	***Adults:*** **OA:** 200mg qd or 100mg bid. **RA:** 100-200mg bid. **AS:** 200mg qd or 100mg bid. **Titrate:** May increase to 400mg/day after 6 weeks. **FAP:** 400mg bid with food. **Acute Pain/ Primary Dysmenorrhea: Day 1:** 400mg, then 200mg if needed. **Maint:** 200mg bid prn. **Moderate Hepatic Insufficiency:** Reduce daily dose by 50%. ***Pediatrics:*** **≥2 yrs: JRA: 10-25kg:** 50mg bid. **>25kg:** 100mg bid.	**BB:** NSAIDs may cause an increased risk of serious cardiovascular thrombotic events, MI, stroke, and serious GI adverse events, including bleeding, ulceration, and perforation of the stomach or intestines. Contraindicated for the treatment of perioperative pain in the setting of coronary artery bypass graft (CABG) surgery. **W/P:** Increased risk of serious adverse cardiovascular thrombotic events, MI, and stroke. May lead to onset of new HTN or worsening of pre-existing HTN; monitor BP closely. Fluid retention and edema reported; caution with fluid retention or heart failure. Renal papillary necrosis and other renal injury reported after long-term use. Not recommended for use with advanced renal disease; if therapy must be initiated, monitor renal function. Greatest risk with those taking diuretics and ACE inhibitors. Anaphylactoid reactions may occur. May cause serious skin adverse events (eg, exfoliative dermatitis, Stevens-Johnson syndrome, and toxic epidermal necrolysis). Avoid in late pregnancy; may cause premature closure of ductus arteriosus. May cause elevations of LFTs; d/c if liver disease develops or systemic manifestations occur. Caution in elderly. Anemia may occur; with long-term use, monitor Hgb/Hct if signs or symptoms of anemia or	Dyspepsia, diarrhea, abdominal pain, nausea, dizziness, headache, sinusitis, upper respiratory infection, rash, fever, **cough**, arthralgia, HTN, insomnia, **pharyngitis**.

†Bold entries denote special dental considerations.
BB = black box warning; **W/P** = warnings/precautions; **Contra** = contraindications; **P/N** = pregnancy category rating and nursing considerations.

Table 3.1. PRESCRIBING INFORMATION FOR ANALGESICS *(cont.)*

NAME	FORM/ STRENGTH	DOSAGE	WARNINGS/PRECAUTIONS & CONTRAINDICATIONS	ADVERSE EFFECTS†
NONOPIOID ANALGESICS *(cont.)*				
NSAIDS *(cont.)*				
Celecoxib (Celebrex) *(cont.)*			blood loss develop. May inhibit platelet aggregation and prolong bleeding time (prolonged APTT); monitor with coagulation disorders. Caution with asthma and avoid with ASA-sensitive asthma. Caution in pediatric patients with systemic onset JRA due to increased possibility of DIC. **Contra:** Sulfonamide hypersensitivity. Asthma, urticaria, or allergic-type reactions after ASA or NSAID use. Treatment of perioperative pain in the setting of CABG surgery. **P/N:** Category C and D (≥30 weeks gestation), not for use in nursing.	
Diclofenac Potassium (Cataflam)	**Tab:** 50mg	***Adults:*** **OA:** 50mg bid-tid. **Max:** 150mg/day. **RA:** 50mg tid-qid. **Max:** 200mg/day. **Pain/Primary Dysmenorrhea: Initial:** 50mg tid or 100mg for 1st dose, then 50mg for subsequent doses.	**BB:** NSAIDs may cause an increased risk of serious cardiovascular thrombotic events, MI, stroke, and serious GI adverse events, including bleeding, ulceration, and perforation of the stomach or intestines. Contraindicated for the treatment of perioperative pain in the setting of coronary artery bypass graft (CABG) surgery. **W/P:** May lead to onset of new HTN or worsening of pre-existing HTN; monitor BP closely. Fluid retention and edema reported; caution with fluid retention or heart failure. Renal papillary necrosis and other renal injury reported after long-term use. Not recommended for use with advanced renal disease; if therapy must be initiated, monitor renal function. Anaphylactoid reactions may occur. May cause serious skin adverse events (eg, exfoliative dermatitis, Stevens-Johnson syndrome, and toxic epidermal necrolysis). Avoid in late pregnancy; may cause premature closure of ductus arteriosis. May cause elevations of LFTs; d/c if liver disease develops or systemic manifestations occur. Caution in elderly. Anemia may occur; with long-term use, monitor Hgb/Hct if signs or symptoms of anemia develop. May inhibit platelet aggregation and prolong bleeding time; monitor with coagulation disorders. Caution with asthma and avoid with ASA-sensitive asthma. **Contra:** ASA or other NSAID allergy that precipitates asthma, urticaria, or allergic reactions. Treatment of perioperative pain in the setting of CABG surgery. **P/N:** Category C, not for use in nursing.	Fluid retention, dizziness, rash, nausea, abdominal cramps, LFT abnormalities, constipation, diarrhea, heartburn, tinnitus, GI ulceration, HTN, insomnia, **stomatitis**, pruritus.
Diclofenac Sodium (Voltaren, Voltaren-XR)	**Tab, Delayed-Release:** (Voltaren) 25mg, 50mg, 75mg; **Tab, Extended-Release:** (Voltaren-XR) 100mg	***Adults:*** (Voltaren) **OA:** 50mg bid-tid or 75mg bid. **Max:** 150mg/day. **RA:** 50mg tid-qid or 75mg bid. **Max:** 200mg/day. **AS:** 25mg qid and 25mg qhs prn. **Max:** 125mg/day. (Voltaren-XR) **OA:** 100mg qd. **RA:** 100mg qd-bid.	**BB:** NSAIDs may cause an increased risk of serious cardiovascular thrombotic events, MI, stroke, and serious GI adverse events, including bleeding, ulceration, and perforation of the stomach or intestines. Contraindicated for the treatment of perioperative pain in the setting of coronary artery bypass graft (CABG) surgery. **W/P:** May lead to onset of new HTN or worsening of pre-existing HTN; monitor BP closely. Fluid retention and edema reported; caution with fluid retention or heart failure. Caution with considerable dehydration.	Fluid retention, dizziness, rash, nausea, abdominal cramps, LFT abnormalities, constipation, diarrhea, heartburn, tinnitus, GI ulceration, flatulence, dyspepsia, anemia, abnormal renal function.

†Bold entries denote special dental considerations.
BB = black box warning; **W/P** = warnings/precautions; **Contra** = contraindications; **P/N** = pregnancy category rating and nursing considerations.

NAME	FORM/ STRENGTH	DOSAGE	WARNINGS/PRECAUTIONS & CONTRAINDICATIONS	ADVERSE EFFECTS†
Diclofenac Sodium (Voltaren, Voltaren-XR) *(cont.)*			Renal papillary necrosis and other renal injury reported after long-term use. Not recommended for use with advanced renal disease; if therapy must be initiated, monitor renal function. Anaphylactoid reactions may occur. May cause serious skin adverse events (eg, exfoliative dermatitis, Stevens-Johnson syndrome, and toxic epidermal necrolysis). Avoid in late pregnancy; may cause premature closure of ductus arteriosis. May cause elevations of LFTs; d/c if liver disease develops or systemic manifestations occur. Caution in elderly. Anemia may occur; with long-term use, monitor Hgb/Hct if signs or symptoms of anemia develop. May inhibit platelet aggregation and prolong bleeding time; monitor with coagulation disorders. Caution with asthma and avoid with ASA-sensitive asthma. Risk of GI ulceration, bleeding, and perforation. **Contra:** ASA or other NSAID allergy that precipitates asthma, urticaria, or allergic-type reactions. Treatment of perioperative pain in the setting of CABG surgery. **P/N:** Category C, not for use in nursing.	
Diclofenac Sodium/ Misoprostol (Arthrotec)	**Tab:** (Diclofenac-Misoprostol) 50mg-0.2mg, 75mg-0.2mg	***Adults:*** **OA:** 50mg tid. **RA:** 50mg tid-qid. **OA/RA:** If not tolerable, give 50-75mg bid (less effective in preventing ulcers). Do not crush, chew, or divide.	**BB:** Contraindicated in pregnancy. Must have negative pregnancy test 2 weeks before therapy. Provide oral and written hazards of misoprostol. Begin on 2nd or 3rd day of the next normal menstrual period. Use reliable contraception. NSAIDs may cause an increased risk of serious cardiovascular thrombotic events, MI, stroke, and serious GI adverse events, including bleeding, ulceration, and perforation of the stomach or intestines. Contraindicated for the treatment of perioperative pain in the setting of coronary artery bypass graft (CABG) surgery. **W/P:** May lead to onset of new HTN or worsening of pre-existing HTN; monitor BP closely. Fluid retention and edema reported; caution with fluid retention or heart failure. Renal papillary necrosis and other renal injury reported after long-term use. Not recommended for use with advanced renal disease; if therapy must be initiated, monitor renal function. May cause elevations of LFTs; d/c if abnormal LFTs persist/worsen, liver disease develops, or systemic manifestations occur. Anaphylactoid reactions may occur. May cause serious skin adverse events (eg, exfoliative dermatitis, Stevens-Johnson syndrome, and toxic epidermal necrolysis). Avoid in late pregnancy; may cause premature closure of ductus arteriosis. Caution in elderly. Anemia may occur; with long-term use, monitor Hgb/Hct if signs or symptoms of anemia. May inhibit platelet aggregation and prolong bleeding time; monitor with coagulation disorders. Caution with asthma and avoid with ASA-sensitive asthma. Aseptic meningitis with fever and coma reported. Avoid with hepatic porphyria. **Contra:** Pregnancy. ASA or other NSAID allergy that precipitates asthma, urticaria, or other allergic reactions. Treatment of perioperative pain in the setting of CABG surgery. **P/N:** Category X, not for use in nursing.	Abdominal pain, diarrhea, dyspepsia, nausea, flatulence, GI disorders.

Table 3.1. PRESCRIBING INFORMATION FOR ANALGESICS *(cont.)*

NAME	FORM/ STRENGTH	DOSAGE	WARNINGS/PRECAUTIONS & CONTRAINDICATIONS	ADVERSE EFFECTS†
NONOPIOID ANALGESICS *(cont.)*				
NSAIDS *(cont.)*				
Diflunisal	**Tab:** 250mg, 500mg	***Adults:* Pain: Initial:** 1g, then 500mg q8-12h. **OA/RA:** 250-500mg bid. **Max:** 1500mg/day. ***Pediatrics:* ≥12 yrs: Pain: Initial:** 1g, then 500mg q12h or 500mg q8h. **OA/RA:** 250-500mg bid. **Max:** 1500mg/day.	**BB:** NSAIDs may cause an increased risk of serious cardiovascular thrombotic events, MI, stroke, and serious GI adverse events, including bleeding, ulceration, and perforation of the stomach or intestines. Contraindicated for the treatment of perioperative pain in the setting of coronary artery bypass graft (CABG) surgery. **W/P:** May lead to onset of new HTN or worsening of pre-existing HTN; monitor BP closely. Fluid retention and edema reported; caution with fluid retention or heart failure. Renal papillary necrosis and other renal injury reported after long-term use. Not recommended for use with advanced renal disease; if therapy must be initiated, monitor renal function. Anaphylactoid reactions may occur. May cause serious skin adverse events (eg, exfoliative dermatitis, Stevens-Johnson syndrome, and toxic epidermal necrolysis). Avoid in late pregnancy; may cause premature closure of ductus arteriosis. May cause elevations of LFTs; d/c if liver disease develops or systemic manifestations occur. Caution in elderly. Anemia may occur; with long-term use, monitor Hgb/Hct if signs or symptoms of anemia develop. May inhibit platelet aggregation and prolong bleeding time; monitor with coagulation disorders. Caution with asthma and avoid with ASA-sensitive asthma. Adverse eye findings reported. Hypersensitivity syndrome reported; d/c if hypersensitivity occurs. Reye's syndrome may develop. **Contra:** ASA or other NSAID allergy that precipitates acute asthmatic attack, urticaria, or rhinitis. Treatment of perioperative pain in the setting of CABG surgery. **P/N:** Category C, not for use in nursing.	Nausea, dyspepsia, GI pain, diarrhea, rash, headache, insomnia, dizziness, tinnitus, fatigue.
Etodolac	**Cap:** 200mg, 300mg; **Tab:** 400mg, 500mg	***Adults:* Acute Pain: Usual:** 200-400mg q6-8h. **Max:** 1000mg/day. **OA/RA: Initial:** 300mg bid-tid, or 400-500mg bid. May give 600mg/day for long-term use. **Titrate:** Lowest effective dose. **Max:** 1000mg/day.	**BB:** NSAIDs may cause an increased risk of serious cardiovascular thrombotic events, MI, stroke, and serious GI adverse events, including bleeding, ulceration, and perforation of the stomach or intestines. Contraindicated for the treatment of perioperative pain in the setting of coronary artery bypass graft (CABG) surgery. **W/P:** May lead to onset of new HTN or worsening of pre-existing HTN; monitor BP closely. Fluid retention and edema reported; caution with fluid retention or heart failure. Renal papillary necrosis and other renal injury reported after long-term use. Not recommended for use with advanced renal disease; if therapy must be initiated, monitor renal function. Anaphylactoid reactions may occur. May cause serious skin adverse events (eg, exfoliative dermatitis, Stevens-Johnson syndrome, and toxic epidermal necrolysis). Avoid in late pregnancy; may cause premature closure of ductus arteriosis. May cause	Dyspepsia, abdominal pain, diarrhea, flatulence, nausea, constipation, gastritis, asthenia, malaise, dizziness, increased bleeding time, GI ulcers, GI bleeding/perforation, heartburn, abnormal renal function.

†Bold entries denote special dental considerations.
BB = black box warning; **W/P** = warnings/precautions; **Contra** = contraindications; **P/N** = pregnancy category rating and nursing considerations.

NAME	FORM/ STRENGTH	DOSAGE	WARNINGS/PRECAUTIONS & CONTRAINDICATIONS	ADVERSE EFFECTS†
Etodolac *(cont.)*			elevations of LFTs; d/c if liver disease develops or systemic manifestations occur. Caution in elderly. Anemia may occur; with long-term use, monitor Hgb/Hct if signs or symptoms of anemia develop. May inhibit platelet aggregation and prolong bleeding time; monitor with coagulation disorders. Caution with asthma and avoid with ASA-sensitive asthma. Risk of GI ulceration, bleeding, and perforation. **Contra:** ASA or other NSAID allergy that precipitates asthma, urticaria, or other allergic type reactions. Treatment of perioperative pain in the setting of CABG surgery. **P/N:** Category C, not for use in nursing.	
Etodolac Extended-Release	**Tab, Extended-Release:** 400mg, 500mg, 600mg	***Adults:* OA/RA: Initial:** 400-1000mg qd. **Titrate:** Lowest effective dose. ***Pediatrics:* 6-16 yrs: JA: >60kg:** 1000mg/day. **46-60kg:** 800mg/day. **31-45kg:** 600mg/day. **20-30kg:** 400mg/day.	**BB:** NSAIDs may cause an increased risk of serious cardiovascular thrombotic events, MI, stroke, and serious GI adverse events, including bleeding, ulceration, and perforation of the stomach or intestines. Contraindicated for the treatment of perioperative pain in the setting of coronary artery bypass graft (CABG) surgery. **W/P:** May lead to onset of new HTN or worsening of pre-existing HTN; monitor BP closely. Fluid retention and edema reported; caution with fluid retention or heart failure. Renal papillary necrosis and other renal injury reported after long-term use. Not recommended for use with advanced renal disease; if therapy must be initiated, monitor renal function. Anaphylactoid reactions may occur. May cause serious skin adverse events (eg, exfoliative dermatitis, Stevens-Johnson syndrome, and toxic epidermal necrolysis). Avoid in late pregnancy; may cause premature closure of ductus arteriosus. May cause elevations of LFTs; d/c if liver disease develops or systemic manifestations occur. Caution in elderly. Anemia may occur; with long-term use, monitor Hgb/Hct if signs or symptoms of anemia develop. May inhibit platelet aggregation and prolong bleeding time; monitor with coagulation disorders. Caution with asthma and avoid with ASA-sensitive asthma. **Contra:** ASA or other NSAID allergy that precipitates asthma, urticaria, or allergic reaction. Treatment of perioperative pain in the setting of CABG surgery. **P/N:** Category C, not for use in nursing.	Dyspepsia, abdominal pain, diarrhea, flatulence, N/V, constipation, GI ulcers, gross bleeding/perforation.
Fenoprofen Calcium (Nalfon)	**Cap:** 200mg; **Tab:** 600mg	***Adults:* OA/RA:** 300-600mg tid-qid. **Max:** 3200mg/day. **Pain:** 200mg q4-6h prn. Take with food or milk with GI upset.	**BB:** NSAIDs may cause an increased risk of serious cardiovascular thrombotic events, MI, stroke, and serious GI adverse events, including bleeding, ulceration, and perforation of the stomach or intestines. Contraindicated for the treatment of perioperative pain in the setting of coronary artery bypass graft (CABG) surgery. **W/P:** May lead to onset of new HTN or worsening of pre-existing HTN; monitor BP closely. Fluid retention and edema reported; caution with fluid retention, compromised cardiac function, or heart failure. Renal papillary necrosis and other renal injury reported after long-term use. Not recommended	Dyspepsia, constipation, N/V, somnolence, dizziness, abdominal pain, headache, diarrhea.

Table 3.1. PRESCRIBING INFORMATION FOR ANALGESICS *(cont.)*

NAME	FORM/ STRENGTH	DOSAGE	WARNINGS/PRECAUTIONS & CONTRAINDICATIONS	ADVERSE EFFECTS†
NONOPIOID ANALGESICS *(cont.)*				
NSAIDS *(cont.)*				
Fenoprofen Calcium (Nalfon) *(cont.)*			for use with advanced renal disease. Anaphylactoid reactions may occur. May cause serious skin adverse events (eg, exfoliative dermatitis, Stevens-Johnson syndrome, and toxic epidermal necrolysis). Avoid in late pregnancy; may cause premature closure of ductus arteriosis. May cause elevations of LFTs; d/c if liver disease develops or systemic manifestations occur. Caution in elderly. Anemia may occur; with long-term use, monitor Hgb/Hct if signs or symptoms of anemia develop. May inhibit platelet aggregation and prolong bleeding time; monitor with coagulation disorders. Caution with asthma and avoid with ASA-sensitive asthma. Perform eye exams if visual disturbances occur. Caution with activities requiring mental alertness. With long-term use, monitor auditory function in hearing-impaired patients. **Contra:** Significantly impaired renal function. ASA or other NSAID allergy that precipitates asthma, rhinitis, or urticaria. Treatment of perioperative pain in the setting of CABG surgery. **P/N:** Category C, not for use in nursing.	
Flurbiprofen (Ansaid)	**Tab:** 50mg, 100mg	***Adults:*** **Initial:** 200-300mg/day in divided doses bid, tid, or qid. **Max:** 300mg/day or 100mg/dose.	**BB:** NSAIDs may cause an increased risk of serious cardiovascular thrombotic events, MI, stroke, and serious GI adverse events, including bleeding, ulceration, and perforation of the stomach or intestines. Contraindicated for the treatment of perioperative pain in the setting of coronary artery bypass graft (CABG) surgery. **W/P:** May lead to onset of new HTN or worsening of pre-existing HTN; monitor BP closely. Fluid retention and edema reported; caution with fluid retention or heart failure. Renal papillary necrosis and other renal injury reported after long-term use. Not recommended for use with advanced renal disease; if therapy must be initiated, monitor renal function. Anaphylactoid reactions may occur. Avoid in late pregnancy; may cause premature closure of ductus arteriosis. May cause elevations of LFTs; d/c if liver disease develops or systemic manifestations occur. Caution in elderly. Anemia may occur; monitor Hgb/Hct with long-term use. May inhibit platelet aggregation and prolong bleeding time; monitor with coagulation disorders. Caution with asthma and avoid with ASA-sensitive asthma. Monitor for visual changes or disturbances. Risk of GI ulceration, bleeding, and perforation. May cause serious skin adverse events (eg, exfoliative dermatitis, Stevens-Johnson syndrome, toxic epidermal necrolysis). **Contra:** ASA, with ASA triad, or other NSAID allergy that precipitates acute asthmatic attack, urticaria, or rhinitis. Treatment of perioperative pain in the setting of CABG surgery. **P/N:** Category C, not for use in nursing.	Dyspepsia, diarrhea, abdominal pain, constipation, headache, nausea, edema.

†Bold entries denote special dental considerations.
BB = black box warning; **W/P** = warnings/precautions; **Contra** = contraindications; **P/N** = pregnancy category rating and nursing considerations.

NAME	FORM/ STRENGTH	DOSAGE	WARNINGS/PRECAUTIONS & CONTRAINDICATIONS	ADVERSE EFFECTS†
Ibuprofen (Motrin)	**Sus:** 100mg/5mL; **Tab:** 400mg, 600mg, 800mg	***Adults:*** **Pain:** 400mg q4-6h prn. **Max:** 2400mg/day. **Dysmenorrhea:** 400mg q4-6h prn. **Max:** 2400mg/day. **OA/RA:** 300mg qid or 400mg, 600mg, or 800mg tid-qid. **Max:** 3200mg/day. **Fever:** 200-400mg q4-6h. **Max:** 1200mg/day. Take with meals/milk. **Renal Impairment:** Reduce dose. ***Pediatrics:*** **Fever: 6 months-12 yrs:** 5mg/kg for temp <102.5°F; 10mg/kg if temp ≥102.5°F q6-8h. **Max:** 40mg/kg/day. **Pain: 6 months-12 yrs:** 10mg/kg q6-8h. **Max:** 40mg/kg/day. **JA:** 30-40mg/kg/day divided into 3 or 4 doses. Milder disease may use 20mg/kg/day.	**BB:** NSAIDs may cause an increased risk of serious cardiovascular thrombotic events, MI, stroke, and serious GI adverse events, including bleeding, ulceration, and perforation of the stomach or intestines. Contraindicated for the treatment of perioperative pain in the setting of coronary artery bypass graft (CABG) surgery. **W/P:** May lead to onset of new HTN or worsening of pre-existing HTN; monitor BP closely. Fluid retention and edema reported; caution with fluid retention or heart failure. Renal papillary necrosis and other renal injury reported after long-term use. Not recommended for use with advanced renal disease; if therapy must be initiated, monitor renal function. Anaphylactoid reactions may occur. May cause serious skin adverse events (eg, exfoliative dermatitis, Stevens-Johnson syndrome, and toxic epidermal necrolysis). Avoid in late pregnancy; may cause premature closure of ductus arteriosis. May cause elevations of LFTs; d/c if liver disease develops or systemic manifestations occur. Caution in elderly. Anemia may occur; with long-term use, monitor Hgb/Hct if signs or symptoms of anemia develop. May inhibit platelet aggregation and prolong bleeding time; monitor with coagulation disorders. Caution with asthma and avoid with ASA-sensitive asthma. D/C if visual disturbances occur. Aseptic meningitis with fever and coma reported. **Contra:** Syndrome of nasal polyps, angioedema, and bronchospastic reactions to ASA or other NSAIDs. Treatment of perioperative pain in the setting of CABG surgery. **P/N:** Category C, not for use in nursing.	Nausea, epigastric pain, heartburn, dizziness, rash.
Ibuprofen (Children's Motrin, Infants' Motrin, Junior Strength Motrin) OTC	**Infant Drops:** 50mg/1.25mL [15mL, 30mL]; **Children's Sus:** 100mg/5mL [60mL, 120mL]; **Children's Tab, Chewable:** 50mg; **Junior Tab/ Tab, Chewable:** 100mg	***Pediatrics:*** **Infant Drops: 6-11 months (12-17 lbs):** 1.25mL q6-8h. **12-23 months (18-23 lbs):** 1.875mL q6-8h. Use only with enclosed dropper. **Sus: 2-3 yrs (24-35 lbs):** 5mL q6-8h. **4-5 yrs (36-47 lbs):** 7.5mL q6-8h. **6-8 yrs (48-59 lbs):** 10mL q6-8h. **9-10 yrs (60-71 lbs):** 12.5mL q6-8h. **11 yrs (72-95 lbs):** 15mL q6-8h. Use only with enclosed measuring cup. **Children's Chewable Tab: 4-5 yrs (36-47 lbs):** 150mg q6-8h. **6-8 yrs (48-59 lbs):** 200mg q6-8h. **9-10 yrs (60-71 lbs):** 250mg q6-8h. **11 yrs (72-95 lbs):** 300mg q6-8h. **Junior Tab/Chewable Tab: 6-8 yrs (48-59 lbs):** 200mg q6-8h. **9-10 yrs (60-71 lbs):** 250mg q6-8h. **11 yrs (72-95 lbs):** 300mg q6-8h. **Max:** 4 doses/24 hrs. Take with food/milk to avoid upset stomach. Take chewable tabs with food/water to avoid mouth/throat burning.	**W/P:** May cause severe allergic reaction (eg, hives, facial swelling, wheezing, shock). Avoid with history of allergic reaction to any other pain reliever/fever reducer. Not for use >10 days; or >2 days if severe/persistent sore throat or sore throat accompanied by high fever, headache, nausea/vomiting; or >3 days if fever/pain persists or gets worse. **P/N:** Safety in pregnancy and nursing not known.	—

Table 3.1. PRESCRIBING INFORMATION FOR ANALGESICS *(cont.)*

NAME	FORM/ STRENGTH	DOSAGE	WARNINGS/PRECAUTIONS & CONTRAINDICATIONS	ADVERSE EFFECTS†
NONOPIOID ANALGESICS *(cont.)*				
NSAIDS *(cont.)*				
Ibuprofen (Motrin IB) OTC	**Tab:** 200mg	***Adults/Pediatrics:*** **≥12 yrs:** 200mg q4-6h. 400mg if symptoms do not respond. **Max:** 1200mg/24 hrs.	**W/P:** Do not take for >10 days for pain or >3 days for fever. May cause severe allergic reaction, especially in people allergic to ASA. Do not use if history of allergic reaction to other pain relievers/ fever reducers or right before or after heart surgery. May cause stomach bleeding; increased risk ≥60 yrs; stomach ulcers or bleeding problems; concomitant blood thinning or steroid drug, and other NSAIDs; ≥3 alcoholic drinks every day; longer course of therapy. Caution if taking ASA for heart attack or stroke; it may decrease this benefit of ASA. **P/N:** Safety in pregnancy and nursing not known.	—
Indomethacin (Indocin)	**Cap:** 25mg, 50mg; **Sus:** 25mg/5mL [237mL]	***Adults/Pediatrics:*** **≥14 yrs: OA/ RA/AS: Initial:** 25mg PO bid-tid. **Titrate:** May increase by 25-50mg/ day at weekly intervals. **Max:** 200mg/ day. **Bursitis/Tendinitis:** 75-150mg/ day given tid-qid for 7-14 days. **Acute Gouty Arthritis:** 50mg PO tid until pain is tolerable, then d/c. Take with food. **2-14 yrs (safety and effectiveness not established): Initial:** 1-2mg/kg/day in divided doses. **Max:** 3mg/kg/day or 150-200mg/day. Take with food.	**BB:** NSAIDs may cause an increased risk of serious cardiovascular thrombotic events, MI, stroke, and serious GI adverse events, including bleeding, ulceration, and perforation of the stomach or intestines. Contraindicated for the treatment of perioperative pain in the setting of coronary artery bypass graft (CABG) surgery. **W/P:** May lead to onset of new HTN or worsening of pre-existing HTN; monitor BP closely. Fluid retention and edema reported; caution with fluid retention or heart failure. Renal papillary necrosis and other renal injury reported after long-term use. Not recommended for use with advanced renal disease; if therapy must be initiated, monitor renal function. Anaphylactoid reactions may occur. May cause serious skin adverse events (eg, exfoliative dermatitis, Stevens-Johnson syndrome, and toxic epidermal necrolysis). Avoid in late pregnancy; may cause premature closure of ductus arteriosis. May cause elevations of LFTs; d/c if liver disease develops or systemic manifestations occur. Caution in elderly. Anemia may occur; with long-term use, monitor Hgb/Hct if signs or symptoms of anemia develop. May inhibit platelet aggregation and prolong bleeding time; monitor with coagulation disorders. Caution with asthma and avoid with ASA-sensitive asthma. Corneal deposits and retinal disturbances reported with prolonged therapy; perform eye exams at periodic intervals during prolonged therapy. May aggravate depression or other psychiatric disturbances, epilepsy, and parkinsonism; use with caution. D/C if severe CNS adverse reactions develop. May impair mental/physical abilities. **Contra:** ASA or other NSAID allergy that precipitates acute asthmatic attack, urticaria, or rhinitis. Do not give suppositories with history of proctitis or recent rectal bleeding. Treatment of perioperative pain in the setting of CABG surgery. **P/N:** Category C, not for use in nursing.	Headache, dizziness, N/V, dyspepsia, diarrhea, abdominal pain, constipation, vertigo, somnolence, depression, fatigue.

†Bold entries denote special dental considerations.
BB = black box warning; **W/P** = warnings/precautions; **Contra** = contraindications; **P/N** = pregnancy category rating and nursing considerations.

NAME	FORM/ STRENGTH	DOSAGE	WARNINGS/PRECAUTIONS & CONTRAINDICATIONS	ADVERSE EFFECTS†
Ketoprofen	**Cap:** 50mg, 75mg **Cap, Extended-Release:** 100mg, 150mg, 200mg	***Adults:*** **(Cap) OA/RA:** 75mg tid or 50mg qid. **Max:** 300mg/day. **Pain/ Dysmenorrhea:** 25-50mg q6-8h. **Max:** 300mg. **Small Patients/ Debilitated/Elderly/Hepatic or Renal Dysfunction:** Reduce dose. **(Cap, Extended-Rlease) OA/RA:** 200mg qd. **Max:** 200mg/day. **Elderly/ Hepatic or Renal Dysfunction:** Reduce dose.	**BB:** NSAIDs may cause an increased risk of serious cardiovascular thrombotic events, MI, stroke, and serious GI adverse events, including bleeding, ulceration, and perforation of the stomach or intestines. Contraindicated for the treatment of perioperative pain in the setting of coronary artery bypass graft (CABG) surgery. **W/P:** May lead to onset of new HTN or worsening of pre-existing HTN; monitor BP closely. Fluid retention and edema reported; caution with fluid retention or heart failure. Renal papillary necrosis and other renal injury reported after long-term use. Not recommended for use with advanced renal disease; if therapy must be initiated, monitor renal function. Anaphylactoid reactions may occur. May cause serious skin adverse events (eg, exfoliative dermatitis, Stevens-Johnson syndrome, and toxic epidermal necrolysis). Avoid in late pregnancy; may cause premature closure of ductus arteriosis. May cause elevations of LFTs; d/c if liver disease develops or systemic manifestations occur. Monitor with chronic liver disease and consider dose reduction. Caution in elderly. Anemia may occur; with long-term use, monitor Hgb/Hct if signs or symptoms of anemia develop. May inhibit platelet aggregation and prolong bleeding time; monitor with coagulation disorders. Caution with asthma and avoid with ASA-sensitive asthma. **Contra:** ASA or other NSAID allergy that precipitates acute asthmatic attack, urticaria, or allergic reactions. Treatment of perioperative pain in the setting of CABG surgery. **P/N:** Category C, not for use in nursing.	Dyspepsia, nausea, abdominal pain, diarrhea, constipation, flatulence, headache, renal dysfunction, LFT abnormalities, CNS effects.
Ketorolac Tromethamine	**Inj:** 15mg/mL, 30mg/mL; **Tab:** 10mg	***Adults:*** **>16 yrs to <65 yrs: Single-Dose:** 60mg IM or 30mg IV. **Multiple-Dose:** 30mg IM/IV q6h. **Max:** 120mg/day. **Transition from IM/IV to PO:** 20mg PO single dose, then 10mg PO q4-6h. **Max:** 40mg/24 hrs. **≥65 yrs/Renal Impairment/<50kg: Single-Dose:** 30mg IM or 15mg IV. **Multiple-Dose:** 15mg IM/IV q6h. **Max:** 60mg/day. **Transition from IM/IV to PO:** 10mg PO q4-6h. **Max:** 40mg/24 hrs. ***Pediatrics:*** **2-16 yrs: Single-Dose: IM:** 1mg/kg. **Max:** 30mg. **IV:** 0.5mg/kg. **Max:** 15mg.	**BB:** For short-term use only (≤5 days). Contraindicated with peptic ulcer disease, GI bleeding/perforation, perioperative pain in coronary artery bypass graft (CABG) surgery, advanced renal impairment, risk of renal failure due to volume depletion, CV bleeding, hemorrhagic diathesis, incomplete hemostasis, high risk of bleeding, intraoperatively when hemostasis is critical, intrathecal/ epidural use, labor & delivery, nursing, and with ASA, NSAIDs, or probenecid. Caution greater risk of GI events with elderly patients. NSAIDs may cause an increased risk of CV thrombotic events (MI, stroke). (PO) Contraindicated in pediatric patients and in minor or chronic painful conditions. **W/P:** Do not exceed 5 days of therapy. Risk of GI ulcerations, bleeding, and perforation. Caution with renal/hepatic dysfunction, dehydration, HTN, CHF, coagulation disorders, debilitated and elderly, pre-existing asthma. Preoperative use prolongs bleeding. CV thrombotic events, fluid retention, edema, NaCl retention, oliguria, anaphylactic reactions, elevated BUN and SrCr, anemia reported. Correct hypovolemia before therapy. **Contra:** Active or history of peptic ulcer, GI bleeding, perioperative pain in CABG surgery, advanced	Nausea, dyspepsia, GI pain, diarrhea, edema, headache, drowsiness, dizziness.

Table 3.1. PRESCRIBING INFORMATION FOR ANALGESICS *(cont.)*

NAME	FORM/ STRENGTH	DOSAGE	WARNINGS/PRECAUTIONS & CONTRAINDICATIONS	ADVERSE EFFECTS†
NONOPIOID ANALGESICS *(cont.)*				
NSAIDS *(cont.)*				
Ketorolac Tromethamine *(cont.)*			renal impairment or risk of renal failure due to volume depletion, labor/delivery, nursing mothers, ASA or NSAID allergy, preoperatively or intraoperatively when hemostasis is critical, cerebrovascular bleeding, hemorrhagic diathesis, incomplete hemostasis, high risk of bleeding, neuraxial (epidural or intrathecal) administration, and concomitant ASA, NSAIDs, probenecid, or pentoxifylline. **P/N:** Category C, not for use in nursing.	
Meclofenamate Sodium	**Cap:** 50mg, 100mg	***Adults/Pediatrics:*** **≥14 yrs: Mild to Moderate Pain:** 50mg q4-6h. **Max:** 400mg/day. **Excessive Menstrual Blood Loss/Primary Dysmenorrhea:** 100mg tid for up to 6 days starting at onset of menstrual flow. **OA/RA:** 200-400mg/day in 3-4 divided doses. **Max:** 400mg/day.	**W/P:** Risk of GI ulcerations, bleeding, and perforation. Borderline LFT elevations may occur. Renal and hepatic toxicity. Extreme caution in the elderly. D/C if visual symptoms occur. **Contra:** ASA or other NSAID allergy that precipitates bronchospasm, allergic rhinitis, or urticaria. **P/N:** Safety in pregnancy is not known. Not for use in nursing.	Diarrhea, N/V, abdominal pain, edema, urticaria, pruritus, headache, dizziness, tinnitus, pyrosis, flatulence, anorexia, constipation, peptic ulcer.
Mefenamic Acid (Ponstel)	**Cap:** 250mg	***Adults/Pediatrics:*** **≥14 yrs: Acute Pain: Usual:** 500mg, then 250mg q6h prn up to 1 week. **Primary Dysmenorrhea: Usual:** 500mg, then 250mg q6h, up to 3 days. Take with food.	**BB:** NSAIDs may cause an increased risk of serious cardiovascular thrombotic events, MI, stroke, and serious GI adverse events, including bleeding, ulceration, and perforation of the stomach or intestines. Contraindicated for the treatment of perioperative pain in the setting of coronary artery bypass graft (CABG) surgery. **W/P:** May lead to onset of new HTN or worsening of pre-existing HTN; monitor BP closely. Fluid retention and edema reported; caution with fluid retention or heart failure. Renal papillary necrosis and other renal injury reported after long-term use. Not recommended for use with advanced renal disease. Anaphylactoid reactions may occur. May cause serious skin adverse events (eg, exfoliative dermatitis, Stevens-Johnson syndrome, and toxic epidermal necrolysis). Avoid in late pregnancy; may cause premature closure of ductus arteriosis. May cause elevations of LFTs; d/c if liver disease develops or systemic manifestations occur. Caution in elderly. Anemia may occur; with long-term use, monitor Hgb/Hct if signs or symptoms of anemia develop. May inhibit platelet aggregation and prolong bleeding time; monitor with coagulation disorders. Caution with asthma and avoid with ASA-sensitive asthma. **Contra:** Pre-existing renal disease, active ulceration, or chronic inflammation of the GI tract. Allergic-type reactions, including asthma and urticaria, after taking ASA or other NSAIDs. Treatment of perioperative pain in the setting of CABG surgery. **P/N:** Category C, not for use in nursing.	Abdominal pain, constipation, diarrhea, dyspepsia, flatulence, gross bleeding/ perforation, heartburn, N/V, GI ulcers, abnormal renal function, anemia, dizziness, edema, elevated liver enzymes, headache, increased bleeding time, pruritus, rash, tinnitus.

†Bold entries denote special dental considerations.
BB = black box warning; **W/P** = warnings/precautions; **Contra** = contraindications; **P/N** = pregnancy category rating and nursing considerations.

NAME	FORM/ STRENGTH	DOSAGE	WARNINGS/PRECAUTIONS & CONTRAINDICATIONS	ADVERSE EFFECTS†
Meloxicam (Mobic)	**Sus:** 7.5mg/5mL; **Tab:** 7.5mg, 15mg	***Adults:*** **≥18 yrs: OA/RA: Initial/ Maint:** 7.5mg qd. **Max:** 15mg/day. ***Pediatrics:*** **>2 yrs: JRA:** 0.125mg/kg qd. **Max:** 7.5mg/day.	**BB:** NSAIDs may cause an increased risk of serious cardiovascular thrombotic events, MI, stroke, and serious GI adverse events, including bleeding, ulceration, and perforation of the stomach or intestines. Contraindicated for the treatment of perioperative pain in the setting of coronary artery bypass graft (CABG) surgery. **W/P:** May lead to onset of new HTN or worsening of pre-existing HTN; monitor BP closely. Fluid retention and edema reported; caution with fluid retention, HTN, or heart failure. Renal papillary necrosis, renal insufficiency, acute renal failure, and other renal injury reported after long-term use. Not recommended for use with advanced renal disease; if therapy must be initiated, monitor renal function. Anaphylactoid reactions may occur. May cause serious skin adverse events (eg, exfoliative dermatitis, Stevens-Johnson syndrome, and toxic epidermal necrolysis). Avoid in late pregnancy; may cause premature closure of ductus arteriosis. May cause elevations of LFTs; d/c if liver disease develops or systemic manifestations occur. Caution with considerable dehydration and in elderly. Anemia may occur; with long-term use, monitor Hgb/ Hct if signs or symptoms of anemia develop. May inhibit platelet aggregation and prolong bleeding time; monitor with coagulation disorders. Caution with asthma and avoid with ASA-sensitive asthma. **Contra:** ASA or other NSAID allergy that precipitates asthma, urticaria, or allergic-type reactions. Treatment of perioperative pain in the setting of CABG surgery. **P/N:** Category C, not for use in nursing.	Abdominal pain, constipation, diarrhea, dyspepsia, N/V, headache, anemia, arthralgia, insomnia, upper respiratory tract infection, UTI.
Nabumetone	**Tab:** 500mg, 750mg	***Adults:*** **Initial:** 1000mg qd. **Max:** 2000mg/day.	**BB:** NSAIDs may cause an increased risk of serious cardiovascular thrombotic events, MI, stroke, and serious GI adverse events, including bleeding, ulceration, and perforation of the stomach or intestines. Contraindicated for the treatment of perioperative pain in the setting of coronary artery bypass graft (CABG) surgery. **W/P:** May lead to onset of new HTN or worsening of pre-existing HTN; monitor BP closely. Fluid retention and edema reported; caution with fluid retention or heart failure. Renal papillary necrosis and other renal injury reported after long-term use. Not recommended for use with advanced renal disease; if therapy must be initiated, monitor renal function. Anaphylactoid reactions may occur. May cause serious skin adverse events (eg, exfoliative dermatitis, Stevens-Johnson syndrome, and toxic epidermal necrolysis). Avoid in late pregnancy; may cause premature closure of ductus arteriosis. May cause elevations of LFTs; d/c if liver disease develops or systemic manifestations occur. Caution in elderly. Anemia may occur; with long-term use, monitor Hgb/ Hct if signs or symptoms of anemia develop. May inhibit platelet aggregation and prolong bleeding time; monitor with	Diarrhea, dyspepsia, abdominal pain, constipation, flatulence, nausea, positive stool guaiac, dizziness, headache, pruritus, rash, tinnitus, edema.

Table 3.1. PRESCRIBING INFORMATION FOR ANALGESICS *(cont.)*

NAME	FORM/ STRENGTH	DOSAGE	WARNINGS/PRECAUTIONS & CONTRAINDICATIONS	ADVERSE EFFECTS†
NONOPIOID ANALGESICS *(cont.)*				
NSAIDS *(cont.)*				
Nabumetone *(cont.)*			coagulation disorders. Caution with asthma and avoid with ASA-sensitive asthma. May induce photosensitivity. Risk of GI ulceration, bleeding, and perforation. **Contra:** Allergy to ASA or other NSAID that precipitates asthma, urticaria, or other allergic-type reaction. Treatment of perioperative pain in the setting of CABG surgery. **P/N:** Category C, not for use in nursing.	
Naproxen (EC-Naprosyn, Naprosyn)	(Naprosyn) **Sus:** 25mg/mL; **Tab:** 250mg*, 375mg, 500mg*; (EC-Naprosyn) **Tab, Delayed-Release:** 375mg, 500mg	***Adults:* OA/RA/AS: Naprosyn:** 250, 375, or 500mg bid; **EC-Naprosyn:** 375 or 500mg bid. **Max:** 1500mg/day. **Acute Gout: Naprosyn:** 750mg, followed by 250mg q8h until attack subsides. **Pain/Dysmenorrhea/ Tendinitis/Bursitis: Naprosyn:** 500mg, followed by 500mg q12h or 250mg q6-8h prn. **Max:** 1250mg on Day 1, then 1000mg/day. EC-Naprosyn should not be chewed, crushed, or broken. ***Pediatrics:* ≥2 yrs: JA: (Sus)** 5mg/kg bid. **Max:** 15mg/kg/day.	**BB:** NSAIDs may cause an increased risk of serious cardiovascular thrombotic events, MI, stroke, and serious GI adverse events, including bleeding, ulceration, and perforation of the stomach or intestines. Contraindicated for the treatment of perioperative pain in the setting of coronary artery bypass graft (CABG) surgery. **W/P:** May lead to onset of new HTN or worsening of pre-existing HTN; monitor BP closely. Fluid retention, edema, and peripheral edema reported; caution with fluid retention, HTN, or heart failure. Renal papillary necrosis and other renal injury reported after long-term use. Not recommended for use with advanced renal disease; if therapy must be initiated, monitor renal function. Anaphylactoid reactions may occur. May cause serious skin adverse events (eg, exfoliative dermatitis, Stevens-Johnson syndrome, and toxic epidermal necrolysis). Avoid in late pregnancy; may cause premature closure of ductus arteriosis. Monitor Hgb levels with long-term therapy if initial Hgb ≤10g. Monitor for visual changes or disturbances. May cause elevations of LFTs; d/c if liver disease develops or systemic manifestations occur. Caution with high doses in chronic alcoholic liver disease and elderly. Anemia may occur; with long-term use, monitor Hgb/Hct if signs or symptoms of anemia develop. May inhibit platelet aggregation and prolong bleeding time; monitor with coagulation disorders. Caution with asthma and avoid with ASA-sensitive asthma. **Contra:** History of ASA or NSAID allergy that cause symptoms of asthma, rhinitis, nasal polyps, and hypotension. Treatment of peri-operative pain in the setting of CABG surgery. **P/N:** Category C, not for use in nursing.	Edema, drowsiness, dizziness, constipation, heartburn, abdominal pain, nausea, headache, tinnitus, dyspnea, pruritus, skin eruptions, ecchymoses.
Naproxen Sodium (Aleve) OTC	**Tab:** 220mg	***Adults:* Initial:** 1-2 tabs, then 1 tab q8-12h. **Max:** 660mg/24 hrs or 440mg/12 hrs. **Elderly: >65 yrs:** 1 tab q12h. ***Pediatrics:* ≥12 yrs: Initial:** 1-2 tabs, then 1 tab q8-12h. **Max:** 660mg/24 hrs or 440mg/12 hrs.	**W/P:** Avoid during last trimester of pregnancy. Do not use >10 days for pain or >3 days for fever. **P/N:** Safety in pregnancy or nursing not known.	—

*Scored. †Bold entries denote special dental considerations.
BB = black box warning; **W/P** = warnings/precautions; **Contra** = contraindications; **P/N** = pregnancy category rating and nursing considerations.

NAME	FORM/ STRENGTH	DOSAGE	WARNINGS/PRECAUTIONS & CONTRAINDICATIONS	ADVERSE EFFECTS†
Naproxen Sodium (Anaprox, Anaprox DS)	(Anaprox) **Tab:** 275mg; (Anaprox DS) **Tab:** 550mg*	***Adults:* OA/RA/AS:** 275mg bid or 550mg bid. **Max:** 1650mg/day. **Acute Gout:** 825mg, followed by 275mg q8h. **Pain/Dysmenorrhea/Tendinitis/ Bursitis:** 550mg, followed by 550mg q12h or 275mg q6-8h prn. **Max:** 1375mg on Day 1, then 1100mg/day.	**BB:** NSAIDs may cause an increased risk of serious cardiovascular thrombotic events, MI, stroke, and serious GI adverse events, including bleeding, ulceration, and perforation of the stomach or intestines. Contraindicated for the treatment of perioperative pain in the setting of coronary artery bypass graft (CABG) surgery. **W/P:** May lead to onset of new HTN or worsening of pre-existing HTN; monitor BP closely. Fluid retention, edema, and peripheral edema reported; caution with fluid retention, HTN, or heart failure. Renal papillary necrosis and other renal injury reported after long-term use. Not recommended for use with advanced renal disease; if therapy must be initiated, monitor renal function. Anaphylactoid reactions may occur. May cause serious skin adverse events (eg, exfoliative dermatitis, Stevens-Johnson syndrome, and toxic epidermal necrolysis). Avoid in late pregnancy; may cause premature closure of ductus arteriosis. Monitor Hgb levels with long-term therapy if initial Hgb ≤10g. Monitor for visual changes or disturbances. May cause elevations of LFTs; d/c if liver disease develops or systemic manifestations occur. Caution with high doses in chronic alcoholic liver disease and elderly. Anemia may occur; with long-term use, monitor Hgb/Hct if signs or symptoms of anemia develop. May inhibit platelet aggregation and prolong bleeding time; monitor with coagulation disorders. Caution with asthma and avoid with ASA-sensitive asthma. **Contra:** History of ASA or NSAID allergy that caused symptoms of asthma, rhinitis, nasal polyps, and hypotension. Treatment of perioperative pain in the setting of CABG surgery. **P/N:** Category C, not for use in nursing.	Edema, drowsiness, dizziness, constipation, heartburn, abdominal pain, nausea, headache, tinnitus, dyspnea, pruritus, skin eruptions, ecchymoses.
Naproxen Sodium (Naprelan)	**Tab, Extended-Release:** 375mg, 500mg	***Adults:* OA/RA/AS: Usual:** 750mg-1g qd. **Max:** 1.5g/day. **Pain/Primary Dysmenorrhea/Tendinitis/Bursitis:** 1g/day or 1.5g for a limited period. **Max:** 1g/day thereafter. **Acute Gout:** 1-1.5g qd for 1 day, then 1g qd until attack subsides.	**BB:** NSAIDs may cause an increased risk of serious cardiovascular thrombotic events, MI, stroke, and serious GI adverse events, including bleeding, ulceration, and perforation of the stomach or intestines. Contraindicated for the treatment of perioperative pain in the setting of coronary artery bypass graft (CABG) surgery. **W/P:** May lead to onset of new HTN or worsening of pre-existing HTN; monitor BP closely. Fluid retention and edema reported; caution with fluid retention or heart failure. Renal papillary necrosis and other renal injury reported after long-term use. Not recommended for use with advanced renal disease; if therapy must be initiated, monitor renal function. Anaphylactoid reactions may occur. May cause serious skin adverse events (eg, exfoliative dermatitis, Stevens-Johnson syndrome, and toxic epidermal necrolysis). Avoid in late pregnancy; may cause premature closure of ductus arteriosis. May cause elevations of LFTs; d/c if liver disease develops or systemic manifestations	Headache, dyspepsia, flu syndrome, pain, infection, nausea, diarrhea, constipation, abdominal pain, heartburn, drowsiness, edema, skin rash, ecchymoses.

Table 3.1. PRESCRIBING INFORMATION FOR ANALGESICS *(cont.)*

NAME	FORM/ STRENGTH	DOSAGE	WARNINGS/PRECAUTIONS & CONTRAINDICATIONS	ADVERSE EFFECTS†
NONOPIOID ANALGESICS *(cont.)*				
NSAIDS *(cont.)*				
Naproxen Sodium (Naprelan) *(cont.)*			occur. Caution in elderly. Anemia may occur; with long-term use, monitor Hgb/Hct if signs or symptoms of anemia develop. May inhibit platelet aggregation and prolong bleeding time; monitor with coagulation disorders. Caution with asthma and avoid with ASA-sensitive asthma. **Contra:** History of angioedema, urticaria, bronchospastic reactivity, nasal polyps. NSAID allergy that precipitates asthma, nasal polyps, urticaria, and hypotension. Treatment of perioperative pain in the setting of CABG surgery. **P/N:** Category C, not for use in nursing.	
Oxaprozin (Daypro)	**Tab:** 600mg*	***Adults:*** **RA:** 1200mg qd. **Max:** 1800mg/day in divided doses (not to exceed 26mg/kg/day). **OA:** 1200mg qd; give 600mg qd for low weight or milder disease. **Max:** 1800mg/day in divided doses (not to exceed 26mg/kg/day). **Renal Dysfunction/ Hemodialysis: Initial:** 600mg qd. ***Pediatrics:*** **6-16yrs: JRA: ≥55kg:** 1200mg qd. **32-54kg:** 900mg qd. **22-31kg:** 600mg qd.	**BB:** NSAIDs may cause an increased risk of serious cardiovascular thrombotic events, MI, stroke, and serious GI adverse events, including bleeding, ulceration, and perforation of the stomach or intestines. Contraindicated for the treatment of perioperative pain in the setting of coronary artery bypass graft (CABG) surgery. **W/P:** May lead to onset of new HTN or worsening of pre-existing HTN; monitor BP closely. Fluid retention and edema reported; caution with fluid retention or heart failure. Renal papillary necrosis and other renal injury reported after long-term use. Not recommended for use with advanced renal disease; if therapy must be initiated, monitor renal function. Anaphylactoid reactions may occur. May cause serious skin adverse events (eg, exfoliative dermatitis, Stevens-Johnson syndrome, and toxic epidermal necrolysis). Avoid in late pregnancy; may cause premature closure of ductus arteriosis. May cause elevations of LFTs; d/c if liver disease develops or systemic manifestations occur. Caution in elderly. Anemia may occur; with long-term use, monitor Hgb/Hct if signs or symptoms of anemia develop. May inhibit platelet aggregation and prolong bleeding time; monitor with coagulation disorders. Caution with asthma and avoid with ASA-sensitive asthma. Rash and/or mild photosensitivity reactions reported. **Contra:** Complete or partial syndrome of nasal polyps, angioedema, and bronchospastic reactivity to ASA or other NSAIDs. Treatment of perioperative pain in the setting of CABG surgery. **P/N:** Category C, not for use in nursing.	Constipation, diarrhea, dyspepsia, flatulence, nausea, rash.
Piroxicam (Feldene)	**Cap:** 10mg, 20mg	***Adults:*** 20mg qd or 10mg bid. **Elderly:** Start at lower end of dosing range.	**BB:** NSAIDs may cause an increased risk of serious cardiovascular thrombotic events, MI, stroke, and serious GI adverse events, including bleeding, ulceration, and perforation of the stomach or intestines. Contraindicated for the treatment of perioperative pain in the setting of coronary artery bypass graft (CABG) surgery. **W/P:** May lead to onset of new HTN or worsening of pre-existing HTN; monitor BP closely. Fluid retention	Edema, dyspepsia, elevated liver enzymes, dizziness, rash, tinnitus, renal dysfunction, **dry mouth**, weight changes, increased bleeding time, GI bleeding/perforation, ulcers, heartburn, anorexia, abdominal pain.

*Scored. †Bold entries denote special dental considerations.
BB = black box warning; **W/P** = warnings/precautions; **Contra** = contraindications; **P/N** = pregnancy category rating and nursing considerations.

NAME	FORM/ STRENGTH	DOSAGE	WARNINGS/PRECAUTIONS & CONTRAINDICATIONS	ADVERSE EFFECTS†
Piroxicam (Feldene) *(cont.)*			and edema reported; caution with fluid retention or heart failure. Renal papillary necrosis and other renal injury reported after long-term use. Not recommended for use with advanced renal disease; if therapy must be initiated, monitor renal function. Anaphylactoid reactions may occur. May cause serious skin adverse events (eg, exfoliative dermatitis, Stevens-Johnson syndrome, and toxic epidermal necrolysis). Avoid in late pregnancy; may cause premature closure of ductus arteriosis. May cause elevations of LFTs; d/c if liver disease develops or systemic manifestations occur. Caution in elderly. Anemia may occur; with long-term use, monitor Hgb/Hct if signs or symptoms of anemia develop. May inhibit platelet aggregation and prolong bleeding time; monitor with coagulation disorders. Caution with asthma and avoid with ASA-sensitive asthma. Adverse eye findings reported. Dermatological and/or allergic signs and symptoms suggestive of serum sickness have occurred. Risk of GI ulceration, bleeding, and perforation. **Contra:** ASA or other NSAID allergy that precipitates asthma, urticaria, or other allergic-type reactions. Treatment of perioperative pain in the setting of CABG surgery. **P/N:** Category C, not for use in nursing.	
Sulindac (Clinoril)	**Tab:** 150mg, 200mg*	***Adults:*** **OA/RA/AS: Initial:** 150mg bid. **Acute Painful Shoulder/Acute Gouty Arthritis:** 200mg bid for 7-14 days. **Max:** 400mg/day. Give with food.	**BB:** NSAIDs may cause an increased risk of serious cardiovascular thrombotic events, MI, stroke, and serious GI adverse events, including bleeding, ulceration, and perforation of the stomach or intestines. Contraindicated for the treatment of perioperative pain in the setting of coronary artery bypass graft (CABG) surgery. **W/P:** May lead to onset of new HTN or worsening of pre-existing HTN; monitor BP closely. Fluid retention and edema reported; caution with fluid retention or heart failure. Renal papillary necrosis and other renal injury reported after long-term use. Not recommended for use with advanced renal disease; if therapy must be initiated, monitor renal function. Anaphylactoid reactions may occur. May cause serious skin adverse events (eg, exfoliative dermatitis, Stevens-Johnson syndrome, and toxic epidermal necrolysis). Avoid in late pregnancy; may cause premature closure of ductus arteriosis. May cause elevations of LFTs; d/c if abnormal LFTs persist/worsen, liver disease develops, or systemic manifestations occur. Caution in elderly. Anemia may occur; monitor Hgb/Hct with long-term use. May inhibit platelet aggregation and prolong bleeding time; monitor with coagulation disorders. Caution with asthma and avoid with ASA-sensitive asthma. Keep patients well-hydrated and caution with renal lithiasis. Pancreatitis reported; if pancreatitis suspected, d/c and do not restart. Adverse eye findings reported. Monitor closely with poor liver function and consider dose reduction.	GI pain, dyspepsia, N/V, diarrhea, constipation, rash, dizziness, headache, tinnitus, edema.

Table 3.1. PRESCRIBING INFORMATION FOR ANALGESICS *(cont.)*

NAME	FORM/ STRENGTH	DOSAGE	WARNINGS/PRECAUTIONS & CONTRAINDICATIONS	ADVERSE EFFECTS†
NONOPIOID ANALGESICS *(cont.)*				
NSAIDS *(cont.)*				
Sulindac (Clinoril) *(cont.)*			Increased risk of aseptic meningitis in patients with systemic lupus erythematosus (SLE) and mixed connective tissue disease. Risk of GI ulceration, bleeding, and perforation. **Contra:** ASA or other NSAID allergy that precipitates acute asthmatic attack, urticaria, or rhinitis. Treatment of perioperative pain in the setting of CABG surgery. **P/N:** Category C, not for use in nursing.	
Tolmetin Sodium	**Cap:** 400mg; **Tab:** 200mg*, 600mg	***Adults:* OA/RA: Initial:** 400mg tid. **Usual:** 200-600mg tid. **Max:** 1800mg/day. Take with antacids other than sodium bicarbonate if GI upset occurs. ***Pediatrics:* JRA: ≥2 yrs: Initial:** 20mg/kg/day given tid-qid. **Usual:** 15-30mg/kg/day. **Max:** 30mg/kg/day. Take with antacids other than sodium bicarbonate if GI upset occurs.	**BB:** NSAIDs may cause an increased risk of serious cardiovascular thrombotic events, MI, stroke, and serious GI adverse events including bleeding, ulceration, and perforation of the stomach or intestines. Contraindicated for the treatment of perioperative pain in the setting of coronary artery bypass graft (CABG) surgery. **W/P:** May cause adverse ocular events. Prolongs bleeding time. Risk of renal toxicity with heart failure, liver dysfunction, and elderly. Caution with compromised cardiac function, HTN, or other conditions predisposing to fluid retention. Borderline LFT elevations may occur. Decreased bioavailability with milk or food. Can cause serious skin adverse reactions such as exfoliative dermatitis, Stevens-Johnson syndrome, and toxic epidermal necrolysis, which can be fatal. Avoid with ASA-sensitive asthma and caution with preexisting asthma. Cannot be expected to substitute for corticosteroids or to treat corticosteroid insufficiency. Notable elevations of ALT or AST reported. Rare cases of severe hepatic reactions, including jaundice and fatal fulminant hepatitis, liver necrosis, and hepatic failure. Patients on long-term treatment should have Hgb or Hct checked if exhibit signs or symptoms of anemia. **Contra:** ASA or other NSAID allergy that precipitates asthma, rhinitis, urticaria, or allergic-type reactions. Treatment of perioperative pain in the setting of CABG surgery. **P/N:** Category C, not for use in nursing.	Dyspepsia, GI distress, diarrhea, flatulence, vomiting, headache, asthenia, elevated blood pressure, dizziness, edema, weight gain/loss.
SALICYLATES				
Aspirin (Bayer Aspirin, Children's Bayer Aspirin, Bayer Aspirin Regimen, Bayer Aspirin Regimen with Calcium, Genuine Bayer Aspirin) OTC	**Tab:** (Genuine Bayer Aspirin) 325mg; **Tab:** (Bayer Aspirin Regimen with Calcium) 81mg; **Tab, Chewable:** (Children's Bayer Aspirin) 81mg; **Tab, Delayed-Release:** (Bayer Aspirin Regimen) 81mg, 325mg	***Adults:* Ischemic Stroke/TIA:** 50-325mg qd. **Suspected Acute MI: Initial:** 160-162.5mg qd as soon as suspect MI. **Maint:** 160-162.5mg qd for 30 days post-infarction; consider further therapy for prevention/recurrent MI. **Prevention or Recurrent MI/Unstable Angina/Chronic Stable Angina:** 75-325mg qd. **CABG:** 325mg qd, start 6 hrs post-surgery. Continue for 1 yr. **PTCA: Initial:** 325mg, 2 hrs pre-surgery. **Maint:** 160-325mg qd. **Carotid Endarterectomy:** 80mg qd to 650mg bid, start pre-surgery. **RA/Arthritis/SLE Pleurisy: Initial:** 3g/day in divided doses. Increase for anti-inflammatory efficacy to 150-300mcg/mL plasma	**W/P:** Increased risk of bleeding with heavy alcohol use (≥3 drinks/day). May inhibit platelet function; can adversely affect inherited (hemophilia) or acquired (hepatic disease, vitamin K deficiency) bleeding disorders. Monitor for bleeding and ulceration. Avoid in history of active peptic ulcer, severe renal failure, severe hepatic insufficiency, and sodium-restricted diets. Associated with elevated LFTs, BUN, and SrCr; hyperkalemia; proteinuria; and prolonged bleeding time. Avoid 1 week before and during labor. **Contra:** NSAID allergy, viral infections in children or teenagers, syndrome of asthma, rhinitis, and nasal polyps. **P/N:** Avoid in 3rd trimester of pregnancy and nursing.	Fever, hypothermia, dysrhythmias, hypotension, agitation, cerebral edema, dehydration, hyperkalemia, dyspepsia, GI bleed, hearing loss, tinnitus, problems in pregnancy.

*Scored. †Bold entries denote special dental considerations.
BB = black box warning; **W/P** = warnings/precautions; **Contra** = contraindications; **P/N** = pregnancy category rating and nursing considerations.

NAME	FORM/ STRENGTH	DOSAGE	WARNINGS/PRECAUTIONS & CONTRAINDICATIONS	ADVERSE EFFECTS†
Aspirin *(cont.)*		salicylate level. **Spondyloarthropathies:** Up to 4g/day in divided doses. **OA:** Up to 3g/day in divided doses. **Pain:** 325-650mg q4-6h. **Max:** 4g/day. ***Pediatrics:*** **JRA: Initial:** 90-130mg/kg/day in divided doses. Increase for anti-inflammatory efficacy to 150-300mcg/mL plasma salicylate level. **Pain: ≥12 yrs:** 325-650mg q4-6h. **Max:** 4g/day.		
Aspirin (Bayer Aspirin Extra Strength) OTC	**Tab:** 500mg	***Adults/Pediatrics:*** **≥12 yrs:** 500-1000mg q4-6h prn. **Max:** 4g/24hrs.	**W/P:** Avoid in children or teenagers for chickenpox or flu symptoms; Reye's syndrome may occur. Do not take >10 days for pain or >3 days for fever. Avoid in asthma, stomach problems that persist or recur, gastric ulcers, or bleeding problems. Stop therapy if ringing in the ears or loss of hearing occurs. **P/N:** Avoid in 3rd trimester of pregnancy; safety in nursing not known.	
Aspirin (Ecotrin) OTC	**Tab, Delayed-Release:** 81mg, 325mg, 500mg	***Adults:*** **Ischemic Stroke/TIA:** 50-325mg qd. **Suspected Acute MI: Initial:** 160-162.5mg qd as soon as suspect MI. **Maint:** 160-162.5mg for 30 days post-infarction; consider further therapy for prevention/ recurrent MI. **Prevention or Recurrent MI/Unstable Angina/Chronic Stable Angina:** 75-325mg qd. **CABG:** 325mg qd, start 6 hrs post-surgery. Continue for 1 yr. **PTCA: Initial:** 325mg, 2 hrs pre-surgery. **Maint:** 160-325mg qd. **Carotid Endarterectomy:** 80mg qd to 650mg bid, start pre-surgery. **RA/Arthritis/SLE Pleurisy: Initial:** 3g/day in divided doses. Increase for anti-inflammatory efficacy to 150-300mcg/mL plasma salicylate level. **Spondyloarthropathies:** Up to 4g/day in divided doses. **OA:** Up to 3g/day in divided doses. ***Pediatrics:*** **JRA: Initial:** 90-130mg/ kg/day in divided doses. Increase for anti-inflammatory efficacy to 150-300mcg/mL plasma salicylate level.	**W/P:** Increased risk of bleeding with heavy alcohol use (≥3 drinks/day). May inhibit platelet function; can adversely affect inherited (hemophilia) or acquired (hepatic disease, vitamin K deficiency) bleeding disorders. Monitor for bleeding and ulceration. Avoid in history of active peptic ulcer, severe renal failure, severe hepatic insufficiency, and sodium-restricted diets. Associated with elevated LFTs, BUN, and SrCr; hyperkalemia; proteinuria; and prolonged bleeding time. Avoid 1 week before and during labor. **Contra:** NSAID allergy, children or teenagers for viral infections with or without fever, syndrome of asthma, rhinitis, and nasal polyps. **P/N:** Avoid in 3rd trimester of pregnancy and nursing.	Fever, hypothermia, dysrhythmias, hypotension, agitation, cerebral edema, dehydration, hyperkalemia, dyspepsia, GI bleed, hearing loss, tinnitus, problems in pregnancy.
Salsalate	**Tab:** 500mg, 750mg*	***Adults:*** **Usual:** 1000mg tid or 1500mg bid.	**W/P:** Competes with thyroid hormone for binding to plasma proteins. Reye's syndrome may develop in viral infections (eg, chickenpox, influenza). Caution in chronic renal impairment and peptic ulcer. Bronchospasm reported with ASA sensitivity. Monitor salicylic acid levels and urinary pH periodically with long-term therapy. **P/N:** Category C, caution in nursing.	Tinnitus, nausea, heartburn, rash, vertigo, hearing impairment.
MISCELLANEOUS				
Botanical/ Mineral Substances (Traumeel Injection)	**Inj:** 2.2mL amps [10^8]	***Adults:*** 1 amp qd for acute disorders or 1-2 amps 1-3 times weekly. May administer IV, IM, SQ, or intradermally. ***Pediatrics:*** **>6 yrs:** 1 amp qd for acute disorders or 1-2 amps 1-3 times weekly. **2-6 yrs:** Use 1/2 of the adult dosage. May administer IV, IM, SQ, or intradermally.	**W/P:** Carefully re-evaluate if pain persists or worsens, if new symptoms occur, or if redness or swelling is present. **P/N:** Category C, caution in nursing.	Allergic reactions, anaphylactic reactions.

Table 3.1. PRESCRIBING INFORMATION FOR ANALGESICS *(cont.)*

NAME	FORM/ STRENGTH	DOSAGE	WARNINGS/PRECAUTIONS & CONTRAINDICATIONS	ADVERSE EFFECTS†
OPIOID-CONTAINING ANALGESICS				
CODEINE COMBINATIONS				
Acetaminophen/ Codeine Phosphate (Acetaminophen w/Codeine Elixir) CV Tylenol with Codeine) CIII	**Elixir:** (Codeine-APAP) (CV) 12-120mg/5mL; **Tab:** (#3) 30-300mg, (#4) 60-300mg	***Adults:*** **(Tab) Usual:** 15-60mg codeine/dose and 300-1000mg APAP/dose, up to q4h prn. **Max:** 60mg codeine/dose, 360mg codeine/day, and 4g APAP/day. **(Elixir):** 15mL q4h prn. ***Pediatrics:*** **(Elixir): Usual: 7-12 yrs:** 10mL tid-qid. **3-6 yrs:** 5mL tid-qid.	**W/P:** Respiratory depressant effects may be exacerbated with head injury or increased ICP. May obscure head injuries, acute abdominal conditions. Caution in the elderly, debilitated, severe hepatic or renal dysfunction, hypothyroidism, Addison's disease, prostatic hypertrophy, or urethral stricture. Potential for physical dependence, tolerance. Tabs contain sulfites. **P/N:** Category C, caution in nursing.	Lightheadedness, dizziness, sedation, SOB, N/V, allergic reactions, euphoria, dysphoria, constipation, abdominal pain, pruritus.
Aspirin/Codeine CIII	**Tab:** (ASA-Codeine) 325mg-30mg, 325mg-60mg	***Adults:*** (325mg-30mg) 1-2 tabs q4h prn. (325mg-60mg) 1 tab q4h prn.	**W/P:** May cause anaphylactic shock, severe allergic reactions. Serious bleeding can occur with peptic ulcer, GI lesions, and bleeding disorders. May prolong bleeding time if given preoperatively. Enhanced respiratory depression and CSF pressure with head injury or intracranial lesion. May obscure signs of acute abdominal conditions or head injury. Caution in children and teenagers with chickenpox or flu. Caution in elderly, debilitated, severe renal/hepatic impairment, gallbladder disease or gallstones, respiratory impairment, arrhythmias, inflammatory GI tract disorders, hypothyroidism, Addison's disease, prostatic hypertrophy, urethral stricture, coagulation disorders, head injuries, or acute abdominal conditions. **Contra:** Severe bleeding, disorders of coagulation or primary hemostasis (eg, hemophilia, hypoprothrombinemia, von Willebrand's disease, thrombocytopenia, thromboasthenia), ill-defined hereditary platelet dysfunction, severe vitamin K deficiency, severe hepatic damage, anticoagulant therapy, peptic ulcer, serious GI lesions. **P/N:** Category C, not for use in nursing.	Lightheadedness, dizziness, drowsiness, N/V, constipation, hearing impairment, tinnitus, diminished vision, headache, respiratory depression, sweating.
DIHYDROCODEINE COMBINATIONS				
Aspirin/Caffeine/ Dihydrocodeine Bitartrate (Synalgos-DC) CIII	**Cap:** (Dihydrocodeine-ASA-Caffeine) 16mg-356.4mg-30mg [Painpak, 12 caps]	***Adults:*** 2 caps q4h prn pain. **Elderly:** Start at low end of dosing range. ***Pediatrics:*** **>12 yrs:** 2 caps q4h prn pain.	**W/P:** Caution in elderly, debilitated, and with peptic ulcer or coagulation abnormalities. May impair mental or physical abilities. Abuse potential. **P/N:** Safety in pregnancy and nursing is not known.	Lightheadedness, dizziness, drowsiness, sedation, N/V, constipation, pruritus, skin reactions.
HYDROCODONE COMBINATIONS				
Acetaminophen/ Hydrocodone Bitartrate CIII	**Tab:** (Hydrocodone-APAP) 5mg-325mg, 7.5mg-325mg, 5mg-500mg, 7.5mg-650mg	***Adults:*** (5-500mg) **Usual:** 1-2 tabs q4-6h prn. **Max:** 8 tabs/day. (7.5-650mg) **Usual:** 1 tab q4-6h prn. **Max:** 6 tabs/day.	**W/P:** Caution in elderly, debilitated, severe hepatic or renal dysfunction, hypothyroidism, Addison's disease, prostatic hypertrophy, urethral stricture, pulmonary disease, and postoperative use. Impairs mental/physical abilities. May obscure diagnosis or clinical course of acute abdominal conditions or head injuries. May produce dose-related respiratory depression. Monitor for tolerance. Suppresses cough reflex. **P/N:** Category C, not for use in nursing.	Lightheadedness, dizziness, sedation, N/V, constipation, rash, respiratory depression.

*Scored. †Bold entries denote special dental considerations.

BB = black box warning; **W/P** = warnings/precautions; **Contra** = contraindications; **P/N** = pregnancy category rating and nursing considerations.

CII = high potential for abuse; CIII = some potential for abuse; CIV = low potential for abuse. For more information on controlled substances categories, see "How to Use This Book" on page iv.

NAME	FORM/ STRENGTH	DOSAGE	WARNINGS/PRECAUTIONS & CONTRAINDICATIONS	ADVERSE EFFECTS†
Acetaminophen/ Hydrocodone Bitartrate (Lorcet, Lorcet 10/650, Lorcet HD, Lorcet Plus) CIII	(Hydrocodone-APAP) **Cap:** (HD) 5mg-500mg; **Tab:** (Plus) 7.5mg-650mg*, (10/650) 10mg-650mg*	***Adults:*** (Plus, 10/650) **Usual:** 1 cap/tab q4-6h prn pain. **Max:** 6 tabs or caps/day. (HD) **Usual:** 1-2 caps q4-6h prn pain. **Max:** 8 caps/day.	**W/P:** May produce dose-related respiratory depression. May obscure acute abdominal conditions or head injuries. Caution in elderly, debilitated, severe hepatic or renal dysfunction, hypothyroidism, Addison's disease, prostatic hypertrophy, urethral stricture, pulmonary disease, and postoperative use. May be habit-forming. Suppresses cough reflex. **P/N:** Category C, not for use in nursing.	Dizziness, drowsiness, N/V, dysphoria, urinary retention, urethral spasm, dyspnea, SOB, rash.
Acetaminophen/ Hydrocodone Bitartrate (Lortab) CIII	(Hydrocodone-APAP) **Sol:** 7.5mg-500mg/15mL; **Tab:** 2.5mg-500mg*, 5mg-500mg*, 7.5mg-500mg*, 10mg-500mg*	***Adults:*** (2.5-500, 5-500) 1-2 tabs q4-6h prn. **Max:** 8 tabs/day. (7.5-500, 10-500) 1 tab q4-6h prn. **Max:** 6 tabs/day. (Sol) 15mL q4-6h prn. **Max:** 90mL/day. ***Pediatrics:*** **≥2 yrs:** (Sol) 12-15kg: 3.75mL. 16-22kg: 5mL. 23-31kg: 7.5mL. 32-45kg: 10mL. ≥46kg: 15mL. May repeat q4-6h prn.	**W/P:** May produce dose-related respiratory depression. May obscure acute abdominal conditions or head injuries. Caution in elderly, debilitated, severe hepatic or renal dysfunction, hypothyroidism, Addison's disease, prostatic hypertrophy, urethral stricture, pulmonary disease, postoperative use. May be habit-forming. Suppresses cough reflex. **P/N:** Category C, not for use in nursing.	Lightheadedness, dizziness, sedation, N/V.
Acetaminophen/ Hydrocodone Bitartrate (Norco) CIII	**Tab:** (Hydrocodone-APAP) 5mg-325mg*, 7.5mg-325mg*, 10mg-325mg*	***Adults:*** (5-325) **Usual:** 1-2 tabs q4-6h prn pain. (7.5-325, 10-325) **Usual:** 1 tab q4-6h prn pain. **Max:** 6 tabs/day.	**W/P:** May produce dose-related respiratory depression. May obscure diagnosis of acute abdominal conditions or head injuries. Caution in elderly, debilitated, severe hepatic or renal dysfunction, hypothyroidism, Addison's disease, prostatic hypertrophy, urethral stricture, pulmonary disease, and postoperative use. May be habit-forming. Suppresses cough reflex. **P/N:** Category C, not for use in nursing.	Lightheadedness, dizziness, sedation, N/V.
Acetaminophen/ Hydrocodone Bitartrate (Vicodin, Vicodin ES, Vicodin HP) CIII	(Hydrocodone-APAP) **Tab:** Vicodin: 5mg-500mg*; Vicodin HP: 10mg-660mg*; Vicodin ES: 7.5mg-750mg*	***Adults:*** **Usual: Vicodin:** 1-2 tabs q4-6h prn. **Max:** 8 tabs/day. **Vicodin HP:** 1 tab q4-6h prn. **Max:** 6 tabs/day. **Vicodin ES:** 1 tab q4-6h prn. **Max:** 5 tabs/day.	**W/P:** Caution in elderly, debilitated, severe hepatic or renal dysfunction, hypothyroidism, Addison's disease, prostatic hypertrophy, urethral stricture, pulmonary disease, and postoperative use. May obscure acute abdominal conditions or head injuries. May produce dose-related respiratory depression. Monitor for tolerance. Suppresses cough reflex. **P/N:** Category C, not for use in nursing.	Lightheadedness, dizziness, sedation, N/V, constipation, rash, respiratory depression.
Acetaminophen/ Hydrocodone Bitartrate (Zydone) CIII	**Tab:** (Hydrocodone-APAP) 5mg-400mg, 7.5mg-400mg, 10mg-400mg	***Adults:*** (5-400): 1-2 tabs q4-6h prn. **Max:** 8 tabs/day. (7.5-400, 10-400): 1 tab q4-6h prn. **Max:** 6 tabs/day.	**W/P:** May produce dose-related respiratory depression. May obscure diagnosis of acute abdominal conditions or head injuries. Caution in elderly, debilitated, severe hepatic or renal dysfunction, hypothyroidism, Addison's disease, prostatic hypertrophy, urethral stricture, pulmonary disease, and postoperative use. May be habit-forming. May impair mental/physical abilities. Suppresses cough reflex. **P/N:** Category C, not for use in nursing.	Lightheadedness, dizziness, sedation, N/V.

Table 3.1. PRESCRIBING INFORMATION FOR ANALGESICS *(cont.)*

NAME	FORM/ STRENGTH	DOSAGE	WARNINGS/PRECAUTIONS & CONTRAINDICATIONS	ADVERSE EFFECTS†
OPIOID-CONTAINING ANALGESICS *(cont.)*				
HYDROCODONE COMBINATIONS *(cont.)*				
Ibuprofen/ Hydrocodone Bitartrate (Reprexain, Vicoprofen) CIII	(Hydrocodone-Ibuprofen) **Tab:** (Vicoprofen) 7.5mg-200mg; (Reprexain) 5mg-200mg, 7.5mg-200mg	***Adults:*** **Usual:** 1 tab q4-6h prn. **Max:** 5 tabs/day. **Elderly:** Use lowest dose or longest interval. ***Pediatrics:*** **≥16 yrs: Usual:** 1 tab q4-6h prn. **Max:** 5 tabs/day.	**W/P:** May produce dose-related respiratory depression. May obscure acute abdominal conditions or head injuries. Avoid with ASA triad, late pregnancy, advanced renal disease, ASA-sensitive asthma. Caution in elderly, debilitated, dehydration, renal disease, intrinsic coagulation defects, severe hepatic dysfunction, asthma, hypothyroidism, Addison's disease, prostatic hypertrophy, urethral stricture, heart failure, HTN, ulcer disease, pulmonary disease, postoperative use. May be habit-forming. Suppresses cough reflex. Risk of GI ulceration, bleeding, perforation. Anemia, fluid retention, edema, severe hepatic reactions reported. Possible risk of aseptic meningitis, especially in SLE patients. Increased risk of serious cardiovascular thrombotic events, MI, and stroke. Fluid retention and edema observed. Skin reactions (eg, exfoliative dermatitis, TEN, SJS) can occur. **Contra:** ASA or other NSAID allergy that precipitates asthma, urticaria, or other allergic reaction. **P/N:** Category C, not for use in nursing.	Headache, somnolence, dizziness, constipation, dyspepsia, N/V, infection, edema, nervousness, anxiety, pruritus, diarrhea, asthenia, abdominal pain, insomnia, **dry mouth**, sweating.
OXYCODONE & COMBINATIONS				
Acetaminophen/ Oxycodone HCl (Endocet, Percocet) CII	**Tab:** (Oxycodone-APAP) 2.5mg-325mg, 5mg-325mg, 7.5mg-325mg, 7.5mg-500mg, 10mg-325mg, 10mg-650mg	***Adults:*** (2.5-325): 1-2 tabs q6h. **Max:** 12 tabs/day. (5-325): 1 tab q6h prn. **Max:** 12 tabs/day. (7.5-325): 1 tab q6h prn. **Max:** 8 tabs/day. (7.5-500): 1 tab q6h prn. **Max:** 8 tabs/day. (10-325): 1 tab q6h prn. **Max:** 6 tabs/day. (10-650) 1 tab q6h prn. **Max:** 6 tabs/day. Do not exceed APAP 4g/day.	**W/P:** May cause drug dependence and tolerance; potential for abuse. Risk of respiratory depression. Capacity to elevate CSF pressure may be exaggerated with head injury, other intracranial lesions, or a pre-existing increase in ICP. May obscure the diagnosis or clinical course with head injuries or with acute abdominal conditions. Caution with severe hepatic impairment, renal dysfunction, hypothyroidism, Addison's disease, prostatic hypertrophy, urethral stricture, the elderly or debilitated. **P/N:** Category C, caution in nursing.	Lightheadedness, dizziness, sedation, N/V, euphoria, dysphoria, constipation, skin rash, pruritus.
Acetaminophen/ Oxycodone HCl (Roxicet) CII	(Oxycodone-APAP) **Sol:** 5mg-325mg/5mL [5mL; 500mL]; **Tab:** 5mg-325mg	***Adults:*** **Usual:** 5mg-325mg (1 tab or 5mL sol) q6h prn. **Titrate:** May need to exceed usual dose based on individual response, pain severity, and tolerance.	**W/P:** May cause drug dependence and tolerance; potential for abuse. Risk of respiratory depression. Capacity to elevate CSF pressure may be exaggerated with head injury, other intracranial lesions, or a pre-existing increase in ICP. May obscure the diagnosis or clinical course with head injuries or with acute abdominal conditions. Caution with severe hepatic impairment, renal dysfunction, hypothyroidism, Addison's disease, prostatic hypertrophy, urethral stricture, the elderly or debilitated. **P/N:** Category C, caution in nursing.	Lightheadedness, dizziness, sedation, N/V, euphoria, dysphoria, constipation, skin rash, pruritus.

*Scored. †Bold entries denote special dental considerations.
BB = black box warning; **W/P** = warnings/precautions; **Contra** = contraindications; **P/N** = pregnancy category rating and nursing considerations.
CII = high potential for abuse; CIII = some potential for abuse; CIV = low potential for abuse. For more information on controlled substances categories, see "How to Use This Book" on page iv.

NAME	FORM/ STRENGTH	DOSAGE	WARNINGS/PRECAUTIONS & CONTRAINDICATIONS	ADVERSE EFFECTS†
Acetaminophen/ Oxycodone HCl (Roxilox, Tylox) CII	**Cap:** (Oxycodone-APAP) 5mg-500mg	***Adults:* Usual:** 1 cap q6h prn.	**W/P:** Contains sulfites. Monitor with head injury; may increase respiratory depressant effects and CSF pressure. Caution in elderly, debilitated, severe hepatic or renal dysfunction, hypothyroidism, Addison's disease, prostatic hypertrophy, or urethral stricture. Potential for physical dependence, tolerance. Inappropriate for intractable/severe pain. **P/N:** Category C, caution in nursing.	Dizziness, sedation, N/V, euphoria, dysphoria, constipation, abdominal pain, pruritus.
Aspirin/ Oxycodone HCl (Endodan, Percodan) CII	**Tab:** (Oxycodone HCl-ASA) 4.8355mg-325mg*	***Adults:* Usual:** 1 tab q6h prn. **Max:** 12 tabs/day or ASA 4g/day.	**W/P:** May cause drug dependence and tolerance; potential for abuse. Risk of respiratory depression. Capacity to elevate CSF pressure may be exaggerated with head injury, other intracranial lesions, or a pre-existing increase in ICP. May obscure the diagnosis or clinical course with head injuries or with acute abdominal conditions. Caution with severe hepatic impairment, renal dysfunction, hypothyroidism, Addison's disease, prostatic hypertrophy, urethral stricture, peptic ulcer, coagulation abnormalities, and the elderly or debilitated. May increase the risk of developing Reye's syndrome in children and teenagers. May impair mental/physical abilities. **P/N:** Category B (Oxycodone) and D (ASA), not for use in nursing.	Lightheadedness, dizziness, sedation, N/V, euphoria, dysphoria, constipation, pruritus.
Ibuprofen/ Oxycodone HCl (Combunox) CII	**Tab:** (Oxycodone-Ibuprofen) 5mg-400mg	***Adults:*** 1 tab/dose. Do not exceed 4 tabs/day and 7 days.	**BB:** NSAIDs may cause an increased risk of serious cardiovascular thrombotic events, MI, stroke, and serious GI adverse events, including bleeding, ulceration, and perforation of the stomach or intestines. Contraindicated for the treatment of perioperative pain in the setting of coronary artery bypass graft (CABG) surgery. **W/P:** May cause drug dependence and tolerance; potential for abuse. Risk of dose-related respiratory depression. May cause severe hypotension. Can lead to HTN or worsening of pre-existing HTN. Fluid retention and edema reported. Capacity to elevate CSF pressure may be exaggerated with head injury, other intracranial lesions, or pre-existing increase in ICP. May obscure diagnosis or clinical course with head injuries or acute abdominal conditions. Risk of GI ulceration, bleeding, and perforation. Risk of anaphylactoid reactions. NSAIDs can cause exfoliative dermatitis, Stevens-Johnson syndrome, and toxic epidermal necrolysis (TEN). Caution with severe hepatic impairment, pulmonary or renal dysfunction, hypothyroidism, Addison's disease, acute alcoholism, convulsive disorders, CNS depression or coma, delirium tremens, kyphoscoliosis associated with respiratory depression, toxic psychosis, prostatic hypertrophy, urethral stricture, biliary tract disease, anemia, pre-existing asthma, elderly or debilitated, aseptic meningitis. **Contra:** Significant respiratory depression, acute or severe bronchial asthma, hypercarbia, paralytic ileus, or in patients who have experienced asthma, urticaria, allergic-type reactions after taking ASA or NSAIDs. Treatment of perioperative pain in the setting of CABG surgery. **P/N:** Category C, caution in nursing.	N/V, somnolence, dizziness, asthenia, fever, headache, vasodilation, constipation.

Table 3.1. PRESCRIBING INFORMATION FOR ANALGESICS *(cont.)*

NAME	FORM/ STRENGTH	DOSAGE	WARNINGS/PRECAUTIONS & CONTRAINDICATIONS	ADVERSE EFFECTS†
OPIOID-CONTAINING ANALGESICS *(cont.)*				
OXYCODONE & COMBINATIONS *(cont.)*				
Oxycodone HCl (OxyContin) CII	**Tab, Extended-Release:** 10mg, 20mg, 40mg, 80mg	***Adults:* Opioid Naive:** 10mg q12h. **Titrate:** May increase to 20mg q12h, then may increase the total daily dose by 25-50% of the current dose. Increase every 1-2 days. **Conversion from Oxycodone:** Divide 24 hr oxycodone dose in half to obtain q12h dose. Round down to appropriate tab strength. **Opioid Tolerant Patients:** May use 80mg tabs. D/C other around-the-clock opioids. **With CNS Depressants:** Reduce dose by 1/3 or 1/2. Swallow whole; do not break, crush, or chew.	**BB:** For continuous analgesia. Abuse potential. 80mg tabs only for opioid-tolerant patients. Swallow tabs whole. **W/P:** Do not break, chew, or crush tabs. Extreme caution with COPD, cor pulmonale, decreased respiratory reserve, hypoxia, hypercapnia, pre-existing respiratory depression. Caution with circulatory shock, delirium tremens, acute alcoholism, adrenocortical insufficiency, CNS depression, myxedema or hypothyroidism, BPH, severe hepatic/renal/ pulmonary impairment, toxic psychosis, biliary tract disease, increased ICP or head injury, elderly or debilitated. May cause severe hypotension. May produce drug dependence; caution in known drug abuse. May aggravate convulsive disorders and mask abdominal disorders. **Contra:** Significant respiratory depression, acute or severe bronchial asthma, hypercarbia, paralytic ileus. **P/N:** Category B, not for use in nursing.	Respiratory depression, constipation, N/V, somnolence, dizziness, pruritus, headache, **dry mouth**, sweating, asthenia.
Oxycodone HCl (OxyIR) CII	**Cap:** 5mg	***Adults:* Usual:** 5mg q6h prn for pain. May add to 30mL of juice or other liquid, applesauce, pudding, or other semi-solid foods.	**W/P:** Extreme caution with COPD, cor pulmonale, decreased respiratory reserve, hypoxia, hypercapnia, pre-existing respiratory depression. Caution with circulatory shock, delirium tremens, acute alcoholism, adrenocortical insufficiency, CNS depression, myxedema or hypothyroidism, BPH, severe hepatic/renal/ pulmonary impairment, toxic psychosis, biliary tract disease, increased ICP, head injury, elderly or debilitated. May cause severe hypotension. May produce drug dependence; caution in known drug abuse. May aggravate convulsive disorders and mask abdominal disorders. May impair mental/physical abilities. **Contra:** Respiratory depression, acute or severe bronchial asthma, hypercarbia, paralytic ileus, situations where opioids are contraindicated. **P/N:** Category B, not for use in nursing.	Lightheadedness, dizziness, N/V, sedation.
Oxycodone HCl (Roxicodone) CII	**Sol:** 5mg/5mL [5mL, 40^{s}; 500mL], (Liquid Concentrate) 20mg/mL [30mL]; **Tab:** 5mg*, 15mg*, 30mg*	***Adults:* Initial: Opioid-Naive:** 5-15mg q4-6h prn. **Titrate:** Based on individual response. For chronic pain or severe chronic pain, use ATC dosing schedule at lowest effective dose.	**W/P:** Potential for physical dependence. May markedly exaggerate respiratory depressant effects in head injuries and increased ICP. May mask symptoms of acute abdominal conditions. Caution with history of drug abuse, the elderly, debilitated, hypothyroidism, Addison's disease, BPH, urethral stricture, severe hepatic and renal impairment. May cause severe hypotension. May impair mental/physical abilities. **Contra:** Significant respiratory depression (in unmonitored settings or the absence of resuscitative equipment), acute or severe bronchial asthma, hypercarbia, paralytic ileus. **P/N:** Category B, not for use in nursing.	Respiratory depression/ arrest, circulatory depression, cardiac arrest, hypotension, shock, N/V, constipation, headache, pruritus, insomnia, dizziness, asthenia, somnolence.

*Scored. †Bold entries denote special dental considerations.
BB = black box warning; **W/P** = warnings/precautions; **Contra** = contraindications; **P/N** = pregnancy category rating and nursing considerations.
CII = high potential for abuse; CIII = some potential for abuse; CIV = low potential for abuse. For more information on controlled substances categories, see "How to Use This Book" on page iv.

NAME	FORM/ STRENGTH	DOSAGE	WARNINGS/PRECAUTIONS & CONTRAINDICATIONS	ADVERSE EFFECTS†
PROPOXYPHENE & COMBINATIONS				
Acetaminophen/ Propoxyphene Napsylate (Darvocet A500) CIV	**Tab:** (Propoxy-phene-APAP) 100mg-500mg	***Adults:*** **Usual:** 1 tab q4h prn for pain. **Max:** 6 tabs/24 hrs. **Elderly:** Increase dosing interval. **Hepatic/Renal Impairment:** Reduce daily dose.	**W/P:** Drug dependence potential. Not for suicidal or addiction-prone patients. Caution with hepatic or renal impairment, elderly. **P/N:** Not for use in pregnancy, safety not known in nursing.	Dizziness, sedation, N/V, liver dysfunction.
Acetaminophen/ Propoxyphene Napsylate (Darvocet-N) CIV	**Tab:** (Propoxy-phene-APAP) 50mg-325mg, 100mg-650mg	***Adults:*** **Usual:** 100mg propoxyphene napsylate and 650mg APAP q4h prn for pain. **Max:** 600mg propoxyphene napsylate/day. **Elderly:** Increase dosing interval. **Hepatic/Renal Impairment:** Reduce daily dose.	**W/P:** Drug dependence potential. Not for suicidal or addiction-prone patients. Caution with hepatic/renal impairment, elderly. May impair mental/physical abilities. **P/N:** Not for use in pregnancy, safety not known in nursing.	Dizziness, sedation, N/V, liver dysfunction.
Propoxyphene HCl (Darvon) CIV	**Cap:** 65mg	***Adults:*** **Usual:** 65mg q4h as needed for pain. **Max:** 390mg/day. **Elderly:** Increase dosing interval. **Hepatic/ Renal Impairment:** Reduce daily dose.	**W/P:** Drug dependence potential. May impair mental/physical ability for operating machinery. Caution with hepatic or renal impairment and the elderly. Not for suicidal or addiction-prone patients. Do not exceed recommended dose. **P/N:** Not for use in pregnancy, unknown use in nursing.	Dizziness, sedation, N/V, liver dysfunction.
Propoxyphene Napsylate (Darvon-N) CIV	**Tab:** 100mg	***Adults:*** **Usual:** 100mg q4h prn pain. **Max:** 600mg/day. **Elderly:** Increase dosing interval. **Hepatic/Renal Impairment:** Reduce daily dose.	**W/P:** Avoid in suicidal or addiction-prone patients. May produce drug dependence in higher-than-recommended doses. May impair mental/physical ability. Caution with hepatic or renal impairment. Do not exceed recommended dose and limit alcohol intake. **P/N:** Safety in pregnancy and nursing not known.	Dizziness, sedation, N/V, constipation, abdominal pain, skin rashes, lightheadedness, headache, weakness, euphoria, dysphoria, hallucination.
TRAMADOL & COMBINATIONS				
Acetaminophen/ Tramadol HCl (Ultracet)	**Tab:** (Tramadol-APAP) 37.5mg-325mg	***Adults:*** 2 tabs q4-6h prn for 5 days or less. **Max:** 8 tabs/24 hrs. **CrCl <30mL/min:** **Max:** 2 tabs q12h.	**W/P:** Seizures and anaphylactic reactions reported. May complicate acute abdominal conditions. Caution with risk of respiratory depression, increased ICP, or head injury. Avoid abrupt withdrawal. Caution in elderly. Avoid use in opioid-dependent patients and with hepatic impairment. **Contra:** Acute intoxication with any of the following: alcohol, hypnotics, narcotics, centrally acting analgesics, opioids, or psychotropic drugs. **P/N:** Category C, not for use in nursing.	Constipation, diarrhea, nausea, somnolence, anorexia, increased sweating, dizziness.
Tramadol HCl (Ultram, Ultram ER)	**Tab:** 50mg*; **Tab, Extended-Release:** 100mg, 200mg, 300mg	***Adults:*** **≥17 yrs: (Tab) Initial:** 25mg qam. **Titrate:** May increase by 25mg every 3 days to 25mg qid, then may increase by 50mg every 3 days to 50mg qid. **Usual:** 50-100mg q4-6h as needed. **Max:** 400mg/day. **Elderly:** Start at low end of dosing range. **>75 yrs: Max:** 300mg/day. **CrCl <30mL/ min:** Dose q12h. **Max:** 200mg/day. **Cirrhosis:** 50mg q12h. **≥18 yrs: (Tab, ER) Initial:** 100mg qd. **Titrate:** May increase by 100mg every 5 days. **Max:** 300mg/day. **Elderly:** Start at low end of dosing range. Avoid in CrCl <30mL/min and severe hepatic impairment (Child-Pugh Class C).	**W/P:** Seizures and anaphylactoid reactions reported. Do not use in opioid-dependent patients. Caution if at risk for respiratory depression, or with increased ICP or head trauma. May complicate acute abdominal conditions. Do not d/c abruptly. Adjust dose with renal or hepatic impairment. **Contra:** Acute intoxication with any of the following: alcohol, hypnotics, narcotics, centrally acting analgesics, opioids, or psychotropic drugs. **P/N:** Category C, not for use in nursing.	Dizziness, N/V, constipation, headache, somnolence, nervousness, sweating, asthenia, dyspepsia, **dry mouth**, diarrhea, CNS stimulation, pruritus.

Table 3.1. PRESCRIBING INFORMATION FOR ANALGESICS *(cont.)*

NAME	FORM/ STRENGTH	DOSAGE	WARNINGS/PRECAUTIONS & CONTRAINDICATIONS	ADVERSE EFFECTS†
OPIOID-CONTAINING ANALGESICS *(cont.)*				
MISCELLANEOUS OPIOIDS				
Alfentanil HCl (Alfenta) CII	**Inj:** 500mcg/mL	***Adults:*** Individualize dose. **Spontaneous Breathing/Assisted Ventilation: Induction:** 8-20mcg/kg. **Maint:** 3-5mcg/kg q 5-20 min or 0.5-1mcg/kg/min. **Total:** 8-40mcg/kg. **Assisted or Controlled Ventilation: Incremental Injection: Induction:** 20-50mcg/kg. **Maint:** 5-15mcg/kg q 5-20 min. **Total:** Up to 75mcg/kg. **Continuous Infusion: Induction:** 50-75mcg/kg. **Maint:** 0.5-3mcg/kg/min (average rate 1-1.5mcg/kg/min). **Total:** Dependent on duration of procedure. **Anesthetic Induction: Induction:** 130-245 mcg/kg. **Maint:** 0.5-1.5mcg/kg/min or general anesthetic. **Total:** dependent on duration of procedure. **Monitored Anesthesia Care (MAC): Induction:** 3-8mcg/kg. **Maint:** 3-5 mcg/kg q 5-20 min or 0.25-1mcg/kg/min. **Total:** 3-40mcg/kg.	**W/P:** May cause delayed respiratory depression, respiratory arrest, bradycardia, asystole, arrhythmias, and hypotension; an opioid antagonist, resuscitative and intubation equipment and oxygen should be readily available. Use in caution with patients with head injury, increased ICP, pulmonary disease, and liver or kidney dysfunction. Initial dose of alfentanil should be appropriately reduced in elderly and debilitated patients. **P/N:** Category C, caution in nursing.	Respiratory depression, skeletal muscle rigidity, N/V, HTN, hypotension, bradycardia, tachycardia, dizziness, skeletal muscle movements, apnea, chest wall rigidity.
Fentanyl (Duragesic) CII	**Patch:** 12.5mcg/hr, 25mcg/hr, 50mcg/hr, 75mcg/hr, 100mcg/hr [5[s]]	***Adults/Pediatrics:*** **≥2 yrs:** Individualize dose. Determine dose based on opioid tolerance. **Initial:** 25mcg/hr for 72 hr.	**BB:** Life-threatening hypoventilation can occur. Contraindicated for acute or post-op pain and mild/intermittent pain. Avoid in patients <2 yrs. Only for use in opioid-tolerant patients. Concomitant use with potent CYP450 3A4 inhibitors may result in an increase in fentanyl plasma concentrations, which may cause potentially fatal respiratory depression. Monitor patients receiving potent CYP450 3A4 inhibitors. **W/P:** Monitor patients with serious adverse events for at least 24 hrs after removal. Avoid exposing application site to direct external heat. Hypoventilation may occur; caution with chronic pulmonary diseases. Caution with brain tumors, bradyarrhythmias, renal/hepatic impairment, pancreatic/biliary tract disease. Avoid with increased ICP, impaired consciousness, or coma. May obscure clinical course of head injury. Tolerance and physical dependence can occur. May impair mental/physical abilities. **Contra:** Non-opioid-tolerant patients, management of acute/post-op pain, mild/intermittent pain. Diagnosis or suspicion of paralytic ileus. Patients who have acute or severe broncial asthma, significant respiratory depression, especially in settings where there is lack of resuscitative equipment. **P/N:** Category C, not for use in nursing.	Hypoventilation, HTN, fever, N/V, constipation, **dry mouth**, somnolence, confusion, asthenia, sweating, nervousness, application site reaction, apnea, dyspnea.
Fentanyl Citrate (Actiq) CII	**Loz:** 0.2mg, 0.4mg, 0.6mg, 0.8mg, 1.2mg, 1.6mg	***Adults/Pediatrics:*** **≥16 yrs: Initial:** 0.2mg (consume over 15 min). **Titrate:** Redose 15 min after previous dose is completed. No more than 2 units per breakthrough pain episode. May increase to next highest available strength if several breakthrough episodes (1-2 days) require more than 1 unit per pain episode. Repeat titration for each new dose	**BB:** May cause life-threatening hypoventilation in opioid nontolerant patients. Only for cancer pain in opioid-tolerant patients with malignancies. Keep out of reach of children and discard properly. Concomitant use with moderate and strong CYP3A4 inhibitors may cause fatal respiratory depression. **W/P:** Caution with COPD, hepatic or renal dysfunction. Risk of clinically significant	

†Bold entries denote special dental considerations.
BB = black box warning; **W/P** = warnings/precautions; **Contra** = contraindications; **P/N** = pregnancy category rating and nursing considerations.
CII = high potential for abuse; CIII = some potential for abuse; CIV = low potential for abuse. For more information on controlled substances categories, see "How to Use This Book" on page iv.

NAME	FORM/ STRENGTH	DOSAGE	WARNINGS/PRECAUTIONS & CONTRAINDICATIONS	ADVERSE EFFECTS†
Fentanyl Citrate (Actiq) CII *(cont.)*		**Max:** 4 units/day. Prescribe 6 units with each new titration. The lozenge should be sucked, not chewed, and consumed over 15 min.	hypoventilation. Extreme caution with evidence of increased ICP or impaired consciousness. Can produce morphine-like dependence. Increased risk of dental decay; ensure proper oral hygiene. Caution with bradyarrhythmias, liver or kidney dysfunction. Patients on concomitant CNS depressants must be monitored for a change in opioid effects. May impair mental and/or physical status. **Contra:** Opioid nontolerant patients and management of acute or postoperative pain. **P/N:** Category C, not for use in nursing.	Respiratory depression, circulatory depression, headache, hypotension, shock, N/V, constipation, dizziness, dyspnea, anxiety, somnolence, **gum hemorrhage, tooth caries, tooth disorder.**
Fentanyl Citrate (Fentora) CII	**Tab, Buccal:** 100mcg, 200mcg, 400mcg, 600mcg, 800mcg	***Adults:*** **Initial: Breakthrough Pain:** 100mcg. Repeat once (30 min after starting dose) during a single pain episode. **Titration Above 100mcg:** Use two 100mcg tabs (one on each side of buccal cavity); if not controlled use two 100mcg tabs on each side (total four 100mcg tabs). **Titration Above 400mcg:** Use 200mcg tab increments. **Max:** Not more than 4 tabs simultaneously. Re-evaluate maintenance (around-the-clock) opioid dose if >4 episodes of breakthrough pain per day occurred. Do not chew, crush, swallow, or dissolve; consume over 14-25 min. Please see the PI for more information on conversion of dosage.	**BB:** Abuse liability. May cause life-threatening respiratory depression in opioid nontolerant patients. Contraindicated in the management of acute or postoperative pain. Do not use in opioid nontolerant patients. Adjust dose appropriately when converting from other oral fentanyl products. See Indications. **W/P:** Caution with concomitant use of other CNS depressants; may cause hypoventilation, hypotension, and profound sedation. Caution wtih COPD, bradyarrhythmias, and hepatic or renal impairment. May cause physical dependence, respiratory depression. Extreme caution with evidence of increased intracranial pressure or impaired consciousness. May cause paresthesia, ulceration, or bleeding at application site. **Contra:** Opioid nontolerant patients and management of acute or postoperative pain. **P/N:** Category C, not for use in nursing.	Respiratory depression, circulatory depression, headache, hypotension, shock, N/V, constipation, dizziness, dyspnea, anxiety, somnolence, **dry mouth, mouth ulceration, tooth abscess, glassodynia.**
Fentanyl Citrate (Onsolis)	**Film, Buccal:** 200mcg, 400mcg, 600mcg, 800mcg, 1200mcg	***Adults:*** **Breakthrough Pain: Initial:** 200mcg. **Titration Above 200mcg:** May titrate by using multiples of 200mcg per episode (for doses of 400mcg, 600mcg, or 800mcg) if adequate pain relief is not achieved after initiation. Do not use more than four 200-mcg films simultaneously. Do not place multiple films on top of each other; may be placed on both sides of the mouth. **Titration Above 800mcg:** Use one 1200mcg-film to treat next episode. **Max:** 1200mcg. Single doses should only be used once per episode, and should be separated by at least 2 hrs. If adequate pain relief is not achieved within 30 mins, use a rescue medication PRN. **Maint:** Once pain relief achieved with an adequate dose, treat with a single film. Re-evaluate dose if >4 episodes of breakthrough pain/day. Do not chew, swallow, cut, or tear film. Place pink side of film against inside of the cheek. Dissolves within 15-30 min; do not eat or drink until film has dissolved.	**BB:** Abuse liability. May cause life-threatening respiratory depression in opioid non-tolerant patients. Contraindicated in the management of acute or postoperative pain (eg, headache/migraine), dental pain, or use in emergency room. Do not use in opioid non-tolerant patients. Adjust dose appropriately when converting from other oral fentanyl products to avoid fatal overdose. **W/P:** Caution with concomitant use of other CNS depressants; may cause hypoventilation, hypotension, and profound sedation. Caution wtih COPD, bradyarrhythmias, and hepatic or renal impairment. May cause physical dependence, respiratory depression. Extreme caution with evidence of increased intracranial pressure or impaired consciousness. May impair physical/mental abilities. **Contra:** Opioid non-tolerant patients and management of acute or postoperative pain. **P/N:** Category C, not for use in nursing.	Respiratory depression, circulatory depression, hypotension, shock, N/V, **dry mouth,** constipation, dehydration, dizziness, dyspnea

Table 3.1. PRESCRIBING INFORMATION FOR ANALGESICS *(cont.)*

NAME	FORM/ STRENGTH	DOSAGE	WARNINGS/PRECAUTIONS & CONTRAINDICATIONS	ADVERSE EFFECTS†
OPIOID-CONTAINING ANALGESICS *(cont.)*				
MISCELLANEOUS OPIOIDS *(cont.)*				
Fentanyl Citrate (Sublimaze) CII	**Inj:** 50mcg/mL	***Adults:* ≥12 yrs:** Individualize dose. **Premedication:** 50-100mcg IM 30-60 min prior to surgery. **Adjunct to General Anesthesia: Low-Dose: Total Dose:** 2mcg/kg for minor surgery. **Maint:** 2mcg/kg. **Moderate Dose: Total Dose:** 2-20mcg/kg for major surgery. **Maint:** 2-20mcg/kg or 25-100mcg IM or IV if surgical stress or lightening of analgesia. **High-Dose: Total Dose:** 20-50mcg/kg for open heart surgery, complicated neurosurgery, or orthopedic surgery. **Maint:** 20-50mcg/kg. **Adjunct to Regional Anesthesia:** 50-100mcg IM or slow IV over 1-2 min. **Post-op:** 50-100mcg IM, repeat q 1-2 hrs as needed. **General Anesthetic:** 50-100mcg/kg with oxygen and a muscle relaxant, up to 150mcg/kg may be used. ***Pediatrics:* 2-12 yrs:** Individualize dose. **Induction/Maint:** 2-3mcg/kg.	**W/P:** Should only be administered by persons specifically trained in the use of IV anesthetics and management of the respiratory effects of potent opioids. An opioid antagonist, resuscitative and intubation equipment, and oxygen should be readily available. Fluids and other countermeasures to manage hypotension should be available with tranquilizers. Initial dose reduction recommended with narcotic analgesia for recovery. May cause muscle rigidity, particularly with muscles used for respiration. Adequate facilities should be available for postoperative monitoring and ventilation. Caution in respiratory depression susceptible patients (eg, comatose patients with head injury or brain tumor). Reduce dose for elderly and debilitated patients. Caution with obstructive pulmonary disease, decreased respiratory reserve, liver and kidney dysfunction, cardiac bradyarrhythmias. Monitor vital signs routinely. **P/N:** Category C, caution with nursing.	Respiratory depression, apnea, rigidity, bradycardia, HTN, hypotension, dizziness, blurred vision, nausea, emesis, diaphoresis, pruritus, urticaria, **laryngospasms,** anaphylaxis, euphoria, miosis, bradycardia, and bronchoconstriction.
Hydromorphone HCl (Dilaudid, Dilaudid-HP) CII	**Inj:** 1mg/mL, 2mg/mL, 4mg/mL, (HP) 10mg/mL, 250mg; **Sol:** 1mg/mL; **Sup:** 3mg; **Tab:** 2mg, 4mg, 8mg*	***Adults:*** Individualize dose. **Initial:** 1-2mg SQ/IM/IV q4-6h prn. (HP) **Range:** 1-14mg IM/SQ; adjust dose based on response. (Sol) 2.5-10mg PO q3-6h prn. (Tab) 2-4mg PO q4-6h prn. (Sup) Insert 1 PR q6-8h prn. **Titrate:** Increase dose as needed. **Elderly:** Start at lower end of dosing range.	**BB:** Contains hydromorphone, a potent Schedule II opioid agonist which has the highest potential for abuse and risk of producing respiratory depression. HP formulation is a highly concentrated solution of hydromorphone; do not confuse with standard parenteral formulations of hydromorphone or other opioids as overdose and death could result. Alcohol, other opioids, CNS depressants potentiate respiratory depressant effects, increasing risk of respiratory depression which may result in death. **W/P:** Increased respiratory depression with head injury and/or increased ICP. May mask acute abdominal conditions. Caution with elderly/debilitated, seizures, biliary tract surgery, renal/hepatic impairment, hypothyroidism, Addison's disease, BPH, and urethral stricture; initial dose should be reduced in these patients. May suppress cough reflex. Potential for physical/psychological tolerance or dependence, especially in patients with alcoholism and drug dependencies; monitor closely. Seizures reported in compromised patients receiving high doses. Dilaudid-HP should only be used in patients already receiving large doses of narcotics. 8mg tab and sol contains sulfites. **Contra:** Intracranial lesions associated with increased ICP, COPD, cor pulmonale, emphysema, kyphoscoliosis, and in status asthmaticus. (HP-Inj) Obstetrical analgesia. **P/N:** Category C, not for use in nursing.	Excessive sedation, lethargy, mental clouding, anxiety, dysphoria, N/V, constipation, urinary retention, respiratory depression. Orthostatic hypotension and fainting reported with injection.

*Scored. †Bold entries denote special dental considerations.
BB = black box warning; **W/P** = warnings/precautions; **Contra** = contraindications; **P/N** = pregnancy category rating and nursing considerations.
CII = high potential for abuse; CIII = some potential for abuse; CIV = low potential for abuse. For more information on controlled substances categories, see "How to Use This Book" on page iv.

NAME	FORM/ STRENGTH	DOSAGE	WARNINGS/PRECAUTIONS & CONTRAINDICATIONS	ADVERSE EFFECTS†
Meperidine HCl (Demerol Injection) CII	**Inj:** 25mg/mL, 50mg/mL, 75mg/mL, 100mg/mL	***Adults:*** **Pain: Usual:** 50-150mg IM/SQ q3-4h prn. **Preoperative: Usual:** 50-100mg IM/SQ 30-90 min before anesthesia. **Anesthesia Support:** Use repeated slow IV inj of fractional doses (eg, 10mg/mL) or continuous IV infusion of a more dilute solution (eg, 1mg/mL). Titrate as needed. **Obstetrical Analgesia: Usual:** 50-100mg IM/SQ when pain is regular, may repeat at 1- to 3-hr intervals. **With Phenothiazines/ Other Tranquilizers:** Reduce dose by 25 to 50%. IM method preferred with repeated use. For IV injection: Reduce dose and administer slowly, preferably using diluted solution. **Elderly:** Start at lower end of dosage range and observe. ***Pediatrics:*** **Pain: Usual:** 0.5-0.8mg/lb IM/SQ, up to 50-150mg, q3-4h prn. **Preoperative: Usual:** 0.5-1mg/lb IM/SQ, up to 50-100mg, 30-90 min before anesthesia. **With Phenothiazines/Other Tranquilizers:** Reduce dose by 25 to 50%. IM method preferred with repeated use. **For IV injection:** Reduce dose and administer slowly, preferably using diluted solution.	**W/P:** May develop tolerance and dependence; abuse potential. Extreme caution with head injury, increased ICP, intracranial lesions, acute asthmatic attack, chronic COPD or cor pulmonale, decreased respiratory reserve, respiratory depression, hypoxia, and hypercapnia. Rapid IV infusion may result in increased adverse reactions. Caution with acute abdominal conditions, atrial flutter, supraventricular tachycardias. May aggravate convulsive disorders. Caution and reduce initial dose with elderly or debilitated, renal/hepatic impairment, hypothyroidism, Addison's disease, prostatic hypertrophy, or urethral stricture. Severe hypotension may occur post-op or if depleted blood volume. Orthostatic hypotension may occur. May impair mental/physical abilities. Not for use in pregnancy prior to labor. May produce depression of respiration and psychophysiologic functions in newborn when used as an obstetrical analgesic. **Contra:** MAOIs during or within 14 days of use. **P/N:** Safety in pregnancy and nursing not known.	Lightheadedness, dizziness, sedation, N/V, sweating, respiratory/ circulatory depression.
Meperidine HCl (Demerol Oral) CII	**Syrup:** 50mg/ 5mL; **Tab:** 50mg*, 100mg*	***Adults:*** **Usual:** 50-150mg q3-4h prn. **Concomitant Phenothiazines/ Other Tranquilizers:** Reduce dose by 25-50%. Dilute syrup in 1/2 glass of water. ***Pediatrics:*** **Usual:** 1.1-1.8mg/kg up to 50-150mg q3-4h prn. **Concomitant Phenothiazines/ Other Tranquilizers:** Reduce dose by 25-50%. Dilute syrup in 1/2 glass of water.	**W/P:** May develop tolerance and dependence; abuse potential. Extreme caution with head injury, increased ICP, intracranial lesions, acute asthma attack, chronic COPD, cor pulmonale, decreased respiratory reserve, respiratory depression, hypoxia, and hypercapnia. Caution with sickle cell anemia, pheochromocytoma, acute alcoholism, Addison's disease, CNS depression or coma, delirium tremens, elderly or debilitated, kyphoscoliosis associated with respiratory depression, myxedema, hypothyroidism, acute abdominal conditions, epilepsy, atrial flutter, other supraventricular tachycardias, renal/ hepatic impairment, prostatic hypertrophy, urethral stricture, drug dependencies, neonates, and young infants. Severe hypotension may occur post-op or if depleted blood volume. Orthostatic hypotension may occur. Not for use in pregnancy prior to labor. **Contra:** MAOI during or within 14 days of use. **P/N:** Category C, not for use in nursing.	Lightheadedness, dizziness, sedation, N/V, sweating, respiratory depression.
Meperidine HCl/ Promethazine HCl (Meprozine) CII	**Cap:** (Meperidine-Promethazine) 50mg-25mg	***Adults:*** 1 cap q4-6h prn.	**W/P:** May cause tolerance and dependence; potential for abuse. Extreme caution with head injury, increased ICP, intracranial lesions, acute asthma, COPD, cor pulmonale, decreased respiratory reserve, respiratory depression, hypoxia, hypercapnia. Severe hypotension may occur with depleted blood volume. Orthostatic hypotension may occur. Caution with atrial flutter and other supraventricular tachycardias. May obscure diagnosis or clinical course of acute abdominal conditions. Reduce initial dose in elderly, debilitated,	Lightheadedness, dizziness, sedation, N/V, sweating.

Table 3.1. PRESCRIBING INFORMATION FOR ANALGESICS *(cont.)*

NAME	FORM/ STRENGTH	DOSAGE	WARNINGS/PRECAUTIONS & CONTRAINDICATIONS	ADVERSE EFFECTS†
OPIOID-CONTAINING ANALGESICS *(cont.)*				
MISCELLANEOUS OPIOIDS *(cont.)*				
Meperidine HCl/ Promethazine HCl (Meprozine) CII *(cont.)*			severe hepatic or renal dysfunction, hypothyroidism, Addison's disease, prostatic hypertrophy, urethral stricture. May aggravate seizure disorders. Not for use in pregnant women prior to labor. **Contra:** During or within 14 days of MAOIs. **P/N:** Safety in pregnancy and nursing not known.	
Methadone HCl (Dolophine) CII	**Tab:** 5mg, 10mg	***Adults:*** **Detoxification: Initial:** 15-20mg/day (up to 40mg/day may be required). Stabilize for 2-3 days, then may decrease every 1-2 days depending on patient symptoms. **Max:** 21 days. May not repeat earlier than 4 weeks after completing previous course. **Pain: Usual:** 2.5-10mg q3-4h PO/IM/SQ prn.	**BB:** Only approved hospitals and pharmacies can dispense oral methadone for the treatment of narcotic addiction. Methadone can be dispensed in any licensed pharmacy when used as an analgesic. Deaths, cardiac and respiratory, have been reported during initiation and conversion of pain patients to methadone treatment from treatment with other opioid agonists. Respiratory depression is the main hazard associated with methadone administration. QT interval prolongation and serious arrhythmias have been observed during treatment with methadone. **W/P:** Do not inject agent. Extreme caution with use of narcotic antagonists in patients physically dependent on narcotics. Can cause respiratory depression and elevate CSF pressure. Caution with head injuries, acute asthma attacks, COPD, cor pulmonale, decreased respiratory reserve, pre-existing respiratory depression, hypoxia, or hypercapnia. Reduce initial dose in elderly, debilitated, severe hepatic or renal impairment, hypothyroidism, Addison's disease, prostatic hypertrophy, or urethral stricture. Risk of tolerance, dependence, and abuse may occur. Impairs physical and mental abilities. Ineffective in relieving anxiety. May mask symptoms of acute abdominal conditions. May produce hypotension. May cause incomplete cross-tolerance and iatrogenic overdose, interactions with other CNS depressants, alcohol, and other drugs of abuse. May cause cardiac conduction effects like prolonged QT interval and serious arrhythmias. **Contra:** Methadone is contraindicated in any patient suspected or having a paralytic ileus, acute bronchial asthma or hypercarbia and respiratory depression. **P/N:** Safety in pregnancy and nursing not known.	Lightheadedness, dizziness, sedation, sweating, N/V, asthenia, cardiomyopathy, ECG abnormalities, abdominal pain, agitation, seizures, confusion, hallucinations, respiratory depression.
Methadone HCl (Methadose) CII	**Oral Concentrate:** 10mg/mL; **Tab:** 5mg, 10mg, 40mg; **Tab, Dispersible:** 40mg	***Adults:*** **Detoxification: Initial/ Induction:** 20-30mg/day. Give 5-10mg 2-4 hrs later if needed. **Max:** 40mg on first day. Adjust dose to control withdrawal symptoms over 1st week. Stabilize for 2-3 days, then may decrease every 1-2 days depending on symptoms. **Maintenance:** Titrate to a dose at which symptoms prevented for 24 hrs. **Usual:** 80-120mg/day. **Pain in**	**BB:** Deaths, cardiac and respiratory, reported during initiation and conversion from other opioid agonists. Respiratory depression and QT prolongation observed. Only certified/approved opioid treatment programs can dispense oral methadone for treatment of narcotic addiction. Use as analgesic should be initiated only if benefits outweigh risks. **W/P:** Do not inject agent. Extreme caution with use of narcotic antagonists	Lightheadedness, dizziness, sedation, sweating, N/V.

†Bold entries denote special dental considerations.
BB = black box warning; **W/P** = warnings/precautions; **Contra** = contraindications; **P/N** = pregnancy category rating and nursing considerations.
CII = high potential for abuse; CIII = some potential for abuse; CIV = low potential for abuse. For more information on controlled substances categories, see "How to Use This Book" on page iv.

NAME	FORM/ STRENGTH	DOSAGE	WARNINGS/PRECAUTIONS & CONTRAINDICATIONS	ADVERSE EFFECTS†
Methadone HCl (Methadose) CII *(cont.)*		**Opioid Nontolerant: Usual:** 2.5-10mg q8-12h, slowly titrated to effect. **Conversion From Parenteral: Initial:** Use a 1:2 dose ratio, parenteral to oral. **Switching From Other Chronic Opioids:** Use caution; see PI for dosing details.	in patients physically dependent on narcotics. Can cause respiratory depression and elevate CSF pressure. Caution with head injuries, acute asthma attacks, COPD, cor pulmonale, decreased respiratory reserve, pre-existing respiratory depression, hypoxia, or hypercapnia. Reduce initial dose in elderly, debilitated, severe hepatic or renal impairment, hypothyroidism, Addison's disease, prostatic hypertrophy, or urethral stricture. Risk of tolerance, dependence, and abuse may occur. Impairs physical and mental abilities. Ineffective in relieving anxiety. May mask symptoms of acute abdominal conditions. May produce hypotension. **Contra:** Respiratory depression. Acute bronchial asthma or hypercarbia. Paralytic ileus. **P/N:** Category C, not for use in nursing.	
Morphine Sulfate (Astramorph PF) CII	**Inj:** 0.5mg/mL, 1mg/mL	***Adults:* IV: Initial:** 2-10mg/70kg. **Epidural Injection: Initial:** 5mg in lumbar region. **Titrate:** If inadequate pain relief within 1 hr, increase by 1-2mg. **Max:** 10mg/24hrs. **Continuous Epidural: Initial:** 2-4mg/24hrs. Give additional 1-2mg if needed. **Intrathecal:** 0.2-1mg single dose, do not repeat; may follow with 0.6mg/hr naloxone infusion to reduce incidence of side effects. **Elderly/ Debilitated: Epidural:** <5mg/24hrs. **Intrathecal:** Lower dose.	**W/P:** Have resuscitation equipment, trained personnel, and narcotic antagonists available; severe respiratory depression may occur. Avoid rapid administration. May be habit-forming. Caution with head injury, increased intracranial/intraocular pressure, decreased respiratory reserve, hepatic/ renal dysfunction, elderly, debilitated. High doses may cause seizures. Smooth muscle hypertonicity may cause biliary colic, urinary difficulty or retention. Orthostatic hypotension may occur with hypovolemia or myocardial dysfunction. Acute respiratory failure reported with COPD or acute asthmatic attack. Limit epidural/intrathecal route to lumbar area. **Contra:** Allergy to opiates, acute bronchial asthma, upper airway obstruction. Epidural/intrathecal routes with injection site infection, anticoagulants, bleeding diathesis, within 2 weeks of IV corticosteroids. **P/N:** Category C, safety in nursing not known.	Respiratory depression, hypotension, pruritus, urinary retention, N/V, constipation, anxiety, **cough reflex depression**, oliguria.
Morphine Sulfate (Avinza) CII	**Cap, Extended-Release:** 30mg, 60mg, 90mg, 120mg	***Adults:* ≥18 yrs: Conversion from Other Oral Morphine Products:** Give total daily morphine dose as a single dose q24h. **Conversion from Parenteral Morphine: Initial:** Give about 3x the previous daily parenteral morphine requirement. **Conversion from Other Parenteral or Oral Non-Morphine Opioids: Initial:** Give 1/2 of estimated daily morphine requirement q24h. Supplement with immediate-release morphine or short-acting analgesics if needed. **Titrate:** Adjust dose as frequently as every other day. **Non-Opioid Tolerant:** 30mg q24h. **Titrate:** Increase by increments ≤30mg every 4 days. The 60, 90, and 120mg caps are for opioid-tolerant patients. **Max:** 1600mg/day. Doses >1600mg/day contain a quantity of fumaric acid, which may cause renal toxicity.	**BB:** Swallow capsules whole or sprinkle contents on applesauce. Do not crush, chew, or dissolve capsule beads. Avoid alcohol and alcohol-containing medications; consumption of alcohol may result in the rapid release and absorption of potentially fatal dose of morphine. **W/P:** Abuse potential. Extreme caution with COPD, cor pulmonale, decreased respiratory reserve (eg, severe kyphoscoliosis), hypoxia, hypercapnia, pre-existing respiratory depression, increased ICP, head injury. May cause orthostatic hypotension, syncope, severe hypotension with depleted blood volume. Caution with circulatory shock, biliary tract disease, severe renal/ hepatic insufficiency, Addison's disease, hypothyroidism, prostatic hypertrophy, urethral stricture, elderly or debilitated, CNS depression, toxic psychosis, acute alcoholism, delirium tremens, seizure	Constipation, N/V, somnolence, dehydration, headache, peripheral edema, diarrhea, abdominal pain, infection, UTI, flu syndrome, back pain, rash, sweating, fever, insomnia, depression, paresthesia, anorexia, **dry mouth**, asthenia, dyspnea.

Table 3.1. PRESCRIBING INFORMATION FOR ANALGESICS *(cont.)*

NAME	FORM/ STRENGTH	DOSAGE	WARNINGS/PRECAUTIONS & CONTRAINDICATIONS	ADVERSE EFFECTS†
OPIOID-CONTAINING ANALGESICS *(cont.)*				
MISCELLANEOUS OPIOIDS *(cont.)*				
Morphine Sulfate (Avinza) CII *(cont.)*			disorders. Avoid with GI obstruction. Withdrawal symptoms with abrupt discontinuation. Tolerance and physical dependence may develop. Potential for severe constipation; use laxatives, stool softeners at onset of therapy. **Contra:** Respiratory depression in the absence of resuscitative equipment, acute or severe bronchial asthma, paralytic ileus. **P/N:** Category C, not for use in nursing.	
Morphine Sulfate (Duramorph) CII	**Inj:** 0.5mg/mL, 1mg/mL, 5mg/mL	***Adults:* IV: Initial:** 2-10mg/70kg. **Epidural Injection: Initial:** 5mg in lumbar region. **Titrate:** If inadequate pain relief within 1 hr, increase by 1-2mg. **Max:** 10mg/24hrs. **Continuous Epidural: Initial:** 2-4mg/24hrs. Give additional 1-2mg if needed. **Intrathecal:** 0.2-1mg single dose, do not repeat; may follow with 0.6mg/hr naloxone infusion to reduce incidence of side effects.	**W/P:** Have resuscitation equipment, oxygen, and antidote (eg, naloxone) available; severe respiratory depression may occur. Avoid rapid administration. May be habit-forming. Caution with head injury, increased intracranial/intraocular pressure, decreased respiratory reserve, hepatic/renal dysfunction, elderly, debilitated. High doses may cause seizures. Smooth muscle hypertonicity may cause biliary colic, urinary difficulty or retention. Orthostatic hypotension may occur with hypovolemia or myocardial dysfunction. Acute respiratory failure reported with COPD or acute asthmatic attack. Limit epidural/intrathecal route to lumbar area. **Contra:** Allergy to opiates, acute bronchial asthma, upper airway obstruction. Severe hypotension may occur in volume-depleted patients or with concurrent administration of phenothiazines or general anesthetics. **P/N:** Category C, safety in nursing not known.	Respiratory depression, convulsions, dysphoric reactions, pruritus, urinary retention, constipation, lumbar puncture-type headache, toxic psychoses.
Morphine Sulfate (Infumorph) CII	**Inj:** 10mg/mL (200mg), 25mg/mL (500mg)	***Adults:* Lumbar Intrathecal: Opioid Intolerant:** 0.2-1mg/day. **Opioid Tolerant:** 1-10mg/day. **Max:** Must be individualized. Caution with >20mg/day. **Epidural: Opioid Intolerant:** 3.5-7.5mg/day. **Opioid Tolerant:** 4.5-10mg/day. May increase to 20-30mg/day. **Max:** Must be individualized. Starting dose must be based on in-hospital evaluation of response to serial single-dose intrathecal/epidural bolus injections of regular morphine sulfate.	**W/P:** Have resuscitation equipment, oxygen, and antidote (eg, naloxone) available; severe respiratory depression may occur. Use only if less invasive means of controlling pain fail. Not for single-dose IV, IM, or SQ administration. May be habit-forming. Observe patient for 24 hours following test dose, and for 1st several days after catheter implantation. Caution with determining refill frequency. Make sure needle is properly placed in the filling port of device. Myoclonic-like spasm of the lower extremities reported if dose >20mg/day; may need detoxification. Caution with head injury, increased ICP, decreased respiratory reserve, hepatic/renal dysfunction (epidural injection), elderly. Avoid with chronic asthma, upper airway obstruction, other chronic pulmonary disorders. Biliary colic reported. May cause micturition disturbances, especially with BPH. Increased risk of orthostatic hypotension with reduced circulating blood volume and impaired myocardial function. Avoid abrupt withdrawal. Risk of withdrawal in patients maintained on parenteral/oral narcotics.	Respiratory depression, myoclonus convulsions, dysphoric reactions, pruritus, urinary retention, constipation, lumbar puncture-type headache, peripheral edema, orthostatic hypotension.

*Scored. †Bold entries denote special dental considerations.
BB = black box warning; **W/P** = warnings/precautions; **Contra** = contraindications; **P/N** = pregnancy category rating and nursing considerations.
CII = high potential for abuse; CIII = some potential for abuse; CIV = low potential for abuse. For more information on controlled substances categories, see "How to Use This Book" on page iv.

NAME	FORM/ STRENGTH	DOSAGE	WARNINGS/PRECAUTIONS & CONTRAINDICATIONS	ADVERSE EFFECTS†
Morphine Sulfate (Infumorph) CII *(cont.)*			Not for routine use in obstetric labor/ delivery. **Contra:** For neuraxial analgesia: Infection at injection site, anticoagulants, uncontrolled bleeding diathesis, any therapy or condition that may render intrathecal or epidural administration hazardous. **P/N:** Category C, safety in nursing not known.	
Morphine Sulfate (Kadian) CII	**Cap, Extended-Release:** 10mg, 20mg, 30mg, 50mg, 60mg, 80mg, 100mg, 200mg	***Adults:*** Individualize dose. **Conversion from Other Oral Morphine:** Give 50% of daily oral morphine dose q12h or give 100% oral morphine dose q24h. Do not give more frequently than q12h. **Conversion from Parenteral Morphine:** Oral morphine 3x the daily parenteral morphine dose may be sufficient in chronic-use settings. **Conversion from Other Parenteral or Oral Opioids: Initial:** Give 50% of estimated daily morphine demand and supplement with immediate-release morphine. May sprinkle contents on small amount of applesauce or in water for gastrostomy tube. Do not chew, crush, or dissolve pellets. Avoid administration through NG-tube.	**BB:** Contains morphine sulfate, an opioid agonist and Schedule II controlled substance, with an abuse liability similar to other opioid analgesics. Indicated for management of moderate-to-severe pain when a continuous, around-the-clock opioid analgesic is needed for an extended period of time. Not for use as a prn analgesic. The 100mg and 200mg capsules are for use in opioid-tolerant patients only. Swallow capsules whole or sprinkle contents on applesauce. Do not crush, chew, or dissolve pellets in capsules. **W/P:** Respiratory depression possible; caution in COPD, cor pulmonale, decreased respiratory reserve. May obscure neurologic signs in head injuries, intracranial lesions, or a pre-existing increase in ICP. May cause severe hypotension. Avoid with GI obstruction. Caution in biliary tract disease, elderly, debilitated, renal/hepatic insufficiency, Addison's disease, myxedema, hypothyroidism, prostatic hypertrophy, urethral stricture, CNS depression, toxic psychosis, acute alcoholism, delirium tremens, and convulsive disorders. Depresses cough reflex. Decreases gastric, biliary, and pancreatic secretions. D/C 24 hrs before procedure that interrupts pain transmission pathways (eg, cordotomy); give short-acting parenteral opioid. **Contra:** Respiratory depression in the absence of resuscitative equipment, acute or severe bronchial asthma, paralytic ileus. **P/N:** Category C, not for use in nursing.	Drowsiness, dizziness, constipation, nausea, anxiety.
Morphine Sulfate CII	**Sol:** 10mg/5mL, 20mg/5mL [100mL, 500mL]; **Tab:** 15mg*, 30mg*	***Adults:*** (Sol) 10-20mg q4h. (Tab) 15-30mg q4h.	**W/P:** May cause tolerance, psychological/ physical dependence; avoid abrupt withdrawal. Caution with head injury, increased ICP, acute asthma attack, chronic COPD or cor pulmonale, decreased respiratory reserve, pre-existing respiratory depression, hypoxia, hypercapnia, elderly, debilitated, severe hepatic/renal impairment, hypothyroidism, Addison's disease, prostatic hypertrophy, or urethral stricture. May cause severe hypotension. May obscure diagnosis or clinical course with abdominal conditions. May impair mental/ physical abilities. **Contra:** Respiratory insufficiency or depression, severe CNS depression, attack of bronchial asthma, heart failure secondary to chronic lung disease, cardiac arrhythmias, increased ICP or CSF pressure, head injuries, brain tumor, acute alcoholism, delirium tremens, convulsive disorders, after biliary tract surgery, suspected surgical abdomen, surgical anastomosis, concomitantly with MAOIs or within 14 days of such treatment. **P/N:** Category C, caution in nursing.	Respiratory depression, lightheadedness, dizziness, sedation, N/V, sweating.

Table 3.1. PRESCRIBING INFORMATION FOR ANALGESICS *(cont.)*

NAME	FORM/ STRENGTH	DOSAGE	WARNINGS/PRECAUTIONS & CONTRAINDICATIONS	ADVERSE EFFECTS†
OPIOID-CONTAINING ANALGESICS *(cont.)*				
MISCELLANEOUS OPIOIDS *(cont.)*				
Morphine Sulfate (MS Contin) CII	**Tab, Extended-Release:** 15mg, 30mg, 60mg, 100mg, 200mg	***Adults:* Conversion from Immediate-Release Oral Morphine:** Give 1/2 of patient's 24-hr requirement as MS Contin q12h or give 1/3 of daily requirement as MS Contin q8h. **Conversion from Parenteral Morphine: Initial:** If daily morphine dose ≤120mg/day, give MS Contin 30mg. **Titrate:** Switch to 60mg or 100mg MS Contin. Swallow whole; do not crush, chew, or break. Taper dose; do not d/c abruptly.	**BB:** Contains morphine sulfate with an abuse liability similar to other opioid analgesics. Not intended for use as a prn analgesic. MS Contin 100mg and 200mg tablets are for use in opioid-tolerant patients only. Tablets are to be swallowed whole; do not break, crush, chew, or dissolve. **W/P:** Extreme caution with COPD, cor pulmonale, decreased respiratory reserve, hypoxia, hypercapnia, respiratory depression. Caution with elderly, debilitated, head injury, increased ICP, circulatory shock, severe hepatic/renal/pulmonary dysfunction, myxedema, hypothyroidism, adrenocortical insufficiency, CNS depression, coma, toxic psychosis, prostatic hypertrophy, urethral stricture, alcoholism, delirium tremens, kyphoscoliosis, inability to swallow, convulsive disorder, acute abdominal problems, biliary tract surgery, acute pancreatitis secondary to biliary tract disease. May cause hypotension and drug dependence. Reserve 200mg tabs for opioid-tolerant patients requiring ≥400mg/day of morphine. May cause neonatal withdrawal syndrome. **Contra:** Paralytic ileus, respiratory depression in the absence of resuscitative equipment, acute or severe bronchial asthma. **P/N:** Category C, not for use in nursing.	Constipation, lightheadedness, dizziness, sedation, N/V, sweating, dysphoria, euphoria, respiratory depression.
Morphine Sulfate (Oramorph SR) CII	**Tab, Extended-Release:** 15mg, 30mg, 60mg, 100mg	***Adults:* Conversion from Parenteral or Immediate Release Oral Morphine:** Daily dose determined by daily requirement of immediate-release formulation. Single dose is 1/2 of daily requirement given q12h. **Initial:** 30mg is recommended if daily morphine requirement is ≤120mg. Use 15mg for low daily morphine requirements. **Titrate:** Increase to 60mg or 100mg after stable dose reached.	**BB:** This is a sustained-release tablet. Swallow tab whole; do not break in half, crush, or chew. **W/P:** Not for initial treatment. Caution with hepatic and renal dysfunction, increased ICP or with head injury, decreased respiratory reserve (eg, emphysema, severe obesity, kyphoscoliosis, or paralysis of the phrenic nerve), chronic asthma, upper airway obstruction, or in other chronic pulmonary disorders. Tolerance, psychological and physical dependence may develop. Avoid abrupt discontinuation. Not for pediatrics or use in women during or immediately before labor. **Contra:** Respiratory depression in the absence of resuscitative equipment, acute or severe bronchial asthma, paralytic ileus. **P/N:** Category C, not for use in nursing.	Constipation, N/V, dizziness, sedation, dysphoria, euphoria, sweating, respiratory depression.
Morphine Sulfate (Roxanol, Roxanol-T) CII	**Sol, Concentrate:** 20mg/mL (Roxanol) [30mL, 120mL, 240mL], (Roxanol-T) [30mL, 120mL]	***Adults:* Usual:** 10-30mg q4h. During first effective pain relief, dose should be maintained for at least 3 days before any dose reduction, if respiratory activity and other vital signs are adequate. **Elderly/Very Ill/ Respiratory Problems/Severe Renal and Hepatic Impairment:** Lower doses may be required.	**BB:** Highly concentrated, check dose carefully. **W/P:** May cause tolerance, psychological, and physical dependence; withdrawal may occur on abrupt discontinuation. Caution with head injury, increased ICP, acute asthmatic attack, COPD, cor pulmonale, decreased respiratory reserve, pre-existing respiratory depression, hypoxia, hypercapnia, elderly, debilitated, severe hepatic/renal impairment, hypothyroidism, Addison's disease, prostatic hypertrophy, or urethral	Respiratory depression, lightheadedness, dizziness, sedation, N/V, sweating, constipation.

†Bold entries denote special dental considerations.
BB = black box warning; **W/P** = warnings/precautions; **Contra** = contraindications; **P/N** = pregnancy category rating and nursing considerations.
CII = high potential for abuse; CIII = some potential for abuse; CIV = low potential for abuse. For more information on controlled substances categories, see "How to Use This Book" on page iv.

NAME	FORM/ STRENGTH	DOSAGE	WARNINGS/PRECAUTIONS & CONTRAINDICATIONS	ADVERSE EFFECTS†
Morphine Sulfate (Roxanol, Roxanol-T) CII *(cont.)*			stricture. May cause orthostatic hypotension in ambulatory patients, severe hypotension with depleted blood volume. May obscure diagnosis/clinical course of acute abdominal conditions. May impair mental/physical abilities. **Contra:** respiratory insufficiency or depression, severe CNS depression, attack of bronchial asthma, heart failure secondary to chronic lung disease, cardiac arrhythmias, increased intracranial or cerebrospinal pressure, head injuries, brain tumor, acute alcoholism, delirium tremens, convulsive disorders, after biliary tract surgery, suspected surgical abdomen, surgical anastomosis, concomitantly with MAOIs or within 14 days of such treatment. **P/N:** Category C, caution in nursing.	
Oxymorphone HCl (Opana, Opana ER) CII	**Tab:** (Opana) 5mg, 10mg; **Tab, Extended-Release:** (Opana ER) 5mg, 7.5mg, 10mg, 15mg, 20mg, 30mg, 40mg	***Adults:*** Individualize dose. **Opana: Opioid-Naive: Initial:** 5-20mg q4-6h. Titrate based on response. **Max:** 20mg/dose. **Conversion from Parenteral Oxymorphone:** Give 10x total daily parenteral oxymorphone dose in 4 or 6 equally divided doses. **Conversion from Other Oral Opioids:** Give half of calculated total daily dose in 4-6 equally divided doses, q4-6h. **Opana ER:** Swallow whole; do not break, chew, crush, or dissolve. **Opioid-Naive: Initial:** 5mg q12h. Titrate based on response. **Usual:** Increase dose by 5-10mg q12h every 3-7 days. **Conversion from Opana:** Divide 24h Opana dose in half to obtain q12h dose. **Conversion from Parenteral Oxymorphone:** Give 10x total daily parenteral oxymorphone dose in 2 equally divided doses. **Conversion from Other Oral Opioids:** Divide calculated 24h Opana dose (refer to PI for conversion ratios) in half to obtain q12h dose. **Mild Hepatic Impairment or Renal Impairment (CrCl <50mL/min):** Start with lowest dose and titrate slowly while carefully monitoring side effects. **With CNS Depressants:** Start at 1/3 to 1/2 of usual dose. **Elderly:** Start at lower end of dosing range.	**BB:** (Opana ER) Abuse liability and potential. For continuous analgesia only; not intended for prn use. To be swallowed whole; not to be broken, chewed, dissolved, or crushed. Must not be taken with alcohol. **W/P:** Schedule II controlled substance with abuse liability. May have additive effects in conjunction with alcohol, other opioids, or illicit drugs that cause CNS depression; respiratory depression, hypotension, and profound sedation or coma may result. Extreme caution with hypoxia, hypercapnia, or decreased respiratory reserve. With head injury, intracranial lesions, or a preexisting increase in ICP, possible respiratory depressant effects and potential to elevate CSF pressure may be markedly exaggerated; effects on pupillary response and consciousness may obscure neurologic signs of further increases in ICP with head injuries. May cause severe hypotension with compromised ability to maintain BP due to depleted blood volume. Caution in elderly or debilitated patients sensitive to CNS depressants. Caution with circulatory shock, acute alcoholism, adrenocortical insufficiency (eg, Addison's disease), CNS depression or coma, delirium tremens, kyphoscoliosis associated with respiratory depression, myxedema or hypothyroidism, prostatic hypertrophy or urethral stricture, severe impairment of pulmonary or renal function, mild/moderate hepatic impairment, and toxic psychosis. May aggravate convulsions with convulsive disorders; may induce or aggravate seizures in some clinical settings. Monitor for decreased bowel motility in post-op patients. May cause spasm of the sphincter of Oddi; caution with biliary tract disease (including acute pancreatitis). May produce tolerance and dependence. Should not abruptly d/c, may cause abstinence syndrome in physically dependent patients. **Contra:** Respiratory depression (except in monitored settings with resuscitative equipment), acute/severe bronchial asthma or hypercarbia, paralytic ileus, moderate/severe hepatic impairment. (Opana ER) Not indicated for pain in	Constipation, N/V, pyrexia, somnolence, headache, dizziness, pruritus, increased sweating, **xerostomia**, sedation, diarrhea, insomnia, fatigue, tachycardia, miosis, biliary colic, hypotension.

Table 3.1. PRESCRIBING INFORMATION FOR ANALGESICS *(cont.)*

NAME	FORM/ STRENGTH	DOSAGE	WARNINGS/PRECAUTIONS & CONTRAINDICATIONS	ADVERSE EFFECTS†
OPIOID-CONTAINING ANALGESICS *(cont.)*				
MISCELLANEOUS OPIOIDS *(cont.)*				
Oxymorphone HCl (Opana, Opana ER) CII *(cont.)*			immediate post-operative period (12-24 hrs following surgery) for patients not previously taking opioids or, if the pain is mild or not expected to persist for extended period of time. **P/N:** Category C, caution with nursing.	
Remifentanil HCl (Ultiva) CII	**Inj:** 1mg, 2mg, 5mg	***Adults:* Continuous IV Infusion: Induction**: 0.5-1mcg/kg/min. **Maint:** 0.4mcg/kg with nitrous oxide 66%; 0.25mcg/kg with isoflurane (0.4 1.25 MAC); 0.25 with propofol (100-200mcg/kg/min). **Post-Op Continuation:** 0.1mcg/kg/min. **CABG: Induction/Maint/Continuation:** 1mcg/kg/min. **Elderly (>65 yrs):** Use 50% of adult dose. Titrate carefully. ***Pediatrics:* Anesthesia Maint: Continuous IV Infusion:** 1-12 yrs: 0.25mcg/kg/min with halothane (0.3-1.5 MAC), sevoflurane (0.3-1.5 MAC), or isoflurane (0.4-1.5 MAC). **Range:** 0.05-1.3mcg/kg/min. **Birth-2 months:** 0.4mcg/kg/min. **Range:** 0.4-1mcg/kg/min.	**W/P:** Administer only with infusion device. IV bolus administration should be used only during the maintenance of general anesthesia. Interruption of infusion will result in rapid offset of effect. Use associated with apnea and respiratory depression. Not for use in diagnostic or therapeutic procedures outside the monitored anesthesia care setting. Resuscitative and intubation equipment, oxygen, and opioid antagonist must be readily available. May cause skeletal muscle rigidity and is related to the dose and speed of administration. Do not administer into the same IV tubing with blood due to potential inactivation by nonspecific esterases in blood products. Continuously monitor vital signs and oxygenation. Bradycardia, hypotension, intraoperative awareness reported. Not recommended as sole agent for induction of anesthesia. **Contra:** Epidural or intrathecal administration, hypersensitivity to fentanyl analogs. **P/N:** Category C, caution in nursing.	N/V, hypotension, muscle rigidity, bradycardia, shivering, fever, dizziness, visual disturbances, respiratory depression, apnea.
OPIOID AGONIST-ANTAGONISTS				
Butorphanol Tartrate (Stadol NS) CIV	**Nasal Spray:** 10mg/mL [2.5mL]	***Adults:* ≥18 yrs: Initial:** 1 spray (1mg) in 1 nostril, may repeat after 60-90 min (after 90-120 min in elderly or renal/hepatic disease) and may repeat in 3-4 hrs after 2nd dose; or may use 1 spray in each nostril, may repeat after 3-4 hrs. **Renal/ Hepatic Disease:** Increase dose interval to no less than 6 hrs.	**W/P:** Not for use in narcotic-dependent patients. May result in physical dependence or tolerance. Avoid abrupt cessation. D/C if severe HTN occurs. Caution with hepatic or renal disease, acute MI, ventricular dysfunction, or coronary insufficiency. May impair ability to operate machinery. Increased respiratory depression with CNS disease or respiratory impairment. Severe risks with head injury. **Contra:** Hypersensitivity to benzethonium chloride. **P/N:** Category C, caution in nursing.	Somnolence, dizziness, N/V, nasal congestion, insomnia.
Nalbuphine HCl	**Inj:** 10mg/mL, 20mg/mL	***Adults:* Pain: Initial:** 10mg/70kg IV/IM/SQ q3-6h prn. Adjust according to severity, physical status, and concomitant agents. **Max:** 20mg/dose or 160mg/day. **Anesthesia Adjunct:** Induction: 0.3-3mg/kg IV over 10-15 min. **Maint:** 0.25-0.5mg/kg IV.	**W/P:** Increased risk of respiratory depression with head injury, intracranial lesions, or pre-existing increased ICP. Only for use by specially trained persons. Naloxone, resuscitative and intubation equipment, and oxygen should be readily available. Caution with emotionally unstable patients, narcotic abuse, impaired respiration, MI with nausea and vomiting, biliary tract surgery. May impair ability to drive or operate machinery. Caution with renal or hepatic dysfunction; reduce dose. Caution during labor and delivery; monitor newborns for respiratory depression, apnea, bradycardia, and arrhythmias. **P/N:** Category B, caution in nursing.	Sedation, sweating, N/V, dizziness/vertigo, **dry mouth,** headache, injection-site reactions.

*Scored. †Bold entries denote special dental considerations.

BB = black box warning; **W/P** = warnings/precautions; **Contra** = contraindications; **P/N** = pregnancy category rating and nursing considerations.

CII = high potential for abuse; CIII = some potential for abuse; CIV = low potential for abuse. For more information on controlled substances categories, see "How to Use This Book" on page iv.

NAME	FORM/ STRENGTH	DOSAGE	WARNINGS/PRECAUTIONS & CONTRAINDICATIONS	ADVERSE EFFECTS†
Pentazocine HCl/ Acetaminophen (Talacen) CIV	**Tab:** (Pentazocine-APAP) 25mg-650mg*	***Adults:*** 1 tab q4h prn. **Max:** 6 tabs/day.	**W/P:** Contains sodium metabisulfite. Caution with head injury, increased ICP, acute CNS manifestations, MI, certain respiratory conditions, renal/hepatic dysfunction, biliary surgery, seizure disorders, and alcohol use. Potential for physical and psychological dependence. **P/N:** Category C, caution in nursing.	N/V, constipation, abdominal distress, anorexia, diarrhea, dizziness, lightheadedness, hallucinations, sedation, euphoria, headache, confusion, disorientation, sweating, tachycardia.
Pentazocine HCl/ Naloxone HCl (Talwin NX) CIV	**Tab:** (Pentazocine-Naloxone) 50mg-0.5mg*	***Adults:*** **Usual:** 1 tab q3-4h. May increase to 2 tabs q3-4h. **Max:** 12 tabs/day. ***Pediatrics:*** **≥12 yrs: Usual:** 1 tab q3-4h. May increase to 2 tabs q3-4h. **Max:** 12 tabs/day.	**BB:** For oral use only. Severe, potentially lethal reactions may result from misuse by injection alone, or in combination with other agents. **W/P:** Caution with elderly, drug dependence, head injury, increased ICP, certain respiratory conditions, acute CNS manifestations, renal or hepatic dysfunction, biliary surgery, and MI. **P/N:** Category C, caution in nursing.	Hypotension, tachycardia, hallucinations, dizziness, sedation, euphoria, sweating, N/V, constipation, diarrhea, anorexia, facial edema, dermatitis, visual problems, chills, insomnia, urinary retention, paresthesia.
OPIOID AGONIST-ANTAGONIST (FOR OPIOID DEPENDENCE, SEE PAGE 50)				
Buprenorphine HCl (Buprenex) CIII	**Inj:** 0.3mg/mL	***Adults:*** 0.3mg IM/IV q6h prn. Repeat if needed, 30-60 min after initial dose and then prn. **High-Risk Patients/ Concomitant CNS Depressants:** Reduce dose by approximately 50%. May use single doses ≤0.6mg IM if not at high-risk. ***Pediatrics:*** **≥13 yrs:** 0.3mg IM/IV q6h prn. Repeat if needed, 30-60 min after initial dose and then prn. **High-Risk Patients/ Concomitant CNS Depressants:** Reduce dose by approximately 50%. May use single doses ≤0.6mg IM if not at high-risk. **2-12 yrs:** 2-6mcg/kg IM/IV q4-6h.	**W/P:** Significant respiratory depression reported; caution with compromised respiratory function. May increase CSF pressure; caution with head injury, intracranial lesions. Caution with debilitated patients , BPH, biliary tract dysfunction, myxedema, hypothyroidism, urethral stricture, acute alcoholism, Addison's disease, CNS disease, coma, toxic psychoses, delirium tremens, elderly, pediatrics, kyphoscoliosis or hepatic/renal/pulmonary impairment. May impair mental or physical abilities. May precipitate withdrawal in narcotic-dependence. May lead to psychological dependence. **P/N:** Category C, not for use in nursing.	Sedation, N/V, dizziness, sweating, hypotension, headache, miosis, hypoventilation.
TOPICAL ANALGESICS				
Botanical/ Mineral Substances (Traumeel Topical) OTC	**Gel:** [50g, 250g]; **Oint:** [50g, 100g]	***Adults/Pediatrics:*** Individualize dose. Apply to affected area(s) 2-3 times daily. **Max:** 5x/day. May apply using mild compression and/or occlusive bandaging. Avoid applying over large areas, over broken skin, or directly into open wounds.	**W/P:** Avoid administration for pain for >10 days for adults or 5 days for children. Persistent or worsening pain, occurrence of new symptoms, or presence of redness or swelling may signify a serious condition. Consult physician before use in children with arthritis pain. **P/N:** Category C, caution in nursing.	Allergic reactions, anaphylactic reactions.
Diclofenac Epolamine (Flector)	**Patch:** 180mg [5^s^]	***Adults:*** Apply 1 patch to most painful area bid.	**BB:** NSAIDs may cause an increased risk of serious cardiovascular thrombotic events, MI, stroke, and serious GI adverse events, including bleeding, ulceration, and perforation of the stomach or intestines. Contraindicated for the treatment of perioperative pain in the setting of coronary artery bypass graft (CABG) surgery. **W/P:** May lead to onset of new HTN or worsening of pre-existing HTN; monitor BP closely. Fluid retention and edema reported; caution with fluid retention or heart failure. Renal papillary necrosis and other renal injury reported after long-term use. Not recommended for use with advanced renal disease; if therapy must be initiated, monitor renal function. Anaphylactoid reactions may occur. May cause serious skin adverse events (eg, exfoliative dermatitis, Stevens-Johnson syndrome, and toxic epidermal necrolysis). Avoid in late pregnancy; may cause premature	Pruritus, dermatitis, burning, nausea, **dysgeusia**, dyspepsia, headache, paresthesia, somnolence.

Table 3.1. PRESCRIBING INFORMATION FOR ANALGESICS *(cont.)*

NAME	FORM/ STRENGTH	DOSAGE	WARNINGS/PRECAUTIONS & CONTRAINDICATIONS	ADVERSE EFFECTS†
TOPICAL ANALGESICS *(cont.)*				
Diclofenac Epolamine (Flector) *(cont.)*			closure of ductus arteriosus. May cause elevations of LFTs; d/c if liver disease develops or systemic manifestations occur. Rare cases of severe hepatic reactions (eg, jaundice, fatal fulminant hepatitis, liver necrosis, hepatic failure) reported. Anemia may occur; with long-term use, monitor Hgb/Hct if signs or symptoms of anemia develop. May inhibit platelet aggregation and prolong bleeding time; monitor with coagulation disorders. Caution with asthma and avoid with ASA-sensitive asthma. Wash hands after applying, handling, or removing patch. Avoid contact with eye and mucosa. **Contra:** ASA or other NSAID allergy that precipitates asthma, urticaria, or allergic-type reactions. Treatment of perioperative pain in the setting of CABG surgery. Application to nonintact or damaged skin (eg, exudative dermatitis, eczema, infected lesion, burns or wounds). **P/N:** Category C, not for use in nursing.	
Diclofenac Sodium (Voltaren Gel)	**Gel:** 1%	***Adults:*** Measure onto enclosed dosing card to appropriate 2g or 4g line. **Lower Extremities:** Apply 4g to affected foot, knee, or ankle qid. **Max:** 16g/day to any single joint. **Upper Extremities:** Apply 2g to affected hand, elbow, or wrist qid. **Max:** 8g/day to any single joint. Total dose should not exceed 32g/day over all affected joints. Avoid showering or bathing for at least 1 hour after application. Avoid open wounds, eyes, mucous membranes, external heat, and/or occlusive dressings. Avoid wearing clothing or gloves for at least 10 min after application.	**BB:** NSAIDs may cause an increased risk of serious cardiovascular thrombotic events, MI, stroke, and serious GI adverse events, including bleeding, ulceration, and perforation of the stomach or intestines. Contraindicated for the treatment of perioperative pain in the setting of coronary artery bypass graft (CABG) surgery. **W/P:** May lead to onset of new HTN or worsening of pre-existing HTN; monitor BP closely. Fluid retention and edema reported; caution with fluid retention or heart failure. Renal papillary necrosis and other renal injury reported after long-term use. Not recommended for use with advanced renal disease; if therapy must be initiated, monitor renal function. Anaphylactoid reactions may occur. May cause serious skin adverse events (eg, exfoliative dermatitis, Stevens-Johnson syndrome, and toxic epidermal necrolysis). Avoid in late pregnancy; may cause premature closure of ductus arteriosis. May cause elevations of LFTs; d/c if liver disease develops or systemic manifestations occur. Caution in elderly. Anemia may occur; with long-term use, monitor Hgb/Hct if signs or symptoms of anemia develop. May inhibit platelet aggregation and prolong bleeding time; monitor with coagulation disorders. Caution with asthma and avoid with ASA-sensitive asthma. Patients should minimize or avoid exposure to natural or artificial sunlight on treated areas. Monitor for signs or symptoms of GI bleeding. **Contra:** ASA or other NSAID allergy that precipitates asthma, urticaria, or allergic-type reactions. Treatment of perioperative pain in the setting of CABG surgery. **P/N:** Category C, not for use in nursing	Application-site reactions, including dermatitis.

†Bold entries denote special dental considerations.
BB = black box warning; **W/P** = warnings/precautions; **Contra** = contraindications; **P/N** = pregnancy category rating and nursing considerations.

NAME	FORM/ STRENGTH	DOSAGE	WARNINGS/PRECAUTIONS & CONTRAINDICATIONS	ADVERSE EFFECTS†
Lidocaine HCl (Xylocaine Jelly)	**Jelly:** 2% [**Tube:** 5mL, 30mL; **Syringe:** 10mL, 20mL]	***Adults:*** **Max:** 600mg/12 hrs. **Surface Anesthesia of Male Urethra:** Instill about 15mL (300mg). Instill an additional dose of not more than 15mL if needed. **Prior to Sounding or Cystoscopy:** A total dose of 30mL (600mg) is usually required. **Prior to Catheterization:** 5-10mL usually adequate. **Surface Anesthesia of Female Urethra:** Instill 3-5mL. **Elderly/Debilitated:** Reduce dose. ***Pediatrics:*** Determine dose by age and weight. **Max:** 4.5mg/kg.	**W/P:** Avoid excessive dosage or frequent administration; may result in serious adverse effects requiring resuscitative measures. Caution with heart block and severe shock. Extreme caution if mucosa traumatized or sepsis is present in the area of application; risk of rapid systemic absorption. **P/N:** Category B, caution in nursing.	Lightheadedness, nervousness, confusion, euphoria, dizziness, drowsiness, blurred vision, tremors, convulsions, respiratory depression, bradycardia, hypotension, urticaria, edema, anaphylactoid reactions.
Lidocaine HCl (Xylocaine Viscous)	**Sol:** 2% [100mL, 450mL]	***Adults:*** **Irritated/Inflamed Mucous Membranes: Usual:** 15mL undiluted. (Mouth) Swish and spit out. (Pharynx) Gargle and may swallow. Do not administer in <3 hr intervals. **Max:** 8 doses/24 hr; (Single Dose) 4.5mg/kg or total of 300mg. ***Pediatrics:*** **>3 yrs: Max:** Determine by age and weight. **Infants <3 yrs:** Apply 1.25mL with cotton-tipped applicator to immediate area. Do not administer in <3 hr intervals. **Max:** 8 doses/24 hr.	**W/P:** Reduce dose in elderly, debilitated, acutely ill, and children. Caution with heart block, severe shock, and known drug sensitivities. Excessive dosage or too-frequent administration may result in high plasma levels and serious adverse effects requiring resuscitative measures. Extreme caution if mucosa traumatized; risk of rapid systemic absorption. Overdose reported in pediatrics due to inappropriate dosing. **P/N:** Category B, caution in nursing.	Lightheadedness, nervousness, confusion, euphoria, dizziness, drowsiness, blurred vision, tremors, convulsions, respiratory depression, bradycardia, hypotension, urticaria, edema, anaphylactoid reactions.
Lidocaine Ointment	**Oint:** 5% [35g]	***Adults:*** Apply up to 5g (6 inches)/application. **Max:** 17-20g/day. ***Pediatrics:*** Determine dose by age and weight. **Max:** 4.5mg/kg.	**W/P:** Reduce dose in elderly, debilitated, acutely ill, and children. Avoid excessive dosage or too-frequent administration; may result in serious adverse effects requiring resuscitative measures. Caution with heart block and severe shock. Extreme caution if mucosa is traumatized or sepsis is present in the area of application; risk of rapid systemic absorption. **P/N:** Category B, caution in nursing.	Lightheadedness, nervousness, confusion, euphoria, dizziness, drowsiness, blurred vision, tremors, convulsions, respiratory depression, bradycardia, hypotension, urticaria, edema, anaphylactoid reactions.
Lidocaine Patch	**Patch:** 5% [30^{s}]	***Adults:*** Apply to intact skin, cover most painful area. Apply up to 3 patches, once for up to 12 hrs within 24-hr period. May cut patches into smaller sizes before removal of the release liner. **Debilitated/Impaired Elimination:** Treat smaller areas. Remove if irritation or burning occurs; may reapply when irritation subsides.	**W/P:** Serious adverse events may occur in children or pets if ingested. Increased risk of toxicity in severe hepatic disease. Avoid broken or inflamed skin, eye contact, larger area or longer duration than recommended. Increased levels with application of >3 patches, small patients. **P/N:** Category B, caution in nursing.	Application site reactions such as: erythema, edema, bruising, papules, vesicles, discoloration, depigmentation, burning sensation, pruritus, dermatitis, petechiae, blisters, exfoliation, abnormal sensation, irritation, allergic reactions (rare).
Lidocaine/ Prilocaine (EMLA)	**Cre:** (Lidocaine-Prilocaine) 2.5%-2.5%	***Adults:*** Apply thick layer of cream to intact skin and cover with occlusive dressing. **Minor Dermal Procedure:** Apply 2.5g (1/2 tube) over 20-25cm^2 of skin surface for at least 1 hr. **Major Dermal Procedure:** Apply 2g/10cm^2 of skin for 2 hrs. **Adult Male Genital Skin:** Apply 1g/10cm^2 of skin surface for 15 min. **Female External Genitalia:** Apply 5-10g for 5-10 min. ***Pediatrics:*** **7-12 yrs and >20kg: Max:** 20g/200cm^2 for up to 4 hrs. **1-6 yrs and >10 kg: Max:** 10g/100cm^2 for up to 4 hrs. **3-12 months and ≥5 kg: Max:** 2g/20cm^2 for up to 4 hrs. **3-12 months and ≥5 kg: Max:** 2g/20cm^2 for up to 4 hrs. **0-3 months or <5kg: Max:** 1g/10cm^2 for up to 1 hr.	**W/P:** Avoid application for longer than recommended times or on large areas. Avoid with methemoglobinemia. Risk of methemoglobinemia in very young or with G6P deficiency. Avoid eye contact, use in ear. Caution with severe hepatic disease, acutely ill, debilitated, elderly, history of drug sensitivities. Avoid in neonates with a gestational age <37 weeks and infants <12 months receiving treatment with methemoglobin-inducing agents. **P/N:** Category B, caution in nursing.	Local reactions such as erythema, edema, abnormal sensations, paleness (pallor or blanching), altered temperature sensations, itching, rash.

Table 3.1. PRESCRIBING INFORMATION FOR ANALGESICS *(cont.)*

NAME	FORM/ STRENGTH	DOSAGE	WARNINGS/PRECAUTIONS & CONTRAINDICATIONS	ADVERSE EFFECTS†
TOPICAL ANALGESICS *(cont.)*				
Lidocaine/ Tetracaine (Synera)	**Patch:** (Lidocaine-Tetracaine) 70mg-70mg	***Adults:*** **Venipuncture or IV Cannulation:** Apply to intact skin for 20-30 min prior to procedure. **Superficial Dermatological Procedures:** Apply to intact skin for 30 min prior to procedure. ***Pediatrics:*** **≥3 yrs: Venipuncture or IV Cannulation:** Apply to intact skin for 20-30 min prior to procedure. **Superficial Dermatological Procedure:** Apply to intact skin for 30 min prior to procedure.	**W/P:** Serious adverse events may occur in children or pets if ingested. Caution in acutely ill or debilitated. Risk of allergic/ anaphylactoid reactions (urticaria, angioedema, bronchospasm, shock). Increased risk of toxicity in severe hepatic disease. Avoid broken or inflamed skin, eye contact, larger area or longer duration than recommended. **Contra:** PABA hypersensitivity. **P/N:** Category B, caution in nursing.	Erythema, blanching, edema, urticaria, **angioedema**, bronchospasm, shock.

†Bold entries denote special dental considerations.
BB = black box warning; **W/P** = warnings/precautions; **Contra** = contraindications; **P/N** = pregnancy category rating and nursing considerations.

Table 3.2. DRUG INTERACTIONS FOR ANALGESICS

NONOPIOID ANALGESICS

Acetaminophen

Acetaminophen (Feverall, Tylenol, Tylenol 8 Hour, Tylenol Arthritis Pain, Tylenol Children's, Tylenol Extra Strength, Tylenol Infants', Tylenol Junior, Tylenol Regular Strength) OTC	
Alcohol	Increases risk of hepatotoxicity with excessive alcohol use (≥3 drinks/day).
NSAIDs	
Celecoxib (Celebrex)	
ACE inhibitors	Decreases antihypertensive effect of ACE inhibitors.
Anticoagulants, coumarin	Increases risk of bleeding complications.
ARBs	Decreases antihypertensive effect of ARBs.
ASA	Increases the risk of GI ulceration and other complications.
CYP2C9 inhibitors	Caution with CYP2C9 inhibitors.
CYP2D6 substrates	Caution with drugs metabolized by CYP2D6.
Fluconazole	Increases plasma levels of celecoxib.
Furosemide	Decreases natriuretic effect of furosemide.
Lithium	Increases plasma levels of lithium.
NSAIDs	Avoid with other NSAIDs; potential for increased adverse reactions.
Thiazides	Decreases natriuretic effect of thiazide diuretics.
Diclofenac Potassium (Cataflam)	
ACE inhibitors	Decreases antihypertensive effect of ACE inhibitors.
ASA	Avoid with ASA; potential for increased adverse reactions.
Cyclosporine	Increases cyclosporine nephrotoxicity with coadministration.
Furosemide	Decreases natriuretic effect of furosemide; monitor for renal failure.
Lithium	May increase plasma levels and decrease clearance of lithium; monitor for toxicity.
Methotrexate	Caution with methotrexate; increases risk of methotrexate toxicity.
Thiazides	Decreases natriuretic effect of thiazide diuretics; monitor for renal failure.
Warfarin	Synergistic effect with warfarin; increases risk of serious GI bleeding.
Diclofenac Sodium (Voltaren, Voltaren-XR)	
ACE inhibitors	Decreases antihypertensive effect of ACE inhibitors.
Anticoagulants, coumarin	Caution with coumarin anticoagulants.
ASA	Avoid with ASA; potential for increased adverse reactions.
Cyclosporine	Increases cyclosporine nephrotoxicity with coadministration.
Digoxin	Increases digoxin toxicity; monitor serum levels.
Diuretics	Decreases natriuretic effect of diuretics; increases serum K^+ levels of K^+-sparing diuretics.
Hypoglycemics, oral	May alter effects of insulin and oral hypoglycemics.

Table 3.2. DRUG INTERACTIONS FOR ANALGESICS *(cont.)*

NONOPIOID ANALGESICS *(cont.)*

NSAIDs

Diclofenac Sodium (Voltaren, Voltaren-XR) *(cont.)*	
Lithium	May increase plasma levels and decrease clearance of lithium; monitor for toxicity.
Methotrexate	Increases methotrexate toxicity with methotrexate.
Diclofenac Sodium/Misoprostol (Arthrotec)	
ACE inhibitors	Decreases antihypertensive effect of ACE inhibitors.
Antacids	Avoid with magnesium-containing antacids.
ASA	Avoid with ASA; potential for increased adverse reactions.
Cyclosporine	Increases cyclosporine toxicity with coadministration; monitor renal function.
Digoxin	Increases plasma levels of digoxin; monitor for digoxin toxicity.
Furosemide	Decreases natriuretic effect of furosemide; monitor for renal failure.
Hypoglycemics	May alter effects of insulin and oral hypoglycemics.
Lithium	May increase plasma levels and decrease clearance of lithium; monitor for toxicity.
Methotrexate	Caution with methotrexate; increases risk of methotrexate toxicity.
Phenobarbital	Phenobarbital toxicity reported with chronic phenobarbital treatment.
Potassium-sparing diuretics	K^+-sparing diuretics may cause hyperkalemia.
Thiazides	Decreases natriuretic effect of thiazide diuretics; monitor for renal failure.
Warfarin	Synergistic effect with warfarin; increases risk of serious GI bleeding.
Diflunisal	
ACE inhibitors	Decreases antihypertensive effect of ACE inhibitors; increases risk of renal impairment.
Acetaminophen	Increases plasma levels of acetaminophen; may cause hepatotoxicity.
Antacids	May decrease plasma levels of diflunisal with a continuous schedule of antacid use.
Anticoagulants, coumarin	Increases risk of serious GI bleeding.
ARBs	Decreases antihypertensive effect of ARBs; increases risk of renal impairment.
ASA	Avoid with ASA; potential for increased adverse reactions.
Cyclosporine	Increases cyclosporine toxicity with coadministration; monitor renal function.
Furosemide	Decreases natriuretic effect of furosemide; monitor for renal failure.
Hydrochlorothiazide	Increases plasma levels of hydrochlorothiazide; decreases hyperuricemic effect.
Indomethacin	Avoid coadministration; increases plasma levels of indomethacin and risk of fatal GI hemorrhage.
Lithium	May increase plasma levels and decrease clearance of lithium; monitor for toxicity.
Methotrexate	Caution with methotrexate; increases risk of methotrexate toxicity.

NONOPIOID ANALGESICS *(cont.)*

NSAIDs

Diflunisal *(cont.)*	
NSAIDs	Avoid with other NSAIDs; potential for increased adverse reactions.
Sulindac	Decreases plasma levels of sulindac active metabolite.
Thiazides	Decreases natriuretic effect of thiazide diuretics; monitor for renal failure.
Etodolac, Etodolac Extended-Release	
ACE inhibitors	Decreases antihypertensive effect of ACE inhibitors.
Antacids	May decrease peak concentration of etodolac.
ASA	Avoid with ASA; potential for increased adverse reactions.
Cyclosporine	Increases cyclosporine toxicity with coadministration; monitor renal function.
Digoxin	Increases plasma levels of digoxin.
Furosemide	Decreases natriuretic effect of furosemide; monitor for renal failure.
Lithium	May increase plasma levels and decrease clearance of lithium; monitor for toxicity.
Methotrexate	Caution with methotrexate; increases risk of methotrexate toxicity.
Phenylbutazone	Avoid with phenylbutazone; may alter plasma levels of etodolac.
Thiazides	Decreases natriuretic effect of thiazide diuretics; monitor for renal failure.
Warfarin	Synergistic effect with warfarin; increases risk of serious GI bleeding.
Fenoprofen Calcium (Nalfon)	
ACE inhibitors	Decreases antihypertensive effect of ACE inhibitors.
ASA	Avoid with ASA; potential for increased adverse reactions.
Furosemide	Decreases natriuretic effect of furosemide; monitor for renal failure.
Lithium	May increase plasma levels and decrease clearance of lithium; monitor for toxicity.
Methotrexate	Caution with methotrexate; increases risk of methotrexate toxicity.
Phenobarbital	Decreases plasma half-life of fenoprofen with chronic phenobarbital therapy.
Protein-bound drugs	May displace or be displaced by highly protein-bound drugs (eg, hydantoins, sulfonamides, sulfonylureas); monitor for increased toxicity.
Thiazides	Decreases natriuretic effect of thiazide diuretics; monitor for renal failure.
Warfarin	Synergistic effect with warfarin; increases risk of serious GI bleeding.
Flurbiprofen (Ansaid)	
ACE inhibitors	Decreases antihypertensive effect of ACE inhibitors.
Anticoagulants, coumarin	Synergistic effect with warfarin and coumarins; increases risk of serious GI bleeding.
ASA	Avoid with ASA; potential for increased adverse reactions.
β-Blockers	May decrease antihypertensive effect of β-blockers.
Furosemide	Decreases natriuretic effect of furosemide; monitor for renal failure.

Table 3.2. DRUG INTERACTIONS FOR ANALGESICS *(cont.)*

NONOPIOID ANALGESICS *(cont.)*

NSAIDs

Flurbiprofen (Ansaid) *(cont.)*	
Lithium	May increase plasma levels and decrease clearance of lithium; monitor for toxicity.
Methotrexate	Caution with methotrexate; increases risk of methotrexate toxicity.
Thiazides	Decreases natriuretic effect of thiazide diuretics; monitor for renal failure.
Ibuprofen (Motrin, Motrin IB, Children's Motrin, Infant's Motrin, Junior Strength Motrin)	
Alcohol	May increase risk of GI bleeding with ≥3 alcoholic drinks/day.
ACE inhibitors	Decreases antihypertensive effect of ACE inhibitors.
Anticoagulants, coumarin	Increases risk of serious GI bleeding with coumarin anticoagulants.
ASA	Avoid with ASA; potential for increased adverse reactions.
Furosemide	Decreases natriuretic effect of furosemide; monitor for renal failure.
Lithium	May increase plasma levels and decrease clearance of lithium; monitor for toxicity.
Methotrexate	Caution with methotrexate; increases risk of methotrexate toxicity.
NSAIDs	Avoid with other NSAIDs; potential for increased adverse reactions.
Thiazides	Decreases natriuretic effect of thiazide diuretics; monitor for renal failure.
Indomethacin (Indocin)	
ACE inhibitors	Decreases antihypertensive effect of ACE inhibitors; increases risk of renal impairment.
Anticoagulants	Caution with anticoagulants; increases risk of GI bleeding.
ARBs	Decreases antihypertensive effect of ARBs; increases risk of renal impairment.
ASA	Avoid with ASA; potential for increased adverse reactions.
β-Blockers	Decreases antihypertensive effect of β-blockers.
Cyclosporine	Increases cyclosporine toxicity with coadministration; monitor renal function.
Diflunisal	Avoid coadministration; increases plasma levels of indomethacin and risk of fatal GI hemorrhage.
Digoxin	Increases plasma levels and prolongs half-life of digoxin.
Lithium	May increase plasma levels and decrease clearance of lithium; monitor for toxicity.
Loop diuretics	Decreases efficacy of loop diuretics.
Methotrexate	Caution with methotrexate; increases risk of methotrexate toxicity.
NSAIDs	Avoid with other NSAIDs; potential for increased adverse reactions.
Potassium-sparing diuretics	Decreases efficacy of K^+-sparing diuretics; may cause hyperkalemia with K^+-sparing diuretics.
Probenecid	Increases plasma levels of indomethacin; may require dose reduction.
Thiazides	Decreases efficacy of thiazide diuretics.

NONOPIOID ANALGESICS *(cont.)*

NSAIDs

Ketoprofen, Ketoprofen Extended-Release	
ACE inhibitors	Decreases antihypertensive effect of ACE inhibitors.
ASA	Avoid with ASA; potential for increased adverse reactions.
Furosemide	Decreases natriuretic effect of furosemide; monitor for renal failure.
Hydrochlorothiazide	Decreases urinary potassium and chloride excretion with coadministration.
Lithium	May increase plasma levels and decrease clearance of lithium; monitor for toxicity.
Methotrexate	Caution with methotrexate; increases risk of methotrexate toxicity.
Probenecid	Avoid with probenecid; decreases plasma clearance of ketoprofen.
Thiazides	Decreases natriuretic effect of thiazide diuretics; monitor for renal failure.
Warfarin	Synergistic effect with warfarin; increases risk of serious GI bleeding.
Ketorolac Tromethamine	
ACE inhibitors	Decreases antihypertensive effect of ACE inhibitors; increases risk of renal impairment.
Anticoagulants	Increases risk of bleeding.
Antiepileptic agents	Seizures reported with concomitant administration.
ARBs	Decreases antihypertensive effect of ARBs; increases risk of renal impairment.
ASA	Avoid with ASA; potential for increased adverse reactions.
Corticosteroids	Increases risk of bleeding.
Furosemide	Decreases natriuretic effect of furosemide; monitor for renal failure.
Lithium	May increase plasma levels and decrease clearance of lithium; monitor for toxicity.
Methotrexate	Caution with methotrexate; increases methotrexate toxicity.
Nondepolarizing muscle relaxants	May cause apnea with nondepolarizing muscle relaxants.
NSAIDs	Avoid with other NSAIDs; potential for increased adverse reactions.
Pentoxifylline	Increases risk of bleeding.
Probenecid	Avoid with probenecid; increases plasma levels of ketorolac.
Psychoactive drugs	Hallucinations reported with concomitant administration.
SSRIs	Caution with SSRIs; increases risk of GI bleeding.
Thiazides	Decreases natriuretic effect of thiazide diuretics; monitor for renal failure.
Meclofenamate Sodium	
ASA	Decreases plasma levels of meclofenamate.
Warfarin	Synergistic effect with warfarin; increases risk of serious GI bleeding.

Table 3.2. DRUG INTERACTIONS FOR ANALGESICS *(cont.)*

NONOPIOID ANALGESICS *(cont.)*

NSAIDs

Mefenamic Acid (Ponstel)	
ACE inhibitors	Decreases antihypertensive effect of ACE inhibitors.
Antacids	May increase plasma levels of mefenamic acid.
Anticoagulants, coumarin	Synergistic effect with warfarin and coumarins; increases risk of serious GI bleeding.
ASA	Avoid with ASA; potential for increased adverse reactions.
CYP2C9 inhibitors	Caution with CYP2C9 inhibitors; possible altered safety and efficacy of mefenamic acid.
Furosemide	Decreases natriuretic effect of furosemide; monitor for renal failure.
Lithium	May increase plasma levels and decrease clearance of lithium; monitor for toxicity.
Methotrexate	Caution with methotrexate; increases risk of methotrexate toxicity.
Thiazides	Decreases natriuretic effect of thiazide diuretics; monitor for renal failure.
Meloxicam (Mobic)	
ACE inhibitors	Decreases antihypertensive effect of ACE inhibitors.
ASA	Avoid with ASA; potential for increased adverse reactions.
Cholestyramine	Increases clearance of meloxicam.
Furosemide	Decreases natriuretic effect of furosemide; monitor for renal failure.
Lithium	May increase plasma levels and decrease clearance of lithium; monitor for toxicity.
Methotrexate	Caution with methotrexate; increases risk of methotrexate toxicity.
Thiazides	Decreases natriuretic effect of thiazide diuretics; monitor for renal failure.
Warfarin	Synergistic effect with warfarin; increases risk of serious GI bleeding.
Nabumetone	
ACE inhibitors	Decreases antihypertensive effect of ACE inhibitors.
ASA	Avoid with ASA; potential for increased adverse reactions.
Furosemide	Decreases natriuretic effect of furosemide; monitor for renal failure.
Lithium	May increase plasma levels and decrease clearance of lithium; monitor for toxicity.
Methotrexate	Caution with methotrexate; increases risk of methotrexate toxicity.
Protein-bound drugs	May displace protein-bound drugs.
Thiazides	Decreases natriuretic effect of thiazide diuretics; monitor for renal failure.
Warfarin	Synergistic effect with warfarin; increases risk of serious GI bleeding.

NONOPIOID ANALGESICS *(cont.)*

NSAIDs

Naproxen (EC-Naprosyn, Naprosyn)	
ACE inhibitors	Decreases antihypertensive effect of ACE inhibitors.
ASA	Avoid with ASA; potential for increased adverse reactions.
β-Blockers	Decreases antihypertensive effect of β-blockers.
Cholestyramine	May delay absorption of naproxen.
Furosemide	Decreases natriuretic effect of furosemide; monitor for renal failure.
GI alkalinizing agents	Avoid coadministration of gastric pH elevating drugs such as H_2-blockers, sucralfate, or intensive antacid therapy with EC-Naprosyn.
Lithium	May increase plasma levels and decrease clearance of lithium; monitor for toxicity.
Methotrexate	Caution with methotrexate; increases risk of methotrexate toxicity.
Probenecid	Increases plasma half-life of naproxen.
Protein-bound drugs	May displace other protein-bound drugs (eg, coumarin anticoagulants, sulfonylureas, hydantoin, other NSAIDs).
SSRIs	Caution with SSRIs; increases risk of GI bleeding.
Thiazides	Decreases natriuretic effect of thiazide diuretics; monitor for renal failure.
Warfarin	Synergistic effect with warfarin; increases risk of serious GI bleeding.
Naproxen Sodium (Aleve, Anaprox, Anaprox DS, Naprelan)	
Alcohol	May increase risk of GI bleeding with ≥3 alcoholic drinks/day.
ACE inhibitors	Decreases antihypertensive effect of ACE inhibitors.
ASA	Avoid with ASA; potential for increased adverse reactions.
β-Blockers	Decreases antihypertensive effect of β-blockers.
Cholestyramine	May delay absorption of naproxen.
Furosemide	Decreases natriuretic effect of furosemide; monitor for renal failure.
GI alkalinizing agents	Avoid coadministration of gastric pH elevating drugs such as H_2-blockers, sucralfate, or intensive antacid therapy.
Lithium	May increase plasma levels and decrease clearance of lithium; monitor for toxicity.
Methotrexate	Caution with coadministration; increases risk of methotrexate toxicity.
NSAIDs	Avoid with other NSAIDs; potential for increased adverse reactions.
Probenecid	Increases plasma half-life of naproxen.
Protein-bound drugs	May displace other protein-bound drugs (eg, coumarin anticoagulants, sulfonylureas, hydantoin, other NSAIDs).
SSRIs	Caution with SSRIs; increases risk of GI bleeding.
Thiazides	Decreases natriuretic effect of thiazide diuretics; monitor for renal failure.
Warfarin	Synergistic effect with warfarin; increases risk of serious GI bleeding.

Table 3.2. DRUG INTERACTIONS FOR ANALGESICS *(cont.)*

NONOPIOID ANALGESICS *(cont.)*

NSAIDs

Oxaprozin (Daypro)	
ACE inhibitors	Decreases antihypertensive effect of ACE inhibitors.
ASA	Avoid with ASA; potential for increased adverse reactions.
β-Blockers	Decreases antihypertensive effect of β-blockers.
Furosemide	Decreases natriuretic effect of furosemide; monitor for renal failure.
H_2-receptor antagonists	Caution with cimetidine or ranitidine; may increase plasma levels of oxaprozin.
Lithium	May increase plasma levels and decrease clearance of lithium; monitor for toxicity.
Methotrexate	Caution with coadministration; increases risk of methotrexate toxicity.
Thiazides	Decreases natriuretic effect of thiazide diuretics; monitor for renal failure.
Warfarin	Synergistic effect with warfarin; increases risk of serious GI bleeding.
Piroxicam (Feldene)	
ACE inhibitors	Decreases antihypertensive effect of ACE inhibitors.
Anticoagulants	Increases risk of GI bleeding with oral anticoagulants.
ASA	Avoid with ASA; potential for increased adverse reactions.
Corticosteroids	Increases risk of GI bleeding with oral corticosteroids.
Furosemide	Decreases natriuretic effect of furosemide; monitor for renal failure.
Lithium	May increase plasma levels and decrease clearance of lithium; monitor for toxicity.
Methotrexate	Caution with coadministration; increases risk of methotrexate toxicity.
NSAIDs	Caution with other NSAIDs; potential for increased adverse reactions.
Protein-bound drugs	May displace protein-bound drugs.
Thiazides	Decreases natriuretic effect of thiazide diuretics; monitor for renal failure.
Sulindac (Clinoril)	
ACE inhibitors	Decreases antihypertensive effect of ACE inhibitors.
Anticoagulants, coumarin	Synergistic effect with warfarin and coumarins; increases risk of serious GI bleeding.
ARBs	Decreases antihypertensive effect of ARBs.
ASA	Avoid with ASA; potential for increased adverse reactions.
Cyclosporine	Increases cyclosporine toxicity with coadministration; monitor renal function.
Diflunisal	Decreases plasma levels of the active metabolite of sulindac.
DMSO	Avoid with DMSO; may reduce efficacy of sulindac and cause peripheral neuropathy.
Furosemide	Decreases natriuretic effect of furosemide; monitor for renal failure.
Lithium	May increase plasma levels and decrease clearance of lithium; monitor for toxicity.

NONOPIOID ANALGESICS *(cont.)*

NSAIDs

Sulindac (Clinoril) *(cont.)*	
Methotrexate	Caution with methotrexate; increases risk of methotrexate toxicity.
NSAIDs	Caution with other NSAIDs; potential for increased adverse reactions.
Probenecid	May increase plasma levels of sulindac; possible reduction in uricosuric action of probenecid.
Thiazides	Decreases natriuretic effect of thiazide diuretics; monitor for renal failure.
Tolmetin Sodium	
ACE inhibitors	Decreases antihypertensive effect of ACE inhibitors.
Anticoagulants, coumarin	Increases risk of serious bleeding.
ASA	Avoid with ASA; potential for increased adverse reactions.
Furosemide	Decreases natriuretic effect of furosemide; monitor for renal failure.
Lithium	May increase plasma levels and decrease clearance of lithium; monitor for toxicity.
Methotrexate	Caution with methotrexate; increases methotrexate toxicity.
Thiazides	Decreases natriuretic effect of thiazide diuretics; monitor for renal failure.

SALICYLATES

Aspirin (Bayer Aspirin, Bayer Aspirin Children's, Bayer Aspirin Regimen, Bayer Aspirin Regimen with Calcium, Bayer Genuine Aspirin, Bayer Aspirin Extra Strength, Ecotrin) OTC	
ACE inhibitors	Decreases antihypertensive effect of ACE inhibitors.
Acetazolamide	Increases plasma levels of acetazolamide.
Alcohol	May increase risk of GI bleeding with ≥3 alcoholic drinks/day.
Anticoagulants	Caution with anticoagulants; increases risk of bleeding.
β-Blockers	Decreases antihypertensive effect of β-blockers.
Hypoglycemic agents	Increases effects of hypoglycemic agents.
Methotrexate	Caution with methotrexate; increases risk of methotrexate toxicity.
NSAIDs	Caution with other NSAIDs; potential for increased adverse reactions.
Phenytoin	Increases plasma levels of phenytoin.
Uricosuric agents	Antagonizes effects of uricosuric agents.
Valproic acid	Increases plasma levels of valproic acid.
Salsalate	
Anticoagulants	Caution with anticoagulants; increases risk of bleeding.
Protein-bound drugs	May displace other protein-bound drugs (eg, corticosteroids, methotrexate, phenytoin).
Salicylates	Avoid with other salicylates.
Sulfonylureas	Potentiation of salsalate effects with sulfonylureas.
Uricosuric agents	Antagonizes effects of uricosuric agents.

Table 3.2. DRUG INTERACTIONS FOR ANALGESICS *(cont.)*

NONOPIOID ANALGESICS *(cont.)*

Salicylates

Salsalate *(cont.)*	
Urinary acidifiers	Potentiation of salsalate effects with urinary acidifiers.
Urinary alkalinizers	Decreases effects of salsalate with drugs that increase urinary pH.

OPIOID-CONTAINING ANALGESICS

Codeine Combinations

Acetaminophen/Codeine Phosphate (Tylenol with Codeine) CIII	
Alcohol	Additive CNS depressant effects.
Anticholinergics	May increase risk of urinary retention and/or severe constipation, which may lead to paralytic ileus.
CNS depressants	Additive CNS depressant effects.
Aspirin/Codeine CIII	
Anticoagulants	Caution with anticoagulants; increases risk of bleeding.
CNS depressants	Additive CNS depressant effects; may require dose reduction.
Corticosteroids	Potentiation of corticosteroid effects.
Furosemide	Caution with furosemide.
Hypoglycemic agents	Increases effects of hypoglycemic agents.
MAOIs	Caution with MAOIs; increases effects of MAOIs.
Methotrexate	Caution with methotrexate; increases risk of methotrexate toxicity.
NSAIDs	Caution with other NSAIDs; potential for increased adverse reactions.
Uricosuric agents	Antagonizes effects of uricosuric agents.

Dihydrocodeine Combinations

Aspirin/Caffeine/Dihydrocodeine Bitartrate (Synalgos-DC) CIII	
Alcohol	Additive CNS depressant effects.
Anticoagulants	Caution with anticoagulants; increases risk of bleeding.
CNS depressants	Additive CNS depressant effects.
Uricosuric agents	Antagonizes effects of uricosuric agents.

Hydrocodone Combinations

Acetaminophen/Hydrocodone Bitartrate (Lorcet, Lorcet 10/650, Lorcet HD, Lorcet Plus, Lortab, Norco, Vicodin, Vicodin ES, Vicodin HP, Zydone) CIII	
Alcohol	Additive CNS depressant effects
CNS depressants	Additive CNS depressant effects; may require dose reduction.
MAOIs	Increases effect of MAOI or hydrocodone with coadministration.
TCAs	Increases effect of TCA or hydrocodone with coadministration.

OPIOID-CONTAINING ANALGESICS *(cont.)*

Hydrocodone Combinations

Hydrocodone Bitartrate/Ibuprofen (Reprexain, Vicoprofen) CIII	
ACE inhibitors	Decreases antihypertensive effect of ACE inhibitors.
Anticholinergics	May increase risk of urinary retention and/or severe constipation, which may lead to paralytic ileus.
ASA	Avoid with ASA; potential for increased adverse reactions.
CNS depressants	Additive CNS depressant effects; may require dose reduction.
Furosemide	Decreases natriuretic effect of furosemide; monitor for renal failure.
Lithium	Increases plasma levels of lithium; may cause toxicity.
MAOIs	Increases effect of MAOI or hydrocodone with coadministration.
Methotrexate	Caution with co administration; increases risk of methotrexate toxicity.
TCAs	Increases effect of TCA or hydrocodone with coadministration.
Thiazides	Decreases natriuretic effect of thiazide diuretics; monitor for renal failure.
Warfarin	Synergistic effect with warfarin; increases risk of serious GI bleeding.

Oxycodone & Combinations

Acetaminophen/Oxycodone HCl (Endocet, Percocet, Roxicet, Roxilox, Tylox) CII	
Alcohol	May cause hepatotoxicity in chronic or heavy alcohol intake.
Anticholinergics	May increase risk of urinary retention and/or severe constipation, which may lead to paralytic ileus; may also delay or decrease the onset of acetaminophen effect.
CNS depressants	Additive CNS depressant effects with other CNS depressants, including alcohol.
Contraceptives, oral	Increases plasma clearance and decreases half-life of acetaminophen.
Lamotrigine	Decreases plasma concentrations of lamotrigine; reduces efficacy.
Loop diuretics	Decreases efficacy of loop diuretics.
Mixed agonist/antagonist opioid analgesics	Mixed agonist/antagonist opioid analgesics (eg, pentazocine, nalbuphine, butorphanol) may reduce analgesic effects and/or precipitate withdrawal symptoms.
Probenecid	Increases effects of acetaminophen.
Propranolol	Increases effects of acetaminophen.
Skeletal muscle relaxants	May enhance skeletal muscle relaxant effects and increase respiratory depression.
Zidovudine	Decreases efficacy of zidovudine.
Aspirin/Oxycodone HCl (Endodan, Percodan) CII	
ACE inhibitors	Decreases antihypertensive effect of ACE inhibitors.
Acetazolamide	Increases plasma levels of acetazolamide.
Alcohol	Increases risk of bleeding with chronic or heavy alcohol intake.
Anticoagulants	Increases risk of bleeding.

Table 3.2. DRUG INTERACTIONS FOR ANALGESICS *(cont.)*

OPIOID-CONTAINING ANALGESICS *(cont.)*

Oxycodone & Combinations

Aspirin/Oxycodone HCl (Endodan, Percodan) CII *(cont.)*	
β-Blockers	Decreases antihypertensive effect of β-blockers.
CNS depressants	Additive CNS depressant effects.
Diuretics	Decreases efficacy of diuretics in patients with renal or cardiovascular disease.
Insulin	Increases glucose-lowering action of insulin; may cause hypoglycemia.
Sulfonylureas	Increases glucose-lowering action of sulfonylureas; may cause hypoglycemia.
Methotrexate	Caution with methotrexate; increases risk of methotrexate toxicity.
Mixed agonist/antagonist opioid analgesics	Mixed agonist/antagonist opioid analgesics (eg, pentazocine, nalbuphine, naltrexone, and butorphanol) may reduce analgesic effects and/or precipitate withdrawal symptoms.
NSAIDs	Caution with other NSAIDs; potential for increased adverse reactions.
Phenytoin	Decreases plasma levels of phenytoin.
Skeletal muscle relaxants	May enhance skeletal muscle relaxant effects and increase respiratory depression.
Uricosuric agents	Antagonizes effect of uricosuric agents (eg, probenecid, sulfinpyrazone).
Valproic acid	Increases plasma levels of valproic acid.
Ibuprofen/Oxycodone HCl (Combunox) CII	
ACE inhibitors	Decreases antihypertensive effect of ACE inhibitors.
Anticholinergics	May increase risk of urinary retention and/or severe constipation, which may lead to paralytic ileus.
ASA	Avoid with ASA; increases risk of adverse reactions.
Coumarins	Caution with coumarins; increases risk of GI bleeding.
CNS depressants	Additive CNS depressant effects with other CNS depressants, including alcohol.
CYP2D6 inhibitors	May interact with CYP2D6 inhibitors (eg, certain cardiovascular drugs and antidepressants).
Diuretics	Decreases efficacy of diuretics; monitor renal function.
Lithium	May increase plasma levels and decrease clearance of lithium; monitor for toxicity.
MAOIs	Avoid within 14 days of MAOIs.
Methotrexate	May enhance methotrexate toxicity.
Mixed agonist/antagonist opioid analgesics	Mixed agonist/antagonist opioid analgesics (eg, pentazocine, nalbuphine, buprenorphine, butorphanol) may reduce analgesic effects and/ or precipitate withdrawal symptoms.
Skeletal muscle relaxants	May enhance skeletal muscle relaxant effects and increase respiratory depression.

OPIOID-CONTAINING ANALGESICS *(cont.)*

Oxycodone & Combinations

Oxycodone HCl (OxyContin, OxyIR, Roxicodone) CII	
CNS depressants	Additive CNS depressant effects with other CNS depressants, including respiratory depression and coma.
CYP2D6 inhibitors	May interact with CYP2D6 inhibitors such as certain cardiovascular drugs (eg, amiodarone, quinidine) and polycyclic antidepressants.
MAOIs	Caution with MAOIs; avoid within 14 days of use.
Mixed agonist/antagonist and partial agonist opioid analgesics	Mixed agonist/antagonist opioid analgesics (eg, pentazocine, nalbuphine, butorphanol, buprenorphine) may reduce analgesic effects and/or precipitate withdrawal symptoms.
Phenothiazines	May cause severe hypotension with phenothiazines.
Skeletal muscle relaxants	May enhance skeletal muscle relaxant effects and increase respiratory depression.
Vasomotor tone, drugs that compromise	May cause severe hypotension with drugs that compromise vasomotor tone.

Propoxyphene & Combinations

Acetaminophen/Propoxyphene Napsylate (Darvocet A500, Darvocet-N) CIV	
Alcohol	Additive CNS depressant effects.
Anticoagulants, coumarin	Increases plasma levels and adverse effects of coumarin anticoagulants.
Anticonvulsants	Increases plasma levels and adverse effects of anticonvulsants.
Antidepressants	Increases plasma levels of antidepressants; may potentiate CNS depressant effects.
Carbamazepine	Severe neurologic signs, including coma reported with carbamazepine.
CNS depressants	Additive CNS depressant effects with other CNS depressants.
Propoxyphene HCl (Darvon) CIV	
Alcohol	Additive CNS depressant effects.
Anticoagulants, coumarin	Increases plasma levels and adverse effects of coumarin anticoagulants.
Anticonvulsants	Increases plasma levels and adverse effects of anticonvulsants.
Antidepressants	Increases plasma levels of antidepressants; may potentiate CNS depressant effects.
Carbamazepine	Severe neurologic signs, including coma, reported with carbamazepine.
CNS depressants	Additive CNS depressant effects.
Propoxyphene Napsylate (Darvon-N) CIV	
Alcohol	Additive CNS depressant effects.
Anticoagulants, coumarin	Increases plasma levels and adverse effects of coumarin anticoagulants.
Anticonvulsants	Increases plasma levels and adverse effects of anticonvulsants.
Antidepressants	Increases plasma levels of antidepressants; may potentiate CNS depressant effects.

Table 3.2. DRUG INTERACTIONS FOR ANALGESICS *(cont.)*

OPIOID-CONTAINING ANALGESICS *(cont.)*

Propoxyphene & Combinations

Propoxyphene Napsylate (Darvon-N) CIV *(cont.)*	
Carbamazepine	Severe neurologic signs, including coma, reported with carbamazepine.
CNS depressants	Additive CNS depressant effects.

Tramadol Combinations

Acetaminophen/Tramadol HCl (Ultracet)	
Acetaminophen-containing products	Avoid other acetaminophen-containing products; potential for hepatotoxicity.
Alcohol	Additive CNS depressant effects.
Carbamazepine	Avoid with carbamazepine due to possible seizure risk of tramadol. Coadministration increases tramadol metabolism and may reduce efficacy.
CNS depressants	Caution with CNS depressants; increased risk of CNS and respiratory depression.
Coumarins	May alter effects of coumarin derivatives (eg, warfarin), including elevation of PT.
CYP2D6 inhibitors	Decreases clearance of tramadol; increases risk of seizure and serotonin syndrome.
CYP3A4 inhibitors	Decreases clearance of tramadol; increases risk of seizure and serotonin syndrome.
Digoxin	Possible digoxin toxicity with coadministration.
Linezolid	Caution with linezolid; potential for serotonin syndrome.
Lithium	Caution with lithium; potential for serotonin syndrome.
MAOIs	Increases risk of seizures and serotonin syndrome with MAOIs.
Neuroleptics	Increases risk of seizures with neuroleptics.
Opioids	Increases risk of seizures with opioids.
Quinidine	Caution with quinidine; may increase plasma levels of tramadol and decrease plasma levels of tramadol metabolite.
Seizure threshold, drugs reducing	Increases the risk of seizures with other drugs that reduce the seizure threshold.
SNRIs	Increases risk of serotonin syndrome with SNRIs.
SSRIs	Increases risk of seizures and serotonin syndrome with SSRIs.
TCAs	Increases risk of seizures and serotonin syndrome with coadministration of TCAs and other tricyclic compounds (eg, cyclobenzaprine).
Triptans	Caution with triptans; potential for serotonin syndrome.
Tramadol HCl (Ultram, Ultram ER)	
Alcohol	Additive CNS depressant effects.
Carbamazepine	Avoid with carbamazepine due to possible seizure risk of tramadol. Coadministration increases tramadol metabolism and may reduce efficacy.

OPIOID-CONTAINING ANALGESICS *(cont.)*

TRAMADOL COMBINATIONS

Tramadol HCl (Ultram, Ultram ER) *(cont.)*	
CNS depressants	Caution with CNS depressants; increased risk of severe CNS and respiratory depression.
Coumarins	May alter effects of coumarin derivatives (eg, warfarin), including elevation of prothrombin time.
CYP2D6 inhibitors	Decreases clearance of tramadol; increases risk of seizure and serotonin syndrome.
CYP3A4 inhibitors	Decreases clearance of tramadol; increases risk of seizure and serotonin syndrome.
Digoxin	Possible digoxin toxicity with coadministration.
Linezolid	Caution with linezolid; potential for serotonin syndrome.
Lithium	Caution with lithium; potential for serotonin syndrome.
MAOIs	Increases risk of seizures and serotonin syndrome with MAOIs.
Neuroleptics	Increases risk of seizures with neuroleptics.
Opioids	Increases risk of seizures with opioids.
Quinidine	Caution with quinidine; may increase plasma levels of tramadol and decrease plasma levels of tramadol metabolite.
Seizure threshold, drugs reducing	Increases the risk of seizures with other drugs that reduce the seizure threshold.
SNRIs	Increases risk of serotonin syndrome with SNRIs.
SSRIs	Increases risk of seizures and serotonin syndrome with SSRIs.
TCAs	Increases risk of seizures and serotonin syndrome with coadministration of TCAs and other tricyclic compounds (eg, cyclobenzaprine).
Triptans	Caution with triptans; potential for serotonin syndrome.

MISCELLANEOUS OPIOIDS

Alfentanil HCl (Alfenta) CII	
Alcohol	Additive CNS depressant effects.
Cimetidine	Decreases clearance and may extend duration of action of alfentanil with coadministration.
CNS depressants	Additive CNS depressant effects.
Erythromycin	Inhibits alfentanil clearance and increases risk of prolonged or delayed respiratory depression.
MAOIs	Caution with MAOIs; avoid within 14 days of use.
Fentanyl (Duragesic) CII	
Alcohol	Additive CNS depressant effects.
CNS depressants	Additive CNS depressant effects, including respiratory depression and coma.
CYP3A4 inducers	Coadministration decreases plasma levels of fentanyl; may reduce efficacy.

Table 3.2. DRUG INTERACTIONS FOR ANALGESICS *(cont.)*

OPIOID-CONTAINING ANALGESICS *(cont.)*

Miscellaneous Opioids

Fentanyl (Duragesic) CII *(cont.)*	
CYP3A4 inhibitors	Caution with CYP3A4 inhibitors (eg, azole antifungals, diltiazem, erythromycin, ritonavir, verapamil); may increase plasma levels of fentanyl, causing severe or prolonged adverse reactions.
MAOIs	Caution with MAOIs; avoid within 14 days of use.
Fentanyl Citrate (Actiq, Fentora, Onsolis, Sublimaze) CII	
Alcohol	Additive CNS depressant effects.
CNS depressants	Additive CNS depressant effects, including respiratory depression and coma.
Conduction anesthesia	May alter respiration with certain forms of conduction anesthesia (eg, spinal anesthesia, some peridural anesthesia).
CYP3A4 inducers	Coadministration decreases plasma levels of fentanyl; may reduce efficacy.
CYP3A4 inhibitors	Caution with CYP3A4 inhibitors (eg, azole antifungals, diltiazem, erythromycin, ritonavir, verapamil); may increase plasma levels of fentanyl, causing severe or prolonged adverse reactions.
MAOIs	Caution with MAOIs; avoid within 14 days of use.
Neuroleptics	May cause elevated blood pressure with neuroleptics; caution in presence of risk factors for development of prolonged QT syndrome and torsades de pointes.
Nitrous oxide	May cause cardiovascular depression with nitrous oxide.
Tranquilizers	May cause a decrease in pulmonary arterial pressure and hypotension with tranquilizers.
Hydromorphone HCl (Dilaudid, Dilaudid-HP) CII	
Alcohol	Additive CNS depressant effects.
CNS depressants	Additive CNS depressant effects.
Mixed agonist/antagonist opioid analgesics	Mixed agonist/antagonist opioid analgesics (eg, pentazocine, nalbuphine, buprenorphine, butorphanol) may reduce analgesic effects and/or precipitate withdrawal symptoms.
Skeletal muscle relaxants	May enhance skeletal muscle relaxant effects and increase respiratory depression.
Meperidine HCl (Demerol Injection) CII	
Alcohol	Additive CNS depressant effects.
Anesthetics	May cause severe hypotension with certain anesthetics.
CNS depressants	Additive CNS depressant effects.
MAOIs	Caution with MAOIs; avoid within 14 days of use.
Phenothiazines	May cause severe hypotension with phenothiazines.
Meperidine HCl (Demerol Oral) CII	
Alcohol	Additive CNS depressant effects.
Acyclovir	Caution with acyclovir; increases plasma levels of meperidine.

OPIOID-CONTAINING ANALGESICS *(cont.)*

Miscellaneous Opioids

Meperidine HCl (Demerol Oral) CII *(cont.)*	
Anesthetics	May cause severe hypotension with certain anesthetics.
Cimetidine	Caution with cimetidine; decreases clearance and volume of distribution of meperidine.
CNS depressants	Additive CNS depressant effects.
MAOIs	Caution with MAOIs; avoid within 14 days of use.
Mixed agonist/antagonist opioid analgesics	Mixed agonist/antagonist opioid analgesics (eg, pentazocine, nalbuphine, buprenorphine, butorphanol) may reduce analgesic effects and/or precipitate withdrawal symptoms.
Phenothiazines	May cause severe hypotension with phenothiazines.
Phenytoin	Decreases half-life and increases clearance of meperidine. Increases plasma levels of meperidine metabolite.
Ritonavir	Avoid with ritonavir; may increase plasma levels of meperidine metabolite.
Skeletal muscle relaxants	May enhance skeletal muscle relaxant effects and increase respiratory depression.
Meperidine HCl/Promethazine HCl (Meprozine) CII	
Anesthetics	Possible severe hypotension with certain anesthetics.
Barbiturates	Potentiates sedative effects; reduce dose of both agents.
CNS depressants	Additive CNS depressant effects; dose reduction required.
MAOIs	Caution with MAOIs; avoid within 14 days of use.
Phenothiazines	May cause severe hypotension with phenothiazines.
Methadone HCl (Dolophine, Methadose) CII	
Alcohol	Additive CNS depressant effects.
Antiretroviral agents	Coadministration may alter plasma levels of antiretroviral agent or methadone.
Arrhythmogenic agents	Caution with drugs associated with drug-induced prolonged QT interval (eg, TCAs, CCBs, class I and III antiarrhythmics).
CNS depressants	Additive CNS depressant effects with other CNS depressants; increases risk of severe CNS and respiratory depression.
CYP3A4 inducers	CYP3A4 inducers (eg, carbamazepine, phenytoin, rifampin) may decrease plasma levels of methadone; monitor for withdrawal symptoms.
CYP3A4 inhibitors	CYP3A4 inhibitors (eg, azole antifungals, macrolide antibiotics, sertraline, fluvoxamine) may increase plasma levels and potentiate adverse effects of methadone.
Desipramine	Increases plasma levels of desipramine.
MAOIs	Caution with MAOIs; may cause severe reactions with concomitant use or within 14 days of use.
Mixed agonist/antagonist opioid analgesics	Mixed agonist/antagonist opioid analgesics (eg, pentazocine, nalbuphine, buprenorphine, butorphanol) may reduce analgesic effects and/or precipitate withdrawal symptoms.

Table 3.2. DRUG INTERACTIONS FOR ANALGESICS *(cont.)*

OPIOID-CONTAINING ANALGESICS *(cont.)*

Miscellaneous Opioids

Methadone HCl (Dolophine, Methadose) CII *(cont.)*	
Opioid antagonists	May precipitate withdrawal symptoms.
Partial opioid agonists	May precipitate withdrawal symptoms.
Morphine Sulfate (Astramorph PF, Avinza, Duramorph, Infumorph, Kadian, MS Contin, Oramorph SR, Roxanol, Roxanol-T) CII	
Acidifying agents	Antagonize the effects of morphine.
Alcohol	Additive CNS depressant effects. (Avinza) Avoid alcoholic beverages and medications containing alcohol. Concomitant use may result in the rapid release and absorption of a potentially fatal dose of morphine.
Alkalizing agents	Potentiates the effects of morphine.
Anticholinergics	May increase risk of urinary retention and/or severe constipation, which may lead to paralytic ileus.
Anticoagulants	Avoid with anticoagulants. May increase anticoagulant activity of coumarin derivatives and other anticoagulants.
Antihistamines	Additive CNS depressant effects.
Chlorpromazine	Potentiates analgesic effects of morphine.
Cimetidine	Increases respiratory and CNS depression with coadministration.
CNS depressants	Additive CNS depressant effects with other CNS depressants, including respiratory depression and coma; dose reduction may be necessary.
Diuretics	May decrease efficacy of diuretics.
MAOIs	Caution with MAOIs; avoid within 14 days of use.
Methocarbamol	Potentiates analgesic effects of morphine.
Mixed agonist/antagonist opioid analgesics	Mixed agonist/antagonist opioid analgesics (eg, pentazocine, nalbuphine, buprenorphine, butorphanol) may reduce analgesic effects and/or precipitate withdrawal symptoms. Avoid concomitant use.
Neuroleptics	Increases risk of respiratory depression, profound sedation, hypotension, and coma.
P-glycoprotein (PGP) inhibitors	PGP inhibitors (eg, quinidine) may increase absorption/exposure of morphine sulfate ~twofold.
Propranolol	Potentiates CNS depressant effects of morphine.
Psychotropic drugs	Additive CNS depressant effects.
Sedatives	Additive CNS depressant effects.
Skeletal muscle relaxants	May enhance skeletal muscle relaxant effects and increase respiratory depression.
Sympatholytic drugs	Increases risk of orthostatic hypotension.
TCAs	Caution with TCAs; increases risk of CNS depressant effects.

OPIOID-CONTAINING ANALGESICS *(cont.)*

Miscellaneous Opioids

Oxymorphone HCl (Opana, Opana ER) CII	
Alcohol	Additive CNS depressant effects.
Anticholinergics	May increase risk of urinary retention and/or severe constipation, which may lead to paralytic ileus.
Cimetidine	Increased CNS toxicity (eg, confusion, disorientation, respiratory depression, apnea, seizures) reported with coadministration of cimetidine.
CNS depressants	Additive CNS depressant effects.
MAOIs	Caution with MAOIs; avoid within 14 days of use.
Mixed agonist/antagonist opioid analgesics	Mixed agonist/antagonist opioid analgesics (eg, pentazocine, nalbuphine, buprenorphine, butorphanol) may reduce analgesic effects and/or precipitate withdrawal symptoms.
Remifentanil HCl (Ultiva) CII	
Anesthetics, inhaled	Synergistic activity with inhaled anesthetics; reduce dose of anesthetic by up to 75%.
Benzodiazepines	Synergistic activity with benzodiazepines; reduce dose of benzodiazepine by up to 75%.
Hypnotics	Synergistic activity with propofol and thiopental; reduce dose of hypnotic by up to 75%.

Opioid Agonist-Antagonists

Butorphanol Tartrate (Stadol NS) CIV	
Alcohol	Additive CNS depressant effects.
Antihistamines	Increased CNS and respiratory depression.
Barbiturates	Increased CNS and respiratory depression.
Erythromycin	May be potentiated by erythromycin.
Hepatic metabolism, drugs affecting	May be potentiated by other drugs affecting hepatic metabolism.
Nasal vasoconstrictors	May decrease the rate of absorption of butorphanol when given with nasal vasoconstrictors (eg, oxymetazoline).
Sumatriptan nasal spray	Diminished analgesic effect if administered shortly after sumatriptan nasal spray.
Theophylline	May be potentiated by theophylline.
Tranquilizers	Increased CNS and respiratory depression.
Nalbuphine HCl	
Anesthetics, general	Possible additive effects with general anesthetics.
CNS Depressants	Possible additive effects with other CNS depressants.
Hypnotics	Possible additive effects with hypnotics.
Ketorolac	Incompatible with ketorolac.

Table 3.2. DRUG INTERACTIONS FOR ANALGESICS *(cont.)*

OPIOID-CONTAINING ANALGESICS *(cont.)*

Opioid Agonist-Antagonists

Nalbuphine HCl *(cont.)*	
Nafcillin	Incompatible with nafcillin.
Opioid analgesics	Possible additive effects with opioid analgesics.
Phenothiazines	Possible additive effects with phenothiazines.
Sedatives	Possible additive effects with sedatives.
Tranquilizers	Possible additive effects with tranquilizers.
Pentazocine HCl/Acetaminophen (Talacen) CIV	
Alcohol	Additive CNS depressant effects.
Narcotics	May experience withdrawal symptoms.
Pentazocine HCl/Naloxone HCl (Talwin NX) CIV	
Alcohol	Additive CNS depressant effects.
Narcotics	May experience withdrawal symptoms with narcotics.

Opioid Agonist-Antagonist (For Opioid Dependence, see page 61.)

Buprenorphine HCl (Buprenex) CIII	
Alcohol	Additive CNS depressant effects.
CNS depressants	Additive CNS depressant effects.
CYP3A4 inducers	CYP3A4 inducers (eg, carbamazepine, phenytoin, rifampin) may induce metabolism and increase clearance of buprenorphine; may require dose adjustment.
CYP3A4 inhibitors	CYP3A4 inhibitors (eg, azole antifungals, macrolide antibiotics, protease inhibitors) may decrease clearance of buprenorphine; may require dose adjustment.
Diazepam	Respiratory and cardiovascular collapse reported with diazepam.
MAOIs	Caution with MAOIs; avoid within 14 days of use.

TOPICAL ANALGESICS

Diclofenac Epolamine (Flector)	
ACE inhibitors	Decreases antihypertensive effect of ACE inhibitors.
Anticoagulants	May increase risk of serious GI bleeding.
ASA	Avoid with ASA; increases risk of adverse effects.
Cyclosporine	Increases cyclosporine nephrotoxicity with coadministration.
Furosemide	Decreases natriuretic effect of furosemide.
Lithium	Increases plasma levels of lithium; monitor for lithium toxicity.
Methotrexate	Caution with methotrexate; increases methotrexate toxicity.
NSAIDs	Avoid with other NSAIDs; potential for increased adverse reactions.
Thiazides	Decreases natriuretic effect of thiazide diuretics.
Topical products	Avoid use with other topical products; may alter absorption and tolerability.

TOPICAL ANALGESICS *(cont.)*

Diclofenac Sodium (Voltaren Gel)	
ACE inhibitors	Decreases antihypertensive effect of ACE inhibitors.
Anticoagulants	May increase risk of serious GI bleeding.
ASA	Avoid with ASA; increases risk of adverse effects.
Cyclosporine	Increases cyclosporine nephrotoxicity with coadministration.
Furosemide	Decreases natriuretic effect of furosemide.
Lithium	Increases plasma levels of lithium; monitor for lithium toxicity.
Methotrexate	Caution with methotrexate; increases methotrexate toxicity.
NSAIDs	Avoid with other NSAIDs; potential for increased adverse reactions.
Thiazides	Decreases natriuretic effect of thiazide diuretics.
Topical products	Avoid use with other topical products; may alter absorption and tolerability.
Lidocaine (Lidoderm Patch)	
Anesthetics, local	Caution with other local anesthetics; consider cumulative doses from all formulations.
Anti-arrhythmics, class I	Caution with class I antiarrhythmic agents; possible additive and synergistic toxic effects.
Lidocaine/Prilocaine (EMLA)	
Anesthetics, local	Caution with other local anesthetics; consider cumulative doses from all formulations.
Antiarrhythmics, class I	Caution with class I antiarrhythmic agents; possible additive and synergistic toxic effects.
Antiarrhythmics, class III	Caution with class III antiarrhythmic agents; additive cardiac effects.
Methemoglobinemia, drugs causing	Increases risk of methemoglobinemia with coadministration.
Lidocaine/Tetracaine (Synera)	
Antiarrhythmics, class I	Caution with class I antiarrhythmic agents; possible additive and synergistic toxic effects.
Anesthetics, local	Caution with other local anesthetics; consider cumulative doses from all formulations.

Chapter 4

Hemostatics, Astringents, Gingival Displacement Products, and Antiseptics

Kenneth H. Burrell, D.D.S., S.M.

HEMOSTATICS

An understanding of hemostasis, how to identify patients with excessive bleeding tendencies, and interventions to stop abnormal bleeding is essential to the provision of safe and appropriate dental care.

Hemostasis can be divided arbitrarily into four phases: a vascular phase and a platelet phase, also referred to as "primary hemostasis;" and a coagulation phase and a fibrinolytic phase, also referred to as "secondary hemostasis."

Defects in any phase of normal hemostasis have characteristic signs and symptoms. Most commonly, dentists performing surgery will be faced with patients who have defects of the platelet and coagulation phases.

People with quantitative or qualitative platelet disorders usually have superficial signs such as petechiae and ecchymosis on the mucosa and skin. Furthermore, patients may report spontaneous gingival bleeding, epistaxis, prolonged postextraction bleeding, or prolonged bleeding after minor trauma. Spontaneous clinical hemorrhage may be present when the platelet count drops below 15,000 to 20,000/mm^3.

The clinical value of a bleeding time for dental procedures is controversial. However, significant prolonged bleeding times beyond 15 to 20 minutes may suggest significant hemorrhage after dental surgery.

Causes of defects of primary hemostasis include congenital as well as acquired disorders. The most common inherited bleeding disorder in the United States is von Willebrand's disease. This disorder is characterized by various degrees of deficiency and qualitative defects of the von Willebrand factor, which is needed primarily for platelet adhesion in high shear areas. In severe cases of von Willebrand's disease, spontaneous bleeding may occur. However, mild cases may be associated with prolonged bleeding only after major trauma. Common acquired dysfunctions of primary hemostasis include idiopathic thrombocytopenic purpura, liver disease, and drug-induced platelet disorders. Also, both acute and chronic leukemia are associated with thrombocytopenia. Some medications are used intentionally to decrease platelet functions in patients with disorders such as coronary artery disease.

Disorders of secondary hemostasis include hemophilia, vitamin K deficiency, and liver disease. Hemophilia is usually classified according to the specific factor deficiency, such as hemophilia A for factor VIII deficiency and hemophilia B for factor IX deficiency. Patients with hemophilia lack the ability to form fibrin and have bleeding episodes, particularly within stress-bearing joints (deep-seated bleeding). This can cause destruction of these joints.

General dentistry can be performed in patients with >50% factor activity, but 100% activity is recommended for surgical procedures. In a 60-kg patient with hemophilia A, a 100% plasma level equals 6,000 units of factor VIII.

Vitamin K deficiency causes decreased activation of factors II, VII, IX, and X, resulting in a defective coagulation cascade and consequent decreased fibrin production. Virtually all coagulation factors are produced in the liver, and vitamin K is stored in the liver. Thus, liver disease may result in increased bleeding tendencies. Medications such as warfarin, an anticoagulant that impairs the action of vitamin K, are used to prevent thrombosis in patients with such disorders as atrial fibrillation, deep vein thrombosis, ischemic cardiovascular disease, and stroke.

A thorough medical history, examination, and laboratory evaluation will identify most patients who have increased bleeding tendencies. The patient assessment should include questions addressing whether the patient has relatives with bleeding problems, has experienced prolonged bleeding after trauma, or takes medications, or has diseases associated with increased bleeding tendencies. The examination should focus on signs of bruising, jaundice, hyperplastic gingival tissue, spontaneous gingival bleeding, and hemarthrosis. Screening tests for impaired hemostasis include platelet count and bleeding time for primary hemostasis, as well as prothrombin time (PT), international normalized ratio (INR), activated partial thromboplastin time (PTT), and thrombin time for secondary hemostasis.

For example, warfarin therapy generally does not need to be modified or discontinued for simple extractions if the INR is ≤3.5. However, modification or discontinuation of warfarin therapy also depends on the outcome of a consultation with the patient's physician, clinical judgment, experience, training, and access to bleeding management resources. A new category of products called fibrin sealants, such as Crosseal and Tisseel, has been developed to promote hemostasis in liver, lung, splenic, and cardiothoracic surgery where conventional methods of hemostasis are not practical. Although research has been conducted using these products in oral surgery, they have not yet been approved for this purpose by the FDA. Fibrin sealants are not used exclusively in patients with bleeding and clotting disorders, since research is showing they promote more rapid postsurgical healing with reduced swelling and ecchymosis. Research may also show these products to be useful in sinus lifts and bone grafting.

Accepted Indications

If blood flow is profuse, mechanical aids such as a compress, hemostatic forceps, a modeling compound splint, or hemostatic ligatures can be used. Mechanical obliteration with cryosurgery, electrocauterization, or laser can also be used. Although these thermal methods are effective, they may be associated with impaired healing. A third kind of mechanically aided hemostasis is the use of chemical glues, such as n-butyl cyanoacrylate and bone wax. These compounds have a mechanical effect without directly affecting the coagulation process.

For slow blood flow and oozing, a combination of hemostatics can be used. The three kinds of hemostatics to be noted here are absorbable hemostatic agents, agents that modify blood coagulation, and vasoconstrictors. The latter act by constricting or closing blood vessels and are used to a limited extent to control capillary bleeding. Vasoconstrictors are described in detail in **Chapter 1**. See **Table 4.1** for a comparison of various hemostatics useful in dentistry.

Absorbable Gelatin Sponge

The absorbable gelatin sponge consists of a tough, porous matrix prepared from purified pork skin gelatin, granules, and water and is indicated as a hemostatic device for control of capillary, venous, or arteriolar bleeding when pressure, ligature, or other conventional procedures are either ineffective or impractical. It can be used in extraction sites and is absorbed in 4 to 6 weeks.

Oxidized Cellulose

Oxidized cellulose is a chemically modified form of surgical gauze or cotton that is used to control moderate bleeding by forming an artificial clot when suturing or ligation is impractical and ineffective. Because it is friable, oxidized cellulose is difficult to place and retain in extraction sockets, but can be used as a sutured implant or temporary packing. The cotton or gauze can be removed before dissolution is complete by irrigation with saline or a mildly alkaline solution.

Absorption of oxidized cellulose ordinarily occurs between the second and seventh day after implantation of material, but complete absorption of large amounts of blood-soaked material may take six weeks or longer.

Oxidized Regenerated Cellulose

Oxidized regenerated cellulose is prepared from alpha-cellulose by reaction with alkali to form viscose, which is then spun into filaments and oxidized. This process results in greater chemical purity and uniformity of physical structure than oxidized cellulose. It is a sterile, absorbable, knitted fabric that is strong enough to be sutured or cut. It has less of a tendency to stick to instruments and gloves and is less friable than oxidized cellulose.

Oxidized regenerated cellulose is used to control capillary, venous, and small arterial hemorrhage when ligature, pressure, or other conventional methods of control are impractical or ineffective. The product can be used as a surface dressing because it does not retard epithelialization. It is bactericidal against numerous gram-negative and gram-positive microorganisms, both aerobic and anaerobic. Additionally, it can be placed over extraction sites.

Microfibrillar Collagen Hemostat

Microfibrillar collagen hemostat is a hemostatically active agent prepared from bovine deep flexor tendon (Achilles tendon) as a water-soluble, partial-acid salt of natural collagen. It reduces bleeding from surgical sites such as those involving cancellous bone and gingival graft donor sites. It should not be left in infected or contaminated spaces because it may prolong or promote infection and delay healing.

Collagen Hemostat

Collagen hemostat is absorbable and composed of purified and lyophilized bovine dermal collagen. Used as an adjunct to hemostasis, collagen absorbable hemostat can be sutured into place. It reduces bleeding when ligation and other conventional methods are ineffective or impractical. Excess material should be removed before the wound is closed.

Aminocaproic Acid

Aminocaproic acid, or ε-aminocaproic acid, is used in patients with excessive bleeding due to underlying conditions such as systemic hyperfibrinolysis and coagulopathies stemming from promyelocytic leukemia. This medication is seldom used for elective oral surgery procedures, but rather during emergency situations in combination with transfusion of fresh frozen blood and fibrinogen.

Desmopressin Acetate

Desmopressin acetate is used primarily to reduce spontaneous bleeding in patients with von Willebrand's disease and in patients with mild-to-moderate hemophilia A (factor VIII levels >5%). It also is used prophylactically during procedures to reduce the incidence of bleeding, as well as after procedures to achieve better hemostasis in these patient populations.

Tranexamic Acid

Tranexamic acid is used primarily to reduce the amount of factor replacement necessary after dental extractions in hemophiliac patients. It is indicated for only two to eight days during and after the dental procedure. It also is used for other patient populations with impaired secondary hemostasis, including patients who are receiving anticoagulation therapy.

Vitamin K

Vitamin K therapy is required when hypoprothrombinemia results from inadequately available vitamins K_1 and K_2. This occurs when there is decreased synthesis by intestinal bacteria, inadequate absorption from the intestinal tract, or increased requirement by the liver for normal synthesis of prothrombin.

Vitamin K, in its various forms, is an essential component of blood coagulation. Vitamins K_1, K_2, or menadione (vitamin K_3) are required for the activation of the functional forms of six coagulation proteins: prothrombin; factors VII, IX, and X; and proteins C and S.

Phytonadione (vitamin K_1)

Phytonadione—known as vitamin K_1—is used for:

- anticoagulant-induced prothrombin deficiency
- prophylaxis and therapy of hemorrhagic disease in newborns
- hypoprothrombinemia resulting from oral antibacterial therapy
- hypoprothrombinemia secondary to factors limiting absorption or synthesis of vitamin K, such as obstructive jaundice, biliary fistula, sprue, ulcerative colitis, celiac disease, intestinal resection, cystic fibrosis of the pancreas, and regional enteritis
- other drug-induced hypoprothrombinemia, such as that resulting from salicylate use

Menadione (vitamin K_3)

Menadione is a synthetic form of vitamin K, which is sometimes referred to as vitamin K_3.

Menadiol sodium diphosphate (vitamin K_4)

Menadiol sodium diphosphate is effective as a hemostatic agent only when bleeding results from prothrombin deficiency.

Thrombin

Thrombin is useful as a topical local hemostatic agent when blood is oozing from accessible capillaries or venules. In certain kinds of hemorrhage, it can be used to wet pledgets of absorbable gelatin sponge and placed on bleeding tissue or in extraction sockets with or without sutures. It is particularly useful whenever blood is flowing from accessible capillaries and small venules.

General Dosing Information

Table 4.1 lists general dosing information for specific hemostatics.

Dosage Adjustments

The actual dose for each patient must be individualized according to factors such as his or her size, age, and physical status. Reduced doses of vitamin K may be indicated for patients who are taking anticoagulants as opposed to those who have malabsorption problems. The other hemostatic agents should be used as needed.

Special Dental Considerations

Cross-Sensitivity

Patients may experience delayed healing using the gelatin, cellulose, and collagen hemostatics. This is more often observed when the surgical site is infected.

Patient Monitoring: Aspects to Watch

Patients receiving vitamin K, especially parenterally, may experience allergic reactions such as rash, urticaria, and anaphylaxis.

Adverse Effects and Precautions

The incidence of adverse reactions to hemostatic agents is relatively low. Many reactions are temporary. Idiosyncratic and allergic reactions account for a small minority of adverse responses. See **Table 4.1**.

Pharmacology

Absorbable Gelatin Sponge

The absorbable gelatin sponge promotes the disruption of platelets and acts as a framework for fibrin, probably because of its physical effect rather than the result of its alteration of the blood-clotting mechanism. It can be placed in dry form or may be moistened with sterile saline or thrombin solution and used in extraction sites.

Oxidized Cellulose

Oxidized cellulose is a chemically modified form of surgical gauze or cotton. Its hemostatic action depends on the formation of an artificial clot by cellulosic acid, which has a marked affinity for hemoglobin.

Oxidized Regenerated Cellulose

Oxidized regenerated cellulose serves as a hemostatic most likely by providing a physical effect rather than altering the normal physiological clotting mechanism.

Microfibrillar Collagen Hemostat

This hemostatic agent is used topically to trigger the adhesiveness of platelets and to stimulate the release phenomenon to produce aggregation of platelets leading to their disintegration and to release coagulation factors that, together with plasma factors, enable fibrin to form. The physical structure of microfibrillar collagen hemostat adds strength to the clot.

Collagen Hemostat

When collagen comes into contact with blood, platelets aggregate and release coagulation factors, which, together with plasma factors, cause the formation of fibrin and a clot.

Aminocaproic Acid

Aminocaproic acid is an antifibrinolytic agent that slows or stops fibrinolysis by inhibiting the action of plasminogen. Consequently, it delays the breakdown of the hemostatic plug. This medication is administered both intravenously and orally in the form of tablets and syrup. Concurrent use of other hemostatic agents in patients with significant bleeding tendencies is recommended.

Desmopressin Acetate

Desamino-D-arginine vasopressin is a synthetic analogue of the natural pituitary hormone 1-8-D-arginine vasopressin. This medication increases plasma levels of von Willebrand factor-VIII complex and factor VIII levels. It is administered 30 minutes before the dental appointment. It facilitates outpatient care for patients with hemophilia, but should always be used in conjunction with other hemostatic agents.

Tranexamic Acid

Tranexamic acid is an antifibrinolytic hemostatic agent that acts by decreasing conversion of plasminogen to plasmin. At much higher doses, it acts as a noncompetitive inhibitor of plasmin. It is indicated for prophylaxis and treatment of patients with hemophilia to prevent or reduce hemorrhage during and after tooth extraction. Unapproved uses include topical use as a mouthwash, along with systemic therapy to reduce bleeding after oral surgery. It is contraindicated for use in patients receiving anticoagulant therapy. This medication is administered both intravenously and orally.

Vitamin K

Two forms of naturally occurring vitamin K have been isolated and prepared synthetically. The naturally occurring forms are designated vitamins K_1 and K_2. Vitamin K_1 is present in most vegetables, particularly in their green leaves. Vitamin K_2 is produced by intestinal bacteria. Menadione has vitamin K activity and is derived from a breakdown of the vitamin K molecule by intestinal bacteria and is sometimes referred to as vitamin K_3. Menadiol sodium diphosphate, or vitamin K_4, is a water-soluble derivative that is converted to menadione in the liver.

Hypoprothrombinemia may result from inadequately available vitamins K_1 and K_2 because of decreased synthesis by intestinal bacteria, inadequate absorption from the intestinal tract or increased requirement by the liver for normal synthesis of prothrombin. Liver dysfunction may also decrease the production of prothrombin, but the hypoprothrombinemia from hepatic cell injury may not respond to the administration of vitamin K as many coagulation proteins are produced in hepatocytes.

Insufficient vitamin K in ingested foods becomes significant only when the synthesis of the vitamin by intestinal bacteria is markedly reduced by the oral administration of antibacterial agents. Biliary obstructions or intestinal disorders may result in an inadequate rate of absorption of vitamin K.

Phytonadione (vitamin K_1)

Vitamin K_1 is required for the production of the functional forms of six coagulation proteins: prothrombin, factors VII, IX and X and proteins C and S.

Menadione (vitamin K_3)

Although it is readily absorbed from the intestine, menadione must be converted to vitamin K_2 by the liver. Therefore, it requires a normal flow of bile into the intestine or the concomitant administration of bile salts.

Menadiol sodium diphosphate (vitamin K_4)

Vitamin K_4, because of its water solubility, is absorbed from the intestinal tract even in the absence of bile salts.

Thrombin

Thrombin is a sterile protein substance that is an essential component of blood coagulation. It activates fibrinogen to form fibrin.

Patient Advice

- Let the patient know that a hemostatic has been used, what kind of hemostatic it is, and why it was used.
- Advise the patient to let you know if bleeding continues from the surgical site.

ASTRINGENTS

Astringents cause contraction of tissues. They accomplish this by constricting small blood vessels, extracting water from tissue, or precipitating protein.

Accepted Indications

Astringents can be applied to gingival tissues before taking impressions, placing Class V or root-surface restorations. They can be used alone or in combination with retraction cords. Aluminum and iron salts are the compounds used as astringents in dentistry.

Aluminum Chloride

Aluminum chloride causes contraction or shrinking of tissue, making it useful in retracting gingival tissue. It also reduces secretions and minor hemorrhage.

Aluminum Potassium Sulfate

Aluminum potassium sulfate, or alum, is not widely used, even though it is relatively innocuous, because its tissue retraction and hemostatic properties are limited.

Aluminum Sulfate

Aluminum sulfate, as with other aluminum salts, serves as an effective astringent for gingival retraction and hemostatic action.

Ferric Sulfate

Ferric sulfate is an effective and safe astringent and hemostatic for use in gingival retraction. It also can be used in vital pulpotomies.

General Dosing Information

Table 4.1 lists general dosing and administration information for specific astringents.

Adverse Effects

The incidence of adverse reactions to astringents is relatively low. Most reactions are temporary. The adverse effects listed in **Table 4.1** apply to all major types of astringents.

Pharmacology

The ability of any astringent to contract or shrink mucous membrane or skin tissue is related to its mode of action involving protein precipitation and water absorption.

GINGIVAL DISPLACEMENT PRODUCTS

Gingival displacement products can be used alone or in combination with astringents or vasoconstrictors. They are usually made of cotton and are woven in various ways to suit the practitioner's preferences. These cotton cords are available in a variety of diameters to accommodate the variation in gingival sulcus width and depth. Gingival displacement pastes are also available. One paste uses kaolin as the vehicle and contains 6.5% aluminum chloride; the other is made of the polymer PVS, which expands into the sulcus as it sets.

Cords can be impregnated with astringents or vasoconstrictors either by the manufacturer or at chairside. Aluminum chloride, aluminum sulfate, and ferric sulfate are the astringents used, while racemic epinephrine is used as the vasoconstrictor.

Epinephrine cord is contraindicated in patients with a history of cardiovascular diseases and dysrhythmias, diabetes, and hyperthyroidism and in those taking rauwolfia and ganglionic blocking agents. Caution is advised in patients taking monoamine oxidase inhibitors.

Some practitioners and educators believe that epinephrine-containing displacement cord and solutions should not be used in dentistry. However, plasma epinephrine concentration increased significantly only after 60 minutes in a study of healthy subjects without a history of high blood pressure. In spite of the elevated plasma epinephrine levels, the subjects' heart rates, mean arterial pressures, and pulse pressure were not significantly different when the same subjects were exposed to a potassium aluminum sulfate– (alum) impregnated cord. The gingival tissues of the subjects were intact, however. Therefore, the patient's medical history, oral health, type of procedure to be done, amount and length of displacement cord, and exposure of the vascular bed should be considered before deciding to use epinephrine-containing retraction cords. **Table 4.1** provides gingival displacement cord information, including adverse effects, precautions and contraindications of a variety of commercially available displacement cords.

Accepted Indications

Gingival displacement cord is used for all kinds of gingival displacement before taking impressions or placing restorations.

General Dosing Information

Dosage Adjustments

The actual maximum dose for each patient must be individualized depending on factors such as oral health and sensitivity.

Adverse Effects and Precautions

The incidence of adverse reactions to gingival displacement cords and paste is relatively low. Most reactions are temporary, but gingival tissue destruction may permanently alter gingival architecture, especially after vigorous cord placement.

Pharmacology

Gingival displacement products work mechanically to widen the gingival sulcus. With the addition of astringents or vasoconstrictors, the gingival tissue is retracted further. The astringents act by constricting blood vessels, extracting water from tissue or precipitating proteins.

ANTISEPTICS

An antiseptic is a broad-spectrum antimicrobial chemical solution that is applied topically to body surfaces to reduce the microbial flora in preparation for surgery or at an injection site. The antimicrobial activity of antiseptics usually is weaker than that of disinfectants and sterilants because less harsh, or weaker, chemicals usually must be applied to body surfaces to avoid irritating the tissues. However, the antimicrobial activity of antiseptics can be lethal to the microbes on the body surfaces. The specific activity depends on the nature of the antiseptic chemical and the microbes involved. In dentistry, antiseptics are grouped into three classes: handwashing agents, skin and mucosal antiseptics, and root canal and cavity preparations (see **Table 4.2** for usage information).

SUGGESTED READING

Aframian DJ, Lalla RV, Peterson DE Management of dental patients taking common hemostasis-altering medications. *Oral Surg Oral Path Oral Radiol Endol*. 2007;103(suppl):S45.e1-11.

Anderson KW, Baker SR. Advances in facial rejuvenation surgery. *Otolaryngol Head Neck Surg*. 2003;11(4):256-260.

Colman RW, Hirsch J, Marder VJ, et al, eds. *Hemostatics and Thrombosis: Basic Principles and Clinical Practice*. 4th ed. Philadelphia: Lippincott Williams & Wilkins; 2000.

Donovan TE, Chee WWL. Current concepts in gingival displacement. *Dent Clin North Am*. 2004;48:433-444.

Fat and water soluble vitamins: vitamin K. In: *Drug Facts and Comparisons*. St Louis: Facts and Comparisons; 2000:12-13.

Garfunkel AA, Galili D, Findler M, et al. Bleeding tendency: a practical approach to dentistry. *Compend Contin Educ Dent*. 1999;20:836-852.

Rossman JA, Rees TD. The use of hemostatic agents in dentistry. *Postgrad Dent*. 1996;3:3-12.

Wahl MJ. Myths of dental surgery in patients receiving anticoagulant therapy. *JADA*. 2000;131:77-81.

Table 4.1. USAGE INFORMATION FOR HEMOSTATICS, ASTRINGENTS, AND GINGIVAL DISPLACEMENT PRODUCTS

NAME	FORM/ STRENGTH	DOSAGE	WARNINGS/PRECAUTIONS & CONTRAINDICATIONS	ADVERSE EFFECTS
HEMOSTATICS				
LOCAL AGENTS THAT MODIFY BLOOD COAGULATION				
Absorbable Gelatin Sponge (Gelfoam)	**Dental Packing Blocks:** 20 x 20 x 7mm; Pow: 1g	Absorbable gelatin sponge may be cut; may be applied to bleeding surfaces to cover area.	**W/P:** Should not be overpacked in extraction sites or surgical defects because it may expand to impinge on neighboring structures.	May form a nidus for infection or abscess formation.
Collagen, Bovine/ Glycosaminoglycans (CollaCote, CollaPlug, CollaTape, Integra Bilayer Matrix Wound Dressing, Integra Dermal Regeneration Template)	**CollaCote, CollaPlug, CollaTape:** 1 x 3, ¾ x 1½, 3/8 x ¾ in	Use as directed.	**W/P:** Do not use on infected or contaminated wounds. Although these dressings will promote hemostasis, they are not intended for use in treating systemic coagulation disorders. **P/N:** Safety during pregnancy unknown.	NA
Collagen Hemostat (Helistat, Instat)	**Pads:** 1 x 2, 3 x 4 in	Should be applied directly to bleeding surface with pressure; is more effective when applied dry, or may be moistened with sterile saline or thrombin solution; may be left in place as necessary; is absorbed 8-10 w after placement.	**W/P:** Incidence of pain has been reported to increase when this material is placed in extraction sockets. Allergic reactions can occur in patients with known sensitivity to bovine material.	Should not be used in mucous membrane closure because it may interfere with healing due to mechanical interposition. Should not be left in infected or contaminated space because of possible delay in healing and increased likelihood of abscess formation. Should not be used in patients with a known sensitivity to bovine material. Should not be overpacked because collagen absorbable hemostat absorbs water and can expand to impinge on neighboring structures. Should not be used in cases where point of hemorrhage is submerged, because collagen must be in direct contact with bleeding site to achieve desired effect.
Microfibrillar Collagen Hemostat (Avitene, Helitene Instat MCH)	**Avitene Flour:** ½-, 1-, 5-g syringes; **Avitene Sheets:** 35 x 35, 70 x 35, 70 x 70 mm; **Instat MCH:** Coherent fibers packaged in 0.5- and 1.0-g containers	Is applied topically and adheres firmly to bleeding surfaces.	**W/P:** Is not intended to treat systemic coagulation disorders. Placement in extraction sites has been reported to increase pain. Should not be left in infected or contaminated spaces because of possible adhesion formation, allergic reaction, foreign body reaction. Interferes with wound margins.	May potentiate abscess formation, hematoma and wound dehiscence.
Oxidized Cellulose (Oxycel)	**Pad:** 3 x 3 in; **Pledget:** 2 x 1 x 1 in; **Strip:** 18 × 2, 5 x ½, 36 x ½ in	Hemostatic effect is greater when material is applied dry as opposed to moistened with water or saline.	**W/P:** Extremely friable and difficult to place. Should not be used at fracture sites because it interferes with bone regeneration. Should not be used as a surface dressing except for the immediate control of hemorrhage, as cellulosic acid inhibits epithelialization. Should not be used in combination with thrombin because the hemostatic action of either alone is greater than that of the combination.	May lead to a foreign-body reaction.

NA = Not available.

This list is not comprehensive. The products shown here are available in various formulations and strengths, not all of which are listed. In addition, the listing of a product does not denote its superiority to any other product that is either listed or not listed, nor does it guarantee its availability or quality.

BB = black box warning; **W/P** = warnings/precautions; **Contra** = contraindications; **P/N** = pregnancy category rating and nursing considerations.

Table 4.1. USAGE INFORMATION FOR HEMOSTATICS, ASTRINGENTS, AND GINGIVAL DISPLACEMENT PRODUCTS *(cont.)*

NAME	FORM/ STRENGTH	DOSAGE	WARNINGS/PRECAUTIONS & CONTRAINDICATIONS	ADVERSE EFFECTS
HEMOSTATICS *(cont.)*				
LOCAL AGENTS THAT MODIFY BLOOD COAGULATION *(cont.)*				
Oxidized Regenerated Cellulose (Surgicel Absorbable Hemostat, Surgicel Nu-Knit Absorbable Hemostat)	**Surgicel sheets:** 2 x 14, 4 x 8, 2 x 3, ½ x 2 in; **Surgicel Nu-Knit sheets:** 1 x 1, 3 x 4, 6 x 9 in	Can be laid over extraction socket for control of bleeding; minimal amounts of the material should be placed on bleeding site; may be held firmly against tissue.	**W/P:** Placement in extraction sites may delay healing; it should not be placed in fracture sites because it may interfere with callus formation and may cause cyst formation. Encapsulation of fluid and foreign bodies possible.	NA
SYSTEMIC AGENTS THAT MODIFY BLOOD COAGULATION				
Aminocaproic Acid (Amicar)	**Inj:** 250mg/mL; **Syr:** 1.25g/5mL; **Tab:** 500mg*, 1000mg*	***Adults:*** **IV:** 16-20mL (4-5g) in 250mL diluent during 1st hr, then 4mL/hr (1g) in 50mL of diluent. **PO:** 5g during 1st hr, then 5mL (syr) or 1g (tabs) per hr. Continue therapy for 8 hrs or until bleeding is controlled.	**W/P:** Avoid in hematuria of upper urinary tract origin due to risk of intrarenal obstruction from glomerular capillary thrombosis or clots in renal pelvis and ureters. Skeletal muscle weakness with necrosis of muscle fibers reported after prolonged therapy. Consider cardiac muscle damage with skeletal myopathy. Avoid rapid IV infusion. Thrombophlebitis may occur. Contains benzyl alcohol; do not administer to neonates due to risk of fatal gasping syndrome. Do not administer without a definite diagnosis of hyperfibrinolysis. **Contra:** Active intravascular clotting process, disseminated intravascular coagulation without concomitant heparin. **P/N:** Category C, caution in nursing.	Edema, headache, anaphylactoid reactions, injection site reactions, pain, bradycardia, hypotension, abdominal pain, diarrhea, nausea, vomiting, agranulocytosis, increased CPK, confusion, dyspnea, pruritus, tinnitus.
Anti-Inhibitor Coagulation Complex (Autoplex T, Feiba-VH)	**Sol:** 1 IU	***Adults/Pediatrics:*** **Autoplex T:** 25 to 100 units/kg, depending on severity of hemorrhage; repeat after 6 hours if no hemostatic improvement. **Feiba-VH:** 50 to 100 units/kg.	**W/P:** Made from human plasma. May contain infectious agents, such as viruses, that can cause disease. The risk that such products will transmit an infectious agent has been reduced by screening plasma donors for prior exposure to certain viruses, by testing for the presence of certain current virus infections, and by inactivating and/or removing certain viruses. Despite these measures, such products can still potentially transmit disease. Because this product is made from human blood, it may carry a risk of transmitting infectious agents, eg, viruses and theoretically, the Creutzfeldt-Jakob disease (CJD) agent. ALL infections thought by a physician possibly to have been transmitted by this product should be reported by the physician or other healthcare provider to the U.S. distributor. **Contra:** Bleeding episodes resulting from coagulation factor deficiencies, eg, disseminated intravascular coagulation, fibrinolysis, normal coagulation mechanism. **P/N:** Category C, caution in nursing.	Tachycardia, hypotension, chest pain, nausea, dizziness, headache, fever.

NA = Not available. *Scored. †Dosage strength not available.

This list is not comprehensive. The products shown here are available in various formulations and strengths, not all of which are listed. In addition, the listing of a product does not denote its superiority to any other product that is either listed or not listed, nor does it guarantee its availability or quality.

BB = black box warning; **W/P** = warnings/precautions; **Contra** = contraindications; **P/N** = pregnancy category rating and nursing considerations.

NAME	FORM/ STRENGTH	DOSAGE	WARNINGS/PRECAUTIONS & CONTRAINDICATIONS	ADVERSE EFFECTS
Desmopressin Acetate (DDAVP)	**Inj:** 4μg/mL; **Nasal Spray:** 10μg/inh [5mL]; **Tab:** 0.1mg*, 0.2mg*; **Rhinal Tube:** 0.01% [2.5mL]	***Adults:*** **Hemophilia A and von Willebrand Disease:** 0.3μg/kg IV. Add 50mL diluent. Give 30 minutes preoperatively. ***Pediatrics:*** **Hemophilia A and von Willebrand Disease: >3 months: (Inj)** 0.3μg/kg IV. Add 50mL diluent if 10kg; add 10mL diluent if >10kg. Give 30 minutes preoperatively.	**W/P:** Mucosal changes with nasal forms may occur; discontinue until resolved. Decrease fluid intake in pediatrics and elderly to decrease risk of water intoxication and hyponatremia; monitor osmolality. Caution with coronary artery insufficiency, hypertensive cardiovascular disease, fluid and electrolyte imbalance (eg, cystic fibrosis). Anaphylaxis reported with IV use. Caution with IV use if history of thrombus formation. For diabetes insipidus, dosage must be adjusted according to diurnal pattern of response; estimate response by adequate duration of sleep and adequate, not excessive, water turnover. **P/N:** Category B, caution in nursing.	**Inj:** Headache, nausea, abdominal cramps, vulval pain, injection site reactions, facial flushing, BP changes. **Spray:** Headache, dizziness, rhinitis, nausea, nasal congestion, sore throat, cough, respiratory infection, epistaxis. **Tab:** Nausea, flushing, abdominal cramps, headache, increased SGOT, water intoxication, hyponatremia.
Epinephrine/Racemic epinephrine (Epidri, Gingi-Pak Pellets,† OroStat, Racellet, Racemistat)	**Sol:** (racemic epinephrine) 8% (OroStat); 25% (Racemistat); **Cotton pellet:** (racemic epinephrine) 0.90- 1.40mg/pellet #2; 0.42-0.68mg/pellet #3 (Racellet); 1.9mg/pellet (Epidri)	Use as directed.	**W/P:** Patient's medical history and oral health, type of procedure to be done, amount and length of retraction, and exposure of the vascular bed should be considered before epinephrine-containing hemostatics are used. **Contra:** Patients with a history of cardiovascular disease, diabetes, hyperthyroidism, hypertension, or arteriosclerosis; and patients taking tricyclic antidepressants, monoamine oxidase inhibitors, rauwolfias, or ganglionic-blocking agents.	May cause irritation or tissue destruction.
Phytonadione (Mephyton, Vitamin K, Vitamin K_1)	**Tab:** 5mg* (Mephyton); **Inj:** 1mg/0.5mL, 10 mg/mL (Vitamin K)	***Adults:*** **Anticoagulant-Induced Prothrombin Deficiency: Initial:** 2.5-10mg up to 25mg (rarely 50mg). May repeat if PT is still elevated 12-48 hrs after initial dose. **Hypoprothrombinemia Due to Other Causes:** 2.5- 25mg or more (rarely up to 50mg). Give bile salts when endogenous bile supply to GIT is deficient.	**W/P:** Does not produce an immediate coagulant effect. Maintain lowest possible dose to prevent original thromboembolic events. Avoid repeated large doses with hepatic disease. Failure to respond may indicate a congenital coagulation defect or a condition unresponsive to vitamin K. Avoid large doses in liver disease. Monitor PT regularly. **P/N:** Category C, caution in nursing.	Severe hypersensitivity reactions (anaphylactoid reactions, death), flushing, peculiar taste sensations, dizziness, rapid and weak pulse, profuse sweating, hypotension, dyspnea, cyanosis.
Tranexamic Acid (Cyklokapron)	**Sol:** 100 mg/mL in 10-mL vials; **Tab:** 500 mg	***Adults/Pediatrics:*** Immediately before surgery, 10mg/kg IV; after surgery, 25mg/kg orally tid or qid for 2-8 days.	**W/P:** Dose should be reduced for patients with renal impairment. Contraindicated in patients with acquired defective color vision and subarachnoid hemorrhage. **P/N:** Category B.	Giddiness, nausea, vomiting, diarrhea, blurred vision; hypotension with IV dose.
Vitamin K_3 or Menadione	**Powder**	***Adults:*** 2-10mg/day, 4-7 days before surgery.	**W/P:** Requires normal flow of bile or administration of bile salts. Patient undergoing prothrombin reduction therapy should not receive vitamin K preparations except under physician supervision.	Adverse reactions are similar to those produced by phytonadione, but incidence is low.
Vitamin K_4 or Menadiol Sodium Diphosphate	**Inj:** 5, 10, 37.5mg/mL; **Tab:** 5mg	**Inj:** 5-10mg q day, 4-7 days. **Oral:** 5mg q day, 4-7 days.	**W/P:** Before administering drug, determine if patient is receiving anticoagulant therapy; a patient undergoing prothrombin reduction therapy should not receive vitamin K preparations except under physician supervision. If patient is taking anticoagulants, this agent may decrease their effectiveness.	Adverse reactions are similar to those produced by phytonadione, but incidence is low.

Table 4.1. USAGE INFORMATION FOR HEMOSTATICS, ASTRINGENTS, AND GINGIVAL DISPLACEMENT PRODUCTS *(cont.)*

NAME	FORM/ STRENGTH	DOSAGE	WARNINGS/PRECAUTIONS & CONTRAINDICATIONS	ADVERSE EFFECTS
HEMOSTATICS *(cont.)*				
THROMBIN (TOPICAL AGENT)				
Thrombin (Recothrom, Thrombin-JMI, Thrombinar, Thrombogen, Thrombostat)	**Pow:** 1,000, 5,000, 10,000, 20,000 units; 50,000 units (Thrombinar only); **Pow (with isotonic saline diluent):** 5,000-, 10,000- and 20,000-unit containers with 5-, 10-, and 20-mL of isotonic saline; **Thrombostat:** Also contains 0.02mg/mL phemerol as a preservative	**Profuse Bleeding (Sol):** 1,000-2,000 units/mL. For bleeding from skin or mucosa—solution: 100 units/mL.	**W/P:** Thrombin must not be injected into blood vessels because it might cause serious or even fatal embolism from extensive intravascular thrombosis; instead, should be applied to surface of bleeding tissue as solution or powder. **P/N:** Category C.	Allergic reactions can occur in patients with known sensitivity to bovine material.
ASTRINGENTS				
Aluminum Chloride (Gingi-Aid, Hemoban, Hemodent, Hemodettes, Hemogin-L, Patterson Buffered Aluminum Chloride, Racestyptine, Retreat Gel 25%, Styptin, Topical Hemostat Solution, ViscoStat Clear)	**Gel:** 20% (Hemodettes), 25% (Retreat Gel 25%; ViscoStat Clear [for use in infuser kit]); **Sol:** 20% (Hemodent, Styptin), 25% (Gingi-Aid, Ultradent); **Oint:** 25% (Hemogin-L); **Retraction cords:** Average concentration of 0.915, 3.5mg/in	***Adults:*** Apply product directly to tissues using a cotton pledget or apply to gingival retraction cords.	None of significance to dentistry.	Concentrated solutions of aluminum chloride are acidic and may have an irritating and even caustic effect on tissues.
Aluminum Potassium Sulfate	**Pow:** 100%, various concentrations, all available and prepared by chemical supply houses	***Adults:*** Any concentration, including 100% powder, can be used.	None of significance to dentistry.	May have an irritating effect.
Aluminum Sulfate (Gel-Cord, Rastringent, Rastringent 2, Tissue Goo Gel)	**Cotton pellet:** 2.20-2.80mg/pellet (Rastringent); **Gel:** In unit-dose cartridge; **Impregnated retraction cord:** Average concentration of 0.48, 0.85, 1.45mg/in; **Topical solution:** 25%	***Adults:*** Apply product directly to tissues using a cotton pledget or apply to gingival retraction cords.	None of significance to dentistry.	May have an irritating and even caustic effect.
Ferric Chloride (ViscoStat Plus)	**Sol:** 22% (for use in infuser kit)	***Adults:*** Apply product directly to tissues using a cotton pledget or apply to gingival retraction cords.	NA	NA

NA = Not available. ‡Retraction cords, braids, and twists come in various diameters. A number of cords are available with epinephrine and racemic epinephrine in concentrations ranging from 0.3-1.45mg/in and varying concentrations of zinc phenolsulfonate or aluminum compounds. Consult the manufacturer's labeling for more information.

This list is not comprehensive. The products shown here are available in various formulations and strengths, not all of which are listed. In addition, the listing of a product does not denote its superiority to any other product that is either listed or not listed, nor does it guarantee its availability or quality.

BB = black box warning; **W/P** = warnings/precautions; **Contra** = contraindications; **P/N** = pregnancy category rating and nursing considerations.

NAME	FORM/ STRENGTH	DOSAGE	WARNINGS/PRECAUTIONS & CONTRAINDICATIONS	ADVERSE EFFECTS
Ferric Sulfate (Astringedent, FS-Hemostatic Liquid, Patterson Ferric Sulfate, Quick-Stat FS, Retreat Gel 20%, Retreat Solution, Stasis, StatGel)	**Gel:** 20% (Retreat Gel 20%; **Sol:** 13.3% (Astringedent), 15.5% (FS-Hemostatic, Retreat Solution), 21% (Stasis)	***Adults:*** Apply product directly to tissues using a cotton pledget or apply to gingival retraction cords.	None of significance to dentistry.	Compound may cause tissue irritation to a greater degree than aluminum compounds.
Ferric Sulfate/ Ferric Subsulfate (Astringedent, Astringedent X, Viscostat, Viscostat Wintermint)	**Sol:** 25%	***Adults:*** Apply product directly to tissues using a cotton pledget or apply to gingival retraction cords.	NA	NA
GINGIVAL DISPLACEMENT PRODUCTS‡				
Retraction cord, plain (Gingibraid, GingiKnit, Gingi-Plain, Gingi-Plain Z-Twist, Hemodent, Knit-Trax, Patterson, Pro/Option, Retrax, Sil-Trax, Soft-Twist, Ultrapak, Whaledent)	NA	Use as directed.	None of significance to dentistry.	None of significance to dentistry.
Retraction cord with aluminum chloride (Gingi-Gel, Hemodent, Retreat, Retreat II, Whaledent)	NA	Use as directed.	**Contra:** History of allergy.	May cause irritation or tissue destruction.
Retraction paste, plain (Magic FoamCord)	PVS	Use as directed.	None of significance to dentistry.	None of significance to dentistry.
Retraction paste with aluminum chloride (Expa-syl, Traxodent Hemodent)	6.5% aluminum chloride	Use as directed.	**Contra:** History of allergy.	May cause irritation or tissue destruction.
Retraction cord with aluminum sulfate (Gingi-Aid Z-Twist, Pascord, Retreat, Sil-Trax AS)	NA	Use as directed.	None of significance to dentistry.	May have an irritating and even caustic effect.
Retraction cord with aluminum potassium sulfate (GingiBraid, GingiKnit, GingiTrac, SulPak, Sultan Ultrax, UniBraid)	NA	Use as directed.	None of significance to dentistry.	May have an irritating effect.
Retraction cord with epinephrine (Gingi-Pak MAX, Patterson, Retreat II w/Epi)	NA	Use as directed.	**W/P:** Patient's medical history and oral health, type of procedure to be done, amount and length of retraction, and exposure of the vascular bed should be considered before epinephrine-containing retraction cords are used. **Contra:** Patients with a history of cardiovascular disease, diabetes, hyperthyroidism, hypertension, or arteriosclerosis; and patients taking tricyclic antidepressants, monoamine oxidase inhibitors, rauwolfias, or ganglionic-blocking agents.	May cause irritation or tissue destruction.

Table 4.1. USAGE INFORMATION FOR HEMOSTATICS, ASTRINGENTS, AND GINGIVAL DISPLACEMENT PRODUCTS *(cont.)*

NAME	FORM/ STRENGTH	DOSAGE	WARNINGS/PRECAUTIONS & CONTRAINDICATIONS	ADVERSE EFFECTS
GINGIVAL DISPLACEMENT PRODUCTS‡ *(cont.)*				
Retraction cord with racemic epinephrine (Racord, Sil-Trax EPI, Sulpak, Sultan, Ultrax)	NA	Use as directed.	**W/P:** Patient's medical history and oral health, type of procedure to be done, amount and length of retraction, and exposure of the vascular bed should be considered before epinephrine-containing retraction cords are used. **Contra:** Patients with a history of cardiovascular disease, diabetes, hyperthyroidism, hypertension, or arteriosclerosis; and patients taking tricyclic antidepressants, monoamine oxidase inhibitors, rauwolfias, or ganglionic-blocking agents.	May cause irritation or tissue destruction.
Retraction cord with racemic epinephrine and aluminum potassium sulfate (GingiBraid, Gingi-Cord, Sulpak, Ultrax, UniBraid)	NA	Use as directed.	**W/P:** Patient's medical history and oral health, type of procedure to be done, amount and length of retraction, and exposure of the vascular bed should be considered before epinephrine-containing retraction cords are used. **Contra:** Patients with a history of cardiovascular disease, diabetes, hyperthyroidism, hypertension, or arteriosclerosis; and patients taking tricyclic antidepressants, monoamine oxidase inhibitors, rauwolfias, or ganglionic-blocking agents.	May cause irritation or tissue destruction.
Retraction cord with racemic epinephrine and zinc phenolsulfonate (Siltrax Plus, Racord Two)	NA	Use as directed.	**W/P:** Patient's medical history and oral health, type of procedure to be done, amount and length of retraction, and exposure of the vascular bed should be considered before epinephrine-containing retraction cords are used. **Contra:** Patients with a history of cardiovascular disease, diabetes, hyperthyroidism, hypertension, or arteriosclerosis; and patients taking tricyclic antidepressants, monoamine oxidase inhibitors, rauwolfias, or ganglionic-blocking agents.	May cause irritation or tissue destruction.
GINGIVAL HEMOSTATIC AGENTS				
Epinephrine/racemic epinephrine (Epidri, Gingi-Pak Pellets,† OroStat, Racellet, Racemistat)	**Sol:** (racemic epinephrine) 8% (OroStat); 25% (Racemistat); **Cotton pellet:** (racemic epinephrine): 0.90- 1.40mg/ pellet #2; 0.42- 0.68mg/pellet #3 (Racellet); 1.9mg/ pellet (Epidri)	Use as directed.	**W/P:** Patient's medical history and oral health, type of procedure to be done, amount and length of retraction, and exposure of the vascular bed should be considered before epinephrine-containing hemostatics are used. **Contra:** Patients with a history of cardiovascular disease, diabetes, hyperthyroidism, hypertension, or arteriosclerosis; and patients taking tricyclic antidepressants, monoamine oxidase inhibitors, rauwolfias, or ganglionic-blocking agents.	May cause irritation or tissue destruction.

NA = Not available. †Dosage strength not available. ‡Retraction cords, braids, and twists come in various diameters. A number of cords are available with epinephrine and racemic epinephrine in concentrations ranging from 0.3-1.45mg/in and varying concentrations of zinc phenolsulfonate or aluminum compounds. Consult the manufacturer's labeling for more information.

This list is not comprehensive. The products shown here are available in various formulations and strengths, not all of which are listed. In addition, the listing of a product does not denote its superiority to any other product that is either listed or not listed, nor does it guarantee its availability or quality.

BB = black box warning; **W/P** = warnings/precautions; **Contra** = contraindications; **P/N** = pregnancy category rating and nursing considerations.

Table 4.2. USAGE INFORMATION FOR TOPICAL ANTISEPTICS, ROOT CANAL MEDICATIONS, AND PERIODONTAL DRESSINGS

NAME	FORM/ STRENGTH	WARNINGS/PRECAUTIONS, CONTRAINDICATIONS & ADVERSE EFFECTS	ACTIONS/ USES
HANDWASHING AGENTS			
Chlorhexidine Gluconate, 4% (BrianCare, Dial, Dyna-Hex 4%, Endure 400, Excelle, Hibiclens, Maxiclens, MetriCare)	**Sol:** 4% chlorhexidine gluconate; 4% isopropyl alcohol	**W/P:** Use only for topical application on the hands. Chlorhexidine is nontoxic on the skin but may cause damage if placed directly into the eye or ear. It has been reported to cause deafness when instilled in the middle ear through perforated eardrums. **A/E:** Irritation, sensitization, and generalized allergic reactions have been reported with chlorhexidine-containing products, especially in the genital area.	Very effective against gram-positive bacteria, moderately effective against gram-negative bacteria, bacteriostatic only against mycobacteria. According to laboratory studies, can eliminate infectivity of lipophilic viruses such as HIV, influenza, and herpes simplex but is not very effective against hydrophilic viruses such as poliovirus and some enteric viruses.
Chlorhexidine Gluconate, 2% (Chlorostat, Dyna-Hex 2%, Endure 420, SaniClenz)	**Sol:** 2% chlorhexidine gluconate; 4% isopropyl alcohol	**W/P:** Use only for topical application on the hands. Chlorhexidine is nontoxic on the skin but may cause damage if placed directly into the eye or ear. It has been reported to cause deafness when instilled in the middle ear through perforated eardrums. **A/E:** Irritation, sensitization, and generalized allergic reactions have been reported with chlorhexidine-containing products, especially in the genital area.	Not as effective as the 4% solution but has similar spectrum of activity.
Chlorhexidine Gluconate, 0.75% (Perfect Care)	**Sol:** 0.75% chlorhexidine gluconate	**W/P:** Use only for topical application on the hands. Chlorhexidine is nontoxic on the skin but may cause damage if placed directly into the eye or ear. It has been reported to cause deafness when instilled in the middle ear through perforated eardrums. **A/E:** Irritation, sensitization, and generalized allergic reactions have been reported with chlorhexidine-containing products, especially in the genital area.	Not as effective as the 4% solution; best for nonsurgical routine handwashing.
Chlorhexidine Gluconate Solution, 0.5% (Hibistat Germicidal Hand Rinse)	**Sol:** 0.5% chlorhexidine gluconate; 70% isopropyl alcohol (4oz, 8oz bottles); **Hand Wipe Towelette:** 5mL solution, 50 per box	**W/P:** Use only for topical application on the hands. Chlorhexidine is nontoxic on the skin but may cause damage if placed directly into the eye or ear. It has been reported to cause deafness when instilled in the middle ear through perforated eardrums. **A/E:** Irritation, sensitization, and generalized allergic reactions have been reported with chlorhexidine-containing products, especially in the genital area.	Not as effective as the 4% solution; best for nonsurgical routine handwashing.
Ethanol (Discovery Hand Sanitizer, Purell Surgical Scrub with Moisturizers)	**Gel:** 62% (Discover); 70% (Purell)	**W/P:** Use only for topical application on the hands. Product is flammable due to alcohol content. **A/E:** No irritation or reaction expected when used on skin. Contact with eyes may cause irritation. If eye contact occurs, do not rub; flush with water for 15 min.	Broad-spectrum activity; meets CDC guidelines for effectiveness at killing the H1N1 virus due to ≥60% alcohol content.
Iodophors (Alphadine, Betadine)	**Sol:** 0.75% (available iodine)	**W/P:** Can cause skin irritation; rinse off after handwashing. **Contra:** Do not use iodophors on infants due to risk of iodine-induced hyperthyroidism. **A/E:** Irritation, allergic reaction.	Very effective against gram-positive bacteria and moderately effective against gram-negative bacteria, the tubercle bacillus, fungi, and many viruses.

This list is not comprehensive. The products shown here are available in various formulations and strengths, not all of which are listed. In addition, the listing of a product does not denote its superiority to any other product that is either listed or not listed, nor does it guarantee its availability or quality.

BB = black box warning; **W/P** = warnings/precautions; **Contra** = contraindications; **A/E** = adverse effects;
P/N = pregnancy category rating and nursing considerations.

Table 4.2. USAGE INFORMATION FOR TOPICAL ANTISEPTICS, ROOT CANAL MEDICATIONS, AND PERIODONTAL DRESSINGS *(cont.)*

NAME	FORM/ STRENGTH	WARNINGS/PRECAUTIONS, CONTRAINDICATIONS & ADVERSE EFFECTS	ACTIONS/ USES
HANDWASHING AGENTS *(cont.)*			
***Para*-chloro-*meta*-xylenol (PCMX) (chloroxylenol)** (Aloe Guard, Derma Cidol 2000, DermAseptic, DisAseptic, DisCide Effect, Lurosep, Medi-Scrub, OmniCare 7, Provon, SaniWash, VioNex, VioNex with Nonoxynol-9, VioNexus)	**PCMX:** 0.5%, 3%, 4%	**A/E:** Irritation, allergic reaction.	Although some studies have shown chlorhexidine and iodophors to be more active than PCMX against skin flora, PCMX is a fairly broad-spectrum antimicrobial agent that is moderately effective against gram-positive bacteria and somewhat effective against gram-negative bacteria, the tubercle bacillus, and some fungi and viruses.
Phenol (Sporicidin Antimicrobial Soap)	**Lotion:** (phenol/sodium phenate) 1.47%	**W/P:** Use only for topical application. **A/E:** No irritation or reaction expected when used on skin. Contact with eyes may cause irritation. If eye contact occurs, do not rub; flush with water for 15 min. **Contra:** Infants <6 months.	Broad-spectrum activity; can use on hands, face, and body.
Triclosan (Bacti-Foam, Bacti-Stat, Cetaphil, Dermasep, Dial, Endure, Lysol I.C., Henry Schein, Oilatum-AD, pHisoderm, Prevacare, Provon, SaniSept, Scrub'n Glove, Septisol, SweetHeart)	**Soap, Sol, Lotion:** 0.2%, 0.25%, 0.3%, 1%	**A/E:** Irritation, allergic reaction.	Moderately effective against gram-positive bacteria and most gram-negative bacteria, but it may be less effective against *Pseudomonas aeruginosa*; somewhat effective against the tubercle bacillus; level of its effectiveness against viruses is unknown.
SKIN AND MUCOSAL ANTISEPTICS			
Chlorhexidine gluconate, subgingival delivery (PerioChip)	**Biodegradable chip:** 2.5mg	**W/P:** Use has not been studied in acutely abscessed periodontal pockets and is not recommended. Rarely, infectious events including abscesses and cellulitis have been reported with adjunctive use of the chip post scaling and root planing. Patient management should include consideration of potentially contributing medical disorders (eg, cancer, diabetes, and immunocompromised status). Patients should avoid dental floss at insertion site for 10 days after placement; all other oral hygiene may be continued as usual. Although sensitivity is normal the first week after placement, patients should promptly report pain, swelling or other problems that occur. Use in pediatric patients has not been studied. **Contra:** Hypersensitivity to chlorhexidine. **P/N:** Category C; safety in nursing unknown. **A/E:** Toothache (including dental, gingival or mouth pain; tenderness; aching; throbbing; soreness; discomfort; and sensitivity), upper respiratory tract infection, headache.	Subgingival delivery of chlorhexidine in a biodegradable hydrolyzed gelatin matrix; FDA-approved as an adjunct to periodontal therapy. Chip maintains antimicrobial concentration in periodontal pocket for at least 7 days. Clinical studies have not demonstrated staining or severe adverse effects using this agent in a local delivery system.
Ethanol/Isopropyl Alcohol (A.B.H.C., Alco-gel, Antiseptic Bio-hand Cleaner, Avagard D, BD Alcohol, Chlorox Anywhere Spray, Citrus II, Derma-Stat, Dial, DisCide XRA Towelettes, Discovery, Endure 450, Epi-Clenz, Henry Schein, Insta-Fresh, Isagel, Kimcare, Quick-Care, Prevacare, Purell, rubbing alcohol, SaniHands, SaniTyze Waterless Gel, Viraguard)	**Liq:** 70% ethyl alcohol; 70% isopropyl alcohol	**W/P:** For external use only; produces serious gastric disturbances if taken internally. Flammable; keep away from fire or flame. **Contra:** Do not use in eyes or on mucous membranes, irritated skin, deep wounds, puncture wounds, or serious burns. **A/E:** Defatting of skin and enhanced exposure of bacteria in hair follicles; painful stinging and burning when applied directly to mucosa and wounds.	Very effective; gives rapid protection against most vegetative gram-positive and gram-negative bacteria; has good activity against the tubercle bacillus, most fungi, and many viruses.

This list is not comprehensive. The products shown here are available in various formulations and strengths, not all of which are listed. In addition, the listing of a product does not denote its superiority to any other product that is either listed or not listed, nor does it guarantee its availability or quality.

BB = black box warning; **W/P** = warnings/precautions; **Contra** = contraindications; **A/E** = adverse effects;
P/N = pregnancy category rating and nursing considerations.

NAME	FORM/ STRENGTH	WARNINGS/PRECAUTIONS, CONTRAINDICATIONS & ADVERSE EFFECTS	ACTIONS/ USES
Iodophors (Betadine)	**Sol:** 1%	**Contra:** Do not use iodophors on infants due to risk of iodine-induced hyperthyroidism. **A/E:** Irritation, allergic reaction.	May be applied to oral mucosa to reduce bacteremias during treatment of patients who are at increased risk of developing endocarditis (as indicated by the American Heart Association) or who may be immunocompromised and have a neutropenia; antiseptic mouthrinses containing chlorhexidine or phenolic compounds also may be used in these instances (see Chapter 9); aqueous iodine preparations or a tincture of iodine (iodine in alcohol) also may be used for skin antisepsis.
***Para*-chloro-*meta*-xylenol (PCMX) (chloroxylenol)** (Discovery Lotion and Gel, p.a.w.s. Personal Wipes, TotalCare, VioNex)	**PCMX:** 0.5%, 3%, 4%	**A/E:** Irritation, allergic reaction.	Although some studies have shown chlorhexidine and iodophors to be more active than PCMX against skin flora, PCMX is a fairly broad-spectrum antimicrobial agent that is moderately effective against gram-positive bacteria and somewhat effective against gram-negative bacteria, the tubercle bacillus, and some fungi and viruses.
Quaternary ammonium compounds (DEFEND + PLUS Wipes, Soft-T-Cleanse Hand Foam, VioNexus No Rinse Spray)	NA	**W/P:** Antiseptic effect is neutralized by dilution or contact with ionic detergents or organic matter.	Bacteriostatic at low concentrations and bactericidal at high concentrations, but certain species of *Pseudomonas* and *Mycobacterium* are resistant.
ROOT CANAL MEDICATIONS AND PERIODONTAL DRESSINGS			
ALDEHYDES			
Formocresol (Buckley's Formo Cresol, Formo Cresol)	**Liq:** (Buckley's) 35% cresol, 19% formaldehyde, 17.5% glycerine, 28.5% water; (Formo) 48.5% cresol, 48.5% formaldehyde, 3% glycerine	**W/P:** Minimize soft-tissue contact. Combined action of cresol, a protein-coagulating phenolic compound, and formaldehyde, an alkylating agent, make formocresol extremely cytotoxic and capable of causing widespread necrosis of vital tissue in the mouth or elsewhere.	Vital pulp therapy in primary teeth.
INTRACANAL MEDICATIONS			
Calcium Hydroxide ($Ca[OH]_2$) (Generic calcium hydroxide powder, Pulpdent TempCanal)	**Pow:** (generic) calcium hydroxide, USP; **Sol:** (Pulpdent) calcium hydroxide in aqueous methylcellulose	**W/P:** Minimize soft-tissue contact.	Used to create an environment for healing pulpal and periapical tissues, to produce antimicrobial effects, to aid in elimination of apical seepage, to induce formation of calcified tissue, and to prevent inflammatory resorption after trauma.
IRRIGANTS			
Ethylenediaminetetra-acetic acid (EDTA) (Generic EDTA, EDTAC, File-EZE, RC Prep, REDTA)	**Sol:** (generic) 17% in aqueous solution, pH 8.0; (EDTA) EDTA with Centrimide; (File-EZE) EDTA in an aqueous solution; (RC) Urea peroxide 10%, EDTA 15% in a special water soluble base; (REDTA) EDTA 17% in an aqueous solution, pH of 8.0	**W/P:** Minimize soft-tissue contact.	In combination with sodium hypochlorite, EDTA removes smear layer; alone, aids in removal of calcified tissue by chelating metal ions.

Table 4.2. USAGE INFORMATION FOR TOPICAL ANTISEPTICS, ROOT CANAL MEDICATIONS, AND PERIODONTAL DRESSINGS *(cont.)*

NAME	FORM/ STRENGTH	WARNINGS/PRECAUTIONS, CONTRAINDICATIONS & ADVERSE EFFECTS	ACTIONS/ USES
ROOT CANAL MEDICATIONS AND PERIODONTAL DRESSINGS *(cont.)*			
IRRIGANTS *(cont.)*			
Hydrogen Peroxide 3% (H_2O_2)	Generic aqueous solution	**W/P:** Minimize soft-tissue contact. Should be used carefully to avoid emphysema of adjacent soft tissue. **A/E:** Irritation, tooth sensitivity, allergic reaction.	Oxidizing power of hydrogen peroxide kills certain anaerobic bacteria in cultures; in contact with tissues, its germicidal power is very limited because it is readily decomposed by organic matter and antimicrobial effect lasts only as long as oxygen is being released; can be used to cleanse and treat infected pulp canals.
Sodium Hypochlorite (NaOCl) (Clorox, Hypogen)	5.25% sodium hypochlorite	**W/P:** Minimize soft-tissue contact. Sodium hypochlorite is caustic and not suitable for application to wounds or areas of infection in soft tissues. **A/E:** Irritation, allergic reaction.	Has a solvent action on pulp tissue and organic debris, is used for irrigation of root canals, and is useful for cleaning dentures; aqueous solutions of 2.5% and 5% sodium hypochlorite are reported to be equally effective in dissolving pulpal debris when used as root canal irrigants.
MISCELLANEOUS PREPARATIONS			
Zinc Oxide (COE-Pak Periodontal Paste; COE-Pak Automix Periodontal Paste; COE-Pak Hard and Fast Set Periodontal Paste; Pulpdent PerioCare Periodontal Dressing; zinc oxide, USP; Zone PerioPak, Zone PerioPutty)	(COE-Pak) **Paste 1:** 45% zinc oxide, 37% magnesium oxide, 11% peanut oil, 6% mineral oil, 1% chloroxylenol, chlorothymol and coumarin, 0.02% Toluidine-Red pigment; **Paste 2:** 43% polymerized rosin, 24% coconut fatty acid, 10% ethyl alcohol, 9% petroleum jelly, 4% gum elemi, 4% lanolin, 3% ethyl cellulose, 1.5% chlorothymol, 1% carnauba, 0.2% zinc acetate, 0.1% spearmint oil; (PerioCare) **Paste:** 38.5% magnesium oxide, 29.8% vegetable oils, 19.2% zinc oxide, 12.5% calcium hydroxide, 0.2% coloring; **Gel:** 63.2% resins, 29.8% fatty acids, 3.5% ethyl cellulose, 3.5% lanolin; (PerioPutty) **Base:** 3.1% polyvinylpyrrolidone-iodine complex, 9% polymer, 5% benzocaine, 82.9% fillers; **Catalyst:** 19.9% zinc oxide, 10.3% magnesium oxide, 12.3% mineral and vegetable oils, 58% inert fillers; **Skin Lubricant:** 95% silicone oils, 5% inert fillers; (Zinc) **Pow:** Zinc oxide; (Zone) **Base:** 3.1% polyvinylpyrrolidone-iodine complex, 38.3% rosin, 2% chlorobutanol, 10% mineral oil, 9.3% isopropyl myristate, 37.3% propylene glycol monoisostearate	**W/P:** Minimize soft-tissue contact.	Periodontal dressing; PerioPutty also has skin lubricant.
Zinc Oxide-Eugenol (various)	NA	**W/P:** Minimize soft-tissue contact.	Periodontal dressing.

This list is not comprehensive. The products shown here are available in various formulations and strengths, not all of which are listed. In addition, the listing of a product does not denote its superiority to any other product that is either listed or not listed, nor does it guarantee its availability or quality.

BB = black box warning; **W/P** = warnings/precautions; **Contra** = contraindications; **A/E** = adverse effects;
P/N = pregnancy category rating and nursing considerations.

NAME	FORM/ STRENGTH	WARNINGS/PRECAUTIONS, CONTRAINDICATIONS & ADVERSE EFFECTS	ACTIONS/ USES
PHENOLIC COMPOUNDS			
Parachlorophenol (PCP) (MCP Root Canal Dressing, Parachlorophenol Liquefied)	(MCP) **Liq:** 25% parachlorophenol, 25% metacresyl acetate, 50% camphor; (parachlorophenol liquefied) **Liq:** 98% parachlorophenol, 2% glycerin	**W/P:** Minimize soft-tissue contact. Phenolic compounds can destroy tissue cells by binding cell membrane lipids and proteins.	Intracanal medicament.
Parachlorophenol, Camphorated (CPC), USP	**Liq:** 35% parachlorophenol and 65% camphor	**W/P:** Minimize soft-tissue contact. Phenolic compounds can destroy tissue cells by binding cell membrane lipids and proteins.	Intracanal medicament.
Eugenol, USP	**Liq:** 100% eugenol	**W/P:** Minimize soft-tissue contact. Phenolic compounds can destroy tissue cells by binding cell membrane lipids and proteins.	Anodyne/oral tissues, teeth.

Chapter 5

Glucocorticoids

Lida Radfar, D.D.S., M.S.; Martha Somerman, D.D.S., Ph.D.

OVERVIEW

Glucocorticoids are hormones secreted by the adrenal gland in response to ultradian and circadian rhythms and to stress. The major effects of glucocorticoids can broadly be defined as influencing the metabolism of carbohydrates, protein, and fat metabolism, as well as water and electrolyte balance. Consequently, glucocorticoids are involved in the deposition of glucose as glycogen and the conversion of glycogen and protein into glucose when needed; the stimulation of protein loss from specific organs; the redistribution of fatty tissue in facial, abdominal, and shoulder regions; and alterations of the filtration rate of specific electrolytes that cause water retention.

Glucocorticoids mainly regulate the metabolic pathways, while mineralocorticoids are involved with electrolyte and water balance. The secretion of glucocorticoids from the adrenal glands is controlled by hormones, such as corticotropin-releasing factor, which is produced by the hypothalamus, and adrenocorticotropic hormone (ACTH), produced by the anterior pituitary gland. This pathway is often referred to as the hypothalamic-pituitary-adrenal (HPA) axis. Glucocorticoid secretion from the adrenal glands is regulated by a negative feedback mechanism; that is, the adrenal glands will diminish glucocorticoid secretion when excess plasma levels of steroids are present. However, the glands cannot distinguish between endogenously and exogenously supplied glucocorticoids. Consequently, administration of supraphysiological levels of exogenous glucocorticoids for long periods may result in secondary adrenal insufficiency.

Glucocorticoids are, among other things, essential for a person's ability to adapt to stressful situations. Adrenal insufficiency or dysfunction, therefore, may predispose a person to inadequate physiological response to stress. Severe adrenal suppression and the subsequent diminished stress response may have clinical significance after seven to 10 days of steroid administration. In stressful situations, cardiovascular collapse may ensue and, if not treated appropriately, can result in a high degree of morbidity and even death. This type of response is rare in patients with adrenal insufficiency owing to exogenous glucocorticoids, but may be a concern for patients with Addison's disease. Dentists need to be able to assess the level of patients' adrenal suppression and provide them with glucocorticoid replacement therapy when necessary.

Assessment of Adrenal Suppression

Many factors play a role in assessing the diminished output of glucocorticoids from the adrenal glands in patients who are prescribed glucocorticoids. These factors include, but are not limited to, the type of glucocorticoids the patient is prescribed, the route of administration, the dosing schedule, the duration of the course of steroids, concomitant systemic disorders, and drug interactions.

Each type and formulation of glucocorticoid has been assigned a specific level of potency that is compared to the potency of hydrocortisone (**Table 5.1**). Thus, prednisone is four times more potent than hydrocortisone, while betamethasone is 25 times more potent. The more potent the drug, the higher the risk of it causing adrenal suppression. The risk of experiencing adverse effects from glucocorticoid administration usually increases with duration of therapy and frequency of administration. Adrenal suppression occurs rapidly and may be present for up to two years, even after as little as two weeks of glucocorticoid therapy. However, although the adrenal function is suppressed, the stress response returns after approximately 11 to 14 days. For the purpose of not causing stress-related adverse events, the return of the stress response is of the essence.

Except for the high-potency topical glucocorticoids, topically applied glucocorticoids—including those used intraorally—have not been associated with adrenal suppression. However, aerosol and systemically administered glucocorticoids have been associated with adrenal suppression and diminished stress response in patients. For patients receiving chronic glucocorticoid therapy, alternate-day therapy is used to reduce potential side effects.

Accepted Indications

Glucocorticoids are used to induce immune suppression in patients with a variety of conditions. Patients who have undergone organ transplantations, for example, often are prescribed high doses of glucocorticoids to prevent organ rejection. Although other conditions such as autoimmune diseases, respiratory diseases, dermatologic diseases, and some hematologic disorders also require long-term glucocorticoid therapy, there is usually no need for such high doses as used with transplant patients.

Glucocorticoids are also used in dental settings. Various oral conditions such as lichen planus, aphthous ulcers, benign mucous membrane pemphigoid, pemphigus, postherpetic neuralgia, and temporomandibular joint disorders benefit from glucocorticoid therapy. Furthermore, glucocorticoids also are used to reduce swelling after major oral-maxillofacial surgical procedures.

General Dosing Information

Table 5.1 provides dosage and prescribing information for systemic glucocorticoids (separated into low-, intermediate-, and high-potency categories); topical glucocorticoids (separated into low-, intermediate-, high-, and very high-potency categories); and inhaled and intranasal glucocorticoids.

When administering glucocorticoids, topical formulations, intralesional, and intra-articular injections or systemic forms may be used. Topical agents are the ones most commonly used by dentists and, if employed for less than one month, usually will not cause significant detrimental effects. However, very high-potency topical glucocorticoids used to treat oral lesions can cause adrenal suppression and should not be used for more than two weeks without a thorough medical evaluation of the patient. Creams, ointments, and gels all can be used intraorally and are applied to lesions two to four times daily. Gels adhere fairly well to the oral mucosa and are applied directly to lesions. To increase penetration and time in contact with lesions, gel formulations also can be placed inside a mouthguard covering the affected area. Ointments usually are mixed with equal amounts of Orabase, a compound that adheres to the oral mucosa, and is placed directly on lesions. Ointments also can be placed inside mouthguards. Although creams can be used for oral lesions, these formulations are not commonly used for this purpose. Dexamethasone elixir and prednisolone syrup are the oral rinses commonly used for topical purposes. The patient is instructed to rinse for 30 seconds with these medications, and then to expectorate them, 2 to 4 times daily.

Intralesional injections commonly are used only intermittently; when used for soft-tissue pathologies, they have not been associated with systemic complications. Triamcinolone hexacetonide is the most frequently used medication for this purpose.

Intra-articular injections, also predominantly performed with triamcinolone hexacetonide, should be performed only in three-week intervals to diminish bone pathology. Stable formulations comprising a mixture of glucocorticoids with an antifungal (Lotrisone cream: clotrimazole 1%/ betamethasone dipropionate 0.064%), an antibiotic (Cortisporin ointment: bacitracin, neomycin, polymyxin B, and hydrocortisone), or a local anesthetic (AnaMantle HC topical: lidocaine and hydrocortisone), are available for topical use.

Systemic glucocorticoid therapy is used in the short term before, during, and after oral surgery to reduce postoperative edema. Oral lesions associated with very high morbidity sometimes are treated with systemic glucocorticoid therapy. High doses of prednisone, up to 60 mg to 80 mg per day for seven to 10 days, can be used for treatment of lichen planus, major aphthous ulcerations, oral pemphigoid, and oral pemphigus. Treatment beyond two weeks should be coordinated with the patient's physician.

Maximum Recommended Doses

The maximum recommended doses for systemic glucocorticoid formulations per procedure or appointment are 5 mg to 20 mg of prednisone for a maintenance dose and 5 mg to 60 mg for continuous or alternate-day therapy, but doses depend on the patient's condition. Dosing schedules and maximum doses are based on the assumption that the dentist has determined (through taking a health history and interviewing) that the patient is in general good health and is not taking any medications that can interact with the glucocorticoid agent (see **Table 5.2**). The main concerns are patients with hyperglycemic conditions and patients who cannot tolerate immunosuppressive therapy. The potential harmful effects of these medications always must be carefully weighed against the benefit.

Dosage Adjustments

The actual maximum dose for each patient must be individualized depending on his or her size, age, and physical status; other drugs he or she may be taking; and duration of existing glucocorticoid therapy (long-term use considerations). Reduced maximum doses may be indicated for pediatric and geriatric patients, patients with serious illness or disability, and patients with medical conditions or who are taking drugs that alter responses to glucocorticoids.

Special Dental Considerations

The effect of glucocorticoids can be divided arbitrarily into two categories that have significance for dentists:

- Dental patients taking glucocorticoids may need modifications and alterations of routine dental therapy, for purposes such as reducing patients' stress response and glucocorticoid replacement.
- Glucocorticoid users may exhibit intraoral manifestations.

Modifications of Routine Dental Therapy

Is there a need for antibiotic coverage?

There are no definitive data regarding the need for patients taking glucocorticoids to receive antibiotic prophylaxis before undergoing dental therapy. However, it is prudent to consider antibiotic prophylaxis in patients taking a combined dose of more than

700 mg of prednisone. No antibiotic prophylaxis is recommended if a patient takes <10 mg of prednisone per day. The same protocol for antibiotic prophylaxis as that put forth by the American Heart Association for prevention of subacute bacterial endocarditis may be chosen (see **Appendix D**). However, the efficacy of this protocol for patients taking glucocorticoids has not been established.

There are two situations in which dentists need to provide patients with extra glucocorticoids.

First, patients with dysfunctional adrenal glands may not be able to produce enough glucocorticoids to respond to the stress associated with dental therapy. The most common condition associated with primary adrenal destruction is Addison's disease, an autoimmune destruction of the adrenal glands. Patients with inadequately functioning adrenal glands will need prophylactic glucocorticoid therapy before undergoing dental procedures. Second, patients who have been taking glucocorticoids for a long period may have iatrogenic adrenal suppression and will need glucocorticoid replacement therapy before undergoing dental procedures.

As the stress response returns within 11 to 14 days after cessation of glucocorticoid therapy, patients do not need replacement therapy after a two- to four-week period of not having taken glucocorticoids. Furthermore, patients being switched from daily therapy to alternate-day therapy can be treated without glucocorticoid replacement therapy on the nonglucocorticoid day. As a rule, patients needing replacement therapy should receive the equivalent of up to 300 mg of hydrocortisone or 60 mg to 75 mg of prednisone the morning of a dental appointment.

The amount of glucocorticoid replacement should be gauged according to the anticipated level of stress. Accordingly, depending on the patient's level of fear and anxiety, oral examinations generally require no replacement therapy, while any procedure requiring local anesthetics warrants additional glucocorticoid coverage.

Oral health care providers should follow this protocol for the management of patients who are receiving glucocorticoid therapy:

- Schedule elective procedures in the morning.
- Use mild sedatives for apprehensive patients.
- Use glucocorticoid replacement therapy when indicated.
- Always use long-acting local anesthetics.
- Monitor blood pressure during the procedure.
- Use medications to alleviate postoperative pain.

As a rule, replacement therapy is indicated for patients who presently are taking more than 30 mg of hydrocortisone equivalent of glucocorticoids for more than two weeks. It also is indicated for patients seeking dental care within the first two to four weeks after having stopped glucocorticoid therapy subsequent to having taken at least 30 mg of hydrocortisone equivalent of glucocorticoids for more than two weeks.

Intraoral Manifestations

Of all the intraoral manifestations caused by glucocorticoids, the most common is oral candidiasis. It has been estimated that up to 75% of people using inhalers that contain glucocorticoids may develop intraoral candidiasis (Table 5.1). These inhalers are used mainly by patients with asthma, but they also can be prescribed for patients with allergies and other respiratory conditions. To diminish the occurrence of candidiasis, properly instruct patients in the use of spacer devices and to rinse their mouths with water after using the inhalers. Resolution of intraoral candidiasis can be accomplished effectively with antifungal troches, lozenges, or oral solutions (**see Chapter 7**).

Long-term systemic administration of glucocorticoids may impair wound healing. This may be the result of the catabolic effect and the reduced inflammatory response induced by these compounds.

The anti-inflammatory property of glucocorticoids may mask a chronic infection. Glucocorticoids will prevent accumulation of neutrophils and monocytes at sites of inflammation (impaired chemotaxis) and further suppress the phagocytic abilities of cells. For this reason, the classic clinical inflammatory response may be greatly blunted.

Intraoral dryness has also been reported in patients taking glucocorticoids, both systemically and in the form of inhalers. An increased caries rate can be anticipated, and patients should be instructed about improved oral hygiene procedures and use of topical fluorides, as well as in-office fluoride therapy.

Drug Interactions of Dental Interest

Table 5.2 lists drug interactions with glucocorticoids and related problems of potential clinical significance in dentistry.

Laboratory Value Alterations

- Low serum cortisol levels, <5 to 10 μg/dL in a specimen obtained between 8 am and 10 am, and increased serum ACTH, 200 to 1,600 μg/dL, are diagnostic for adrenal insufficiency. Requesting a complete blood count may be warranted, as neutropenia and lymphocytosis may be present.

Special Patients

Pregnant and nursing women

All systemic glucocorticoid preparations are classified in pregnancy risk category C (potential risk of fetal harm) and may cause birth defects such as cleft lip and palate. Consequently, glucocorticoid administration during pregnancy and during breastfeeding should be avoided.

Pediatric, geriatric, and other special patients

Administration of as little as 5 mg of prednisone may cause growth retardation in children. However, if glucocorticoid therapy ceases before the epiphyses close, catch-up growth may take place.

Pediatric patients may have a greater susceptibility to topical glucocorticoids-induced adrenal suppression than that of adults because children have thinner skin and their ratio of skin surface area to body weight is larger than that of adults. Topical glucocorticoids should be used with caution in children.

Geriatric patients exhibit a propensity to develop hypertension and osteoporosis while receiving glucocorticoid therapy. Glucocorticoid dosage also needs to be adjusted in younger and older patients to minimize damage to kidney and liver functions.

Patient Monitoring: Aspects to Watch

- Symptoms of blood dyscrasias (such as infection, bleeding, and poor healing); for patients with these symptoms, the dentist should request a medical consultation for blood studies and postpone dental treatment until normal values are re-established
- Vital signs; check at every appointment. Necessary to monitor possible cardiovascular side effects
- Salivary flow; a factor in caries, periodontal disease, and candidiasis
- Dose and duration of glucocorticoid therapy; to assess stress tolerance and risk of immunosuppression
- Need for medical consultation; to assess disease control and patient's stress tolerance

Adverse Effects and Precautions

The multitude of potential side effects of systemic glucocorticoids necessitates complete disclosure of the risks to patients (see **Table 5.1**). Withdrawal of glucocorticoids after patients are treated for more than 10 consecutive days should be accomplished gradually to diminish side effects. Patients taking daily doses of 60 mg of prednisone should reduce their daily intake by 10 mg every day before completely stopping therapy. Withdrawing glucocorticoid therapy too rapidly may result in a flare-up of the underlying condition or even adrenal crisis. If it is necessary that a patient continue to receive glucocorticoid therapy for longer than two weeks, a consultation with a physician is appropriate.

Severe hepatic disease may prevent prednisone metabolism; when treating such patients, the active form of the medication, prednisolone, may have to be administered to achieve a clinical effect. Furthermore, patients with severe liver disease may not be able to take glucocorticoids with acetaminophen, as acetaminophen toxicity may ensue.

Concurrent administration of other medications such as barbiturates, phenytoin, and rifampin may double the clearance of prednisolone. Interactions also may occur with other medications and need to be considered when prescribing glucocorticoids (see **Table 5.2**).

The most common adverse signs of glucocorticoid therapy include changes in skin (such as acne, ecchymosis, thinning, violaceous abdominal striae), weight gain, truncal obesity, "buffalo hump" (adipose tissue accumulation on the back of the neck), thin extremities, decreased muscle mass, and "moon face." These features appear in 13% of patients after as little as 60 days of glucocorticoid use and in up to 50% of patients treated for five to eight years. Patients with these signs need to be encouraged to keep a low-fat, low-calorie diet and to exercise.

Skeletal fractures may occur in 11% to 20% of patients treated with daily doses of 7.5 mg to 10 mg of prednisone for more than one year. The major underlying cause of these osteoporotic changes may be decreased osteoblastic activity and maturation. The most rapid loss of trabecular bone loss occurs within the first two months of high-dose glucocorticoid therapy, with an average of 5% bone mass loss within the first year. It is prudent to give calcium and vitamin D supplements and hormone replacements and to initiate weight-bearing exercise programs for patients receiving long-term glucocorticoid therapy. Another complication, more commonly found with patients taking long-term glucocorticoids, is osteonecrosis, which specifically affects the hip joint.

Patients taking a total dose of >1,000 mg of prednisone are more predisposed than patients taking lesser doses to develop peptic ulcers. This side effect is aggravated in patients already taking other potentially ulcerogenic medications. Administration of an H_2-antagonist may be beneficial as a prophylactic measure to reduce the incidence of peptic ulcerations.

Glucocorticoids initially may induce a psychological state of well-being, which subsequently may become a state of glucocorticoid-induced depression when the glucocorticoids are withdrawn.

Increased incidence of accelerated atherosclerosis has been noted in patients with systemic lupus erythematosus or rheumatoid arthritis who are treated with long-term glucocorticoids. Furthermore, patients with pre-existing hypertension may experience a worsening of their hypertensive control when treated with glucocorticoids.

Glucocorticoid-induced glucose intolerance is not associated with serious complications, but caution should be heeded when treating diabetic patients.

Progression of carcinoma of the breast and Kaposi's sarcoma has been reported in patients receiving glucocorticoid therapy. Although renewed development of Kaposi's sarcoma may occur, this lesion usually disappears after cessation of glucocorticoid therapy.

Pharmacology

Mechanism of action/effect

The effectiveness of glucocorticoid hormones is based on their ability to bind to cytosolic receptors in target tissues and subsequently enter the nucleus, where the glucocorticoid-receptor complex interacts with nuclear chromatin. This results in a cascade of events, including the expression of hormone-specific ribonucleic acids, or RNAs, which in turn increases synthesis of specific proteins that mediate distinct physiological functions. The glucocorticoid cortisol is a normal circulating hormone secreted by the adrenal gland that functions in regulating normal metabolism and providing resistance to stress. In addition, at high levels whether the result of disease or drug intake glucocorticoids can have one or more physiological effects. These include:

- altering levels of blood cells in the plasma (that is, decreasing eosinophils, basophils, monocytes, and lymphocytes and increasing levels of hemoglobin, erythrocytes, and neutrophils), which decreases circulating levels of cells involved in fighting off infections and results in increased susceptibility to infections
- reducing the inflammatory response as a result of a decrease in lymphocytes as well as altering lymphocytes' ability to inhibit the enzyme phospholipase A_2, which is required for production of prostaglandins and leukotrienes
- suppressing the HPA axis, thus inhibiting further synthesis of glucocorticoids

Therefore, patients taking glucocorticoids warrant special attention as discussed in the introduction to this chapter.

Absorption

Systemically, most glucocorticoids are rapidly and readily absorbed from the GI tract because of their lipophilic character. Also, absorption occurs via synovial and conjunctival spaces.

Topically, absorption through the skin is very slow. However, chronic use in a nasal spray (for seasonal rhinitis, for example) can lead to pulmonary epithelial atrophy. Furthermore, excessive or prolonged use of topical glucocorticoids can result in sufficient absorption to cause systemic effects.

Both cortisone and prednisone contain a keto group at position II that must be hydroxylated in the liver to become activated. Thus, these drugs should be avoided in patients with abnormal liver function. Also, topical application of position II ketocorticoids is ineffective as a result of inactivity of this form of the glucocorticoid.

Distribution

In general, circulating cortisol is bound to plasma proteins: about 80% to 90% bound to transcortin—a cortisol-binding globulin with high affinity—while about 5% to 10% binds loosely to albumin. About 3% to 10% remains in the free (bioactive) form. Transcortin can bind to most synthetic glucocorticoids as well. However, some glucocorticoids, such as dexamethasone, do not bind to transcortin and, thus, are almost 100% in free form.

Biotransformation

Inactivation occurs primarily in the liver and also in the kidney, mostly to inactive metabolites. However, cortisone and prednisone are activated only after being metabolized to hydrocortisone and prednisolone, respectively. Fluorinated glucocorticoids are metabolized more slowly than the other members of this group.

Elimination

About 30% of inactive metabolite is metabolized further and then excreted in the urine.

Patient Advice

- Emphasize the importance of good oral hygiene to prevent soft-tissue inflammation.
- Caution the patient to prevent injury when using oral hygiene aids; he or she

should use a soft toothbrush and have the dentist or hygienist evaluate his or her brushing and flossing techniques.
- Suggest the use of daily home fluoride preparations if chronic xerostomia occurs.
- Suggest the use of sugarless gum, frequent sips of water, or artificial saliva substitutes if chronic xerostomia occurs.
- Caution against using mouthrinses with high alcohol content, as they have drying effects on the oral mucosa.
- The patient should use a topical glucocorticoid after brushing and eating and at bedtime for optimal effect.
- Use of topical glucocorticoids on oral herpetic ulcerations is contraindicated.
- The patient should apply the agent with a cotton-tipped applicator by pressing, not rubbing, the paste on the lesion.
- When a topical glucocorticoid is used to treat oral lesions, a tissue response should be noted within seven to 14 days. If not, the patient should return for oral evaluation. If glucocorticoids are used chronically, the patient should return for frequent recall visits.
- If irritation, infection, or sensitization occurs at site, the patient should discontinue use and return for evaluation.
- The patient should avoid exposing the affected area to sunlight; burns may occur.
- Topical glucocorticoids are for external use only.
- The patient should prevent the topical glucocorticoid from coming in contact with his or her eyes.
- The patient should not bandage or wrap the affected area unless directed to do so.
- The patient should report adverse reactions.
- The patient should avoid taking anything by mouth for 30 or 60 minutes after topical use in the mouth (as a mouthrinse or an ointment, respectively).

SUGGESTED READING

Barnes PJ. Molecular mechanisms and cellular effects of glucocorticosteroids. *Immunol Allergy Clin North Am.* 2005;25:451-468.

Effect of corticosteroids for fetal maturation on perinatal outcomes. *NIH Consens Statement.* 1994;12(2):1-24.

Ference JD, Last AR. Choosing topical corticosteroids. *Am Fam Physician.* 2009;79(2):135-140.

Lester RS, Knowles SR, Shear NH. The risks of systemic corticosteroid use. *Dermatol Clin.* 1998;16(2):277-286.

Miller CS, Little JW, Falace DA. Supplemental corticosteroids for dental patients with adrenal insufficiency: reconsideration of the problem. *JADA.* 2001;132:1570-1579.

Siegel MA, Silverman Jr S, Sollecito TP, eds. *Clinician's Guide to Treatment of Common Oral Conditions.* 6th ed. Hamilton, Ontario: BC Decker Inc; 2005.

Table 5.1. PRESCRIBING INFORMATION FOR GLUCOCORTICOIDS

NAME	FORM/ STRENGTH	DOSAGE	WARNINGS/PRECAUTIONS & CONTRAINDICATIONS	ADVERSE EFFECTS†
INHALED CORTICOSTEROIDS				
Beclomethasone Dipropionate (Qvar)	**MDI:** 40mcg/ inh, 80mcg/inh [7.3g]	***Adults:* Previous Bronchodilator Only:** 40-80mcg bid. **Max:** 320mcg bid. **Previous Inhaled Corticosteroid (CS) Therapy:** 40-160mcg bid. **Max:** 320mcg bid. **Maintained on Systemic CS:** May attempt gradual reduction of systemic CS dose after 1 week on inhaled therapy. ***Pediatrics:* Adolescents: Previous Bronchodilator Only:** 40-80mcg bid. **Max:** 320mcg bid. **Previous Inhaled Corticosteroid (CS) Therapy:** 40-160mcg bid. **Max:** 320mcg bid. **5-11 yrs: Previous Bronchodilator Only or Inhaled CS Therapy:** 40mcg bid. **Max:** 80mcg bid. **≥5 yrs: Maintained on Systemic CS:** May attempt gradual reduction of systemic CS dose after 1 week on inhaled therapy.	**W/P:** Deaths due to adrenal insufficiency have occurred with transfer from systemic corticosteroids to inhaled corticosteroids. Resume oral corticosteroids during stress or severe asthma attack. Risk of adrenal insufficiency and withdrawal symptoms when replacing systemic corticosteroids. May unmask allergic conditions previously suppressed by systemic steroid therapy. Caution with TB, ocular herpes simplex, or untreated systemic bacterial, fungal, parasitic, or viral infections. May suppress growth in children. Exposure to chickenpox or measles requires prophylactic treatment. Not for rapid relief of bronchospasm. **Contra:** Primary treatment of status asthmaticus or other acute episodes of asthma where intensive measures are required. **P/N:** Category C, not for use in nursing.	Headache, **pharyngitis**, upper respiratory tract infection, rhinitis, increased asthma symptoms, sinusitis.
Budesonide (Pulmicort Flexhaler, Pulmicort Respules)	**Powder, Inhalation:** (Flexhaler) 90mcg/dose, 180mcg/dose; **Sus, Inhalation:** (Respules) 0.25mg/2mL, 0.5mg/2mL, 1mg/2mL [2mL, 30^s]	***Adults:* (Flexhaler) Initial:** 180-360mcg bid. **Max:** 720mcg bid. Individualize dose. ***Pediatrics:* (Flexhaler) 6-17 yrs: Initial:** 180-360mcg bid. **Max:** 360mcg bid. Individualize dose. **(Respules) 1-8 yrs: Previous Bronchodilator Only: Initial:** 0.5mg qd or 0.25mg bid. Administer via jet nebulizer. **Max:** 0.5mg/ day. **Previous Inhaled Corticosteroid:** 0.5mg qd or 0.25mg bid. **Max:** 1mg/ day. **Previous Oral Corticosteroid:** 1mg qd or 0.5mg bid. **Max:** 1mg/day. Gradually reduce PO corticosteroid after 1 week of budesonide.	**W/P:** Deaths due to adrenal insufficiency have occurred with transfer from systemic corticosteroids to inhaled corticosteroids. Resume oral corticosteroids during stress or severe asthma attack. Transferring from oral to inhalation therapy may unmask allergic conditions (eg, rhinitis, conjunctivitis, arthritis, eosinophilic conditions, eczema). Observe for adrenal insufficiency, systemic corticosteroid withdrawal effects, and growth suppression (children). Increased susceptibility to infections. Not for acute bronchospasm. D/C if bronchospasm occurs after dosing. Caution with TB of respiratory tract; untreated systemic fungal, bacterial, viral or parasitic infections; or ocular herpes simplex. *Candida* infection of mouth and pharynx reported. Patients requiring oral corticosteroids should be weaned slowly from systemic corticosteroid use. **Contra:** Primary treatment of status asthmaticus or other acute episodes of asthma where intensive measures are required. **P/N:** (Flexhaler) Category B, caution in nursing; (Respules) Category B, caution in nursing.	**Nasopharyngitis, pharyngitis,** headache, fever, sinusitis, pain, bronchospasm, bronchitis, respiratory infection, moniliasis.
Budesonide/ Formoterol Fumarate Dihydrate (Symbicort)	**MDI** (Budesonide-Formoterol): 80mcg-4.5mcg/ inh, 160mcg-4.5mcg/inh [10.2g]	***Adults/Pediatrics:* ≥12 yrs: Asthma: Current Medium-High Dose Inhaled CS:** 2 inh bid of 160/4.5. **Current Low to Medium Dose Inhaled CS:** 2 inh bid of 80/4.5. **No Current Inhaled CS:** 2 inh bid of 80/4.5 or 160/4.5 depending on asthma severity. **Max:** 640mcg/18mcg (2 inh bid of 160/4.5). Patients not responding to the starting dose after 1-2 weeks of therapy with 80/4.5, replace with 160/4.5 for better asthma control. Rinse mouth after use. ***Adults:* COPD** (160/4.5mcg only): 2 inh bid. Rinse mouth after use.	**BB:** Long-acting β_2-adrenergic agonists (formoterol) may increase the risk of asthma-related death. **W/P:** Do not use in patients with significantly worsening or acutely deteriorating asthma. Not for acute treatment of symptoms. Monitor for increasing use of inhaled, short-acting β_2-agonists. Deaths due to adrenal insufficiency have occurred with transfer from systemic corticosteroids to inhaled corticosteroids. Resume oral corticosteroids during stress or severe asthma attack. Transferring from oral to inhalation therapy may unmask allergic conditions (eg, rhinitis, conjunctivitis, eczema). Observe for adrenal insufficiency, systemic corticosteroid withdrawal effects, and growth suppression	**Nasopharyngitis,** headache, upper respiratory tract infections, sinusitis, back pain, nasal/ sinus congestion, **oral candidiasis,** influenza, rhinitis, **pharyngolaryngeal pain,** vomiting.

†Bold entries denote special dental considerations.
BB = black box warning; **W/P** = warnings/precautions; **Contra** = contraindications; **P/N** = pregnancy category rating and nursing considerations.

Table 5.1. PRESCRIBING INFORMATION FOR GLUCOCORTICOIDS *(cont.)*

NAME	FORM/ STRENGTH	DOSAGE	WARNINGS/PRECAUTIONS & CONTRAINDICATIONS	ADVERSE EFFECTS†
INHALED CORTICOSTEROIDS *(cont.)*				
Budesonide/ Formoterol Fumarate Dihydrate (Symbicort) *(cont.)*			(pediatrics). Increased susceptibility to infections. Not for acute bronchospasm. Do not use any additional inhaled long-acting β_2-agonist for prevention of exercise-induced bronchospasm or the maintenance treatment of asthma. D/C if paradoxical bronchospasm occurs. Immediate hypersensitivity and upper airway symptom reactions reported. Caution with cardiovascular disorder (eg, coronary insufficiency, arrhythmia, HTN), seizures, thyroid and hepatic problems, diabetes, osteoporosis. QTc interval prolongation reported. Glaucoma, increased IOP, and cataracts reported. Caution in patients with active or quiescent tuberculosis infection, untreated systemic fungal, bacterial, viral, or parasitic infections, or ocular herpes simplex. Localized infections with *Candida albicans* may occur in the mouth and pharynx. **Contra:** Primary treatment of status asthmaticus or other acute asthma attacks. **P/N:** Category C, not for use in nursing.	
Ciclesonide (Alvesco)	**MDI:** 80mcg/ actuation [60 actuations], 160mcg/ actuation [60 or 120 actuations]	***Adults/Pediatrics:*** **≥12 yrs: Previous Bronchodilator Alone: Initial:** 80mcg bid. **Max:** 160mcg bid. **Previous Inhaled Corticosteroid Therapy: Initial:** 80mcg bid. **Max:** 320mcg bid. **Previous Oral Corticosteroid Therapy: Initial:** 320mcg bid. **Max:** 320mcg bid.	**W/P:** *Candida albicans* infections of mouth and pharynx may occur; examine periodically and treat accordingly. Advise to rinse mouth after inhalation. Caution with active or quiescent TB infections, untreated local/systemic bacterial/fungal infections, systemic viral or parasitic infections, or ocular herpes simplex. Risk for more severe/fatal course of infections (eg, chickenpox, measles); avoid exposure in patients who have not had the disease or been properly immunized. Risk of adrenal insufficiency and withdrawal symptoms when replacing oral corticosteroids with inhaled corticosteroids; monitor closely. Taper dose if symptoms of hypercorticism and adrenal suppression occur. May cause reduced growth velocity in pediatrics. May decrease bone mineral density with prolonged treatment; monitor and treat accordingly. Caution with history of glaucoma, increased IOP, and cataracts; monitor closely. Acute asthma episodes or bronchospasm may occur; d/c use and institute alternative treatment if occur.	Headache, **nasopharyngitis**, sinusitis, **pharyngolaryngeal pain**, upper respiratory infection, arthralgia, nasal congestion, pain in extremity, back pain.
Flunisolide (Aerobid, Aerobid-M)	**MDI:** 0.25mg/ inh [7g]	***Adults:*** **Initial:** 2 inh bid. **Max:** 4 inh bid. Rinse mouth after use. ***Pediatrics:*** **6-15 yrs:** 2 inh bid. Rinse mouth after use.	**W/P:** Deaths due to adrenal insufficiency have occurred with transfer from systemic corticosteroids to inhaled corticosteroids. Resume oral corticosteroids during stress or severe asthma attack. Observe for adrenal insufficiency, systemic corticosteroid withdrawal effects, and growth suppression (children). More susceptible to infections. Not for acute bronchospasm. D/C if bronchospasm occurs after dosing. Caution with TB of the respiratory tract; untreated systemic fungal, bacterial, viral, or parasitic infections; or ocular herpes simplex. *Candida* infection of the mouth and pharynx reported. **Contra:** Primary treatment of status asthmaticus or other acute asthma attacks. **P/N:** Category C, caution with nursing.	Upper respiratory infection, diarrhea, stomach upset, cold symptoms, nasal congestion, headache, N/V, **sore throat, unpleasant taste.**

†Bold entries denote special dental considerations.
BB = black box warning; **W/P** = warnings/precautions; **Contra** = contraindications; **P/N** = pregnancy category rating and nursing considerations.

NAME	FORM/ STRENGTH	DOSAGE	WARNINGS/PRECAUTIONS & CONTRAINDICATIONS	ADVERSE EFFECTS†
Fluticasone Proprionate (Flovent Diskus)	**Disk, Inhalation** (Fluticasone Propionate): 50mcg, 100mcg, 250mcg [60 blisters]	***Adults/Pediatrics:*** **≥12 yrs: Previous Bronchodilator Only: Initial:** 100mcg bid. **Max:** 500mcg bid. **Previous Inhaled Corticosteroids: Initial:** 100-250mcg bid. **Max:** 500mcg bid. **Previous Oral Corticosteroids: Initial:** 500-1000mcg bid. **Max:** 1000mcg bid. **4-11yrs: Initial:** 50mcg bid. **Max:** 100mcg bid.	**W/P:** Deaths due to adrenal insufficiency have occurred with transfer from systemic corticosteroids to inhaled corticosteroids. Resume oral corticosteroids during stress or severe asthma attack. Wean slowly from systemic corticosteroid therapy. Observe for adrenal insufficiency, systemic corticosteroid withdrawal effects, hypercorticism, adrenal suppression (including adrenal crisis), reduction in growth velocity (children and adolescents). May increase susceptibility to infections. Not for acute bronchospasm. D/C if bronchospasm occurs after dosing. Caution with TB of respiratory tract; untreated systemic fungal, bacterial, viral or parasitic infections; or ocular herpes simplex. *Candida* infection of mouth and pharynx reported. Glaucoma, increased IOP and cataracts reported. Rare cases of eosinophilic conditions. **Contra:** Primary treatment of status asthmaticus or other acute asthma attacks. **P/N:** Category C, not for use in nursing.	Upper respiratory tract infection, headache, **throat irritation**, sinusitis/ sinus infection, **candidiasis mouth/ throat** & non-site specific, and **cough**.
Fluticasone Propionate (Flovent HFA)	**MDI:** 44mcg/ inh [10.6g], 110mcg/inh [12g], 220mcg/ inh [12g]	***Adults/Pediatrics:*** **≥12 yrs: Previous Bronchodilator Only: Initial:** 88mcg bid. **Max:** 440mcg bid. **Previous Inhaled Corticosteroids: Initial:** 88-220mcg bid. **Max:** 440mcg bid. **Previous Oral Corticosteroids: Initial:** 440mcg bid. **Max:** 880mcg bid. **4-11yrs: Inital/Max:** 88mcg bid. Reduce PO prednisone no faster than 2.5 to 5mg/day weekly, beginning at least 1 week after starting fluticasone. Rinse mouth after use. Reduce PO prednisone no faster than 2.5 to 5mg/day weekly, beginning at least 1 week after starting fluticasone. Rinse mouth after use.	**W/P:** Deaths due to adrenal insufficiency have occurred with transfer from systemic corticosteroids to inhaled corticosteroids. Resume oral corticosteroids during stress or severe asthma attack. Wean slowly from systemic corticosteroid therapy. Observe for adrenal insufficiency, systemic corticosteroid withdrawal effects, hypercorticism, adrenal suppression (including adrenal crisis), reduction in growth velocity (children and adolescents). May increase susceptibility to infections. Not for acute bronchospasm. D/C if bronchospasm occurs after dosing. Caution with TB of respiratory tract; untreated systemic fungal, bacterial, viral or parasitic infections; or ocular herpes simplex. *Candida* infection of mouth and pharynx reported. Glaucoma, increased IOP and cataracts reported. Rare cases of eosinophilic conditions. **Contra:** Primary treatment of status asthmaticus or other acute asthma attacks. **P/N:** Category C, not for use in nursing.	Upper respiratory tract infection, headache, **throat irritation**, sinusitis/ sinus infection, **candidiasis mouth/ throat** & non-site specific, and **cough**.

Table 5.1. PRESCRIBING INFORMATION FOR GLUCOCORTICOIDS *(cont.)*

NAME	FORM/ STRENGTH	DOSAGE	WARNINGS/PRECAUTIONS & CONTRAINDICATIONS	ADVERSE EFFECTS†
INHALED CORTICOSTEROIDS *(cont.)*				
Fluticasone Propionate/ Salmeterol Xinafoate (Advair Diskus)	**Disk, Inhalation (Fluticasone-Salmeterol):** (100/50) 0.1mg-0.05mg/ inh, (250/50) 0.25mg-0.05mg/ inh, (500/50) 0.5mg-0.05mg/ inh [60 blisters]	*Adults/Pediatrics:* >12 yrs: **Asthma:** 1 inh q12h. **Without Prior Inhaled Corticosteroid (CS) Therapy/Inadequate Control on Current Inhaled CS: Initial:** 100/50 or 250/50 bid. **Max:** 500/50 bid. If no response within 2 weeks, may increase to higher strength. **COPD: (250/50 only):** 1 inh q12h. Rinse mouth after use. **4-11 yrs: (100/50 only): Symptomatic on Inhaled CS:** 1 inh q12h. Rinse mouth after use.	**BB:** Long-acting β_2-adrenergic agonists, such as salmeterol, may increase risk of asthma-related deaths. Use of diskus should be reserved for patients not adequately controlled on other medications or whose disease severity warrants initiation with 2 maintenance therapies. **W/P:** Deaths due to adrenal insufficiency have occurred with transfer from systemic corticosteroids to inhaled corticosteroids. Resume oral corticosteroids during stress or severe asthma attack. Observe for adrenal insufficiency, systemic corticosteroid withdrawal effects, hypercorticism, reduction in growth velocity (pediatrics). More susceptible to infection. Not for acute bronchospasm. D/C if bronchospasm occurs after dosing. Caution with TB; untreated systemic fungal, bacterial, viral, or parasitic infections; or ocular herpes simplex. *Candida* infection of mouth and pharynx, glaucoma, hypersensitivity reactions, increased IOP, cataracts reported. Monitor for increasing use of β_2-agonists. QTc interval prolongation reported with large doses. D/C if paradoxical bronchospasm occurs. Caution with cardiovascular or CNS disorders, convulsive disorders, thyrotoxicosis, DM, and ketoacidosis. May produce hypokalemia, hyperglycemia, and eosinophilic conditions. **Contra:** Status asthmaticus, other acute asthma or COPD episodes, and hypersensitivity to milk proteins. **P/N:** Category C, caution in nursing.	Upper respiratory tract inflammation, **pharyngitis**, sinusitis, **cough**, hoarseness, headaches, GI effects, musculoskeletal pain, palpitations.
Fluticasone Propionate/ Salmeterol Xinafoate (Advair HFA)	**MDI (Fluticasone-Salmeterol):** (45/21) 0.045mg-0.021mg/ inh, (115/21) 0.115mg-0.021mg/ inh, (230/21) 0.230mg-0.021mg/inh [120 inhalations]	*Adults/Pediatrics:* ≥12 yrs: **Asthma:** 2 inh q12h. **Without Prior Inhaled Corticosteroid (CS): Initial:** 2 inh of 45/21 bid or 1 inh of 115/21 bid. **Max:** 2 inh of 230/21 bid. **Current Inhaled CS: Beclomethasone:** ≤160mcg/day use 2 inh of 45/21 bid, 320mcg/day use 2 inh of 115/21 bid, 640mcg/day use 2 inh of 230/21 bid. **Budesonide:** ≤400mcg/day use 2 inh of 45/21 bid, 800-1200mcg/ day use 2 inh of 115/21 bid, 1600mcg/ day use 2 inh of 230/21 bid. **Flunisolide:** ≤1000mcg/day use 2 inh of 45/21 bid, 1250-2000mcg/day use 2 inh of 115/21 bid. **Flunisolide HFA:** ≤320mcg/ day use 2 inh of 45/21 bid, 640mcg/day use 2 inh of 115/21 bid. **Fluticasone Aerosol:** ≤176mcg/day use 2 inh of 45/21 bid, 440mcg/day use 2 inh of 115/21 bid, 660-880mcg/day use 2 inh of 230/21 bid. **Fluticasone Powder:** ≤200mcg/day use 2 inh of 45/21 bid, 500mcg/day use 2 inh of 115/21 bid, 1000mcg/day use 2 inh of 230/21 bid. **Mometasone Powder:** 220mcg/day use 2 inh of 45/21 bid, 440mcg/day use 2 inh of 115/21 bid, 880mcg/day use 2 inh of 230/21 bid. **Triamcinolone:**	**BB:** Long-acting β_2-adrenergic agonists, such as salmeterol, may increase risk of asthma-related deaths. **W/P:** May increase the risk of asthma-related death. Should only be given to patients not adequately controlled by other asthma-controller medications (eg, low or medium-dose inhaled corticosteroids) or patient's disease severity needs to start 2 maintenance therapies. Should not be given to rapidly deteriorating or potentially life-threatening episodes of asthma. Not be used to treat acute symptoms. Should not be used for transferring patients from systemic corticosteroid therapy. Should not be coadministered with inhaled, long-acting β_2-agonist and strong CYP3A4 inhibitors (eg, ketoconazole, ritonavir). Should not exceed recommended dosage. Life-threatening paradoxical bronchospasm reported; d/c therapy immediately; start alternative therapy. Immediate hypersensitivity reactions (eg, urticaria, angioedema, rash, and bronchospasm) may occur. Upper airway symptoms (eg, laryngeal spasm, irritation, or swelling, stridor, and choking) and lower respira-	Upper respiratory tract infection, **throat irritation**, upper respiratory tract inflammation, headaches, dysphonia, N/V, musculoskeletal pain, menstruation symptoms.

†Bold entries denote special dental considerations.
BB = black box warning; **W/P** = warnings/precautions; **Contra** = contraindications; **P/N** = pregnancy category rating and nursing considerations.

NAME	FORM/ STRENGTH	DOSAGE	WARNINGS/PRECAUTIONS & CONTRAINDICATIONS	ADVERSE EFFECTS†
Fluticasone Propionate/ Salmeterol Xinafoate (Advair HFA) *(cont.)*		≤1000mcg/day use 2 inh of 45/21 bid, 1100-1600mcg/day use 2 inh of 115/21 bid. If no response within 2 weeks, increase to higher strength.	tory tract infections (eg, pneumonia) reported. Caution in CVD, convulsive disorders, thyrotoxicosis, active or quiescent TB, untreated systemic fungal, bacterial, viral, or parasitic infection, and ocular herpes simplex. Prolonged use may affect bone metabolism and bone mineral density. *Candida* infection of mouth and pharynx, glaucoma, hypersensitivity reactions, increased IOP, cataracts reported. Cases of eosinophilic conditions reported. Caution in elderly. **Contra:** Status asthmaticus or other acute asthma. **P/N:** Category C, caution in nursing.	
Mometasone Furoate (Asmanex)	**Twisthaler:** 110mcg/inh, 220mcg/inh	***Adults/Pediatrics:*** **≥12 yrs: Previous Therapy with Bronchodilators Alone or Inhaled Corticosteroids: Initial:** 220mcg qpm. **Max:** 440mcg qpm or 220mcg bid. **Previous Therapy with Oral Corticosteroids: Initial:** 440mcg bid. **Max:** 880mcg/day. Titrate to lowest effective dose once asthma stability achieved. **4-11 yrs:** 110mcg qpm regardless of prior therapy. Titrate to lowest effective dose once asthma stability achieved.	**W/P:** Deaths due to adrenal insufficiency have occurred with transfer from systemic corticosteroids to inhaled corticosteroids. Wean slowly from systemic corticosteroid therapy. Resume oral corticosteroids during stress or severe asthma attack. May unmask allergic conditions previously suppressed by systemic corticosteroid therapy. May increase susceptibility to infections. Not for rapid relief of bronchospasm or other acute episodes of asthma. D/C if bronchospasm occurs after dosing. Observe for systemic corticosteroid withdrawal effects, hypercorticism, reduced bone mineral density, and adrenal suppression; reduce dose slowly if needed. Decreased growth velocity may occur in pediatrics. *Candida* infections in the mouth and pharynx reported. Caution with active or quiescent TB infection of respiratory tract; untreated systemic fungal, bacterial, viral, or parasitic infections; or ocular herpes simplex. Glaucoma, increased IOP, and cataracts reported. **Contra:** Primary treatment of status asthmaticus or other acute episodes of asthma where intensive measures are required. **P/N:** Category C, caution in nursing.	Headache, allergic rhinitis, **pharyngitis**, upper respiratory tract infection, sinusitis, **oral candidiasis**, dysmenorrhea, musculoskeletal pain, back pain, dyspepsia, myalgia, abdominal pain, nausea.
Triamcinolone Acetonide (Azmacort)	**MDI:** 75mcg/inh [20g]	***Adults/Pediatrics:*** **>12 yrs:** 2 inh (150mcg) tid-qid or 4 inh (300mcg) bid. **Severe Asthma: Initial:** 12-16 inh/day. **Max:** 16 inh/day (1200mcg). Rinse mouth after use. **6-12 yrs:** 1-2 inh (75-150mcg) tid-qid or 2-4 (150-300mcg) inh bid. **Max:** 12 inh/day (900mcg). Rinse mouth after use.	**W/P:** Deaths due to adrenal insufficiency have occurred with transfer from systemic corticosteroids to inhaled corticosteroids. Resume oral corticosteroids during stress or severe asthma attack. Observe for adrenal insufficiency, systemic corticosteroid withdrawal effects, hypercorticism and growth suppression (children). More susceptible to infections. Not for acute bronchospasm. D/C if bronchospasm occurs after dosing. Caution with TB of respiratory tract; untreated systemic fungal, bacterial, viral or parasitic infections; or ocular herpes simplex. *Candida* infection of mouth and pharynx reported. **Contra:** Primary treatment of status asthmaticus or other acute asthma attacks. **P/N:** Category C, caution in nursing.	**Pharyngitis**, sinusitis, headache, flu syndrome.

Table 5.1. PRESCRIBING INFORMATION FOR GLUCOCORTICOIDS *(cont.)*

NAME	FORM/ STRENGTH	DOSAGE	WARNINGS/PRECAUTIONS & CONTRAINDICATIONS	ADVERSE EFFECTS†
INTRANASAL CORTICOSTEROIDS				
Beclomethasone Dipropionate Monohydrate (Beconase AQ)	**Spray:** 42mcg/ spray [25g]	***Adults/Pediatrics:*** **>12 yrs:** 1-2 sprays per nostril bid. **6-12 yrs: Initial:** 1 spray per nostril bid. **Titrate:** May increase to 2 sprays per nostril bid. Decrease to 1 spray per nostril bid once adequate control achieved. **Max:** 2 sprays per nostril bid.	**W/P:** Risk of adrenal insufficiency and withdrawal symptoms when replacing systemic corticosteroids with topical corticosteroids. Caution with active or quiescent TB, ocular herpes simplex, or untreated bacterial, fungal, and systemic viral infections. Avoid with recent nasal trauma/surgery or septum ulcers. Risk for more severe/fatal course of infections (eg, chickenpox, measles) and for *Candida* infections of nose and pharynx. Potential for reduced growth velocity in pediatrics. **P/N:** Category C, caution in nursing.	**Nasopharyngeal irritation,** sneezing, headache, nausea, lightheadedness, nose and **throat irritation/dryness, unpleasant taste/ smell.**
Budesonide (Rhinocort Aqua)	**Spray:** 32mcg/ spray [8.6g]	***Adults/Pediatrics:*** **>12 yrs:** 1 spray per nostril qd. **Max:** 4 sprays/nostril/day. **6-12 yrs:** 1 spray per nostril qd. **Max:** 2 sprays per nostril/day	**W/P:** Risk of adrenal insufficiency and withdrawal symptoms when replacing systemic corticosteroids with a topical corticosteroid. Caution with active or quiescent TB, ocular herpes simplex, or untreated bacterial, fungal, and systemic viral infections. Avoid with recent nasal trauma, surgery, or septum ulcers. Risk of more severe/fatal course of infections (eg, chickenpox, measles) and for *Candida* infections of the nose and pharynx. Potential for reduced growth velocity in pediatrics. Should not delay or interfere with infant feeding. Immediate and/or delayed hypersensitivity reactions may occur rarely. Larger than recommended doses should be avoided; may cause hypercorticism and adrenal suppression. D/C slowly if such changes occur. Caution with hepatic dysfunction. **P/N:** Category B, caution in nursing.	Nasal irritation, **pharyngitis, cough,** epistaxis, bronchospasm.
Ciclesonide (Omnaris)	**Spray:** 50mcg/ spray [12.5g]	***Adults/Pediatrics:*** **≥6 yrs: Seasonal Allergic Rhinitis/≥12 yrs: Perennial Allergic Rhinitis:** 2 sprays (50mcg/ spray) each nostril qd.	**W/P:** Risk of acute adrenal insufficiency and withdrawal symptoms when replacing systemic corticosteroids with topical corticosteroids; monitor closely. Risk for more severe/fatal course of infections (eg, chickenpox, measles); avoid exposure in patients who have not had the disease or been properly immunized. May cause reduced growth velocity in pediatrics; routinely monitor growth. May impair wound healing; avoid in recent nasal septal ulcers, nasal surgery, or nasal trauma until healed. *Candida* infections of nose or pharynx may occur; examine periodically and treat accordingly. Caution with active or quiescent TB infections, untreated local or systemic fungal or bacterial infections, systemic viral or parasitic infections, or ocular herpes simplex. Taper dose if symptoms of hypercorticism occur. Caution with history of glaucoma and/or cataracts; monitor IOP accordingly.	Headache, epistaxis, **nasopharyngitis,** ear pain, **pharyngolaryngeal pain.**

†Bold entries denote special dental considerations.
BB = black box warning; **W/P** = warnings/precautions; **Contra** = contraindications; **P/N** = pregnancy category rating and nursing considerations.

NAME	FORM/ STRENGTH	DOSAGE	WARNINGS/PRECAUTIONS & CONTRAINDICATIONS	ADVERSE EFFECTS†
Flunisolide Nasal Spray	**Spray:** 25mcg/ spray [25mL]	***Adults:*** **Initial:** 2 sprays per nostril bid. **Titrate:** May increase to 2 sprays per nostril tid. **Max:** 8 sprays per nostril/ day. ***Pediatrics:*** **6-14 yrs: Initial:** 1 spray per nostril tid or 2 sprays per nostril bid. **Max:** 4 sprays per nostril/ day.	**W/P:** Risk of adrenal insufficiency and withdrawal symptoms when replacing systemic corticosteroids with topical corticosteroids. Caution with active or quiescent TB, ocular herpes simplex, or untreated bacterial, fungal, and systemic viral infections. Avoid with recent nasal trauma, surgery, or septum ulcers. Risk for more severe/fatal course of infections (eg, chickenpox, measles) and for *Candida* infections of the nose and pharynx. **Contra:** Untreated localized infection of the nasal mucosa. **P/N:** Category C, caution in nursing.	Nasal congestion, sneezing, epistaxis, bloody mucous, nasal irritation, watery eyes, **sore throat**, N/V, headache.
Flunisolide (Nasarel)	**Spray:** 29mcg/ spray [25mL]	***Adults:*** **Initial:** 2 sprays per nostril bid. **Titrate:** May increase to 2 sprays per nostril tid. **Max:** 8 sprays per nostril/ day. ***Pediatrics:*** **6-14 yrs: Initial:** 1 spray per nostril tid or 2 sprays per nostril bid. **Max:** 4 sprays per nostril/ day.	**W/P:** Risk of adrenal insufficiency and withdrawal symptoms when replacing systemic corticosteroids with topical corticosteroids. Caution with active or quiescent TB, ocular herpes simplex, or untreated bacterial, fungal, and systemic viral infections. Avoid with recent nasal trauma, surgery, or septum ulcers. Risk for more severe/fatal course of infections (eg, chickenpox, measles) and for *Candida* infections of the nose and pharynx. Potential for reduced growth velocity in pediatrics. **Contra:** Untreated localized infection of the nasal mucosa. **P/N:** Category C, caution in nursing.	**After-taste**, nasal burning/dryness/ stinging, **cough**, epistaxis, **pharyngitis**, sinusitis.
Fluticasone Furoate (Veramyst)	**Spray:** 27.5mcg/ spray [10g]	***Adults/Pediatrics:*** **≥12 yrs: Initial:** 2 sprays per nostril qd. **Maint:** 1 spray per nostril qd. **2-11 yrs: Initial:** 1 spray per nostril qd. **Titrate:** If inadequate response, may increase to 2 sprays per nostril.	**W/P:** Excessive use may cause hypercorticism and adrenal suppression. Risk of adrenal insufficiency and withdrawal symptoms when replacing systemic corticosteroids with topical corticosteroids. Caution with active or quiescent TB, ocular herpes simplex, or untreated bacterial, fungal, and systemic viral infections. Risk for more severe/fatal course of infections (eg, chickenpox, measles); avoid exposure in patients who have not had disease or have not been properly immunized. Epistaxis and nasal ulcerations may occur. *Candida* infection of nose reported. Avoid with recent nasal trauma, ulcers, or surgery. May result in glaucoma and cataracts. Potential for reduced growth velocity in pediatrics. **P/N:** Category C, caution in nursing.	Headache, epistaxis, **nasopharyngitis**, pyrexia, **pharyngolaryngeal pain, cough,** nasal ulceration, back pain
Fluticasone Propionate (Flonase)	**Spray:** 50mcg/ spray [16g]	***Adults/Pediatrics:*** **≥12 yrs: Initial:** 2 sprays per nostril qd or 1 spray per nostril bid. **Maint:** 1 spray per nostril qd. May dose as 2 sprays per nostril qd as needed for seasonal allergic rhinitis. ***Pediatrics:*** **≥4 yrs: Initial:** 1 spray per nostril qd. If inadequate response, may increase to 2 sprays per nostril. **Maint:** 1 spray per nostril qd. **Max:** 2 sprays per nostril/day.	**W/P:** Risk of adrenal insufficiency and withdrawal symptoms when replacing systemic corticosteroids with topical corticosteroids. Caution with active or quiescent TB, ocular herpes simplex, or untreated bacterial, fungal, and systemic viral infections. Avoid with recent nasal trauma, surgery, or septum ulcers. Risk for more severe/fatal course of infections (eg, chickenpox, measles); avoid exposure in patients who have not had disease or have not been properly immunized. *Candida* infection of nose and pharynx reported (rare). Potential for reduced growth velocity in pediatrics. Excessive use may cause signs of hypercorticism or HPA suppression. **P/N:** Category C, caution in nursing.	Headache, **pharyngitis**, epistaxis, nasal burning/ irritation, asthma symptoms, N/V, **cough**.

Table 5.1. PRESCRIBING INFORMATION FOR GLUCOCORTICOIDS *(cont.)*

NAME	FORM/ STRENGTH	DOSAGE	WARNINGS/PRECAUTIONS & CONTRAINDICATIONS	ADVERSE EFFECTS†
INTRANASAL CORTICOSTEROIDS *(cont.)*				
Mometasone Furoate Monohydrate (Nasonex)	**Spray:** 50mcg/ spray [17g]	***Adults/Pediatrics:*** **≥12 yrs: Allergic Rhinitis: Treatment/Prophylaxis:** 2 sprays per nostril qd. For prophylaxis, start 2-4 weeks before allergy season. **Nasal Polyps:** 2 sprays per nostril bid. **2-11 yrs: Treatment:** 1 spray per nostril qd.	**W/P:** Risk of adrenal insufficiency and withdrawal symptoms when replacing systemic corticosteroids with topical corticosteroids. Caution with active or quiescent TB, ocular herpes simplex, or untreated bacterial, fungal, and systemic viral infections. Avoid with recent nasal trauma, surgery, or septum ulcers. Risk for more severe/fatal course of infections (eg, chickenpox, measles) and for *Candida* infections of nose and pharynx. Potential for reduced growth velocity in pediatrics. **P/N:** Category C, caution with nursing.	Headache, viral infection, **pharyngitis**, epistaxis, **cough**, upper respiratory tract infection, dysmenorrhea, myalgia, sinusitis.
Triamcinolone Acetonide (Nasacort AQ)	**Spray:** 55mcg/ spray [16.5g]	***Adults/Pediatrics:*** **≥12 yrs: Initial/ Max:** 2 sprays per nostril qd. With improvement, may reduce dose to 1 spray per nostril qd. **6-12 yrs: Initial:** 1 spray per nostril qd. **Max:** 2 sprays per nostril qd. **2-5 yrs: Initial/Max:** 1 spray per nostril qd.	**W/P:** Risk of adrenal insufficiency and withdrawal symptoms when replacing systemic corticosteroids with topical corticosteroids. Caution with active or quiescent TB, ocular herpes simplex, or untreated bacterial, fungal, and systemic viral infections. Avoid with recent nasal trauma, surgery, or septum ulcers. Risk for more severe/fatal course of infections (eg, chickenpox, measles) and for *Candida* infections of nose and pharynx. Potential for reduced growth velocity in pediatrics. **P/N:** Category C, caution in nursing.	**Pharyngitis**, epistaxis, infection, otitis media, headache, sneezing, rhinitis, nasal irritation, **cough**, sinusitis, vomiting.
SYSTEMIC CORTICOSTEROIDS (LOW POTENCY)				
Hydrocortisone (Cortef)	**Sus:** (Hydrocortisone Cypionate) 10mg/5mL [120mL]; **Tab:** (Hydrocortisone) 5mg, 10mg, 20mg	***Adults/Pediatrics:*** **Initial:** 20-240mg/ day depending on disease. Adjust until a satisfactory response. **Maint:** Decrease in small amounts to lowest effective dose. **MS Exacerbations:** (Tab) 200mg/day of prednisolone for 1 week, then 80mg every other day for 1 month (20mg hydrocortisone=5mg prednisolone).	**W/P:** May need to increase dose before, during, and after stressful situations. May mask signs of infections. Avoid abrupt withdrawal. Prolonged use may produce glaucoma, optic nerve damage, secondary ocular infections. Increases BP, salt/water retention, potassium excretion. More severe/fatal course of infections reported with chickenpox, measles. Caution with TB, hypothyroidism, cirrhosis, ocular herpes simplex, HTN, diverticulitis, fresh intestinal anastomosis, ulcerative colitis, osteoporosis, myasthenia gravis, renal insufficiency, and peptic ulcer disease. Growth and development of children on prolonged therapy should be monitored. Monitor for psychic disturbances. Kaposi's sarcoma reported. **Contra:** Systemic fungal infections. **P/N:** Safety in pregnancy and nursing not known.	Fluid/electrolyte disturbances, HTN, osteoporosis, muscle weakness, cushingoid state, menstrual irregularities, nervousness, insomnia, impaired wound healing, DM, ulcerative esophagitis, excessive sweating, increased ICP, carbohydrate intolerance, glaucoma, cataracts.

†Bold entries denote special dental considerations.
BB = black box warning; **W/P** = warnings/precautions; **Contra** = contraindications; **P/N** = pregnancy category rating and nursing considerations.

NAME	FORM/ STRENGTH	DOSAGE	WARNINGS/PRECAUTIONS & CONTRAINDICATIONS	ADVERSE EFFECTS†
SYSTEMIC CORTICOSTEROIDS (LOW POTENCY)				
Hydrocortisone Sodium Succinate (Solu-Cortef)	**Inj:** 100mg, 250mg, 500mg, 1g	***Adults:*** **Initial:** 100-500mg IV/IM, depending on condition severity. May repeat dose at 2, 4, or 6 hrs based on clinical response. High-dose therapy usually not >48-72 hrs; may use antacids prophylactically. ***Pediatrics:*** Use lower adult doses. Determine dose by severity of condition and response. Dose should not be <25mg/day	**W/P:** May need to increase dose before, during, and after stressful situations. May mask signs of infection or cause new infections. Prolonged use may produce glaucoma, optic nerve damage, secondary ocular infections. Increases BP, salt/water retention, potassium and calcium excretion. More severe/ fatal course of infections reported with chickenpox, measles. Enhanced effect with hypothyroidism or cirrhosis. Caution with *Strongyloides*, latent TB, ocular herpes simplex, HTN, diverticulitis, fresh intestinal anastomoses, ulcerative colitis, osteoporosis, myasthenia gravis, renal insufficiency, and peptic ulcer disease. Kaposi's sarcoma reported. Monitor for psychic disturbances. Acute myopathy with high doses. Avoid abrupt withdrawal. Monitor growth and development of children on prolonged therapy. Hypernatremia may occur with high-dose therapy >48-72 hrs. **Contra:** Premature infants, systemic fungal infections. **P/N:** Safety in pregnancy and nursing not known.	Fluid/electrolyte disturbances, HTN, osteoporosis, muscle weakness, cushingoid state, menstrual irregularities, vertigo, headache, impaired wound healing, DM, ulcerative esophagitis, peptic ulcer, pancreatitis, increased sweating, increased ICP, carbohydrate intolerance, glaucoma, cataracts.
SYSTEMIC CORTICOSTEROIDS (INTERMEDIATE POTENCY)				
Fludrocortisone Acetate	**Tab:** 0.1mg*	***Adults:*** **Addison's Disease: Usual:** 0.1mg/day with concomitant cortisone 10-37.5mg/day or hydrocortisone 10-30mg/day in divided doses. **Dose Range:** 0.1mg three times weekly to 0.2mg/day. If HTN develops, reduce to 0.05mg/day. **Salt-Losing Adrenogenital Syndrome:** 0.1-0.2mg/day.	**W/P:** May need to increase dose before, during, and after stressful situations. Caution with hypothyroidism, cirrhosis, ocular herpes simplex, HTN, ulcerative colitis, diverticulitis, peptic ulcer, osteoporosis, myasthenia gravis, renal impairment, and elderly. May mask signs of infection or cause new infection. Avoid exposure to chickenpox or measles. Marked effect on sodium retention; monitor electrolytes. May need salt restriction and potassium supplements. Monitor for psychic disturbances. Risk of glaucoma, cataracts, and eye infections. Avoid abrupt withdrawal. **Contra:** Systemic fungal infections. **P/N:** Category C, caution in nursing.	HTN, CHF, edema, convulsions, hypokalemia, hypokalemic alkalosis, muscle weakness, impaired wound healing, menstrual irregularities, cataracts, suppression of growth, hyperglycemia, HPA-suppression, acne, rash.
Methylprednisolone (Medrol, Medrol Dosepak)	**Tab:** 2mg*, 4mg*, 8mg*, 16mg*, 32mg*; (Dosepak) 4mg* [21 tablets]	***Adults/Pediatrics:*** **Initial:** 4-48mg/day depending on disease and response. **Maint:** Decrease dose by small amounts to lowest effective dose. **MS Exacerbations:** 160mg/day for 1 week, then 64mg every other day for 1 month. **Alternate Day Therapy:** Twice the usual dose every other day for long-term therapy.	**W/P:** May need to increase dose before, during, and after stressful situations. May mask signs of infection or cause new infections. Prolonged use may produce glaucoma, optic nerve damage, secondary ocular infections. Increases BP, salt/water retention, potassium excretion. More severe/fatal course of infections reported with chickenpox and measles. Caution with *Strongyloides,* latent TB, hypothyroidism, cirrhosis, ocular herpes simplex, HTN, diverticulitis, fresh intestinal anastomoses, ulcerative colitis, osteoporosis, myasthenia gravis, renal insufficiency, peptic ulcer disease. Kaposi's sarcoma reported. Growth and development of children on prolonged therapy should be monitored. Monitor for psychic disturbances. Avoid abrupt withdrawal. The 24mg tabs contain tartrazine; caution with tartrazine sensitivity. **Contra:** Systemic fungal infections. **P/N:** Safety in pregnancy and nursing not known.	Fluid/electrolyte disturbances, HTN, osteoporosis, muscle weakness, cushingoid state, menstrual irregularities, nervousness, insomnia, impaired wound healing, DM, ulcerative esophagitis, excessive sweating, increased ICP, carbohydrate intolerance, glaucoma, cataracts, weight gain, nausea, malaise.

Table 5.1. PRESCRIBING INFORMATION FOR GLUCOCORTICOIDS *(cont.)*

NAME	FORM/ STRENGTH	DOSAGE	WARNINGS/PRECAUTIONS & CONTRAINDICATIONS	ADVERSE EFFECTS†
SYSTEMIC CORTICOSTEROIDS (INTERMEDIATE POTENCY) *(cont.)*				
Methylprednisolone Acetate (Depo-Medrol)	**Inj:** 20mg/mL, 40mg/mL, 80mg/mL	***Adults:* Local Effect: OA/RA: Large Joint:** 20-80mg. **Medium Joint:** 10-40mg. **Small Joint:** 4-10mg. Administer intra-articularly into synovial space every 1-5 weeks or more depending on relief. **Ganglion/Tendinitis/Epicondylitis:** 4-30mg into cyst/area of greatest tenderness. May repeat if necessary. **Dermatologic Conditions:** Inject 20-60mg into lesion. Distribute 20-40mg doses by repeated injections into large lesions. **Usual:** 1-4 injections. **Systemic Effect: Substitute for Oral Therapy:** IM dose should equal total daily PO methylprednisolone dose q24h. **Prolonged Therapy:** Administer weekly PO dose as single IM injection. **Androgenital Syndrome:** 40mg IM every 2 weeks. RA: 40-120mg IM weekly. **Dermatologic Lesions:** 40-120mg IM weekly for 1-4 weeks. **Acute Severe Dermatitis (Poison Ivy):** 80-120mg IM single dose. **Chronic Contact Dermatitis:** May repeat injections every 5-10 days. **Seborrheic Dermatitis:** 80mg IM weekly. **MS Exacerbations:** 200mg/day prednisolone for 1 week, then 80mg every other day for 1 month (4mg methylprednisolone=5mg prednisolone). **Asthma/Allergic Rhinitis:** 80-120mg IM. ***Pediatrics:*** Use lower adult doses. Determine dose by severity of condition and response.	**W/P:** Dermal and subdermal atrophy reported; do not exceed recommended doses. May need to increase dose before, during, and after stressful situations. May mask signs of infection or cause new infections. Prolonged use may produce cataracts, glaucoma, secondary ocular infections. Increases BP, salt/water retention, potassium and calcium excretion. More severe/fatal course of infections reported with chickenpox, measles. Caution with *Strongyloides,* latent TB, hypothyroidism, cirrhosis, ocular herpes simplex, HTN, diverticulitis, fresh intestinal anastomoses, ulcerative colitis, osteoporosis, myasthenia gravis, renal insufficiency, peptic ulcer disease. Kaposi's sarcoma reported. Growth and development of children on prolonged therapy should be monitored. Monitor for psychic disturbances. Avoid abrupt withdrawal. Do not use intra-articularly, intrabursally, or for intratendinous administration in acute infection. Avoid injection into unstable and previously infected joints. Monitor urinalysis, blood sugar, BP, weight, chest X-ray, and upper GI X-ray (if ulcer history) regularly during prolonged therapy. **Contra:** Intrathecal administration, systemic fungal infections. **P/N:** Safety in pregnancy and nursing not known.	Fluid/electrolyte disturbances, HTN, osteoporosis, muscle weakness, Cushingoid state, menstrual irregularities, impaired wound healing, DM, ulcerative esophagitis, excessive sweating, increases ICP, carbohydrate intolerance, glaucoma, cataracts, urticaria, subcutaneous/cutaneous atrophy.
Methylprednisolone Sodium Succinate (Solu-Medrol)	**Inj:** 40mg, 125mg	***Adults:* Usual: Initial:** 10-40mg IV over several min. May repeat IV/IM dose at intervals based on clinical response. **High-Dose Therapy:** 30mg/kg IV over at least 30 min, may repeat q4-6h for 48 hrs. High-dose therapy usually not >48-72 hrs. Give antacids prophylactically. **MS Exacerbations:** 200mg/day prednisolone for 1 week, then 80mg every other day for 1 month (4mg methylprednisolone=5mg prednisolone). ***Pediatrics:*** Use lower adult doses. Determine dose by severity of condition and response. Dose should not be <0.5mg/kg q24h.	**W/P:** May need to increase dose before, during, and after stressful situations. May mask signs of infection or cause new infections. Prolonged use may produce cataracts, glaucoma, secondary ocular infections. Increases BP, salt/water retention, calcium/potassium excretion. More severe/fatal course of infections reported with chickenpox, measles. Caution with latent TB, hypothyroidism, cirrhosis, ocular herpes simplex, HTN, diverticulitis, fresh intestinal anastomoses, ulcerative colitis, osteoporosis, myasthenia gravis, renal insufficiency, peptic ulcer disease. Kaposi's sarcoma reported. Growth and development of children on prolonged therapy should be monitored. Monitor for psychic disturbances. Avoid abrupt withdrawal. Reports of cardiac arrhythmias, circulatory collapse, cardiac arrest following rapid administration of large IV doses. Effectiveness not established for the treatment of sepsis syndrome and septic shock. Bradycardia reported with high doses. **Contra:** Premature infants (due to benzyl alcohol diluent) and systemic fungal infections. **P/N:** Safety in pregnancy and nursing not known.	Fluid/electrolyte disturbances, HTN, osteoporosis, muscle weakness, cushingoid state, menstrual irregularities, insomnia, impaired wound healing, DM, ulcerative esophagitis, excessive sweating, increases ICP, carbohydrate intolerance, glaucoma, cataracts, nausea.

†Bold entries denote special dental considerations.
BB = black box warning; **W/P** = warnings/precautions; **Contra** = contraindications; **P/N** = pregnancy category rating and nursing considerations.

NAME	FORM/ STRENGTH	DOSAGE	WARNINGS/PRECAUTIONS & CONTRAINDICATIONS	ADVERSE EFFECTS†
Prednisolone	**Syrup:** 5mg/5mL [120mL], 15mg/5mL [240mL, 480mL]	***Adults/Pediatrics:* Initial:** 5-60mg/day depending on disease and response. **Maint:** Decrease dose by small amounts to lowest effective dose.	**W/P:** Adjust dose during stress or change in thyroid status. May mask signs of infection or cause new infections. Prolonged use may produce glaucoma, optic nerve damage, secondary ocular infections. Increases BP, salt/water retention, and potassium excretion. Avoid exposure to chickenpox, and measles. Caution with latent TB, hypothyroidism, cirrhosis, ocular herpes simplex, HTN, diverticulitis, fresh intestinal anastomosis, ulcerative colitis, osteoporosis, myasthenia gravis, renal insufficiency, and peptic ulcer disease. Growth and development of children on prolonged therapy should be monitored. Monitor for psychic disturbances. Avoid abrupt withdrawal. **Contra:** Systemic fungal infections. **P/N:** Safety in pregnancy and nursing not known.	Fluid/electrolyte disturbances, osteoporosis, muscle weakness, cushingoid state, menstrual irregularities, nervousness, insomnia, impaired wound healing, excessive sweating, carbohydrate intolerance, glaucoma, cataracts, weight gain, nausea, malaise.
Prednisolone Sodium Phosphate (Orapred, Orapred ODT, Pediapred)	**Sol:** (Orapred) 15mg/5mL [237mL]; (Pediapred) 5mg/mL [120mL]; **Tab, Orally Disintegrating:** (Orapred ODT): 10mg, 15mg, 30mg	**Adults: Initial:** (Sol) 5-60mg/day depending on disease and response. (Tab) 10-60mg/day depending on disease and response. **Maint:** Decrease dose by small amounts to lowest effective dose. **MS Exacerbations:** (Sol/Tab) 200mg qd for 1 week, then 80mg every other day for 1 month. ***Pediatrics:* Initial:** (Sol/Tab) 0.14-2mg/kg/day, depending on disease and response, given tid-qid. **Nephrotic Syndrome:** 60mg/m^2/day given in 3 divided doses for 4 weeks, then 40mg/m^2/day single-doses every other day for 4 weeks. **Uncontrolled Asthma:** 1-2mg/kg/day in single or divided doses until peak expiratory flow rate of 80% is achieved (usually 3-10 days).	**W/P:** May produce reversible HPA axis suppression. Adjust dose during stress or change in thyroid status. May mask signs of infection or cause new infections. May activate latent amebiasis. Avoid with cerebral malaria. Avoid exposure to chickenpox or measles. Not for treatment of optic neuritis or active ocular herpes simplex. May cause elevation of BP or IOP, cataracts, glaucoma, optic nerve damage, Kaposi's sarcoma, psychic derangements, salt/water retention, increased excretion of potassium and/or calcium, osteoporosis, growth suppression in children, secondary ocular infections. Caution with *Strongyloides*, CHF, diverticulitis, HTN, renal insufficiency, fresh intestinal anastomoses, active or latent peptic ulcer, ulcerative colitis. Enhanced effect in hypothyroidism or cirrhosis. Avoid abrupt withdrawal. Use with caution in elderly, increased risk of corticosteroid-induced side effects; start at low end of dosing range; monitor bone mineral density. **Contra:** Systemic fungal infections. **P/N:** Category C, caution in nursing.	Edema, fluid/electrolyte disturbances, osteoporosis, muscle weakness, pancreatitis, peptic ulcer, impaired wound healing, increased ICP, cushingoid state, hirsutism, menstrual irregularities, growth suppression in children, glaucoma, nausea, weight gain.
Prednisone	**Sol:** 5mg/mL, 5mg/5mL; **Tab:** 1mg, 2.5mg*, 5mg*, 10mg*, 20mg*, 50mg*	***Adults/Pediatrics:* Initial:** 5-60mg/day depending on disease and response. **Maint:** Decrease dose by small amounts to lowest effective dose.	**W/P:** May need to increase dose before, during, and after stressful situations. May mask signs of infection or cause new infections. Prolonged use may produce glaucoma, optic nerve damage, and secondary ocular infections. Increases BP, salt/water retention, and potassium excretion. More severe/fatal course of infections reported with chickenpox, measles. Caution with latent TB, hypothyroidism, cirrhosis, ocular herpes simplex, HTN, diverticulitis, fresh intestinal anastomosis, ulcerative colitis, osteoporosis, myasthenia gravis, renal insufficiency, and peptic ulcer disease. Growth and development of children on prolonged therapy should be monitored. Monitor for psychic disturbances. Avoid abrupt withdrawal. **Contra:** Systemic fungal infections. **P/N:** Safety in pregnancy and nursing not known.	Fluid/electrolyte disturbances, HTN, osteoporosis, muscle weakness, cushingoid state, menstrual irregularities, nervousness, insomnia, impaired wound healing, DM, **ulcerative esophagitis**, excessive sweating, increased ICP, carbohydrate intolerance, glaucoma, cataracts, weight gain, nausea, malaise.

Table 5.1. PRESCRIBING INFORMATION FOR GLUCOCORTICOIDS *(cont.)*

NAME	FORM/ STRENGTH	DOSAGE	WARNINGS/PRECAUTIONS & CONTRAINDICATIONS	ADVERSE EFFECTS†
SYSTEMIC CORTICOSTEROIDS (HIGH POTENCY)				
Betamethasone (augmented) Sodium Phosphate/ Betamethasone Acetate (Celestone Soluspan)	**Inj (Betamethasone Acetate-Betamethasone Sodium Phosphate):** 3mg-3mg/mL	***Adults:*** **Initial:** 0.25-9mg/day depending on the specific disease. **Maint:** Decrease in small increments at appropriate time intervals until lowest effective dose. D/C gradually. **Bursitis:** 0.25-1mL intrabursal injection (site-specific; see PI). May give several injections for recurrence/acute exacerbations. **Chronic Bursitis:** Reduce initial dose once controlled. **Tenosynovitis/ Tendinitis:** Give 3-4 injections of 0.5 mL into tendon sheaths q3 days-2 weeks (site specific; see PI). **Ganglion Cysts:** 0.5mL-injection directly into cysts. **Dermatologic Conditions:** 0.2mL/cm² intradermally. **Max:** 1mL/ week. **MS Exacerbations:** 30mg/day for 1 week, then 12mg every other day for 1 month. **OA/RA:** 0.5-2mL intra-articularly (site-specific; see PI). **Acute Gouty Arthritis:** 0.5-1mL q3 days-2 weeks. ***Pediatrics:*** **Initial:** 0.02-0.3 mg/kg/day in 3 or 4 divided doses depending on the specific disease. **Maint:** Decrease in small increments at appropriate time intervals until reach lowest dose that sustains response. D/C gradually.	**W/P:** May need to increase dose before, during, and after stressful situations. May mask signs of infection or cause new infections. Prolonged use may produce posterior subcapsular cataracts, glaucoma, optic nerve damage, and secondary ocular infections. Increases BP, salt/water retention, potassium and calcium excretion. More severe/ fatal course of infections reported with chickenpox, measles. Caution with threadworm infestation, latent TB, hypothyroidism, cirrhosis, ocular herpes simplex, HTN, diverticulitis, fresh intestinal anastomosis, ulcerative colitis, osteoporosis, myasthenia gravis, renal insufficiency, peptic ulcer disease. Growth and development of children on prolonged therapy should be monitored. Monitor for psychic disturbances. Avoid abrupt withdrawal. **(Intra-articular)** Examine joint fluid to rule out a septic process. Avoid injection into previously infected joint. **Contra:** Systemic fungal infections. **P/N:** Safety in pregnancy and nursing not known.	Sodium retention, fluid retention, potassium loss, muscle weakness, myopathy, peptic ulcer, impaired wound healing, thin fragile skin, convulsions, menstrual irregularities, cataracts.
Betamethasone (Celestone)	**Sol:** 0.6mg/5mL [118mL]	***Adults:*** **Initial:** 0.6-7.2mg/day depending on disease. Maintain until sufficient response. **Maint:** Decrease dose by small amounts to lowest effective dose. D/C gradually. **MS Exacerbations:** 30mg/day for 1 week, then 12mg every other day for 1 month. ***Pediatrics:*** **Initial:** 0.02-0.3mg/kg/day in 3 or 4 divided doses depending on the disease and clniical response. **Maint:** Decrease dose by small amounts to lowest effective dose. D/C gradually.	**W/P:** May need to increase dose before, during, and after stressful situations. May mask signs of infection or cause new infections. Prolonged use may produce posterior subcapsular cataracts, glaucoma, optic nerve damage, secondary ocular infections. Increases BP, salt/ water retention, potassium and calcium excretion. More severe/fatal course of infections reported with chickenpox, measles. Caution with threadworm infestation, latent TB, hypothyroidism, cirrhosis, ocular herpes simplex, HTN, diverticulitis, fresh intestinal anastomosis, ulcerative colitis, osteoporosis, myasthenia gravis, renal insufficiency, and peptic ulcer disease. Growth and development of children on prolonged therapy should be monitored. Monitor for psychic disturbances. Avoid abrupt withdrawal. **Contra:** Systemic fungal infections. **P/N:** Safety in pregnancy and nursing not known.	Sodium retention, fluid retention, potassium loss, muscle weakness, myopathy, peptic ulcer, impaired wound healing, thin fragile skin, convulsions, menstrual irregularities, cataracts.

*Scored. †Bold entries denote special dental considerations.
BB = black box warning; **W/P** = warnings/precautions; **Contra** = contraindications; **P/N** = pregnancy category rating and nursing considerations.

NAME	FORM/ STRENGTH	DOSAGE	WARNINGS/PRECAUTIONS & CONTRAINDICATIONS	ADVERSE EFFECTS†
Dexamethasone	**Inj (Dexamethasone Sodium Phosphate):** 4mg/mL, 10mg/mL; **Sol (Dexamethasone):** 0.5mg/5mL; **Concentrated Sol (Dexamethasone Intensol):** 1mg/mL; **Tab (Dexamethasone):** 0.5mg*, 0.75mg*, 1mg*, 1.5mg*, 2mg*, 4mg*, 6mg*	***Adults:*** Individualize for disease and patient response. Withdraw gradually. **(Tab, Sol) Initial:** 0.75-9mg/day PO. **Maint:** Decrease in small amounts to lowest effective dose. **Acute Allergic Disorders:** 4 or 8mg IM on 1st day, then 2 tabs of 0.75mg PO bid on days 2-3, then 1 tab of 0.75mg PO bid on day 4, then 1 tab of 0.75mg PO qd on days 5-6. **MS Exacerbations:** 30mg/day for 1 week, then 4-12mg every other day for 1 month. **(Inj) Initial:** 0.5-9mg IV/IM depending on the disease being treated. **Cerebral Edema: Initial:** 10mg IV, then 4mg IM q6h until edema subsides. Reduce dose after 2-4 days and gradually d/c over 5-7 days. **Palliative Management of Recurrent/ Inoperable Brain Tumors: Maint:** 2mg IV/PO bid-tid. **Intra-Articular/ Intralesional/Soft Tissue Injection: Usual:** 0.2-6mg once every 3-5 days to once every 2-3 weeks (sidte-specific). See PI for Shock Treatment. Mix Intensol with liquid or semi-solid food. ***Pediatrics:*** Individualize for disease and patient response. Withdraw gradually. **(Tab, Sol) Initial:** 0.02-0.3mg/kg/day in 3 or 4 divided doses. **Maint:** Decrease in small amounts to lowest effective dose.	**W/P:** Increase dose before, during, and after stressful situations. Avoid abrupt withdrawal. May mask signs of infection, activate latent amebiasis, elevate BP, cause salt/water retention, increase excretion of potassium and calcium. Prolonged use may produce cataracts, glaucoma, and secondary ocular infections. Caution with recent MI, ocular herpes simplex, emotional instability, nonspecific ulcerative colitis, diverticulitis, peptic ulcer, renal insufficiency, HTN, osteoporosis, myasthenia gravis, threadworm infection, and active tuberculosis. Enhanced effect with hypothyroidism and cirrhosis. Consider prophylactic therapy if exposed to measles or chickenpox. Risk of glaucoma, cataracts, and eye infections. False negative dexamethasone suppression test with indomethacin. **Contra:** Systemic fungal infections. **P/N:** Category C, not for use in nursing.	Fluid/electrolyte disturbances, muscle weakness, osteoporosis, peptic ulcer, pancreatitis, **ulcerative esophagitis**, impaired wound healing, headache, psychic disturbances, growth suppression (pediatrics), glaucoma, hyperglycemia, weight gain, nausea, malaise.
TOPICAL CORTICOSTEROIDS (LOW POTENCY)				
Alclometasone Dipropionate (Aclovate)	**Cre, Oint:** 0.05% [15g, 45g, 60g]	***Adults/Pediatrics:*** **≥1 yr:** Apply bid-tid. Reassess if no improvement after 2 weeks.	**W/P:** May produce reversible HPA axis suppression, manifestations of Cushing's syndrome, hyperglycemia, and glucosuria. Use appropriate antifungal or antibacterial agent with dermatological infections. Peds may be more susceptible to systemic toxicity. Avoid occlusive dressings. Avoid diaper area. Not for use in diaper dermatitis. D/C if irritation occurs. Caution in peds. **P/N:** Category C, caution in nursing.	Itching, burning, erythema, dryness, irritation, papular rash, folliculitis, acneiform eruptions, hypopigmentation, **perioral dermatitis**, allergic contact dermatitis, secondary infection, skin atrophy, striae.
Desonide (DesOwen)	**Cre, Oint:** 0.05% [15g, 60g]; **Lot:** 0.05% [60mL, 120mL]	***Adults:*** Apply bid-tid, depending on severity. Reassess if no improvement after 2 weeks.	**W/P:** May produce reversible HPA axis suppression, manifestations of Cushing's syndrome, hyperglycemia, and glucosuria. D/C if irritation occurs. Use appropriate antifungal or antibacterial agent with dermatological infections. Peds may be more susceptible to systemic toxicity. Caution when applied to large surface areas. Avoid occlusive dressings. **P/N:** Category C, caution in nursing.	Stinging, burning, irritation, erythema, contact dermatitis, worsening condition, skin peeling, dryness/scaliness.
Desonide (Desonate)	**Gel:** 0.05% [15g, 30g, 60g]	***Adults/Pediatrics:*** **≥3 months:** Apply thin layer bid to affected area(s) and rub in gently. Not recommended beyond 4 consecutive weeks.	**W/P:** May produce reversible HPA axis suppression, manifestations of Cushing's syndrome, hyperglycemia, and glucosuria. D/C if irritation occurs. Pediatrics may be more susceptible to systemic toxicity. Caution when applied to large surface areas. Avoid occlusive dressings. Avoid use beyond 4 wks. **P/N:** Category C, caution in nursing.	Burning, rash, application site pruritus.

Table 5.1. PRESCRIBING INFORMATION FOR GLUCOCORTICOIDS *(cont.)*

NAME	FORM/ STRENGTH	DOSAGE	WARNINGS/PRECAUTIONS & CONTRAINDICATIONS	ADVERSE EFFECTS†
TOPICAL CORTICOSTEROIDS (LOW POTENCY) *(cont.)*				
Desonide (Verdeso)	**Foam:** 0.05% [100g]	***Adults/Pediatrics:*** **≥3 months:** Apply thin layer to affected area(s) bid. **Max Duration:** 4 consecutive weeks. Not to dispense directly on face; use hands to gently massage. Avoid occlusive dressings.	**W/P:** May produce reversible HPA axis suppression, manifestations of Cushing's syndrome, hyperglycemia, and glucosuria. D/C if irritation occurs. Caution when applied to large surface areas. Pediatrics may be more susceptible to systemic toxicity. Use appropriate antifungal or antibacterial with concomitant skin infections; d/c if infection does not clear. **P/N:** Category C, caution in nursing.	Application site burning, upper respiratory tract infection, **cough**.
TOPICAL CORTICOSTEROIDS (MEDIUM POTENCY)				
Betamethasone Valerate (Luxiq)	**Foam:** 0.12% [50g, 100g]	***Adults:*** Place foam onto saucer or other cool surface first, then apply in small amounts to scalp. Gently massage into affected area bid (am and pm) until foam disappears. Reassess if no improvement after 2 weeks.	**W/P:** May produce reversible HPA axis suppression, manifestations of Cushing's syndrome, hyperglycemia, and glucosuria. Caution when applied to large surface areas, for prolonged use, or under occlusive dressings. Use appropriate antifungal or antibacterial agent with dermatological infections; d/c if infection does not clear. Pediatrics may be more susceptible to systemic toxicity. Avoid eyes. D/C if irritation occurs. **P/N:** Category C, caution in nursing.	Burning, stinging, pruritus, paresthesia, acne, alopecia, conjunctivitis.
Fluocinolone Acetonide	**Cre:** 0.01%, 0.025% [15g, 60g]; **Oint:** 0.025% [15g, 60g], **Shampoo: (Capex)** 0.01% [180mL]; **Sol:** 0.01% [60mL]	***Adults/Pediatrics:*** (Cre, Oint, Sol) Apply tid-qid. May use occlusive dressings for psoriasis or recalcitrant conditions; d/c dressings if infection develops. ***Adults:*** (Shampoo) Apply up to 1oz to scalp qd. Work into lather, rinse after 5 min.	**W/P:** May produce reversible HPA axis suppression, manifestations of Cushing's syndrome, hyperglycemia, and glucosuria. Caution when applied to large surface areas or under occlusive dressings. Use appropriate antifungal or antibacterial agent with dermatological infections; d/c if infection does not clear. Peds may be more susceptible to systemic toxicity. Avoid eyes. D/C if irritation occurs. **P/N:** Category C, caution with nursing.	Burning, itching, irritation, dryness, folliculitis, hypertrichosis, acneiform eruptions, hypopigmentation, **perioral dermatitis**, allergic dermatitis, skin maceration, secondary infection, skin atrophy, striae, miliaria.
Flurandrenolide (Cordran, Cordran SP)	**Cre (SP):** 0.05% [15g, 30g, 60g]; **Lot:** 0.05% [15mL, 60mL]; **Tape:** 4mcg/cm[24"x3", 80"x3'"]	***Adults/Pediatrics:*** (Cre, Lot) Apply qd-qid depending on severity. For moist lesions, apply cream bid-tid. Apply lotion bid-tid. (Tape) Clean and dry skin. Shave or clip hair. Apply tape q12-24h.	**W/P:** Systemic absorption may produce reversible HPA axis suppression, manifestations of Cushing's syndrome, hyperglycemia, and glucosuria. Application of more potent steroids, use on large surfaces, prolonged use, or occlusive dressings may augment systemic absorption. Evaluate periodically for HPA suppression if large dose applied to large area or with occlusive dressings. Pediatrics are more susceptible to toxicity. D/C if irritation develops. May use occlusive dressing for psoriasis or recalcitrant conditions. **Contra: (Tape)** Not for lesions exuding serum or in intertriginous areas. **P/N:** Category C, caution in nursing.	Burning, itching, irritation, dryness, folliculitis, hypertrichosis, acneiform eruptions, hypopigmentation, dermatitis. Occlusive dressing may cause skin maceration, secondary infection, skin atrophy, miliaria.

†Bold entries denote special dental considerations.
BB = black box warning; **W/P** = warnings/precautions; **Contra** = contraindications; **P/N** = pregnancy category rating and nursing considerations.

NAME	FORM/ STRENGTH	DOSAGE	WARNINGS/PRECAUTIONS & CONTRAINDICATIONS	ADVERSE EFFECTS†
Fluticasone Propionate (Cutivate)	**Cre:** 0.05% [30g, 60g]; **Lot:** 0.05% [120mL]; **Oint:** 0.005% [30g, 60g]	***Adults:* Atopic Dermatitis:** (Cre) Apply qd-bid. (Lot) Apply qd. **Other Dermatoses:** (Cre) Apply bid. (Oint) Apply bid. (Cre, Lot, Oint) Avoid occlusive dressings and re-evaluate if no improvement after 2 weeks. ***Pediatrics:* ≥3 months: Atopic Dermatitis:** (Cre) Apply qd-bid. **Other Dermatoses:** (Cre) Apply bid. Avoid in diaper area. **≥1 yr: Atopic Dermatitis:** (Lot) Apply qd. (Cre, Lot) Avoid occlusive dressings and re-evaluate if no improvement after 2 weeks. Oint not approved in peds.	**W/P:** Caution with cream in peds. May produce reversible HPA axis suppression, manifestations of Cushing's syndrome, hyperglycemia, and glucosuria. D/C if irritation occurs. Use appropriate antifungal or antibacterial agent with dermatological infections. Peds may be more susceptible to systemic toxicity. Caution when applied to large surface areas. Avoid with pre-existing skin atrophy. Not for use in rosacea or perioral dermatitis. **P/N:** Category C, caution in nursing.	(Cre) Pruritus, dryness, numbness of fingers, burning. (Oint) Pruritus, burning, hypertrichosis, increased erythema, hives, irritation, lightheadedness. (Lot) Burning, stinging, dryness, common cold, upper respiratory tract infection, **cough**, fever.
Halcinonide (Halog)	**Cre:** 0.1% [30g, 60g], **Oint:** 0.1% [15g, 30g, 60g]; **Sol:** 0.1% [20mL, 60mL]	***Adults:*** (Cre, Oint, Sol) Apply bid-tid. May use occlusive dressings for psoriasis and recalcitrant conditions. ***Pediatrics:*** Limit to least amount compatible with an effective therapeutic regimen.	**W/P:** May produce reversible HPA axis suppression, manifestations of Cushing's syndrome, hyperglycemia, and glucosuria. Occlusive dressings and application to large surface areas may augment systemic absorption. Pediatrics may be more susceptible to systemic toxicity. D/C if irritation occurs. **P/N:** Category C, caution in nursing.	Burning, itching, irritation, dryness, folliculitis, hypertrichosis, acneiform eruptions, hypopigmentation, **perioral dermatitis,** contact dermatitis, skin maceration, secondary infection.
Hydrocortisone Acetate/Pramoxine HCl (Epifoam, Novacort, Pramosone, Proctofoam HC)	**Cre (Hydrocortisone-Pramoxine):** (Pramosone)1%-1%, 1%-2.5% [30g, 60g]; **Foam:** (Epifoam, Proctofoam HC) 1%-1% [10g]; **Gel:** (Novacort) 2%-1% [29g]; **Lot:** (Pramosone) 1%-1% [60mL, 120mL, 240mL], 1%-2.5% [60mL, 120mL]; **Oint:** (Pramosone) 1%-1%, 1%-2.5% [30g]	***Adults:*** Apply to affected area(s) tid-qid. May use occlusive dressings for psoriasis or recalcitrant conditions. D/C dressings if infection develops. ***Pediatrics:*** Use least amount necessary for effective regimen. May use occlusive dressings for psoriasis or recalcitrant conditions. D/C dressings if infection develops.	**W/P:** May produce reversible HPA axis suppression, manifestations of Cushing's syndrome, hyperglycemia, and glucosuria. Caution when applied to large surface areas, under occlusive dressings, or with prolonged use. Use appropriate antifungal or antibacterial agent with dermatological infections; d/c if infection does not clear. Pediatrics may be more susceptible to systemic toxicity. D/C if irritation develops. Avoid eyes. **P/N:** Category C, caution in nursing	Burning, itching, irritation, dryness, folliculitis, hypertrichosis, acneiform eruptions, hypopigmentation, **perioral dermatitis**, allergic dermatitis, skin maceration, secondary infection, skin atrophy, striae, miliaria.
Hydrocortisone Butyrate (Locoid)	**Cre, Oint:** 0.1% [15g, 45g]; **Sol:** 0.1% [20mL, 60mL]	***Adults:*** (Cre, Oint) Apply bid-tid. May use occlusive dressings for psoriasis or recalcitrant conditions. D/C dressings if infection develops. (Sol) Apply bid-tid. ***Pediatrics:*** (Cre, Oint): Use least amount necessary for effective regimen. May use occlusive dressings for psoriasis or recalcitrant conditions. D/C dressings if infection develops. (Sol) Use least amount necessary for effective regimen.	**W/P:** May produce reversible HPA axis suppression, manifestations of Cushing's syndrome, hyperglycemia, and glucosuria. D/C if irritation occurs. Use appropriate antifungal or antibacterial agent with dermatological infections. Peds may be more susceptible to systemic toxicity. Caution when applied to large surface areas. Avoid contact with eyes. Limit to least amount compatible with an effective therapeutic regimen. Chronic corticosteroid therapy may interfere with the growth and development of children. **P/N:** Category C, caution in nursing.	Burning, itching, irritation, dryness, folliculitis, hypertrichosis, acneiform eruptions, hypopigmentation, **perioral dermatitis**, allergic dermatitis, skin maceration, secondary infection, skin atrophy, striae, miliaria.

Table 5.1. PRESCRIBING INFORMATION FOR GLUCOCORTICOIDS *(cont.)*

NAME	FORM/ STRENGTH	DOSAGE	WARNINGS/PRECAUTIONS & CONTRAINDICATIONS	ADVERSE EFFECTS†
TOPICAL CORTICOSTEROIDS (MEDIUM POTENCY) *(cont.)*				
Hydrocortisone Probutate (Pandel)	**Cre:** 0.1% [15g, 45g, 80g]	***Adults:*** Apply qd-bid depending on severity of condition. May use occlusive dressing for refractory lesions of psoriasis and other deep-seated dermatoses.	**W/P:** May produce reversible HPA axis suppression, manifestations of Cushing's syndrome, hyperglycemia, and glucosuria. D/C if irritation occurs. Use appropriate antifungal or antibacterial agent with dermatological infections. Pediatrics may be more susceptible to systemic toxicity. Caution when applied to large surface areas. Avoid eyes. **P/N:** Category C, caution in nursing.	Burning, stinging, moderate paresthesia, itching, dryness, folliculitis, hypertrichosis, acneiform eruptions, hypopigmentation, **perioral dermatitis**, skin atrophy, secondary infections, striae, millaria.
Hydrocortisone Valerate (Westcort)	**Cre, Oint:** 0.2% [15g, 45g, 60g]	***Adults/Pediatrics:*** Apply bid-tid.	**W/P:** May produce reversible HPA axis suppression, manifestations of Cushing's syndrome, hyperglycemia, and glucosuria. Caution when applied to large surface areas or under occlusive dressings. Use appropriate antifungal or antibacterial agent with dermatological infections; d/c if infection does not clear. Pediatrics may be more susceptible to systemic toxicity. Avoid eyes. D/C if irritation occurs. **P/N:** Category C, caution in nursing.	Burning, itching, dryness, irritation, folliculitis, hypertrichosis, acneiform eruptions, hypopigmentation, allergic contact dermatitis, skin maceration, secondary infection, skin atrophy, striae, miliaria.
Mometasone Furoate (Elocon)	**Cre, Oint:** 0.1% [15g, 45g]; **Lot:** 0.1% [30mL, 60mL]	***Adults:*** (Cre, Oint) Apply qd. (Lot) Apply a few drops qd. Re-assess if no improvement within 2 weeks. ***Pediatrics:*** **≥2 yrs:** (Cre, Oint) Apply qd for up to 3 weeks max. Avoid in diaper area. Re-assess if no improvement within 2 weeks. **≥12 yrs:** (Lot) Apply a few drops qd. Re-assess if no improvement within 2 weeks.	**W/P:** May produce reversible HPA axis suppression, manifestations of Cushing's syndrome, hyperglycemia, and glucosuria. D/C if irritation occurs. Use appropriate antifungal or antibacterial agent with dermatological infections. Pediatrics may be more susceptible to systemic toxicity. Caution when applied to large surface areas or with occlusive dressings. **P/N:** Category C, caution in nursing.	Burning, pruritus, skin atrophy, rosacea, acneiform reaction, tingling, stinging, furunculosis, folliculitis.
Prednicarbate (Dermatop)	**Cre, Oint:** 0.1% [15g, 60g]	***Adults:*** (Cre, Oint) Apply bid. ***Pediatrics:*** **≥1 yr:** (Cre) Apply bid. **Max:** 3 weeks of therapy. **≥10 yrs:** (Oint) Apply bid.	**W/P:** May produce reversible HPA axis suppression, manifestations of Cushing's syndrome, hyperglycemia, and glucosuria. D/C if irritation occurs. Use appropriate antifungal or antibacterial agent with dermatological infections. Pediatrics may be more susceptible to systemic toxicity. Re-evaluate if no improvement after 2 weeks. Avoid eyes, occlusive dressings. Not for treatment of diaper dermatitis. **P/N:** Category C, caution in nursing.	Stinging, burning, dry skin, pruritus, urticaria, allergic contact dermatitis, edema, paresthesia, rash, skin atrophy.
Triamcinolone Acetonide	**Cre:** 0.025%, 0.1% [15g, 80g], 0.5% [15g]; **Lot:** 0.025%, 0.1% [60mL]; **Oint:** 0.025% [80g],0.1% [15g, 80g]; **Spray:** (Kenalog) 0.147mg/g [63g]	***Adults:*** (Cre, Lot, Oint) Apply 0.025% bid-qid. Apply 0.1% or 0.5% bid-tid. (Spray) Apply tid-qid. May use occlusive dressings for psoriasis or recalcitrant conditions. D/C dressings if infection develops.	**W/P:** May produce reversible HPA axis suppression, manifestations of Cushing's syndrome, hyperglycemia, and glucosuria. D/C if irritation occurs. Pediatrics may be more susceptible to systemic toxicity. Monitor for HPA suppression if applied to large surface areas or under occlusive dressings. Avoid eyes. **P/N:** Category C, caution in nursing.	Burning, itching, irritation, dryness, folliculitis, hypertrichosis, acneiform eruptions, hypopigmentation, **perioral dermatitis**, allergic contact dermatitis.

†Bold entries denote special dental considerations.
BB = black box warning; **W/P** = warnings/precautions; **Contra** = contraindications; **P/N** = pregnancy category rating and nursing considerations.

NAME	FORM/ STRENGTH	DOSAGE	WARNINGS/PRECAUTIONS & CONTRAINDICATIONS	ADVERSE EFFECTS†
TOPICAL CORTICOSTEROIDS (HIGH POTENCY)				
Amcinonide	**Cre:** 0.1% [15g, 30g, 60g]; **Oint:** 0.1% [60g] **Lot:** 0.1% [60mL]	***Adults:*** Apply bid-tid depending on severity. ***Pediatrics:*** Use least amount necessary for effective regimen.	**W/P:** Systemic absorption may produce reversible HPA axis suppression, manifestations of Cushing's syndrome, hyperglycemia, and glucosuria. D/C if irritation occurs. Use appropriate antifungal or antibacterial agent with dermatological infections. Pediatrics may be more susceptible to systemic toxicity. Caution when applied to large surface areas or with occlusive dressings. **P/N:** Category C, not for use in nursing.	Itching, stinging, soreness, burning, irritation, folliculitis, hypertrichosis, hypopigmentation, **perioral dermatitis**, skin maceration, striae, miliaria, skin atrophy, secondary infection, contact dermatitis.
Betamethasone (augmented) Dipropionate (Diprolene, Diprolene AF)	**Cre (AF), Oint:** 0.05% [15g, 50g]; **Lot:** 0.05% [30mL, 60mL]	***Adults:*** (Lot) Apply qd-bid for no more than 2 weeks. **Max:** 50mL/week. (Cre, Oint) Apply qd-bid. **Max:** (Cre) 50g/week, (Oint) 50g/week. ***Pediatrics:*** (Cre) Apply qd-bid for no more than 2 weeks. Limit to 50g/week. **≥13 yrs:** (Lot) Apply qd-bid for no more than 2 weeks. Limit to 50mL/week. (Oint) Apply qd-bid, up to 50g/week.	**W/P:** May produce reversible HPA axis suppression, manifestations of Cushing's syndrome, hyperglycemia, and glucosuria. D/C if irritation occurs. Use appropriate antifungal or antibacterial agent with dermatological infections. Pediatrics may be more susceptible to systemic toxicity. Caution when applied to large surface areas. Not for use with occlusive dressings. Gel is not for use in rosacea, perioral dermatitis, on the face, on the groin, or in the axillae. **P/N:** Category C, caution in nursing.	Stinging, burning, dry skin, pruritus, folliculitis, acneiform papules, irritation, hypopigmentation, skin maceration, secondary infection, skin atrophy, striae, miliaria.
Betamethasone Dipropionate	**Cre, Oint:** 0.05% [15g, 45g]; **Lot:** 0.05% [60mL]	***Adults:*** (Cre, Oint) Apply qd-bid. (Lot) Apply a few drops bid, am and pm. ***Pediatrics:*** Use least amount necessary for effective regimen.	**W/P:** May produce reversible HPA axis suppression, manifestations of Cushing's syndrome, hyperglycemia, and glucosuria. Avoid occlusive dressings. Pediatrics are more prone to systemic toxicity. D/C if irritation occurs. Avoid eyes. **P/N:** Category C, caution in nursing.	Burning, itching, irritation, dryness, folliculitis, hypertrichosis, acneiform eruptions, hypopigmentation, **perioral dermatitis**, allergic contact dermatitis, skin maceration, secondary infection, skin atrophy, striae, miliaria.
Desoximetasone (Topicort, Topicort LP)	**Cre:** (LP) 0.05% [15g, 60g], 0.25% [15g, 60g, 100g]; **Gel:** 0.05% [15g, 60g]; **Oint:** 0.25% [15g, 60g]	***Adults:*** Apply bid. ***Pediatrics:*** (Cre, Gel) Use least amount necessary for effective regimen. **≥10 yrs:** (Oint) Use least amount necessary for effective regimen.	**W/P:** May produce reversible HPA axis suppression, manifestations of Cushing's syndrome, hyperglycemia, and glucosuria. Caution when applied to large surface areas or under occlusive dressings. Use appropriate antifungal or antibacterial agent with dermatological infections; d/c if infection does not clear or if irritation occurs. Peds may be more susceptible to systemic toxicity. Avoid eyes. **P/N:** Category C, caution in nursing.	Burning, itching, irritation, dryness, folliculitis, hypertrichosis, acneiform eruptions, hypopigmentation, **perioral dermatitis**, allergic contact dermatitis, skin maceration, secondary infection, skin atrophy, striae, miliaria.
Fluocinonide (Fluocinonide, Fluocinonide-E, Lidex, Lidex-E)	**Cre, Gel, Oint (Fluocinonide):** 0.05% [15g, 30g, 60g]; **Sol:** 0.05% [60mL]; **Cre (Fluocinonide-E):** 0.05% [15g, 30g, 60g]	***Adults:*** Apply bid-qid. ***Pediatrics:*** Use least amount necessary for effective regimen. May use occlusive dressing for psoriasis or recalcitrant conditions; d/c dressings if infection develops.	**W/P:** May produce reversible HPA axis suppression, manifestations of Cushing's syndrome, hyperglycemia, and glucosuria. Caution when applied to large surface areas or under occlusive dressings. Use appropriate antifungal or antibacterial agent with dermatological infections; d/c if infection does not clear. Pediatrics may be more susceptible to systemic toxicity. Avoid eyes. D/C if irritation occurs. **P/N:** Category C, caution in nursing.	Burning, itching, irritation, dryness, folliculitis, hypertrichosis, acneiform eruptions, hypopigmentation, **perioral dermatitis**, allergic contact dermatitis, skin maceration, secondary infection, skin atrophy, striae, miliaria.

Table 5.1. PRESCRIBING INFORMATION FOR GLUCOCORTICOIDS *(cont.)*

NAME	FORM/ STRENGTH	DOSAGE	WARNINGS/PRECAUTIONS & CONTRAINDICATIONS	ADVERSE EFFECTS†
TOPICAL CORTICOSTEROIDS (HIGH POTENCY) *(cont.)*				
Fluocinonide (Vanos)	**Cre:** 0.1% [30g, 60g]	***Adults/Pediatrics:*** **≥12 yrs:** Apply thin layer to affected area qd-bid no more than two weeks. **Max:** 60g/week.	**W/P:** May produce reversible HPA axis suppression, manifestations of Cushing's syndrome, hyperglycemia, and glucosuria. Caution when applied to large surface areas or under occlusive dressings. Use appropriate antifungal or antibacterial agent with dermatological infections. D/C if infection does not clear or irritation develops. Do not use for more than 2 weeks at a time. **P/N:** Category C, not for use in nursing.	Headache, application site burning, **nasopharyngitis**, nasal congestion, unspecified application site reaction.
TOPICAL CORTICOSTEROIDS (VERY HIGH POTENCY)				
Clobetasol Propionate (Clobevate)	**Gel:** 0.05% [45g]	***Adults/Pediatrics:*** **≥12 yrs:** Apply thin layer bid. Limit treatment to 2 consecutive weeks. **Max:** 50g/week. Avoid with occlusive dressings.	**W/P:** May produce reversible HPA axis suppression, manifestations of Cushing's syndrome, hyperglycemia, and glucosuria. Pediatrics may be more susceptible to systemic toxicity. D/C if irritation occurs. Use appropriate antifungal or antibacterial with concomitant skin infections; d/c if infection does not clear. Should not be used to treat rosacea or perioral dermatitis. Avoid use on face, groin, or axillae. **P/N:** Category C, caution in nursing.	Burning, stinging, irritation, pruritus, erythema, folliculitis, cracking and fissuring of the skin, numbness of fingers, skin atrophy, telangiectasia.
Clobetasol Propionate (Clobex)	**Lot:** 0.05% [30mL, 59mL]; **Shampoo:** 0.05% [118mL]; **Spray:** 0.05% [2oz, 4.25oz]	***Adults:*** **≥18 yrs:** (Lot) Apply bid for up to 2 consecutive weeks for no more than 2 weeks. **Psoriasis:** May repeat for additional 2 weeks. **Max:** 50g/week or 50mL/week. (Shampoo) Apply thin film daily to dry scalp for up to 4 consecutive weeks. Leave in place for 15 mins before lathering and rinsing. (Spray) Spray on affected area(s) bid. Rub in gently and completely. Reassess after 2 weeks; may repeat for additional 2 weeks. Limit treatment to 4 weeks. **Max:** 50g/week.	**W/P:** Not for use on the face, groin, axillae, eyes, lips, or for the treatment of rosacea or perioral dermatitis. May produce reversible HPA axis suppression, manifestations of Cushing's syndrome, hyperglycemia, and glucosuria. D/C if irritation occurs. Use appropriate antifungal or antibacterial agent with dermatological infections. Use in patients under 18 years of age is not recommended. **P/N:** Category C, caution in nursing.	Burning/stinging, pruritus, folliculitis, skin dryness, skin atrophy, telangiectasia.
Clobetasol Propionate (Cormax, Cormax Scalp)	**Cre:** 0.05% [15g, 30g, 45g]; **Oint:** 0.05% [15g, 45g]; **Sol (Scalp):** 0.05% [25mL, 50mL]	***Adults/Pediatrics:*** **≥12 yrs:** (Cre, Oint, Sol) Apply bid, am and pm. Limit treatment to 2 consecutive weeks. **Max:** 50g/week or 50mL/week.	**W/P:** Not for treatment of rosacea or perioral dermatitis. May produce reversible HPA axis suppression, manifestations of Cushing's syndrome, hyperglycemia, and glucosuria. Reassess diagnosis if no improvement after 2 weeks. D/C if irritation occurs. Pediatrics may be more susceptible to systemic toxicity. Use appropriate antifungal or antibacterial agent with dermatological infections. Avoid occlusive dressings. **Contra:** Primary infections of the scalp with solution. **P/N:** Category C, caution in nursing.	Burning, stinging, pruritus, skin atrophy, cracking/fissuring of skin, irritation, tingling (Sol), folliculitis (Sol).
Clobetasol Propionate (Olux)	**Foam:** 0.05% [50g, 100g]	***Adults/Pediatrics:*** **≥12 yrs:** Apply to affected area bid (am and pm). No more than 1.5 capfuls/application. Limit to 2 consecutive weeks. Avoid with occlusive dressings. **Max:** 50g/week.	**W/P:** May produce reversible HPA axis suppression, manifestations of Cushing's syndrome, hyperglycemia, and glucosuria. Caution when applied to large surface areas or under occlusive dressings. Use appropriate antifungal or antibacterial agent with dermatological infections; d/c if infection does not clear. Pediatrics may be more susceptible to systemic toxicity. Avoid eyes. D/C if irritation occurs. **P/N:** Category C, caution in nursing.	Burning/stinging, pruritus, irritation, erythema, folliculitis, cracking/fissuring of skin, numbness of fingers, telangiectasia, skin atrophy.

†Bold entries denote special dental considerations.
BB = black box warning; **W/P** = warnings/precautions; **Contra** = contraindications; **P/N** = pregnancy category rating and nursing considerations.

NAME	FORM/ STRENGTH	DOSAGE	WARNINGS/PRECAUTIONS & CONTRAINDICATIONS	ADVERSE EFFECTS†
Clobetasol Propionate (Olux-E)	**Foam:** 0.05% [50g,100g]	***Adults/Pediatrics:*** **≥12 yrs:** Apply thin layer to affected area bid (am and pm). No more than the size of a golf ball. Limit to 2 consecutive weeks. Avoid with occlusive dressings. **Max:** 50g/week.	**W/P:** May produce reversible HPA axis suppression, manifestations of Cushing's syndrome, hyperglycemia, and glucosuria. Caution when applied to large surface area or under occlusive dressings. Use appropriate antifungal or antibacterial agent with dermatological infections; d/c if infection does not clear. Pediatrics may be more susceptible to systemic toxicity. D/C if irritation occurs. Should not be used to treat rosacea or perioral dermatitis. Avoid use on face, groin, axillae, or other intertriginous areas. **P/N:** Category C, caution in nursing.	Folliculitis, acneiform eruptions, hypopigmentation, **perioral dermatitis**, allergic contact dermatitis, secondary infection, irritation, striae, miliaria.
Clobetasol Propionate (Temovate, Temovate Scalp, Temovate-E)	**(Temovate) Cre, Oint:** 0.05% [15g, 30g, 45g, 60g]; **Gel:** 0.05% [15g, 30g, 60g]; **Sol:** 0.05% [25mL]; **(Temovate-E) Cre:** 0.05% [15g, 30g, 60g]; **(Temovate Scalp) Sol:** 0.05% [25mL, 50mL]	***Adults/Pediatrics:*** **≥12 yrs:** Apply bid. **Max:** 50g/week or 50mL/week. **Moderate-Severe Psoriasis:** (Temovate-E) Apply bid for up to 4 weeks. May use on 5-10% of BSA. **Max:** 50g/week. Limit treatment to 2 consecutive weeks. Avoid with occlusive dressings.	**W/P:** Not for use on face, groin, or axillae, or for treatment of rosacea or perioral dermatitis. May produce reversible HPA axis suppression, manifestations of Cushing's syndrome, hyperglycemia, and glucosuria. Use appropriate antifungal or antibacterial agent with dermatological infections; d/c if infection does not clear. Peds may be more susceptible to systemic toxicity. Avoid eyes. D/C if irritation occurs. **Contra: (Scalp Sol)** Primary scalp infections. **P/N:** Category C, caution in nursing.	Burning, stinging, pruritus, skin atrophy, cracking/fissuring of the skin, erythema, folliculitis, numbness of fingers, telangiectasia, tingling (Sol), folliculitis (Sol).
Diflorasone Diacetate	**Cre, Oint:** 0.05% [15g, 30g, 60g]	***Adults:*** (Cre) Apply bid. (Oint) Apply qd-tid depending on the severity of the condition.	**W/P:** May produce reversible HPA axis suppression, manifestations of Cushing's syndrome, hyperglycemia, and glucosuria. Caution when applied to large surface areas or under occlusive dressings. Use appropriate antifungal or antibacterial agent with dermatological infections; d/c if infection does not clear. Pediatrics may be more susceptible to systemic toxicity. Avoid eyes. D/C if irritation occurs. Avoid occlusive dressings.Cream has an increased risk of producing adrenal suppression than ointment. Cream should not be used in the treatment of rosacea or perioral dermatitis; avoid face, groin, or axillae. **P/N:** Category C, caution in nursing.	Burning, itching, irritation, dryness, folliculitis, hypertrichosis, acneiform eruptions, hypopigmentation, **perioral dermatitis**, allergic contact dermatitis, skin maceration, secondary infection, skin atrophy, striae, miliaria.
Halobetasol Propionate (Ultravate)	**Cre, Oint:** 0.05% [15g, 50g]	***Adults/Pediatrics:*** **≥12 yrs:** Apply qd-bid. Rub in gently. Limit treatment to 2 weeks. **Max:** 50g/week.	**W/P:** Avoid face, groin, or axillae. Not for treatment of rosacea or perioral dermatitis. May produce reversible HPA axis suppression, manifestations of Cushing's syndrome, hyperglycemia, and glucosuria. Caution when applied to large surface areas. Avoid occlusive dressings. Use appropriate antifungal or antibacterial agent with dermatological infections; d/c if infection does not clear. Pediatrics may be more susceptible to systemic toxicity. Avoid eyes. D/C if irritation occurs. Re-assess if no improvement after 2 weeks. **P/N:** Category C, caution in nursing.	Stinging, burning, itching, irritation, dryness, folliculitis, hypertrichosis, acneiform eruptions, hypopigmentation, **perioral dermatitis**, allergic contact dermatitis, skin maceration, secondary infection, skin atrophy, striae, miliaria.

Table 5.2. DRUG INTERACTIONS FOR GLUCOCORTICOIDS

INHALED CORTICOSTEROIDS	
Beclomethasone Dipropionate (Qvar)	
Corticosteroids, systemic	Concomitant systemic corticosteroids (eg, prednisone) may increase the risk of hypercorticism and/or HPA axis suppression.
Budesonide (Pulmicort Flexhaler, Pulmicort Respules)	
Cimetidine	May decrease clearance and increase bioavailability of budesonide (respules).
Corticosteroids, systemic	Concomitant systemic corticosteroids (eg, prednisone) may increase the risk of hypercorticism and/or HPA axis suppression.
CYP3A4 inhibitors	CYP3A4 inhibitors (eg, azole antifungals, macrolide antibiotics) may increase plasma levels of budesonide.
Budesonide/Formoterol Fumarate Dihydrate (Symbicort)	
β-Blockers	Avoid or use with caution. May cause severe bronchospasm in asthmatics.
Corticosteroids, systemic	Concomitant systemic corticosteroids (eg, prednisone) may increase the risk of hypercorticism and/or HPA axis suppression.
CYP3A4 inhibitors	CYP3A4 inhibitors (eg, azole antifungals, macrolide antibiotics) may increase plasma levels of budesonide.
Diuretics	Caution with loop and thiazide diuretics; may potentiate ECG changes and/or hypokalemia.
MAOIs	Caution within 14 days of MAOI use; potentiation of vascular system effects.
TCAs	Caution within 14 days of TCA use; potentiation of vascular system effects.
Ciclesonide (Alvesco)	
Ketoconazole	Coadminister with caution; ketoconazole may increase levels of the pharmacologically active metabolite des-ciclesonide.
Flunisolide (Aerobid, Aerobid-M)	
Corticosteroids, systemic	Concomitant systemic corticosteroids (eg, prednisone) may increase the risk of hypercorticism and/or HPA axis suppression.
Fluticasone Propionate (Flovent Diskus, Flovent HFA)	
Corticosteroids, systemic	Concomitant systemic corticosteroids (eg, prednisone) may increase the risk of hypercorticism and/or HPA axis suppression.
CYP3A4 inhibitors	Caution with potent CYP3A4 inhibitors (eg, azole antifungals, macrolide antibiotics). Avoid use with ritonavir. May increase plasma levels of fluticasone and decrease serum cortisol.
Fluticasone Propionate/Salmeterol Xinafoate (Advair Diskus, Advair HFA)	
β-Blockers	Avoid or use with caution. May cause severe bronchospasm in asthmatics.
Corticosteroids, systemic	Concomitant systemic corticosteroids (eg, prednisone) may increase the risk of hypercorticism and/or HPA axis suppression.
CYP3A4 inhibitors	Avoid concomitant use with strong CYP3A4 inhibitors (eg, azole antifungals, macrolide antibiotics, ritonavir, saquinavir). May increase plasma levels of fluticasone and decrease serum cortisol. May increase plasma levels of salmeterol and increase cardiovascular adverse effects.
Diuretics	Caution with loop and thiazide diuretics; may potentiate ECG changes and/or hypokalemia.

Table 5.2. DRUG INTERACTIONS FOR GLUCOCORTICOIDS *(cont.)*

INHALED CORTICOSTEROIDS *(cont.)*

Fluticasone Propionate/Salmeterol Xinafoate (Advair Diskus, Advair HFA) *(cont.)*	
MAOIs	Caution within 14 days of MAOI use; potentiation of vascular system effects.
TCAs	Caution within 14 days of TCA use; potentiation of vascular system effects.
Mometasone Furoate (Asmanex)	
Corticosteroids, systemic	Concomitant systemic corticosteroids (eg, prednisone) may increase the risk of hypercorticism and/or HPA axis suppression.
CYP3A4 inhibitors	Strong CYP3A4 inhibitors (eg, azole antifungals, macrolide antibiotics) may increase plasma levels of mometasone.
Triamcinolone Acetonide (Azmacort)	
Corticosteroids, systemic	Concomitant systemic corticosteroids (eg, prednisone) may increase the risk of hypercorticism and/or HPA axis suppression.

INTRANASAL CORTICOSTEROIDS

Beclomethasone Dipropionate Monohydrate (Beconase AQ)	
Corticosteroids, systemic	Concomitant systemic corticosteroids (eg, prednisone) may increase the risk of hypercorticism and/or HPA axis suppression.
Budesonide (Rhinocort Aqua)	
Cimetidine	May decrease clearance and increase bioavailability of budesonide.
Corticosteroids, systemic	Concomitant systemic corticosteroids (eg, prednisone) may increase the risk of hypercorticism and/or HPA axis suppression.
CYP3A4 inhibitors	CYP3A4 inhibitors (eg, azole antifungals, macrolide antibiotics) may increase plasma levels of budesonide.
Ciclesonide (Omnaris)	
Ketoconazole	Coadminister with caution; ketoconazole may increase levels of the pharmacologically active metabolite des-ciclesonide.
Flunisolide (Nasarel)	
Corticosteroids, systemic	Concomitant systemic corticosteroids (eg, prednisone) may increase the risk of hypercorticism and/or HPA axis suppression.
Fluticasone Furoate (Veramyst)	
Corticosteroids, systemic	Concomitant systemic corticosteroids (eg, prednisone) may increase the risk of hypercorticism and/or HPA axis suppression.
CYP3A4 inhibitors	Caution with potent CYP3A4 inhibitors (eg, azole antifungals, macrolide antibiotics). Avoid use with ritonavir. May increase plasma levels of fluticasone and decrease serum cortisol.
Fluticasone Propionate (Flonase)	
Corticosteroids, systemic	Concomitant systemic corticosteroids (eg, prednisone) may increase the risk of hypercorticism and/or HPA axis suppression.
CYP3A4 inhibitors	Caution with potent CYP3A4 inhibitors (eg, azole antifungals, macrolide antibiotics). Avoid use with ritonavir. May increase plasma levels of fluticasone and decrease serum cortisol.

INTRANASAL CORTICOSTEROIDS *(cont.)*

Mometasone Furoate Monohydrate (Nasonex)	
Corticosteroids, systemic	Concomitant systemic corticosteroids (eg, prednisone) may increase the risk of hypercorticism and/or HPA axis suppression.
Triamcinolone Acetonide (Nasacort AQ)	
Corticosteroids, systemic	Concomitant systemic corticosteroids (eg, prednisone) may increase the risk of hypercorticism and/or HPA axis suppression.

SYSTEMIC CORTICOSTEROIDS (LOW-POTENCY)

Hydrocortisone (Cortef)	
Anticoagulants	Caution with anticoagulants; may increase or decrease anticoagulant effects. Monitor PT/INR.
ASA, high-dose	May increase clearance of chronic high-dose ASA; possible salicylate toxicity when corticosteroid withdrawn. Caution with concomitant use in hypoprothrombinemia.
CYP450 inducers	CYP450 inducers (eg, phenobarbital, phenytoin, rifampin) may increase clearance of hydrocortisone; may require increased corticosteroid dose.
CYP450 inhibitors	CYP450 inhibitors (eg, ketoconazole) may decrease clearance of hydrocortisone; titrate corticosteroid dose.
Diuretics	Increases risk of hypokalemia with K^+-depleting diuretics.
Hypoglycemic agents	May increase insulin and oral hypoglycemic requirements in diabetics.
Vaccines, killed or inactivated	May decrease response to killed or inactivated vaccines with immunosuppressive doses of corticosteroids.
Vaccines, live	Live vaccines contraindicated with immunosuppressive doses of corticosteroids.
Hydrocortisone Sodium Succinate (Solu-Cortef)	
Anticoagulants	Caution with anticoagulants; may increase or decrease anticoagulant effects. Monitor PT/INR.
ASA, high-dose	May increase clearance of chronic high-dose ASA; possible salicylate toxicity when corticosteroid withdrawn. Caution with concomitant use in hypoprothrombinemia.
CYP450 inducers	CYP450 inducers (eg, phenobarbital, phenytoin, rifampin) may increase clearance of hydrocortisone; may require increased corticosteroid dose.
CYP450 inhibitors	CYP450 inhibitors (eg, ketoconazole) may decrease clearance of hydrocortisone; titrate corticosteroid dose.
Diuretics	Increases risk of hypokalemia with K^+-depleting diuretics.
Hypoglycemic agents	May increase insulin and oral hypoglycemic requirements in diabetics.
Vaccines, killed or inactivated	May decrease response to killed or inactivated vaccines with immunosuppressive doses of corticosteroids.
Vaccines, live	Live vaccines contraindicated with immunosuppressive doses of corticosteroids.

Table 5.2. DRUG INTERACTIONS FOR GLUCOCORTICOIDS *(cont.)*

SYSTEMIC CORTICOSTEROIDS (INTERMEDIATE-POTENCY)	
Fludrocortisone Acetate	
Amphotericin B	Coadministration increases risk of hypokalemia.
Anabolic steroids	Increases tendency toward edema with concomitant anabolic steroids (eg, oxymetholone, methandrostenolone, norethandrolone)
Anticoagulants	Caution with anticoagulants; may increase or decrease anticoagulant effects. Monitor PT/INR.
ASA, high-dose	May increase clearance of chronic high-dose ASA; possible salicylate toxicity when corticosteroid withdrawn. Caution with concomitant use in hypoprothrombinemia.
CYP450 inducers	CYP450 inducers (eg, phenobarbital, phenytoin, rifampin) may increase clearance of fludrocortisone; may require increased corticosteroid dosage.
Digitalis glycosides	Increases risk of digitalis toxicity or arrhythmias due to hypokalemia.
Diuretics	Coadministration with K^+-depleting diuretics increases risk of hypokalemia.
Estrogens	Increases effect of fludrocortisone; may require reduction in corticosteroid dose.
Hypoglycemic agents	May increase insulin and oral hypoglycemic requirements in diabetics.
Vaccines, live	Avoid live virus vaccines and immunization procedures.
Methylprednisolone (Medrol)	
Anticoagulants	Caution with anticoagulants; may increase or decrease anticoagulant effects. Monitor PT/INR.
ASA, high-dose	May increase clearance of chronic high-dose ASA; possible salicylate toxicity when corticosteroid withdrawn. Caution with concomitant use in hypoprothrombinemia.
Cyclosporine	Mutual inhibition of metabolism with coadministration. Increases risk of drug specific adverse reactions, including convulsions.
CYP450 inducers	CYP450 inducers (eg, phenobarbital, phenytoin, rifampin) may increase clearance of methylprednisolone; may require increased corticosteroid dose.
CYP450 inhibitors	CYP450 inhibitors (eg, ketoconazole) may decrease clearance of methylprednisolone; titrate corticosteroid dose.
Hypoglycemic agents	May increase insulin and oral hypoglycemic requirements in diabetics.
Vaccines, killed or inactivated	May decrease response to killed or inactivated vaccines with immunosuppressive doses of corticosteroids.
Vaccines, live	Live vaccines contraindicated with immunosuppressive doses of corticosteroids.
Methylprednisolone Acetate (Depo-Medrol)	
Aminoglutethimide	May decrease corticosteroid-induced adrenal suppression.
Amphotericin B	Coadministration increases risk of hypokalemia.
Anticholinesterase agents	May produce severe weakness in myasthenia gravis patients on anticholinesterase agents.
Anticoagulants	Caution with anticoagulants; may increase or decrease anticoagulant effects. Monitor PT/INR.

SYSTEMIC CORTICOSTEROIDS (INTERMEDIATE-POTENCY) *(cont.)*

Methylprednisolone Acetate (Depo-Medrol) *(cont.)*	
ASA, high-dose	May increase clearance of chronic high-dose ASA; possible salicylate toxicity when corticosteroid withdrawn. Caution with concomitant use in hypoprothrombinemia.
Cholestyramine	Coadministration may increase clearance of corticosteroids.
Cyclosporine	Mutual inhibition of metabolism with coadministration. Increases risk of drug-specific adverse reactions, including convulsions.
CYP450 inducers	CYP450 inducers (eg, phenobarbital, phenytoin, rifampin) may increase clearance of methylprednisolone; may require increased corticosteroid dose.
CYP450 inhibitors	CYP450 inhibitors (eg, ketoconazole, macrolide antibiotics) may decrease clearance of methylprednisolone; titrate corticosteroid dose.
Digitalis glycosides	Increases risk of digitalis toxicity or arrhythmias due to hypokalemia.
Diuretics	Coadministration with K^+-depleting diuretics increases risk of hypokalemia.
Estrogens	Increase effect of methylprednisolone; may require reduction in corticosteroid dose.
Hypoglycemic agents	May increase insulin and oral hypoglycemic requirements in diabetics.
Isoniazid	Coadministration may increase concentration of isoniazid.
Vaccines, killed or inactivated	May decrease response to killed or inactivated vaccines with immunosuppressive doses of corticosteroids.
Vaccines, live	Live vaccines contraindicated with immunosuppressive doses of corticosteroids.
Methylprednisolone Sodium Succinate (Solu-Medrol)	
Anticoagulants	Caution with anticoagulants; may increase or decrease anticoagulant effects. Monitor PT/INR.
ASA, high-dose	May increase clearance of chronic high-dose ASA; possible salicylate toxicity when corticosteroid withdrawn. Caution with concomitant use in hypoprothrombinemia.
Cyclosporine	Mutual inhibition of metabolism with coadministration. Increases risk of drug-specific adverse reactions, including convulsions.
CYP450 inducers	CYP450 inducers (eg, phenobarbital, phenytoin, rifampin) may increase clearance of methylprednisolone; may require increased corticosteroid dose.
CYP450 inhibitors	CYP450 inhibitors (eg, ketoconazole) may decrease clearance of methylprednisolone; titrate corticosteroid dose.
Hypoglycemic agents	May increase insulin and oral hypoglycemic requirements in diabetics.
Vaccines, killed or inactivated	May decrease response to killed or inactivated vaccines with immunosuppressive doses of corticosteroids.
Vaccines, live	Live vaccines contraindicated with immunosuppressive doses of corticosteroids.
Prednisolone	
ASA, high-dose	May increase the clearance of chronic high-dose ASA; possible salicylate toxicity when corticosteroid withdrawn. Caution with concomitant use in hypoprothrombinemia.

Table 5.2. DRUG INTERACTIONS FOR GLUCOCORTICOIDS *(cont.)*

SYSTEMIC CORTICOSTEROIDS (INTERMEDIATE-POTENCY) *(cont.)*	
Prednisolone *(cont.)*	
Hypoglycemic agents	May increase insulin and oral hypoglycemic requirements in diabetics.
Vaccines	Avoid live virus vaccines and immunization procedures.
Prednisolone Sodium Phosphate (Orapred, Orapred ODT, Pediapred)	
Amphotericin B	Coadministration increases risk of hypokalemia.
Anticholinesterase agents	May produce severe weakness in myasthenia gravis patients on anticholinesterase agents.
Anticoagulants	Caution with anticoagulants; may increase or decrease anticoagulant effects. Monitor PT/INR.
ASA, high-dose	May increase clearance of chronic high-dose ASA; possible salicylate toxicity when corticosteroid withdrawn. Caution with concomitant use in hypoprothrombinemia.
Cyclosporine	Mutual inhibition of metabolism with coadministration. Increases risk of drug-specific adverse reactions, including convulsions.
CYP450 inducers	CYP450 inducers (eg, phenobarbital, phenytoin, rifampin) may increase clearance of prednisolone; may require increased corticosteroid dose.
CYP450 inhibitors	CYP450 inhibitors (eg, ketoconazole) may decrease clearance of prednisolone; titrate corticosteroid dose.
Digitalis glycosides	Increases risk of digitalis toxicity or arrhythmias due to hypokalemia.
Diuretics	Coadministration with K^+-depleting diuretics increases risk of hypokalemia.
Estrogens	Increase effect of prednisolone; may require reduction in corticosteroid dose.
Hypoglycemic agents	May increase insulin and oral hypoglycemic requirements in diabetics.
Neuromuscular blockers	May cause acute myopathy with neuromuscular blockers (eg, pancuronium).
Vaccines, killed or inactivated	May decrease response to killed or inactivated vaccines with immunosuppressive doses of corticosteroids.
Vaccines, live	Live vaccines contraindicated with immunosuppressive doses of corticosteroids.
Prednisone	
Anticoagulants	Caution with anticoagulants; may increase or decrease anticoagulant effects. Monitor PT/INR.
ASA, high-dose	May increase clearance of chronic high-dose ASA; possible salicylate toxicity when corticosteroid withdrawn. Caution with concomitant use in hypoprothrombinemia.
CYP450 inducers	CYP450 inducers (eg, phenobarbital, phenytoin, rifampin) may increase clearance of prednisone; may require increased corticosteroid dose
CYP450 inhibitors	CYP450 inhibitors (eg, ketoconazole) may decrease clearance of prednisone; titrate corticosteroid dose.
Hypoglycemic agents	May increase insulin and oral hypoglycemic requirements in diabetics.
Vaccines, killed or inactivated	May decrease response to killed or inactivated vaccines with immunosuppressive doses of corticosteroids.

SYSTEMIC CORTICOSTEROIDS (INTERMEDIATE-POTENCY) *(cont.)*

Prednisone *(cont.)*	
Vaccines, live	Live vaccines contraindicated with immunosuppressive doses of corticosteroids.

SYSTEMIC CORTICOSTEROIDS (HIGH-POTENCY)

Betamethasone (augmented) Sodium Phosphate/Betamethasone Acetate (Celestone Soluspan)	
Aminoglutethimide	Coadministration may lead to a loss of corticosteroid-induced adrenal suppression.
Amphotericin B	Coadministration increases risk of hypokalemia.
Anticholinesterase agents	May produce severe weakness in myasthenia gravis patients on anticholinesterase agents.
Anticoagulants	Caution with anticoagulants; may increase or decrease anticoagulant effects. Monitor PT/INR.
ASA, high-dose	May increase clearance of chronic high-dose ASA; possible salicylate toxicity when corticosteroid withdrawn. Caution with concomitant use in hypoprothrombinemia.
Cholestyramine	May increase the clearance of betamethasone.
Cyclosporine	Mutual inhibition of metabolism with coadministration. Increases risk of drug-specific adverse reactions, including convulsions.
CYP450 inducers	CYP450 inducers (eg, phenobarbital, phenytoin, rifampin) may increase clearance of betamethasone; may require increased corticosteroid dose.
CYP450 inhibitors	CYP450 inhibitors (eg, ketoconazole, macrolide antibiotics) may decrease clearance of betamethasone; titrate corticosteroid dose.
Digitalis glycosides	Increases risk of arrhythmias due to hypokalemia.
Diuretics	Coadministration with K^+-depleting diuretics increases risk of hypokalemia.
Estrogens	Increase effect of betamethasone; may require reduction in corticosteroid dose.
Hypoglycemic agents	May increase insulin and oral hypoglycemic requirements in diabetics.
Isoniazid	May decrease plasma levels of isoniazid.
Neuromuscular blockers	May cause acute myopathy with neuromuscular blockers (eg, pancuronium).
Vaccines, killed or inactivated	May decrease response to killed or inactivated vaccines with immunosuppressive doses of corticosteroids.
Vaccines, live	Live vaccines contraindicated with immunosuppressive doses of corticosteroids.
Betamethasone (Celestone)	
Aminoglutethimide	Coadministration may lead to a loss of corticosteroid-induced adrenal suppression.
Amphotericin B	Coadministration increases risk of hypokalemia.
Anticholinesterase agents	May produce severe weakness in myasthenia gravis patients on anticholinesterase agents.

Table 5.2. DRUG INTERACTIONS FOR GLUCOCORTICOIDS *(cont.)*

SYSTEMIC CORTICOSTEROIDS (HIGH-POTENCY) *(cont.)*	
Betamethasone (Celestone) *(cont.)*	
Anticoagulants	Caution with anticoagulants; may increase or decrease anticoagulant effects. Monitor PT/INR.
ASA, high-dose	May increase clearance of chronic high-dose ASA; possible salicylate toxicity when corticosteroid withdrawn. Caution with concomitant use in hypoprothrombinemia.
Cholestyramine	May increase the clearance of betamethasone.
Cyclosporine	Mutual inhibition of metabolism with coadministration. Increases risk of drug-specific adverse reactions, including convulsions.
CYP450 inducers	CYP450 inducers (eg, phenobarbital, phenytoin, rifampin) may increase clearance of betamethasone; may require increased corticosteroid dose.
CYP450 inhibitors	CYP450 inhibitors (eg, ketoconazole, macrolide antibiotics) may decrease clearance of betamethasone; titrate corticosteroid dose.
Digitalis glycosides	Increases risk of arrhythmias due to hypokalemia.
Diuretics	Coadministration with K^+-depleting diuretics increases risk of hypokalemia.
Estrogens	Increases effect of betamethasone; may require reduction in corticosteroid dose.
Hypoglycemic agents	May increase insulin and oral hypoglycemic requirements in diabetics.
Isoniazid	May decrease plasma levels of isoniazid.
Vaccines, killed or inactivated	May decrease response to killed or inactivated vaccines with immunosuppressive doses of corticosteroids.
Vaccines, live	Live vaccines contraindicated with immunosuppressive doses of corticosteroids.
Dexamethasone	
Aminoglutethimide	Coadministration may lead to a loss of corticosteroid-induced adrenal suppression.
Amphotericin B	Coadministration increases risk of hypokalemia.
Anticholinesterase agents	May produce severe weakness in myasthenia gravis patients on anticholinesterase agents.
Anticoagulants	Caution with anticoagulants; may increase or decrease anticoagulant effects. Monitor PT/INR.
ASA, high-dose	May increase clearance of chronic high-dose ASA; possible salicylate toxicity when corticosteroid withdrawn. Caution with concomitant use in hypoprothrombinemia.
Cholestyramine	May increase the clearance of dexamethasone.
Cyclosporine	Mutual inhibition of metabolism with coadministration. Increases risk of drug-specific adverse reactions, including convulsions.
CYP450 inducers	CYP450 inducers (eg, phenobarbital, phenytoin, rifampin) may increase clearance of dexamethasone; may require increased corticosteroid dose.

SYSTEMIC CORTICOSTEROIDS (HIGH-POTENCY) *(cont.)*

Dexamethasone *(cont.)*	
CYP450 inhibitors	CYP450 inhibitors (eg, ketoconazole, macrolide antibiotics) may decrease clearance of dexamethasone; titrate corticosteroid dose.
Digitalis glycosides	Increases risk of arrhythmias due to hypokalemia.
Diuretics	Coadministration with K^+-depleting diuretics increases risk of hypokalemia.
Ephedrine	Increases clearance of dexamethasone; may require increased dexamethasone dosage.
Estrogens	Increases effect of dexamethasone; may require reduction in corticosteroid dose.
Hypoglycemic agents	May increase insulin and oral hypoglycemic requirements in diabetics.
Isoniazid	May decrease plasma levels of isoniazid.
Phenytoin	Effects on phenytoin are variable; may result in alterations in seizure control.
Thalidomide	Caution with thalidomide; toxic epidermal necrolysis reported with coadministration.
Vaccines, killed or inactivated	May decrease response to killed or inactivated vaccines with immunosuppressive doses of corticosteroids.
Vaccines, live	Live vaccines contraindicated with immunosuppressive doses of corticosteroids.

Chapter 6

Antibiotics

Clay Walker, Ph.D.; Luciana M. Shaddox, D.D.S., Ph.D.

OVERVIEW

The term "antibiotic" initially was used to refer to any compound produced by a microorganism that inhibited another microorganism. Through common usage, this definition has evolved to include any natural, semisynthetic or, in some cases, totally man-made antimicrobial agent that inhibits bacterial growth. An antibiotic can be classified as either bactericidal or bacteriostatic. Bactericidal drugs, such as penicillins, directly kill an infecting organism; bacteriostatic drugs, such as tetracyclines and erythromycin, inhibit the proliferation of bacteria by interfering with an essential metabolic process, resulting in the elimination of bacteria by the host's immune defense system.

Antibiotics are used commonly in dentistry for both therapeutic and preventive measures involving oral bacterial infections. Oral infections can occur for a number of reasons and primarily involve pulpal and periodontal tissues. Secondary infections of the soft tissues pose special therapeutic challenges. Regardless of the oral infection being treated, monitoring the course of the infection with observation of the patient between 24 and 72 hours is recommended to ensure efficacy of the drug selected. Although culturing oral infections is not always possible or necessary, consideration of this procedure followed by antibiotic sensitivity testing should be included in the treatment of patients who do not respond to the antibiotic used initially.

Before undertaking the therapeutic use of any antibiotic, the clinician should determine an established need for antibiotic therapy; take a careful history to determine if the patient has experienced any previous adverse reactions or developed a sensitivity to a specific antibiotic; determine which antibiotic is or is most likely to be effective against specific organism(s); and ensure that he or she has a thorough knowledge of the side effects and drug interactions.

Penicillin is still the drug of choice for treatment of infections in and around the oral cavity. In patients allergic to penicillin, erythromycin or clindamycin may be an appropriate alternative. Finally, if there is no response to penicillin V, then amoxicillin with clavulanic acid may be a good alternative in patients not allergic to penicillin, as the spectrum of sensitivity is altered. In general, there is no advantage in selecting a bactericidal rather than a bacteriostatic antibiotic for the treatment of healthy people. However, if the patient is immunocompromised, either by concurrent treatment (such as cancer chemotherapy or drugs associated with a bone-marrow transplant) or by a preexisting disease (such as HIV infection), a bactericidal antibiotic would be indicated.

Prophylactic Use of Antibiotics

Prophylactic use of antibiotics is recommended before performing invasive dental procedures on patients who are at risk of developing bacterial endocarditis (see **Appendix D**) and late prosthetic joint infections (those occurring six or more months after placement of the prosthesis). Injudicious use of antibiotics can have dire consequences, and the clinician must carefully consider, and discuss with the patient, the advantages and disadvantages of prescribing an antibiotic.

Antibiotics and Oral Contraceptives

With regard to possible drug interactions with antibiotics, and the common use of oral steroid contraceptives, it is important to recognize an American Dental Association report. Dental practitioners have been advised to discuss a possible reduction in efficacy of oral steroid contraceptives during antibiotic therapy with all women of childbearing age. Furthermore, these patients should be advised to use additional forms of contraception during short-term antibiotic use. The American Medical Association also concluded that women should be informed of the possible interaction, as an interaction could not be completely discounted and could not be predicted. It is the opinion of the ADA Council of Scientific Affairs that, considering the possible consequences of an unwanted pregnancy, when prescribing antibiotics to a patient using oral contraceptives, dentists should make sure to do the following:

- advise the patient of the potential risk that the antibiotic may reduce the effectiveness of the oral contraceptive
- recommend that the patient discuss with her physician the use of an additional nonhormonal means of contraception
- advise the patient to maintain compliance with oral contraceptives when concurrently using antibiotics

PENICILLINS AND CEPHALOSPORINS

Antibiotics belonging to these two classes are referred to as "β-lactam antibiotics" owing to the presence of the β-lactam ring common to all drugs in these classes. These drugs are considered bactericidal because they directly result in the death of bacteria by inhibiting specific bacterial enzymes required for the assembly of the bacterial cell wall. Many of the β-lactam antibiotics are rendered inactive by the bacterial production of β-lactamase, an enzyme that hydrolyzes the β-lactam ring and renders the antibiotic inactive. The bacterial production of β-lactamase is the primary reason that treatment with penicillins or cephalosporins can fail.

The cephalosporins and the closely related cephamycins normally are listed together as a single related group and are similar to the penicillins in structure and action. Although penicillins are usually superior for treating dental-related infections, the cephalosporins/cephamycins are included in this chapter because they are used frequently in medical practice and may be encountered in patients seeking dental treatment. Additionally, they may be indicated in the prevention of infections arising from bacteremias of an oral nidus, as in prophylaxis against late prosthetic joint infections.

Accepted Indications

Table 6.1 lists common indications for penicillins and cephalosporins.

General Dosing and Dosage Adjustments

These are the dosages more frequently recommended for the treatment of dental-related infections (see **Table 6.2**). Other semisynthetic penicillins (eg, piperacillin, ticarcillin) as well as most of the cephalosporins/cephamycins (eg, cefazolin, cefoxitin, cefotaxime, ceftazidime) are available only IM or IV owing to poor oral absorption and instability in the presence of gastric acids. These are generally reserved for the treatment of severe infections and diseases that require hospitalization (see **Table 6.2**).

Under normal circumstances, penicillins and cephalosporins are rapidly eliminated from the body primarily through the kidneys and, partly, in the bile and by other routes. In the case of patients with reduced renal function, dosages should be adjusted downward relative to creatinine clearance rates in consultation with the patient's physician. In patients undergoing peritoneal dialysis, an alternative antibiotic should be considered because most penicillins and cephalosporins are effectively removed from the bloodstream by hemodialysis.

Special Dental Considerations

Drug Interactions of Dental Interest

Table 6.3 lists possible interactions between penicillins and cephalosporins and other drugs.

Cross-Sensitivity

Before initiating therapy with any penicillin or cephalosporin, careful inquiry should be made concerning previous hypersensitivity reactions to any penicillin, cephalosporin, or other allergens. Serious and occasionally fatal hypersensitivity (anaphylactoid) reactions have been reported in patients receiving penicillin or cephalosporin therapy. These reactions are more apt to occur in people with a history of penicillin and/or cephalosporin hypersensitivity and/or a history of sensitivity to multiple allergens. Penicillins and cephalosporins should be used with caution in patients who have a history of significant allergies and/or asthma. Because of the similarity in the structure of the penicillins and cephalosporins, patients allergic to one class may manifest cross-reactivity to members of the other class. Cross-reactivity to cephalosporins may occur in as many as 20% of the patients who are allergic to penicillins. Patients with a history or suspected history of hypersensitivity to a penicillin or cephalosporin, if given any antibiotic in this class, should be observed for any difficulty in breathing or other sign of allergic reaction for a minimum of 1 hour before being released.

Special Patients

Pregnant and nursing women

Penicillins and cephalosporins are secreted in human breast milk, and caution should be exercised when a drug from either group is administered to nursing women, as it may lead to sensitization, diarrhea, and candidiasis. Clinical experience with the penicillins and cephalosporins during pregnancy has not shown any evidence of adverse effects on the fetus. However, there have been no adequate and well-controlled studies in pregnant women that show conclusively that harmful effects of these drugs on the fetus can be ruled out. Therefore, penicillins and cephalosporins should be used during pregnancy only if clearly needed.

Pharmacology

See **Table 6.4** for pharmacologic information on penicillins and cephalosporins.

Patient Advice

- In case of the development of any adverse effect (rash; nausea; vomiting; diarrhea; swelling of lips, tongue or face; fever and so forth), advise the patient to stop taking the medication and promptly inform the dentist.
- Encourage compliance with the full course of therapy despite improvement in clinical signs and symptoms of an infection.
- There have been reports of reduced oral contraceptive effectiveness in women taking ampicillin, amoxicillin, and penicillin, resulting in unplanned pregnancy. Although the association is weak, advise

patients of this information and encourage them to use an alternate or additional method of contraception while taking any of these penicillins.

MACROLIDES

The macrolide group of antibiotics contains approximately 40 compounds, but only a limited few have clinical use. Erythromycin has generally been the most effective and is widely used as an alternative to penicillins for the treatment and prevention of infections caused by gram-positive microorganisms. Clarithromycin, a semisynthetic macrolide antibiotic, is similar to erythromycin, but has a broader spectrum of activity. Both antibiotics have good activity against most gram-positive bacteria associated with the mouth. Unlike erythromycin, clarithromycin has relatively good activity against a number of gram-negative bacteria.

In recent years, a novel class of antibiotics called the azalides has surfaced. These new macrolide derivatives appear superior to erythromycin and clarithromycin in that they offer better pharmacokinetic properties, excellent tissue distribution, longer therapeutic half-life and activity against many gram-negative and gram-positive bacteria. Of the azalides, azithromycin has received extensive clinical use.

Azithromycin has been used extensively in the past few years as an adjunct to periodontal scaling and root planing in the treatment of both chronic and aggressive periodontitis. Although this is a broad-spectrum antibiotic, it has little effect against obligate anaerobes including those frequently associated with chronic periodontitis. Its use in the treatment of periodontitis should probably be limited to aggressive periodontitis where *Aggregatibacter actinomycetemcomitans* is likely to be involved. It exerts little or no effect against the obligate anaerobes associated with the "red" complex, eg, *P. gingivalis*, *T. forsythsis*, and *T. denticola*.

Accepted Indications

Table 6.1 lists common indications for macrolides.

General Dosing and Dosage Adjustments

See **Table 6.2** for general dosage and prescribing information. Erythromycin and azithromycin are principally eliminated from the body via the liver. Therefore, dosages and/or the dosage interval should be adjusted when these drugs are administered to a patient with impaired hepatic function. Clarithromycin is eliminated via the liver and kidney and may be administered without dosage adjustment in patients with hepatic impairment and normal renal function. However, in the presence of severe renal impairment with or without coexisting hepatic impairment, decreased dosage or prolonged dosage intervals may be appropriate. Hepatotoxicity has been associated rarely with all erythromycin salts, but more frequently with erythromycin estolate.

Special Dental Considerations

Drug Interactions of Dental Interest

Table 6.3 lists possible interactions between macrolides and other drugs.

Cross-Sensitivity

Erythromycin, azithromycin, or clarithromycin are contraindicated in patients with known hypersensitivity to any of the macrolide antibiotics.

Special Patients

Pregnant and nursing women

Clarithromycin should not be used in pregnant women except in clinical circumstances in which no alternative therapy is appropriate. If pregnancy occurs while taking the drug, the patient should be advised that clarithromycin has demonstrated teratogenicity in animals, but as of yet not in humans. Although no evidence of impaired fertility or harm to the fetus has been found with either erythromycin or azithromycin, these drugs should be used during pregnancy only if needed.

Erythromycin is secreted in human breast milk and should be used with caution in nursing mothers. As it is not known if azithromycin and clarithromycin are secreted in human breast milk, the same cautions should be applied to these drugs as well.

Pediatric, geriatric, and other special patients

The safety of clarithromycin and azithromycin has not been established for children <6 months.

Dosage adjustment does not appear to be necessary in elderly patients who have normal renal and hepatic function.

Pharmacology

See **Table 6.4** for pharmacologic information on macrolides.

TETRACYCLINES

The tetracyclines, which include tetracycline, doxycycline, and minocycline, all have essentially the same broad-spectrum of activity and are frequently indicated in the treatment of gram-positive and gram-negative bacterial infections of the head and neck as well as other regions of the body. They are considered to be bacteriostatic at normal dosages and inhibit bacterial protein synthesis in sensitive bacteria by binding to the 30S ribosomal subunits and preventing the addition of amino acids to the growing peptide chain. At high concentrations, the tetracyclines are bactericidal and may inhibit protein synthesis in mammalian cells. The advantage of using doxycycline or minocycline rather than tetracycline, is that the former two antibiotics are absorbed better after oral administration. This greater absorption results in higher serum levels and a lesser need for frequent dosing. Unfortunately, resistance to one tetracycline often indicates resistance to all tetracyclines.

Accepted Indications

Dental applications include the adjunctive treatment of refractory periodontitis and juvenile periodontitis, dental abscesses, soft tissue abscesses, and as an alternative when penicillins are contraindicated or when β-lactamase-producing microorganisms are involved. Due to bacterial resistance, the tetracyclines are not indicated in the treatment of streptococcal or staphylococcal infections unless the organisms have been shown to be susceptible.

Resistance to tetracycline hydrochloride has become so widespread that this drug is rarely used in clinical medicine. However, the drug still appears to be beneficial in the treatment of certain dental infections, including periodontitis that do not respond favorably to conventional periodontal therapy. See **Table 6.1** for indications.

Subantimicrobial-Dose Doxycycline

The U.S. Food and Drug Administration has approved the use of a subantimicrobial dose of doxycycline hyclate (20 mg bid, available generically and as the brand Periostat) as an adjunct to periodontal therapy. Although this drug is classified as an antibiotic, it does not act as one because of its low dose. The major mechanism of action of this drug is the suppression of collagenase, particularly that which is produced by polymorphonuclear leukocytes. As the dose is too low to affect bacteria, resistance to this medication does not seem to develop. The therapeutic objective is to modulate the inflammatory host response, not necessarily kill bacteria. Since a subantimicrobial dose of doxycycline hyclate has no antibacterial properties, it is important that it be used as an adjunct to mechanical therapy. Note: A nonantibacterial dose of doxycycline hyclate is available in a slow-release tablet (Oracea, 40 mg qd) for treating rosacea.

Treatment with a subantimicrobial dose of doxycycline hyclate, 20 mg q12h, in conjunction with either dental debridement or scaling and root planing, significantly and consistently improved clinical signs of periodontal disease in clinical trials. A subantimicrobial dose of doxycycline hyclate represents the application of the concept of host modulation to the treatment of periodontal disease.

Safety studies showed that use of a subantimicrobial dose of doxycycline hyclate twice daily was well-tolerated for up to 12 months, and that the rates and types of adverse events were not different than those associated with placebos. Furthermore, the dose demonstrated neither an antimicrobial effect on the periodontal microflora nor a shift in normal flora. Lastly, there was no evidence of the development of multiantibiotic resistance.

General Dosing and Dosage Adjustments

See **Table 6.2** for dosage and prescribing information.

Because tetracyclines have been shown to depress plasma prothrombin activity, patients receiving anticoagulant therapy may require downward adjustment of the anticoagulant dosage.

If renal impairment exists, the recommended doses for any tetracycline may lead to excessive systemic accumulation of the antibiotic and, possibly, liver toxicity. The antianabolic action of the tetracyclines may cause an increase in blood urea nitrogen. In patients with significant renal insufficiency, this may lead to azotemia, hyperphosphatemia, and acidosis. Total dosages of any tetracycline should therefore be decreased in patients with renal impairment by reduction of recommended individual doses and/or by extending the time between doses.

Special Dental Considerations

Drug Interactions of Dental Interest

Table 6.3 lists possible interactions between tetracyclines and other drugs.

Special Patients

Pregnant and nursing women

All tetracyclines cross the placenta and form a stable calcium complex in bone-forming tissue. Consequently, use of tetracyclines is not recommended during the last half of pregnancy, as the drugs may cause permanent discoloration of teeth, enamel hypoplasia, and inhibition of skeletal growth in the fetus.

Although previous recommendations advised against prescribing tetracycline in nursing mothers, the latest statement of the American Academy of Pediatrics considers tetracycline safe in this patient population.

Pediatric, geriatric, and other special patients

Tetracycline drugs should not be used in children ≤8 years because these drugs may cause permanent discoloration of the teeth.

Concurrent, long-term use of tetracyclines with estrogen-containing oral contraceptives may result in reduced contraceptive reliability. Patients should be advised of this possibility and encouraged to use an alternative or additional method of contraception while taking any tetracycline.

Pharmacology

See **Table 6.4** for pharmacologic information on tetracylines.

LOCALLY DELIVERED ANTIBIOTICS

There is evidence that locally delivered, controlled-release antimicrobial agents—such as doxycycline hyclate gel (10%; Atridox) and minocycline HCl microspheres (1 mg; Arestin)—are effective in the treatment of periodontal pockets. The general benefit of locally delivered, controlled-release antibiotics is the achievement of high site concentrations of antibiotic with low systemic drug levels. Accordingly, one is able to reduce the putative pathogenic bacteria while minimizing the risk of adverse systemic side effects.

Accepted Indications

Clinical studies suggest that subgingival delivery of doxycycline hyclate 10% (Atridox) has a potential periodontal benefit. Doxycycline hyclate gel is injected into a periodontal pocket through a syringe system that is intended to deliver an antibacterial concentration for 7 to 14 days and is biodegradable. The effects of doxycycline hyclate on attachment-level gain and probing depth reduction have been shown to be equivalent to those of scaling and root planing alone and also, when used in combination with mechanical instrumentation, it shows better results than instrumentation alone.

In a recent multicenter study, the adjunctive effect of the local delivery of 10% doxycycline hyclate and subantimicrobial-dose doxycycline (20 mg bid) in combination with scaling and root planing was evaluated against scaling and root planing alone in a subject cohort with moderate to severe chronic periodontitis. The combined therapy was reported to yield significantly greater clinical benefits than scaling and root planing alone.

Clinical trials suggest that minocycline HCl 1 mg microspheres (Arestin) as an adjunct to scaling and root planing are more effective in reducing pocket depths than scaling and root planing alone. The minocycline HCl microsphere is a bioadhesive, biodegradable polymer in powder form that is injected into the periodontal pocket to maintain a therapeutic drug concentration for 10 to 14 days.

Reapplication of both of these drugs may be indicated at certain intervals.

Recently, there have been reports of the use of azithromycin at a 0.5% concentration in a bioabsorbable controlled-release gel. This preparation is reported to provide antimicrobial activity for up to 28 days. When used in combination with scaling and root planing, it enhanced both the clinical and microbiologic results relative to scaling and root planing alone. The data supporting its use as an adjunct in the treatment of chronic periodontitis are limited at this time.

A meta-analysis of various treatments for peri-implantitis, which included topical or local delivery of metronidazole, doxycycline, or chlorhexidine as an adjunct to subgingival debridement, failed to demonstrate any convincing clinical differences relative to subgingival debridement alone.

Adverse Effects and Precautions

The most common side effect of controlled-release antibiotic agents is localized erythema. There are also rare occurrences of localized candidiasis. The potential side effects of antibiotics described earlier should be kept in mind—such as development of resistant strains or increased growth of opportunistic organisms—when considering prescription of local controlled-release antibiotics for periodontal pocket delivery.

Patient Advice

- Until more evidence becomes available, it is prudent to advise patients receiving locally delivered antibiotics in the same manner as he or she would those taking the antibiotic in its oral form. Please refer to the section on Patient Advice for each antibiotic.

CLINDAMYCIN

Clindamycin is a semisynthetic derivative of lincomycin. Although not structurally related to erythromycin, it shares the same primary mode of action in that it binds to the 50S ribosomal subunits and inhibits bacterial protein synthesis in sensitive organisms (bacteriostatic). At higher concentrations, clindamycin can be bactericidal. Clindamycin is relatively active against gram-positive and gram-negative anaerobic bacteria, including most of those associated with the mouth. Essentially, all gram-negative aerobic bacteria are resistant.

Accepted Indications

Clindamycin is generally reserved for the treatment of serious infections of the respiratory tract, skin and soft tissue, female genital tract, intra-abdominal infections and abscesses, and septicemia involving gram-positive and/or gram-negative anaerobes, streptococci, staphylococci, and mixed infections involving anaerobes and facultative gram-positive bacteria.

However, clindamycin is indicated as a prophylactic antibiotic for dental patients at risk of developing bacterial endocarditis and who are allergic to penicillin and unable to take oral medications. Additionally, clindamycin is effective as adjunctive treatment of chronic and acute osteomyelitis caused by staphylococcus and is an alternative to penicillin V potassium and erythromycin for treatment of orofacial infections. See **Table 6.1**.

General Dosing and Dosage Adjustments

See **Table 6.2** for dosing and prescribing information. In patients with severe renal and/or hepatic impairment, clindamycin should be administered only for very severe infections, with the dosages and dosage intervals adjusted accordingly.

Special Dental Considerations

Drug Interactions of Dental Interest

Table 6.3 lists possible interactions between clindamycin and other drugs.

Cross-Sensitivity

There are no cross-sensitivities reported between clindamycin and any other antibiotic group. However, the 75- and 150-mg capsules of clindamycin HCl contain FD&C Yellow no. 5 (tartrazine), which may cause allergic reactions in some patients with hypersensitivity to aspirin.

Special Patients

Pregnant and nursing women

Clindamycin is secreted in breast milk in sufficient concentrations to cause disturbances of the intestinal flora of infants and should not be administered to nursing mothers unless warranted by clinical circumstances. Jaundice and abnormalities in liver function tests also may occur.

The safety of clindamycin for use during pregnancy has not been established.

Pediatric, geriatric, and other special patients

Clindamycin use should be carefully monitored in older patients who have an associated severe illness that may render them more susceptible to diarrhea.

The drug should be administered with caution to any patient with a history of gastrointestinal disease, particularly colitis, or to a patient with severe renal disease and/or severe hepatic disease.

Pharmacology

See **Table 6.4** for pharmacologic information on clindamycin.

METRONIDAZOLE

Metronidazole's primary use is in the bactericidal treatment of obligate anaerobic bacteria associated with the mouth, the intestinal tract, and the female genital tract.

As an adjunct to periodontal therapy, metronidazole and amoxicillin are often used in combination at dosages consisted of 250 mg of metronidazole and 250 mg to 500 mg of amoxicillin given concurrently at 8-hour intervals (tid) for a period of 7 to 10 days.

Note: The combined use of metronidazole with amoxicillin or amoxicillin/clavulanic acid has not been approved for this use.

Accepted Indications

Metronidazole is generally reserved for the treatment of serious infections of the lower respiratory tract, skin and soft tissue, female genital tract, intra-abdominal infections and abscesses, bones and joints, and bacterial septicemia involving obligate gram-positive anaerobic cocci, gram-negative anaerobic bacilli and *Clostridium* species.

The drug is indicated in the treatment of symptomatic and asymptomatic trichomoniasis in both females and males, amebic dysentery, antibiotic-associated colitis, and in pseudomembraneous colitis due to infection by *Clostridium difficile* (see **Table 6.1**).

Metronidazole has been used with considerable success as an adjunct to the treatment of periodontitis; this probably is related to its high activity against the gram-negative anaerobic bacilli that are often associated with the disease. The concurrent oral administration of metronidazole with amoxicillin has been used with considerable success in the treatment of both juvenile and adult forms of periodontitis and in the treatment of refractory periodontitis that has not responded favorably to other forms of periodontal therapy. It has been reported to be particularly effective in the treatment of *Actinobacillus actinomycetemcomitans*-associated periodontitis. Additionally, the use of metronidazole and penicillin V for severe mixed odontogenic infections has been a successful adjunct in clinically resolving these infections.

General Dosing and Dosage Adjustments

See **Table 6.2** for dosage and prescribing information. Patients with severe hepatic disease or impairment metabolize metronidazole slowly, with a resultant accumulation in the plasma. For such patients, the drug should be given with caution and the dosages adjusted downward from those normally given. However, for patients receiving renal dialysis, adjustment is not necessary because metronidazole is rapidly removed by dialysis.

In elderly patients, the pharmacokinetics of the drug may be altered and monitoring of serum levels may be necessary to adjust the dosage.

Special Dental Considerations

Drug Interactions of Dental Interest

Table 6.3 lists possible interactions between metronidazole and other drugs.

Cross-Sensitivity

Metronidazole is contraindicated in patients with a history of hypersensitivity to metronidazole or any other nitroimidazole derivative.

Special Patients

Pregnant and nursing women

Metronidazole should be used with caution in pregnant women. Animal reproduction studies have failed to demonstrate teratogenic effects on the fetus, and there are no adequate, well-controlled studies in pregnant women. Metronidazole is distributed in breast milk and has been shown in some animal studies to have a carcinogenic effect and possibly adverse effects in infants. Therefore, its use is not recommended in nursing mothers.

Pediatric, geriatric, and other special patients

As the pharmacokinetics of metronidazole may be altered in elderly patients, the drug should be given with caution and only when an alternative antibiotic is not available.

Drug serum levels should be watched in elderly patients as well as in patients with severe hepatic disease or impairment to avoid toxicity.

The safety and effectiveness of metronidazole has not been established in children except for the treatment of amebiasis.

Patients with Crohn's disease should not be treated with metronidazole, as the drug may potentiate the tendency for the formation of gastrointestinal and certain extraintestinal cancers.

Pharmacology

See **Table 6.4** for pharmacologic information on metronidazole.

QUINOLONES

The quinolones are a group 1,8-naphthyridine synthetic derivatives that are not chemically related to any other antibacterial agents. These drugs may be divided into the older quinolones, such as nalidixic acid, that have limited antibacterial activity, and the newer fluoroquinolones, which are characterized as having a broad spectrum of activity. Examples of the latter are ciprofloxacin and levofloxacin. Both of these have excellent activity against a wide range of gram-negative and gram-positive bacteria, including many that are resistant to third-generation cephalosporins, broad-spectrum semisynthetic penicillins, and the newer semisynthetic aminoglycosides. Most anaerobic bacteria, including those of the oral cavity, are resistant to these drugs. Due to their widespread usage in the treatment of upper respiratory tract and urinary tract infections as well as a host of other bacterial infections, it is very likely that some patients presenting for dental treatment may be taking one of these drugs. Fortunately, neither ciprofloxacin nor levofloxacin are reported to cross-react with most other classes of antibiotics.

Accepted Indications

Both ciprofloxacin and levofloxacin are indicated in the treatment of infections caused by aerobic or facultative gram-negative rods or by *Staphylococcus aureus* (including methacillin-resistant *S aureus*), *Staphylococcus epidermidis, Escherichia coli, Streptococcus pyogenes*, or *Enterococcus faecalis*, as well as other bacteria involving infections of the sinuses, the respiratory tract, the skin and skin structures, the bones and joints, and the urinary tract. Neither drug is indicated in the treatment of infections caused by obligate anaerobic bacteria. See **Table 6.1**.

General Dosing and Dosage Adjustments

See **Table 6.2** for dosing and prescribing information. In patients who have impaired renal clearance and are not undergoing renal dialysis, dosage intervals should be adjusted based on serum creatinine levels. For patients who are undergoing renal dialysis, dosages of 250 mg to 500 mg should be given either qd or should be based on serum creatinine levels.

For patients with changing renal function or for patients with both renal and hepatic insufficiency, adjusted dosages should be based on serum concentrations of ciprofloxacin.

Special Dental Considerations

Drug Interactions of Dental Interest

Table 6.3 lists possible interactions between quinolones and other drugs.

Cross-Sensitivity

A history of hypersensitivity to ciprofloxacin, levofloxacin, or to any other quinolone is a contraindication to its use.

Special Patients

Pregnant and nursing women

The safety and effectiveness of ciprofloxacin and levofloxacin in pregnant or lactating women has not been established. The drug should be used during pregnancy only if the potential benefit justifies the potential risk to the fetus.

Both drugs are excreted in human milk. Owing to the potential for serious adverse reactions in nursing infants, nursing should be discontinued if it is necessary to administer either ciprofloxacin or levofloxacin to the mother.

Pediatric, geriatric, and other special patients
Although ciprofloxacin is indicated for use in patients ≥1 year and levofloxacin is indicated in patients ≥6 months (for anthrax only), an increased incidence of adverse events compared to controls, including events related to joints and/or surrounding tissues, has been observed in pediatric patients.

Patient Monitoring: Aspects to Watch

Monitor serum creatinine levels in patients receiving ciprofloxacin who have severe renal impairment.

Owing to the potential for serious adverse reactions, monitor serum levels of theophylline closely if it is necessary to administer either drug to patients receiving theophylline.

Adverse Effects and Precautions

The most common side effects are nausea, diarrhea, vomiting, abdominal pain/discomfort, headache, restlessness, and rash (see **Table 6.2**). Each of these has been reported in 1% to 5% of patients receiving quinolones.

Pharmacology

See **Table 6.4** for pharmacologic information on quinolones (ciprofloxacin and levofloxacin).

SUGGESTED READING

American Academy of Pediatrics Committee on Drugs. The transfer of drugs and other chemicals into human milk. *Pediatrics*. 1994;93(1):137-150.

American Dental Association Council on Scientific Affairs. Antibiotic interference with oral contraceptives. *JADA*. 2002;133:880. Available at: http://www.ada.org/prof/resources/pubs/jada/reports/report_antibiotic.pdf.

American Medical Association Council on Scientific Affairs. Report 8 of the Council on Scientific Affairs (A-00): drug interactions between oral contraceptives and antibiotics. Available at: http://www.ama-assn.org/ama1/pub/upload/mm/443/csaa-00.pdf.

Consensus reports from the 1996 World Workshop in Periodontics. *JADA*. 1998;29(suppl):1S-69S.

Liu P, Muller M, Derendorf H. Rational dosing of antibiotics: the use of plasma concentrations versus tissue concentrations. *Int J Antimicrob Agents*. 2002;19(4):285-290.

Novak MJ, Dawson DR 3rd, Magnusson I, et al. Combining host modulation and topical antimicrobial therapy in the management of moderate to severe periodontitis: a randomized multicenter trial. *J Periodontol*. 2008;79:33-41.

Ramgoolam A, Steele R. Formulations of antibiotics for children in primary care: effects on compliance and efficacy. *Paediatr Drugs*. 2002;4(5):323-333.

United States Pharmacopeial Convention, Inc. *Drug Information for the Health Care Professional*. 18th ed. Rockville, Md.: United States Pharmacopeial Convention, Inc.; 1998.

Walker CB. Antimicrobial agents and chemotherapy. In: Slots J, Taubman M, eds. *Contemporary Oral Microbiology and Immunology*. St. Louis: Mosby; 1992:242-264.

Walker CB. Selected antimicrobial agents: Mechanisms of action, side effects, and drug interactions. In: Slots J, Rams T, eds. *Periodontology 2000*. Vol. 10: Systemic and topical antimicrobial therapy in periodontics. Copenhagen: Munksgaard; 1996:12-28.

Table 6.1. COMMON USES FOR ANTIBIOTICS

NAME	CHARACTERISTICS	COMMON INDICATIONS FOR USE
CLINDAMYCIN		
	Active against most gram-positive bacteria, including many staphylococcal and streptococcal species Excellent activity against both gram-positive and gram-negative anaerobic bacteria	Treatment of severe infections caused by anaerobic bacteria Adjunct to treatment of adult refractory periodontitis Adjunct to treatment of chronic and acute osteomyelitis caused by staphylococcus Alternative to penicillin and erythromycin for treating orofacial infections Alternative prophylactic antibiotic for dental patients allergic to penicillin and unable to take oral medication
MACROLIDES		
Azithromycin	Broad spectrum of activity for both gram-positive and gram-negative bacteria Given once daily	Indicated in the treatment of patients ≥ age 16 y who have mild-to-moderate infections Alternative prophylactic antibiotic for dental patients at risk of bacterial endocarditis and allergic to penicillin Alternative to penicillin G and other penicillins for treatment of gram-positive coccoid infections in patients with hypersensitivity to penicillins
Clarithromycin	Active against gram-positive and many gram-negative bacteria	Treatment of mild-to-moderate respiratory infections and uncomplicated skin infections Alternative prophylactic antibiotic for dental patients at risk of bacterial endocarditis and allergic to penicillin Alternative to penicillin G and other penicillins for treatment of gram-positive coccoid infections in patients with hypersensitivity to penicillins
Erythromycin Base	Active against gram-positive bacteria, particularly gram-positive cocci Provides only limited activity against gram-negative bacteria Yields irregular and unpredictable serum levels Given during a fasting state	Treatment of upper and lower respiratory tract, skin and soft tissue infections of mild-to-moderate severity Alternative to penicillin G and other penicillins for treatment of gram-positive coccoid infections in patients with hypersensitivity to penicillins
Erythromycin Ethylsuccinate	Activity same as for erythromycin base	Uses same as for erythromycin base
Erythromycin Stearate	Activity same as for erythromycin base Less subject to gastric acids than erythromycin base Yields more predictable serum levels	Uses same as for erythromycin base
METRONIDAZOLE		
	Antibacterial activity against all anaerobic cocci and both gram-negative bacilli and gram-positive spore-forming bacilli Nonsporulating gram-positive bacilli are often resistant, as are most facultative bacteria	Indicated in treatment of trichomoniasis, amebiasis, and giardiasis as well as a variety of infections caused by obligate anaerobic bacteria Indicated in treatment of obligate anaerobic bacterial infections associated with mouth, intestinal tract, and female genital tract Has been used as adjunct in treatment of periodontitis

Table 6.1. COMMON USES FOR ANTIBIOTICS *(cont.)*

NAME	CHARACTERISTICS	COMMON INDICATIONS FOR USE
PENICILLINS AND CEPHALOSPORINS		
Amoxicillin	Similar to ampicillin but yields higher serum levels More rapidly and completely absorbed from stomach than ampicillin Penetrates gingival crevicular fluid well but is hydrolyzed rapidly if significant levels of β-lactamases are present	Has same uses as ampicillin Designed specifically for oral administration Recommended as a prophylactic antibiotic to prevent bacterial endocarditis and late prosthetic joint infections following invasive dental procedures in at-risk patients
Amoxicillin/Clavulanic Acid	Has same properties as amoxicillin but is resistant to wide range of β-lactamases Penetrates gingival crevicular fluid well Resistant to most β-lactamases produced by oral bacteria	Broad-spectrum antibiotic with excellent activity against many β-lactamase-producing oral and nonoral bacteria Recommended as a prophylactic antibiotic to prevent late prosthetic joint infections following invasive dental procedures in at-risk patients
Ampicillin	Provides broad-spectrum activity against both gram-negative and gram-positive bacteria Stable to stomach acids and readily absorbed from the stomach Susceptible to β-lactamases	Broad-spectrum penicillin for use against a variety of bacteria that do not produce β-lactamase (for example, *Escherichia coli,* as well as *Neisseria, Haemophilus,* and *Proteus* species) For dental patients at risk for bacterial endocarditis and unable to take oral medication, the IM or IV route is recommended
QUINOLONES (CIPROFLOXACIN AND LEVOFLOXACIN)		
	Bactericidal Broad spectrum of activity against both gram-positive and gram-negative bacteria Inactive against most anaerobic bacteria	Indicated in treatment of infections of the lower respiratory tract, skin, bone and joints, and urinary tract, and for the treatment of infectious diarrhea As a single agent or in combination with metronidazole in the treatment of periodontitis associated with *Actinobacillus actinomycetemcomitans*
TETRACYCLINES		
Doxycycline Hyclate	Has the same characteristics as tetracycline except that it is absorbed more completely following oral administration and yields higher serum levels	Adjunctive treatment of adult periodontitis and juvenile periodontitis Treatment of acute necrotizing ulcerative gingivitis and dental abscesses Alternative to penicillins for treatment of actinomycosis and other oral infections
Minocycline Hydrochloride	Has the same characteristics as tetracycline except that it is absorbed more completely following oral administration and yields higher serum levels More lipophilic than doxycycline and provides better tissue penetration	Uses same as for doxycycline (above)
Tetracycline Hydrochloride	Broad-spectrum antibiotic with activity against gram-positive and gram-negative bacteria, mycoplasmas, rickettsial and chlamydial infections	Uses same as for doxycycline (above)

Table 6.2. PRESCRIBING INFORMATION FOR ANTIBIOTICS

NAME	FORM/ STRENGTH	DOSAGE	WARNINGS/PRECAUTIONS & CONTRAINDICATIONS	ADVERSE EFFECTS†
AMINOGLYCOSIDES				
Amikacin Sulfate	**Inj:** 50mg/mL, 250mg/mL	***Adults/Pediatrics:*** **IM/IV:** 15mg/kg/day given q8h or q12h. **Max:** 15mg/kg/day. **Heavier Wt Patients: Max:** 1.5g/day. **Recurrent Uncomplicated UTI:** 250mg bid. **Usual Duration:** 7-10 days. D/C therapy if no response after 3-5 days. D/C if azotemia increases or if progressive decrease in urinary output occurs. **Renal Impairment:** Reduce dose. ***Newborns:*** **LD:** 10mg/kg. **Maint:** 7.5mg/kg q12h.	**BB:** Potential for ototoxicity and nephrotoxicity. Neuromuscular blockade, respiratory blockade reported. Avoid prolonged peak levels >35mcg/mL. Monitor renal and eight cranial nerve function, urine, BUN, serum creatinine, and CrCl. Obtain serial audiograms. Avoid potent diuretics and other neurotoxic, nephrotoxic, and ototoxic drugs. **W/P:** May aggravate muscle weakness; caution with muscular disorders (eg, myasthenia gravis, parkinsonism). May cause fetal harm in pregnancy. Contains sodium metabisulfite, allergic reactions may occur especially in asthmatics. Maintain adequate hydration. Assess kidney function before therapy, then daily. **P/N:** Category D, not for use in nursing.	Ototoxicity, neuromuscular blockage, nephrotoxicity, skin rash, drug fever, headache, paresthesia, tremor, nausea, arthralgia, anemia, hypotension.
Gentamicin Sulfate	**Inj:** 10mg/mL, 40mg/mL	***Adults:*** **IM/IV: Serious Infections:** 3mg/kg/day given q8h. **Life-Threatening Infections:** 5mg/kg/day tid-qid; reduce to 3mg/kg/day as soon as clinically indicated. Treat for 7-10 days; may need longer course in difficult and complicated infections. **Renal Impairment:** Reduced dose given q8h or usual dose given at prolonged intervals based on either CrCl or SrCr. **Dialysis:** 1-1.7mg/kg, depending on severity of infection, at end of each dialysis period. **Obese Patients:** Calculate dose based on estimated lean body mass. ***Pediatrics:*** 6-7.5mg/kg/day (2-2.5mg/kg given q8h). **Infants and Neonates:** 7.5mg/kg/day (2.5mg/kg given q8h). **Premature and Full-Term Neonates ≤1 Week:** 5mg/kg/day (2.5mg/kg given q12h). Treat for 7-10 days; may need longer course in difficult and complicated infections. **Renal Impairment:** Reduced dose given q8h or usual dose given at prolonged intervals based on either CrCl or SrCr. **Dialysis:** 2mg/kg at end of each dialysis period. **Obese Patients:** Calculate dose based on estimated lean body mass.	**BB:** Potential nephrotoxicity, neurotoxicity, ototoxicity. Risk of toxicity is greater with impaired renal function, high dosage, or prolonged therapy. Monitor serum concentrations closely. Avoid prolonged peak levels >12mcg/mL and trough levels >2mcg/mL. Monitor renal and eight cranial nerve function, urine, BUN, serum creatinine, and CrCl. Obtain serial audiograms. Advanced age and dehydration increase risk of toxicity. Adjust dose or D/C use with evidence of ototoxicity or nephrotoxicity. May cause fetal harm during pregnancy. Avoid concurrent and/or sequential systemic or topical use of other potentially neurotoxic and/or nephrotoxic drugs such as cisplatin, cephaloridine, kanamycin, amikacin, neomycin, polymyxin B, colistin, paromomycin, streptomycin, tobramycin, vancomycin, and viomycin. Avoid concurrent use with potent diuretics such as ethacrynic acid or furosemide. **W/P:** Contains metabisulfite. Neuromuscular blockade, respiratory paralysis, ototoxicity, and nephrotoxicity may occur after local irrigation or topical application during surgical procedures. Caution with neuromuscular disorders (eg, myasthenia gravis, parkinsonism). Caution in elderly; monitor renal function. Keep patients well-hydrated during treatment. May cause fetal harm when administered to pregnant women. **P/N:** Category D, safety not known in nursing.	Nephrotoxicity, neurotoxicity, rash, fever, urticaria, N/V, headache, lethargy, confusion, depression, decreased appetite, weight loss, BP changes, blood dyscrasias, elevated LFTs.
Streptomycin Sulfate	**Inj:** 1g	***Adults:*** IM only. **TB:** 15mg/kg/day (**Max:** 1g), or 25-30mg/kg twice weekly (**Max:** 1.5g), or 25-30mg/kg three times weekly (**Max:** 1.5g). Do not exceed a total dose of 120g over the course of therapy unless no other therapeutic options exist. **Elderly (>60 yrs):** Reduce dose. Treat for minimum of 1 year if possible.	**BB:** Risk of severe neurotoxic reactions (eg, vestibular and cochlear disturbances) increased significantly with renal dysfunction or pre-renal azotemia. Optic nerve dysfunction, peripheral neuritis, arachnoiditis, and encephalopathy may occur. Monitor renal function; reduce dose with renal impairment and/or nitrogen retention. Do not exceed	Vestibular ototoxicity (N/V, vertigo), paresthesia of face, rash, fever, urticaria, angioneurotic edema, eosinophilia, nephrotoxicity (rare).

†Bold entries denote special dental considerations.
BB = black box warning; **W/P** = warnings/precautions; **Contra** = contraindications; **P/N** = pregnancy category rating and nursing considerations.
Note: See the Miscellaneous listing at the end of this table if a drug name does not appear under a particular therapeutic category.

Table 6.2. PRESCRIBING INFORMATION FOR ANTIBIOTICS *(cont.)*

NAME	FORM/ STRENGTH	DOSAGE	WARNINGS/PRECAUTIONS & CONTRAINDICATIONS	ADVERSE EFFECTS†
AMINOGLYCOSIDES *(cont.)*				
Streptomycin Sulfate *(cont.)*		**Tularemia:** 1-2g/day in divided doses for 7-14 days until afebrile for 5-7 days. **Plague:** 1g bid for minimum of 10 days. **Streptococcal Endocarditis:** With PCN, 1g bid for week 1, then 500mg bid for week 2. **Elderly (>60 yrs):** 500mg bid for 2 weeks. **Enterococcal Endocarditis:** With PCN, 1g bid for 2 weeks, then 500mg bid for 4 weeks. **Renal Impairment:** Reduce dose. **Moderate/Severe Infections:** 1-2g/day in divided doses q6-12h. **Max:** 2g/day. ***Pediatrics:*** IM only. **TB:** 20-40mg/kg/day (**Max:** 1g), or 25-30mg/kg twice weekly (**Max:** 1.5g), or 25-30mg/kg three times weekly (**Max:** 1.5g). Do not exceed a total dose of 120g over the course of therapy unless no other therapeutic options exist. Treat for minimum of 1 year if possible. **Moderate/Severe Infections:** 20-40mg/kg/day (8-20mg/lb/day) in divided doses q6-12h.	peak serum level of 20-25mcg/mL with kidney damage. Avoid other neurotoxic and/or nephrotoxic drugs (eg, neomycin, kanamycin, gentamicin, cephaloridine, paromomycin, viomycin, polymyxin B, colistin, tobramycin, cyclosporine). Respiratory paralysis can occur, especially if given soon after anesthesia or muscle relaxants. Reserve parenteral form when adequate lab and audiometric testing is available. **W/P:** Vestibular and auditory dysfunction may occur. Contains sodium metabisulfite. Can cause fetal harm in pregnancy. Caution with dose selection in renal impairment. Alkalinize urine to minimize or prevent renal irritation with prolonged therapy. CNS depression (eg, stupor, flaccidity) reported in infants with higher than recommended doses. If syphilis is suspected when treating venereal infections, perform dark field exam before initiate treatment, and monthly serologic tests for at least 4 months. Overgrowth of nonsusceptible organisms may occur. Terminate therapy when toxic symptoms appear, when impending toxicity is feared, when organisms become resistant, or when full treatment effect has been obtained. Contains sodium metabisulfite, a sulfite that may cause allergic-type reactions including anaphylaxis. **P/N:** Category D, not for use in nursing	
Tobramycin (TOBI)	**Sol:** 60mg/mL (300mg/amp)	***Adults/Pediatrics:* ≥6 yrs:** Inhale via nebulizer 300mg q12h for 28 days, then stop for 28 days. Resume therapy for next 28-day on/28-day off cycle.	**W/P:** Caution with muscular disorders (eg, myasthenia gravis, Parkinson's disease), and renal, auditory, vestibular, or neuromuscular dysfunction. May cause hearing loss, bronchospasm. Can cause fetal harm in pregnancy. D/C if nephrotoxicity occurs until serum level <2mcg/mL. **P/N:** Category D, not for use in nursing.	Voice alteration, **taste perversion**, tinnitus.
Tobramycin Sulfate	**Inj:** 10mg/mL, 40mg/mL, 1.2g	***Adults:* IM/IV: Serious Infections:** 3mg/kg/day given q8h. **Life-Threatening Infections:** Up to 5mg/kg/day given tid-qid. Reduce to 3mg/kg/day as soon as clinically indicated. **Max:** 5mg/kg/day unless serum levels monitored. Treat for 7-10 days; may need longer course in difficult and complicated infections. **Severe Cystic Fibrosis: Initial:** 10mg/kg/day given qid. Measure levels to determine subsequent doses. **Renal Impairment: LD:** 1mg/kg, followed by reduced doses given q8h or normal doses given at prolonged intervals based on either CrCl or SrCr. Do not use either method during dialysis. **Obese Patients:** Calculate dose based on estimated LBW plus 40% of excess as basic wt on which to figure mg/kg. ADD-Vantage vials not for IM use. ***Pediatrics:*** **>1 week: IM/IV:** 6-7.5mg/kg/day given tid-qid (eg, 2-2.5mg/kg q8h or	**BB:** Potential ototoxicity, nephrotoxicity, and neurotoxicity. Monitor peak and trough serum levels to avoid toxicity. Avoid prolonged serum levels >12mcg/mL. Rising trough levels (>2mcg/mL) may indicate tissue accumulation. Tissue accumulation, excessive peak levels, advanced age, and cumulative dose may contribute to ototoxicity and nephrotoxicity. Monitor urine, BUN, SrCr, and CrCl periodically. Obtain serial audiograms. D/C or adjust dose with renal, vestibular, or auditory dysfunction. Caution in premature and neonatal infants, advanced age, and dehydration. Avoid other neurotoxic or nephrotoxic agents, particularly other aminoglycosides, cephaloridine, viomycin, polymyxin B, colistin, cisplatin, and vancomycin. Avoid potent diuretics (eg, ethacrynic acid, furosemide). Risk of fetal harm during pregnancy.	Neurotoxicity (eg, dizziness, tinnitus, hearing loss, numbness, skin tingling, muscle twitching, convulsions), nephrotoxicity (eg, rising BUN/nonprotein nitrogen/serum creatinine, oliguria, cylindruria, increased proteinuria), blood dyscrasias, fever, rash, exfoliative dermatitis, urticaria, N/V, diarrhea, headache, lethargy, injection-site pain, confusion, disorientation, increased serum transaminases.

†Bold entries denote special dental considerations.
BB = black box warning; **W/P** = warnings/precautions; **Contra** = contraindications; **P/N** = pregnancy category rating and nursing considerations.

NAME	FORM/ STRENGTH	DOSAGE	WARNINGS/PRECAUTIONS & CONTRAINDICATIONS	ADVERSE EFFECTS†
Tobramycin Sulfate *(cont.)*		1.5-1.89mg/kg q6h). **≤1 week:** Up to 2mg/kg q12h. Treat for 7-10 days; may need longer course in difficult and complicated infections. **Severe Cystic Fibrosis: Initial:** 10mg/kg/day given qid. Measure levels to determine subsequent doses. **Renal Impairment: LD:** 1mg/kg, followed by reduced doses given q8h or normal doses given at prolonged intervals based on either CrCl or SrCr. Do not use either method during dialysis. **Obese Patients:** Calculate dose based on estimated LBW plus 40% of excess as basic wt on which to figure mg/kg. ADD-Vantage vials not for IM use.	**W/P:** Increased risk of ototoxicity, nephrotoxicity, and neurotoxicity if treatment >10 days. Contains sodium bisulfite. D/C if allergic reaction occurs. Monitor serum calcium, magnesium, and sodium. For peak levels, measure about 30 min after IV infusion or 1 hr after IM injection. For trough levels, measure at 8 hrs or just before next dose. Prolonged or secondary apnea may occur with massive transfusions of citrated blood. Caution with muscular disorders (eg, myasthenia gravis, parkinsonism). Increased risk of neurotoxicity and nephrotoxicity after absorption from body surfaces with local irrigation or application. Not for intraocular and/or subconjunctival use. Overgrowth of nonsusceptible organisms may occur. **P/N:** Category D, safety not known in nursing.	
CARBAPENEMS				
Doripenem (Doribax)	**Inj:** 500mg	***Adults:*** **≥18 yrs:** 500mg IV q8h for 5-14 days (intra-abdominal) or 10 days (UTI). Infuse over 1 hour. **Renal Impairment: CrCl: >50mL/min:** No dose adjustment. **CrCl 30-50mL/min:** 250mg IV q8h. **CrCl >10 to <30mL/min:** 250mg IV q12h.	**W/P:** Serious hypersensitivity (anaphylactic) reactions reported. *Clostridium difficile*-associated diarrhea reported (ranging from mild diarrhea to fatal colitis); evaluate if diarrhea occurs. **P/N:** Category B, caution in nursing.	Headache, nausea, diarrhea, rash, phlebitis, anemia, pruritus.
Ertapenem Sodium (Invanz)	**Inj:** 1g (IM, IV)	***Adults/Pediatrics:*** **≥13yrs:** 1g IM/IV qd. **Treatment Duration: Complicated Intra-Abdominal Infections:** 5-14 days. **Complicated SSSI:** 7-14 days. **CAP/UTI:** 10-14 days. **Acute Pelvic Infections:** 3-10 days. May give IV for up to 14 days and IM for up to 7 days. **Prophylaxis Following Colorectal Surgery:** 1g IV as single dose given 1 hr prior to surgical incision. **CrCl ≤30mL/min/1.73m²:** 500mg IM/IV qd. **Hemodialysis:** Give 150mg IM/IV after dialysis only if 500mg dose was given within 6 hrs prior to dialysis. ***Pediatrics:*** **3 months-12 yrs:** 15mg/kg IM/IV bid (**Max:** 1g/day). **Treatment Duration: Complicated Intra-Abdominal Infections:** 5-14 days. **Complicated SSSI:** 7-14 days. **CAP/UTI:** 10-14 days. **Pelvic Infections:** 3-10 days. May administer IV for up to 14 days and IM for up to 7 days.	**W/P:** Serious, sometimes fatal, hypersensitivity reported with β-lactam therapy. *Clostridium difficile*-associated diarrhea (CDAD) reported. D/C if CDAD confirmed. Seizures and CNS adverse experiences reported. Increased risk of seizures with CNS disorders and/or compromised renal function. Use lidocaine HCl as diluent for IM use. Monitor renal, hepatic, hematopoietic functions during prolonged therapy. Do not inject into blood vessel. **P/N:** Category B, caution in nursing.	Diarrhea, infused vein complication, N/V, headache, edema/swelling, fever, abdominal pain, constipation, altered mental status, headache, insomnia, rash, pruritis, vaginitis, phlebitis/thrombophlebitis.
Imipenem/ Cilastatin (Primaxin I.M.)	**Inj:** (Imipenem-Cilastatin) 500mg-500mg, 750mg-750mg	***Adults/Pediatrics:*** **≥12 yrs:** Dose according to imipenem. **Mild to Moderate LRTI/SSSI/Gynecologic Infection:** 500mg or 750mg IM q12h depending on severity. **Intra-Abdominal Infection:** 750mg IM q12h. Continue for at least 2 days after symptoms resolve. **Elderly:** Start at low end of dosing range. Continue for at least 2 days after symptoms resolve; do not treat for >14 days. **Max:** 1500mg/day. Avoid if CrCl <20mL/min.	**W/P:** Serious, sometimes fatal, hypersensitivity reactions reported with β-lactam therapy. *Clostridium difficile*-associated diarrhea reported. Prolonged use may result in overgrowth of non-susceptible organisms. Avoid injection into blood vessel. Caution in elderly. CNS adverse events (eg, myoclonic activity, confusion, seizures) reported most commonly with CNS disorders and renal dysfunction; d/c if any occur. Positive Coombs test reported. **P/N:** Category C, caution in nursing.	Injection site pain, N/V, diarrhea, fever, rash, hypotension, seizures, dizziness, pruritus, urticaria, somnolence.

Table 6.2. PRESCRIBING INFORMATION FOR ANTIBIOTICS *(cont.)*

NAME	FORM/ STRENGTH	DOSAGE	WARNINGS/PRECAUTIONS & CONTRAINDICATIONS	ADVERSE EFFECTS†
CARBAPENEMS *(cont.)*				
Imipenem/ Cilastatin (Primaxin I.V.)	**Inj:** (Imipenem-Cilastatin) 250mg-250mg, 500mg-500mg	***Adults:* ≥70kg and CrCl >70mL/min:** Dose based on imipenem component. **Uncomplicated UTI:** 250mg q6h. **Complicated UTI:** 500mg q6h. **Mild Infection:** 250-500mg q6h. **Moderate Infection:** 500mg q6-8h or 1g q8h. **Severe, Life-Threatening Infection:** 500mg-1g q6h or 1g q8h. **Max:** 50mg/kg/day or 4g/day, whichever lower. **Renal Impairment and/or <70kg:** Refer to PI. **CrCl 6-20mL/min:** 125-250mg q12h. **CrCl ≤5mL/min:** Administer hemodialysis within 48 hrs of dose. ***Pediatrics:* ≥3 months:** Dose based on imipenem component. **Non-CNS Infections:** 15-25mg/kg q6h. **Max:** 2g/day if susceptible or 4g/day if moderately susceptible. May use up to 90mg/kg/day in older cystic fibrosis children. **4 weeks-3 months and ≥1500g:** 25mg/kg q6h. **1-4 weeks and ≥1500g:** 25mg/kg q8h. **<1 week and ≥1500g:** 25mg/kg q12h. Not recommended with CNS infection, and <30kg with impaired renal function.	**W/P:** Serious, sometimes fatal, hypersensitivity reactions reported with β-lactam therapy. *Clostridium difficile*-associated diarrhea reported. Prolonged use may result in overgrowth of nonsusceptible organisms. CNS adverse events (eg, myoclonic activity, confusion, seizures) reported most commonly with CNS disorders and renal dysfunction. **P/N:** Category C, caution in nursing.	Phlebitis/thrombophlebitis, N/V, diarrhea, rash, fever, hypotension, seizures, dizziness, pruritus, urticaria, somnolence, hepatitis (including fulminant hepatitis), hepatic failure.
Meropenem (Merrem)	**Inj:** 500mg, 1g	***Adults:* IV: Intra-Abdominal:** 1g q8h. **CrCl 26-50mL/min:** 1g q12h. **CrCl 10-25mL/min:** 500mg q12h. **CrCl <10mL/min:** 500mg q24h. **cSSSI:** 500mg q8h. **CrCl 26-50mL/min:** 500mg q12h. **CrCl 10-25mL/min:** 250mg q12h. **CrCl <10mL/min:** 250mg q24h. ***Pediatrics:* IV: ≥3 months: >50kg: Intra-Abdominal:** 1g q8h. **Meningitis:** 2g q8h. **cSSSI:** 500mg q8h. **≤50kg: Intra-Abdominal:** 20mg/kg q8h. **Max:** 1g q8h. **Meningitis:** 40mg/kg q8h. **Max:** 2g q8h. **cSSSI:** 10mg/kg q8h. **Max:** 500mg q8h.	**W/P:** Severe and fatal hypersensitivity reactions reported; increased risk with allergens and/or PCN sensitivity. *Clostridium difficile*-associated diarrhea reported; if CDAD suspected d/c therapy. Seizures and other CNS effects reported, particularly with pre-existing CNS disorders, bacterial meningitis, and renal dysfunction. Thrombocytopenia reported with severe renal impairment. Prolonged use may result in superinfection. Use as monotherapy for meningitis caused by penicillin nonsusceptible strains of *Streptococcus pneumoniae* has not been established. **P/N:** Category B, caution in nursing.	Headache, rash, local reactions, diarrhea, N/V, constipation.
CEPHALOSPORINS				
1ST GENERATION CEPHALOSPORINS				
Cefadroxil Monohydrate	**Cap:** 500mg; **Sus:** 250mg/5mL [100mL], 500mg/5mL [75mL, 100mL]; **Tab:** 1g*	***Adults:* Uncomplicated Lower UTI:** 1-2g/day given qd or bid. **Other UTI:** 1g bid. **SSSI:** 1g qd or 500mg bid. **Group A β-hemolytic Strep Pharyngitis/Tonsillitis:** 1g qd or 500mg bid for 10 days. **CrCl ≤50mL/min: Initial:** 1g. **Maint: CrCl 25-50mL/min:** 500mg q12h; **CrCl 10-25mL/min:** 500mg q24h; **CrCl 0-10mL/min:** 500mg q36h. ***Pediatrics:* UTI/SSSI:** 15mg/kg q12h. **Pharyngitis/Tonsillitis/Impetigo:** 30mg/kg qd or 15mg/kg q12h. Treat β-hemolytic strep infections for at least 10 days.	**W/P:** Caution with markedly impaired renal function, history of GI disease. Cross-sensitivity with cephalosporins and PCNs. False (+) direct Coombs' tests, colitis, and *Clostridium difficile*-associated diarrhea (CDAD) reported. **P/N:** Category B, caution in nursing.	Diarrhea, rash, hypersensitivity reactions, pruritus, hepatic dysfunction, genital moniliasis, vaginitis, fever, superinfection (prolonged use).
Cefazolin	**Inj:** 500mg, 1g, 10g, 20g	***Adults:* Moderate-Severe Infections:** 500mg-1g q6-8h. **Mild Gram-Positive Cocci Infection:** 250-500mg q8h. **Acute, Uncomplicated UTI:** 1g q12h. **Pneumococcal Pneumonia:** 500mg q12h. **Severe Life-Threatening Infection**	**W/P:** Prolonged use may result in overgrowth of nonsusceptible organisms. Possible cross-sensitivity between PCNs, cephalosporins, and other β-lactam antibiotics. Pseudomembranous colitis	Diarrhea, oral candidiasis, N/V, stomach cramps, anorexia, allergic reactions, blood

*Scored. †Bold entries denote special dental considerations.
BB = black box warning; **W/P** = warnings/precautions; **Contra** = contraindications; **P/N** = pregnancy category rating and nursing considerations.

NAME	FORM/ STRENGTH	DOSAGE	WARNINGS/PRECAUTIONS & CONTRAINDICATIONS	ADVERSE EFFECTS†
Cefazolin *(cont.)*		**(eg, Endocarditis, Septicemia):** 1-1.5g q6h; **Max:** 12g/day (rare). **Perioperative Prophylaxis:** 1g IM/IV 0.5-1 hr before surgery. **For Procedures ≥2 hrs:** 500mg-1g IM/IV during surgery. **Maint:** 500mg-1g IM/IV q6-8h for 24 hrs post-op. Continue for 3-5 days post-op for devastating procedures (eg, open-heart surgery and prosthetic arthroplasty). **Renal Impairment: CrCl 35-54mL/min:** Full dose q8h. **CrCl 11-34mL/min:** 1/2 usual dose q12h. **CrCl <10mL/min:** 1/2 usual dose q18-24h. Apply reduced dosage recommendations after initial LD is given. ***Pediatrics:*** **Mild-Moderately Severe Infection:** 25-50mg/kg/day in 3-4 equal doses. **Severe Infection:** 100mg/kg/day in divided doses. **Renal Impairment: CrCl 40-70mL/min:** 60% of normal daily dose in equally divided doses q12h. **CrCl 20-40mL/min:** 25% of normal daily dose in equally divided doses q12h. **CrCl 5-20mL/min:** 10% of normal daily dose q24h. Apply reduced dosage recommendations after initial LD is given.	reported. Elevated levels with renal insufficiency can lead to seizures. Caution with colitis and other GI diseases. Safety in premature infants and neonates not established. **P/N:** Category B, caution in nursing.	dyscrasias, renal failure, transient rise in SGOT/SGPT/BUN/SCr/alkaline phosphatase, local reactions.
Cephalexin (Keflex)	**(Keflex) Cap:** 250mg, 500mg, 750mg; **(Generic) Cap:** 250mg, 500mg; **Sus:** 125mg/ 5mL [100mL, 200mL], 250mg/5mL [100mL, 200mL]	***Adults:*** **Usual:** 250mg q6h. **Streptococcal Pharyngitis/SSSI/Uncomplicated Cystitis (>15 yrs):** 500mg q12h. Treat cystitis for 7-14 days. **Max:** 4g/day. ***Pediatrics:*** **Usual:** 25-50mg/kg/day in divided doses. **Streptococcal Pharyngitis (>1 yr)/SSSI:** May divide dose and give q12h. **Otitis Media:** 75-100mg/kg/day in divided doses. Administer for ≥10 days in β-hemolytic streptococcal infections.	**W/P:** Caution with markedly impaired renal function, history of GI disease. Cross-sensitivity with cephalosporins and PCNs. *Clostridium difficile*-associated diarrhea reported. Positive direct Coombs' tests reported. False (+) for urine glucose with Benedict's or Fehling's solution, and Clinitest tabs. May result in overgrowth of nonsusceptible bacteria. **P/N:** Category B, caution in nursing.	Diarrhea, allergic reactions, dyspepsia, gastritis, abdominal pain, superinfection (prolonged use).
2ND GENERATION CEPHALOSPORINS				
Cefaclor	**Cap:** 250mg, 500mg; **Sus:** 125mg/ 5mL [75mL, 150mL], 187mg/ 5mL [50mL, 100mL], 250mg/ 5mL [75mL, 150mL], 375mg/5mL [50mL, 100mL]	***Adults:*** **Usual:** 250mg q8h. **Severe Infections/Pneumonia:** 500mg q8h. Treat β-hemolytic strep for 10 days. ***Pediatrics:*** **≥1 month: Usual:** 20mg/kg/day given q8h. **Otitis Media/Serious Infections/Infections caused by Less Susceptible Organisms:** 40mg/kg/day. **Max:** 1g/day. May administer q12h for otitis media and pharyngitis. Treat β-hemolytic strep for 10 days.	**W/P:** Cross-sensitivity to PCNs and other cephalosporins may occur. *Clostridium difficile*-associated diarrhea reported. Positive direct Coombs' test reported. Caution with markedly impaired renal function, history of GI disease. False (+) for urine glucose with Benedict's or Fehling's solution, and Clinitest tabs. **P/N:** Category B, caution in nursing.	Hypersensitivity reactions, diarrhea, eosinophilia, genital pruritus and vaginitis, serum-sickness-like reactions, superinfection.
Cefaclor ER	**Tab, Extended-Release:** 500mg	***Adults/Pediatrics:*** **≥16 yrs: ABECB/Acute Bronchitis:** 500mg q12h for 7 days. **Pharyngitis/Tonsillitis:** 375mg q12h for 10 days. **SSSI:** 375mg q12h for 7-10 days. Take with meals. Do not crush, cut, or chew tab.	**W/P:** Cross-sensitivity to PCNs and other cephalosporins may occur. *Clostridium difficile*-associated diarrhea reported. Positive direct Coombs' test reported. Caution with markedly impaired renal function, history of GI disease. False (+) for urine glucose with Benedict's or Fehling's solution, and Clinitest tabs. **P/N:** Category B, caution in nursing.	Headache, rhinitis, diarrhea, nausea, vaginitis, abdominal pain, **pharyngitis**, increased cough, pruritus, back pain, serum-sickness-like reactions, superinfection (prolonged use).

Table 6.2. PRESCRIBING INFORMATION FOR ANTIBIOTICS *(cont.)*

NAME	FORM/ STRENGTH	DOSAGE	WARNINGS/PRECAUTIONS & CONTRAINDICATIONS	ADVERSE EFFECTS†
CEPHALOSPORINS *(cont.)*				
2ND GENERATION CEPHALOSPORINS *(cont.)*				
Cefotetan Disodium	**Inj:** 1g, 2g	***Adults:* Usual:** 1-2g IM/IV q12h for 5-10 days. **UTI:** 1-4g/day IM/IV given q12h or q24h. **SSSI: Mild-Moderate:** 2g IV q24h or 1g IM/IV q12h; *K. pneumoniae* 1g or 2g IM/IV q12h. **Severe:** 2g IV q12h. **Other Sites:** 1g or 2 g IM/IV q12h. **Severe:** 2g IV q12h. **Life-Threatening:** 3g IV q12h. **Max:** 6g/day. **Surgical Prophylaxis:** 1g or 2g IV single dose 30-60 minutes before surgery. **CrCl >30mL/min:** Usual dose q12h. **CrCl 10-30mL/min:** Usual dose q24h or 50% usual dose q12h. **CrCl <10mL/min:** Usual dose q48h or 25% usual dose q12h. **Hemodialysis:** 25% usual dose q24h on days between dialysis and 50% usual dose on dialysis days.	**W/P:** Possible cross-sensitivity between PCNs, cephalosporins, and other β-lactam antibiotics. Pseudomembranous colitis reported; caution with history of GI disease (eg, colitis). Possible decrease in PT; caution with renal or hepatic impairment, poor nutritional state, the elderly, and cancer; monitor PT and give vitamin K if needed. Caution with colitis and other GI diseases. Severe cases of immune-mediated hemolytic anemia reported. D/C if anemia develops within 2-3 weeks after initiation of therapy; monitor hematological parameters with prolonged use. Increased risk of seizures especially with renal impairment when dose is not reduced; d/c if seizures occur. Galaxy plastic container not for IM injection. ADD-Vantage vial for IV infusion only. **Contra:** History of cephalosporin-associated hemolytic anemia. **P/N:** Category B, caution in nursing.	Diarrhea, nausea, hematologic abnormalities, hepatic enzyme elevations, hypersensitivity reactions, superinfection (prolonged use).
Cefoxitin Sodium (Mefoxin)	**Inj:** 1g, 1g/50mL, 2g, 2g/50mL, 10g	***Adults:* Usual:** 1-2g IV q6-8h. **Uncomplicated Infections:** 1g IV q6-8h. **Moderate-Severe:** 1g IV q4h or 2g IV q6-8h. **Gas Gangrene/Other Infections Requiring Higher Dose:** 2g IV q4h or 3g IV q6h. **Renal Insufficiency: LD:** 1-2g IV. **Maint: CrCl 30-50mL/min:** 1-2g IV q8-12h. **CrCl 10-29mL/min:** 1-2g IV q12-24h. **CrCl 5-9mL/min:** 0.5-1g IV q12-24h. **CrCl <5mL/min:** 0.5-1g IV q24-48h. **Hemodialysis: LD:** 1-2g IV after dialysis. **Maint:** See renal insufficiency doses above. **Prophylaxis: Uncontaminated GI Surgery/Hysterectomy:** 2g IV 0.5-1 hr prior to surgery (1/2-1 hr before initial incision), then 2g IV q6h after 1st dose up to 24 hrs. **C-Section:** 2g IV single dose as soon as umbilical cord is clamped, or 2g IV as soon as umbilical cord is clamped, followed by 2g IV at 4 and 8 hrs after initial dose. ***Pediatrics:* ≥3 months:** 80-160mg/kg/day divided into 4-6 equal doses. **Max:** 12g/day. **Prophylaxis: Uncontaminated GI Surgery/Hysterectomy:** 30-40mg/kg IV 0.5-1 hr prior to surgery, then 30-40mg/kg IV q6h after first dose for up to 24 hrs.	**W/P:** Possible cross-sensitivity between PCNs and cephalosporins. *Clostridium difficile*-associated diarrhea reported. Caution with allergies, GI disease, particularly colitis. Prolonged use may result in overgrowth of nonsusceptible organisms. Monitor renal, hepatic, hematopoietic functions, especially with prolonged therapy. False (+) for urine glucose with Clinitest tabs. **P/N:** Category B, caution in nursing.	Thrombophlebitis, rash, pseudomembranous colitis, pruritus, fever, dyspnea, hypotension, diarrhea, blood dyscrasias, elevated LFTs, changes in renal function tests, exacerbation of myasthenia gravis.
Cefprozil (Cefzil)	**Sus:** 125mg/5mL [50mL, 75mL, 100mL], 250mg/5mL [50mL, 75mL, 100mL]; **Tab:** 250mg, 500mg	***Adults/Pediatrics:* ≥13 yrs: Pharyngitis/Tonsillitis:** 500mg q24h for 10 days. **Acute Sinusitis:** 250-500mg q12h for 10 days. **ABECB/Acute Bronchitis:** 500mg q12h for 10 days. **SSSI:** 250-500mg q12h or 500mg q24h for 10 days. **CrCl <30mL/min:** 50% of standard dose. ***Pediatrics:* 2-12 yrs: Pharyngitis/Tonsillitis:** 7.5mg/kg q12h for 10 days. **SSSI:** 20mg/kg q24h for 10 days. **6 months-12 yrs: Otitis Media:** 15mg/kg q12h for 10 days. **Acute Sinusitis:** 7.5-15mg/kg q12h for 10 days. Do not exceed adult dose. **CrCl <30mL/min:** 50% of standard dose.	**W/P:** Cross-sensitivity with cephalosporins and PCNs. False (+) direct Coombs' tests reported. *Clostridium difficile*-associated diarrhea reported. Caution with GI disease, renal impairment, elderly. False (+) for urine glucose with Benedict's or Fehling's solution, and Clinitest tabs. Sus contains phenylalanine. **P/N:** Category B, caution in nursing.	Diarrhea, nausea, hepatic enzyme elevations, eosinophilia, genital pruritus, vaginitis, superinfection (prolonged use).

†Bold entries denote special dental considerations.
BB = black box warning; **W/P** = warnings/precautions; **Contra** = contraindications; **P/N** = pregnancy category rating and nursing considerations.

NAME	FORM/ STRENGTH	DOSAGE	WARNINGS/PRECAUTIONS & CONTRAINDICATIONS	ADVERSE EFFECTS†
Cefuroxime (Zinacef)	**Inj:** 750mg, 1.5g, 7.5g, 750mg/50mL, 1.5g/50mL	***Adults:*** **Usual:** 750mg-1.5g q8h for 5-10 days. **Uncomplicated Pneumonia and UTI/SSSI/Disseminated Gonococcal Infections:** 750mg q8h. **Severe/ Complicated Infections:** 1.5g q8h. **Bone and Joint Infections:** 1.5g q8h. **Life-Threatening Infections/Infections With Susceptible Organisms:** 1.5g q6h. **Meningitis: Max:** 3g q8h. **Uncomplicated Gonococcal Infection:** 1.5g IM single dose at 2 different sites with 1g PO probenecid. **Surgical Prophylaxis:** 1.5g IV 0.5-1 hr before incision, then 750mg IM/IV q8h with prolonged procedure. **Open Heart Surgery (Perioperative):** 1.5g IV at induction of anesthesia and q12h thereafter, for total of 6g. **Renal Impairment: CrCl 10-20mL/min:** 750mg q12h. **CrCl <10mL/min:** 750mg q24h. **Hemodialysis:** Give further dose at end of dialysis. ***Pediatrics:*** **>3 months: Usual:** 50-100mg/kg/day in divided doses q6-8h. **Severe Infections:** 100mg/kg/day (not to exceed max adult dose). **Bone and Joint Infections:** 150mg/kg/day in divided doses q8h (not to exceed max adult dose). **Meningitis:** 200-240mg/kg/day IV in divided doses q6-8h. **Renal Dysfunction:** Modify dosing frequency consistent with adult recommendations.	**W/P:** Cross-sensitivity to PCNs and other cephalosporins may occur. *Clostridium difficile*-associated diarrhea reported, ranging in severity from mild diarrhea to fatal colitis. Monitor renal function. May result in overgrowth of nonsusceptible organisms. Caution with history of GI disease, particularly colitis. Hearing loss in peds being treated for meningitis. Risk of decreased prothrombin activity with renal or hepatic impairment, poor nutritional state, or protracted course of therapy. False (+) urine glucose with copper reduction tests and false (-) with ferricyanide test. **P/N:** Category B, caution in nursing.	Thrombophlebitis, GI symptoms, decreased Hgb and Hct, eosinophilia. Transient rise in SGOT, SGPT, alkaline phosphatase, bilirubin, and LDH.
Cefuroxime Axetil (Ceftin)	**Sus:** 125mg/5mL [100mL], 250mg/5mL [50mL, 100mL]; **Tab:** 250mg, 500mg	***Adults/Pediatrics:*** **≥13 yrs: (Tab) Pharyngitis/Tonsillitis/Sinusitis:** 250mg bid for 10 days. **ABECB/SSSI:** 250-500mg bid for 10 days. **Acute Bronchitis:** 250-500mg bid for 5-10 days. **UTI:** 250mg bid for 7-10 days. **Gonorrhea:** 1000mg single dose. **Lyme Disease:** 500mg bid for 20 days. ***Pediatrics:*** **3 months-12 yrs: (Sus) Pharyngitis/Tonsillitis:** 10mg/kg bid for 10 days. **Max:** 500mg/day. **Otitis Media/Sinusitis/ Impetigo:** 15mg/kg bid for 10 days. **Max:** 1000mg/day. **(Tab-if can swallow whole) Otitis Media/Sinusitis:** 250mg bid for 10 days.	**W/P:** Tabs are not bioequivalent to sus. Caution with colitis, renal impairment. Cross-sensitivity with cephalosporins and PCNs. False (+) for urine glucose with Benedict's or Fehling's solution, and Clinitest tabs. May cause fall in PT; risk in patients stable on anticoagulants, if receiving protracted course of antibiotics, renal/hepatic impairment, or a poor nutritional state; give vitamin K as needed. Watery, bloody stools (with or without stomach cramps and fever) may develop after starting treatment; notify physician. *Clostridium difficile*-associated diarrhea (CDAD) reported. **P/N:** Category B, not for use in nursing.	Diarrhea, N/V, vaginitis, **taste aversion** (suspension in peds), superinfection (prolonged use).
3RD GENERATION CEPHALOSPORINS				
Cefdinir (Omnicef)	**Cap:** 300mg; **Sus:** 125mg/5mL, 250mg/5mL [60mL, 100mL]	***Adults/Pediatrics:*** **≥13 yrs: (Cap) SSSI/ CAP:** 300mg q12h for 10 days. **AECB/ Pharyngitis/Tonsillitis:** 300mg q12h for 5-10 days or 600mg q24h for 10 days. **Sinusitis:** 300mg q12h or 600mg q24h for 10 days. **CrCl <30mL/min:** 300mg qd. ***Pediatrics:*** **6 months-12 yrs: (Sus) Otitis Media/Pharyngitis/Tonsillitis:** 7mg/kg q12h for 5-10 days or 14mg/ kg q24h for 10 days. **Sinusitis:** 7mg/ kg q12h or 14mg/kg q24h for 10 days. **SSSI:** 7mg/kg q12h or 14mg/kg q24h for 10 days.	**W/P:** Cross-sensitivity to PCNs and other cephalosporins may occur. *Clostridium difficile*-associated diarrhea has been reported. Positive direct Coombs' tests may occur. Caution with renal dysfunction, history of colitis. Sus contains 2.86g/5mL of sucrose; caution in diabetes. False (+) for urine glucose with Clinitest and Benedict's or Fehling's solution. **P/N:** Category B, safe in nursing.	Diarrhea, vaginal moniliasis, nausea, headache, abdominal pain, superinfection (prolonged use).

Table 6.2. PRESCRIBING INFORMATION FOR ANTIBIOTICS *(cont.)*

NAME	FORM/ STRENGTH	DOSAGE	WARNINGS/PRECAUTIONS & CONTRAINDICATIONS	ADVERSE EFFECTS†
CEPHALOSPORINS *(cont.)*				
3RD GENERATION CEPHALOSPORINS *(cont.)*				
Cefditoren Pivoxil (Spectracef)	**Tab:** 200mg	***Adults/Pediatrics:*** **≥12: ABECB:** 400mg bid for 10 days. **Pharyngitis/Tonsillitis/ SSSI:** 200mg bid for 10 days. **CAP:** 400mg bid for 14 days. **CrCl 30-49mL/ min:** 200mg bid. **CrCl <30mL/min:** 200mg qd. Take with meals.	**W/P:** Cross sensitivity to PCNs and other cephalosporins may occur. Pseudomembranous colitis reported. Not recommended for prolonged antibiotic therapy. Prolonged therapy may cause superinfection. May decrease PT. **Contra:** Milk protein hypersensitivity, carnitine deficiency. **P/N:** Category B, caution in nursing.	Diarrhea, nausea, vaginal moniliasis, headache.
Cefixime (Suprax)	**Tab:** 400mg; **Sus:**100mg/5mL [50mL, 75mL, 100mL]	***Adults:*** **Usual:** 400mg qd. **Gonorrhea:** 400mg single dose. **CrCl 21-60mL/min/ Hemodialysis:** Give 75% of standard dose. **CrCl <20mL/min/CAPD:** Give 50% of standard dose. ***Pediatrics:*** **>12 yrs or >50kg: (Tab/Sus) Usual:** 400mg qd. **≥6 months: (Sus)** 8mg/kg qd or 4mg/ kg bid. Treat for at least 10 days with *S.pyogenes.* **CrCl 21-60mL/min/ Hemodialysis:** Give 75% of standard dose. **CrCl <20mL/min/CAPD:** Give 50% of standard dose.	**W/P:** Caution with PCN or other allergy, GI disease (eg, colitis). Anaphylactic/ anaphylactoid reactions, pseudomembranous colitis reported. May cause false (+) direct Coombs' test or false (+) reaction for urinary glucose using Benedict's/ Fehling's solution or Clinitest. **P/N:** Category B, not for use in nursing.	Diarrhea, abdominal pain, nausea, dyspepsia, flatulence, superinfection.
Cefotaxime Sodium (Claforan)	**Inj:** 500mg, 1g, 2g, 10g	***Adults/Pediatrics:*** **≥50kg: Gonococcal Urethritis/Cervicitis (Males/Females):** 500mg single dose IM. **Rectal Gonorrhea:** 0.5g (females) or 1g (males) single dose IM. **Uncomplicated Infections:** 1g IM/IV q12h. **Moderate-Severe Infections:** 1-2g IM/IV q8h. **Septicemia:** 2g IV q6-8h. **Life-Threatening Infections:** 2g IV q4h. **Max:** 12g/day. **Surgical Prophylaxis:** 1g IM/IV 30-90 min before surgery. **Cesarean Section:** 1g IV when umbilical cord is clamped, then 1g IV at 6 and 12 hrs after 1st dose. **CrCl <20mL/min/1.73m²:** Give 1/2 of usual dose. ***Pediatrics:*** **1 month-12 yrs and ≤50kg:** 50-180mg/kg/day IM/IV divided in 4-6 doses. **1-4 weeks:** 50mg/ kg IV q8h. **0-1 week:** 50mg/kg IV q12h. **CrCl <20mL/min/1.73m²:** Give 1/2 of usual dose.	**W/P:** Cross sensitivity to PCNs and other cephalosporins may occur. *Clostridium difficile*-associated diarrhea reported. May result in overgrowth of nonsusceptible organisms. Caution with history of GI disease. Reduce dose with renal dysfunction. Granulocytopenia may occur with long-term use. Monitor blood counts if therapy >10 days. Monitor injection site for tissue inflammation. False (+) direct Coombs' tests reported. **P/N:** Category B, caution in nursing.	Injection site reactions, rash, pruritus, fever, eosinophilia, colitis, diarrhea.
Cefpodoxime Proxetil (Vantin)	**Sus:** 50mg/5mL [50mL, 75mL, 100mL], 100mg/5mL [50mL, 75mL, 100mL]; **Tab:** 100mg, 200mg	***Adults/Pediatrics:*** **≥12 yrs:** Take tabs with food. **Pharyngitis/Tonsillitis:** 100mg q12h for 5-10 days. **CAP:** 200mg q12h for 14 days. **ABECB:** 200mg q12h for 10 days. **Uncomplicated Gonorrhea (Men/Women)/Rectal Gonococcal Infections (Women):** 200mg single dose. **SSSI:** 400mg q12h for 7-14 days. **Sinusitis:** 200mg q12h for 10 days. **UTI:** 100mg q12h for 7 days. **CrCl <30mL/min:** Increase interval to q24h. **Hemodialysis:** Dose 3 times weekly after dialysis. ***Pediatrics:*** **2 months-12 yrs: Otitis Media:** 5mg/kg q12h for 5 days. **Max:** 200mg/dose. **Pharyngitis/ Tonsillitis:** 5mg/kg q12h for 5-10 days. **Max:** 100mg/dose. **Sinusitis:** 5mg/kg q12h for 10 days. **Max:** 200mg/dose. **CrCl <30mL/min:** Increase interval to q24h. **Hemodialysis:** Dose 3 times weekly after dialysis.	**W/P:** Cross-sensitivity to PCNs and other cephalosporins may occur. *Clostridium difficile*-associated diarrhea reported. Positive direct Coombs' tests reported. Caution with renal impairment; dose reduction may be needed. May result in overgrowth of nonsusceptible organisms. **P/N:** Category B, not for use in nursing.	Diarrhea, nausea.

†Bold entries denote special dental considerations.
BB = black box warning; **W/P** = warnings/precautions; **Contra** = contraindications; **P/N** = pregnancy category rating and nursing considerations.

NAME	FORM/ STRENGTH	DOSAGE	WARNINGS/PRECAUTIONS & CONTRAINDICATIONS	ADVERSE EFFECTS†
Ceftazidime	**Inj:** 500mg, 1g, 2g, 6g	***Adults/ Pediatrics:* >12 yrs: Usual:** 1g IM/IV q8-12h. **Uncomplicated UTI:** 250mg IM/IV q12h. **Complicated UTI:** 500mg IM/IV q8-12h. **Bone and Joint Infection:** 2g IV q12h. **Uncomplicated Pneumonia/SSSI:** 500mg-1g IM/IV q8h. **Gynecological/Intra-Abdominal/ Meningitis/Severe Life-Threatening Infection:** 2g IV q8h. **Lung Infection Caused by *Pseudomonas spp.* in Cystic Fibrosis (Normal Renal Function):** 30-50mg/kg IV q8h. **Max:** 6g/day. **CrCl 31-50mL/min:** 1g q12h. **CrCl 16-30mL/ min:** 1g q24h. **CrCl 6-15mL/min:** 500mg q24h. **CrCl <5mL/min:** 500mg q48h. For severe infections (6g/day), increase renal impairment dose by 50% or increase dosing interval. Apply reduced dosage recommendations after initial 1g LD is given. **Hemodialysis:** Give 1g before, then 1g after each hemodialysis. **Intra-Peritoneal Dialysis/Continuous Ambulatory Peritoneal Dialysis:** Give 1g followed by 500mg q24h, or add to fluid at 250mg/2L. ***Pediatrics:* 1 month-12 yrs:** 30-50mg/kg IV q8h. **Max:** 6g/day. **Neonates (0-4 weeks):** 30mg/ kg IV q12h. Higher doses for cystic fibrosis or meningitis. **CrCl 31-50mL/ min:** 1g q12h. **CrCl 16-30mL/min:** 1g q24h. **CrCl 6-15mL/min:** 500mg q24h. **CrCl <5mL/min:** 500mg q48h. For severe infections (6g/day), increase renal impairment dose by 50% or increase dosing interval. Apply reduced dosage recommendations after initial 1g LD is given. Hemodialysis: Give 1g before, then 1g after each hemodialysis. **Intra-Peritoneal Dialysis/Continuous Ambulatory Peritoneal Dialysis:** Give 1g followed by 500mg q24h, or add to fluid at 250mg/2L.	**W/P:** Monitor renal function; potential for nephrotoxicity. Prolonged use may result in overgrowth of nonsusceptible organisms. Possible cross-sensitivity between PCNs, cephalosporins, and other β-lactam antibiotics. Pseudomembranous colitis reported. Elevated levels with renal insufficiency can lead to seizures, encephalopathy, asterixis, coma, and neuromuscular excitability. Possible decrease in PT; caution with renal or hepatic impairment, poor nutritional state; monitor PT and give vitamin K if needed. Caution with colitis and other GI diseases. Distal necrosis can occur after inadvertent intra-arterial administration. Continue therapy for 2 days after the signs and symptoms of infection have disappeared, but in complicated infections longer therapy may be required. False positive for urine glucose with Benedict's or Fehling's solution, and Clinitest tabs. **P/N:** Category B, not for use in nursing.	Phlebitis and inflammation at injection site, pruritus, rash, fever, diarrhea.
Ceftazidime (Fortaz)	**Inj:** 500mg, 1g, 1g/50mL, 2g, 2g/50mL, 6g	***Adults/ Pediatrics:* >12 yrs: Usual:** 1g IM/IV q8-12h. **Uncomplicated UTI:** 250mg IM/IV q12h. **Complicated UTI:** 500mg IM/IV q8-12h. **Bone and Joint Infection:** 2g IV q12h. **Uncomplicated Pneumonia/SSSI:** 500mg-1g IM/IV q8h. **Gynecological/Intra-Abdominal/ Meningitis/Severe Life-Threatening Infection:** 2g IV q8h. **Lung Infection Caused by *Pseudomonas spp.* in Cystic Fibrosis (Normal Renal Function):** 30-50mg/kg IV q8h. **Max:** 6g/day. **CrCl 31-50mL/min:** 1g q12h. **CrCl 16-30mL/ min:** 1g q24h. **CrCl 6-15mL/min:** 500mg q24h. **CrCl <5mL/min:** 500mg q48h. For severe infections (6g/day), increase renal impairment dose by 50% or increase dosing interval. Apply reduced dosage recommendations after initial 1g LD is given. **Hemodialysis:**	**W/P:** Monitor renal function; potential for nephrotoxicity. Prolonged use may result in overgrowth of nonsusceptible organisms. Possible cross-sensitivity between PCNs, cephalosporins, and other β-lactam antibiotics. *Clostridium difficile*-associated diarrhea reported and may range in severity from mild diarrhea to fatal colitis. Elevated levels with renal insufficiency can lead to seizures, encephalopathy, coma, asterixis, and neuromuscular excitability. Possible decrease in PT; caution with renal/ hepatic impairment, poor nutritional state; monitor PT and give vitamin K if needed. Caution with colitis, other GI diseases, and elderly. Distal necrosis may occur after inadvertent intra-arterial administration. Continue therapy for 2 days after the signs and symptoms of	Phlebitis and inflammation at injection site, pruritus, rash, fever, diarrhea.

Table 6.2. PRESCRIBING INFORMATION FOR ANTIBIOTICS *(cont.)*

NAME	FORM/ STRENGTH	DOSAGE	WARNINGS/PRECAUTIONS & CONTRAINDICATIONS	ADVERSE EFFECTS†
CEPHALOSPORINS *(cont.)*				
3RD GENERATION CEPHALOSPORINS *(cont.)*				
Ceftazidime (Fortaz) *(cont.)*		Give 1g before, then 1g after each hemodialysis. **Intra-Peritoneal Dialysis/ Continuous Ambulatory Peritoneal Dialysis:** Give 1g followed by 500mg q24h, or add to fluid at 250mg/2L. ***Pediatrics:* 1 month-12 yrs:** 30-50mg/ kg IV q8h. **Max:** 6g/day. **Neonates (0-4 weeks):** 30mg/kg IV q12h. Higher doses for cystic fibrosis or meningitis. **CrCl 31-50mL/min:** 1g q12h. **CrCl 16-30mL/ min:** 1g q24h. **CrCl 6-15mL/min:** 500mg q24h. **CrCl <5mL/min:** 500mg q48h. For severe infections (6g/day), increase renal impairment dose by 50% or increase dosing interval. Apply reduced dosage recommendations after initial 1g LD is given. **Hemodialysis:** Give 1g before, then 1g after each hemodialysis. **Intra-Peritoneal Dialysis/Continuous Ambulatory Peritoneal Dialysis:** Give 1g followed by 500mg q24h, or add to fluid at 250mg/2L.	infection have disappeared, but in complicated infections longer therapy may be required. False (+) for urine glucose with Benedict's or Fehling's solution, and Clinitest tabs. **P/N:** Category B, caution in nursing.	
Ceftazidime (Tazicef)	**Inj:** 500mg, 1g, 2g, 6g	***Adults:* Usual:** 1g IV q8-12h. **Uncomplicated UTI:** 250mg IM/IV q12h. **Complicated UTI:** 500mg IM/IV q8-12h. **Bone and Joint Infections:** 2g IV q12h. **Uncomplicated Pneumonia/SSSI:** 500mg-1g IM/IV q8h. **Gynecological/ Intra-Abdominal/Meningitis/Severe Life-Threatening Infection:** 2g IV q8h. **Lung Infection caused by *Pseudomonas* in Cystic Fibrosis (normal renal function):** 30-50mg/kg IV q8h. **Max:** 6g/ day. **Renal Impairment: CrCl 31-50mL/ min:** 1g q12h. **CrCl 16-30mL/min:** 1g q24h. **CrCl 6-15mL/min:** 500mg q24h. **CrCl <5mL/min:** 500mg q48h. For severe infections (6g/day), increase renal impairment dose by 50% or increase dosing interval. Apply reduced dosage recommendations after initial 1g LD is given. **Hemodialysis:** Give 1g LD before and 1g after each hemodialysis period. **Intra-Peritoneal Dialysis/Continuous Ambulatory Peritoneal Dialysis:** Give 1g LD followed by 500mg q24h, or add to fluid at 250mg/2L. ***Pediatrics:* Neonates (0-4 weeks):** 30mg/kg IV q12h. **1 month-12 yrs:** 30-50mg/kg IV q8h. **Max:** 6g/day. Higher doses for patients with cystic fibrosis or when treating meningitis. **Renal Impairment: CrCl 31-50mL/min:** 1g q12h. **CrCl 16-30mL/ min:** 1g q24h. **CrCl 6-15mL/min:** 500mg q24h. **CrCl <5mL/min:** 500mg q48h. **Hemodialysis:** Give 1 g before and 1g after each hemodialysis. For severe infections (6g/day), increase renal impairment dose by 50% or increase dosing interval. Apply reduced dosage recommendations after initial 1g LD is given. **Hemodialysis:** Give 1g LD before and 1g after each hemodialysis period. **Intra-Peritoneal Dialysis/Continuous Ambulatory Peritoneal Dialysis:** Give 1g followed by 500mg q24h, or add to fluid at 250mg/2L.	**W/P:** Monitor renal function; potential for nephrotoxicity. May result in overgrowth of nonsusceptible organisms. Possible cross-sensitivity between PCNs, cephalosporins, and other β-lactams. Pseudomembranous colitis reported. Elevated levels with renal insufficiency can lead to seizures, encephalopathy, asterixis, and neuromuscular excitability. Possible decrease in PT; caution with renal or hepatic impairment, poor nutritional state; monitor PT and give vitamin K if needed. Caution with colitis and other GI diseases. Distal necrosis may occur after inadvertent intra-arterial administration. Continue for 2 days after signs/symptoms of infection resolve; may require longer therapy with complicated infections. Caution in elderly. **P/N:** Category B, caution in nursing.	Phlebitis and inflammation at injection site, pruritus, rash, fever, diarrhea, N/V.

†Bold entries denote special dental considerations.
BB = black box warning; **W/P** = warnings/precautions; **Contra** = contraindications; **P/N** = pregnancy category rating and nursing considerations.

NAME	FORM/ STRENGTH	DOSAGE	WARNINGS/PRECAUTIONS & CONTRAINDICATIONS	ADVERSE EFFECTS†
Ceftibuten (Cedax)	**Cap:** 400mg; **Sus:** 90mg/5mL [30mL, 60mL, 90mL, 120mL]	***Adults/Pediatrics:*** **≥12 yrs: ABECB/ Otitis Media/Pharyngitis/Tonsillitis:** 400mg qd for 10 days. **Max:** 400mg/ day. **CrCl 30-49mL/min:** 4.5mg/kg or 200mg qd. **CrCl 5-29mL/min:** 2.25mg/ kg or 100mg qd. Take 2 hrs before or at least 1 hr after a meal. ***Pediatrics:*** **≥6 months: Pharyngitis/Tonsillitis/ Otitis Media:** 9mg/kg qd for 10 days. **Max:** 400mg.	**W/P:** Pseudomembranous colitis (toxin produced by *Clostridium difficile* is the primary cause) reported. Caution with history of GI disease. Cross-sensitivity with cephalosporins and penicillins. **P/N:** Category B, caution in nursing.	Diarrhea, N/V, abdominal pain, anorexia, dizziness, dyspepsia, **dry mouth**, dyspnea, dysuria, fatigue, flatulence, loose stools, headache, pruritus, rash, rigors, urticaria, superinfection (prolonged use).
Ceftriaxone Sodium (Rocephin)	**Inj:** (Rocephin) 500mg, 1g; (Generic) 250mg, 500mg, 1g, 2g, 10g, 1g/50mL, 2g/50mL	***Adults:*** **Usual:** 1-2g/day IV/IM given qd-bid. **Max:** 4g/day. **Gonorrhea:** 250mg IM single dose. **Surgical Prophylaxis:** 1g IV 1/2-2 hrs before surgery. Avoid diluents containing calcium. ***Pediatrics:*** **Skin Infections:** 50-75mg/kg/day IV/ IM given qd-bid. **Max:** 2g/day. **Otitis Media:** 50mg/kg (up to 1g) IM single dose. **Serious Infections:** 50-75mg/ kg/day IM/IV given q12h. **Max:** 2g/day. **Meningitis: Initial:** 100mg/kg (up to 4g), then 100mg/kg/day given qd-bid for 7-14 days. **Max:** 4g/day. Avoid diluents containing calcium.	**W/P:** Cross-sensitivity to PCNs and other cephalosporins may occur. *Clostridium difficile*-associated diarrhea reported. May result in overgrowth of nonsusceptible organisms. Altered PT, transient BUN, and serum creatinine elevations may occur. Do not exceed 2g/day and monitor blood levels with both hepatic dysfunction and significant renal disease. Caution with history of GI disease. D/C if gallbladder disease develops. May alter PT; monitor with impaired vitamin K synthesis or low vitamin K stores. **Contra:** Avoid use in hyperbilirubinemic neonates esp. prematures. Avoid concurrent use with calcium-containing solutions/products in newborns. **P/N:** Category B, caution in nursing.	Injection-site reactions, eosinophilia, thrombocytosis, diarrhea, SGOT and SGPT elevations.
4TH GENERATION CEPHALOSPORIN				
Cefepime HCl (Maxipime)	**Inj:** 500mg, 1g, 2g	***Adults:*** **Moderate-Severe Pneumonia:** 1-2g IV q12h for 10 days. **Febrile Neutropenia Emperic Therapy:** 2g IV q8h for 7 days or until neutropenia resolved. **Mild-Moderate UTI:** 0.5-1g IM/IV q12h for 7-10 days. **Severe UTI/ Moderate-Severe SSSI:** 2g IV q12h for 10 days. **Complicated Intra-Abdominal Infections:** 2g IV q12h for 7-10 days. **Renal Impairment: Initial:** Normal dose. **Maint: CrCl >60mL/min:** Normal dose. **CrCl 30-60mL/min:** 500mg-2g q24h or 2g q12h. **CrCl 11-29mL/min:** 500mg-2g q24h. **CrCl <11mL/min:** 250mg-1g q24h. **CAPD:** 500mg-2g q48h. **Hemodialysis:** 1g on Day 1, then 500mg q24h. ***Pediatrics:*** **2 months-16 yrs: ≤40kg: UTI/SSSI/Pneumonia:** 50mg/kg IV q12h. **Febrile Neutropenia:** 50mg/kg IV q8h. **Max:** Do not exceed adult dose.	**W/P:** Caution with PCN sensitivity; cross hypersensitivity may occur. *Clostridium difficile*-associated diarrhea reported. Treatment may result in overgrowth of nonsusceptible organisms. Caution with renal impairment or history of GI disease especially colitis. Encephalopathy, myoclonus, seizures, and/or renal failure reported. D/C if seizure occurs. Associated with a fall in PT; monitor PT with renal or hepatic impairment, poor nutritional state, and protracted course of antimicrobials; give vitamin K as indicated. Associated with (+) direct Coombs' test. **P/N:** Category B, caution in nursing.	Local reactions (eg, phlebitis), rash, diarrhea.
FLUOROQUINOLONES				
Ciprofloxacin (Cipro IV)	**Inj:** 10mg/mL, 200mg/100mL, 400mg/200mL	***Adults:*** **≥18 yrs: IV: UTI: Mild-Moderate:** 200mg q12h for 7-14 days. **Complicated/ Severe:** 400mg q12h for 7-14 days. **LRTI/SSSI: Mild-Moderate:** 400mg q12h for 7-14 days. **Complicated/ Severe:** 400mg q8h for 7-14 days. **Bone and Joint: Mild-Moderate:** 400mg q12h for ≥4-6 weeks. **Complicated/Severe:** 400mg q8h for ≥4-6 weeks. **Nosocomial Pneumonia:** 400mg q8h for 10-14 days. **Complicated Intra-Abdominal:** 400mg q12h (w/metronidazole) for 7-14 days. **Acute Sinusitis:** 400mg q12h for 10	**BB:** Fluoroquinolones are associated with an increased risk of tendinitis and tendon rupture in all ages. Risk further increased in patients >60 yrs, patients taking corticosteroid drugs, and patients with kidney, heart, or lung transplants. **W/P:** Convulsions, increased ICP, and toxic psychosis reported. Caution with CNS disorders or if predisposed to seizures. Severe, fatal hypersensitivity reactions may occur. *Clostridium difficile*-associated diarrhea, achilles and other tendon ruptures reported. D/C at	Nausea, diarrhea, CNS disturbances, local IV site reactions, hepatic enzyme abnormalities, eosinophilia, headache, restlessness, and rash.

Table 6.2. PRESCRIBING INFORMATION FOR ANTIBIOTICS *(cont.)*

NAME	FORM/ STRENGTH	DOSAGE	WARNINGS/PRECAUTIONS & CONTRAINDICATIONS	ADVERSE EFFECTS†
FLUOROQUINOLONES *(cont.)*				
Ciprofloxacin (Cipro IV) *(cont.)*		days. **Chronic Bacterial Prostatitis:** 400mg q12h for 28 days. **Febrile Neutropenia:** 400mg q8h (w/piperacillin 50mg/kg q4h) for 7-14 days. **Max:** 24g/day. **Inhalational Anthrax:** 400mg q12h for 60 days. Administer over 60 min. **CrCl 5-29mL/min:** 200-400mg q18-24h. ***Pediatrics:*** **<18 yrs: Inhalational Anthrax:** 10mg/kg q12h for 60 days. **Max:** 400mg/dose. **1-17 yrs: Complicated UTI/Pyleonephritis:** 6-10mg/kg q8h for 10-21 days. **Max:** 400mg/dose.	first sign of rash/hypersensitivity or if pain, inflammation, or ruptured tendon occur. May permit overgrowth of clostridia. Maintain hydration; avoid alkaline urine. Avoid excessive sunlight and UV light. Do not give via feeding tube. Monitor renal, hepatic, and hematopoietic function with prolonged use. Adjust dose with renal dysfunction. Caution with concomitant drugs that may result in prolongation of QT interval or in patients with risk factors for torsade de pointes. Caution in elderly taking corticosteroids. **Contra:** Concomitant administration with tizanidine. **P/N:** Category C, not for use in nursing.	
Ciprofloxacin (Cipro XR)	**Tab, Extended-Release:** 500mg, 1000 mg	***Adults:*** **≥18 yrs: Uncomplicated UTI:** 500mg qd for 3 days. **Complicated UTI:** 1000mg qd for 7-14 days. **CrCl <30mL/min:** 500 mg qd. **Acute Uncomplicated Pyelonephritis:** 1000mg qd for 7-14 days. **CrCl <30mL/min:** 500mg qd. Take with fluids. Administer at least 2 hrs before or 6 hrs after magnesium or aluminum containing antacids, sucralfate, Videx (didanosine) chewable/buffered tablets or pediatric powder, metal cations (eg, iron), multivitamins with zinc. Avoid concomitant administration with dairy products alone, or with calcium-fortified products. Space concomitant calcium intake (>800mg) by at least 2 hrs. Do not split, crush, or chew. Swallow tab whole. **Dialysis:** Give after procedure is completed.	**BB:** Fluoroquinolones are associated with an increased risk of tendinitis and tendon rupture in all ages. Risk further increased in patients >60 yrs, patients taking corticosteroid drugs, and patients with kidney, heart, or lung transplants. **W/P:** Convulsions, increased ICP, and toxic psychosis reported. Caution with CNS disorders or if predisposed to seizures. Severe, sometimes fatal, hypersensitivity reactions may occur. *Clostridium difficile*-associated diarrhea, colitis, achilles and other tendon ruptures reported. D/C at first sign of rash or if pain, inflammation, or ruptured tendon occurs. Maintain hydration; avoid alkaline urine. Avoid excessive sunlight and UV light. Not interchangeable with immediate-release tablets. To d/c treatment, rest and refrain from exercise. Caution with concomitant drugs that may result in prolongation of the QT interval or in patients with risk factors for torsade de pointes. Caution in elderly taking corticosteroids. **Contra:** Concomitant administration with tizanidine. **P/N:** Category C, not for use in nursing.	Nausea, headache, diarrhea, pain, swelling, tendon tears.
Ciprofloxacin HCl (Cipro Oral)	**Sus:** 250mg/5mL, 500mg/5mL [100mL]; **Tab:** 250mg, 500mg, 750mg	***Adults:*** **≥18 yrs: Acute Sinusitis/Typhoid Fever:** 500mg q12h for 10 days. **LRTI/SSSI: Mild-Moderate:** 500mg q12h for 7-14 days. **Severe/Complicated:** 750mg q12h for 7-14 days. **Cystitis/Acute Uncomplicated UTI:** 250mg q12h for 3 days. **Mild-Moderate UTI:** 250mg q12h for 7-14 days. **Severe/Complicated UTI:** 500mg q12h for 7-14 days. **Chronic Bacterial Prostatitis:** 500mg q12h for 28 days. **Intra-Abdominal:** 500mg q12h (w/metronidazole) for 7-14 days. **Bone and Joint: Mild-Moderate:** 500mg q12h for ≥4-6 weeks. **Severe/Complicated:** 750mg q12h for ≥4-6 weeks. **Infectious Diarrhea:** 500mg q12h for 5-7 days. **Uncomplicated Urethral/Cervical Gonococcal Infections:** 250mg single dose. **Inhalational Anthrax:** 500mg q12h for 60 days. **CrCl 30-50mL/min:** 250-500mg q12h. **CrCl 5-29mL/min:** 250-500mg q18h. **Hemodialysis/Peritoneal Dialysis:** 250-500mg q24h	**BB:** Fluoroquinolones are associated with an increased risk of tendinitis and tendon rupture in all ages. Risk further increased in patients >60 yrs, patients taking corticosteroid drugs, and patients with kidney, heart, or lung transplants. **W/P:** Convulsions, increased ICP, and toxic psychosis reported. Caution with CNS disorders or if predisposed to seizures. Severe, fatal hypersensitivity reactions may occur. *Clostridium difficile*-associated diarrhea, colitis, achilles and other tendon ruptures reported. D/C at first sign of rash or if pain, inflammation, or ruptured tendon occurs. Maintain hydration; avoid alkaline urine. Avoid excessive sunlight and UV light. Do not give via feeding tube. Monitor renal, hepatic, and hematopoietic function with prolonged use. Adjust dose with renal dysfunction. Caution with concomitant drugs that may result in prolongation of the QT interval or in patients with	N/V, dizziness, headache, CNS disturbances, diarrhea, rash, abdominal pain/discomfort, pain, swelling, tendon tears.

†Bold entries denote special dental considerations.
BB = black box warning; **W/P** = warnings/precautions; **Contra** = contraindications; **P/N** = pregnancy category rating and nursing considerations.

NAME	FORM/ STRENGTH	DOSAGE	WARNINGS/PRECAUTIONS & CONTRAINDICATIONS	ADVERSE EFFECTS†
Ciprofloxacin HCl (Cipro Oral) *(cont.)*		(after dialysis). Administer at least 2 hrs before or 6 hrs after magnesium- or aluminum-containing antacids, sucralfate, Videx (didanosine) chewable/ buffered tablets or pediatric powder, or other products containing calcium, iron, or zinc. ***Pediatrics:* <18 yrs: Inhalational Anthrax:** 15mg/kg q12h for 60 days. **Max:** 500mg/dose. **1-17 yrs: Complicated UTI/Pyelonephritis:** 10-20mg/kg q12h for 10-21 days. **Max:** 750mg/dose.	risk factors for torsades de pointes. Caution in elderly taking corticosteroids. **Contra:** Concomitant administration with tizanidine. **P/N:** Category C, not for use in nursing.	
Ciprofloxacin HCl (Proquin XR)	**Tab, Extended-Release:** 500mg	***Adults:*** 500mg qd with pm meal for 3 days. Administer at least 4 hrs before or 2 hrs after magnesium-or aluminum-containing antacids, sucralfate, Videx (didanosine) chewable/buffered tablets of pediatric powder, metal cations (eg, iron), multivitamins with zinc. Do not split, crush, or chew. Swallow tab whole.	**BB:** Fluoroquinolones are associated with an increased risk of tendinitis and tendon rupture in all ages. Risk further increased in patients >60 yrs, patients taking corticosteroid drugs, and patients with kidney, heart, or lung transplants. **W/P:** Convulsions, increased ICP and toxic psychosis reported. D/C if dizziness, confusion, tremors, hallucinations, depression, or suicidal thoughts/ acts. Caution with CNS disorders or if predisposed to seizures. May cause CNS events (eg, agitation, insomnia, anxiety, nightmares, or paranoia). Severe, fatal hypersensitivity reactions may occur. *Clostridium difficile*-associated diarrhea, colitis, achilles, and other tendon ruptures reported. D/C at first sign of rash, jaundice or if pain, inflammation, or ruptured tendon occurs. Maintain hydration; avoid alkaline urine. Avoid excessive sunlight and UV light. Not interchangeable with immediate-release or other extended-release oral formulations. D/C if symptoms of peripheral neuropathy occur. Caution in elderly taking corticosteroids. **P/N:** Category C, not for use in nursing.	Fungal infection, **nasopharyngitis**, headache, micturition urgency.
Gemifloxacin Mesylate (Factive)	**Tab:** 320mg	***Adults:* ≥18 yrs: ABECB:** 320mg qd for 5 days. **CAP:** 320mg qd for 5 days *(S.pneumoniae, H.influenzae, M.pneumoniae, or C.pneumoniae)* or 7 days (MDRSP, *K.pneumoniae, or M.catarrhalis*). **Renal Impairment: CrCl ≤40mL/min or Dialysis:** 160mg qd. Take with fluids.	**BB:** Fluoroquinolones are associated with an increased risk of tendinitis and tendon rupture in all ages. Risk further increased in patients >60 yrs, patients taking corticosteroid drugs, and patients with kidney, heart, or lung transplants. **W/P:** May prolong QT interval; avoid in patients with a history of prolonged QTc interval, uncontrolled electrolyte disorders. Caution with proarrhythmic conditions, epilepsy, or if predisposed to convulsions. D/C at first sign of hypersensitivity (eg, rash). CNS effects, photosensitivity reactions, hypersensitivity reactions (some fatal) reported; d/c if any of these occur. *Clostridium difficile*-associated diarrhea, achilles and other tendon rupture reported. D/C therapy if rash, pain, inflammation, or ruptured tendon occurs. Caution in elderly patients taking corticosteroids. Avoid excessive sunlight and UV light. Maintain hydration. Increases of International Normalized Ratio (INR), or prothrombin time (PT), and/or clinical episodes of bleeding have been noted with concurrent administration with warfarin or derivatives. **P/N:** Category C, not for use in nursing.	Diarrhea, rash, N/V, headache, abdominal pain, dizziness.

Table 6.2. PRESCRIBING INFORMATION FOR ANTIBIOTICS *(cont.)*

NAME	FORM/ STRENGTH	DOSAGE	WARNINGS/PRECAUTIONS & CONTRAINDICATIONS	ADVERSE EFFECTS†
FLUOROQUINOLONES *(cont.)*				
Levofloxacin (Levaquin)	**Inj:** 5mg/mL, 25mg/mL; **Sol:** 25mg/mL; **Tab:** 250mg, 500mg, 750mg [Leva-pak, 5[s]]	***Adults:* ≥18 yrs: IV/PO: ABECB:** 500mg qd for 7 days. **CAP:** 500mg qd for 7-14 days or 750mg qd for 5 days. **Sinusitis:** 500mg qd for 10-14 days or 750mg qd for 5 days. **CBP:** 500mg qd for 28 days. **Uncomplicated SSSI:** 500mg qd for 7-10 days. **Complicated SSSI/ Nosocomial Pneumonia:** 750mg qd for 7-14 days. **Inhalational Anthrax:** 500mg qd for 60 days. **Complicated SSSI/ Nosocomial Pneumonia/CAP/Sinusitis: CrCl 20-49mL/min:** 750mg, then 750mg q48h. **CrCl 10-19mL/min/Hemodialysis/ CAPD:** 750mg, then 500mg q48h. **ABECB/CAP/Sinusitis/Uncomplicated SSSI/CBP/Inhalational Anthrax: CrCl 20-49mL/min:** 500mg, then 250mg q24h. **CrCl 10-19mL/min/Hemodialysis/ CAPD:** 500mg, then 250mg q48h. **Complicated UTI/Acute Pyelonephritis:** 250mg qd for 10 days or 750mg qd for 5 days. **CrCl 10-19mL/min:** 250mg, then 250mg q48h or 750mg, then 500mg q48h. **Hemodialysis:** 750mg, then 500mg q48h. **Uncomplicated UTI:** 250mg qd for 3 days. Take oral solution 1 hr before or 2 hrs after eating. ***Pediatrics:* ≥6 months: >50kg:** 500mg q24h for 60 days. **<50kg:** 8mg/kg (not to exceed 250mg per dose) q12h for 60 days.	**BB:** Fluoroquinolones are associated with an increased risk of tendinitis and tendon rupture in all ages. Risk further increased in patients >60 yrs, patients taking corticosteroid drugs, and patients with kidney, heart, or lung transplants. **W/P:** Only administer injection via IV infusion over period of not less than 60 or 90 min, depending on dosage. Convulsions, toxic psychoses, increased ICP, CNS stimulation reported; d/c if any occur. Caution with CNS disorders that may predispose to seizures/lower seizure threshold (eg, epilepsy, renal insufficiency, drug therapy). Moderate to severe phototoxicity can occur. Serious/ fatal hypersensitivity reactions; d/c at first sign of rash. Colitis reported. May permit overgrowth of Clostridia. *Clostridium difficile*-associated diarrhea reported. Liver, hematologic (including agranulocytosis, thrombocytopenia) and renal toxicities may occur after multiple doses. Caution in renal insufficiency. Severe hepatotoxicity (eg, acute hepatitis) reported; d/c if signs and symptoms of hepatitis occur. Prolongation of QT interval and torsades de pointes reported; caution with any factors that may predispose to QTc prolongation or proarrhythmic conditions. Peripheral neuropathy, Stevens-Johnson syndrome reported. Causes musculoskeletal disorder in pediatrics and arthropathic effects in animals. More susceptible to QT interval prolongation and caution in elderly taking corticosteroids. **P/N:** Category C, not for use in nursing.	Nausea, diarrhea, headache, insomnia, constipation, pain, swelling, tendon tears.
Lomefloxacin HCl (Maxaquin)	**Tab:** 400mg*	***Adults:* ≥18 yrs: ABECB:** 400mg qd for 10 days. **Uncomplicated Cystitis:** 400mg qd for 3 days (*E.coli*) or 10 days (*K.pneumoniae, P.mirabilis, or S.saprophyticus*). **Complicated UTI:** 400mg qd for 14 days. **Hemodialysis/ CrCl >10 to <40mL/min: LD:** 400mg. **Maint:** 200mg qd. **Preoperative Prevention: TRPB:** 400mg single dose 1-6 hrs before procedure. **TUSP:** 400mg single dose 2-6 hrs before procedure.	**W/P:** Rare cases of torsades de pointes have been reported; avoid with known prolongation of the QT interval, uncorrected hypokalemia, concomitant treatment with Class IA (quinidine, procainamide) or class III (amiodarone, sotalol) antiarrhythmic agents. Moderate to severe phototoxicity, convulsions, pseudomembranous colitis, serious fatal hypersensitivity reactions reported. Avoid in pregnancy and nursing. Not for empiric treatment of *Pseudomonas* bacteremia or ABECB caused by *S.pneumoniae*. Caution with CNS disorder or those predisposed to seizures. Adjust dose in renal impairment. D/C if pain, inflammation, or tendon rupture occur. Increased risk of tendon rupture in patients receiving concomitant corticosteroids. Maintain adequate hydration. Rare cases of sensory or sensorimotor axonal polyneuropathy reported; d/c if symptoms of neuropathy occur. **P/N:** Category C, not for use in nursing.	Headache, nausea, photosensitivity, dizziness, diarrhea, abdominal pain.

*Scored. †Bold entries denote special dental considerations.
BB = black box warning; **W/P** = warnings/precautions; **Contra** = contraindications; **P/N** = pregnancy category rating and nursing considerations.

NAME	FORM/ STRENGTH	DOSAGE	WARNINGS/PRECAUTIONS & CONTRAINDICATIONS	ADVERSE EFFECTS†
Moxifloxacin HCl (Avelox)	**Inj:** 400mg/ 250mL; **Tab:** 400mg	***Adults:* ≥18 yrs: Sinusitis:** 400mg PO/ IV q24h for 10 days. **ABECB:** 400mg PO/IV q24h for 5 days. **Uncomplicated SSSI:** 400mg PO/IV q24h for 7 days. **Complicated SSSI:** 400mg PO/IV q24h for 7-21 days. **CAP:** 400mg PO/ IV q24h for 7-14 days. **Complicated Intra-Abdominal Infections:** 400mg PO/ IV q24h for 5-14 days.	**BB:** Fluoroquinolones are associated with an increased risk of tendinitis and tendon rupture in all ages. Risk further increased in patients >60 yrs, patients taking corticosteroid drugs, and patients with kidney, heart, or lung transplants. **W/P:** QT prolongation risk may increase if >65 yrs and may be dose or infusion-rate dependent; do not exceed recommended dose. Avoid with known QT interval prolongation, and uncorrected hypokalemia. Caution with ongoing proarrhythmic conditions (eg, significant bradycardia, acute MI). *Clostridium difficile*-associated diarrhea reported. Caution with CNS disorders (eg, severe cerebral arteriosclerosis, epilepsy). Tendon ruptures reported. D/C if convulsions, CNS effects, hypersensitivity reaction, or tendon rupture occurs. Rare cases of peripheral neuropathy reported. **P/N:** Category C, not for use in nursing.	Nausea, diarrhea, dizziness.
Norfloxacin (Noroxin)	**Tab:** 400mg	***Adults:* ≥18 yrs: Uncomplicated UTI Due To *E.coli, K.pneumonia, P.mirabilis*:** 400mg q12h for 3 days. **Uncomplicated UTI Due To Other Organisms:** 400mg q12h for 7-10 days. **Complicated UTI:** 400mg q12h for 10-21 days. **GFR ≤30mL/min/1.73m²:** 400mg qd for the duration listed above. **Uncomplicated Gonorrhea:** 800mg single dose. **Acute/Chronic Prostatitis:** 400mg q12h for 28 days. Take 1 hr before or 2 hrs after meals or milk/dairy products.	**BB:** Fluoroquinolones are associated with an increased risk of tendinitis and tendon rupture in all ages. Risk further increased in patients >60 yrs, patients taking corticosteroid drugs, and patients with kidney, heart, or lung transplants. **W/P:** Pseudomembranous colitis, convulsions, phototoxicity, peripheral neuropathy, and ruptures of the shoulder, hand, and Achilles tendons reported. Avoid in pregnancy and nursing mothers. Convulsions reported. Caution with renal dysfunction. D/C if CNS stimulation, increase in ICP, or toxic psychoses occurs. Not effective for treatment of syphilis. May exacerbate myasthenia gravis. Hemolytic reactions reported with G6P deficiency. *Clostridium difficile*-associated diarrhea reported. Caution in elderly taking corticosteroids. **Contra:** History of tendinitis or tendon rupture associated with use of quinolones. **P/N:** Category C, not for use in nursing.	Dizziness, nausea, headache, abdominal pain, asthenia.
Ofloxacin (Floxin)	**Tab:** 200mg, 300mg, 400mg	***Adults:* ≥18 yrs: ABECB/CAP/SSSI:** 400mg q12h for 10 days. **Cervicitis/ Urethritis:** 300mg q12h for 7 days. **Gonorrhea:** 400mg single dose. **PID:** 400mg q12h for 10-14 days. **Uncomplicated Cystitis:** 200mg q12h for 3 days (*E.coli* or *K.pneumoniae*) or 7 days (other pathogens). **Complicated UTI:** 200mg q12h for 10 days. **Prostatitis:** (*E.coli*) 300mg q12h for 6 weeks. **CrCl 20-50mL/min:** Dose q24h. **CrCl <20mL/ min:** After regular initial dose, give 50% of normal dose q24h. **Severe Hepatic Impairment: Max:** 400mg/day.	**BB:** Fluoroquinolones are associated with an increased risk of tendinitis and tendon rupture in all ages. Risk further increased in patients >60 yrs, patients taking corticosteroid drugs, and patients with kidney, heart or lung transplants. **W/P:** Convulsions, increased ICP, toxic psychosis, CNS stimulation, and serious, sometimes fatal, hypersensitivity reactions reported; d/c if any occur. *Clostridium difficile*-associated diarrhea and ruptures of shoulder, hand, and Achilles tendon reported. Not shown to be effective for syphilis. Safety and efficacy unknown in patients <18 yrs old, pregnancy, and nursing. Maintain adequate hydration. Caution with renal or hepatic dysfunction, risk for seizures, CNS disorder with predisposition to seizures. Avoid excessive sunlight. Monitor blood, renal, and hepatic function with prolonged therapy. Tendon ruptures	N/V, insomnia, headache, dizziness, diarrhea, external genital pruritus in women, vaginitis.

Table 6.2. PRESCRIBING INFORMATION FOR ANTIBIOTICS *(cont.)*

NAME	FORM/ STRENGTH	DOSAGE	WARNINGS/PRECAUTIONS & CONTRAINDICATIONS	ADVERSE EFFECTS†
FLUOROQUINOLONES *(cont.)*				
Ofloxacin (Floxin) *(cont.)*			reported. D/C immediately at the first appearance of skin rash, jaundice, or any other sign of hypersensitivity and supportive measures instituted. Drug therapy should be d/c if photosensitivity/ phototoxicity occurs. Medications should be avoided in patients with known prolongation of the QT interval, patients with uncorrected hypokalemia, and patients receiving Class IA (quinidine, procainamide), or Class III (amiodarone, sotalol) antiarrhythmic agents. Caution in elderly taking corticosteroids. **P/N:** Category C, not for use in nursing.	
MACROLIDES				
Azithromycin (Zithromax, Zmax)	(Zithromax) **Inj:** 500mg; **Sus:** 100mg/5mL [15mL], 200mg/5mL [15mL, 22.5mL, 30mL], 1g/pkt [3[s], 10[s]]; **Tab:** 250mg [Z-PAK, 6[s]], 500mg [TRI-PAK, 3[s]], 600mg; (Zmax) **Sus, Extended-Release:** 2g (27mg/mL)	***Adults:*** (Zithromax) **PO: CAP/Pharyngitis/Tonsillitis (2nd-line therapy)/SSSI:** 500mg on Day 1, then 250mg qd on Days 2-5. **COPD:** 500mg qd for 3 days or 500 mg on Day 1, then 250ng qd on Days 2-5. **ABS:** 500mg qd for 3 days. **Genital Ulcer Disease and Nongonococcal Urethritis/Cervicitis:** 1g single dose. **Gonococcal Urethritis/Cervicitis:** 2g single dose. **MAC Prophylaxis:** 1200mg once weekly. **MAC Treatment:** 600mg qd with ethambutol 15mg/kg/ day. **IV: CAP:** 500mg qd for at least 2 days, then 500mg PO qd to complete 7-10 day course. **PID:** 500mg qd for 1-2 days, then 250mg PO qd to complete 7 day course. (Zmax) **CAP/ Sinusitis:** 2g single dose. Take on empty stomach (1 hr before or 2 hrs after a meal). ***Pediatrics:*** **≥6 months: Otitis Media:** 30mg/kg single dose; 10mg/ kg qd for 3 days; or 10mg/kg qd on Day 1, then 5mg/kg qd on Days 2-5. **ABS:** 10mg/kg qd for 3 days. **CAP:** 10mg/kg qd on Day 1, then 5mg/kg qd on Days 2-5. **≥2 yrs: Pharyngitis/Tonsillitis:** 12mg/kg qd for 5 days. 1g sus not for pediatric use. (Zmax) **CAP/Sinusitis:** 60mg/kg (1ml/lb) single dose. Take on empty stomach (1 hr before or 2 hrs after a meal). **Max:** 2g single dose. Patients weighing >34kg should receive the adult dose.	**W/P:** Rare reports of angioedema, anaphylaxis, and dermatologic reactions including Stevens-Johnson syndrome and toxic epidermal necrolysis. D/C if allergic reaction occurs. Hypersensitivity reactions may recur after initial successful symptomatic treatment. *Clostridium difficile*-associated diarrhea reported. Caution with renal/hepatic dysfunction and patients with increased risk for prolonged cardiac repolarization. Exacerbation and new onset of symptoms of myasthenia gravis reported. Higher incidence of GI disturbance in patients with a GFR <10mL/min. Prolonged cardiac repolarization and QT interval, imparting a risk of developing cardiac arrhythmia and torsades de pointes, have been seen in treatment with other macrolides. Use in the absence of a proven or strongly suspected bacterial infection is unlikely to provide benefit to the patient and increases the risk of the development of drug-resistant bacteria. **P/N:** Category B, caution in nursing.	Diarrhea/loose stools, nausea, abdominal pain, smell/ **taste perversion.**
Clarithromycin (Biaxin, Biaxin XL)	(Biaxin) **Sus:** 125mg/5mL, 250mg/5mL [50mL, 100mL]; **Tab:** 250mg, 500mg; (Biaxin XL) **Tab, Extended-Release:** 500mg [PAC 14[s]]	***Adults:*** (Biaxin) **Pharyngitis/Tonsillitis:** 250mg q12h for 10 days. **Sinusitis:** 500mg q12h for 14 days. **ABECB:** 250-500mg q12h for 7-14 days. **SSSI/CAP:** 250mg q12h for 7-14 days. **MAC Prophylaxis/Treatment:** 500mg bid. **CrCl <30mL/min:** Give 50% dose or double interval. ***H.pylori:*** **Triple Therapy:** 500mg + amoxicillin 1g + omeprazole 20mg, all q12h for 10 days; or 500mg + amoxicillin 1g + lansoprazole 30mg, all q12h for 10-14 days. Give additional omeprazole 20mg qd for 18 days with active ulcer. **Dual Therapy:** 500mg q8h + omeprazole 40mg qd for 14 days (give additional omeprazole 20mg qd for 14 days with active ulcer); or 500mg q8h or q12h + ranitidine bismuth citrate	**W/P:** Avoid in pregnancy. *Clostridium difficile*-associated diarrhea reported. Adjust dose with severe renal impairment. Colchicine toxicity reported; avoid concomitant use especially in elderly. **Contra:** Concomitant cisapride, pimozide, astemizole, terfenadine, ergotamine or dihydroergotamine, or other macrolide antibiotics. **P/N:** Category C, caution in nursing.	Diarrhea, N/V, **abnormal taste**, dyspepsia, abdominal pain, headache, rash.

*Scored. †Bold entries denote special dental considerations.

BB = black box warning; **W/P** = warnings/precautions; **Contra** = contraindications; **P/N** = pregnancy category rating and nursing considerations.

NAME	FORM/ STRENGTH	DOSAGE	WARNINGS/PRECAUTIONS & CONTRAINDICATIONS	ADVERSE EFFECTS†
Clarithromycin (Biaxin, Biaxin XL) *(cont.)*		400mg q12h for 14 days (give additional ranitidine bismuth citrate 400mg bid for 14 days with active ulcer). Avoid combination with ranitidine bismuth citrate if CrCl <25mL/min. (Biaxin XL) **Sinusitis:** 1000mg qd for 14 days. **ABECB/CAP:** 1000mg qd for 7 days. **CrCl <30mL/min:** Give 50% dose or double interval. Take with food. ***Pediatrics:* ≥6 months:** (Biaxin) **Usual:** 7.5mg/kg q12h for 10 days. **≥20 months: MAC Prophylaxis/ Treatment:** 7.5mg/kg bid, up to 500mg bid. **CrCl <30mL/min:** Give 50% dose or double interval.		
Erythromycin (ERYC, Ery-Tab, PCE) **Erythromycin Stearate** (Erythrocin)	**Cap, Delayed-Release:** (ERYC) 250mg; **Tab:** (Erythrocin) 250mg, 500mg; **Tab, Delayed-Release:** (Ery-Tab) 250mg, 333mg, 500mg; **Tab, Extended-Release:** (PCE) 333mg, 500mg	***Adults:* Usual:** 250mg q6h, 333mg q8h, or 500mg q12h without food. **Max:** 4g/day. Do not take bid when dose is ≥1g/day. Treat strep infections for at least 10 days. **Streptococcal Infection Long-Term Prophylaxis of Rheumatic Fever:** 250mg bid. **Chlamydial Urogenital Infection During Pregnancy:** 500mg qid or 666mg q8h for at least 7 days, or 500mg q12h, 333mg q8h, or 250mg qid for at least 14 days. **Urethral/Endocervical/Rectal Chlamydial Infections and Nongonococcal Urethritis:** 500mg qid or 666mg q8h for at least 7 days. **Primary Syphilis:** 30-40g in divided doses over 10-15 days. **Acute PID:** 500mg (erythromycin lactobionate) IV q6h for 3 days, then 250mg PO q6h, 333mg PO q8h, or 500mg PO q12h for 7 days. **Intestinal Amebiasis:** 500mg q12h, 333mg q8h, or 250mg q6h for 10-14 days. **Pertussis:** 40-50mg/kg/day in divided doses for 5-14 days. **Legionnaires' Disease:** 1-4g/day in divided doses. ***Pediatrics:* Usual:** 30-50mg/kg/day in divided doses without food. **Severe Infections:** May double dose. **Max:** 4g/day. Treat strep infections for at least 10 days. **Streptococcal Infection Long-Term Prophylaxis of Rheumatic Fever:** 250mg bid. **Chlamydial Conjunctivitis of Newborns/Chlamydial Pneumonia in Infancy: (Sus)** 12.5mg/kg qid for 2 weeks and 3 weeks, respectively. **Intestinal Amebiasis:** 30-50mg/kg/day in divided doses for 10-14 days.	**W/P:** *Clostridium difficile*-associated diarrhea, hepatic dysfunction, and prolonged QT syndrome reported. Caution with impaired hepatic function. May aggravate weakness of patients with myasthenia gravis. Erythromycin does not reach adequate concentrations in fetus to prevent congenital syphilis. **Contra:** Concomitant terfenadine, astemizole, pimozide, or cisapride. **P/N:** Category B, caution in nursing.	Abdominal pain, N/V, diarrhea, anorexia, abnormal LFTs, allergic reactions, hepatic dysfunction, superinfection (prolonged use).
Erythromycin Ethylsuccinate (E.E.S., EryPed)	**Sus:** (E.E.S.) 200mg/5mL, 400mg/5mL; (EryPed) 100mg/2.5mL [50mL], 200mg/5mL, 400mg/5mL [5mL, 100mL, 200mL]; **Tab:** (E.E.S.) 400mg; **Tab, Chewable:** (EryPed) 200mg*	***Adults:* Usual:** 1600mg/day in divided doses given q6h, q8h, or q12h. **Max:** 4g/day. Treat strep infections for at least 10 days. **Streptococcal Infection Prophylaxis with Rheumatic Heart Disease:** 400mg bid. **Urethritis (*C.trachomatis or U.urealyticum*):** 800mg tid for 7 days. **Primary Syphilis:** 48-64g in divided doses over 10-15 days. **Intestinal Amebiasis:** 400mg qid for 10-14 days. **Pertussis:** 40-50mg/kg/day in divided doses for 5-14 days. **Legionnaires' Disease:** 1.6-4g/day in divided doses. ***Pediatrics:* Usual:** 30-50mg/kg/day in divided doses q6h, q8h, or q12h. **Severe Infections:** May double dose. Treat strep infections for at least 10 days. **Streptococcal Infection Prophylaxis with Rheumatic Heart Disease:** 400mg bid. **Intestinal Amebiasis:** 30-50mg/kg/day in divided doses for 10-14 days.	**W/P:** *Clostridium difficile*-associated diarrhea, hepatic dysfunction reported. Caution with impaired hepatic function. May aggravate weakness of patients with myasthenia gravis. **Contra:** Concomitant terfenadine, astemizole, cisapride, or pimozide. **P/N:** Category B, caution in nursing.	N/V, abdominal pain, diarrhea, anorexia, hepatic dysfunction, abnormal LFTs, allergic reactions, superinfection (prolonged use).

Table 6.2. PRESCRIBING INFORMATION FOR ANTIBIOTICS *(cont.)*

NAME	FORM/ STRENGTH	DOSAGE	WARNINGS/PRECAUTIONS & CONTRAINDICATIONS	ADVERSE EFFECTS†
MACROLIDE/SULFONAMIDE				
Erythromycin Ethylsuccinate/ Sulfisoxazole Acetyl (Pediazole)	**Sus:** (Erythromycin Ethylsuccinate/Sulfisoxazole Acetyl) 200mg-600mg/5mL [100mL, 150mL, 200mL]	***Pediatrics:*** **≥2 months:** Dose based on 50mg/kg/day erythromycin or 150mg/kg/day sulfisoxazole given tid-qid for 10 days. **Max:** 6g/day sulfisoxazole.	**W/P:** Pseudomembranous colitis, hepatic dysfunction reported. Severe, fatal allergic reactions reported with sulfonamides. Caution with hepatic or renal dysfunction, bronchial asthma, and severe allergies. May aggravate myasthenia gravis. Erythromycin does not reach adequate concentrations in fetus to prevent congenital syphilis. Hemolysis may occur in G6P-deficiency patients. Sulfonamides not for treatment of group A β-hemolytic infections. **Contra:** Pediatrics <2 months old, pregnant women at term, mothers nursing infants <2 months old, concomitant terfenadine. **P/N:** Category C, not for use in nursing.	N/V, abdominal pain, diarrhea, anorexia, hepatic dysfunction, abnormal LFTs, allergic reactions, tachycardia, syncope, blood dyscrasias, BUN elevation, edema, superinfection.
NITROIMIDAZOLES				
Metronidazole (Flagyl ER)	**Tab, Extended-Release:** 750mg	***Adults:*** 750mg qd for 7 days. Take 1 hr before or 2 hrs after meals. **Elderly:** Adjust dose based on serum levels. **Hepatic Disease:** Give lower dose cautiously; monitor levels.	**BB:** Metronidazole has been shown to be carcinogenic in mice and rats. Unnecessary use of the drug should be avoided. **W/P:** Seizures and peripheral neuropathy reported. D/C if abnormal neurological signs occur. Caution with severe hepatic impairment, blood dyscrasias, or CNS diseases. Monitor leukocytes before and after therapy. **Contra:** Treatment during 1st trimester of pregnancy. **P/N:** Category B, not for use in nursing.	Headache, vaginitis, N/V, metallic taste, dizziness, seizures, peripheral neuropathy, leukopenia, urticaria, rash, dysuria, vaginal candidiasis.
Metronidazole (Flagyl)	**Cap:** 375mg; **Tab:** 250mg, 500mg	***Adults:*** **Trichomoniasis (Female/Male Sex Partner): Seven-Day Treatment: (Cap/Tab)** 375mg bid or 250mg tid for 7 days. **One-Day Therapy: (Tab)** 2g as single dose or in two divided doses of 1g each given in the same day. If repeat course needed, reconfirm diagnosis and allow 4-6 weeks between courses. **Acute Intestinal Amebiasis:** 750mg PO tid for 5-10 days. **Amebic Liver Abscess:** 500mg or 750mg PO tid for 5-10 days. **Anaerobic Bacterial Infection:** Usually IV therapy initially if serious. 7.5mg/kg PO q6h for 7-10 days or longer. **Max:** 4g/24 hrs. **Elderly:** Adjust dose based on serum levels. **Hepatic Disease:** Give lower dose cautiously; monitor levels. ***Pediatrics:*** **Amebiasis:** 35-50mg/kg/24 hrs given tid for 10 days.	**BB:** Metronidazole has been shown to be carcinogenic in mice and rats. Unnecessary use of the drug should be avoided. **W/P:** Seizures and peripheral neuropathy reported. D/C if abnormal neurological signs occur. Caution with severe hepatic impairment, blood dyscrasias, or CNS diseases. Monitor leukocytes before and after therapy. **Contra:** Treatment during 1st trimester of pregnancy. **P/N:** Category B, not for use in nursing.	Seizures, peripheral neuropathy, N/V, headache, anorexia, urticaria, rash, metallic taste, dysuria, vaginal candidiasis, dizziness, leukopenia.
Metronidazole HCl (Flagyl IV)	**Inj:** 500mg/ 100mL	***Adults:*** **Anaerobic Infections: LD:** 15mg/kg IV. **Maint:** 7.5mg/kg IV q6h, starting 6 hrs after LD. Usual duration is 7-10 days or longer. **Max:** 4g/24 hrs. **Surgical Prophylaxis:** 15mg/kg given 1 hr before surgery, then 7.5mg/kg given 6 hrs and 12 hrs after initial dose.	**BB:** Metronidazole has been shown to be carcinogenic in mice and rats. Unnecessary use of the drug should be avoided. **W/P:** Seizures and peripheral neuropathy reported. D/C if abnormal neurological signs occur. Caution with severe hepatic impairment, blood dyscrasias, or CNS diseases. Monitor leukocytes before and after therapy. Metronidazole IV is effective in *B.fragilis* infections resistant to clindamycin, chloramphenicol, or PCN. **P/N:** Category B, not for use in nursing.	Convulsive seizures, peripheral neuropathy, N/V, headache, leukopenia, rash, vaginal candidiasis, thrombophlebitis.

*Scored. †Bold entries denote special dental considerations.
BB = black box warning; **W/P** = warnings/precautions; **Contra** = contraindications; **P/N** = pregnancy category rating and nursing considerations.

NAME	FORM/ STRENGTH	DOSAGE	WARNINGS/PRECAUTIONS & CONTRAINDICATIONS	ADVERSE EFFECTS†
PENICILLINS				
AMINOPENICILLIN/β-LACTAMASE INHIBITORS				
Amoxicillin/ Clavulanate Potassium (Augmentin)	**(Amoxicillin-Clavulanate) Sus:** 125-31.25mg/ 5mL [75mL, 100mL, 150mL], 200-28.5mg/ 5mL [50mL, 75mL, 100mL], 250-62.5mg/ 5mL [75mL, 100mL, 150mL], 400-57mg/ 5mL [50mL, 75mL, 100mL]; **Tab:** 250-125mg, 500-125mg, 875-125mg*; **Tab, Chewable:** 200-28.5mg, 250-62.5mg, 400-57mg	***Adults/Pediatrics:* ≥40kg:** (Dose based on amoxicillin) 500mg q12h or 250mg q8h. **Severe Infections/RTI:** 875mg q12h or 500mg q8h. May use 125mg/5mL or 250mg/5mL sus in place of 500mg tab and 200mg/5mL sus or 400mg/5mL sus in place of 875mg tab. **CrCl <30mL/min:** Do not give 875mg tab. **CrCl 10-30mL/min:** 250-500mg q12h. **CrCl <10mL/min:** 250-500mg q24h. **Hemodialysis:** 250-500mg q24h, give additional dose during and at end of dialysis. ***Pediatrics:*** (Dose based on amoxicillin) **≥12 weeks: Sinusitis/ Otitis Media/LRTI/Severe Infections:** (Sus/Tab, Chewable) 45mg/kg/day given q12h or 40mg/kg/day given q8h. Treat otitis media for 10 days. **Less Severe Infections:** 25mg/kg/day given q12h or 20mg/kg/day given q8h. **<12 weeks:** 15mg/kg q12h (use 125mg/5mL sus).	**W/P:** Serious, sometimes fatal, hypersensitivity reactions reported with PCN therapy. *Clostridium difficile*-associated diarrhea reported. Possibility of superinfection. Caution with hepatic dysfunction. Monitor renal, hepatic, and hematopoietic functions with prolonged use. Avoid with mononucleosis. Take with food to reduce GI upset. The 200mg and 400mg chewable tabs and 200mg/5mL and 400mg/5mL sus contain phenylalanine. The 250mg tab and chewable tab are not interchangeable due to unequal clavulanic acid amounts. Only use 250mg tab in pediatrics ≥40kg. False (+) for urine glucose with Clinitest and Benedict's or Fehling's solution. **P/N:** Category B, caution in nursing.	Diarrhea/loose stools, N/V, skin rashes, urticaria, vaginitis.
Amoxicillin/ Clavulanate Potassium (Augmentin ES-600)	**Sus:** (Amoxicillin-Clavulanate) 600mg-42.9mg/ 5mL [75mL, 125mL, 200mL]	***Pediatrics:* 3 months-12 yrs: <40kg:** (Dose based on amoxicillin) 45mg/kg q12h for 10 days.	**W/P:** Serious, sometimes fatal, hypersensitivity reactions reported with PCN therapy. *Clostridium difficile*-associated diarrhea reported. Possibility of superinfection. Caution with hepatic dysfunction. Monitor renal, hepatic, and hematopoietic functions with prolonged use. Avoid with mononucleosis. Contains phenylalanine. False (+) for urine glucose with Clinitest and Benedict's or Fehling's solution. **P/N:** Category B, caution in nursing.	Diaper rash, diarrhea, vomiting, moniliasis, rash.
Amoxicillin/ Clavulanate Potassium (Augmentin XR)	**Tab, Extended-Release:** (Amoxicillin-Clavulanate) 1000mg-62.5mg	***Adults:* Sinusitis:** 2 tabs q12h for 10 days. **CAP:** 2 tabs q12h for 7-10 days. Take at start of a meal. ***Pediatrics:* ≥16 yrs: Sinusitis:** 2 tabs q12h for 10 days. **CAP:** 2 tabs q12h for 7-10 days. Take at the start of a meal.	**W/P:** Serious, sometimes fatal, hypersensitivity reactions reported with PCN therapy. Clostridium difficile-associated diarrhea reported. Possibility of superinfection. Caution with hepatic dysfunction. Monitor renal, hepatic, and hematopoietic functions with prolonged use. Avoid with mononucleosis. Not interchangeable with other Augmentin products due to unequal clavulanic acid amounts. False (+) for urine glucose with Clinitest and Benedict's or Fehling's solution. **Contra:** Severe renal impairment (CrCl <30mL/min), hemodialysis. **P/N:** Category B, caution in nursing.	Diarrhea, nausea, genital moniliasis, abdominal pain, vaginal mycosis.
BROAD-SPECTRUM PENICILLINS				
Piperacillin Sodium	**Inj:** 2g, 3g, 4g	***Adults/Pediatrics:* ≥12 yrs: Usual:** 3-4g IM/IV q4-6h. **Max:** 24g/day; **IM:** 2g/ site. **Serious Infections:** 200-300mg/kg/ day IV divided q4-6h. **Complicated UTI:** 125-200mg/kg/day IV divided q6-8h. **Uncomplicated UTI/CAP:** 100-125mg/ kg/day IM/IV divided q6-12h. **Uncomplicated Gonorrhea:** 2g IM single dose with 1g PO probenecid 1/2 hr before injection. **Surgical Prophylaxis:** 2g IV 20-30 min just prior to anesthesia (See PI for follow-up dosing). **Renal Impairment: Uncomplicated/Complicated UTI: CrCl <20mL/min:** 3g q12h. **Complicated UTI: CrCl 20-40mL/min:** 3g q8h.	**W/P:** Serious, sometimes fatal, hypersensitivity reactions reported with PCN therapy. *Clostridium difficile*-associated diarrhea reported. Cross-sensitivity to cephalosporins. Monitor renal, hepatic, and hematopoietic functions with prolonged use. D/C if bleeding manifestations occur; increased risk with renal failure. Prolonged use may cause superinfections. May experience neuromuscular excitability or convulsions with higher than recommended doses. Contains 1.85mEq/g sodium; caution with salt restriction. Monitor electrolytes periodically with low potassium levels.	Thrombophlebitis, erythema and pain at injection site, diarrhea, headache, dizziness, anaphylaxis, rash, superinfections.

Table 6.2. PRESCRIBING INFORMATION FOR ANTIBIOTICS *(cont.)*

NAME	FORM/ STRENGTH	DOSAGE	WARNINGS/PRECAUTIONS & CONTRAINDICATIONS	ADVERSE EFFECTS†
PENICILLINS *(cont.)*				
BROAD-SPECTRUM PENICILLINS *(cont.)*				
Piperacillin Sodium *(cont.)*		**Serious Infection: CrCl 20-40mL/min:** 4g q8h. **CrCl <20mL/min:** 4g q12h. **Hemodialysis:** Give 1g additional dose after each dialysis. **Max:** 2g q8h. Usual treatment is for 7-10 days; treat gynecologic infections for 3-10 days; treat *S.pyogenes* infections for at least 10 days.	Increased incidence of rash and fever in cystic fibrosis. Continue treatment for at least 48-72 hrs after patient becomes asymptomatic. **P/N:** Category B, caution in nursing.	
BROAD-SPECTRUM PENICILLINS/β-LACTAMASE INHIBITORS				
Piperacillin Sodium/ Tazobactam (Zosyn)	**Inj:** (Piperacillin-Tazobactam) 40mg-5mg/mL, 60mg-7.5mg/mL, 2g-0.25g, 3g-0.375g, 4g-0.5g, 2g-0.25g/50mL, 3g-0.375g/50mL, 4g-0.5g/100mL, 36g-4.5g	***Adults/Pediatrics*** **>40kg: Usual:** 3.375g q6h for 7-10 days. **CrCl 20-40mL:** 2.25g q6h. **CrCl <20mL/min:** 2.25g q8h. **Hemodialysis/CAPD:** 2.25g q12h. Give 1 additional 0.75g dose after each dialysis period. **Nosocomial Pneumonia:** 4.5g q6h for 7-14 days plus aminoglycoside. **CrCl 20-40mL/min:** 3.375g q6h. **CrCl <20mL/min:** 2.25g q6h. **Hemodialysis/CAPD: Max:** 2.25g q8h. Give 1 additional 0.75g dose after each dialysis period. ***Pediatrics:*** **>9 months: ≤40kg: Appendicitis/Peritonitis:** 100mg piperacillin-12.5mg tazobactam/kg q8h. **2-9 months:** 80mg piperacillin-10mg tazobactam/kg q8h.	**W/P:** Serious, fatal hypersensitivity reactions may occur with PCN allergy. *Clostridium difficile*-associated diarrhea reported. D/C if bleeding manifestations occur. May experience neuromuscular excitability or convulsions with higher doses. Contains 2.79mEq/g Na; caution with restricted salt intake. Increased incidence of rash and fever in cystic fibrosis. Monitor electrolyte periodically with low K^+ reserves. Therapy may lead to emergence of resistant organisms that can cause superinfections. Caution with renal impairment (CrCl <40mL/min). **P/N:** Category B, caution in nursing.	Diarrhea, headache, constipation, N/V, insomnia, rash, dyspepsia, pruritus.
Ticarcillin Disodium/ Clavulanate Potassium (Timentin)	**Inj:** (Ticarcillin-Clavulanate) 3g-100mg, 3g-100mg/100mL, 30g-1g	***Adults:*** **≥60kg: UTI/Systemic Infection:** 3g-100mg (3.1g vial) IV q4-6h. **Gynecologic Infections: Moderate:** 200mg/kg/day ticarcillin IV given q6h. **Severe:** 300mg/kg/day ticarcillin IV given q4h. **<60kg: Usual:** (based on ticarcillin) 200-300mg/kg/day ticarcillin IV given q4-6h. **Renal Impairment: LD:** 3.1g. **Maint: CrCl >60mL/min:** 3.1g q4h. **CrCl 30-60mL/min:** 2g IV q4h. **CrCl 10-30mL/min:** 2g IV q8h. **CrCl <10mL/min:** 2g IV q12h (2g IV q24h with hepatic dysfunction). **Peritoneal Dialysis:** 3.1g IV q12h. **Hemodialysis:** 2g IV q12h, and 3.1g after each dialysis. ***Pediatrics:*** **≥3 months: ≥60kg: Mild to Moderate:** 3g-100mg (3.1g vial) IV q6h. **Severe:** 3g-100mg (3.1g vial) IV q4h. **<60 kg:** (based on ticarcillin) **Mild to Moderate:** 50mg/kg ticarcillin IV q6h. **Severe:** 50mg/kg ticarcillin IV q4h.	**W/P:** Serious, sometimes fatal, hypersensitivity reactions reported with PCN therapy. *Clostridium difficile*-associated diarrhea reported. Prolonged use may result in overgrowth of nonsusceptible organisms. Risk of convulsions with high doses, especially with renal impairment. Monitor renal, hepatic, hematopoietic functions, and serum K^+ with prolonged therapy. Caution with fluid and electrolyte imbalance; hypokalemia reported. Clotting time, platelet aggregation, and PT abnormalities may occur especially with renal impairment; d/c therapy. Continue therapy for at least 2 days after signs/symptoms disappear. Caution in elderly patients with impaired renal function. **P/N:** Category B, caution in nursing.	Hypersensitivity reactions, headache, giddiness, **taste/ smell disturbances**, stomatitis, flatulence, N/V, diarrhea, hematologic disturbances, hepatic/ renal function tests abnormalities, local reactions.
PENICILLINS				
Dicloxacillin Sodium (Dicloxacillin)	**Cap:** 250mg, 500mg	***Adults:*** **Mild-Moderate Infection:** 125mg q6h. **Severe Infection:** 250mg q6h for at least 14 days. ***Pediatrics:*** **<40kg: Mild-Moderate Infection:** 12.5mg/kg/day in divided doses q6h. **Severe Infection:** 25mg/kg/day in divided doses q6h for at least 14 days.	**W/P:** Serious, fatal hypersensitivity reactions reported. Pseudomembranous colitis has been reported; toxin produced by *Clostridium difficile* is the primary cause. Caution with history of allergy and/or asthma. Monitor renal, hepatic, and hematopoietic function with prolonged use. Not for use as initial therapy with serious, life-threatening infections, or with N/V, gastric dilation, cardiospasm, or intestinal hypermotility. **P/N:** Category B, caution in nursing.	Allergic reactions, N/V, diarrhea, stomatitis, **black or hairy tongue**, superinfection (prolonged use), hepatotoxicity.
Penicillin G Benzathine (Bicillin L-A)	**Inj:** 600,000U/mL	***Adults:*** **Group A Strep: URTI:** 1.2MU IM single dose. **Primary/Secondary/Latent Syphilis:** 2.4MU IM single dose. **Late Syphilis (Tertiary/Neurosyphilis):**	**BB:** Not for IV use nor for admix with other IV solutions. Cardiorespiratory arrest and death reported with inadvertent IV administration. **W/P:** Serious, fatal	Maculopapular/ exfoliative dermatitis, urticaria, **laryngeal edema**, fever,

†Bold entries denote special dental considerations.
BB = black box warning; **W/P** = warnings/precautions; **Contra** = contraindications; **P/N** = pregnancy category rating and nursing considerations.

NAME	FORM/ STRENGTH	DOSAGE	WARNINGS/PRECAUTIONS & CONTRAINDICATIONS	ADVERSE EFFECTS†
Penicillin G Benzathine (Bicillin L-A) *(cont.)*		2.4MU IM every 7 days for 3 doses. **Yaws/Bejel/Pinta:** 1.2MU IM single dose. **Rheumatic Fever/Glomerulonephritis Prophylaxis:** 1.2MU IM once a month or 600,000U IM every 2 weeks. Administer IM into upper, outer quadrant of buttock. ***Pediatrics:*** **Group A Strep: URTI: Older Pediatrics:** 900,000U IM single dose. **Infants & <60 lbs:** 300,000-600,000U IM single dose. **Congenital Syphilis: 2-12 yrs:** Adjust dose based on adult schedule. **<2 yrs:** 50,000U/kg IM single dose. **Rheumatic Fever/Glomerulonephritis Prophylaxis:** 1.2MU IM once a month or 600,000U every 2 weeks. Administer IM into upper, outer quadrant of buttock. Use the midlateral aspect of thigh in neonates, infants, and small children.	anaphylactic reactions reported; increased risk with hypersensitivity to PCNs, cephalosporins, and other allergens. Pseudomembranous colitis reported. Avoid IV, intra-arterial administration, or injection into/near major peripheral nerves or blood vessels; may cause severe neurovascular and neurological damage. IM administration into anterolateral thigh may cause quadriceps femoris fibrosis and atrophy. Caution with asthma. May result in overgrowth of nonsusceptible organisms. Monitor culture after therapy completion to determine eradication. **Contra:** Do not inject into or near an artery or nerve. **P/N:** Category B, caution in nursing.	pseudomembranous colitis, hemolytic anemia, leukopenia, thrombocytopenia, neuropathy, nephropathy.
Penicillin G Benzathine (Permapen)	**Inj:** 600,000 U/mL	***Adults:*** **Streptococcal Infection:** 1.2 MU IM single dose. **Primary/Secondary/Latent Syphilis:** 1 MU IM single dose. **Late (Tertiary/Neurosyphilis) Syphilis:** 3 MU IM every 7 days for total of 6-9 MU. **Yaws/Bejel/Pinta:** 1.2 MU IM single dose. **Rheumatic Fever/Glomerulonephritis Prophylaxis:** 1.2 MU IM once monthly or 600,000 U IM twice monthly. Use upper outer quadrant of buttock. Rotate inj site. ***Pediatrics:*** **≤12 yrs:** Adjust dose according to age and wt and severity of infection. **Streptococcal Infection:** 900,000 U IM single dose in older children. **Congenital Syphilis: <2 yrs:** 50,000 U/kg IM single dose. **2-12 yrs:** Adjust dose based on adult schedule. Use midlateral aspect of thigh in infants and small children. May divide dose between 2 buttocks in peds <2 yrs. Rotate inj site.	**W/P:** Caution in newborns; evaluate organ system function frequently. Evaluate renal, hepatic, and hematopoietic systems with prolonged therapy. Serious, fatal anaphylactic reactions reported; increased risk with hypersensitivity to PCNs, cephalosporins, and other allergens. Avoid IV, intra-arterial administration, or injection into/near major peripheral nerves or blood vessels as this may cause severe neurovascular damage. May result in overgrowth of nonsusceptible organisms. Avoid subcutaneous and fat-layer injections. Take culture after therapy completion to determine streptococci eradication. **P/N:** Category B, caution in nursing.	Skin eruptions, urticaria, **laryngeal edema**, anaphylaxis, fever, eosinophilia.
Penicillin G Benzathine/ Penicillin G Procaine (Bicillin C-R 900/300)	**Inj:** (Penicillin G Benzathine-Penicillin G Procaine) 900,000-300,000U/ 2mL	***Pediatrics:*** **Group A Strep: URTI/SSTI/ Scarlet Fever/Erysipelas:** 1.2MU IM single dose. **Pneumococcal Infections (Except Meningitis):** 1.2MU IM every 2-3 days until temperature is normal for 48 hrs. Administer IM into upper, outer quadrant of buttock. Use midlateral aspect of thigh in neonates, infants, and small children.	**BB:** Not for IV use nor for admix with other IV solutions. Cardiorespiratory arrest and death reported with inadvertent IV administration. **W/P:** Serious, fatal anaphylactic reactions reported; increased risk with hypersensitivity to penicillin, cephalosporins, and other allergens. *Clostridium difficile*-associated diarrhea reported. Avoid IV, intra-arterial administration, or injection into/near major peripheral nerves or blood vessels as this may cause severe neurovascular and neurological damage. IM administration into anterolateral thigh may cause quadriceps femoris fibrosis and atrophy. Caution with asthma. Avoid with procaine sensitivity. May result in overgrowth of nonsusceptible organisms. Monitor culture after therapy completion to determine eradication. Monitor renal and hematopoietic systems periodically with prolonged and high-dose therapy. **Contra:** Do not inject into or near an artery or nerve. **P/N:** Category B, caution in nursing.	Maculopapular/ exfoliative dermatitis, urticaria, **laryngeal edema**, fever, pseudomembranous colitis, hemolytic anemia, leukopenia, thrombocytopenia, neuropathy, nephropathy.

Table 6.2. PRESCRIBING INFORMATION FOR ANTIBIOTICS *(cont.)*

NAME	FORM/ STRENGTH	DOSAGE	WARNINGS/PRECAUTIONS & CONTRAINDICATIONS	ADVERSE EFFECTS†
PENICILLINS *(cont.)*				
PENICILLINS *(cont.)*				
Penicillin G Benzathine/ Penicillin G Procaine (Bicillin C-R)	**Inj:** (Penicillin G Benzathine-Penicillin G Procaine) 300,000-300,000U/mL [2mL]	***Adults:*** **Group A Strep: URTI/SSTI/ Scarlet Fever/Erysipelas:** 2.4MU IM. Treat at a single session using multiple IM sites, or use an alternative schedule and give 1/2 of the total dose on Day 1 and 1/2 on Day 3. **Pneumococcal Infections (Except Meningitis):** 1.2MU IM, repeat every 2-3 days until temperature is normal for 48 hrs. Administer IM into upper, outer quadrant of buttock. ***Pediatrics:*** **Group A Strep: URTI/SSTI/Scarlet Fever/Erysipelas: >60 lbs:** 2.4MU IM. **30-60 lbs:** 900,000U-1.2MU IM. **<30 lbs:** 600,000U IM. Treat at a single session using multiple IM sites, or use an alternative schedule and give 1/2 of the total dose on Day 1 and 1/2 on Day 3. **Pneumococcal Infections (Except Meningitis):** 600,000U IM, repeat every 2-3 days until temperature is normal for 48 hrs. Administer IM into upper, outer quadrant of buttock. Use the midlateral aspect of thigh in neonates, infants, and small children.	**BB:** Not for IV use nor for admix with other IV solutions. Cardiorespiratory arrest and death reported with inadvertent IV administration. **W/P:** Serious, fatal anaphylactic reactions reported; increased risk with hypersensitivity to PCNs, cephalosporins, and other allergens. *Clostridium difficile*-associated diarrhea reported. Avoid IV, intra-arterial administration, or injection into/near major peripheral nerves or blood vessels as this may cause severe neurovascular and neurological damage. IM administration into anterolateral thigh may cause quadriceps femoris fibrosis and atrophy. Caution with asthma. Avoid with procaine sensitivity. May result in overgrowth of nonsusceptible organisms. Monitor culture after therapy completion to determine eradication. Monitor renal and hematopoietic systems periodically with prolonged and high-dose therapy. **Contra:** Do not inject into or near an artery or nerve. **P/N:** Category B, caution in nursing.	Maculopapular/ exfoliative dermatitis, urticaria, **laryngeal edema**, fever, pseudomembranous colitis, hemolytic anemia, leukopenia, thrombocytopenia, neuropathy, nephropathy.
Penicillin G Potassium (Pfizerpen)	**Inj:** 1MU, 5MU, 20MU	***Adults:*** **Anthrax/Gonorrheal Endocarditis/Severe Infections (Streptococci, Pneumococci, Staphylococci):** Minimum of 5MU/day. **Syphilis:** Administer in hospital. Determine dose and duration based on age and wt. **Meningococcic Meningitis:** 1-2MU IM q2h or 20-30MU/ day continuous IV. **Actinomycosis:** 1-6MU/day for cervicofacial cases; 10-20MU/day for thoracic and abdominal disease. **Clostridial Infections:** 20MU/ day (adjunct to antitoxin). **Fusospirochetal Severe Infections:** 5-10MU/ day for oropharynx, lower respiratory tract, and genital area infection. **Rat-bite Fever:** 12-15MU/day for 3-4 weeks. **Listeria Endocarditis:** 15-20MU/day for 4 weeks. **Pasteurella Bacteremia/ Meningitis:** 4-6MU/day for 2 weeks. **Erysipeloid Endocarditis:** 2-20MU/ day for 4-6 weeks. **Gram Negative Bacillary Bacteremia:** 20-80MU/day. **Diphtheria (carrier state):** 0.3-0.4MU/ day in divided doses for 10-12 days. **Endocarditis Prophylaxis:** 1MU IM mixed with 0.6MU procaine penicillin G 0.5-1 hr before procedure. **Renal/Cardiac/ Vascular Dysfunction:** Consider dose reduction. For streptococcal infection, treat for minimum 10 days. ***Pediatrics:*** **Listeria Infections: Neonates:** 0.5-1MU/ day. **Congenital Syphilis:** Administer in hospital. Determine dose and duration based on age and wt. **Endocarditis Prophylaxis:** 30,000U/kg IM mixed with 0.6MU procaine penicillin G 0.5-1 hr before procedure. For streptococcal infection, treat for minimum 10 days.	**W/P:** Serious, fatal anaphylactic reactions reported; increased risk with hypersensitivity to PCNs, cephalosporins, and other allergens. Avoid IV, intra-arterial administration, or injection into/near major peripheral nerves or blood vessels; may cause severe neurovascular damage. Take culture after therapy completion to determine streptococci eradication. Caution with history of significant allergies or asthma. May result in overgrowth of nonsusceptible organisms. Evaluate renal, hepatic, and hematopoietic systems with prolonged therapy. Administer slowly to avoid electrolyte imbalance from potassium or sodium content; monitor electrolytes and consider dose reductions with renal, cardiac, or vascular dysfunction. Caution in newborns; evaluate organ system function frequently. **P/N:** Category B, caution in nursing.	Skin rash (eg, maculopapular eruption, exfoliative dermatitis) urticaria, chills, fever, edema, arthralgia, prostration, anaphylaxis, arrhythmias, cardiac arrest, Jarisch-Herxheimer reaction.

†Bold entries denote special dental considerations.
BB = black box warning; **W/P** = warnings/precautions; **Contra** = contraindications; **P/N** = pregnancy category rating and nursing considerations.

NAME	FORM/ STRENGTH	DOSAGE	WARNINGS/PRECAUTIONS & CONTRAINDICATIONS	ADVERSE EFFECTS†
Penicillin V Potassium (Veetids)	**Sus:** 125mg/5mL, 250mg/5mL [100mL, 200mL]; **Tab:** 250mg, 500mg	***Adults:*** **Usual: Streptococcal Infections (Scarlet Fever/Erysipelas/Upper Respiratory Tract):** 125-250mg q6-8h for 10 days. **Pneumococcal Infections (Otitis Media/Respiratory Tract):** 250-500mg q6h until afebrile for at least 2 days. **Staphylococcus Infections (Skin/Soft Tissue):** 250-500mg q6-8h. **Fusospirochetosis Infections (Oropharnyx):** 250-500mg q6-8h. **Rheumatic Fever/Chorea Prevention:** 125-250mg bid. ***Pediatrics:*** **≥12 yrs: Usual: Streptococcal Infections (Scarlet Fever/Erysipelas/Upper Respiratory Tract):** 125-250mg q6-8h for 10 days. **Pneumococcal Infections (Otitis Media/Respiratory Tract):** 250-500mg q6h until afebrile for at least 2 days. **Staphylococcus Infections (Skin/ Soft Tissue):** 250-500mg q6-8h. **Fusospirochetosis Infections (Oropharnyx):** 250-500mg q6-8h. **Rheumatic Fever/ Chorea Prevention:** 125-250mg bid.	**W/P:** Not for severe pneumonia, empyema, bacteremia, pericarditis, meningitis, and arthritis during the acute stage. Serious, fatal anaphylactic reactions reported. Pseudomembranous colitis reported. Oral administration may not be effective with severe illnesses, N/V, gastric dilation, cardiospasm, intestinal hypermotility. Cross-sensitivity with cephalosporins. Caution with asthma and allergies. **P/N:** Category B, caution in nursing.	Epigastric distress, N/V, diarrhea, hypersensitivity reactions, **black hairy tongue**, anaphylaxis, superinfection (prolonged use).
SEMISYNTHETIC AMPICILLIN DERIVATIVE				
Amoxicillin (Amoxil)	**(Amoxil) Cap:** 500mg; **Sus:** 50mg/mL [30mL], 250mg/ 5mL [100mL, 150mL], 400mg/ 5mL [100mL]. **(Generic) Cap:** 250mg, 500mg; **Sus:** 125mg/ 5mL [80mL, 100mL, 150mL], 200mg/ 5mL [50mL, 75mL, 100mL], 250mg/ 5mL [80mL,100mL, 150mL], 400mg/ 5mL [50mL, 75mL, 100mL]; Tab: 500mg, 875mg; **Tab, Chewable:** 125mg, 200mg, 250mg, 400mg	***Adults/Pediatrics*** **>40kg: Ear/Nose/ Throat/SSSI/GU: Mild/Moderate:** 500mg q12h or 250mg q8h. **Severe:** 875mg q12h or 500mg q8h. **LRTI:** 875mg q12h or 500mg q8h. **Gonorrhea:** 3g as single dose. ***H.pylori:*** **(Dual Therapy)** 1g + 30mg lansoprazole, both tid x 14 days. **(Triple Therapy)** 1g + 30mg lansoprazole + 500mg clarithromycin, all q12h x 14 days. **(Amoxicillin) CrCl 10-30mL/min:** 250-500mg q12h. **CrCl <10mL/min:** 250-500mg q24h. **Hemodialysis:** 250-500mg or 250mg q24h, additional dose during and at end of dialysis. ***Pediatrics:*** **Neonates: ≤12 weeks: Max:** 30mg/kg/day divided q12h. **>3 months: Ear/Nose/Throat/ SSSI/GU: (Mild/Moderate)** 25mg/kg/day given q12h or 20mg/kg/day given q8h. **(Severe):** 45mg/kg/day given q12h or 40mg/kg/day given q8h. **LRTI:** 45mg/kg/ day given q12h or 40mg/kg/day given q8h. **Gonorrhea: (Prepubertal)** 50mg/kg with 25mg/kg probenecid as single dose (Not for <2yrs).	**W/P:** Serious, sometimes fatal, hypersensitivity reactions reported with PCN therapy. *Clostridium difficile*-associated diarrhea has been reported. Monitor renal, hepatic, and blood with prolonged use. The 200mg and 400mg chewable tabs contain phenylalanine. **P/N:** Category B, caution in nursing.	N/V, diarrhea, pseudomembranous colitis, hypersensitivity reactions, blood dyscrasias, superinfection (prolonged use).
SEMISYNTHETIC PENICILLIN DERIVATIVES				
Ampicillin	**Cap:** 250mg, 500mg; **Sus:** 125mg/5mL, 250mg/5mL [100mL, 200mL]	***Adults:*** **GI/GU:** 500mg qid. Use larger doses in chronic or severe infections. **Gonorrhea:** 3.5g single dose with 1g probenecid. **Respiratory:** 250mg qid. Treat minimum 48-72 hrs after eradication. Treat minimum 10 days for hemolytic strains of strep. ***Pediatrics:*** **>20kg: GI/GU:** 500mg qid. **Respiratory:** 250mg qid. **<20kg: GI/GU:** 25mg/kg qid. **Respiratory:** 50mg/kg/day given tid-qid. Do not exceed adult doses. Use larger doses in chronic or severe infections. Treat minimum 48-72 hrs after eradication. Treat minimum 10 days for hemolytic strains of strep.	**W/P:** Possible cross-sensitivity with cephalosporins. Pseudomembranous colitis and anaphylatic reactions may occur. **Contra:** Infections caused by penicillinase-producing organisms. **P/N:** Category B, not for use in nursing.	Stomatitis, N/V, diarrhea, rash, SGOT elevation, blood dyscrasias, eosinophilia, thrombocytopenic purpura, hypersensitivity reactions, superinfection (prolonged use).

Table 6.2. PRESCRIBING INFORMATION FOR ANTIBIOTICS *(cont.)*

NAME	FORM/ STRENGTH	DOSAGE	WARNINGS/PRECAUTIONS & CONTRAINDICATIONS	ADVERSE EFFECTS†
PENICILLINS *(cont.)*				
SEMISYNTHETIC PENICILLIN DERIVATIVES *(cont.)*				
Ampicillin Sodium	**Inj:** 250mg, 500mg, 1g, 2g	***Adults:* IM/IV: Respiratory Tract/Soft Tissues: ≥40kg:** 250-500mg q6h. **<40kg:** 25-50mg/kg/day given q6-8h. **GI/GU: ≥40kg:** 500mg q6h. **<40kg:** 50mg/kg/day given q6-8h. **Urethritis (Caused by *N.gonorrhoeae* in Males):** 500mg q8-12h for 2 doses; may retreat if needed. **Bacterial Meningitis:** 150-200mg/kg/day given q3-4h. **Septicemia:** 150-200mg/kg/day IV for 3 days, continue with IM q3-4h. Treatment of all infections should be continued for a minimum of 48-72 hrs after becoming asymptomatic. Minimum of 10 days treatment recommended for Group A β-hemolytic streptococci. ***Pediatrics:* Bacterial Meningitis:** 150-200mg/kg/day given q3-4h. **Septicemia:** 150-200mg/kg/day IV given q3-4h for 3 days, continue with IM q3-4h. Treatment of all infections should be continued for a minimum of 48-72 hrs after becoming asymptomatic. Minimum of 10 days treatment recommended for Group A β-hemolytic streptococci.	**W/P:** Serious, sometimes fatal, hypersensitivity reactions reported with PCN therapy. Caution with renal impairment. Cross-sensitivity with other β-lactams. May cause skin rash, especially in mononucleosis; avoid use. Pseudomembranous colitis reported. May result in overgrowth of nonsusceptible organisms. **P/N:** Category B, caution in nursing.	Headache, N/V, vaginal and **oral candidiasis**, diarrhea, urticaria, allergic reactions, anaphylaxis, serum sickness-like reactions, exfoliative dermatitis.
SEMISYNTHETIC PENICILLIN/β-LACTAMASE INHIBITOR				
Ampicillin Sodium/ Sulbactam Sodium (Unasyn)	**Inj:** (Ampicillin-Sulbactam) 1g-0.5g, 2g-1g, 10g-5g	***Adults/Pediatrics:* ≥40kg:** 1.5-3g (ampicillin+sulbactam) IM/IV q6h. **Max:** 4g sulbactam/day. **Renal Impairment: CrCl ≥30mL/min:** 1.5-3g q6-8h. **CrCl 15-29mL/min:** 1.5-3g q12h. **CrCl 5-14mL/min:** 1.5-3g q24h. ***Pediatrics:* ≥1 yr:** 300mg/kg/day (ampicillin+sulbactam) IV in equally divided doses q6h. **Max:** 4g sulbactam/day.	**W/P:** Serious, sometimes fatal, hypersensitivity reactions reported with PCN therapy. *Clostridium difficile*-associated diarrhea reported. Increased risk of skin rash with mononucleosis; use alternate agent. **P/N:** Category B, caution in nursing.	Injection site pain, thrombophlebitis, diarrhea.
SULFONAMIDES				
Sulfisoxazole (Gantrisin Pediatric)	**Sus:** 500mg/5mL	***Pediatrics:* >2 months: Initial:** 1/2 of 24hr dose. **Maint:** 150mg/kg/24hr or 4g/m²/24hr given q4-6h. **Max:** 6g/24hr.	**W/P:** Fatalities reported due to Stevens-Johnson syndrome, toxic epidermal necrolysis, fulminant hepatic necrosis, agranulocytosis, aplastic anemia, and other blood dyscrasias. D/C if skin rash or sign of an adverse reaction develops. Hypersensitivity reactions of the respiratory tract reported. Do not use in group A β-hemolytic streptococcal infections. Pseudomembranous colitis reported. Caution with renal/hepatic impairment, severe allergy, or bronchial asthma. Hemolysis may occur in G6PD-deficient patients. **Contra:** Infants <2 months (except in congenital toxoplasmosis treatment), pregnancy at term, mothers nursing infants <2 months old. **P/N:** Category C, not for use in nursing.	Anaphylaxis, erythema multiforme, toxic epidermal necrolysis, tachycardia, hepatitis, nausea, anorexia, hematuria, crystalluria, BUN and creatinine elevations, blood dyscrasias, dizziness, psychosis, cough.
SULFONAMIDE/TETRAHYDROFOLIC ACID INHIBITORS				
Sulfamethoxazole/ Trimethoprim (Bactrim, Bactrim DS, Septra, Septra DS, Sulfatrim Pediatric)	Sulfamethoxazole (SMX)-Trimethoprim (TMP): **Sus:** (Sulfatrim Pediatric, Septra) 200mg-40mg/5mL	***Adults:* UTI:** 800mg SMX-160mg TMP q12h for 10-14 days. **Shigellosis:** 800mg SMX-160mg TMP q12h for 5 days. **AECB:** 800mg SMX-160mg TMP q12h for 14 days. **PCP Treatment:** 75-100mg/kg SMX and 15-20mg/kg TMP per 24 hrs given q6h for 14-21 days	**W/P:** Fatal hypersensitivity reactions (eg, Stevens-Johnson syndrome, toxic epidermal necrolysis, fulminant hepatic necrosis, agranulocytosis, aplastic anemia) may occur. Pseudomembranous colitis, cough, SOB, and pulmonary infiltrates reported. Avoid with group	Anorexia, N/V, rash, urticaria, cough, SOB, cholestatic jaundice, agranulocytosis, anemia, hyperkalemia, renal failure, interstitial

*Scored. †Bold entries denote special dental considerations.
BB = black box warning; **W/P** = warnings/precautions; **Contra** = contraindications; **P/N** = pregnancy category rating and nursing considerations.

NAME	FORM/ STRENGTH	DOSAGE	WARNINGS/PRECAUTIONS & CONTRAINDICATIONS	ADVERSE EFFECTS†
Sulfamethoxazole/ Trimethoprim (Bactrim, Bactrim DS, Septra, Septra DS, Sulfatrim Pediatric) *(cont.)*	[100mL, 473mL]; **Tab:** (Bactrim, Septra) 400mg-80mg*; **Tab, DS:** (Bactrim DS, Septra DS) 800mg-160mg*	**PCP Prophylaxis:** 800mg SMX-160mg TMP qd. **Traveler's Diarrhea:** 800mg SMX-160mg TMP q12h for 5 days. **CrCl: 15-30mL/min:** 50% usual dose. **CrCl: <15mL/min:** Not recommended. ***Pediatrics:* ≥2 months: UTI/Otitis Media:** 20mg/kg SMX-4mg/kg TMP q12h for 10 days. **Shigellosis:** 20mg/kg SMX-4mg/kg TMP q12h for 5 days. **PCP Treatment:** 75-100mg/kg SMX and 15-20mg/kg TMP per 24 hrs given q6h for 14-21 days. **PCP Prophylaxis:** 750mg/m²/day SMX and 150mg/m²/day TMP given bid, on 3 consecutive days/week. **Max:** 1600mg SMX-320mg TMP/day. **CrCl: 15-30mL/min:** 50% usual dose. **CrCl: <15mL/min:** Not recommended.	A β-hemolytic streptococcal infections. *Clostridium difficile*-associated diarrhea reported. Caution with hepatic/renal impairment, elderly, folate deficiency (eg, chronic alcoholics, anticonvulsants, malabsorption, malnutrition), bronchial asthma, and other allergies. In G6PD deficiency, hemolysis may occur. Increased incidence of adverse events with AIDS. Ensure adequate fluid intake and urinary output. Caution with porphyria, thyroid dysfunction. **Contra:** Megaloblastic anemia due to folate deficiency, pregnancy, nursing, infants <2 months, marked hepatic damage, severe renal insufficiency if cannot monitor renal status. **P/N:** Category C, contraindicated in nursing.	nephritis, hyponatremia, convulsions.
TETRACYCLINE DERIVATIVES				
Demeclocycline HCl (Declomycin)	**Tab:** 150mg, 300mg	***Adults:* Usual:** 150mg qid or 300mg bid. **Gonorrhea:** 600mg followed by 300mg q12h for 4 days to a total of 3g. **Renal/Hepatic Impairment:** Reduce dose and/or extend dose intervals. Continue therapy for at least 24-48 hrs after symptoms subside. Treat strep infections for at least 10 days. Take at least 1 hr before or 2 hrs after meals with plenty of fluids. ***Pediatrics:* >8 yrs: Usual:** 7-13mg/kg/day divided bid-qid. **Max:** 600mg/day.	**W/P:** May cause fetal harm during pregnancy. Use during tooth development (last half of pregnancy, infancy, <8 yrs), or long-term use, or repeated short-term use may cause permanent discoloration of the teeth. Pseudotumor cerebri (adults), bulging fontanels (infants) reported. Caution with renal or hepatic impairment. Long-term use may cause reversible, nephrogenic diabetes insipidus syndrome. May result in overgrowth of nonsusceptible organisms; d/c if superinfection develops. CNS symptoms may occur; caution when operating machinery. May decrease bone growth in premature infants. Monitor hematopoietic, renal, and hepatic function with long-term use. D/C at first evidence of skin erythema after sun/UV light exposure. **P/N:** Category D, not for use in nursing.	GI problems, rash, esophageal ulceration, hypersensitivity reactions, dizziness, headache, tinnitus, blood dyscrasias, photosensitivity reactions, **enamel hypoplasia**, elevated BUN, acute renal failure.
Doxycycline (Atridox, Doryx, Doxycycline IV, Periostat, Vibramycin, Vibra-Tabs)	**Cap:** (Monodox) Doxycycline Monohydrate: 50mg, 75mg, 100mg; (Vibramycin) Doxycycline Hyclate: 50mg, 100mg. **Gel syringe:** (Atridox) 10% Doxycycline Hycalate: 50mg in a 500mg-blended formulation. **Inj:** 100mg. **Syrup:** (Vibramycin) Doxycycline Calcium: 50mg/5mL. **Sus:** (Vibramycin) Doxycycline Monohydrate: 25mg/5mL [60mL]. **Tab:** (Periostat) 20mg; (Vibra-Tabs) 100mg. **Tab, Delayed-Release:** (Doryx) 75mg, 100mg	***Adults:* (Atridox) Periodontitis:** Prepare the gel and inject it into the periodontal pocket; cover the pocket with either Coe-Pak periodontal dressing or a cyanoacrylate dental adhesive. May repeat four months after initial treatment. **(Periostat) Periodontitis:** Following scaling and root planing, 20mg bid, 1 hour prior to morning and evening meals for up to 9 months. Maintain adequate fluid intake with caps to reduce risk of esophageal irritation and ulceration. ***Adults/Pediatrics:* >8 yrs: >100 lbs: (Doxycycline IV) Usual:** 200mg IV divided qd-bid on Day 1 then 100-200mg/day IV depending on severity, with 200mg administered in 1 or 2 infusions. **Primary/Secondary Syphilis:** 300mg/day IV for at least 10 days. **Inhalational Anthrax (post-exposure):** 100mg IV bid. Institute oral therapy as soon as possible and continue therapy for a total of 60 days. **(Doryx, Vibramycin, Vibra-Tabs) Usual:** 100mg q12h on 1st day, followed by 100mg/day (single dose or as 50mg q12h). **Severe Infections/Chronic UTI:** 100mg q12h. **Uncomplicated Gonococcal Infections (Men, except anorectal infections):** 100mg bid for 7 days, or 300mg	**W/P:** *Clostridium difficile*-associated diarrhea reported. May decrease bone growth in premature infants, and cause fetal harm during pregnancy. May cause permanent discoloration of the teeth or enamel hypoplasia if used in last half of pregnancy, infancy, or <8 yrs. Photosensitivity, increased BUN, superinfection may occur. Monitor hematopoietic, renal, and hepatic values periodically with long-term therapy. Bulging fontanels in infants and benign intracranial HTN in adults reported. May increase incidence of vaginal candidiasis. Take adequate fluids with caps or tabs to reduce esophageal irritation. Take with food or milk if GI irritation occurs. **(Atridox)** Use has not been evaluated in pregnant women, patients with severe periodontal defects and immunocompromised patients. Atridox has not been tested for use in the regeneration of alveolar bone. Use with caution in patients with a history of or predisposition to oral candidiasis. May result in overgrowth of nonsusceptible organisms; effects of prolonged treatment (>6 mo) have not been studied. Mechanical oral hygiene procedures (ie, tooth brushing, flossing) should be avoided on treated areas for	Anorexia, N/V, diarrhea, dysphagia, enterocolitis, rash, inflammatory lesions, exfoliative dermatitis, renal toxicity, photosensitivity, increased BUN, hypersensitivity reactions, hemolytic anemia, GI effects, thrombocytopenia, neutropenia, eosinophilia, blood dyscrasias, **tooth discloration (<8 yrs).** (Atridox) **Pressure sensitivity of tooth, toothache.** (Periostat) common cold, flu symptoms, **toothache, periodontal abscess, tooth disorder,** sinusitis, dyspepsia, sore throat, joint pain, diarrhea, sinus congestion, coughing.

Table 6.2. PRESCRIBING INFORMATION FOR ANTIBIOTICS *(cont.)*

NAME	FORM/ STRENGTH	DOSAGE	WARNINGS/PRECAUTIONS & CONTRAINDICATIONS	ADVERSE EFFECTS†
TETRACYCLINE DERIVATIVES *(cont.)*				
Doxycycline (Atridox, Doryx, Doxycycline IV, Periostat, Vibramycin, Vibra-Tabs) *(cont.)*		followed 300mg 1 hr later. **Acute Epididymo-Orchitis:** 100mg bid for at least 10 days. **Early Syphilis:** 100mg bid for 14 days. **Syphilis >1 yr:** 100mg bid for 28 days. **Primary/Secondary Syphilis (Monodox):** 300mg/day in divided dose for at least 10 days. **Nongonococcal Urethritis, Uncomplicated Urethral/ Endocervical/Rectal Infection:** 100mg bid for at least 7 days. **Inhalational Anthrax (post-exposure):** 100mg bid for 60 days. Treat Strep infections for 10 days. ***Pediatrics:* >8 yrs: ≤100lbs: (Doxycycline IV) Usual:** 2mg/lb IV divided qd-bid on Day 1 then 1-2mg/lb/ day IV divided qd-bid depending on severity. **Inhalational Anthrax (post-exposure):** 1 mg/lb IV bid. Institute oral therapy as soon as possible and continue therapy for total of 60 days. **(Doryx, Vibramycin, Vibra-Tabs) Severe Infections/Chronic UTI:** 2mg/lb in divided doses bid on Day 1, followed by 1mg/lb/day (single dose or divided bid) thereafter. **Severe Infections:** Up to 2mg/lb. **Inhalational Anthrax (post-exposure):** 1mg/lb bid for 60 days.	7 days **P/N:** Category D, not for use in nursing.	
Minocycline HCl (Arestin, Dynacin, Minocin)	**Cartridge:** (Arestin) 1mg; **Tab:** (Dynacin) 50mg, 75mg, 100mg; (Minocin) **Cap:** (Minocin) 50mg, 100mg; **Inj:** (Minocin) 100mg; **Sus:** (Minocin) 50mg/5mL [60mL]	***Adults:*** (Arestin) **Periodontitis:** Single injection of one unit dosage into periodontal pocket, 5mm or deeper, after scaling and root planing. One dose delivers antibacterial concentrations for 10-14 days. **Max:** 1 injection per pocket every 3 mo. (Dynacin, Minocin) **Usual:** 200mg initially, then 100mg q12h; alternative is 100-200mg initially, then 50mg qid. **Uncomplicated Gonococcal Infection (Men, Other Than Urethritis and Anorectal Infections):** 200mg initially, then 100mg q12h for minimum 4 days. **Uncomplicated Gonococcal Urethritis (Men):** 100mg q12h for 5 days. **Syphilis:** Administer usual dose for 10-15 days. **Meningococcal Carrier State:** 100mg q12h for 5 days. ***Mycobacterium marinum:*** 100mg q12h for 6-8 weeks. **Uncomplicated Urethral, Endocervical, or Rectal Infection Caused by *Chlamydia trachomatis* or *Ureaplasma urealyticum:*** 100mg q12h for at least 7 days. **Gonorrhea in Patients Sensitive to PCN:** 200mg initially, then 100mg q12h for at least 4 days, with post-therapy cultures within 2-3 days. Take with plenty of fluids. **Renal Dysfunction:** Reduce dose and/or extend dose intervals. **Max:** 200mg/24 hrs. ***Pediatrics:* >8 yrs:** 4mg/kg initially followed by 2mg/kg q12h. Take with plenty of fluids.	**W/P:** (Dynacin, Minocin) May cause fetal harm during pregnancy. Use during tooth development (last half of pregnancy, infancy, <8 yrs) may cause permanent discoloration of the teeth or enamel hypoplasia; avoid use during this period. Renal toxicity, hepatotoxicity, photosensitivity, increased BUN, superinfection, pseudotumor cerebri may occur; perform hematopoietic, renal, and hepatic monitoring. May impair mental/ physical abilities. Use alternate form of contraception other than oral contraceptives. May decrease bone growth in premature infants. If *Clostridium difficile*-associated diarrhea (CDAD) develops, appropriate therapy should be initiated. (Arestin) Caution in patients with history or predisposition to oral candidiasis. May result in overgrowth of nonsusceptible organisms; effects of prolonged treatment (>6 mo) have not been studied. Use has not been studied in acutely abscessed periodontal pockets and is not recommended. Arestin has not been tested in pregnant women or immunocompromised patients; or for use in regeneration of alveolar bone. Advise patients of the following: avoid hard, crunchy, or sticky foods 1 wk after treatment; wait 12 hrs after treatment before brushing teeth; postpone use of interproximal cleaning devices for 10 days after treatment; do not touch treated areas. Although sensitivity is normal the first week after treatment, patients should promptly report pain, swelling, or other problems that occur. **P/N:** Category D, not for use in nursing.	(Dynacin, Minocin) Anorexia, N/V, diarrhea, dysphagia, enterocolitis, pancreatitis, increased LFTs, renal toxicity, rash, exfoliative dermatitis, Stevens-Johnson syndrome, skin and mucous membrane pigmentation, blood dyscrasias, headache, tooth discoloration. (Arestin) **Swelling of gums, toothache.**

†Bold entries denote special dental considerations.
BB = black box warning; **W/P** = warnings/precautions; **Contra** = contraindications; **P/N** = pregnancy category rating and nursing considerations.

NAME	FORM/ STRENGTH	DOSAGE	WARNINGS/PRECAUTIONS & CONTRAINDICATIONS	ADVERSE EFFECTS†
MISCELLANEOUS ANTIBIOTICS				
Aztreonam (Azactam)	**Inj:** 1g, 2g, 1g/50mL, 2g/50mL	***Adults:*** **GFR ≥30mL/min/1.73m²: UTI:** 500mg-1g IV q8-12h. **Moderately Severe Infections:** 1-2g IV q 8-12h. **Severe/Life-Threatening Infections:** 2g IV q6-8h. **Max:** 8g/day. **GFR <30mL/min/1.73m²: Initial: LD:** 1 or 2g. **Maint:** 50% of usual dose. **GFR <10mL/min/1.73m²: Initial: LD:** 500mg, 1g or 2g. **Maint:** 25% of usual initial dose at usual intervals. **Serious/Life-Threatening Infections:** In addition to maint dose, give 1/8 initial dose after each hemodialysis session. ***Pediatrics:*** **9 months-16 yrs: Mild-Moderate Infections:** 30mg/kg IV q8h. **Moderate-Severe Infections:** 30mg/kg IV q6-8h. **Max:** 120mg/kg/day. IV route is recommended for single doses >1g or for bacterial septicemia, localized parenchymal abscess (eg, intra-abdominal abscess), peritonitis, or other severe systemic or life-threatening infections. Continue for at least 48 hrs after patient is asymptomatic or evidence of bacterial eradication.	**W/P:** Caution with hypersensitivity to other β-lactams or allergens. *Clostridium difficile*-associated diarrhea reported. May promote overgrowth of nonsusceptible organisms. Monitor with renal or hepatic impairment. Toxic epidermal necrolysis reported (rarely) in bone marrow transplant with multiple risk factors including sepsis. **P/N:** Category B, not for use in nursing.	Diarrhea, N/V, rash, abdominal cramps, vaginal candidiasis, discomfort/swelling at injection site, hypersensitivity reaction.
Bacitracin (Bacitracin Injection)	**Inj:** 50,000U	***Pediatrics:*** **<2500g:** 900U/kg/24h IM. **>2500g:** 1000U/kg/24h IM. Administer in 2-3 divided doses. Inject in upper outer quadrant of buttocks.	**BB:** May cause renal failure due to tubular and glomerular necrosis. Monitor renal function prior to, and daily during therapy. Fluid intake and urinary output should be maintained at proper levels to avoid kidney toxicity. Discontinue if renal toxicity occurs. Avoid other nephrotoxic drugs. **W/P:** Use appropriate therapy if superinfection occurs. **P/N:** Safety in pregnancy or nursing not known.	Albuminuria, cylindruria, azotemia, N/V, pain at injection site, skin rashes, rising blood levels without increase in dosage.
Clindamycin HCl (Cleocin)	**Cap:** (HCl) 75mg, 150mg, 300mg; **Inj:** (Phosphate) 150mg/mL, 300mg/50mL, 600mg/50mL, 900mg/50mL; **Sus:** (Palmitate HCl) 75mg/5mL [100mL]	***Adults:*** **Serious Infection:** 150-300mg PO q6h or 600-1200mg/day IM/IV given bid-qid. **More Severe Infection:** 300-450mg PO q6h or 1200-2700mg/day IM/IV given bid-qid. **Life-Threatening Infections:** Up to 4800mg/day IV. **Max:** 600mg per IM injection. Take caps with full glass of water. Treat β-hemolytic strep for at least 10 days. ***Pediatrics:*** Give tid or qid. **Cap: Serious Infections:** 8-16mg/kg/day. More **Severe Infections:** 16-20mg/kg/day. **Sol: Serious Infections:** 8-12mg/kg/day. **Severe Infections:** 13-16mg/kg/day. **More Severe Infections:** 17-25mg/kg/day. **IM/IV: 1 month-16 yrs:** 20-40mg/kg/day; use the higher dose for more severe infections. **<1 month:** 15-20mg/kg/day. Take caps with full glass of water. Treat β-hemolytic strep for at least 10 days.	**BB:** *Clostridium difficile*-associated diarrhea (CDAD) reported with use of nearly all antibacterial agents, including clindamycin, and may range in severity from mild diarrhea to fatal colitis. If CDAD is suspected or confirmed, ongoing antibiotic use not directed against *C.difficile* may need to be discontinued. **W/P:** May permit overgrowth of clostridia. Not for treatment of meningitis. Caution with atopic patients, GI disease (eg, colitis), hepatic disease, and the elderly. Monitor blood, hepatic, and renal function with long-term use. Do not give injection undiluted as bolus. The 75mg and 100mg caps contain tartrazine. **P/N:** Category B, not for use in nursing.	Abdominal pain, colitis, esophagitis, N/V, diarrhea, hypersensitivity reactions, jaundice, blood dyscrasias, pruritus, vaginitis, superinfection (prolonged use).
Colistimethate Sodium (Coly-Mycin M)	**Inj:** 150mg	***Adults/Pediatrics:*** **Usual:** 2.5-5mg/kg/day IV/IM in 2-4 divided doses. **Max:** 5mg/kg/day. **SCr 1.3-1.5mg/dL:** 2.5-3.8mg/kg/day IV/IM in 2 divided doses. **SCr 1.6-2.5mg/dL:** 2.5mg/kg/day IV/IM in 1-2 divided doses. **SCr 2.6-4mg/dL:** 1.5mg/kg/day IV/IM q36h. **Obesity:** Base dose on IBW.	**W/P:** Transient neurological disturbances may occur; dose reduction may alleviate symptoms. Respiratory arrest reported after IM administration. Increased risk of apnea and neuromuscular blockade with renal impairment. Reversible dose-dependent nephrotoxicity reported. Pseudomembranous colitis reported. May permit overgrowth of clostridia. Use extreme caution with renal impairment; d/c with further impairment. **P/N:** Category C, caution in nursing.	GI upset, **tingling of tongue** and extremities, **slurred speech**, dizziness, vertigo, paresthesia, itching, urticaria, rash, fever, increased BUN and creatinine, decreased creatinine clearance, respiratory distress, apnea, nephrotoxicity, decreased urine output.

Table 6.2. PRESCRIBING INFORMATION FOR ANTIBIOTICS *(cont.)*

NAME	FORM/ STRENGTH	DOSAGE	WARNINGS/PRECAUTIONS & CONTRAINDICATIONS	ADVERSE EFFECTS†
MISCELLANEOUS ANTIBIOTICS *(cont.)*				
Dalfopristin/ Quinupristin (Synercid)	**Inj:** (Dalfopristin-Quinupristin) 350mg-150mg per 500mg vial	***Adults/Pediatrics:*** **≥16 yrs: VREF:** 7.5mg/kg IV q8h. Duration depends on site and severity of infection. **cSSSI:** 7.5mg/kg IV q12h for at least 7 days. **Hepatic Cirrhosis (Child Pugh A or B):** May need dose reduction.	**W/P:** Pseudomembranous colitis reported. Flush vein with 5% dextrose after infusion to minimize venous irritation. Arthralgia, myalgia, and bilirubin elevation reported. **P/N:** Category B, caution in nursing.	Infusion site reactions (inflammation, pain, edema), nausea, diarrhea, rash.
Daptomycin (Cubicin)	**Inj:** 500mg	***Adults:*** **≥18 yrs:** Administer as IV infusion over 30 min. **Complicated SSSI:** 4mg/kg q24h for 7-14 days. ***S.aureus*** **Bacteremia:** 6mg/kg q24h for minimum 2-6 weeks. **Renal impairment: CrCl <30mL/min, HD, or CAPD:** 4mg/kg (Complicated SSSI) or 6mg/kg (*S.aureus* bacteremia) once q48h.	**W/P:** *Clostridium difficile*-associated diarrhea reported. D/C if CDAD confirmed. Monitor CPK levels weekly; d/c with unexplained signs and symptoms of myopathy and CPK elevation >1000 U/L (~5x ULN), or with CPK levels ≥10x ULN. Persisting or relapsing *S.aureus* infection or poor clinical response should have repeat blood cultures. **P/N:** Category B, caution in nursing.	Constipation, N/V, injection site reactions, headache, diarrhea, insomnia, rash, abnormal LFTs, superinfection, **pharyngolaryngeal pain**, pain in extremity and pulmonary eosinophilia.
Lincomycin HCl (Lincocin)	**Inj:** 300mg/mL	***Adults:*** **IM: Serious Infection:** 600mg q24h. **More Severe Infection:** 600mg q12h or more often. **IV:** Dose depends on severity. **Serious Infection:** 600mg-1g q8-12h. **More Severe Infection:** Increase dose. Infuse over ≥1 hr. **Life-Threatening Situation:** Up to 8g/day has been given. **Max:** 8g/day. **Severe Renal Dysfunction:** 25-30% of normal dose. ***Pediatrics:*** **>1 month: IM: Serious Infection:** 10mg/kg q24h. **More Severe Infection:** 10mg/kg q12h or more often. **IV:** 10-20mg/kg/day, depending on severity infused in divided doses as described for adults. **Severe Renal Dysfunction:** 25-30% of normal dose.	**BB:** Diarrhea, colitis, pseudomembranous colitis reported; may begin up to several weeks after discontinuation. Reserve for serious infections where less toxic antimicrobials are inappropriate. **W/P:** May be inadequate for meningitis treatment. Contains benzyl alcohol. Monitor elderly for change in bowel frequency. Caution with severe renal/hepatic dysfunction, or with history of GI disease (eg, colitis), asthma, significant allergies. Superinfections may occur. Perform periodic CBC, LFTs, and renal function tests with prolonged therapy. Do not administer undiluted as IV bolus. Cardiopulmonary arrest and hypotension with too rapid IV administration. **Contra:** Clindamycin hypersensitivity. **P/N:** Category C, not for use in nursing.	**Glossitis**, stomatitis, N/V, diarrhea, colitis, pruritus, blood dyscrasias, hypersensitivity reactions, rash, urticaria, vaginitis, tinnitus, vertigo.
Linezolid (Zyvox)	**Inj:** 2mg/mL [100mL, 200mL, 300mL]; **Sus:** 100mg/5mL [150mL]; **Tab:** 400mg, 600mg	***Adults:/Pediatrics:*** **≥12yrs: Complicated SSSI/CAP/Nosocomial Pneumonia:** 600mg IV/PO q12h for 10-14 days. **VRE:** 600mg IV/PO q12h for 14-28 days. **Uncomplicated SSSI:** 400mg PO q12h for 10-14 days; **≥12yrs:** 600mg PO q12h for 10-14 days. ***Pediatrics:*** **Birth-11 yrs: Complicated SSSI/CAP/Nosocomial Pneumonia:** 10mg/kg IV/PO q8h for 10-14 days. **VRE:** 10mg/kg IV/PO q8h for 14 to 28 days. **Uncomplicated SSSI: 5-11 yrs:** 10mg/kg PO q12h for 10 to 14 days; **<5 yrs:** 10mg/kg PO q8h for 10 to 14 days. **Neonates <7 days:** Initiate with dosing regimen of 10mg/kg q12h; may increase to 10mg/kg q8h if suboptimal response. All neonatal patients should receive 10mg/kg q8h by 7 days of life.	**W/P:** Myelosuppression, including anemia, thrombocytopenia, pancytopenia, and leukopenia reported; monitor CBC weekly. *Clostridium difficile*-associated diarrhea reported. Oral sus contains phenylalanine. Peripheral and optic neuropathy reported; monitor visual function if on for extended periods (≥3 months). Lactic acidosis and convulsions reported. May promote overgrowth of nonsusceptible organisms. **P/N:** Category C, caution in nursing.	Diarrhea, headache, N/V.
Telithromycin (Ketek)	**Tab:** 300mg, 400mg [Ketek Pak, 20[s]]	***Adults:*** 800mg qd for 7-10 days. **Severe Renal Impairment (CrCl <30mL/min):** 600mg qd. **Hemodialysis:** Give after dialysis session on dialysis days. **Severe Renal Impairment (CrCl <30mL/min) with Hepatic Impairment:** 400mg qd.	**BB:** Contraindicated with myasthenia gravis. **W/P:** Acute hepatic failure and severe liver injury, including fulminant hepatitis and hepatic necrosis reported; monitor closely and d/c if any signs/symptoms of hepatitis occur. Visual disturbances and loss of consciousness reported; minimize hazardous activities such as driving and operating heavy machinery. May prolong QTc interval; avoid with congenital prolongation,	Diarrhea, N/V, headache, dizziness, visual disturbances.

†Bold entries denote special dental considerations.
BB = black box warning; **W/P** = warnings/precautions; **Contra** = contraindications; **P/N** = pregnancy category rating and nursing considerations.

NAME	FORM/ STRENGTH	DOSAGE	WARNINGS/PRECAUTIONS & CONTRAINDICATIONS	ADVERSE EFFECTS†
Telithromycin (Ketek) *(cont.)*			ongoing proarrhythmic conditions (eg, uncorrected hypokalemia or hypomagnesemia), significant bradycardia. Torsades de pointes reported. *Clostridium difficile*-associated diarrhea reported. Reduce dose with severe renal impairment. **Contra:** Myasthenia gravis. History of hepatitis and/or jaundice associated with use of telithromycin or any macrolide antibiotic. Hypersensitivity to macrolide antibiotics; concomitant use with cisapride or pimozide. **P/N:** Category C, caution in nursing.	
Tigecycline (Tygacil)	**Inj:** 50mg/5mL	***Adults:*** 100mg IV over 30-60 min then 50mg q12h over 30-60 min for 5-14 days. **Severe Hepatic Impairment (Child-Pugh C):** 100mg IV over 30-60 min then 25mg q12h.	**W/P:** Structurally similar to tetracyclines and may have similar adverse effects: photosensitivity, pseudotumor cerebri, pancreatitis, and anti-anabolic action (may lead to increased BUN, azotemia, acidosis, and hyperphosphatemia). Caution with known hypersensitivity to tetracyclines. May cause fetal harm and permanent tooth discoloration (yellow-gray-brown) when administered during tooth development (last half of pregnancy to 8 yrs). *Clostridium difficile*-associated diarrhea reported. Caution when used for cIAI secondary to clinical apparent intestinal perforations. **P/N:** Category D, caution in nursing.	N/V, diarrhea, abdominal pain, infection, fever, headache, HTN, thrombocythemia, anemia, hypoproteinemia, increased lactic dehydrogenase, increased SGOT, increased SGPT.
Trimethoprim HCl (Primsol)	**Sol:** 50mg/5mL	***Adults:*** **UTI: Usual:** 100mg q12h or 200mg q24h for 10 days. **CrCl: 15-30mL/min:** Give 50% of usual dose. ***Pediatrics:*** **Otitis Media: >6 months:** 5mg/kg q12h for 10 days. **CrCl: 15-30mL/min:** Give 50% of usual dose.	**W/P:** May interfere with hematopoiesis. Serious blood disorders; monitor for sore throat, fever, pallor, and purpura. Caution with folate deficiency and renal/hepatic impairment, diarrhea, rash. **Contra:** Megaloblastic anemia due to folate deficiency. **P/N:** Category C, caution in nursing.	Epigastric distress, N/V, anemia, methemoglobinemia, hyperkalemia, hyponatremia, fever, elevation of serum transaminases and bilirubin, increases BUN and serum creatinine.
Vancomycin HCl	**Inj:** 500mg, 1g, 5g, 500mg/100mL, 1g/200mL	***Adults:*** **Inj: Usual:** 500mg IV q6h or 1g IV q12h. Administer at no >10mg/min or over at least 60 min, whichever is longer. **Max Conc:** 5mg/mL. **Max Rate:** 10mg/min. **Renal Impairment: Initial:** Not <15mg/kg. Dosage per day in mg is about 15x the GFR in mL/min (refer to table in PI). **Elderly:** Require greater dose reductions than expected. **Functionally Anephric: Initial:** 15mg/kg, then 1.9mg/kg/24 hrs. **Marked Renal Impairment:** 250-1000mg every several days. **Anuria:** 1000mg every 7-10 days. **PO:** 500-2000mg/day in 3-4 divided doses for 7-10 days. **Max:** 2000mg/day. May dilute in 1oz of water. ***Pediatrics:*** **Inj: Usual:** 10mg/kg IV q6h. **Infants/Neonates: Initial:** 15mg/kg, then 10mg/kg q12h for neonates in 1st week of life and q8h thereafter until 1 month of age. Administer over at least 60 min. **Renal Impairment: Initial:** Not <15mg/kg. Dosage per day in mg is about 15x the GFR in mL/min (refer to table in PI). **Premature Infants:** Require greater dose reduction. ADD-Vantage vials should not be used in neonates, infants, and pediatrics who require doses <500mg. **PO:** 40mg/kg/day in 3-4 divided doses for 7-10 days. **Max:** 2000mg/day. May dilute in 1oz of water.	**W/P:** Rapid bolus administration may cause hypotension and cardiac arrest (rare); administer in diluted solution over ≥60 min. Frequency of infusion-related events may increase with concomitant use of anesthetic agents. Ototoxicity reported; monitor auditory function. Caution with renal insufficiency and adjust dose with renal dysfunction. Pseudomembranous colitis reported. Alters the normal flora of the colon and may permit overgrowth of clostridia. Prolonged use may result in overgrowth of nonsusceptible organisms. Reversible neutropenia reported; monitor leukocyte count. Administer via IV route; pain, avoid IM route. Thrombophlebitis may occur; rotate injection sites. Safety and efficacy of administration via the intraperitoneal and intrathecal (intralumbar and intraventricular) routes has not been established. Administration via intraperitoneal route during CAPD has resulted in a syndrome of chemical peritonitis. Adjust dosing schedules in elderly. **P/N:** Category C, not for use in nursing.	Infusion-related events, hypotension, wheezing, pruritus, pain, chest and head muscle spasm, dyspnea, urticaria, "Red Man" syndrome, nephrotoxicity, pseudomembranous colitis, ototoxicity, neutropenia, phlebitis.

Table 6.3. DRUG INTERACTIONS FOR ANTIBIOTICS

AMINOGLYCOSIDES

Amikacin Sulfate	
Aminoglycosides	Avoid with other aminoglycosides; potential for additive nephrotoxicity and neurotoxicity.
Amphotericin B	Avoid with amphotericin B; potential for additive nephrotoxicity and neurotoxicity.
Anesthetics	May increase risk of neuromuscular blockade and respiratory paralysis with anesthetics.
Bacitracin	Avoid with bacitracin; potential for additive nephrotoxicity.
β-Lactams	Significant mutual inactivation may occur with β-lactams (eg, penicillin, cephalosporins).
Cephalosporins	Avoid with cephalosporins; may increase risk of nephrotoxicity.
Cisplatin	Avoid with cisplatin; potential for additive nephrotoxicity and neurotoxicity.
Colistin	Avoid with colistin; potential for additive nephrotoxicity and neurotoxicity.
Diuretics	Avoid with potent diuretics (eg, ethacrynic acid, furosemide); potential for additive ototoxicity. Intravenous diuretics may enhance aminoglycoside toxicity.
Nephrotoxic drugs	Avoid with nephrotoxic drugs; potential for additive nephrotoxicity.
Neuromuscular blockers	May increase risk of neuromuscular blockade and respiratory paralysis with neuromuscular blockers (tubocurarine, succinylcholine, decamethonium).
Neurotoxic drugs	Avoid with neurotoxic drugs; potential for additive neurotoxicity.
Polymyxin B	Avoid with polymyxin B; potential for additive nephrotoxicity and neurotoxicity.
Vancomycin	Avoid with vancomycin; potential for additive nephrotoxicity and neurotoxicity.
Gentamicin Sulfate	
Aminoglycosides	Avoid with other aminoglycosides; potential for additive nephrotoxicity and neurotoxicity.
Anesthetics	May increase risk of neuromuscular blockade and respiratory paralysis with anesthetics.
Cephalosporins	Avoid with cephalosporins; may increase risk of nephrotoxicity.
Cisplatin	Avoid with cisplatin; potential for additive nephrotoxicity and neurotoxicity.
Colistin	Avoid with colistin; potential for additive nephrotoxicity and neurotoxicity.
Diuretics	Avoid with potent diuretics (eg, ethacrynic acid, furosemide); potential for additive ototoxicity. Intravenous diuretics may enhance aminoglycoside toxicity.
Nephrotoxic drugs	Avoid with nephrotoxic drugs; potential for additive nephrotoxicity.
Neuromuscular blockers	May increase risk of neuromuscular blockade and respiratory paralysis with neuromuscular blockers (tubocurarine, succinylcholine, decamethonium).
Neurotoxic drugs	Avoid with neurotoxic drugs; potential for additive neurotoxicity.
Polymyxin B	Avoid with polymyxin B; potential for additive nephrotoxicity and neurotoxicity.
Vancomycin	Avoid with vancomycin; potential for additive nephrotoxicity and neurotoxicity.

Note: See the Miscellaneous listing at the end of this table if a drug name does not appear under a particular therapeutic category.

Table 6.3. DRUG INTERACTIONS FOR ANTIBIOTICS *(cont.)*

AMINOGLYCOSIDES *(cont.)*

Streptomycin Sulfate	
Aminoglycosides	Avoid with other aminoglycosides; potential for additive nephrotoxicity and neurotoxicity.
Anesthetics	May increase risk of neuromuscular blockade and respiratory paralysis with anesthetics.
Colistin	Avoid with colistin; potential for additive nephrotoxicity and neurotoxicity.
Cyclosporine	Avoid with cyclosporine; potential for additive nephrotoxicity and neurotoxicity.
Diuretics	Potential for additive ototoxicity with ethacrynic acid, furosemide, mannitol, and possibly other diuretics.
Muscle relaxants	May increase risk of neuromuscular blockade and respiratory paralysis with muscle relaxants.
Nephrotoxic drugs	Avoid with nephrotoxic drugs; potential for additive nephrotoxicity.
Neurotoxic drugs	Avoid with neurotoxic drugs; potential for additive neurotoxicity.
Polymyxin B	Avoid with polymyxin B; potential for additive nephrotoxicity and neurotoxicity.
Tobramycin (TOBI)	
Aminoglycosides	Avoid with other aminoglycosides; potential for additive nephrotoxicity and neurotoxicity.
Diuretics	Avoid with diuretics (eg, ethacrynic acid, furosemide, urea, mannitol); may enhance aminoglycoside toxicity, including neurotoxicity.
Nephrotoxic drugs	Avoid with nephrotoxic drugs; potential for additive nephrotoxicity.
Neurotoxic drugs	Avoid with neurotoxic drugs; potential for additive neurotoxicity.
Tobramycin Sulfate	
Aminoglycosides	Avoid with other aminoglycosides; potential for additive nephrotoxicity and neurotoxicity.
Cephalosporins	Avoid with cephalosporins; may increase risk of nephrotoxicity.
Cisplatin	Avoid with cisplatin; potential for additive nephrotoxicity and neurotoxicity.
Colistin	Avoid with colistin; potential for additive nephrotoxicity and neurotoxicity.
Neuromuscular blockers	Possibility of prolonged or secondary apnea in anesthetized patients receiving neuromuscular blockers (eg, succinylcholine, tubocurarine, decamethonium).
Polymyxin B	Avoid with polymyxin B; potential for additive nephrotoxicity and neurotoxicity.
Vancomycin	Avoid with vancomycin; potential for additive nephrotoxicity and neurotoxicity.

CARBAPENEMS

Doripenem (Doribax)	
Probenecid	May increase plasma levels of doripenem; avoid coadministration.
Valproic acid	May decrease plasma levels of valproic acid, which may result in loss of seizure control; monitor serum valproic levels frequently after initiation of therapy.

CARBAPENEMS *(cont.)*

Ertapenem Sodium (Invanz)	
Probenecid	May decrease clearance and increase plasma levels of ertapenem.
Valproic acid	May decrease serum levels of valproic acid when coadministered.
Imipenem/Cilastatin (Primaxin I.M.)	
Antibiotics	Do not mix with or physically add to other antibiotics.
Probenecid	Coadministration produces only minimal increases in plasma levels and half-life of imipenem; concomitant use not recommended.
Valproic acid	May decrease plasma levels of valproic acid, which may result in loss of seizure control.
Imipenem/Cilastatin (Primaxin IV)	
Antibiotics	Do not mix with or physically add to other antibiotics.
Ganciclovir	Seizures reported with ganciclovir; avoid concomitant use.
Probenecid	Coadministration produces only minimal increases in plasma levels and half-life of imipenem; concomitant use not recommended.
Valproic acid	May decrease plasma levels of valproic acid, which may result in loss of seizure control.
Meropenem (Merrem)	
Probenecid	May increase plasma levels and half-life of meropenem; avoid concomitant use.
Valproic acid	May decrease plasma levels of valproic acid.

CEPHALOSPORINS

1ST GENERATION CEPHALOSPORINS

Cefazolin	
Probenecid	May increase and prolong plasma levels of cefazolin.
Cephalexin (Keflex)	
Probenecid	May inhibit renal excretion of cephalexin.

2ND GENERATION CEPHALOSPORINS

Cefaclor, Cefaclor ER	
Antacids	May decrease absorption of cefaclor ER with magnesium or aluminum hydroxide-containing antacids taken within 1 hour of administration.
Anticoagulants	May potentiate anticoagulant effects with coadministration; monitor PT/INR.
Probenecid	May inhibit renal excretion of cefaclor.
Cefotetan Disodium	
Alcohol	Possible disulfiram-like reaction if alcohol is ingested within 72 hours after cefotetan administration.
Aminoglycosides	May increase risk of nephrotoxicity with aminoglycosides; monitor renal function.
Cefoxitin Sodium (Mefoxin)	
Aminoglycosides	May increase risk of nephrotoxicity with aminoglycosides.

Table 6.3. DRUG INTERACTIONS FOR ANTIBIOTICS *(cont.)*

CEPHALOSPORINS *(cont.)*

2ND GENERATION CEPHALOSPORINS *(cont.)*

Cefprozil (Cefzil)	
Aminoglycosides	May increase risk of nephrotoxicity with aminoglycosides.
Diuretics	Caution with potent diuretics; may adversely affect renal function.
Probenecid	May increase plasma levels of cefprozil.
Cefuroxime (Zinacef)	
Aminoglycosides	May increase risk of nephrotoxicity with aminoglycosides.
Contraceptives, oral	May reduce efficacy of combined estrogen/progesterone oral contraceptives.
Diuretics	Caution with potent diuretics; may adversely affect renal function.
Probenecid	May increase plasma levels and half-life of cefuroxime.
Cefuroxime Axetil (Ceftin)	
Contraceptives, oral	May reduce efficacy of combined estrogen/progesterone oral contraceptives.
Diuretics	Caution with potent diuretics; may adversely affect renal function.
Gastric acidity, drugs lowering	May lower bioavailability of cefuroxime with drugs that lower gastric acidity.
Probenecid	May increase plasma levels of cefuroxime.
3RD GENERATION CEPHALOSPORINS	
Cefdinir (Omnicef)	
Antacids	May decrease absorption of cefdinir with aluminum- or magnesium-containing antacids; separate doses by 2 hours.
Iron	May decrease absorption of cefdinir with iron-fortified foods and iron supplements; separate doses by 2 hours. Reddish stools reported with concomitant iron-containing products.
Probenecid	May increase plasma levels of cefdinir.
Cefditoren Pivoxil (Spectracef)	
Antacids	May decrease absorption of cefditoren with aluminum- or magnesium-containing antacids; avoid concomitant use.
H_2-blockers	May decrease absorption of cefditoren; avoid concomitant use.
Probenecid	May increase plasma levels and half-life of cefditoren.
Cefixime (Suprax)	
Anticoagulants	May increase prothrombin time with coadministration.
Carbamazepine	May increase plasma levels of carbamazepine; monitor plasma levels.
Cefotaxime Sodium (Claforan)	
Aminoglycosides	May increase risk of nephrotoxicity with aminoglycosides.
Nephrotoxic drugs	May potentiate the renal toxicity of nephrotoxic drugs.
Probenecid	May decrease clearance and increase plasma levels of cefotaxime.
Cefpodoxime Proxetil (Vantin)	
Antacids	May reduce absorption of cefpodoxime with high doses of antacids.
Anticholinergics	Anticholinergics may delay peak plasma levels.

CEPHALOSPORINS *(cont.)*

3RD GENERATION CEPHALOSPORINS *(cont.)*

Cefpodoxime Proxetil (Vantin) *(cont.)*	
H_2-blockers	May decrease absorption and plasma levels of cefpodoxime with H_2 blockers.
Nephrotoxic agents	Closely monitor renal function with concomitant nephrotoxic agents.
Probenecid	May inhibit renal excretion and increase plasma levels of cefpodoxime.
Ceftazidime (Fortaz, Tazicef)	
Aminoglycosides	May increase risk of nephrotoxicity with aminoglycosides.
Chloramphenicol	Avoid with chloramphenicol; may decrease effect of β-lactam antibiotics.
Contraceptives, oral	May reduce efficacy of oral contraceptives.
Diuretics	Nephrotoxicity reported with potent diuretics (eg, furosemide).
Ceftriaxone Sodium (Rocephin)	
Calcium-containing products	Calcium-containing infusions, such as parenteral nutrition, should not be mixed or coadministered. Contrainidicated in neonates; risk of precipitation of ceftriaxone-calcium salt.

4TH GENERATION CEPHALOSPORIN

Cefepime HCl (Maxipime)	
Aminoglycosides	May increase risk of nephrotoxicity and ototoxicity with aminoglycosides.
Diuretics	May increase risk of nephrotoxicity with concomitant potent diuretics (eg, furosemide).

FLUOROQUINOLONES

Ciprofloxacin (Cipro IV)	
Anticoagulants, coumarin	May enhance the effects of oral coumarin anticoagulants; monitor PT/INR.
Caffeine	May reduce clearance and prolong half-life of caffeine.
Corticosteroids	Coadministration may increase risk of tendinitis and tendon rupture.
Cyclosporine	Transient elevations in serum creatinine with cyclosporine.
CYP1A2 substrates	May increase plasma levels of drugs metabolized by CYP1A2 (eg, theophylline, methylxanthines, tizanidine).
Diuretics	Risk of nephrotoxicity with potent diuretics (eg, furosemide).
Glyburide	Severe hypoglycemia reported with concomitant glyburide (rare).
Methotrexate	May increase plasma levels of methotrexate.
NSAIDs	NSAIDs (except ASA) may increase risk of convulsions with very high dose ciprofloxacin.
Phenytoin	May increase or decrease plasma levels of phenytoin.
Probenecid	May increase plasma levels of ciprofloxacin.
QT interval, drugs prolonging	May increase risk of QT prolongation with other drugs that prolong the QT interval (eg, class IA and III antiarrhythmics).

Table 6.3. DRUG INTERACTIONS FOR ANTIBIOTICS *(cont.)*

FLUOROQUINOLONES *(cont.)*	
Ciprofloxacin (Cipro IV) *(cont.)*	
Seizure threshold, drugs lowering	May increase risk of seizure with drugs that lower seizure threshold.
Theophylline	May increase plasma levels and prolong half-life of theophylline. Avoid concomitant use if possible; serious and fatal reactions including cardiac arrest, seizure, and respiratory failure reported.
Tizanidine	Concomitant use contraindicated; may increase plasma levels and potentiate hypotensive and sedative effects of tizanidine.
Ciprofloxacin HCl (Cipro Oral, Cipro XR, Proquin XR)	
Antacids	May reduce absorption and decrease levels of ciprofloxacin with magnesium/aluminum antacids; administer 2 hours before or 6 hours after antacids. Proquin XR should be administered at least 4 hours before or 2 hours after these products.
Anticoagulants, coumarin	May enhance the effects of oral coumarin anticoagulants; monitor PT/INR.
Buffered drugs	May reduce absorption and decrease levels of ciprofloxacin; administer 2 hours before or 6 hours after highly buffered drugs. Proquin XR should be administered at least 4 hours before or 2 hours after these products.
Caffeine	May reduce clearance and prolong half-life of caffeine.
Calcium-containing products	May reduce absorption and decrease levels of ciprofloxacin; administer 2 hours before or 6 hours after calcium-containing products. Proquin XR should be administered at least 4 hours before or 2 hours after these products.
Corticosteroids	Coadministration may increase risk of severe tendon disorder.
Cyclosporine	Transient elevations in serum creatinine with cyclosporine.
Didanosine	May reduce absorption and decrease levels of ciprofloxacin with didanosine (chewable/buffered tablets, pediatric powder); administer 2 hours before or 6 hours after didanosine. Proquin XR should be administered at least 4 hours before or 2 hours after didanosine.
Glyburide	Severe hypoglycemia reported with concomitant glyburide (rare).
Iron	May reduce absorption and decrease levels of ciprofloxacin; administer 2 hours before or 6 hours after iron. Proquin XR should be administered at least 4 hours before or 2 hours after iron products.
Methotrexate	May increase plasma levels of methotrexate.
NSAIDs	NSAIDs (except ASA) may increase risk of convulsions with very high dose ciprofloxacin.
Phenytoin	May increase or decrease plasma levels of phenytoin.
Probenecid	May increase plasma levels of ciprofloxacin.
QT interval, drugs prolonging	May increase risk of QT prolongation with other drugs that prolong the QT interval (eg, class IA and III antiarrhythmics).
Seizure threshold, drugs lowering	May increase risk of seizure with drugs that lower seizure threshold.

FLUOROQUINOLONES *(cont.)*

Ciprofloxacin HCl (Cipro Oral, Cipro XR, Proquin XR) *(cont.)*	
Sucralfate	May reduce absorption and decrease plasma levels of ciprofloxacin; administer 2 hours before or 6 hours after sucralfate. Proquin XR should be administered at least 4 hours before or 2 hours after sucralfate.
Theophylline	May increase plasma levels and prolong half-life of theophylline. Avoid concomitant use if possible; serious and fatal reactions including cardiac arrest, seizure, and respiratory failure reported.
Tizanidine	Concomitant use contraindicated; may increase plasma levels and potentiate hypotensive and sedative effects of tizanidine.
Zinc	May reduce absorption and decrease levels of ciprofloxacin; administer 2 hours before or 6 hours after zinc. Proquin XR should be administered at least 4 hours before or 2 hours after zinc products.
Gemifloxacin Mesylate (Factive)	
Antacids	May decrease absorption of gemifloxacin with magnesium/aluminum antacids; avoid administration within 3 hours before or 2 hours after gemifloxacin.
Antiarrhythmics	Avoid Class IA (eg, quinidine, procainamide) or III (eg, amiodarone, sotalol) antiarrhythmics.
Anticoagulants, coumarin	Increased PT/INR and bleeding episodes reported with concomitant coumarin anticoagulants.
Didanosine	May decrease absorption of gemifloxacin with didanosine (chewable/buffered tablets, pediatric powder); avoid administration within 3 hours before or 2 hours after gemifloxacin.
Iron	May decrease absorption of gemifloxacin; avoid administration within 3 hours before or 2 hours after gemifloxacin.
Probenecid	May increase systemic exposure of gemifloxacin with probenecid.
QT interval, drugs prolonging	May increase risk of QT prolongation with other drugs that prolong the QT interval (eg, class IA and III antiarrhythmics, erythromycin, antipsychotics, TCAs).
Zinc	May decrease absorption of gemifloxacin; avoid administration within 3 hours before or 2 hours after gemifloxacin.
Sucralfate	May decrease absorption of gemifloxacin; avoid administration within 2 hours of gemifloxacin.
Levofloxacin (Levaquin)	
Antacids	May decrease absorption of oral levofloxacin with magnesium/aluminum antacids; separate dosing by 2 hours.
Anticoagulants, coumarin	May enhance anticoagulant effects of warfarin; monitor PT/INR.
Antidiabetic agents	Blood glucose disturbances, including hyperglycemia and hypoglycemia reported with coadministration.
Corticosteroids	Coadministration may increase risk of tendinitis and tendon rupture.
Didanosine	May decrease absorption of oral levofloxacin; separate dosing by 2 hours.
Iron	May decrease absorption of oral levofloxacin; separate dosing by 2 hours.

Table 6.3. DRUG INTERACTIONS FOR ANTIBIOTICS *(cont.)*

FLUOROQUINOLONES *(cont.)*	
Levofloxacin (Levaquin) *(cont.)*	
NSAIDs	May increase risk of CNS stimulation and convulsive seizures.
QT interval, drugs prolonging	May increase risk of QT prolongation with other drugs that prolong the QT interval (eg, class IA and III antiarrhythmics).
Sucralfate	May decrease absorption of oral levofloxacin; separate dosing by 2 hours.
Theophylline	May increase plasma levels and prolong half-life of theophylline; monitor levels.
Zinc (multivitamins)	May decrease absorption of oral levofloxacin; separate dosing by 2 hours.
Lomefloxacin HCl (Maxaquin)	
Antacids	May decrease bioavailability of lomefloxacin with magnesium/aluminum antacids; administer 4 hours before or 2 hours after lomefloxacin.
Anticoagulants, coumarin	May enhance effects of coumarin anticoagulants; monitor PT/INR.
Cimetidine	May increase AUC and half-life of lomefloxacin.
Cyclosporine	May increase plasma levels of cyclosporine.
Didanosine	May decrease bioavailability of lomefloxacin; administer 4 hours before or 2 hours after lomefloxacin.
Multivitamins (minerals/iron)	May decrease bioavailability of lomefloxacin; separate dosing by 2 hours.
Probenecid	May increase plasma levels of lomefloxacin.
Sucralfate	May decrease bioavailability of lomefloxacin; administer 4 hours before or 2 hours after lomefloxacin.
Moxifloxacin HCl (Avelox)	
Antacids	May decrease absorption of moxifloxacin with magnesium/aluminum antacids; administer moxifloxacin 4 hours before or 8 hours after these products.
Anticoagulants, coumarin	May enhance effects of coumarin anticoagulants; monitor PT/INR.
Corticosteroids	Coadministration may increase risk of tendinitis and tendon rupture.
Didanosine	May decrease absorption of moxifloxacin; administer moxifloxacin 4 hours before or 8 hours after these products.
Multivitamin	May decrease absorption of moxifloxacin with iron/zinc-containing multivitamins; administer moxifloxacin 4 hours before or 8 hours after these products.
NSAIDs	May increase risk of CNS stimulation and convulsive seizures.
QT interval, drugs that prolong	May increase risk of QT prolongation with other drugs that prolong the QT interval (eg, class IA and III antiarrhythmics, erythromycin, antipsychotics, TCAs).
Sucralfate	May decrease absorption of moxifloxacin; administer moxifloxacin 4 hours before or 8 hours after these products.
Norfloxacin (Noroxin)	
Antacids	May decrease absorption of norfloxacin; separate dosing by 2 hours.
Anticoagulants, coumarin	May enhance effects of coumarin anticoagulants; monitor PT/INR.
Caffeine	May reduce clearance and prolong half-life of caffeine.
Corticosteroids	Coadministration may increase risk of tendinitis and tendon rupture.

FLUOROQUINOLONES *(cont.)*

Norfloxacin (Noroxin) *(cont.)*	
Cyclosporine	May increase plasma levels of cyclosporine; monitor levels.
CYP1A2 substrates	May increase plasma levels of drugs metabolized by CYP1A2 (eg, caffeine, clozapine, ropinirole, tacrine, theophylline, tizanidine).
Didanosine	May decrease absorption of norfloxacin with didanosine (chewable/buffered tablets, pediatric powder); separate dosing by 2 hours.
Glyburide	Severe hypoglycemia reported with concomitant glyburide (rare).
Iron	May decrease absorption of norfloxacin; separate dosing by 2 hours.
Multivitamins	May decrease absorption of norfloxacin; separate dosing by 2 hours.
Nitrofurantoin	May antagonize the antibacterial effect of norfloxacin in the urinary tract; concomitant use not recommended.
NSAIDs	May increase risk of CNS stimulation and convulsive seizures.
Probenecid	May decrease urinary excretion of norfloxacin.
Sucralfate	May decrease absorption of norfloxacin; separate dosing by 2 hours.
Theophylline	May increase plasma levels of theophylline; monitor levels.
Zinc	May decrease absorption of norfloxacin; separate dosing by 2 hours.
Ofloxacin (Floxin)	
Antacids	May decrease absorption of ofloxacin; separate dosing by 2 hours.
Anticoagulants, coumarin	May enhance effects of coumarin anticoagulants; monitor PT/INR.
Antidiabetic agents	Blood glucose disturbances, including hyperglycemia and hypoglycemia reported with coadministration.
Cimetidine	Increased AUC and half-life reported with some quinolones; caution with coadministration.
Corticosteroids	Coadministration may increase risk of tendinitis and tendon rupture.
Cyclosporine	Increased plasma levels of cyclosporine reported with some quinolones; caution with coadministration.
CYP450 substrates	Increased plasma levels of drugs metabolized by CYP450 enzymes observed with some quinolones.
Didanosine	May decrease absorption of ofloxacin; separate dosing by 2 hours.
Iron	May decrease absorption of ofloxacin; separate dosing by 2 hours.
Multivitamins	May decrease absorption of ofloxacin with zinc-containing multivitamins; separate dosing by 2 hours.
NSAIDs	May increase risk of CNS stimulation and convulsive seizures.
Probenecid	Decreased elimination of some quinolones observed with probenecid; caution with probenecid.
Sucralfate	May decrease absorption of ofloxacin; separate dosing by 2 hours.
Theophylline	May increase plasma levels of theophylline; monitor levels.

Table 6.3. DRUG INTERACTIONS FOR ANTIBIOTICS *(cont.)*

MACROLIDES

Azithromycin (Zithromax, Zmax)	
Antacids	May decrease plasma levels with aluminum/magnesium antacids.
Carbamazepine	May increase carbamazepine levels.
Cyclosporine	Monitor cyclosporine levels.
Digoxin	May increase plasma levels of digoxin.
Ergot derivatives	Acute ergot toxicity may occur with concomitant ergotamine or dihydroergotamine.
Hexobarbital	Monitor with hexobarbital.
Nelfinavir	May increase plasma levels of azithromycin; monitor for adverse events.
Phenytoin	Monitor phenytoin levels.
Terfenadine	Monitor with terfenadine.
Uricosuric drugs	Uricosuric drugs (eg, probenecid and sulfinpyrazone) increase nitrofurantoin levels.
Warfarin	May enhance anticoagulant effects of warfarin.
Clarithromycin (Biaxin, Biaxin XL)	
Antiarrhythmics	Torsades de pointes reported with concurrent use of clarithromycin and quinidine or disopyramide; monitor serum concentrations and EKG for QT prolongation.
Anticoagulants	May potentiate the effects of oral anticoagulants; monitor PT.
Astemizole	Concomitant use contraindicated; potential for cardiac arrhythmias due to inhibition of astemizole metabolism.
Benzodiazepines	May increase plasma levels of benzodiazepines metabolized by CYP3A [eg, alprazolam, midazolam (oral), triazolam]. Coadministration with oral midazolam should be avoided. CNS effects, including somnolence and confusion reported with concomitant triazolam.
Carbamazepine	May increase plasma levels of carbamazepine.
Cisapride	Concomitant use contraindicated; potential for cardiac arrhythmias due to inhibition of cisapride metabolism.
Colchicine	May increase plasma levels of colchicine; monitor for colchicine toxicity.
CYP3A substrates	May increase plasma levels of drugs metabolized by CYP3A (eg, PDE5 inhibitors, carbamazepine); caution with drugs having a narrow safety margin.
CYP450 inducers	CYP450 inducers (eg, efavirenz, nevirapine, rifampicin, rifabutin, and rifapentine) may increase metabolism of clarithromycin and possibly decrease efficacy.
Digoxin	May increase plasma levels of digoxin; monitor serum concentrations.
Ergot derivatives	Concomitant use contraindicated; potential for ergot toxicity.
Fluconazole	May increase plasma levels of fluconazole.
HMG-CoA reductase inhibitors (statins)	May increase plasma levels of statins (eg, lovastatin, simvastatin); rare reports of rhabdomyolysis with coadministration.

MACROLIDES *(cont.)*

Clarithromycin (Biaxin, Biaxin XL) *(cont.)*	
Omeprazole	May increase plasma levels of omeprazole.
Pimozide	Concomitant use contraindicated; potential for cardiac arrhythmias due to inhibition of pimozide metabolism.
Ranitidine	Avoid coadministration with ranitidine bismuth citrate if CrCl <25 mL/min or history of porphyria.
Ritonavir	May increase plasma levels of clarithromycin; reduce dose with coadministration in renal impairment if CrCl <60 mL/min.
Terfenadine	Concomitant use contraindicated; potential for cardiac arrhythmias due to inhibition of terfenadine metabolism.
Theophylline	May increase plasma levels of theophylline.
Triazolam	May decrease clearance of triazolam.
Verapamil	Hypotension, bradyarrhythmias, and lactic acidosis observed with concomitant verapamil.
Zidovudine	May decrease plasma levels of zidovudine in HIV-infected adults; separate dosing.
Erythromycin (ERYC, Ery-Tab, Erythromycin Base, Erythromycin Delayed-Release, PCE, E.E.S., EryPed, Erythrocin)	
Anticoagulants, oral	May increase effects of oral anticoagulants.
Astemizole	Concomitant use contraindicated; potential for cardiac arrhythmias due to inhibition of astemizole metabolism.
Benzodiazepines	May decrease clearance of midazolam and triazolam; possible increased benzodiazepine effect.
Cisapride	May inhibit metabolism of cisapride; cardiac arrhythmias reported with coadministration.
CYP450 substrates	May increase plasma levels of drugs metabolized by CYP450 enzymes (eg, carbamazepine, cyclosporine, hexobarbital, phenytoin, tacrolimus).
Digoxin	May increase plasma levels of digoxin.
Ergot derivatives	Acute ergot toxicity may occur with concomitant ergotamine or dihydroergotamine.
HMG-CoA reductase inhibitors (statins)	May increase plasma levels of statins; rhabdomyolysis reported with coadministration.
Quinidine	Caution with quinidine; QT prolongation, torsades de pointes, and cardiac arrest reported with coadministration.
Sildenafil	May increase plasma levels of sildenafil; consider sildenafil dose reduction.
Terfenadine	Concomitant use contraindicated; potential for cardiac arrhythmias due to inhibition of terfenadine metabolism.
Theophylline	May increase plasma levels of theophylline; potential for theophylline toxicity.

Table 6.3. DRUG INTERACTIONS FOR ANTIBIOTICS *(cont.)*

MACROLIDE/SULFONAMIDE	
Erythromycin Ethylsuccinate/Sulfisoxazole Acetyl (Pediazole)	
Anticoagulants, oral	May increase effects of oral anticoagulants.
Benzodiazepines	May decrease clearance of midazolam and triazolam; possible increased benzodiazepine effect.
CYP450 substrates	May increase plasma levels of drugs metabolized by CYP450 enzymes (eg, carbamazepine, cyclosporine, hexobarbital, phenytoin, tacrolimus).
Digoxin	May increase plasma levels of digoxin.
Diuretics	Cross-sensitivity with thiazides and acetazolamide.
Ergot derivatives	Acute ergot toxicity may occur with concomitant ergotamine or dihydroergotamine.
Hypoglycemics, oral	Cross-sensitivity with oral hypoglycemics.
Lovastatin	Rhabdomyolysis reported with coadministration; monitor creatine kinase and serum transaminase levels.
Methotrexate	May displace methotrexate from plasma protein-binding sites, thereby increasing free methotrexate concentrations.
Sildenafil	May increase AUC of sildenafil; consider dose reduction of sildenafil.
Terfenadine	Concomitant use contraindicated; potential for cardiac arrhythmias due to inhibition of terfenadine metabolism.
Theophylline	May increase plasma levels of theophylline; potential for theophylline toxicity.
Thiopental	May require less thiopental for anesthesia with sulfisoxazole.
NITROIMIDAZOLE	
Metronidazole (Flagyl, Flagyl ER, Flagyl IV)	
Alcohol	Avoid alcohol during metronidazole therapy and for 3 days after.
Anticoagulants, coumarin	May potentiate the effects of coumarin anticoagulants; may prolong PT.
Disulfiram	Avoid within 2 weeks of disulfiram; may increase risk of psychotic reactions.
Hepatic enzyme inducers	May decrease plasma levels of metronidazole with hepatic enzyme inducers (eg, phenytoin, phenobarbital).
Hepatic enzyme inhibitors	May decrease metronidazole clearance and prolong half-life with hepatic enzyme inhibitors (eg, cimetidine).
Lithium	May increase plasma levels of lithium.
Phenytoin	Coadministration may impair phenytoin clearance and decrease plasma levels of metronidazole.
PENICILLINS	
AMINOPENICILLIN/β-LACTAMASE INHIBITOR	
Amoxicillin/Clavulanate Potassium (Augmentin, Augmentin ES-600, Augmentin XR)	
Allopurinol	May increase incidence of rash.
Anticoagulants	May increase PT with anticoagulant therapy.

PENICILLINS *(cont.)*

AMINOPENICILLIN/β-LACTAMASE INHIBITOR *(cont.)*

Amoxicillin/Clavulanate Potassium (Augmentin, Augmentin ES-600, Augmentin XR) *(cont.)*	
Contraceptives, oral	May reduce efficacy of oral contraceptives.
Probenecid	Avoid coadministration with probenecid; may decrease the renal tubular secretion of amoxicillin resulting in increased and prolonged plasma levels of amoxicillin.

BROAD-SPECTRUM PENICILLIN

Piperacillin Sodium	
Aminoglycosides	Do not mix with aminoglycoside in parenteral solution; may cause inactivation of aminoglycoside.
Anticoagulants	Closely monitor coagulation parameters with concomitant anticoagulants.
Cytotoxic therapy	May increase risk of hypokalemia with cytotoxic therapy.
Diuretics	May increase risk of hypokalemia with diuretics.
Methotrexate	May decrease clearance of methotrexate; monitor methotrexate serum levels to avoid toxicity.
Muscle relaxants, non-depolarizing	May prolong neuromuscular blockade of non-depolarizing muscle relaxants (eg, vecuronium).
Probenecid	May increase plasma levels of piperacillin.

BROAD-SPECTRUM PENICILLINS/β-LACTAMASE INHIBITORS

Piperacillin Sodium/Tazobactam (Zosyn)	
Aminoglycosides	Do not mix with aminoglycoside in parenteral solution; may cause inactivation of aminoglycosides.
Anticoagulants	Closely monitor coagulation parameters with concomitant anticoagulants.
Cytotoxic therapy	May increase risk of hypokalemia with cytotoxic therapy.
Diuretics	May increase risk of hypokalemia with diuretics.
Methotrexate	May decrease clearance of methotrexate; monitor methotrexate serum levels to avoid toxicity.
Muscle relaxants, non-depolarizing	May prolong neuromuscular blockade of non-depolarizing muscle relaxants (eg, vecuronium).
Probenecid	May prolong half-life of piperacillin and tazobactam.
Ticarcillin Disodium/Clavulanate Potassium (Timentin)	
Aminoglycosides	Do not mix with aminoglycoside in parenteral solution; may cause inactivation of aminoglycoside.
Contraceptives, oral	May reduce efficacy of combined oral estrogen/progesterone contraceptives.
Probenecid	May increase plasma levels and prolong half-life with probenecid.

Table 6.3. DRUG INTERACTIONS FOR ANTIBIOTICS *(cont.)*

PENICILLINS	
Dicloxacillin Sodium	
Anticoagulants, coumarin	May decrease the anticoagulant response to coumarin anticoagulants.
Probenecid	May increase and prolong plasma dicloxacillin levels.
Tetracycline	Tetracycline may antagonize the bactericidal effects of dicloxacillin; avoid concomitant use.
Penicillin G Benzathine (Bicillin L-A, Permapen)	
Antibiotics, bacteriostatic	Bacteriostatic antibiotics (eg, tetracycline, erythromycin) may decrease the bactericidal activity of penicillins.
Probenecid	May increase and prolong plasma levels of penicillins.
Penicillin G Benzathine/Penicillin G Procaine (Bicillin C-R, Bicillin C-R 900/300)	
Antibiotics, bacteriostatic	Bacteriostatic antibiotics (eg, tetracycline, erythromycin) may decrease the bactericidal activity of penicillins.
Probenecid	May increase and prolong plasma levels of penicillins.
Penicillin G Potassium (Pfizerpen)	
Antibiotics, bacteriostatic	Bacteriostatic antibiotics (eg, tetracycline, erythromycin) may decrease the bactericidal activity of penicillins.
Probenecid	May increase and prolong plasma levels of penicillins.
SEMISYNTHETIC AMPICILLIN DERIVATIVE	
Amoxicillin (Amoxil)	
Antibiotics, bacteriostatic	Bacteriostatic antibiotics (eg, chloramphenicol, macrolides, sulfonamides, tetracyclines) may interfere with bactericidal effects of amoxicillin.
Probenecid	May increase and prolong plasma levels of amoxicillin.
SEMISYNTHETIC PENICILLIN DERIVATIVES	
Ampicillin Oral	
Allopurinol	May increase risk of rash with allopurinol.
Antibiotics, bacteriostatic	Bacteriostatic antibiotics (eg, chloramphenicol, erythromycins, sulfonamides, tetracyclines) may decrease the bactericidal activity of ampicillin.
Contraceptives, oral	May decrease the efficacy of oral contraceptives.
Probenecid	May increase plasma levels of ampicillin.
Ampicillin Sodium Injection	
Allopurinol	May increase risk of rash with allopurinol.
Contraceptives, oral	May decrease the efficacy of oral contraceptives.
Probenecid	May increase plasma levels of ampicillin.
SEMISYNTHETIC PENICILLIN/β-LACTAMASE INHIBITOR	
Ampicillin Sodium/Sulbactam Sodium (Unasyn)	
Allopurinol	May increase risk of rash with allopurinol.
Probenecid	May increase and prolong plasma levels of ampicillin and sulbactam.

SULFONAMIDE

Sulfisoxazole (Gantrisin Pediatric)	
Anticoagulants	May prolong PT with anticoagulants.
Methotrexate	May displace methotrexate from plasma protein-binding sites, thereby increasing free methotrexate concentrations.
Sulfonylureas	May potentiate glucose-lowering effect of sulfonylureas.
Thiopental	May require less thiopental for anesthesia with sulfisoxazole.

SULFONAMIDE/TETRAHYDROFOLIC ACID INHIBITORS

Sulfamethoxazole/Trimethoprim (Bactrim, Bactrim DS)	
ACE inhibitors	Hyperkalemia reported in elderly patients with concomitant ACE inhibitors (rare).
Amantadine	Single case of toxic delirium reported with amantadine.
Anticoagulants, coumarin	May prolong PT; caution with coadministration.
Cyclosporine	Marked but reversible nephrotoxicity reported with cyclosporine.
Digoxin	May increase plasma levels of digoxin (especially in elderly); monitor levels.
Diuretics	May increase risk of thrombocytopenia with purpura in elderly patients receiving concomitant diuretics, primarily thiazides.
Hypoglycemics, oral	May potentiate glucose-lowering effect of oral hypoglycemics.
Indomethacin	May increase plasma levels of sulfamethoxazole.
Methotrexate	May displace methotrexate from plasma protein-binding sites, thereby increasing free methotrexate concentrations.
Phenytoin	May decrease clearance and increase half-life of phenytoin; monitor for phenytoin toxicity.
Pyrimethamine	Megaloblastic anemia reported with concomitant pyrimethamine >25 mg/week.
Tricyclic antidepressants (TCAs)	May decrease efficacy of TCAs.
Sulfamethoxazole/Trimethoprim (Septra, Septra DS, Sulfatrim Pediatric)	
ACE inhibitors	Hyperkalemia reported in elderly patients with concomitant ACE inhibitors (2 cases).
Anticoagulants, coumarin	May prolong PT; caution with coadministration.
Diuretics	May increase risk of thrombocytopenia with purpura in elderly patients receiving concomitant diuretics, primarily thiazides.
Methotrexate	May displace methotrexate from plasma protein-binding sites, thereby increasing free methotrexate concentrations.
Phenytoin	May decrease clearance and increase half-life of phenytoin; monitor for phenytoin toxicity.

Table 6.3. DRUG INTERACTIONS FOR ANTIBIOTICS *(cont.)*

TETRACYCLINE DERIVATIVES

Demeclocycline HCl (Declomycin)	
Antacids	May decrease absorption of demeclocycline with antacids containing aluminum, calcium, or magnesium.
Contraceptives, oral	May decrease efficacy of oral contraceptives.
Food	Foods/dairy products may interfere with absorption; administer at least 1 hour before or 2 hours after meals.
Iron-containing products	May decrease absorption of demeclocycline.
Methoxyflurane	Fatal renal toxicity reported with methoxyflurane.
Penicillin	May interfere with the bactericidal action of penicillin; avoid concurrent use.
Doxycycline (Doryx, Monodox, Periostat, Vibramycin, Vibra-Tabs)	
Antacids	May decrease absorption of doxycycline with antacids containing aluminum, calcium, or magnesium.
Anticoagulants, oral	May decrease PT, adjust oral anticoagulant doses.
Barbiturates	May decrease half-life of doxycycline.
Bismuth subsalicylate	May impair absorption of doxycycline.
Carbamazepine	May decrease half-life of doxycycline.
Contraceptives, oral	May decrease efficacy of oral contraceptives.
Iron-containing products	May impair absorption of doxycycline.
Methoxyflurane	Fatal renal toxicity reported with methoxyflurane.
Penicillin	May interfere with the bactericidal action of penicillin; avoid concurrent use.
Phenytoin	May decrease half-life of doxycycline.
Minocycline HCl (Dynacin, Minocin)	
Antacids	May decrease absorption of minocycline with antacids containing aluminum, calcium, or magnesium.
Contraceptives, oral	May decrease efficacy of oral contraceptives.
Ergot alkaloids	May increase risk of ergotism with concomitant ergot alkaloids/derivatives (Minocin).
Hepatotoxic drugs	Caution with other hepatotoxic drugs (Minocin).
Iron-containing products	May impair absorption of minocycline.
Isotretinoin	Avoid isotretinoin shortly before, during, and after minocycline therapy; risk of pseudotumor cerebri.
Methoxyflurane	Fatal renal toxicity reported with methoxyflurane.
Penicillin	May interfere with the bactericidal action of penicillin; avoid concurrent use.
Tetracycline HCl (Sumycin)	
Antacids	Absorption of tetracycline is impaired by antacids containing aluminum, calcium, or magnesium.
Bactericidal agents	May interfere with the bactericidal action of penicillin and other bactericidal agents; avoid concomitant use.

TETRACYCLINE DERIVATIVES *(cont.)*

Tetracycline HCl (Sumycin) *(cont.)*	
Contraceptives, oral	May decrease efficacy of oral contraceptives.
Dairy products	Dairy products may interfere with absorption; administer tetracycline 1 hour before or 2 hours after dairy products.
Iron-containing products	Absorption of tetracycline is impaired by iron-containing products.
Methoxyflurane	Fatal renal toxicity reported with concurrent methoxyflurane.

MISCELLANEOUS ANTIBIOTICS

Aztreonam (Azactam)	
Aminoglycosides	May increase risk of nephrotoxicity and ototoxicity with aminoglycosides; monitor renal function.
Toxic epidermal necrolysis, drugs causing	May increase risk of toxic epidermal necrolysis.
Bacitracin Injection	
Nephrotoxic drugs	May potentiate renal toxicity with other nephrotoxic drugs (eg, streptomycin, kanamycin, polymyxin B, polymyxin E, neomycin).
Clindamycin HCl (Cleocin)	
Erythromycin	Antagonism may occur between erythromycin and clindamycin; avoid coadministration.
Neuromuscular blockers	May enhance the action of other neuromuscular blockers; caution with coadministration.
Colistimethate Sodium (Coly-Mycin M)	
Antibiotics	Avoid certain antibiotics (eg, aminoglycosides, polymyxin); may interfere with nerve transmission at neuromuscular junction.
Muscle relaxants	Extreme caution with curariform muscle relaxants (eg, tubocurarine), succinylcholine, gallamine, decamethonium, and sodium citrate; may potentiate neuromuscular blocking effect.
Sodium cephalothin	Avoid with sodium cephalothin; may enhance nephrotoxicity.
Dalfopristin/Quinupristin (Synercid)	
Cyclosporine	May increase plasma levels of cyclosporine; monitor levels.
CYP3A4 substrates	May increase plasma levels of drugs metabolized by CYP3A4 (eg, cyclosporin A, tacrolimus, midazolam, nifedipine, verapamil, diltiazem, astemizole, terfenadine, delaviridine, nevirapine, indinavir, ritonavir, vinca alkaloids, docetaxel, paclitaxel, diazepam, HMG-CoA reductase inhibitors, methylprednisolone, carbamazepine, quinidine, lidocaine, disopyramide).
Digoxin	May inhibit gut metabolism of digoxin.
Daptomycin (Cubicin)	
HMG-CoA reductase inhibitors (statins)	Limited data with statins; consider temporarily suspending these agents with daptomycin therapy.
Tobramycin	Coadministration may alter levels of tobramycin and daptomycin; caution with concomitant use.

Table 6.3. DRUG INTERACTIONS FOR ANTIBIOTICS ***(cont.)***

MISCELLANEOUS ANTIBIOTICS *(cont.)*	
Daptomycin (Cubicin) *(cont.)*	
Warfarin	Limited data with warfarin; monitor anticoagulant activity for several days after initiating daptomycin therapy.
Lincomycin HCl (Lincocin)	
Erythromycin	Possible antagonism between erythromycin and lincomycin; avoid concomitant use.
Kaolin-pectin	Kaolin-pectin inhibits oral lincomycin.
Neuromuscular blockers	May enhance the action of neuromuscular blockers; caution with coadministration.
Linezolid (Zyvox)	
Adrenergic agents	May enhance pressor response to sympathomimetics, vasopressors, and dopaminergic agents; caution with dopamine, epinephrine, pseudoephedrine, and phenylpropanolamine.
Serotonergic agents	Serotonin syndrome may occur with concomitant serotonergic agents, including antidepressants such as SSRIs.
Tyramine	Avoid large quantities of tyramine-containing foods or beverages; may induce significant pressor response.
Telithromycin (Ketek)	
Antiarrhythmics	May increase risk of QT prolongation with Class IA (eg, quinidine, procainamide) and Class III (eg, dofetilide) antiarrhythmics; avoid concomitant use.
Anticoagulants, oral	May enhance effects of oral anticoagulants.
Antifungals	May increase plasma levels of telithromycin with ketoconazole/itraconazole.
Cisapride	Contraindicated; do not use concomitantly.
CYP3A4 inducers	May decrease plasma levels and efficacy of telithromycin with CYP3A4 inducers (eg, rifampin, phenytoin, carbamazepine, phenobarbital).
CYP450 substrates	May increase plasma levels of drugs metabolized by the CYP450 system (eg, carbamazepine, cyclosporine, tacrolimus, sirolimus, hexobarbital, phenytoin, midazolam, triazolam, metoprolol), especially CYP3A4.
Digoxin	May increase plasma levels of digoxin; monitor levels.
Ergot alkaloid derivatives	Avoid ergot alkaloid derivatives; acute ergot toxicity reported with coadministration.
HMG-CoA reductase inhibitors (statins)	May increase plasma levels of statins due to CYP3A4 inhibition. May increase risk of myopathy; avoid concomitant use.
Pimozide	Contraindicated; do not use concomitantly.
Sotalol	May decrease plasma levels of sotalol.
Theophylline	Coadministration may increase plasma levels of theophylline and worsen GI side effects. Separate dosing by 1 hour to decrease GI side effects.
Tigecycline (Tygacil)	
Contraceptives, oral	May decrease efficacy of oral contraceptives.
Warfarin	Monitor PT with warfarin.

MISCELLANEOUS ANTIBIOTICS *(cont.)*

Trimethoprim HCl (Primsol)	
Phenytoin	May decrease clearance and increase half-life of phenytoin; monitor for phenytoin toxicity.
Vancomycin HCl Injection	
Anesthetics	Concomitant use of anesthetic agents has been associated with erythema, histamine-like flushing, and anaphylactoid reactions.
Nephrotoxic/neurotoxic drugs	Concurrent and/or sequential systemic or topical use of other potentially neurotoxic and/or nephrotoxic drugs (eg, amphotericin B, aminoglycosides, bacitracin, polymyxin B, colistin, viomycin, cisplatin) requires careful monitoring.

Table 6.4. PHARMACOLOGIC PROPERTIES OF ANTIBIOTICS

DRUG	ACTION	ABSORPTION	DISTRIBUTION	EXCRETION
CLINDAMYCIN				
	Bacteriostatic: inhibits bacterial protein synthesis. At higher concentrations, clindamycin can be bactericidal.	Nearly completely absorbed from the stomach after oral administration; absorption is not appreciably influenced by the presence of food.	The drug is widely distributed to many fluids and tissues, including bone. It crosses the placental barrier and enters the fetal circulation.	The drug is excreted in the urine and the feces. Antimicrobial activity may persist in the colonic contents for up to 1 week after therapy.
MACROLIDES				
	Inhibit bacterial protein synthesis by binding reversibly to the 50S ribosomal subunits of sensitive bacteria.	Food in stomach delays drug's ultimate absorption. Clarithromycin and azithromycin are better absorbed than erythromycin and yield higher serum levels.	Diffuse readily into intracellular fluids, and antibacterial activity can be achieved at essentially all body sites with the exception of the brain and cerebrospinal fluid.	Erythromycin and azithromycin are mainly eliminated via the liver. Clarithromycin is eliminated via the liver and kidneys.
METRONIDAZOLE				
	Bactericidal: inhibits DNA synthesis; it also modifies cell-mediated immunity, thereby normalizing excessive immune reactions.	Usually completely and promptly absorbed after oral administration and achieves therapeutic levels in the serum about 1 hour after the first dosage.	Penetrates well into body tissues and fluids, including vaginal secretions, saliva, breast milk, and cerebrospinal fluid; passes the placental barrier and enters fetal circulation.	The liver accounts for more than 50% of the drug's systemic clearance. However, unchanged metronidazole and its metabolites are excreted in various proportions in the urine.
PENICILLINS AND CEPHALOSPORINS				
	Bactericidal: inhibit specific bacterial enzymes required for the assembly of the bacterial cell wall.	Excellent absorption; more predictable blood levels can be obtained if given on an empty stomach.	Widely distributed throughout the body, including the saliva and gingival crevicular fluid; crosses the placenta.	Rapidly eliminated from plasma by the kidneys.
QUINOLONES (CIPROFLOXACIN AND LEVOFLOXACIN)				
	Bactericidal: inhibit DNA synthesis.	Rapidly absorbed from the stomach after oral administration; maximum serum concentrations are obtained 1-2 hours after oral administration.	Present in antibacterial concentrations in saliva, nasal and bronchial secretions, sputum, breast milk, skin blister fluid, lymphatic and peritoneal fluid, and prostatic secretions.	In patients with reduced renal function, drug half-life is slightly prolonged and dosage adjustments may be required.
TETRACYCLINES				
	Bacteriostatic: inhibit bacterial protein synthesis. Bactericidal at high concentrations; may inhibit protein synthesis in mammalian cells.	Doxycycline and minocycline possess greater absorption than tetracycline. Absorption is greater in the fasting state.	Tetracyclines penetrate soft tissues, the CNS, and the brain, cross the placenta, and enter fetal circulation and amniotic fluid. High concentrations are also present in breast milk.	Excretion is via the urine and feces. Renal clearance of minocycline is lower than tetracycline. Doxycycline does not accumulate significantly in the blood of patients with renal failure.

Chapter 7

Antifungal and Antiviral Agents

Brian C. Muzyka, D.M.D., M.S., M.B.A.;
Martha Somerman, D.D.S., Ph.D.

ANTIFUNGAL AGENTS

The most common oral fungal infection is caused by *Candida* species. Oral *Candida* infections may have four clinical presentations. 1) Pseudomembranous candidiasis (thrush) appears as white or yellow plaque on mucosal surfaces and may be wiped away easily; 2) erythematous (atrophic) candidiasis appears as red patches on any mucosal surface. When found on the tongue, it may cause depapillation; 3) hyperplastic (chronic) candidiasis is similar to the pseudomembranous variant, but the plaques cannot readily be removed; and 4) angular chelitis (perleche), the last variant of oral *Candida* infection, is a mixed *Candida* and bacterial infection. Angular chelitis appears as red radiating fissures from the corners of the mouth and is often accompanied by a pseudomembranous covering.

Candida infections may be diagnosed empirically or through oral cultures or cytological smears. As *Candida* is a normal constituent of the oral cavity, use care to interpret findings of oral *Candida* species.

Pharmacological treatment for oral fungal infections is limited to three classes of antifungal agents: azoles, polyenes, and echinocandins. The azole group is further subdivided into imidazole and triazole groups. Echinocandins are a newer class of antifungals that inhibit synthesis of β (1-3)-d-glucan, an integral part of fungal cell walls. β (1-3)-d-glucan is not found in mammalian cells and, therefore, limited adverse effects have been reported.

Superficial oral fungal infections are most commonly treated with topical antifungal agents. These agents are available in several forms, such as rinses, troches, and creams. Cutaneous fungal infections are most often treated with topical agents such as creams and ointments. Systemic fungal infections with an oral presentation are treated with systemic medications.

Table 7.1 provides dosing and prescribing information on antifungal drugs.

Azole Antifungal Agents

These drugs are divided into the following subgroups:

- Imidazoles: clotrimazole, miconazole, ketoconazole, and sertaconazole.
- Triazoles: fluconazole, itraconazole, and posaconazole.

Many of the azoles are used to treat oropharyngeal candidiasis. They are also used for other fungal infections, such as aspergillosis, blastomycosis, chromomycosis, coccidioidomycosis, cryptococcosis, and histoplasmosis.

Polyene Antifungal Agents

Polyenes are amphotericin B and nystatin. Polyenes are used for local treatment of fungal infections of the mouth caused by

Candida albicans and other *Candida* species. Intravenous formulations of amphotericin B are used for treatment of severe systemic fungal infections.

The pharmacokinetics of the different formulations of amphotericin can differ substantially. In general, usual dosages of amphotericin B cholesteryl sulfate complexes (ABCD), amphotericin B lipid complexes (ABLC), and liposomal amphotericin B (L-AmB) are tolerated better than the conventional formulation of amphotericin B.

ABCD is labeled for treatment of invasive aspergillosis in people who are nonresponsive to amphotericin and in those who are unable to tolerate amphotericin secondary to renal impairment or toxicity. It also is being investigated for treatment of other invasive fungal infections, including *Candida*.

ABLC is labeled for the use of invasive fungal infections in people who are intolerant of or refractory to treatment with conventional amphotericin B.

L-AmB is labeled for the use of cryptococcal meningitis in people with HIV infection and in empiric therapy of presumed fungal infections in people with febrile neutropenia.

Echinocandins

Echinocandins are sometimes referred to as glucan synthesis inhibitors because they inhibit synthesis of β (1-3)-d-glucan, an integral component of the yeast cell wall. Echinocandins are used for the treatment of nonresponsive or refractory aspergillosis, esophageal candidiasis, and candidemia.

General Dosing Information

General dosing information is provided in **Table 7.1**. The selection of agent and dosage depends on the extent of the oral fungal infection. Topical forms of treatment are recommended for superficial infections in patients who are immunocompetent; systemic medications are recommended for deep fungal infections or for the treatment of immunocompromised patients.

Special Dental Considerations

- Examine the oral mucosa for signs of fungal infection, such as white plaque, erythematous areas, ulcerations, and nodules or granulomas.
- Consider laboratory confirmation for deep fungal or superficial fungal disease in immunocompromised patients.
- Disinfect removable dental prosthetics and oral appliances with an antifungal solution or appropriate disinfection solution during the treatment period for superficial disease.
- Replace toothbrushes, denture brushes, and other oral hygiene devices that may be contaminated with fungal organisms.
- Consider systemic formulations of antifungal medications for use with dentate patients who have poor oral hygiene or a high Caries Index, as the troche formulations have high sugar content.
- Consider the use of topical solutions, topical creams, or systemic treatment with patients with xerostomia who may have difficulty using troches.

Drug Interactions of Dental Interest

Table 7.2 lists potential interactions with antifungal drugs.

Azoles

- Absorption of itraconazole and ketoconazole can be affected by concomitant use of antacids. If concomitant administration of sulcralfate or other drugs that affect gastric acidity is necessary, administer these drugs at least 2 hours after or 1 hour before ketoconazole or itraconazole administration.
- Other drug classes that may affect absorption of itraconazole and fluconazole include anticholinergics, antispasmodics, antimuscarinics, H_2-histamine receptor agonists, omeprazole, and sulcralfate.
- Posaconazole serum concentrations may be decreased with coadministration of

UDP glucuronidation or P-gp inducers, which are rifabutin, phenytoin, and cimetidine.

- Increased anticoagulant effects may occur in patients who are taking antifungal agents in conjunction with coumadin. Closely monitor anticoagulation levels and adjust anticoagulation medication dosages accordingly.
- Concomitant use of antihistamines such as terfenadine and astemizole—neither of which is available in most countries—with itraconazole and ketoconazole has led to cardiac dysrhythmias and is contraindicated.
- Concomitant use of cisapride (available in the United States to certain patients who meet manufacturer eligibility criteria through a special program) and ketoconazole is contraindicated and has resulted in serious cardiovascular effects.
- Concomitant use of ketoconazole and rifampin has resulted in decreased serum concentrations of ketoconazole. These drugs should not be administered concomitantly.
- Concomitant use of ketoconazole with cyclosporine or phenytoin may increase plasma levels of cyclosporine and phenytoin. Patients taking these drugs should be monitored closely.
- Concomitant administration of ketoconazole and the steroids methylprednisolone or prednisolone may result in increased plasma levels of the steroids.
- Concomitant use of alcohol and antifungal drugs may increase liver damage. Patients should be counseled not to drink alcohol while taking antifungal medications. Additionally, a disulfiram-type reaction (such as flushing, rash, peripheral edema, nausea, or headache) has occurred in patients ingesting alcohol while receiving ketoconazole therapy.
- Concomitant use of ketoconazole and the benzodiazepines midazolam or triazolam may result in increased plasma concentration of the benzodiazepine agents. Because of the potentiated hypnotic and sedative effects, these agents should not be used concomitantly with ketoconazole.
- Itraconazole and ketoconazole may increase serum digoxin levels; therefore, digoxin levels should be closely monitored when administered with itraconazole or ketoconazole.

Polyenes

- Nephrotoxic effects of certain drugs (such as aminoglycosides, capreomycin, cisplatin, colistin, cyclosporine, methoxyflurane, pentamidine, polymixin B, and vancomycin) may be additive with the concurrent or sequential use of IV amphotericin B and should be avoided. Intensive monitoring of renal function is recommended if amphotericin B is used in conjunction with any nephrotoxic agent.
- Monitor serum potassium concentrations closely in patients receiving any amphotericin B formulation concomitantly with a cardiac glycoside or skeletal muscle relaxant.
- Corticosteroids may enhance potassium depletion caused by amphotericin B and should not be used concomitantly.

Echinocandins

Clinicians should be cautious when using echinocandins in people with hepatic impairment. Dosage reduction may be required for those with moderate hepatic impairment.

Limited data suggest that coadministration of drug clearance—inducers, inducer/inhibitors, or both--with caspofungin acetate may result in reduced doses of caspofungin acetate. These inducer and inducer/inhibitors include efavirenz, nelfinavir, nevaripine, phenytoin, rifampin, dexamethasone, and carbamazepine. Consider increasing the dosage of caspofungin acetate to 70 mg in nonresponsive patients who are coadministered one or more of the inducer or inducer/inhibitor agents.

Concomitant use of caspofungin acetate with cyclosporine is not recommended secondary to elevated hepatic transaminase levels unless the benefit of using the drug outweighs the risk.

Concomitant use of micafungin sodium with nifedipine may cause increased nifedipine levels. Use of micafungin sodium with sirolimus may increase sirolimus levels.

Special Patients

Pregnant and nursing women

Most antifungal drugs are classified in pregnancy risk category B or C (see Appendix B). Use caution in prescribing these agents to pregnant women as well as to women who are breastfeeding, as some antifungal agents may enter breast milk.

Pediatric, geriatric and, other special patients

Many antifungal agents can alter kidney and liver function, which may be severely damaging to older and younger patients. Therefore, dentists may need to adjust doses of antifungal agents accordingly.

Adverse Effects and Precautions

Table 7.1 lists adverse effects and precautions related to antifungal agents.

Pharmacology

The azole antifungal agents interfere with cytochrome P450 activity, which is necessary for the demethylation of 14-α methylsterol to ergosterol. Ergosterol is the major sterol associated with fungal cell membranes. This interference in ergosterol causes changes in the cell membrane permeability and allows fungal cell elements to escape from the cell.

The polyenes inhibit fungal growth by binding with sterol in the fungal cell wall to interfere with cell membrane permeability, resulting in cell lysis.

The class of echinocandins inhibits the synthesis of β (1-3)-d-glucan, an integral part of fungal cell walls. This class at present is limited to caspofungin acetate, micafungin sodium, and anidulafungin; they do not inhibit the enzymes in the cytochrome P450 system.

Patient Advice

The following advice can be given to all patients diagnosed with oral fungal infections.

- Long-term therapy may be indicated to clear the infection and prevent relapse.
- Take the medication as prescribed and complete the course of the medication.
- Do not use commercial alcohol-based mouthrinses during treatment unless they are prescribed by the dentist.
- Removable oral appliances and dental prosthetics should be treated daily with an antifungal solution or appropriate disinfection solution during the treatment period for superficial disease.
- Oral hygiene devices (such as toothbrushes and denture brushes) that may be contaminated should be replaced.

ANTIVIRAL AGENTS

Viruses are among the simplest and smallest forms of life and must use a living host to replicate. Human viral infections have a wide spectrum of presentation, from subclinical infection to lethal infection. Viruses that affect the oral cavity, however, usually are self-limiting and heal spontaneously in a host with an intact immune system. Oral viral infections encountered in dental practice are usually limited to Coxsackie-type viruses (such as herpangina, acute lymphonodular pharyngitis, and hand-foot-and-mouth disease) and treatment is usually supportive. Other viral infections commonly encountered in the dental practice include herpes-type viruses (eg, herpes labialis, chickenpox, and shingles) and human papilloma viruses (HPV).

Viral diseases that affect the delivery of dental care include all forms of viral hepatitis and human immunodeficiency virus (HIV) disease. As a comprehensive description of these disease processes would be lengthy, the reader may learn more about these diseases by reviewing the "Suggested Reading" later in this chapter.

Coxsackie virus infection

Coxsackie viruses are a group of RNA viruses responsible for herpangina, acute lymphonodular, and hand-foot-and-mouth disease. Herpangina occurs in epidemics with symptoms a bit milder than those of herpetic infections.

Herpes virus infection

Clinical signs of herpes-type viruses often are preceded by a prodromal period in which a sharp burning or shooting pain occurs along the affected nerve distribution. Vesicles appear and rupture, leaving a raw ulcerated hemorrhagic surface that is quite painful. Multiple intraoral lesions may interfere with the ability to maintain adequate nutritional status, and supportive therapy will be required. Diagnosis of herpetic infections can be difficult, and a cytological smear or biopsy of the affected site may be necessary to rule out other disease processes such as aphthous ulcerations, pemphigus, pemphigoid, or lichen planus.

The most common viral disease encountered in dental practices is recurrent herpes labialis, which is caused by the herpes simplex virus (HSV) and is estimated to affect up to 40% of the U.S. population annually. Treatment for herpes labialis has usually been relegated to formulations that contain an anesthetic and/or a moistening agent. Improved treatment outcomes, such as reduced healing time, have been observed with newer agents.

One such agent used in the treatment of recurrent herpes labialis is docosanol. Docosanol is reported to reduce herpes labialis symptoms and reduces healing time by 0.72 days.

Valacyclovir, an acyclovir analogue, also is used in the treatment of herpes labialis. In a study where the majority of patients initiated treatment within 2 hours of onset of symptoms, the mean duration of herpes labialis episodes was about 1 day shorter in subjects treated with 2 g twice daily for 1 day.

Oral herpetic infections usually are self-limiting, and treatment consists mainly of nutritional support and pain palliation. Patients with compromised immune function are at increased risk of reactivation of viral disease, and often the reactivated disease will be more involved and more difficult to control. Patients with HIV may develop severe HSV infections that affect the oral cavity. These infections can be life-threatening, and appropriate diagnosis and treatment are crucial. Acyclovir and acyclovir analogues are most commonly used for the treatment of HSV infection in this population.

Aphthous ulcers

Quite often, recurrent aphthous ulcers are misdiagnosed as herpes. Recurrent aphthous ulcers (RAUs) are characterized by periodic ulcerations confined to the oral mucosa. No single etiologic agent has been implicated for RAUs; however, many theories have been put forward, suggesting multifactorial causes including stress, vitamin deficiency, diet, hormonal changes, allergies, trauma and immune dysfunction.

Minor aphthous ulcers (ulcers less than 1 cm in diameter) usually are found on the less keratinized tissues in the oral cavity such as the buccal mucosa, the floor of the mouth and the ventral surface of the tongue. In certain susceptible individuals, the use of dentifrices formulated without sodium lauryl sulfate may decrease the incidence of aphthous ulcers.

A prescription drug called amlexanox (Aphthasol) is approved for the treatment of aphthous ulcerations. Amlexanox is a potent inhibitor of the formation and release of inflammatory mediators from mast cells. A number of nonprescription products also are available for treatment of aphthous ulcers and other oral ulcerative conditions. Strategies used in the treatment of aphthous ulcer include barrier products (eg, pastes, gels, dissolvable patches), local anesthetic agents, oxygenating agents (used to debride ulcerations in an effort to promote healing), and others, including herbal extracts. Other agents exert their major effect by providing a protective coating over the ulcer to decrease pain and promote healing. These agents are commonly found in most drug stores.

Human papilloma virus (HPV)

Presently, 17 different subtypes of HPV have been isolated from oral mucosa. HPV lesions in the oral cavity may present as verrucous, hyperplastic, or papillomatous growths that are asymptomatic. Various modalities of treatment for HPV have been employed with limited success. These treatments include excision, laser ablation, cryotherapy, application of keratinolytic agents, and injection of antiviral agents.

Hepatitis B and C (HBV, HCV)

Although vaccination for hepatitis B virus (HBV) is recommended by the Centers for Disease Control and Prevention (CDC) Advisory Committee on Immunization Practices, HBV is still a highly prevalent disease, with 350 million chronic cases worldwide. Despite immunization efforts, 4,713 incident cases of hepatitis B were diagnosed in the United States in 2006. Because many HBV infections are either asymptomatic or never reported, the actual number of new infections is estimated to be approximately 10-fold higher. An estimated 2,000 to 4,000 deaths per year in the United States are related to chronic hepatitis B liver diseases, including liver cirrhosis and hepatocellular carcinoma.

Treatment of HBV infection remains focused on nucleoside analogs such as lamivudine, and adefovir, or the nucleotide analog dipivoxil entecavir.

Hepatitis C virus (HCV) infection is a leading cause of chronic liver disease in the United States; the estimated prevalence of antibodies to HCV is 3.9 million individuals nationwide. Chronic HCV is typically a slow process, no symptoms or physical signs may be noted for decades after the infection. Chronic HCV leads to cirrhosis in about 20% of patients within 20 years of infection.

Interferon alfa was licensed for treatment of chronic HBV in 1992 and is the standard therapy for patients who do not have evidence of decompensated liver disease. Ribavirin is a nucleoside analogue with a broad spectrum of antiviral activity, particularly against RNA viruses. Ribavirin has been used with interferon alfa in treatment of patients with chronic HCV.

Interferon alfa (Intron A, Roferon-A, Peg Intron). The interferons are a group of naturally occurring biologic response modifiers. These agents have antiviral properties and they also have some antiproliferative, immune enhancing, and differentiating effects. There are three main types of interferons: alpha and beta interferons (type 1), and gamma interferon (type 2), which is different in structure and function from both the alpha and beta interferons.

Accepted Indications

Because of substantial toxicity and side effects, antiviral agents usually are reserved for immunocompromised patients with mucocutaneous HSV-associated lesions. Studies in immunocompetent patients have shown little clinical benefit of using topical acyclovir in treatment of herpes labialis. Application of penciclovir to herpes labialis lesions decreased the duration of pain, viral shedding and time required for healing.

The clinical benefit of penciclovir is modest, however; on average, it shortens the duration of pain and viral shedding by less than one day.

General Dosing Information

Dosing and prescribing information for antiviral agents and aphthous ulcer medications can be found in **Table 7.1**.

Special Dental Considerations

Drug Interactions of Dental Interest

Table 7.2 presents information regarding drug interactions with antiviral agents.

- Systemic acyclovir, ganciclovir, and valacyclovir are nephrotoxic and should be used with caution in patients who have renal disease or in patients who are receiving other nephrotoxic medications.
- Concomitant administration of acyclovir and probenecid may delay the urinary excretion and renal clearance of acyclovir. Probenecid also may interfere with the renal clearance and urinary excretion of ganciclovir.
- Concomitant use of acyclovir and zidovudine (AZT) may increase CNS symptoms such as drowsiness or lethargy; therefore, monitor patients closely.
- Famciclovir and valacyclovir are eliminated by the kidneys. Adjust its dosage accordingly for patients with renal impairment.
- Foscarnet has a high toxic profile and should be used with care, especially in patients with a history of renal impairment.

Adjunctive Therapy

For relief of pain associated with viral lesions and aphthous ulcers, typical anesthetic agents bring temporary relief. Lidocaine viscous, 2%, can be of value. Diphenhydramine elixir, an antihistamine containing 12.5 mg of diphenhydramine per milliliter, also can be used for its topical anesthetic properties. Lidocaine viscous sometimes is mixed with equal parts of antacids and diphenhydramine elixir to improve adherence to the oral mucosa.

If patients are experiencing difficulty in eating, liquid dietary supplements may be recommended.

Adverse Effects and Precautions

Table 7.1 lists adverse effects, precautions, and contraindications associated with antiviral agents.

Pharmacology

Viral resistance to antiviral agents has become an increasing problem. Drug resistance has many causes and, depending on the specific drug, can have many mechanisms. With acyclovir, it is believed that resistant herpes simplex viruses have developed because of alterations in either the viral thymidine kinase or the viral DNA polymerase. Viral thymidine kinase starts the process through which acyclovir is transformed to its active derivative, acyclovir triphosphate. This process does not occur in uninfected cells to any great extent, and because acyclovir is taken up selectively by infected cells, the concentration of acyclovir triphosphate in infected cells is 40 to 100 times greater than in uninfected cells. Clinically, acyclovir-resistant HSV infections are seen in patients whose immunodeficiency is increasing. Other antiviral medications, such as foscarnet, must be used to treat such acyclovir-resistant patients.

Interferons bind to specific cell receptors, activating the synthesis of different proteins including 2′-5′ oligoadenylate synthetase and protein kinase. This interaction causes an interference with viral replication, assembly and release. Included is a change in cellular glycosylation that produces a glycoprotein-deficient virus that shows lower infectivity. Interferons also exert their actions by immune modulation, thereby increasing the lytic effects of cytotoxic T lymphocytes.

Effects of interferon alpha can include fever, myalgia, lethargy, headaches (flulike syndrome), central nervous system dysfunction, gastrointestinal disturbances, and bone marrow suppression.

Currently, interferon alpha has FDA approval for the treatment of hairy cell leukemia, Kaposi's sarcoma (HHV-8), condylomata acuminata (HPV), chronic HBV or HCV infection, and melanoma after wide local excision. Pegylated interferon has proved more effective than standard interferon therapy for HCV infection.

Patient Advice

- Apply topical acyclovir and penciclovir using a finger cot or some type of protective covering.
- Patients who have oral viral disease should avoid using mouthrinses with a high alcohol content.
- Patients who have oral viral disease should dispose of toothbrushes used during periods of infection.
- Amlexanox paste should be applied using a finger cot. If a protective finger covering is not used, wash the hands immediately after applying the medication.

SUGGESTED READING

Arduino PG, Porter SR. Herpes simplex virus type 1 infection: overview on relevant clinico-pathological features. *J Oral Pathol Med*. 2008;37(2):107-121.

Barnett JA. A history of research on yeasts 12: medical yeasts part 1, *Candida albicans*. *Yeast*. 2008;25(6):385-417.

Hairston BR, Bruce AJ, Rogers III RS. Viral diseases of the oral mucosa. *Dermatol Clin*. 2003;21:17-32.

Letsinger JA, McCarty MA, Jorizzo JL. Complex aphthosis: a large case series with evaluation algorithm and therapeutic ladder from topicals to thalidomide. *J Am Acad Dermatol*. 2005;52:500-508.

Muzyka BC. Oral fungal infections. *Dent Clin North Am*. 2005;49:49-65.

Pallasch TJ. Antifungal and antiviral chemotherapy. *Periodontology 2000*. 2002;28:240-255.

Patton LL. HIV disease. *Dent Clin North Am*. 2003;47:467-492.

Pienaar ED, Young T, Holmes H. Interventions for the prevention and management of oropharyngeal candidiasis associated with HIV infection in adults and children. *Cochrane Database Syst Rev*. 2006;3: CD003940.

Preiser W, Doerr HW, Vogel JU. Virology and epidemiology of oral herpesvirus infections. *Med Microbiol Immunol*. 2003;192(3):133-136.

Scully C, Porter S. Oral mucosal disease: recurrent aphthous stomatitis. *Br J Oral Maxillofac Surg*. 2008;46(3):198-206.

Worthington HV, Clarkson JE, Eden TOB. Interventions for treating oral candidiasis for patients with cancer receiving treatment. *Cochrane Database Syst Rev*. 2007;(2): CD001972.

Yotsuyanagi H, Koike K. Drug resistance in antiviral treatment for infections with hepatitis B and C viruses. *J Gastroenterol*. 2007;42(5):329-335.

Table 7.1. PRESCRIBING INFORMATION FOR ANTIFUNGAL AND ANTIVIRAL AGENTS

NAME	FORM/ STRENGTH	DOSAGE	WARNINGS/PRECAUTIONS & CONTRAINDICATIONS	ADVERSE EFFECTS†
ANTIFUNGALS				
Amphotericin B (Fungizone)	**Inj:** 50mg	***Adults:*** Administer by slow IV infusion. **Test Dose:** 1mg in 20mL of D5W over 20-30 min. **Treatment: Initial:** 0.25mg/kg. **Severe Infection: Initial:** 0.3mg/kg. Give smaller initial dose if impaired cardio-renal function or severe reaction to test dose. **Titrate:** May increase by 5-10mg/day, depending on cardio-renal status, up to 0.5-0.7mg/kg/day. **Max:** 1mg/kg/day or 1.5mg/kg/day when given on alternate days. **Sporotrichosis:** Therapy has ranged up to 9 months with total dose up to 2.5g. **Aspergillosis:** Has been treated up to 11 months with total dose up to 3.6g. **Rhinocerebral Phycomycosis:** Cumulative dose of at least 3g is recommended. Whenever therapy is interrupted for >7 days, resume with lowest dose.	**BB:** Treatment primarily for progressive and potentially life-threatening fungal infections. Not for noninvasive fungal infections (eg, oral thrush, vaginal and esophageal candidiasis) in patients with normal neutrophil counts. Exercise caution to prevent inadvertent OD; verify product name and dose if dose >1.5mg/kg. **W/P:** Acute reactions (eg, fever, shaking chills, hypotension, anorexia, N/V, tachypnea) 1-3 hrs after starting infusion may occur. Avoid rapid infusion. Caution with renal impairment. Decreased risk of nephrotoxicity with hydration and sodium repletion. Acute pulmonary reactions reported with leukocyte infusions; separate infusions and monitor pulmonary function. Leukoencephalopathy reported. Monitor renal function, LFTs, electrolytes, blood counts, Hgb. **P/N:** Category B, not for use in nursing.	Fever, malaise, weight loss, hypotension, tachypnea, anorexia, N/V, diarrhea, dyspepsia, normochromic normocytic anemia, injection-site pain, renal dysfunction.
Amphotericin B Cholesteryl Sulfate (Amphotec)	**Inj:** 50mg, 100mg	***Adults/Pediatrics:*** **Test Dose:** Infuse small amount over 15-30 min. **Treatment:** 3-4mg/kg/day IV at 1mg/kg/hr.	**W/P:** Anaphylaxis may occur. D/C if severe respiratory distress occurs. Acute reactions (eg, fever, shaking chills, hypotension, nausea, tachypnea) 1-3 hrs after starting infusion may occur. Monitor renal/hepatic function, electrolytes, CBC, PT during therapy. **P/N:** Category B, not for use in nursing.	Chills, fever, headache, hypotension, tachycardia, HTN, N/V, thrombocytopenia, increased creatinine, hypokalemia, dyspnea, hypoxia.
Amphotericin B Lipid Complex (Abelcet)	**Inj:** 5mg/mL	***Adults/Pediatrics:*** **≥16 yrs:** 5mg/kg IV at 2.5mg/kg/hr.	**W/P:** Anaphylaxis reported. D/C if respiratory distress occurs. Monitor SCr, LFTs, serum electrolytes, CBC during therapy. **P/N:** Category B, not for use in nursing.	Chills, fever, increased SCr, multiorgan failure, N/V, hypotension, respiratory failure, dyspnea, sepsis, diarrhea, headache, heart arrest, HTN, hypokalemia, infection, kidney failure, pain, thrombocytopenia.
Amphotericin B Liposome (AmBisome)	**Inj:** 50mg	***Adults/Pediatrics:*** **1 month-16 yrs: Empiric Therapy:** 3mg/kg/day IV. **Systemic Infections *(Aspergillus, Candida, Cryptococcus):*** 3-5mg/kg/day IV. **Cryptococcal Meningitis in HIV:** 6mg/kg/day IV. **Visceral Leishmaniasis: Immunocompetent:** 3mg/kg/day IV on Days 1-5, 14, 21. May repeat course if needed. **Immunocompromised:** 4mg/kg/day IV on Days 1-5, 10, 17, 24, 31, 38.	**W/P:** If anaphylaxis occurs, d/c all further infusions. Significantly less toxic than amphotericin B deoxycholate. Monitor renal, hepatic, and hematopoietic function, and electrolytes (especially K^+, Mg^{++}). **P/N:** Category B, not for use in nursing.	Chills, asthenia, back pain, pain, infection, chest pain, HTN, hypotension, tachycardia, GI hemorrhage, diarrhea, N/V, hyperglycemia, hypokalemia, dyspnea.
Anidulafungin (Eraxis)	**Inj:** 50mg, 100mg	***Adults:*** **Candidemia/*Candida* Infections: LD:** 200mg on Day 1. Follow with 100mg qd thereafter. Continue therapy for at least 14 days after last positive culture. **Esophageal Candidiasis: LD:** 100mg on Day 1. Follow with 50mg qd thereafter. Treat for minimum of 14 days and for at least 7 days after symptoms resolve.	**W/P:** Hepatic abnormalities may occur; monitor hepatic function if abnormal LFTs develop during therapy. **P/N:** Category C, caution in nursing.	Diarrhea, nausea, rash, hypokalemia, headache, increased LFTs, neutropenia.

†Bold entries denote special dental considerations.
BB = black box warning; **W/P** = warnings/precautions; **Contra** = contraindications; **P/N** = pregnancy category rating and nursing considerations.

Table 7.1. PRESCRIBING INFORMATION FOR ANTIFUNGAL AND ANTIVIRAL AGENTS *(cont.)*

NAME	FORM/ STRENGTH	DOSAGE	WARNINGS/PRECAUTIONS & CONTRAINDICATIONS	ADVERSE EFFECTS†
ANTIFUNGALS *(cont.)*				
Caspofungin Acetate (Cancidas)	**Inj:** 50mg, 70mg	***Adults:*** **Empirical Therapy: LD:** 70mg IV on Day 1. **Maint:** 50mg IV qd. If 50mg is well tolerated but does not provide adequate clinical response, daily dose can be increased to 70mg. Fungal infections should be treated for a minimum of 14 days. Continue treatment 7 days after neutropenia and clinical symptoms are resolved. **Candidemia/*Candida* Infections: LD:** 70mg IV on Day 1. **Maint:** 50mg IV qd. **Esophageal Candidiasis:** 50mg IV qd. Consider PO suppressive therapy with HIV. **Invasive Aspergillosis: LD:** 70mg IV on Day 1. **Maint:** 50mg IV qd. **Moderate Hepatic Insufficiency (Child-Pugh Score 7-9): LD:** 70mg IV on Day 1. **Maint:** 35mg IV qd. **Concomitant Rifampin:** 70mg IV qd. **Concomitant Nevirapine/Efavirenz/ Carbamazepine/Dexamethasone/ Phenytoin:** May need to increase dose to 70mg IV qd. Base duration of treatment on severity of disease, clinical response, microbiological response, and recovery from immunosuppression. ***Pediatrics:*** **3 months-17 yrs: LD:** 70mg/m^2 IV on Day 1. **Maint:** 50mg/m^2 IV qd. If 50mg/m^2 is well tolerated but does not provide adequate clinical response, daily dose can be increased to 70mg/m^2. **Max:** 70mg/day. **Concomitant Rifampin/Nevirapine/ Efavirenz/Carbamazepine/ Dexamethasone/Phenytoin:** 70mg/m^2 IV qd. **Max:** 70mg/day.	**W/P:** LFT abnormalities may be seen; if abnormal LFTs develop, monitor for evidence of worsening hepatic function and re-evaluate. **P/N:** Category C, caution in nursing.	Fever, chills, hypotension, diarrhea, N/V, abdominal pain, edema, headache, rash, pneumonia, **cough,** erythema, anaphylaxis.
Clotrimazole (Mycelex Troche)	**Tab:** 10mg	***Adults/Pediatrics:*** **≥3 yrs: Treatment:** Slowly dissolve 1 troche in mouth 5 times/day for 14 days. **Prophylaxis:** Slowly dissolve 1 troche in mouth tid for duration of chemotherapy or until steroids reduced to maint levels.	**W/P:** Not for systemic mycoses. May cause abnormal LFTs; monitor hepatic function. Only use in patients mentally and physically able to dissolve the troche. Confirm diagnosis by KOH smear and/or culture. **P/N:** Category C, safety in nursing is not known.	Abnormal LFTs, N/V, **unpleasant mouth sensations**, pruritus.
Fluconazole (Diflucan)	**Inj:** 200mg/ 100mL, 400mg/200mL; **Sus:** 50mg/5mL, 200mg/5mL [35mL]; **Tab:** 50mg, 100mg, 150mg, 200mg	***Adults:*** **Vaginal Candidiasis:** 150mg PO single dose. **IV/PO: Oropharyngeal Candidiasis:** 200mg on Day 1, then 100mg qd for at least 2 weeks. **Esophageal Candidiasis:** 200mg on Day 1, then 100mg qd for at least 3 weeks and for at least 2 weeks following resolution of symptoms. **Max:** 400mg/day. **Systemic *Candida* Infections:** Up to 400mg/day. **UTI/ Peritonitis:** 50-200mg/day. **Cryptococcal Meningitis:** 400mg on Day 1, then 200mg qd for 10-12 weeks after negative CSF culture. **Suppression of Cryptococcal Meningitis Relapse in AIDS:** 200mg qd. **Prophylaxis in BMT:** 400mg qd. **Renal Impairment: CrCl ≤50mL/min (no dialysis): Initial: LD:** 50-400mg.	**W/P:** Monitor LFTs. D/C if hepatic dysfunction develops or exfoliative skin disorder progresses. Anaphylaxis reported. Rare cases of QT prolongation and torsades de pointes reported. **Contra:** Coadministration with cisapride or terfenadine (with multiple fluconazole doses of ≥400mg). Caution if hypersensitive to other azoles. **P/N:** Category C, not for use in nursing.	Headache, N/V, abdominal pain, diarrhea, skin rash.

*Scored. †Bold entries denote special dental considerations.
BB = black box warning; **W/P** = warnings/precautions; **Contra** = contraindications; **P/N** = pregnancy category rating and nursing considerations.

NAME	FORM/ STRENGTH	DOSAGE	WARNINGS/PRECAUTIONS & CONTRAINDICATIONS	ADVERSE EFFECTS†
Fluconazole (Diflucan) *(cont.)*		**Maint:** Give 50% of recommended dose. **Dialysis:** Give 100% of dose after each dialysis. ***Pediatrics:* IV/PO: Oropharyngeal Candidiasis:** 6mg/kg on Day 1, then 3mg/kg/day for at least 2 weeks. **Esophageal Candidiasis:** 6mg/kg on 1st day, then 3mg/kg/day for at least 3 weeks and for at least 2 weeks following resolution of symptoms. **Max:** 12mg/kg/day. **Systemic *Candida* Infections:** 6-12mg/kg/day. **Cryptococcal Meningitis:** 12mg/kg on Day 1, then 6mg/kg/day for 10-12 weeks after negative CSF culture. **Suppression of Cryptococcal Meningitis Relapse in AIDS:** 6mg/kg qd. **Renal Impairment: CrCl ≤50mL/min (no dialysis): Initial: LD:** 50-400mg. **Maint:** Give 50% of recommended dose. **Dialysis:** Give 100% of dose after each dialysis.		
Flucytosine (Ancobon)	**Cap:** 250mg, 500mg	***Adults:*** 50-150mg/kg/day given q6h. **Renal Impairment:** Reduce initial dose. Take a few caps over 15 min to reduce N/V.	**BB:** Extreme caution with renal dysfunction. Monitor hematologic, renal, and hepatic status closely. **W/P:** Caution with renal dysfunction and bone marrow depression. Bone marrow depression can be irreversible and fatal. **P/N:** Category C, not for use in nursing.	Myocardial toxicity, chest pain, dyspnea, rash, pruritus, urticaria, photosensitivity, N/V, jaundice, renal failure, pyrexia, crystalluria, anemia, leukopenia, eosinophilia, thrombocytopenia, ataxia, hearing loss, neuropathy.
Griseofulvin (Grifulvin V)	**Sus:** 125mg/5mL [120mL]; **Tab:** 250mg, 500mg	***Adults:* Tinea Capitis:** 500mg qd for 4-6 weeks. **Tinea Corporis:** 500mg qd for 2-4 weeks. **Tinea Pedis:** 1g qd for 4-8 weeks. **Tinea Cruris:** 500mg qd. **Tinea Unguium:** 1g qd for at least 4 months (fingernail) or at least 6 months (toenail). ***Pediatrics:* Usual:** 5mg/lb/day. **30-50lb:** 125-250mg qd. **>50lb:** 250-500mg qd. **Tinea Capitis:** Treat for 4-6 weeks. **Tinea Corporis:** Treat for 2-4 weeks. **Tinea Pedis:** Treat for 4-8 weeks. **Tinea Unguium:** Treat for at least 4 months (fingernail) or at least 6 months (toenail).	**W/P:** Confirm diagnosis. Not for prophylactic use. Monitor renal, hepatic, and hematopoietic functions periodically with prolonged therapy. Cross-sensitivity with PCN may exist. Photosensitivity reported. D/C if granulocytopenia occurs. **Contra:** Porphyria, hepatocellular failure, pregnancy. **P/N:** Not for use in pregnancy and in nursing.	Rash, urticaria, **oral thrush**, N/V, epigastric distress, diarrhea, headache, dizziness, insomnia, mental confusion.
Griseofulvin (Gris-PEG)	**Tab:** 125mg*, 250mg*	***Adults:* Tinea Capitis:** 375mg qd in single or divided doses for 4-6 weeks. **Tinea Corporis:** 375mg qd in single or divided doses for 2-4 weeks. **Tinea Pedis:** 375mg bid for 4-8 weeks. **Tinea Cruris:** 375mg qd in single or divided doses. **Tinea Unguium:** 375mg bid for at least 4 months (fingernail) or at least 6 months (toenail). ***Pediatrics:* Usual:** 3.3mg/lb/day. **35-60lb:** 125-187.5mg qd. **>60lb:** 187.5-375mg qd. **Tinea Capitis:** Treat for 4-6 weeks. **Tinea Corporis:** Treat for 2-4 weeks. **Tinea Pedis:** Treat for 4-8 weeks. **Tinea Unguium:** Treat for at least 4 months (fingernail) or at least 6 months (toenail).	**W/P:** Not for prophylactic use. Periodically monitor renal, hepatic, and hematopoietic functions in prolonged therapy. Cross-sensitivity with PCN may exist. Photosensitivity reported. D/C if granulocytopenia occurs. **Contra:** Porphyria, hepatocellular failure, pregnancy. **P/N:** Not for use in pregnancy and in nursing.	Rash, urticaria, **oral thrush**, N/V, epigastric distress, diarrhea, headache, dizziness, insomnia, mental confusion.

Table 7.1. PRESCRIBING INFORMATION FOR ANTIFUNGAL AND ANTIVIRAL AGENTS *(cont.)*

NAME	FORM/ STRENGTH	DOSAGE	WARNINGS/PRECAUTIONS & CONTRAINDICATIONS	ADVERSE EFFECTS†
ANTIFUNGALS *(cont.)*				
Itraconazole (Sporanox)	**Cap:** 100mg [Blister, 3 x 10 caps], [PulsePak, 7 blisters x 4 caps]; **Inj:** 10mg/mL [25mL]; **Sol:** 10mg/mL [150mL]	***Adults:*** (Cap) Take with full meal. If patient has achlorhydria or is taking gastric acid suppressors, give with cola beverage. **Onychomycosis: Toenail:** 200mg qd for 12 consecutive weeks. **Fingernail:** (PulsePak) 200mg bid for 1 week, skip 3 weeks, then repeat. **Blastomycosis/ Histoplasmosis:** 200mg qd. May increase by 100mg increments if no improvement. **Max:** 400mg/day. Give bid if dose >200mg/day. **Aspergillosis:** 200-400mg/day. **Life-Threatening Infections: LD:** 200mg tid for first 3 days. Continue for at least 3 months and until infection subsides. (IV) **Empiric Therapy in Febrile Neutropenia (ETFN):** 200mg bid over 1 hr infusion for four doses, followed by 200mg qd for 14 days. Continue with oral solution 200mg bid until resolution of clinically significant neutropenia. **Blastomycosis/ Histoplasmosis/Aspergillosis:** 200mg bid over 1 hr infusion for four doses, followed by 200mg qd. Continue for at least 3 months until active fungal infection subsides. (Sol) Take on empty stomach. Swish 10mL at a time for several seconds, then swallow. **Candidiasis: Oropharyngeal:** 200mg/day for 1-2 weeks. If refractory to fluconazole, give 100mg bid (response in 2-4 weeks; may relapse shortly after d/c). **Esophageal:** 100-200mg/day for at least 3 weeks. Continue for 2 weeks after symptoms resolve.	**BB:** Contraindicated with cisapride, pimozide, quinidine, dofetilide, or levacetylmethadol. Serious cardiovascular events (eg, QT prolongation, torsades de pointes, ventricular tachycardia, cardiac arrest, and/or sudden death) reported with cisapride, pimozide, quinidine, and other CYP3A4 inhibitors. Do not use caps for onychomycosis with ventricular dysfunction. **W/P:** Rare cases of hepatotoxicity reported. Monitor LFTs; d/c if hepatic dysfunction develops. Avoid with liver disease. D/C if neuropathy or CHF occurs. Sol and caps not interchangeable. Consider alternative therapy if unresponsive in patients with cystic fibrosis. Avoid with ventricular dysfunction. Caution with ischemic/ valvular disease, pulmonary disease, renal failure, other edematous disorders. Avoid injection if CrCl <30mL/min. **Contra:** (Cap, Sol) Concomitant cisapride, oral midazolam, pimozide, quinidine, dofetilide, triazolam, and HMG-CoA reductase inhibitors metabolized by CYP3A4 (eg, lovastatin, simvastatin). (Cap) Treatment of onychomycosis if pregnant or contemplating pregnancy, ventricular dysfunction (eg, CHF). **P/N:** Category C, not for use in nursing.	N/V, diarrhea, abdominal pain, fever, cough, rash, increased sweating, headache, hypokalemia.
Ketoconazole (Nizoral)	**Tab:** 200mg*	***Adults:*** **Initial:** 200mg qd. **Max:** 400mg qd. ***Pediatrics:*** **>2 yrs:** 3.3-6.6mg/kg/day.	**BB:** Risk of fatal hepatotoxicity. Concomitant terfenadine, astemizole, and cisapride are contraindicated due to serious cardiovascular adverse events. **W/P:** Hepatotoxicity reported. Monitor LFTs prior to therapy and periodically thereafter. Serum testosterone levels may be lowered. Hypersensitivity reactions reported. Tablets require acidity for dissolution. Not for use in children unless benefit outweighs risk. **Contra:** Concomitant terfenadine, astemizole, cisapride, or oral triazolam. **P/N:** Category C, not for use in nursing.	N/V, abdominal pain, pruritus.
Micafungin Sodium (Mycamine)	**Inj:** 50mg, 100mg	***Adults:*** **Candidemia/Acute Disseminated Candidiasis/*Candida* Peritonitis/Abscesses:** 100mg IV qd (usual range 10-47 days). **Esophageal Candidiasis:** 150mg IV qd (usual range 10-30 days). ***Candida*** **Infection Prophylaxis in HSCT:** 50mg IV qd (usual range 6-51 days). Do not mix or co-infuse with other drugs.	**W/P:** Reports of serious hypersensitivity reactions (eg, anaphylaxis, anaphylactoid shock); d/c drug and administer appropriate treatment. LFT abnormalities, monitor for evidence of worsening. Reports of significant renal dysfunction, acute renal failure, and elevations in BUN and creatinine. Reports of acute intravascular hemolysis, hemolytic anemia, and hemoglobinuria. **P/N:** Category C, caution in nursing.	Hyperbilirubinemia, neutropenia, headache, rash, phlebitis, N/V, diarrhea, pyrexia, hypokalemia, thrombocytopenia.

*Scored. †Bold entries denote special dental considerations.
BB = black box warning; **W/P** = warnings/precautions; **Contra** = contraindications; **P/N** = pregnancy category rating and nursing considerations.

NAME	FORM/ STRENGTH	DOSAGE	WARNINGS/PRECAUTIONS & CONTRAINDICATIONS	ADVERSE EFFECTS†
Nystatin	**Sus:** 100,000 U/mL [60mL, 480mL]; **Tab:** 500,000 U	***Adults:* Oral Candidiasis:** (Sus) 4-6mL qid. Retain in mouth as long as possible before swallowing. **GI Candidiasis:** (Tab) 500,000-1,000,000 U tid. ***Pediatrics:* Oral Candidiasis:** (Sus) 4-6mL qid. **Infants:** 2mL qid. Retain in mouth as long as possible before swallowing.	**W/P:** Not for systemic mycoses. D/C if irritation/hypersensitivity occurs. Confirm diagnosis with KOH smear and/or cultures if symptoms persist after course of therapy. Continue at least 48 hrs after clinical response. **P/N:** Category C, caution in nursing.	Diarrhea, N/V, GI distress, rash, urticaria, Stevens-Johnson syndrome, **oral irritation.**
Posaconazole (Noxafil)	**Sus:** 40mg/mL	***Adults/Pediatrics:* ≥13 yrs: Prophylaxis of Invasive Fungal Infections:** 200mg (5mL) tid. Base duration of therapy on recovery from neutropenia or immunosuppression. **Oropharyngeal Candidiasis: LD:** 100mg (2.5mL) bid on Day 1, then 100mg qd for 13 days. **Oropharyngeal Candidiasis Refractory to Itraconazole and/or Fluconazole:** 400mg (10mL) bid. Base duration of therapy on severity of underlying disease and clinical response. Give each dose with full meal or nutritional supplement.	**W/P:** Hepatic reactions (eg, mild-to-moderate elevations in ALT, AST, alkaline phosphatase, total bilirubin, and/or clinical hepatitis) reported; monitor LFTs at start of and during therapy. Caution with hepatic impairment. Monitor closely with severe renal impairment. Prolongation of QT interval reported; caution with potentially proarrhythmic conditions. **Contra:** Concomitant ergot alkaloids, terfenadine, astemizole, cisapride, pimozide, halofantrine, quinidine, or sirolimus. **P/N:** Category C, not for use in nursing.	Fever, headache, rigors, HTN, anemia, neutropenia, diarrhea, N/V, abdominal pain, constipation, hypokalemia, thrombocytopenia, coughing, dyspnea.
Terbinafine HCl (Lamisil)	**Granules:** 125mg/pkt, 187.5mg/pkt; **Tab:** 250mg	***Adults:*** (Tabs) **Fingernail:** 250mg qd for 6 weeks. **Toenail:** 250mg qd for 12 weeks. ***Adults/Pediatrics:* ≥4 yrs: (Granules)** Take qd with food for 6 weeks. **<25 kg:** 125mg/day. **25-35kg:** 187.5mg/day. **>35kg:** 250mg/day.	**W/P:** Liver disease and serious skin reactions reported; d/c therapy if these develop. Avoid with liver disease or renal impairment (CrCl ≤50 mL/min). Check serum transaminases before therapy. Monitor CBC if immunocompromised and taking terbinafine >6 weeks. Severe neutropenia reported; d/c therapy if neutrophil count ≤1,000 cells/mm^3. Changes in ocular lens and retina reported (unknown significance). **P/N:** Category B, not for use in nursing.	**(Granules) Nasopharyngitis,** headache, pyrexia, **cough,** vomiting, upper respiratory tract infection, upper abdominal pain, diarrhea, liver enzyme abnormalities, rash. **(Tabs)** Headache, diarrhea, dyspepsia, abdominal pain, liver enzyme abnormalities, rash.
Voriconazole (Vfend)	**Inj:** 200mg; **Sus:** 40mg/mL; **Tab:** 50mg, 200mg	***Adults:*** (Inj) **LD:** 6mg/kg IV q12h x 2 doses. **Maint:** 4mg/kg IV q12h. Switch to PO when appropriate. (PO) **Maint: ≥40kg:** 200mg q12h; 300mg q12h if inadequate response. **<40kg:** 100mg q12h; 150 mg q12h if inadequate response. **Esophageal Candidiasis:** (PO) **≥40kg:** 200mg q12h. **<40kg:** 100mg q12h. Treat for minimum of 14 days and at least 7 days following resolution of symptoms. **Intolerant:** (Inj/PO) **Maint:** IV: 3mg/kg q12h. PO: Reduce by 50mg steps to minimum of 200mg q12h for >40kg or 100mg q12h for <40kg. **Concomitant Phenytoin: Maint:** IV: 5mg/kg q12h. PO: **≥40kg:** 400mg q12h. **<40kg:** 200mg q12h. **Concomitant Efavirenz: Maint:** 400mg q12h and efavirenz should be decreased to 300mg q24h. **Mild to Moderate Hepatic Cirrhosis: Maint:** 1/2 of maint dose. **CrCl <50mL/min:** Use PO. Give PO 1 hr before or 1 hr after a meal. Base duration on severity of underlying disease, recovery from immunosuppression, and clinical response.	**W/P:** Monitor visual function with treatment >28 days. Hepatic reactions (eg, clinical hepatitis, cholestasis, fulminant hepatic failure) reported; monitor LFTs at initiation and during therapy. D/C if liver dysfunction occurs. Tabs contain lactose; avoid with galactose intolerance, Lapp lactase deficiency, or glucose-galactose malabsorption. Anaphylactoid-type reactions reported with infusion. Avoid strong, direct sunlight. Monitor renal function. May prolong QT interval; caution with proarrhythmic conditions. Correct electrolyte disturbances before starting therapy. If rash develops, monitor closely and consider discontinuation of voriconazole. **Contra:** Concomitant CYP3A4 substrates (terfenadine, astemizole, cisapride, pimozide, quinidine), sirolimus, rifampin, carbamazepine, long-acting barbiturates, high-dose ritonavir (400mg q12h), low-dose ritonavir (100mg q12h; assess benefit/risk), rifabutin, ergot alkaloids, St. John's wort. **P/N:** Category D, not for use in nursing.	Visual disturbances, fever, chills, rash, headache, N/V, sepsis, peripheral edema, abdominal pain, respiratory disorder, increased LFTs, and alkaline phosphatase.

Table 7.1. PRESCRIBING INFORMATION FOR ANTIFUNGAL AND ANTIVIRAL AGENTS *(cont.)*

NAME	FORM/ STRENGTH	DOSAGE	WARNINGS/PRECAUTIONS & CONTRAINDICATIONS	ADVERSE EFFECTS†
ANTIVIRALS				
Acyclovir (Zovirax Cream, Ointment)	**Cre:** 5% [2g, 5g]; **Oint:** 5% [15g]	***Adults/Pediatrics:* ≥12 yrs: Recurrent Herpes Labialis:** (Cre) Apply 5x/day for 4 days. Initiate with 1st sign/symptom. ***Adults:* Initial Genital Herpes/Limited Non-Life-threatening Mucocutaneous Herpes Simplex Infections in Immunocompromised:** (Oint) Apply to all lesions q3h, 6x/day for 7 days. Apply with finger cot or rubber glove to prevent autoinoculation and transmission. Initiate with 1st sign/symptom.	**W/P:** (Cre) Cutaneous use only; not for use in the eye, mouth, or nose. (Oint) Not for use for the prevention of recurrent HSV infections. Cutaneous use only; avoid eyes. **P/N:** Category B, caution in nursing.	**Dry lips**, skin desquamation, dryness/burning/flakiness/stinging of skin, **cracked lips**, pruritus.
Acyclovir (Zovirax Oral)	**Cap:** 200mg, **Sus:** 200mg/5mL; **Tab:** 400mg, 800mg	***Adults:* Herpes Zoster:** 800mg q4h, 5x/day for 7-10 days. Start within 72 hrs after onset of rash. **Genital Herpes: Initial:** 200mg q4h, 5x/day for 10 days. **Chronic Therapy:** 400mg bid or 200mg 3-5x/day up to 12 months, then re-evaluate. **Intermittent Therapy:** 200mg q4h, 5x/day for 5 days. Start with 1st sign/symptom of recurrence. **Chickenpox:** 800mg qid for 5 days. **CrCl 10-25mL/min:** For a dose of 800mg q4h, give 800mg q8h. **CrCl 0-10mL/min:** For a dose of 200mg q4h, give 200mg q12h. For a dose of 400mg q12h, give 200mg q12h. For a dose of 800mg q4h, give 800mg q12h. **Elderly:** Reduce dose. ***Pediatrics:* ≥2 yrs: ≤40kg: Chickenpox:** 20mg/kg qid for 5 days. **>40kg:** 800mg qid for 5 days.	**W/P:** Adjust dose in renal impairment, elderly. Renal failure and death reported. Thrombotic thrombocytopenic purpura/hemolytic uremic syndrome in immunocompromised patients reported. **Contra:** Hypersensitivity to valacyclovir. **P/N:** Category B, caution in nursing.	N/V, diarrhea, headache, malaise, renal dysfunction.
Acyclovir Sodium (Zovirax Injection)	**Inj:** 500mg, 1000mg	***Adults/Adolescents:* ≥12 yrs:** Initiate with first sign/symptom. **Max:** 20mg/kg q8h for any patient. **Mucosal/Cutaneous Herpes Simplex Infections:** 5mg/kg q8h for 7 days. **Herpes Genitalis:** 5mg/kg q8h for 5 days. **Herpes Simplex Encephalitis:** 10mg/kg q8h for 10 days. **Varicella Zoster:** 10mg/kg q8h for 7 days. **Obese Patients:** Dose according to IBW. **CrCl 25-50mL/min:** Give 100% of recommended dose q12h. **CrCl 10-25mL/min:** Give 100% of recommended dose q24h. **CrCl 0-10mL/min:** Give 50% of recommended dose q24h. **Elderly:** Reduce dose and monitor renal function. ***Pediatrics:*** Initiate with first sign/symptom. **Max:** 20mg/kg q8h for any patient. **Mucosal/Cutaneous Herpes Simplex: <12yrs:** 10mg/kg q8h for 7 days. **Herpes Simplex Encephalitis: 3 months-12 yrs:** 20mg/kg q8h for 10 days. **Neonatal Herpes Simplex: Birth-3 months:** 10mg/kg q8h for 10 days. **Varicella Zoster: <12 yrs:** 20mg/kg q8h for 7 days. **Obese Patients:** Dose according to IBW. **CrCl 25-50mL/min:** Give 100% of recommended dose q12h. **CrCl 10-25mL/min:** Give 100% of recommended dose q24h. **CrCl 0-10mL/min:** Give 50% of recommended dose q24h.	**W/P:** Do not administer topically, IM, PO, SQ, or in the eye. Adjust dose in renal impairment and the elderly. Renal failure and death reported. Thrombotic thrombocytopenic purpura/hemolytic uremic syndrome in immunocompromised patients reported. Patient must be adequately hydrated. Caution with underlying neurologic abnormalities, electrolyte abnormalities, significant hypoxia, and serious renal or hepatic abnormalities. Infusion must not be given over <1 hr. **Contra:** Hypersensitivity to valacyclovir. **P/N:** Category B, caution in nursing.	Injection-site inflammation, phlebitis, transient serum creatinine and BUN elevations, N/V.

†Bold entries denote special dental considerations.
BB = black box warning; **W/P** = warnings/precautions; **Contra** = contraindications; **P/N** = pregnancy category rating and nursing considerations.

NAME	FORM/ STRENGTH	DOSAGE	WARNINGS/PRECAUTIONS & CONTRAINDICATIONS	ADVERSE EFFECTS†
Adefovir Dipivoxil (Hepsera)	**Tab:** 10mg	***Adults/Pediatrics:*** **≥12 yrs: Chronic HBV:** 10mg qd. **Renal Impairment: CrCl 30-49mL/min:** 10mg q48h. **CrCl 10-29mL/min:** 10mg q72h. **Hemodialysis Patients:** 10mg every 7 days following dialysis.	**BB:** Discontinuation may result in severe acute exacerbations of hepatitis. Chronic use may result in nephrotoxicity in patients at risk of or having underlying renal dysfunction. HIV resistance may occur with unrecognized or untreated HIV infection. May cause lactic acidosis and severe hepatomegaly with steatosis. **W/P:** Monitor hepatic function at repeated intervals upon discontinuation. Monitor renal function in patients with pre-existing or risk factors for renal dysfunction; adjust dosage appropriately. May require HIV antibody testing prior to treatment. Suspend treatment if lactic acidosis and severe hepatomegaly are suspected. **P/N:** Category C, caution in nursing.	Asthenia, headache, abdominal pain, nausea, flatulence, diarrhea, dyspepsia, increased creatinine, hypophosphatemia.
Amantadine HCl (Symmetrel)	**Syrup:** 50mg/ 5mL; **Tab:** 100mg	***Adults:*** **Influenza A Virus Prophylaxis/ Treatment:** 200mg qd or 100mg bid. **Elderly: ≥65 yrs:** 100mg qd. **Parkinsonism: Initial:** 100mg bid. **Serious Associated Illness/ Concomitant High-Dose Antiparkinson Agent: Initial:** 100mg qd. **Titrate:** May increase to 100mg bid after 1 to several weeks. **Max:** 400mg/day. **Drug-Induced Extrapyramidal Reactions:** 100mg bid. **Titrate:** May increase to 300mg/day in divided doses. **CrCl 30-50mL/min:** 200mg on Day 1, then 100mg qd. **CrCl 15-29mL/min:** 200mg on Day 1, then 100mg every other day. **CrCl <15mL/min/Hemodialysis:** 200mg every 7 days. ***Pediatrics:*** **Influenza A Virus Prophylaxis/Treatment: 9-12 yrs:** 100mg bid. **1-9 yrs:** 4.4-8.8mg/ kg/day. **Max:** 150mg/day.	**W/P:** Deaths reported from overdose. Suicide attempts, NMS reported. Caution with CHF, peripheral edema, orthostatic hypotension, renal or hepatic dysfunction, recurrent eczematoid rash, uncontrolled psychosis, or severe psychoneurosis. Avoid in untreated angle-closure glaucoma. Do not d/c abruptly in Parkinson's disease. May increase seizure activity. **P/N:** Category C, not for use in nursing.	Nausea, dizziness, insomnia, depression, anxiety, hallucinations, confusion, anorexia, **dry mouth**, constipation, ataxia, livedo reticularis, peripheral edema, orthostatic hypotension, agranulocytosis.
Cidofovir (Vistide)	**Inj:** 75mg/mL	***Adults:*** **IV: Induction:** 5mg/kg once weekly for 2 weeks. **Maint:** 5mg/kg once every 2 weeks. Reduce maint from 5mg/kg to 3mg/kg for an increase in SCr of 0.3-0.4mg/dL above baseline. D/C with increase in SCr ≥0.5mg/dL above baseline or ≥3+ proteinuria. Administer probenecid 2g PO 3 hrs before cidofovir, then 1g at 2 hrs and 8 hrs after completion of cidofovir infusion. Administer at least 1L 0.9% normal saline (NS) immediately before infusion. If tolerated, give second liter at start of or immediately after infusion.	**BB:** Renal impairment is a major toxicity; prehydrate with IV NS and administer probenecid with each dose. Monitor serum creatinine (SCr) and urine protein within 48 hrs prior to each dose. Modify dose with renal function changes. Contraindicated with nephrotoxic agents. Neutropenia reported; monitor neutrophils. Carcinogenic, teratogenic, and hypospermatic in animal studies. **W/P:** Dose-dependent nephrotoxicity. Monitor IOP, visual acuity, ocular symptoms, uveitis/iritis, and renal function periodically. Monitor WBC with differential before each dose. Avoid during pregnancy. Adequate contraception for both sexes during and following treatment is advised. May cause male infertility. Potentially carcinogenic. **Contra:** SCr >1.5mg/dL, CrCl ≤55mL/min, or urine protein ≥100mg/dL (≥2+ protein-uria) with therapy initiation. Nephrotoxic agents (discontinue at least 7 days before therapy), severe hypersensitivity to probenecid or other sulfa-containing agents, direct intraocular use. **P/N:** Category C, not for use in nursing.	N/V, neutropenia, proteinuria, decreased IOP/ocular hypotonia, anterior uveitis/iritis, metabolic acidosis, nephrotoxicity, pneumonia, dyspnea, infection, fever, creatinine ≥2mg/ dL, decreased sodium bicarbonate.
Docosanol (Abreva) OTC	**Cre:** 10% [2g]	***Adults/Pediatrics:*** **≥12 yrs: Herpes Labialis:** Apply to affected area on face or lips at 1st sign of cold sore/ fever blister (tingle). Use 5x/day until healed.	**W/P:** Avoid in or near eyes, and inside mouth. D/C if sore worsens or does not heal in 10 days. **P/N:** Safety in pregnancy and nursing not known.	

Table 7.1. PRESCRIBING INFORMATION FOR ANTIFUNGAL AND ANTIVIRAL AGENTS *(cont.)*

NAME	FORM/ STRENGTH	DOSAGE	WARNINGS/PRECAUTIONS & CONTRAINDICATIONS	ADVERSE EFFECTS†
ANTIVIRALS *(cont.)*				
Entecavir (Baraclude)	**Sol:** 0.05mg/mL; **Tab:** 0.5mg, 1mg	***Adults/Pediatrics:* ≥16 yrs: Chronic HBV: Nucleoside-Treatment-Naive:** 0.5mg qd. **CrCl 30 to <50mL/min:** 0.25mg qd or 0.5mg q48h. **CrCl 10 to <30mL/min:** 0.15mg qd or 0.5mg q72h. **CrCl <10mL/min:** 0.05mg qd or 0.5mg q7 days. **Lamivudine-Refractory:** 1mg qd. **CrCl 30 to <50mL/min:** 0.5mg qd or 1mg q48h. **CrCl 10 to <30mL/min:** 0.3mg qd or 1mg q72h. **CrCl <10mL/min:** 0.1mg qd or 1mg q7 days. Take on empty stomach.	**BB:** Lactic acidosis and severe, possibly fatal, hepatomegaly with steatosis reported. Reports of severe acute exacerbations of hepatitis B upon discontinuation of therapy. Follow-up liver function monitoring required. Limited clinical experience suggests that there is potential for the development of resistance to HIV nucleoside reverse transcriptase inhibitors if baraclude is used to treat chronic hepatitis B virus infection in patients with HIV infection that is not being treated. Not recommended for HIV/HBV coinfected who are not receiving highly active antiretroviral therapy (HAART). **W/P:** See BlackBox Warning. Reduce dose in renal dysfunction (CrCl <50mL/min), including patients on hemodialysis or continuous ambulatory peritoneal dialysis (CAPD). Exacerbations of hepatitis after discontinuation of treatment. Caution with known risk factors of liver disease. D/C with lactic acidosis and hepatotoxicity. **P/N:** Category C, not for use in nursing.	Headache, fatigue, dizziness, nausea, hyperglycemia, ALT >5.0 X ULN, lipase ≥2.1 X ULN, glycosuria, and hematuria.
Famciclovir (Famvir)	**Tab:** 125mg, 250mg, 500mg	***Adults:* ≥18 yrs: Herpes Zoster: Usual:** 500mg q8h for 7 days; start within 72 hrs after rash onset. **CrCl 40-59mL/min:** 500mg q12h. **CrCl 20-39mL/min:** 500mg q24h. **CrCl <20mL/min:** 250mg q24h. **Hemodialysis:** 250mg following dialysis. **Recurrent Genital Herpes:** 1000mg bid for 1 day; start within 6 hrs of onset of symptom. **CrCl 40-59mL/min:** 500mg q12h; **CrCl 20-39mL/min:** 500mg as single dose; **CrCl <20mL/min:** 250mg as a single dose; **Hemodialysis:** 250mg following dialysis. **Suppression of Recurrent Genital Herpes:** 250mg bid for up to 1 yr. **CrCl 20-39mL/min:** 125mg q12h; **CrCl <20mL/min:** 125mg q24h; **Hemodialysis:** 125mg following dialysis. **Recurrent Orolabial or Genital Herpes in HIV:** 500mg bid for 7 days. **CrCl <20mL/min:** 250mg q24h. **Hemodialysis:** 250mg following dialysis. **Recurrent Herpes Labialis:** 1500mg as a single dose; **CrCl 40-59mL/min:** 750mg single dose; **CrCl 20-39mL/min:** 500mg single dose; **CrCl <20mL/min:** 250mg single dose; **Hemodialysis:** 250mg following dialysis.	**W/P:** Prodrug of penciclovir. Dose adjustment in renal disease. Not indicated for initial episode of genital herpes infection, ophthalmic zoster, disseminated zoster, or in immunocompromised patients with herpes zoster. **Contra:** Hypersensitivity to penciclovir cream. **P/N:** Category B, safety not known in nursing.	Headache, migraine, N/V, diarrhea, fatigue, urticaria, hallucinations, confusion.

†Bold entries denote special dental considerations.
BB = black box warning; **W/P** = warnings/precautions; **Contra** = contraindications; **P/N** = pregnancy category rating and nursing considerations.

NAME	FORM/ STRENGTH	DOSAGE	WARNINGS/PRECAUTIONS & CONTRAINDICATIONS	ADVERSE EFFECTS†
Foscarnet Sodium	**Inj:** 24mg/mL	***Adults:*** **Induction: CMV Retinitis:** 90mg/kg q12h or 60mg/kg q8h for 2-3 weeks. **Maint:** 90-120mg/kg/day. **Acyclovir-Resistant HSV:** 40mg/kg q8-12h for 2-3 weeks or until healed. Administer 750-1000mL of NS or D5W prior to first infusion to establish diuresis. Then, 750-1000mL with 90-120 mg/kg dose and 500mL with 40-60 mg/kg dose. Use infusion pump to control rate of infusion. See PI for renal impairment dosing.	**BB:** Renal impairment, seizures reported. Monitor SrCr and adjust dose for any changes in renal function. For use only in immunocompromised patients with CMV retinitis and mucocutaneous acyclovir-resistant HSV infections. **W/P:** Hydration reduces risk of nephrotoxicity. Anemia, granulocytopenia, serum electrolyte alterations, decrease in ionized serum calcium reported. Infuse into veins with adequate blood flow to avoid local irritation. Avoid rapid administration. Cases of male and female genital irritation/ulceration reported. **P/N:** Category C, safety in nursing not known.	Fever, N/V, diarrhea, anemia, renal impairment, hypocalcemia, hypophosphatemia, hyperphosphatemia, hypomagnesemia, hypokalemia, seizures, paresthesia, fatigue.
Ganciclovir (Cytovene)	**Cap:** 250mg, 500mg; **Inj:** 500mg	***Adults:*** **CMV Retinitis Treatment: Initial:** 5mg/kg IV q12h for 14-21 days. **Maint:** 5mg/kg IV qd for 7 days or 6mg/kg IV qd for 5 days/ week or 1000mg PO tid or 500mg PO 6 times daily q3h, while awake. **CMV Retinitis Prevention in HIV Patients:** 1000mg PO tid. **CMV Retinitis Prevention in Transplant Patients: Initial:** 5mg/kg IV q12h for 7-14 days. **Maint:** 5mg/kg IV qd for 7 days or 6mg/kg IV for 5 days/ week or 1000mg PO tid. **Renal Impairment:** See PI for details. Take caps with food.	**BB:** Risk of granulocytopenia, anemia, and thrombocytopenia. More rapid rate of CMV retinitis progression with caps; only use as maintenance treatment when the risk is balanced by the benefit of avoiding daily IV infusions. **W/P:** Avoid if ANC <500 cells/microliter, or platelets <25,000 cells/microliter. Caution in preexisting cytopenias and history of cytopenic reactions to drugs, chemicals, and irradiation. Reduce dose in renal impairment. High frequency of renal dysfunction in transplant recipients. Women of childbearing potential should use effective contraception during treatment due to fetal mutagenic/teratogenic potential. Men should practice barrier contraception during and ≥90 days after therapy. **Contra:** Hypersensitivity to acyclovir. **P/N:** Category C, not for use in nursing.	Fever, diarrhea, anorexia, vomiting, leukopenia, anemia, sweating.
Interferon alfa-2b (Intron A)	**Inj:** 10 MIU, 18 MIU, 50 MIU, 10 MIU/mL, 3 MIU/0.2mL, 5 MIU/0.2mL, 10 MIU/0.2mL	***Adults:*** **≥18 yrs: Hairy Cell Leukemia:** 2 MIU/m^2 IM/SQ 3x/week up to 6 months. Reduce dose by 50% or stop therapy with severe reactions. **Malignant Melanoma: Initial:** 20 MIU/m^2 IV for 5 consecutive days/ week for 4 weeks. **Maint:** 10 MIU/m^2 SQ 3x/week for 48 weeks. **Follicular Lymphoma:** 5 MIU SQ 3x/ week up to 18 months. **Condylomata Acuminata:** 1 MIU into lesion 3x/ week alternating days for 3 weeks. **Max:** 5 lesions/course. **Kaposi's Sarcoma:** 30 MIU/m^2 3x/week IM/ SQ. **Hepatitis C:** 3 MIU IM/SQ 3x/ week for 18-24 months. **Hepatitis B:** 5 MIU qd IM/SQ or 10 MIU IM/ SQ 3x/week for 16 weeks. Dose adjust according to severe adverse reactions and laboratory abnormalities (see PI for more information). ***Pediatrics:*** **≥1 yr: Hepatitis B:** 3 MIU/m^2 SQ 3x/week for 1 week, then 6 MIU/m^2 3x/week for total therapy of 16-24 weeks. **Max:** 10 MIU/ m^2 3x/week. Reduce dose by 50% or stop therapy with severe reactions. Adjust based on WBC, granulocyte, and/or platelet counts. Dose adjust according to severe adverse reactions and laboratory abnormalities (see PI for more information).	**BB:** May cause or aggravate fatal or life-threatening neuropsychiatric, autoimmune, ischemic, and infectious disorders. Monitor closely with periodic clinical and laboratory evaluations. **W/P:** Do not give IM if platelet count is less than 50,000 cells/mm^3. Hepatotoxicity, retinal hemorrhages, autoimmune diseases, pulmonary infiltrates, pneumonitis, thyroid abnormalities, and pneumonia reported. Avoid with immunosuppressed transplant, autoimmune disorders, decompensated liver disease. Caution with cardiac disease, coagulation disorders, severe myelosuppression, pulmonary disease, thyroid disorders, or DM prone to ketoacidosis. Avoid with preexisting psychiatric condition; depression, suicidal behavior, and aggressive behavior; monitor during treatment and in the 6-month follow-up period. D/C if psychiatric symptoms worsen or suicidal ideation is identified. Cases of encephalopathy observed in elderly treated with higher doses. Dental and periodontal disorders have been reported with ribavirin and interferon combination therapy. May exacerbate psoriasis or sarcoidosis. Do not interchange brands. **Contra:** Autoimmune hepatitis, decompensated liver disease. **P/N:** Category C, Category X when used with ribavirin, not for use in nursing.	Fever, headache, chills, fatigue, myalgia, GI disturbances, alopecia, dyspnea, depression.

Table 7.1. PRESCRIBING INFORMATION FOR ANTIFUNGAL AND ANTIVIRAL AGENTS *(cont.)*

NAME	FORM/ STRENGTH	DOSAGE	WARNINGS/PRECAUTIONS & CONTRAINDICATIONS	ADVERSE EFFECTS†
ANTIVIRALS *(cont.)*				
Interferon alfacon-1 (Infergen)	**Inj:** 9mcg/0.3mL, 15mcg/0.5mL	***Adults:* ≥18 yrs:** 9mcg 3x/week SQ for 24 weeks; wait 48 hrs between doses. **If No Response or Relapse:** 15mcg 3x/week for up to 48 weeks. Hold dose temporarily in severe adverse effects and reduce to 7.5mcg.	**BB:** May cause or aggravate fatal or life-threatening neuropsychiatric, autoimmune, ischemic, and infectious disorders. Monitor closely with periodic clinical and laboratory evaluations. **W/P:** Severe psychiatric adverse events (eg, depression, suicidal ideation, suicide attempt) may occur. Avoid in decompensated hepatic disease. Monitor CBC, platelets, and clinical chemistry tests before therapy and periodically thereafter. D/C if severe decrease in neutrophils or platelets, or serious hypersensitivity reaction occurs. Caution with cardiac disease, history of endocrine disorders, or low peripheral blood cell counts. Decrease/loss of vision and retinopathy reported; perform eye examination at baseline, if any ocular symptoms develop, and periodically with preexisting disorder. May exacerbate autoimmune disorders. Neutropenia, thrombocytopenia, hypertriglyceridemia, and thyroid disorders reported. Caution in elderly. Pancreatitis, pneumonia, interstitial pneumonitis, colitis reported; d/c when signs and symptoms develop. **Contra:** Decompensated hepatic disease, autoimmune hepatitis. **P/N:** Category C, caution in nursing.	Flu-like symptoms, depression, leukopenia, granulocytopenia, hot flushes, malaise, insomnia, dizziness, headache, myalgia, abdominal pain, N/V, diarrhea, anorexia, thrombocytopenia, nervousness.
Lamivudine (Epivir-HBV)	**Sol:** 5mg/mL [240mL]; **Tab:** 100mg	***Adults:* Chronic HBV:** 100mg qd. **CrCl 30-49mL/min:** 100mg Day 1, then 50mg qd. **CrCl 15-29mL/min:** 100mg Day 1, then 25mg qd. **CrCl 5-14mL/min:** 35mg Day 1, then 15mg qd. **CrCl <5mL/min:** 35mg Day 1, then 10mg qd. ***Pediatrics:* 2-17 yrs:** 3mg/kg qd. **Max:** 100mg/day.	**BB:** Lactic acidosis and severe, possibly fatal, hepatomegaly reported. If prescribed for patients with unrecognized or untreated HIV infection, rapid emergence of HIV resistance is likely; Epivir-HBV contains a lower dose of lamiviudine than Epivir, which is used to treat HIV. Severe acute exacerbations of hepatitis B reported upon discontinuation of therapy; follow-up liver function monitoring required. **W/P:** Reduce dose in renal dysfunction. Caution in elderly. This formulation is not appropriate in both HBV and HIV infections. Post-treatment exacerbations of hepatitis reported. Pancreatitis reported, especially in HIV-infected pediatrics with prior nucleoside exposure. Monitor patient regularly during treatment. Safety and efficacy of treatment after 1 yr is not known. Suspend therapy if lactic acidosis or pronounced hepatotoxicity develops. Emergence of resistance-associated HBV mutations. **P/N:** Category C, not for use in nursing.	Pancreatitis, lactic acidosis, severe hepatomegaly, GI complaints, **sore throat**, infections, elevated LFTs, arthralgia.
Oseltamivir Phosphate (Tamiflu)	**Cap:** 30mg, 45mg, 75mg; **Sus:** 12mg/mL [25mL]	***Adults:* Prophylaxis:** Begin within 2 days of exposure to infection. 75mg qd for at least 10 days, up to 6 weeks with community outbreak. **CrCl 10-30mL/min:** 75mg every other day or 30mg qd. **Treatment:** Begin therapy within 2 days of symptom onset. 75mg bid for 5 days. **CrCl 10-30mL/min:** 75mg qd for 5 days. ***Pediatrics:* Prophylaxis: ≥13 yrs:** Begin within 2 days of exposure to infection. 75mg qd for at least 10 days, up to 6 weeks with community outbreak. **≥1 yr:**	**W/P:** Efficacy not known with chronic cardiac disease, respiratory disease, and immunocompromised. Not a substitute for influenza vaccine. Adjust dose with renal dysfunction. Postmarketing neuropsychiatric events (self-injury and delirium) reported. Caution with kidney, heart, or respiratory disease, or any serious health condition. Sorbitol in Tamiflu may cause upset stomach and diarrhea in patients with history of fructose intolerance. **P/N:** Category C, caution in nursing.	N/V, diarrhea, **cough**, headache, fatigue, abdominal pain, bronchitis, dizziness.

†Bold entries denote special dental considerations.
BB = black box warning; **W/P** = warnings/precautions; **Contra** = contraindications; **P/N** = pregnancy category rating and nursing considerations.

NAME	FORM/ STRENGTH	DOSAGE	WARNINGS/PRECAUTIONS & CONTRAINDICATIONS	ADVERSE EFFECTS†
Oseltamivir Phosphate (Tamiflu) *(cont.)*		(Sus) **≤15kg:** 30mg qd. **>15-23kg:** 45mg qd. **>23-40kg:** 60mg qd. **>40kg:** 75mg qd. **Duration:** 10 days. **Treatment: ≥13 yrs:** Begin therapy within 2 days of symptom onset. 75mg bid for 5 days. **≥1 yr:** (Sus) **≤15kg:** 30mg bid. **>15-23kg:** 45mg bid. **>23-40kg:** 60mg bid. **>40kg:** 75mg bid. **Duration:** 5 days.		
Palivizumab (Synagis)	**Inj:** 50mg, 100mg	***Pediatrics:*** 15mg/kg IM; give first dose before start of RSV season (November-April), then monthly throughout season. Give monthly if develop RSV infection. Safety and efficacy established in infants with bronchopulmonary dysplasia (BPD) and infants with history of prematurity (≤35 weeks gestational age).	**W/P:** Anaphylactoid reactions reported. Caution with thrombocytopenia or any coagulation disorder due to IM injection. Safety and efficacy not demonstrated for treatment of established RSV disease. **P/N:** Category C, safety in nursing not known.	Upper respiratory infection, otitis media, rash, **cough,** diarrhea, vomiting, liver function abnormality, fever, rhinitis, hernia, gastroenteritis, wheezing.
Peginterferon alfa-2a (Pegasys)	**Inj: Syringe:** 180mcg/0.5mL; **Single-Dose Vial:** 180mcg/mL	***Adults:*** **≥18 yrs: HCV: Monotherapy:** 180mcg SQ (in abdomen or thigh) once weekly for 48 weeks. **Combination Therapy With Copegus:** 180mcg SQ once weekly for 24 weeks with genotypes 2 and 3 or 48 weeks with genotypes 1 and 4. **HCV with HIV: Monotherapy:** 180mcg SQ once weekly for 48 weeks. **Combination Therapy with Copegus:** 180mcg SQ once weekly for 48 weeks, regardless of genotype. **HBV: Monotherapy:** 180mcg SQ once weekly for 48 weeks. Adjust dose based on hematological parameters and depression severity (see PI for dose modifications).	**BB:** May cause or aggravate fatal or life-threatening neuropsychiatric, autoimmune, ischemic, and infectious disorders. Monitor closely with periodic clinical and laboratory evaluations. D/C with persistently severe or worsening signs or symptoms of these conditions. When used with ribavirin, refer to the individual monograph. **W/P:** Life-threatening neuropsychiatric reactions may occur; extreme caution with history of depression. Risk of bone marrow suppression; obtain CBCs prior to initiation and routinely thereafter. HTN, arrhythmias, chest pain, and MI reported; caution with preexisting cardiac disease. Decrease/loss of vision and retinopathy reported; perform eye exam at baseline (periodically with preexisting disorder); d/c if patient develops new or worsening of ophthalmologic disorders. Monitor for signs/symptoms of toxicity with impaired renal function and caution with CrCl <50mL/min. Development or exacerbation of autoimmune disorders reported. Caution in elderly. May induce or aggravate dyspnea, pulmonary infiltrates, pneumonia, bronchiolitis obliterans, interstitial pneumonitis, and sarcoiditis; d/c if persistent or unexplained pulmonary infiltrates or pulmonary function impairment. Hypersensitivity reactions, hemorrhagic/ischemic colitis, and pancreatitis reported; d/c if any of these develop. May cause or aggravate hypothyroidism or hyperthyroidism. Hypoglycemia, hyperglycemia, and DM reported. Avoid if failed other alpha interferon treatments, liver or other organ transplant recipients, or with HIV or HBV coinfection. Monitor for severe viral, bacterial, fungal infections. Exacerbation of hepatitis B reported. Chronic hepatitis C patients with cirrhosis may be at risk for hepatic decompensation; monitor hepatic function and serum ALTs. **Contra:** Autoimmune hepatitis, hepatic decompensation; neonates and infants (contains benzyl alcohol). When used with ribavirin, refer to the individual monograph. **P/N:** Category C (monotherapy) and Category X (with ribavirin), not for use in nursing.	Injection-site reaction, fatigue/asthenia, pyrexia, rigors, N/V, neutropenia, myalgia, headache, irritability/anxiety/ nervousness, insomnia, depression, alopecia.

Table 7.1. PRESCRIBING INFORMATION FOR ANTIFUNGAL AND ANTIVIRAL AGENTS *(cont.)*

NAME	FORM/ STRENGTH	DOSAGE	WARNINGS/PRECAUTIONS & CONTRAINDICATIONS	ADVERSE EFFECTS†
ANTIVIRALS *(cont.)*				
Peginterferon alfa-2b (PEG-Intron)	**Inj:** 50mcg/0.5mL, 80mcg/0.5mL, 120mcg/0.5mL, 150mcg/0.5mL	***Adults:* ≥18 yrs:** Administer SQ once weekly for 1 yr. **Monotherapy:** 1mcg/kg/week. **Combination Therapy With Rebetol:** 1.5mcg/kg/week plus Rebetol 800mg/day in 2 divided doses. **CrCl <50mL/min:** D/C ribavirin. **Monotherapy or With Rebetol:** D/C if HCV levels remain high after 6 months. Adjust dose based on hematological parameters and depression severity. **Renal Impairment: CrCl 30-50mL/min:** reduce dose by 25%. **CrCl 10-29mL/min:** reduce dose by 50%. D/C if renal function decreases.	**BB:** May cause or aggravate fatal or life-threatening neuropsychiatric, autoimmune, ischemic, and infectious disorders. Monitor closely with periodic clinical and laboratory evaluations. D/C with severe or worsening signs or symptoms of these conditions. When used with Rebetol, refer to the individual monograph. **W/P:** Life-threatening neuropsychiatric reactions may occur; caution with history of depression or psychiatric symptoms/disorders. Risk of bone marrow suppression; monitor CBCs and blood chemistry at initiation and periodically thereafter. Hypotension, arrhythmia, tachycardia, angina pectoris, MI reported; caution with cardiovascular disease. Conduct baseline eye exam in all patients and periodic exams with preexisting ophthalmologic disorders; d/c if new or worsening ophthalmologic disorders occur. Caution with CrCl <50mL/min, autoimmune disorders, and the elderly. D/C if persistent or unexplained pulmonary infiltrates, or pulmonary dysfunction, or hypersensitivity reaction occurs, or if hemorrhagic/ischemic colitis or pancreatitis develops. May cause or aggravate hypothyroidism/hyperthyroidism. Hyperglycemia and DM reported. Avoid if failed other alpha interferon treatments, liver or other organ transplant recipients, or with HIV or HBV coinfection. May elevate triglyceride levels. Monitor renal impairment for toxicity. **Contra:** Autoimmune hepatitis, decompensated liver disease. When used with Rebetol, refer to the individual monograph. **P/N:** Category C, safety in nursing not known.	Headache, fatigue, rigors, dizziness, nausea, anorexia, depression, insomnia, irritability, myalgia, arthralgia, weight loss, alopecia, pruritus, decreased platelets/Hgb/neutrophils.
Penciclovir (Denavir)	**Cre:** 1% [1.5g]	***Adults/Pediatrics:* ≥12 yrs: Herpes Labialis:** Apply q2h while awake, for 4 days. Start with earliest sign or symptom.	**W/P:** Only use on herpes labialis on the lips and face. Avoid mucous membranes or near the eyes. Effectiveness not established in immunocompromised patients. **P/N:** Category B, not for use in nursing.	Headache, application site reaction, local anesthesia, **taste perversion**, rash.
Ribavirin (Copegus)	**Tab:** 200mg	***Adults:* HCV:** Give bid in divided doses. Treat for 24-48 weeks with Pegasys 180mcg. **Genotypes 1 and 4: <75kg:** 1000mg/day for 48 weeks. **≥75kg:** 1200mg/day for 48 weeks. **Genotypes 2 and 3:** 800mg/day for 24 weeks. **HCV/HIV:** 800mg qd. Treat for 48 weeks with Pegasys 180mcg. **Dose Modifications:** Reduce to 600mg/day if Hgb <10g/dL with no cardiac history, or if Hgb decreases by ≥2g/dL during a 4-week period with stable cardiac disease. D/C if Hgb <8.5g/dL with no cardiac history or if Hgb <12g/dL after 4 weeks of dose reduction with stable cardiac disease. After dose modification, may restart at 600mg/day, then may increase to 800mg/day. **CrCl <50mL/min:** Avoid use.	**BB:** Not for monotherapy treatment of chronic hepatitis C. Primary toxicity is hemolytic anemia. Avoid with significant or unstable cardiac disease. Contraindicated in pregnancy and male partners of pregnant women. Use two forms of contraception during therapy and for 6 months after discontinuation. **W/P:** D/C with hepatic decompensation, confirmed pancreatitis, and hypersensitivity reaction. Severe depression, suicidal ideation, hemolytic anemia, bone marrow suppression, autoimmune and infectious disorders, pancreatitis, and diabetes reported. Pulmonary symptoms reported; monitor closely with evidence of pulmonary infiltrates or pulmonary function impairment and d/c if appropriate. Assess for underlying cardiac disease (obtain EKG); fatal and nonfatal	Injection-site reaction, fatigue/asthenia, pyrexia, rigors, N/V, neutropenia, anorexia, myalgia, headache, irritability/anxiety/nervousness, insomnia, alopecia.

†Bold entries denote special dental considerations.
BB = black box warning; **W/P** = warnings/precautions; **Contra** = contraindications; **P/N** = pregnancy category rating and nursing considerations.

NAME	FORM/ STRENGTH	DOSAGE	WARNINGS/PRECAUTIONS & CONTRAINDICATIONS	ADVERSE EFFECTS†
Ribavirin (Copegus) *(cont.)*			MI reported with anemia. Caution with cardiac disease, d/c if cardiovascular status deteriorates. Hemolytic anemia reported; monitor Hgb or Hct initially then at week 2 and 4 (or more if needed) of therapy. Suspend therapy if symptoms of pancreatitis arise. Avoid if CrCl <50mL/min. Obtain negative pregnancy test prior to initiation then monthly, and for 6 months post-therapy. **Contra:** Pregnancy, male partners of pregnant women, hemoglobinopathies (eg, thalassemia major, sickle cell anemia). Autoimmune hepatitis and hepatic decompensation (Child-Pugh score greater than 6, Class B and C) in cirrhotic CHC patients, and in cirrhotic CHC patients coinfected with HIV before or during treatment when used in combination with Pegasys. **P/N:** Category X, not for use in nursing.	
Ribavirin (Rebetol)	**Cap:** 200mg; **Sol:** 40mg/mL [100mL]	***Adults:*** **≥18 yrs: With Intron A: ≤75kg:** 400mg qam and 600mg qpm. **>75kg:** 600mg qam and 600mg qpm. Treat for 24-48 weeks interferon-naive; 24 weeks in relapse. **With Peg-Intron:** 400mg bid, qam and qpm with food. Reduce to 600mg qd if Hgb <10g/dL with no cardiac history, or if Hgb decreases by ≥2g/dL during a 4-week period with a cardiac history. D/C if Hgb <8.5g/dL with no cardiac history or if Hgb <12g/dL after 4 weeks of dose reduction with a cardiac history. **CrCl <50mL/min:** Avoid use. ***Pediatrics:*** **≥3 yrs:** 15mg/kg/day in divided doses qam and qpm. Use sol if ≤25kg or cannot swallow caps. **With Intron A: 25-36kg:** 200mg bid, qam and qpm. **37-49kg:** 200mg qam and 400mg qpm. **50-61kg:** 400mg bid, qam and qpm. **>61kg:** Dose as adult. **Genotype 1:** Treat for 48 weeks. **Genotypes 2 and 3:** Treat for 24 weeks. Reduce to 7.5mg/day if Hgb <10g/dL with no cardiac history, or if Hgb decreases by ≥2g/dL during a 4-week period with a cardiac history. D/C if Hgb <8.5g/dL with no cardiac history or if Hgb <12g/dL after 4 weeks of dose reduction with a cardiac history.	**BB:** Not for monotherapy treatment of chronic hepatitis C. Primary toxicity is hemolytic anemia. Avoid with significant or unstable cardiac disease. Contraindicated in pregnancy and male partners of pregnant women. Use two forms of contraception during therapy and for 6 months after discontinuation. **W/P:** Severe depression, suicidal ideation, bone marrow suppression, autoimmune and infectious disorders, pulmonary dysfunction, pancreatitis, and DM reported. Assess for underlying cardiac disease (obtain EKG); fatal and nonfatal MI reported with anemia. Hemolytic anemia reported; monitor Hgb or Hct initially then at Week 2 and 4 (or more if needed) of therapy. Suspend therapy if symptoms of pancreatitis arise. Avoid if CrCl <50mL/min. Obtain negative pregnancy test prior to initiation then monthly, and for 6 months post-therapy. **Contra:** Pregnancy, male partners of pregnant women, hemoglobinopathies (eg, thalassemia major, sickle cell anemia). When used with Intron A or PEG-Intron, refer to individual monograph. **P/N:** Category X, not for use in nursing.	Hemolytic anemia, headache, fatigue, rigors, fever, nausea, anorexia, myalgia, arthralgia, insomnia, irritability, depression, dyspnea, alopecia.
Rimantadine HCl (Flumadine)	**Syrup:** 50mg/5mL [240mL]; **Tab:** 100mg	***Adults:*** **Prophylaxis/Treatment:** 100mg bid. **Elderly/Severe Hepatic Dysfunction/CrCl ≤10mL/min:** 100mg qd. Initiate treatment within 48 hrs of onset of symptoms. Treat for 7 days from initial onset of symptoms. ***Pediatrics:*** **Prophylaxis: 1-9 yrs:** 5mg/kg qd. **Max:** 150mg qd. **≥10 yrs:** 100mg bid.	**W/P:** Caution with a history of epilepsy. D/C if seizures develop. Caution with renal or hepatic dysfunction. **P/N:** Category C, not for use in nursing.	Insomnia, dizziness, nervousness, N/V, anorexia, **dry mouth,** abdominal pain, asthenia.

Table 7.1. PRESCRIBING INFORMATION FOR ANTIFUNGAL AND ANTIVIRAL AGENTS *(cont.)*

NAME	FORM/ STRENGTH	DOSAGE	WARNINGS/PRECAUTIONS & CONTRAINDICATIONS	ADVERSE EFFECTS†
ANTIVIRALS *(cont.)*				
Valacyclovir HCl (Valtrex)	**Tab:** 500mg, 1g	***Adults:* Herpes Zoster:** 1g q8h for 7 days. Start within 48-72 hrs after onset of rash. **CrCl 30-49mL/min:** 1g q12h. **CrCl 10-29mL/min:** 1g q24h. **CrCl <10mL/min:** 500mg q24h. **Genital Herpes: Initial:** 1g q12h for 10 days. Start within 48-72 hrs after onset of symptoms. **CrCl 10-29mL/min:** 1g q24h. **CrCl <10mL/min:** 500mg q24h. **Recurrent Episodes: Treatment:** 500mg bid for 3 days. Start within 24 hrs after onset of symptoms. **CrCl ≤29mL/min:** 500mg q24h. **Suppressive Therapy with Normal Immune Function:** 1g q24h. **CrCl ≤29mL/min:** 500mg q24h. **Alternative:** (≤9 episodes/yr) 500mg q24h. **CrCl ≤29mL/min:** 500mg q48h. **Suppressive Therapy with HIV and CD4 ≥100cells/mm^3:** 500mg q12h. **CrCl ≤29mL/min:** 500mg q24h. **Herpes Labialis:** 2g q12h for 1 day. Start at earliest symptom of cold sore. **CrCl 30-49mL/min:** 1g q12h. **CrCl 10-29mL/min:** 500mg q12h. **CrCl <10mL/min:** 500mg single dose. Administer therapy for 1 day. Initiate at earliest symptoms of a cold sore. ***Pediatrics:* ≥12 yrs: Herpes Labialis:** 2g q12h for 1 day. Start at earliest symptom of cold sore. **2 to <18 yrs: Chickenpox:** 20mg/kg tid for 5 days **Max:** 1g q8h. Initiate at earliest sign or symptom.	**W/P:** Thrombotic thrombocytopenic purpura/hemolytic uremic syndrome reported with advanced HIV disease, allogenic bone marrow or renal transplants. Reduce dose with renal dysfunction. Possible renal and CNS toxicity in elderly. **Contra:** Acyclovir hypersensitivity. **P/N:** Category B, caution in nursing.	N/V, headache, dizziness, abdominal pain.
Valganciclovir HCl (Valcyte)	**Tab:** 450mg	***Adults:* Treatment of CMV Retinitis: Initial:** 900mg bid for 21 days. **Maint:** 900mg qd. **Prevention of CMV Disease:** 900mg qd starting within 10 days of transplantation until 100 days post-transplantation. **CrCl 40-59mL/min: Initial:** 450mg bid. **Maint:** 450mg qd. **CrCl 25-39mL/min: Initial:** 450mg qd. **Maint:** 450mg every 2 days. **CrCl 10-24mL/min: Initial:** 450mg every 2 days. **Maint:** 450mg twice weekly. **CrCl <10mL/min:** Not recommended. Take with food.	**BB:** Granulocytopenia, anemia, and thrombocytopenia reported. Carcinogenic, teratogenic, and may cause aspermatogenesis based on animal studies. **W/P:** Avoid if the neutrophils <500cells/mcL, platelet count <25,000/mcL or Hgb >8g/dL. Severe leukopenia, neutropenia, anemia, thrombocytopenia, pancytopenia, bone marrow depression, and aplastic anemia observed. Adjust dose in renal impairment. Do not substitute with ganciclovir caps. May cause temporary or permanent inhibition of spermatogenesis. **Contra:** Hypersensitivity to ganciclovir. **P/N:** Category C, not for use in nursing.	Diarrhea, N/V, graft rejection, abdominal pain, pyrexia, headache, neutropenia, leukopenia, anemia, insomnia, peripheral neuropathy, HTN.
Zanamivir (Relenza)	**Inh:** 5mg/inh [20 blisters]	***Adults/Pediatrics:* Influenza: Treatment: ≥7 yrs: Usual:** 2 inh (10mg) q12h for 5 days. Take 2 doses at least 2 hrs apart on first day. **Prophylaxis: ≥5 yrs: Household Setting:** 2 inh (10mg) qd for 10 days. **Community Outbreaks:** 2 inh (10mg) qd for 28 days. Administer at same time every day.	**W/P:** Not recommended for use with underlying airways disease (eg, asthma, COPD). Serious cases of bronchospasm reported during treatment; d/c if bronchospasm or decline in respiratory function develops. D/C if allergic reaction occurs. Postmarketing neuropsychiatric events (seizures, delirium, hallucinations) reported. **P/N:** Category C, caution in nursing.	Dizziness, headaches, diarrhea, nausea, sinusitis, bronchitis, **cough, ear/nose/throat infections**, nasal symptoms.
MISCELLANEOUS APHTHOUS MEDICATION				
Amlexanox (Aphthasol) OTC	**Paste:** 5% [5g]	***Adults:*** Begin at 1st sign of aphthous ulcer. Apply 1/4 inch qid, pc and qhs, following oral hygiene. Use until ulcer heals. Re-evaluate if healing or pain reduction has not occurred after 10 days of use.	**W/P:** Wash hands immediately after applying paste. D/C if rash or contact mucositis occurs. Re-evaluate if healing or pain reduction has not occurred after 10 days. Avoid eyes. **P/N:** Category B, caution in nursing.	Transient pain, stinging, burning.

†Bold entries denote special dental considerations.
BB = black box warning; **W/P** = warnings/precautions; **Contra** = contraindications; **P/N** = pregnancy category rating and nursing considerations.

Table 7.2. DRUG INTERACTIONS FOR ANTIFUNGAL AND ANTIVIRAL AGENTS

ANTIFUNGALS

Amphotericin B (Fungizone)	
Antineoplastics	May potentiate renal toxicity, bronchospasm, hypotension.
Azole antifungals	May induce fungal resistance with azole antifungals (eg, ketoconazole, clotrimazole, miconazole, fluconazole).
Corticosteroids	May potentiate hypokalemia.
Corticotropin	May potentiate hypokalemia.
Flucytosine	May increase flucytosine toxicity.
Nephrotoxic drugs	May increase risk of renal toxicity with nephrotoxic drugs (eg, aminoglycosides, cyclosporine, pentamidine).
Skeletal muscle relaxants	May enhance curariform effect of skeletal muscle relaxants (eg, tubocurarine).
Amphotericin B Cholesteryl Sulfate (Amphotec)	
Antineoplastics	May potentiate renal toxicity, bronchospasm, hypotension.
Azole antifungals	May induce fungal resistance with azole antifungals (eg, ketoconazole, clotrimazole, miconazole, fluconazole).
Corticosteroids	May potentiate hypokalemia.
Corticotropin	May potentiate hypokalemia.
Flucytosine	May increase flucytosine toxicity.
Nephrotoxic drugs	May increase risk of renal toxicity (eg, aminoglycosides, cyclosporine, pentamidine).
Skeletal muscle relaxants	May enhance curariform effect of skeletal muscle relaxants (eg, tubocurarine).
Amphotericin B Lipid Complex (Abelcet)	
Antineoplastics	May potentiate renal toxicity, bronchospasm, and hypotension.
Corticosteroids	May potentiate hypokalemia, predisposing patients to cardiac dysfunction.
Corticotropin	May potentiate hypokalemia, predisposing patients to cardiac dysfunction.
Cyclosporine	May be associated with nephrotoxicity if given within several days of bone marrow ablation.
Digitalis glycosides	May potentiate digitalis toxicity.
Flucytosine	Increases risk of flucytosine toxicity.
Leukocyte transfusions	May result in acute pulmonary toxicity.
Nephrotoxic drugs	May increase risk of renal toxicity (eg, aminoglycosides, cyclosporine, pentamidine).
Skeletal muscle relaxants	May enhance curariform effect of skeletal muscle relaxants (eg, tubocurarine).
Zidovudine	May increase risk of myelotoxicity and nephrotoxicity with coadministration.
Amphotericin B Liposome (AmBisome)	
Antineoplastics	May potentiate renal toxicity, bronchospasm, hypotension.
Azole antifungals	May induce fungal resistance with azole antifungals (eg, ketoconazole, miconazole, clotrimazole, fluconazole); caution with combination therapy, especially in immunocompromised patients.

Table 7.2. DRUG INTERACTIONS FOR ANTIFUNGAL AND ANTIVIRAL AGENTS *(cont.)*

ANTIFUNGALS *(cont.)*	
Amphotericin B Liposome (AmBisome) *(cont.)*	
Corticosteroids	May potentiate hypokalemia.
Corticotropin	May potentiate hypokalemia.
Digitalis glycosides	May potentiate digitalis toxicity.
Flucytosine	May increase flucytosine toxicity.
Leukocyte transfusions	May result in acute pulmonary toxicity.
Nephrotoxic drugs	May enhance potential for renal toxicity.
Skeletal muscle relaxants	May enhance curariform effect of skeletal muscle relaxants due to hypokalemia.
Anidulafungin (Eraxis)	
Cyclosporine	Slightly increases levels with cyclosporine.
Caspofungin Acetate (Cancidas)	
Carbamazepine	May decrease levels of caspofungin.
Cyclosporine	May increase levels of caspofungin.
Dexamethasone	May decrease levels of caspofungin.
Dextrose-containing diluents	Do not use with diluents containing dextrose.
Efavirenz	May decrease levels of caspofungin.
Nevirapine	May decrease levels of caspofungin.
Phenytoin	May decrease levels of caspofungin.
Rifampin	May decrease levels of caspofungin.
Tacrolimus	May reduce blood levels of tacrolimus.
Fluconazole (Diflucan)	
Astemizole	Increases levels of astemizole.
Cimetidine	May decrease fluconazole levels.
Cisapride	Increases levels of cisapride; concomitant use contraindicated due to prolongation of QTc interval and cardiac events (torsades de pointes).
Contraceptives, oral	May increase or decrease levels of ethinyl estradiol- and levonorgestrel-containing oral contraceptives.
Coumarin-like drugs	May increase PT with concomitant administration.
Cyclosporine	Increases levels of cyclosporine.
HCTZ	May increase fluconazole levels.
Hypoglycemics, oral	May increase risk of severe hypoglycemia with oral hypoglycemic agents (eg, tolbutamide, glyburide, glipizide).
Phenytoin	Increases levels of phenytoin.
Rifabutin	May cause uveitis with coadministration.
Rifampin	Enhances metabolism of fluconazole.
Tacrolimus	Nephrotoxicity reported with concomitant administration.

ANTIFUNGALS *(cont.)*

Fluconazole (Diflucan) *(cont.)*	
Terfenadine	Contraindicated due to prolongation of QTc interval.
Theophylline	Increases the serum concentration of theophylline.
Zidovudine	Increases levels of zidovudine.
Flucytosine (Ancobon)	
Cytosine	Antagonized by cytosine.
Glomerular filtration, drugs that impair	May prolong half-life of flucytosine.
Polyene antibiotics	Antifungal synergism with polyene antibiotics (eg, amphotericin B).
Griseofulvin (Grifulvin V, Gris-PEG)	
Alcohol	Increases effects of alcohol.
Anticoagulants, coumarin	May require dosage adjustment of coumarin anticoagulants during and after griseofulvin therapy.
Barbiturates	Decreases effects of griseofulvin.
Contraceptives, oral	Decreases efficacy and increases incidence of breakthrough bleeding.
Itraconazole (Sporanox)	
Alfentanil	Increases levels of alfentanil.
Alprazolam	Increases levels of alprazolam.
Astemizole	Increases levels of astemizole.
Budesonide	Increases levels of budesonide.
Buspirone	Increases levels of buspirone.
Busulfan	Increases levels of busulfan.
Carbamazepine	Increases levels of carbamazepine.
CCBs, dihydropyridine	Increases levels of dihydropyridine CCBs; concurrent use with nisoldipine contraindicated.
Cilostazol	Increases levels of cilostazol.
Cisapride	Contraindicated; increases levels of cisapride
CYP3A4 inducers	CYP3A4 inducers (eg, carbamazepine, phenobarbital, phenytoin, isoniazid, rifabutin, rifampin, nevirapine) decrease levels of itraconazole.
CYP3A4 inhibitors	CYP3A4 inhibitors (eg, erythromycin, clarithromycin, indinavir, ritonavir) may increase itraconazole levels.
Dexamethasone	Increases levels of dexamethasone.
Diazepam	Increases levels of diazepam.
Digoxin	Increases levels of digoxin.
Disopyramide	Increases levels of disopyramide.
Docetaxel	Increases levels of docetaxel.
Dofetilide	Contraindicated; increases levels of dofetilide.

Table 7.2. DRUG INTERACTIONS FOR ANTIFUNGAL AND ANTIVIRAL AGENTS *(cont.)*

ANTIFUNGALS *(cont.)*	
Itraconazole (Sporanox) *(cont.)*	
Eletriptan	Increases levels of eletriptan.
Ergot alkaloids	Increases levels of ergot alkaloids (dihydroergotamine, ergometrine [ergonovine], ergotamine, and methylergometrine [methylergonovine]); concurrent use contraindicated.
Fentanyl	Increases levels of fentanyl.
Fluticasone	Increases levels of fluticasone.
Gastric acid suppressors/ neutralizers	Antacids, H_2-receptor antagonists, and proton pump inhibitors may decrease absorption of itraconazole capsules.
Halofantrine	Increases levels of halofantrine.
HMG-CoA reductase inhibitors (statins)	Increases levels of statins; concurrent use with lovastatin and simvastatin contraindicated.
Hypoglycemics, oral	Increases levels of oral hypoglycemics; severe hypoglycemia.
Immunosuppressants	Increases levels of immunosuppressants (eg, cyclosporine, sirolimus, tacrolimus).
Levacetylmethadol	Contraindicated; increases levels of levacetylmethadol (levomethadyl).
Methylprednisolone	Increases levels of methylprednisolone.
Midazolam, oral	Contraindicated; increases levels of oral midazolam.
Pimozide	Contraindicated; increases levels of pimozide.
Protease inhibitors	Increases levels of protease inhibitors.
Quinidine	Contraindicated; increases levels of quinidine.
Rifabutin	Increases levels of rifabutin.
Triazolam	Contraindicated; increases levels of triazolam.
Trimetrexate	Increases levels of trimetrexate.
Verapamil	Increases levels of verapamil.
Vinca alkaloids	Increases levels of vinca alkaloids.
Warfarin	Increases levels of warfarin.
Ketoconazole (Nizoral)	
Antacids	Possible drug-induced achlorhydria may decrease ketoconazole absorption; administer antacids at least 2 hrs after ketoconazole.
Anticholinergics	May decrease ketoconazole absorption; administer anticholinergics at least 2 hrs after ketoconazole.
Astemizole	Contraindicated; avoid coadministration with ketoconazole.
Cisapride	Contraindicated; avoid coadministration with ketoconazole.
Coumarin-like drugs	May enhance anticoagulant effect.
Cyclosporine	Ketoconazole may alter metabolism of cyclosporine.

ANTIFUNGALS *(cont.)*

Ketoconazole (Nizoral) *(cont.)*	
CYP3A4 substrates	Ketoconazole may alter metabolism of CYP3A4 substrates.
Digoxin	Rare cases of elevated plasma levels of digoxin reported; monitor digoxin levels with coadministration.
H_2-blockers	Possible drug-induced achlorhydria may decrease ketoconazole absorption; administer H_2-blockers at least 2 hrs after ketoconazole.
Hypoglycemics, oral	May potentiate effects and result in severe hypoglycemia.
Isoniazid	Avoid concomitant use; may adversely affect ketoconazole levels.
Methylprednisolone	May alter metabolism resulting in elevated plasma concentrations of methylprednisolone.
Midazolam	May potentiate effects of midazolam.
Phenytoin	Concomitant administration may alter metabolism of phenytoin and/or ketoconazole; monitor plasma levels of both drugs.
Rifampin	Avoid concomitant use; may reduce plasma levels of ketoconazole.
Tacrolimus	May alter metabolism resulting in elevated plasma concentrations of tacrolimus.
Terfenadine	Contraindicated; avoid coadministration with ketoconazole.
Triazolam	May potentiate effects of triazolam.
Micafungin Sodium (Mycamine)	
Itraconazole	May increase risk of itraconazole toxicity.
Nifedipine	May increase risk of nifedipine toxicity.
Sirolimus	May increase risk of sirolimus toxicity.
Posaconazole (Noxafil)	
Benzodiazepines	Monitor adverse events of benzodiazepines; consider dose reduction with benzodiazepines metabolized by CYP3A4.
CCBs	Monitor for adverse events and toxicity of CCBs; may require dose reduction of CCBs.
Cimetidine	Avoid concurrent use unless benefit outweighs risks.
Cyclosporine	May elevate levels of cyclosporine, consider dose reduction and more frequent monitoring.
CYP3A4 substrates	Coadministration with the CYP3A4 substrates (terfenadine, astemizole, cisapride, pimozide, halofantrine, or quinidine) is contraindicated, may result in increased plasma concentrations of substrates leading to QTc prolongation and rare occurrences of torsades de pointes.
Efavirenz	Avoid concurrent use unless benefit outweighs risk.
Ergot alkaloids	May increase plasma levels of ergot alkaloids (ergotamine and dihydroergotamine); avoid concomitant use.
HMG-CoA reductase inhibitors (statins)	Consider dose reduction of statins metabolized by CYP3A4; may increase risk of rhabdomyolysis with increased plasma levels of statins.

Table 7.2. DRUG INTERACTIONS FOR ANTIFUNGAL AND ANTIVIRAL AGENTS *(cont.)*

ANTIFUNGALS *(cont.)*	
Posaconazole (Noxafil) *(cont.)*	
Phenytoin	Avoid concurrent use unless benefit outweighs risk; monitor closely and consider dose reduction.
Rifabutin	Avoid concurrent use unless benefit outweighs risk; monitor CBC and adverse events.
Sirolimus	Contraindicated; avoid coadministration with posaconazole.
Tacrolimus	May elevate tacrolimus levels, consider dose reduction and more frequent monitoring.
Vinca alkaloids	May increase vinca alkaloid levels.
Terbinafine HCl (Lamisil)	
β-Blockers	May potentiate drug levels of β-blockers.
Caffeine	Decreases clearance of caffeine.
Cimetidine	Decreases clearance of terbinafine.
Cyclosporine	Increases clearance of cyclosporine.
MAO-B Inhibitors	May potentiate drug levels of MAO-B inhibitors.
Rifampin	Increases clearance of terbinafine.
SSRIs	May potentiate drug levels of SSRIs.
TCAs	May potentiate drug levels of TCAs.
Voriconazole (Vfend)	
Benzodiazepines	May increase levels of benzodiazepines, monitor for adverse events and toxicity.
CCBs, dihydropyridine	May increase levels of dihydropyridine CCBs, monitor for adverse events and toxicity.
Carbamazepine	Contraindicated; avoid coadministration with voriconazole.
Contraceptives, oral	May increase levels of oral contraceptives containing ethinyl estradiol and norethindrone.
Cyclosporine	May increase levels of cyclosporine; monitor levels. Reduce cyclosporine to half of original dose with initiation of voriconazole therapy.
CYP3A4 substrates	Coadministration of the CYP3A4 substrates (terfenadine, astemizole, cisapride, pimozide or quinidine) are contraindicated since increased plasma concentrations of these drugs can lead to QT prolongation and rare occurrences of torsades de pointes.
Efavirenz	Reduces levels of efavirenz.
Ergot alkaloids	Contraindicated; do not administer with voriconazole.
HMG-CoA reductase inhibitors (statins)	May increase levels of statins; monitor for adverse events and toxicity.
Hypoglycemics	May increase levels of hypoglycemics; monitor blood glucose levels.
Methadone	May increase levels of methadone and enhance toxicity, including QT interval prolongation; may require dose reduction of methadone.

ANTIFUNGALS *(cont.)*

Voriconazole (Vfend) *(cont.)*	
NNRTIs	May increase levels of NNRTIs; monitor for adverse events and toxicity.
Omeprazole	Coadministration may increase levels of omeprazole; reduce omeprazole dose by half when initiating voriconazole in patients already receiving ≥40mg omeprazole.
Phenytoin	May increase levels of phenytoin; monitor levels.
Protease inhibitors	May increase levels of protease inhibitors; monitor for adverse events and toxicity.
Proton pump inhibitors (PPIs)	May increase levels of PPIs that are CYP2C19 substrates.
Rifabutin	Contraindicated; avoid coadministration with voriconazole.
Rifampin	Contraindicated; avoid coadministration with voriconazole.
Ritonavir	Avoid with low-dose ritonavir (100mg q12h) unless an assessment of the benefit/risk to the patient justifies the use of voriconazole. Concomitant administration with high-dose ritonavir (400mg q12h) is contraindicated.
Sirolimus	Contraindicated; avoid coadministration with voriconazole.
St. John's wort	Contraindicated; avoid coadministration with voriconazole.
Tacrolimus	May increase levels of tacrolimus; monitor levels. Reduce tacrolimus to 1/3 of original dose with initiation of voriconazole therapy.
Vinca alkaloids	May increase levels of vinca alkaloids; monitor for adverse events and toxicity.
Warfarin	May increase levels of warfarin; monitor levels.

ANTIVIRALS

Acyclovir, Acyclovir Sodium (Zovirax Oral, Injection)	
Nephrotoxic agents	Caution with potentially nephrotoxic agents; concomitant use may increase the risk of renal impairment and/or the risk of reversible CNS symptoms.
Probenecid	May increase acyclovir (IV) half-life and AUC with probenecid.
Adefovir Dipivoxil (Hepsera)	
Nephrotoxic agents	Coadministration with drugs that reduce renal function or compete for active tubular secretion may increase concentrations of adefovir or the coadministered drugs.
Amantadine HCl (Symmetrel)	
Anticholinergic agents	May potentiate anticholinergic side effects of amantadine.
CNS stimulants	Caution with concomitant use.
Influenza vaccine, attenuated	Avoid use of attenuated influenza vaccine within 2 wks before or 48 hrs after administration of amantadine.
Quinidine	May increase plasma levels of amantadine with quinidine.
Quinine	May increase plasma levels of amantadine with quinine.
Thioridazine	Increased tremor reported in elderly Parkinson's patients with concomitant thioridazine.
TMP/SMX	May increase plasma levels of amantadine with TMP/SMX.

Table 7.2. DRUG INTERACTIONS FOR ANTIFUNGAL AND ANTIVIRAL AGENTS *(cont.)*

ANTIVIRALS *(cont.)*	
Cidofovir (Vistide)	
Nephrotoxic agents	Avoid nephrotoxic agents (eg, aminoglycosides, amphotericin B, foscarnet, IV pentamidine, vancomycin, and NSAIDs); discontinue nephrotoxic agents at least 7 days before therapy.
Zidovudine	Temporarily discontinue zidovudine or decrease dose by 50% on days of cidofovir administration as probenecid reduces metabolic clearance of zidovudine.
Entecavir (Baraclude)	
Renal function, drugs reducing	May increase serum concentrations of entecavir or coadministered drug with drugs that reduce renal function or compete for active tubular secretion.
Famciclovir (Famvir)	
Active tubular secretion, drugs eliminated by	May increase plasma levels of active metabolite penciclovir with drugs that are significantly eliminated by active renal tubular secretion (eg, probenecid).
Aldehyde oxidase, drugs metabolized by	Potential interaction with drugs metabolized by aldehyde oxidase.
Foscarnet Sodium	
Calcium, drugs affecting	Caution with drugs that affect plasma calcium levels.
Nephrotoxic drugs	Avoid potentially nephrotoxic drugs (eg, aminoglycosides, amphotericin B, pentamidine IV).
Pentamidine	Possible hypocalcemia with pentamidine.
Ritonavir	Renal dysfunction reported with ritonavir.
Saquinavir	Renal dysfunction reported with saquinavir.
Ganciclovir (Cytovene)	
Adriamycin	Caution with adriamycin; potential additive toxicity.
Amphotericin B	Caution with amphotericin B; potential additive toxicity.
Cyclosporine	Caution with cyclosporine; potential additive toxicity.
Dapsone	Caution with dapsone; potential additive toxicity.
Didanosine	Increases plasma levels of didanosine.
Flucytosine	Caution with flucytosine; potential additive toxicity.
Imipenem-cilastatin	Avoid imipenem-cilastatin; may precipitate seizures.
Nucleoside analogues	Caution with other nucleoside analogues.
Pentamidine	Caution with pentamidine; potential additive toxicity.
Probenecid	May increase AUC and decrease clearance of ganciclovir.
TMP/SMX	Caution with TMP/SMX; potential additive toxicity.
Vinblastine	Caution with vinblastine; potential additive toxicity.
Vincristine	Caution with vincristine; potential additive toxicity.
Zidovudine	Coadministration may decrease levels of ganciclovir and increase levels of zidovudine. May increase risk of neutropenia and anemia with concomitant use.

ANTIVIRALS *(cont.)*

Interferon alfa-2b (Intron A)	
Myelosuppressive agents	Caution with other myelosuppressive agents (eg, zidovudine).
Ribavirin	Hemolytic anemia, cardiac and pulmonary events reported with concomitant ribavirin.
Theophylline	May decrease clearance of theophylline; may result in 100% increase in theophylline levels.
Interferon alfacon-1 (Infergen)	
CYP450 substrates	Caution with drugs that are metabolized by the CYP450 pathway; monitor for changes in therapeutic and/or toxic levels of concomitant drugs.
Myelosuppressive drugs	Caution with agents that cause myelosuppression.
Lamivudine (Epivir-HBV)	
Combinations of abacavir, lamivudine, and zidovudine	Avoid with fixed-dose combinations of abacavir, lamivudine, and zidovudine.
Emtricitabine-, efavirenz-, and tenofovir-containing drugs	Avoid emtricitabine and fixed-dose combinations of emtricitabine, efavirenz, and tenofovir.
TMP/SMX	TMP/SMX increases levels of lamivudine.
Zalcitabine	Avoid with zalcitabine.
Zidovudine	Avoid with zidovudine.
Oseltamivir Phosphate (Tamiflu)	
Influenza vaccine, live attenuated	Avoid administration within 2 wks before or 48 hrs after administration of oseltamivir; may inhibit replication of live vaccine virus.
Peginterferon alfa-2a (Pegasys)	
Methadone	May increase methadone levels; monitor for methadone toxicity.
Nucleoside reverse transcriptase inhibitors (NRTIs)	May increase risk of hepatic decompensation with concomitant use of peginterferon alfa-2a +/- ribavirin.
Theophylline	Coadministration may increase theophylline AUC; monitor theophylline serum levels.
Peginterferon alfa-2b (PEG-Intron)	
CYP2C8, 2C9 substrates	Caution with medications metabolized by CYP2C8, 2C9 (eg, warfarin and phenytoin); may decrease therapeutic effects of these substrates.
CYP2D6 substrates	Caution with medications metabolized by CYP2D6 (eg, flecainide); may decrease therapeutic effects of these substrates.
Methadone	May increase plasma levels of methadone; monitor for increased narcotic effect.
Ribavirin	Closely monitor for hepatic decompensation and anemia with concomitant interferon with ribavirin and NRTIs.
Ribavirin (Copegus, Rebetol)	
Didanosine	Avoid with didanosine; fatal hepatic failure, peripheral neuropathy, pancreatitis, and symptomatic hyperlactatemia/lactic acidosis reported with coadministration.
NRTIs	May increase risk of hepatic decompensation with concomitant use of NRTIs and ribavirin

Table 7.2. DRUG INTERACTIONS FOR ANTIFUNGAL AND ANTIVIRAL AGENTS *(cont.)*

ANTIVIRALS *(cont.)*	
Ribavirin (Copegus, Rebetol) *(cont.)*	
Stavudine	May antagonize antiviral activity of stavudine; caution with coadministration.
Zidovudine	Avoid concomitant use with zidovudine; may increase risk of severe neutropenia and anemia with coadministration.
Rimantadine HCl (Flumadine)	
APAP	APAP may decrease levels of rimantadine.
ASA	ASA may decrease levels of rimantadine.
Cimetidine	May decrease clearance of rimantadine.
Influenza virus vaccine, live attenuated	Avoid administration within 2 wks before or 48 hrs after administration of rimantadine; potential for interference between products.
Valacyclovir HCl (Valtrex)	
Nephrotoxic drugs	May cause renal and CNS toxicity.
Valganciclovir HCl (Valcyte)	
Didanosine	May increase plasma levels of didanosine; monitor for didanosine toxicity.
Mycophenolate mofetil	Coadministration in renal impairment may increase plasma levels of metabolites of both drugs.
Probenecid	May decrease clearance and increase AUC of ganciclovir with probenecid; monitor for ganciclovir toxicity.
Zidovudine	Coadministration may increase risk for neutropenia and anemia.
Zanamivir (Relenza)	
Influenza vaccine, live attenuated	Avoid administration within 2 wks before or 48 hrs after zanamivir therapy.

Chapter 8

Agents Affecting Salivation

John A. Yagiela, D.D.S., Ph.D.

ANTICHOLINERGIC DRUGS

Saliva plays a vital role in protecting the health of soft and hard tissues of the mouth and in such functions as taste, mastication, and deglutition. Excessive salivation, however, can complicate the performance of dental procedures such as the taking of impressions and the placement of restorations. If chronic, hypersalivation can cause psychosocial problems and both local and systemic disorders.

A number of anticholinergic drugs—otherwise referred to as cholinergic antagonists, antimuscarinic agents, or parasympatholytics—are effective antisialogogues and are used by dentists and physicians for treating inappropriate salivary secretions and for reducing normal salivation to facilitate the performance of intraoral procedures. Because none of these agents is selective in action, they all have a tendency to produce side effects, and this must be considered before proceeding with antisialogogue therapy. The anticholinergic drugs included in this chapter are limited to agents that have been approved for use to control salivation or that are used in dentistry for that purpose.

Accepted Indications

The control of salivation for dental procedures is a generally recognized but not officially accepted indication for these drugs. Atropine, glycopyrrolate, hyoscyamine (the active isomer of atropine), propantheline, and scopolamine are the most commonly used agents. These drugs also have several medical indications. For example, parenteral atropine has been approved for these uses:

- the control of bradycardia and first-degree heart block associated with excessive vagal activity or administration of succinylcholine
- to inhibit salivation and respiratory tract secretions during general anesthesia
- to minimize the muscarinic side effects of cholinesterase inhibitors used to reverse the action of neuromuscular blocking drugs

Parenteral glycopyrrolate and hyoscyamine have been approved for the same purposes, except for the prophylaxis of succinylcholine-induced bradydysrhythmias. Glycopyrrolate and hyoscyamine are also indicated before general anesthesia to reduce secretion of gastric acid and to minimize the danger of pulmonary aspiration. Parenteral scopolamine has been approved for the control of secretions during general anesthesia and as a preanesthetic sedative and anesthetic adjunct in conjunction with opioid analgesics.

Anticholinergic drugs also have been approved for the management of peptic ulcers and various gastrointestinal, biliary, and genitourinary disorders. For most drugs and conditions, these indications are considered obsolete. Transdermal scopolamine remains a useful agent for the prophylaxis and treatment of motion sickness. Selected anticholinergic drugs also are used to treat parkinsonism and as mydriatics and cycloplegics in ophthalmology. Atropine and hyoscyamine are recognized antidotes for the muscarinic toxicity of mushrooms, parasympathomimetic agonists and anticholinesterase drugs, insecticides, and nerve gases.

Atropine usually is the anticholinergic of choice for most uses in dentistry. Oral dosage forms of atropine are not widely available in neighborhood pharmacies, however, so the dentist should be familiar with the use of other antisialogogues. By parenteral injection, glycopyrrolate is excellent for the control of salivation; scopolamine is a suitable parenteral choice when its sedative, amnestic, and antiemetic effects are desired.

General Dosing Information

Low doses of the anticholinergic drugs described in this chapter for blocking excessive salivary secretion, properly adjusted for route of administration, are relatively selective in effect. Larger doses, such as those required to treat vagally induced bradydysrhythmias, uniformly produce side effects, including pronounced dryness of the mouth. General dosing guidelines for the control of salivation are provided in **Table 8.1**.

To control salivation when performing restorative dentistry, the dentist should time drug administration so that the peak effect occurs when a dry operative field is most needed. Thus, atropine, hyoscyamine, or scopolamine tablets should be given to the patient 60 to 90 minutes prior to taking impressions or placing composite restorations. The analogous interval for oral glycopyrrolate or propantheline is 45 to 75 minutes.

Maximum Recommended Doses

Maximum recommended doses have not been established for single administrations of anticholinergics beyond the usual doses indicated in **Table 8.1**.

Dosage Adjustments

Within the recommended range, the dose of an anticholinergic drug may be adjusted according to need. For control of salivation, a low dose may be adequate when only moderation of salivation is required, whereas a larger dose may be necessary if secretions are preventing the successful accomplishment of a procedure, such as an impression. Reduced doses should be considered for infants, geriatric patients, and those with medical conditions that alter their responses to anticholinergic drugs.

Special Dental Considerations

Drug Interactions of Dental Interest

Drug interactions and related problems involving anticholinergic antisialogogues listed in **Table 8.2** are potentially of clinical significance in dentistry.

Laboratory Value Alterations

- Gastric acid secretion tests are impaired by anticholinergic drugs because they decrease stimulation of gastric acids.
- Radionuclide gastric emptying tests are impaired by anticholinergic drugs because of delayed gastric emptying.
- Phenolsulfonphthalein excretion tests are impaired by atropine because the two agents compete for the same transport mechanism.
- Serum uric acid is decreased in patients with hyperuricemia or gout who are receiving glycopyrrolate.

Cross-Sensitivity

A person with sensitivity to any belladonna alkaloid may also have sensitivity to atropine, hyoscyamine, or scopolamine.

Special Patients

Pregnant and nursing women

Atropine, hyoscyamine, and scopolamine cross the placenta. Although there is no evidence of teratogenic effects, intravenous atropine can cause tachycardia in the fetus, and parenteral scopolamine given during labor may adversely affect the neonate by depressing the CNS and reducing vitamin K-dependent clotting factors. Glycopyrrolate and propantheline are quaternary ammonium compounds, and it is unlikely that they reach the fetal circulation in large amounts.

All anticholinergic drugs may inhibit lactation. In addition, atropine, hyoscyamine, and scopolamine are distributed into breast milk. Although single doses to control salivation have not been associated with any health problem, it may be advisable for nursing mothers to collect sufficient milk to cover the 8-hour period after taking an anticholinergic drug.

Pediatric, geriatric, and other special patients

Pediatric patients. Infants and small children are especially sensitive to the toxic effects of anticholinergic drugs, even when the dose is corrected for body size. Because of their high metabolic rate, children generate relatively large amounts of heat and must dissipate that heat in a warm environment by sweating. Blockade of acetylcholine-mediated perspiration by these agents can quickly lead to grossly elevated temperatures. Flushing of the skin is an important early visual cue that steps must be taken to improve heat loss. Young children may also be especially sensitive to the CNS effects of atropine, hyoscyamine, and scopolamine.

Geriatric patients. Geriatric patients are particularly susceptible to the parasympatholytic effects of anticholinergic drugs on visceral smooth muscle. Although single doses, as used in dentistry for control of salivation, are generally well tolerated by elderly people, large doses of atropine and scopolamine have been associated with excessive depressant and excitatory CNS reactions. Repeated doses can cause constipation and, especially in men, urinary retention. Xerostomia and associated increased dental caries and fungal infections are dental concerns linked to chronic use of these drugs in elderly patients. In addition, patients older than 40 are at increased risk of an acute attack of previously undiagnosed angle-closure glaucoma.

Patients with medical problems. Patients with certain medical problems are especially susceptible to the adverse effects of anticholinergic drugs. These include patients with obstructive or paralytic gastrointestinal and urinary tract disorders, cardiac disease, and angle-closure glaucoma. Specific recommendations regarding these patients are listed in **Table 8.1**.

Patient Monitoring: Aspects to Watch

- Cardiovascular status (arterial blood pressure, heart rate, electrocardiogram) with parenteral anticholinergic drugs

Adverse Effects and Precautions

The adverse effects of the anticholinergic drugs are the predictable consequences of the inhibition of various physiological actions of acetylcholine. Single oral doses of agents used to control salivation are usually well tolerated, but large parenteral doses invariably induce a host of side effects. Although these effects may be unpleasant, they are virtually never life-threatening except in small children and medically compromised patients. The adverse effects, precautions, and contraindications listed in **Table 8.1** apply to all routes of administration.

Pharmacology

Anticholinergic drugs competitively block the effects of acetylcholine and cholinergic drugs at muscarinic receptor sites. Muscarinic receptors mediate tissue responses to parasympathetic nervous system stimulation and cholinergic-induced sweating and vasodilation. Tertiary amines, such as atropine and especially scopolamine, may produce CNS effects because of their ability to cross the blood-brain barrier. Quaternary amines, such as glycopyrrolate and propantheline, are largely excluded from the brain and do not act directly on the CNS. The existence of muscarinic receptor subtypes (designated M_1 through M_5) also accounts for some of the differences in peripheral effects among the anticholinergic drugs because of different relative affinities of the drugs for these subtypes. It has been determined that the M_3 receptor supports serous salivary gland secretion and the M_2 receptor is responsible for parasympathomimetic cardiac effects. In tissues where acetylcholine release at muscarinic receptors is chronically active, anticholinergic drugs will exert pronounced antimuscarinic effects. If acetylcholine or other cholinergic drugs are absent, anticholinergic drugs will elicit little or no observable effect.

Atropine, hyoscyamine, and scopolamine, all naturally occurring belladonna alkaloids, are well absorbed from the gastrointestinal tract; however, absorption is less complete with the synthetic quaternary ammonium drugs. Atropine is partially metabolized in the liver and excreted in the urine as both the parent compound and metabolites. A similar fate presumably occurs with the other anticholinergic agents. **Table 8.3** lists the time to effect and duration of effect of anticholinergic drugs used orally for control of salivation.

Patient Advice

- Patients should be aware of the potential common side effects, such as dryness of the mouth, nose, and throat; difficulty in swallowing; and inhibition of sweating.
- Parents should be warned of the potential for hyperthermia in small children, especially when the children are overdressed, physically active, or in a warm environment.
- Because of the possibility of psychomotor impairment after use of scopolamine, driving or other tasks requiring alertness and coordination should be avoided or performed with added caution, as appropriate, on the day of treatment. It is also desirable to avoid the use of alcohol or other CNS depressants during this time.

SUGGESTED READING

Anticholinergics. *JADA*. 2001;132:1021–1022.

Dowd FJ. Antimuscarinic drugs. In: Yagiela JA, Dowd FJ, Neidle EA, eds. *Pharmacology and Therapeutics for Dentistry*. 5th ed. St. Louis: Mosby; 2004:139-146.

Sherman CR, Sherman BR. Atropine sulfate—a current review of a useful agent for controlling salivation during dental procedures. *Gen Dent*. 1999;47(1):56-60.

CHOLINERGIC DRUGS

In contrast to the anticholinergic agents, cholinergic drugs produce effects that mimic those of acetylcholine, the natural ligand for cholinergic receptors. Additional terms used to identify cholinergic drugs include cholinergic agonists, cholinomimetics, parasympathomimetics, and muscarinic agonists. The only recognized use for these drugs in dentistry is in the management of xerostomia. Diseases or conditions that cause xerostomia commonly result in opportunistic infection, increased caries, and difficulty in speaking and in maintaining normal dietary intake. Although pilocarpine, a naturally occurring cholinergic agonist, has been used as a sialogogue since the early 1900s, it was approved for this purpose by the FDA only in 1994, after being developed under the provisions of the Orphan Drug Act of 1983. Cevimeline, a cholinergic agonist chemically unrelated to pilocarpine, received approval for clinical use in 2000.

Successful stimulation of salivary secretion by cholinergic drugs requires the presence of intact salivary gland tissue and nerve supply. In the case of radiation therapy, this requirement may be met by residual active tissue in the irradiated field or healthy tissue outside the field.

Accepted Indications

Pilocarpine has been approved for the relief of xerostomia caused by radiation therapy of the head and neck and for the management of xerostomia and keratoconjunctivitis sicca in patients with Sjögren's syndrome. In its topical forms, pilocarpine has also been approved for treating various types of glaucoma and producing pupillary constriction (miosis) after surgery or ocular examination. Cevimeline is approved only for the treatment of xerostomia associated with Sjögren's syndrome.

General Dosing Information

As shown in **Table 8.1**, the usual adult daily dose of pilocarpine is 5 mg tid, usually 30 minutes before meals. A dose of 10 mg tid may be tried in refractory cases; however, the incidence of dose-related side effects increases at this dosage and, as a general rule, the dentist should use the lowest effective dose that is tolerated by the patient. Cevimeline generally is prescribed as a dose of 30 mg tid. Absorption is best if the drug is taken on an empty stomach. Pilocarpine and cevimeline have not been tested in children.

Special Dental Considerations

Drug Interactions of Dental Interest

Table 8.2 lists possible drug interactions and related problems involving cholinergic drugs that are potentially of clinical significance in dentistry.

Cross-Sensitivity

Patients sensitive to other forms of pilocarpine dosage (that is, ophthalmic) should be considered sensitive to oral pilocarpine.

Special Patients

Pregnant and nursing women

There are no data regarding the influence of pilocarpine on reproduction and fetal development. High doses of cevimeline decrease fertility in female rats. Both drugs have been designated as FDA pregnancy category C. It has not been determined if these drugs are excreted into breast milk, and there are no reports of related problems in humans. However, the potential for adverse effects in nursing infants must be considered.

Pediatric, geriatric, and other special patients

These cholinergic drugs have not been tested for, nor are they indicated for, use in children. There appears to be no special concern regarding pilocarpine and cevimeline and the geriatric population, although elderly people are more likely to have specific medical problems (such as angle-closure glaucoma, pulmonary disease, or cardiovascular disease) that may complicate therapy.

Adverse Effects and Precautions

Most of the adverse effects observed with cholinergic agonists (**Table 8.1**) are dose-dependent extensions of the drugs' ability to stimulate cholinergic muscarinic receptors. Hypertension may be an important exception to this generalization. Excessive secretions (sweating, bronchial secretions, rhinitis) are the most common side effects associated with oral cholinergic agonists.

Pharmacology

Pilocarpine and cevimeline stimulate muscarinic receptors to elicit most of their effects. Muscarinic receptors are linked to specific G proteins that mediate intracellular signaling in response to drug-receptor binding. For the M_3 receptor involved in salivary secretion, stimulation of its G protein causes the intracellular formation of inositol 1,4,5-trisphosphate and diacylglycerol, which promote secretion and smooth muscle contraction. Stimulation of muscarinic receptors in the central nervous system contributes to the sialogogic effect. Anomalous hypertensive responses to these drugs may result, at least in part, from central stimulation of M_1 receptors.

Pilocarpine is readily absorbed from the gastrointestinal tract. Peak drug effects occur within 1 hour and last 3 to 5 hours. Pilocarpine is partially metabolized, possibly in the plasma or at neuronal synapses, and is then excreted in the urine. Cevimeline is similarly absorbed when taken between meals but is longer lasting. Most of the drug is metabolized in the liver (elimination half-life: 5 hours) before being excreted by the kidneys.

Patient Advice

- Because adverse effects are dose-dependent, patients should be cautioned to take the medication as directed.
- If dizziness, lightheadedness, or blurred vision occurs, patients should refrain from driving or other tasks requiring alertness, coordination, and visual acuity until the problem is resolved.

SUGGESTED READING

Borella TL, De Luca LA, Jr, Colombari DS, et al. Central muscarinic receptor subtypes involved in pilocarpine-induced salivation, hypertension and water intake. *Br J Pharmacol.* 2008;155(8):1256-1263.

Chambers MS, Garden AS, Kies MS, et al. Radiation-induced xerostomia in patients with head and neck cancer: pathogenesis, impact on quality of life, and management. *Head Neck.* 2004;26(9):796-807.

Davies AN, Daniels C, Pugh R, et al. A comparison of artificial saliva and pilocarpine in the management of xerostomia in patients with advanced cancer. *Palliative Med.* 1998;12(2):105-111.

Porter SR, Scully C, Hegarty AM. An update of the etiology and management of xerostomia. *Oral Surg Oral Med Oral Pathol Oral Radiol Endod.* 2004(1);97:28-46.

Vivino FB, Al-Hashimi I, Khan Z, et al. Pilocarpine tablets for the treatment of dry mouth and dry eye symptoms in patients with Sjögren syndrome: a randomized, placebo-controlled, fixed-dose, multicenter trial. *Arch Intern Med.* 1999;159(2):174-181.

SALIVA SUBSTITUTES

When salivary function is absent or minimal, cholinergic drug therapy with pilocarpine or related agents is ineffective. Replacement of missing saliva is a natural therapeutic alternative. Water is most commonly used by patients afflicted with chronic xerostomia because of its unique advantages of availability and low cost. Water is a poor substitute for saliva, however, because it lacks necessary ions, buffering capacity, lubricating mucins, and protective proteins. Saliva substitutes, or artificial salivas, are designed to more closely match the chemical and physical characteristics of saliva. These preparations often contain complex mixtures of salts, with cellulose derivatives or animal mucins added to increase viscosity (often to a viscosity greater than that of natural saliva, in an attempt to improve retention within the mouth). Flavoring agents, usually sorbitol or xylitol, generally are added to improve taste, and parabens are sometimes included to inhibit bacterial growth. A general deficiency of artificial salivas is their complete lack of anti-infective proteins, such as secretory immunoglobulin A, histatins, and lysozyme. A saliva substitute in the form of a long-lasting moisturizing gel or liquid (Oral*balance*; see **Table 8.4**) contains various ingredients that are claimed to be biologically active, but data supporting their clinical effectiveness are limited.

Accepted Indications

Saliva substitutes are indicated for the symptomatic relief of dry mouth and dry throat in patients with xerostomia.

General Dosing Information

Saliva substitutes are meant to be taken ad libitum throughout the day, usually in the form of sprays, to keep the oral mucosa moist. There are no specific dosing guidelines, nor are there specific recommendations for special patients. **Table 8.4** lists, by manufacturer's brand name, the ingredients of some commercially available preparations.

Special Dental Considerations

Patients with severe xerostomia who use a saliva substitute containing sorbitol on a regular basis may be at increased risk of caries associated with a very limited fermentation of sorbitol. A proper, professionally designed topical fluoride treatment program undertaken to protect from caries the teeth of the patient with xerostomia should also overcome any problem posed by sorbitol. Use of sugarless chewing gum, some of which may contain a remineralizing agent, and sugarless citrus-flavored lozenges may increase salivary flow. Some patients have claimed benefits from use of Biotene products (e.g., Oral*balance*), but there is little information from properly controlled trials to substantiate these claims.

There are no known drug interactions involving saliva substitutes, nor any need for patient monitoring pertaining to these products. Laboratory tests are likewise unaffected.

Cross-Sensitivity

Saliva substitutes containing parabens pose a risk of cross-sensitivity in patients allergic to parabens, para-aminobenzoic acid, or its derivatives, such as ester local anesthetics. Some products contain other ingredients that pose additional risks of allergic cross-reactions.

Adverse Effects and Precautions

Aside from the allergic potential of parabens or other components of selected preparations and the possibility of increased caries incidence with sorbitol, there are few potential adverse effects or precautions associated with saliva substitutes. Microbial contamination is a possibility with multiple-dose formulations, but this risk is partially offset by the inclusion of paraben preservatives.

Pharmacology

Saliva substitutes are physically active agents. When used regularly, they help minimize the sequelae of xerostomia by keeping the oral mucosa moist and lubricated. Surface abrasion is reduced, and patients are more able to perform the everyday activities of speaking, eating, and sleeping. Long-term compliance, however, is a problem with these products because of their perceived inconvenience and relatively high cost.

Because saliva substitutes are quickly swallowed and their activity is of limited duration, they must be administered repeatedly. The components of the ingested solution undoubtedly undergo gastrointestinal absorption; however, there is no information on the pharmacokinetics of the currently available saliva substitutes.

Patient Advice

- Patients should be informed of the necessity of the continual use of saliva substitutes.
- Patients with chronic xerostomia should be educated on the need for regular professional care and for a high degree of compliance with the dental professional's recommendations for minimizing caries and soft-tissue pathology.

SUGGESTED READING

Alves MB, Motta AC, Messina WC, et al. Saliva substitute in xerostomic patients with primary Sjogren's syndrome: a single-blind trial. *Quintessence Int*. 2004;35(5):392-396.

Dodds MWJ, Johnson DA, Yeh C-K. Health benefits of saliva: a review. *J Dent*. 2005;33(3): 223-233.

Fox PC. Management of dry mouth. *Dent Clin North Am*. 1997;41(4):863-875.

Levine MJ. Development of artificial salivas. *Crit Rev Oral Biol Med*. 1993;4:279-286.

Meyer-Lueckel H, Schulte-Monting J, Kielbassa AM. The effect of commercially available saliva substitutes on predemineralized bovine dentin in vitro. *Oral Dis*. 2002;8(4):192-198.

Table 8.1. PRESCRIBING INFORMATION FOR ANTICHOLINERGIC AND CHOLINERGIC DRUGS

NAME	FORM/ STRENGTH	DOSAGE	WARNINGS/PRECAUTIONS & CONTRAINDICATIONS	ADVERSE EFFECTS*
Atropine Sulfate (Anticholinergic) (Sal-Tropine)	**Inj:** Atropine sulfate 0.05mg/ mL, 0.1mg/ mL, 0.4mg/mL, 0.5mg/mL,1mg/ mL; **Tab:** Sal-Tropine 0.4mg	***Adults:*** **Inj: Usual:** 0.4-0.6mg IM/IV/ SC. **Range:** 0.3-1.2mg. **Tab: Usual:** 0.4mg. **Range:** 0.4-1.2mg. ***Pediatrics:*** **Sol, Inj: Usual:** 0.01mg/kg up to 0.4mg. **Range:** 0.1mg (newborn) to 0.6mg (>12 yrs). **Tab: Usual:** 0.01mg/kg up to 0.4mg.	**W/P:** Avoid overdose. Increased susceptibility to toxic effects in children. Caution in patients >40 yrs. Conventional doses may precipitate acute angle-closure glaucoma in susceptible patients, convert partial organic pyloric stenosis into complete obstruction, lead to complete urinary retention in patients with prostatic hypertrophy, or cause inspissations of bronchial secretions and formation of dangerous viscid plugs in patients with chronic lung disease. **Contra:** Hypersensitivity to atropine or other naturally occurring belladonna alkaloids, angle-closure glaucoma, pyloric stenosis or prostatic hypertrophy except in doses used for preanesthetic medication. **P/N:** Category C, safety in nursing not known.	**Dry mouth,** nose, throat, eyes, skin; urinary hesitancy and retention, blurred vision, photophobia, tachycardia, palpitation, anhidrosis, hyperthermia, drowsiness, dizziness, confusion, hallucinations, delirium.
Cevimeline HCl (Cholinergic) (Evoxac)	**Cap:** 30mg	***Adults:*** 30mg tid.	**W/P:** Caution with significant cardiovascular disease, night driving, performing hazardous activities in reduced lighting, nephrolithiasis, cholelithiasis, biliary tract disease, controlled asthma, chronic bronchitis, or COPD requiring pharmacotherapy. Monitor for toxicity and dehydration. Possible dose-related CNS effects. **Contra:** Uncontrolled asthma, when miosis is undesirable (eg, acute iritis, narrow-angle glaucoma). **P/N:** Category C, safety in nursing not known.	Excessive sweating, nausea, rhinitis, diarrhea, headache, sinusitis, upper respiratory tract infection, **cough, pharyngitis,** vomiting, injury, back pain, rash, conjunctivitis, dizziness, bronchitis, arthralgia, fatigue, pain.
Glycopyrrolate (Anticholinergic) (Robinul, Robinul Forte)	**Inj:** Robinul 0.2mg/mL **Tab:** Robinul 1mg, Robinul Forte 2mg	***Adults:*** **Inj: Range:** 0.1-0.2 mg. **Maint:** q6-8h up to 0.8mg/day. ***Adults and adolescents:*** **Tab: Usual:** 1mg. **Range:** 1-2mg. **Maint:** 1mg bid up to 8mg/day. ***Pediatrics:*** **Sol, Inj: Range:** 4-10mcg/kg up to 0.2 mg. **Maint:** q3-4h up to 0.8 mg/day.	**W/P:** May produce drowsiness and blurred vision; avoid operating machinery. Risk of heat prostration with high environmental temperature. Diarrhea may be early symptom of incomplete intestinal obstruction especially with ileostomy or colostomy. Caution in elderly, autonomic neuropathy, hepatic/ renal disease, ulcerative colitis, hyperthyroidism, coronary heart disease, CHF, tachyarrhythmias, tachycardia, HTN, prostatic hypertrophy, hiatal hernia associated with reflux esophagitis. **Contra:** Hypersensitivity to glycopyrrolate, angle-closure glaucoma, obstructive uropathy, GI tract obstruction, paralytic ileus, intestinal atony of elderly/debilitated, unstable cardiovascular status in acute hemorrhage, severe ulcerative colitis, toxic megacolon complicating ulcerative colitis, myasthenia gravis. **P/N:** Category C, caution in nursing.	Blurred vision, **dry mouth,** urinary retention and hesitancy, increased ocular tension, tachycardia, decreased sweating, hyperthermia, **loss of taste,** headache.

*Bold entries denote special dental considerations.
BB = black box warning; **W/P** = warnings/precautions; **Contra** = contraindications; **P/N** = pregnancy category rating and nursing considerations.

Table 8.1. PRESCRIBING INFORMATION FOR ANTICHOLINERGIC AND CHOLINERGIC DRUGS *(cont.)*

NAME	FORM/ STRENGTH	DOSAGE	WARNINGS/PRECAUTIONS & CONTRAINDICATIONS	ADVERSE EFFECTS*
Hyoscyamine Sulfate (Anticholinergic) (Anaspaz, Hyosyne, Levbid, Levsin, Levsinex, NuLev, Symax)	**Cap ER:** Levsinex 0.375mg; **Drops:** Hyosyne 0.125mg/mL, Levsin 0.125mg/mL; **Elixir:** Hyosyne 0.125mg/5mL, Levsin 0.125mg/5mL; **Inj:** Levsin 0.5mg/mL; **Tab:** Anaspaz 0.125mg, Levsin 0.125mg; **Tab ER:** Levbid 0.375mg, Levsin 0.375mg; Symax-SR 0.375mg; **Tab ODT:** NuLev 0.125mg; **Tab SL:** Levsin 0.125mg, Symax-SL 0.125mg	***Adults and adolescents:*** **Cap ER, Tab ER:** 0.375-0.75mg q12h, or 1 cap/tab may be given q8h. Do not crush or chew. **Drops, Elixir, Tab, Tab ODT, Tab SL** (may also chew or swallow SL tabs): **Usual:** 0.125-0.25mg. **Range:** 0.125-0.5mg. **Maint:** q4-6h. **Max:** 1.5mg/day. **Solution, Inj:** 0.25-0.5mg IM/IV/SC. **Maint:** q4h. ***Pediatrics:*** **Drops, Elixir: 2.3-3.3kg:** 12.5mcg. **3.4-4.4kg:** 15.6mcg. **4.5-6.7kg:** 18.8mcg. **6.8-9kg:** 25mcg. **9.1-13.5kg:** 31.3mcg. **13.6-22.6kg:** 63mcg. **22.7-33kg:** 94-125mcg. **34-36kg:** 125-187mcg. **Tab, Tab ODT, Tab SL: 2-12 yrs:** 0.0625-0.125mg. **Maint:** q4-6h. **Inj: 2-12 yrs:** 5mcg/kg IM/IV/SC.	**W/P:** Risk of heat prostration with high environmental temperature. Avoid activities requiring mental alertness. Psychosis has been reported. Caution with diarrhea, autonomic neuropathy, hyperthyroidism, coronary heart disease, CHF, dysrhythmias/tachycardia, HTN, renal disease and hiatal hernia associated with reflux esophagitis. **Contra:** Angle-closure glaucoma, obstructive uropathy, GI tract obstructive disease, paralytic ileus, intestinal atony of elderly/debilitated, unstable cardiovascular status in acute hemorrhage, severe ulcerative colitis, toxic megacolon, myasthenia gravis. **P/N:** Category C, caution in nursing.	**Dry mouth,** nose, throat, eyes, skin; urinary hesitancy and retention, blurred vision, photophobia, tachycardia, palpitation, anhidrosis, hyperthermia, drowsiness, dizziness, confusion, hallucinations, delirium.
Pilocarpine HCl (Cholinergic) (Salagen)	**Tab:** 5mg, 7.5mg	***Adults:*** **Cancer Patients: Initial:** 5mg tid. **Usual:** 15-30mg/day. **Max:** 10mg/dose. **Sjögren's Syndrome: Usual:** 5mg qid.	**W/P:** Caution with significant cardiovascular disease, night driving, performing hazardous activities in reduced lighting, cholelithiasis, biliary tract disease, controlled asthma, chronic bronchitis, or COPD requiring pharmacotherapy. Monitor for toxicity and dehydration. May cause renal colic. Possible dose-related CNS effects. **Contra:** Uncontrolled asthma, when miosis is undesirable (eg, acute iritis, narrow-angle glaucoma). **P/N:** Category C, not for use in nursing.	Sweating, nausea, rhinitis, diarrhea, chills, flushing, urinary frequency, dizziness, asthenia, headache, dyspepsia, lacrimation, edema, amblyopia, vomiting, **pharyngitis,** HTN, bradycardia, tachycardia.
Propantheline Bromide (Anticholinergic)	**Tab:** 7.5mg, 15mg	***Adults and adolescents:*** **Usual:** 15-30mg. **Range:** 7.5-60mg. **Maint:** tid-qid up to 120mg/day.	**W/P:** In presence of a high environmental temperature, heat prostration can occur, diarrhea may be an early symptom of incomplete intestinal obstruction; in this instance, treatment with propantheline would be inappropriate and possibly harmful with heart disease, may increase heart rate, autonomic neuropathy, cardiac tachyarrhythmias, caution when operating motor vehicle or other machinery, congestive heart failure, coronary heart disease, hepatic or renal disease, hiatal hernia associated with reflux esophagitis, hypertension, hyperthyroidism. **Contra:** Hypersensitivity to other anticholinergics, angle-closure glaucoma, intestinal atony of elderly or debilitated patients, myasthenia gravis, obstructive disease of gastrointestinal tract, obstructive uropathy, severe ulcerative colitis/toxic megacolon, unstable cardiovascular adjustment in acute hemorrhage. **P/N:** Category C, caution in nursing.	Diminished sweating, constipation, **dry mouth,** dizziness, drowsiness, confusion, blurred vision, hyperthermia, headache, N/V.

*Bold entries denote special dental considerations.
BB = black box warning; **W/P** = warnings/precautions; **Contra** = contraindications; **P/N** = pregnancy category rating and nursing considerations.

NAME	FORM/ STRENGTH	DOSAGE	WARNINGS/PRECAUTIONS & CONTRAINDICATIONS	ADVERSE EFFECTS*
Scopolamine Hydrobromide (Anticholinergic) (Scopace, Transderm Scop)	**Patch:** Transderm Scop 0.33mg/ 24 hrs; **Inj:** scopolamine hydrobromide 0.4mg/mL; **Tab:** Scopace 0.4mg	***Adults:*** **Patch: Motion Sickness:** Apply 1 patch 4 hrs before travel. Replace after 3 days; **Post-OP N/V:** Apply 1 patch the evening before surgery. Keep in place for 24 hrs. Apply patch to a hairless area behind the ear. Do not cut patch in half. **Sol, Inj: Anesthesia: Excessive Salivation:** 0.2-0.6mg IM 30-60 min before induction of anesthesia; **Preoperative Sedation:** 0.32-0.65mg IM/IV/ SC; **Vomiting:** 0.6-1mg SC. **Tab: Usual:** 0.4mg. **Range:** 0.4-0.8mg. ***Pediatrics:*** **Inj: Anesthesia: Excessive Salivation: 4-7 months:** 0.1mg IM 45-60 min before anesthesia. **7 months-3 yrs:** 0.15mg IM 45-60 min before anesthesia. **3-8 yrs:** 0.2mg IM 45-60 min before anesthesia. **8-12 yrs:** 0.3mg IM 45-60 min before anesthesia; **Vomiting:** 6mcg/ kg/dose SC.	**W/P:** Monitor IOP with open-angle glaucoma. Not for dental use in children. Caution with pyloric obstruction, urinary bladder neck or intestinal obstruction, elderly. Increased CNS effects with liver or kidney dysfunction. May aggravate seizures or psychosis. Idiosyncratic reactions reported (rare). **Contra:** Angle-closure glaucoma, hypersensitivity to belladonna alkaloids. **P/N:** Category C, caution in nursing.	**Dry mouth,** drowsiness, blurred vision, dilation of pupils, dizziness, disorientation, confusion.

Table 8.2. DRUG INTERACTIONS FOR ANTICHOLINERGIC AND CHOLINERGIC DRUGS

ALL ANTICHOLINERGIC DRUGS	
Antacids or absorbent antidiarrheal drugs	May impair absorption of anticholinergic drug. Avoid administration within 2-3 hours.
Antimyasthenics	Muscarinic effects are blocked by anticholinergic drugs, possibly obscuring early signs of an antimyasthenic overdose. Use cautiously.
CNS depressants	Summation of CNS depression with scopolamine; hallucination and behavioral disturbances have been reported with parenteral lorazepam and scopolamine. Use cautiously.
Drugs with anticholinergic side effects	Additive anticholinergic effects. Use cautiously with antiparkinson drugs, antipsychotic agents, carbamazepine, digoxin, dronabinol, orphenadrine, procainamide, quinidine, sedative antihistamines, and tricyclic antidepressants.
Haloperidol	Antipsychotic effects of haloperidol may be impaired. Use cautiously.
Ketoconazole	Absorption may be impaired by increased gastric pH. Take ketoconazole at least 2 hours before the anticholinergic drug.
Metoclopramide	Effect of hastening gastric emptying may be blocked. Use cautiously.
Opioid analgesics	Summation of constipating effects. Use cautiously.
Potassium chloride	Delayed absorption may increase gastrointestinal toxicity of potassium chloride. Avoid concurrent use.
ALL CHOLINERGIC DRUGS	
β-Adrenergic blocking drugs	Summation of drug effects on cardiac automaticity and conduction. Use cautiously.
Drugs with anticholinergic activity	Antagonistic drug effects. Use cautiously when the anticholinergic effect of the interacting drug is not the goal of therapy; consult with a physician to optimize drug treatment. Drugs requiring caution include anticholinergics, antiparkinson drugs, antipsychotic agents, carbamazepine, digoxin, dronabinol, orphenadrine, procainamide, quinidine, sedative antihistamines, and tricyclic antidepressants.
Drugs with cholinergic activity	Summation of drug effects. Use cautiously with cholinergic antiglaucoma drugs, antimyasthenic agents, and bethanechol.
Hepatic enzyme inhibitors	Inhibition of cevimeline metabolism. Use cautiously with azole antifungals, erythromycins, nefazodone, protease inhibitors, and selective serotonin reuptake inhibitors.

Table 8.3. PHARMACOKINETIC PARAMETERS OF ANTICHOLINERGIC DRUGS

DRUG	TIME OF ONSET (MIN)	DURATION OF EFFECT (HRS)	AMINE STRUCTURE
Atropine	30-60	4-6	Tertiary
Hyoscyamine	30-60	4-6	Tertiary
Scopolamine	30-60	4-6	Tertiary
Glycopyrrolate	30-45	6-8	Quaternary
Propantheline	30-45	6	Quaternary

Table 8.4. SALIVA SUBSTITUTES PRODUCT INFORMATION

BRAND NAME(S)	FORM/INGREDIENTS
GC Dry Mouth Gel	**Gel:** sodium carboxymethylcellulose, carrageenan, polyglycerol (diglycerol), ethyl p-hydroxybenzoate, sodium citrate, flavor, water in 35-mL tubes
Entertainer's Secret	**Solution:** sodium carboxymethylcellulose, dibasic sodium phosphate, potassium chloride, parabens, aloe vera gel, glycerin, flavor, water in 60-mL spray
Moi-Stir	**Solution:** sodium carboxymethylcellulose; dibasic sodium phosphate; calcium, magnesium, potassium, and sodium chlorides; parabens; sorbitol; water in 4-oz spray
MouthKote	**Solution:** Yerba Santa, citric acid, ascorbic acid, sodium benzoate, flavor, sodium saccharin, sorbitol, xylitol, water in 2- and 8-oz spray
Oasis Moisturizing Mouth Spray	**Solution:** glycerin, sodium benzoate, xanthum gum, PEG-60 hydrogenated castor oil, copovidone, cetylpyridinium chloride, methylparaben, propylparaben, sodium saccharin, xylitol, flavor, water in 1-oz spray
Oral*balance*	**Gel:** hydroxyethylcellulose, hydrogenated starch, glycerate polyhydrate, potassium thiocyanate, glucose oxidase, lactoperoxidase, lysozyme, lactoferrin, aloe vera, xylitol in 1.5-oz tubes
Orajel Dry Mouth Moisturizing Gel	**Gel:** glycerin, xanthan gum, calcium disodium EDTA, citric acid, disodium phosphate, methylparaben, propylparaben, sucralose, thione complex (antioxidants), flavor, water in 1.5-oz tubes
Oralube	**Solution:** potassium, sodium, magnesium, calcium, chloride, phosphate, fluoride, methyl hydroxybenzoate, sorbitol, flavor, water in 125-mL spray
Rain Dry Mouth Spray	**Solution:** glycerin, aloe vera concentrate, cellulose gum, calcium glycerophosphate, grapefruit seed extract, xylitol, flavoring, water in 1- and 3.5-oz spray bottles
Saliva Substitute	**Solution:** sodium carboxymethylcellulose, flavor, sorbitol, water in 120-mL squeeze bottles
Salivart Oral Moisturizer	**Solution:** sodium carboxymethylcellulose; dibasic potassium phosphate; calcium, magnesium, potassium, and sodium chlorides; sorbitol; water; nitrogen propellant in 1- and 2.48-oz spray cans
Thayers Dry Mouth Spray	**Solution:** glycerin, Tris Amino (buffers), citric acid, potassium chloride, calcium gluconate, flavor, water in 4-oz spray

Chapter 9

Mouthrinses and Dentifrices

Angelo J. Mariotti, D.D.S., Ph.D.; Kenneth H. Burrell, D.D.S., S.M.

MOUTHRINSES

Depending on the formulation, mouthrinses are designed to control or reduce halitosis, reduce or prevent gingivitis, help prevent caries, aid in the discomfort of xerostomia, act as a cleaning/debridement agent, reduce the rate of supragingival calculus formation, offer topical pain relief, and serve as a tooth whitener.

The major components of mouthrinses are water, flavoring, humectant, surfactant, alcohol, and the active ingredients. Water is the major vehicle used to solubilize the ingredients. The flavor is designed to make the mouthrinse pleasant to use. The humectant adds substance or "body" to the product and inhibits crystallization around the opening of the container. The surfactant is used to solubilize the flavoring agent and provide foaming action. In addition, the surfactant helps remove oral debris and has some limited antimicrobial properties. If the formulation requires an antimicrobial agent, the surfactant must be compatible with it. Alcohol also helps solubilize some of the ingredients present in the formulation. Although alcohol can denature bacterial cell walls, it serves as a nontherapeutic vehicle in most mouthrinses. There has been some concern about the association between mouthrinses containing alcohol and oral cancers, but current findings do not establish a causal relationship.

Accepted Indications

Gingivitis

Mouthrinses to control gingivitis contain active ingredients that are antimicrobial (for example, essential oils, chlorhexidine gluconate, cetylpyridinium chloride). Clinical trials should demonstrate that these agents are effective when used as directed for six months without the development of opportunistic infections.

Prebrushing rinses are claimed to remove or loosen plaque responsible for gingivitis by employing surface-active agents (for example, sodium lauryl sulfate and sodium benzoate) to make plaque easier to remove while toothbrushing.

Delmopinol hydrochloride is a plaque formation inhibitor. At press time, this product has not been marketed (in the United States as Impede; in Canada as Decapinol).

To receive the ADA Seal of Acceptance, a mouthrinse used for the control of gingival inflammation must demonstrate a statistically significant reduction in gingival inflammation that represents a proportionate reduction of at least 15% in favor of the mouthrinse in any one study and an average of 20% reduction in two studies. To see the ADA's evaluation guidelines for mouthrinses useful for the prevention and reduction of plaque and gingivitis, go to *www.ada.org/ada/seal/standards/index.asp*.

Halitosis

Mouthrinses thought to be useful in the control of halitosis either contain agents that limit the growth of bacteria responsible for common mouth odors or that inactivate the malodorous, volatile sulfur-containing compounds that are present because of amino acid degradation. The antimicrobial agents include chlorhexidine, chlorine dioxide, cetylpyridinium chloride, and oral rinses based on a mixture of essential oils (such as eucalyptol, menthol, thymol, and methyl salicylate). Examples of agents that inhibit odor-causing compounds are zinc salts, ketone, terpene, and ionone, a compound found in tomato juice.

At press time, there were no ADA-accepted mouthrinses for the control of halitosis. Although several ADA-accepted mouthrinses can substantiate their claims using criteria that are currently used by the oral-care industry, these criteria may not reflect the ADA-established guidelines for evaluating products' effectiveness against oral malodor.

Xerostomia

Several formulations are available to reduce the discomfort of xerostomia. They contain salts, enzymes, cellulose derivatives, and/or animal mucins that mimic the composition and mouth feel of saliva (see **Chapter 8**).

Caries

Fluoride-containing mouthrinses are available to augment the benefits of fluoride toothpastes (see **Chapter 10**).

Cleaning/Debridement

The bubbling action of hydrogen peroxide in these mouthrinses helps to physically remove necrotic tissue and food particles to facilitate healing. Oxygenating compounds with concentrations of ≥3% hydrogen peroxide should not be considered for frequent and extended use, as this could result in damage to oral tissues. In solutions containing carbamide peroxide, one-third of the carbamide peroxide is converted to hydrogen peroxide, which with long-term use has the potential to damage oral tissue if the dose exceeds 3% hydrogen peroxide. A solution of 10% carbamide peroxide releases approximately 3% hydrogen peroxide into the mouth.

Topical Pain Relief

Most of the mouthrinses for pain relief contain topical local anesthetics such as lidocaine, benzocaine/butamin/tetracaine hydrochloride, or dyclonine hydrochloride (see **Chapter 1**). A phenol-containing mouthrinse is also available. The low concentration of phenol it contains acts as a mild topical anesthetic.

A mouthrinse containing sodium hyaluronate, polyvinylpyrrolidine, and glycyrrhetinic acid acts as a physical barrier to relieve pain secondary to oral soft tissue lesions, including aphthous ulcers.

Tooth Whitening

Mouthrinses containing 1.5% to 2% hydrogen peroxide have been shown to bleach teeth.

Supragingival Calculus Accumulation (Antitartar)

An antimicrobial mouthrinse containing essential oils and zinc chloride has been shown to reduce the rate of supragingival calculus accumulation. This product has been clinically shown to have plaque-, gingivitis-, and calculus-reducing properties.

General Dosing Information

The usual adult dosage (and often the geriatric dosage) for mouthrinses (see **Table 9.1**) is 10 to 20 mL for therapeutic rinses; a typical dosage has not been established for cosmetic and prebrushing rinses and so can be dictated by individual choice. For oxygenating agents, dosage regimens are more restrictive in terms of frequency and duration of usage. Duration of rinsing varies by the type of agent used.

Safety and efficacy typically have not been established for antigingivitis mouthrinses used by pediatric patients.

Maximum Recommended Doses

Maximum recommended doses for mouthrinses are typically what can be held in the mouth comfortably (10 to 20 mL). The exception is an oxygenating agent of 1.5% hydrogen peroxide (Peroxyl), which is used in 10-mL quantities. Depending on whether the formulations are purchased over the counter (with directions on packaging) or are prescribed (with directions on the enclosed label), additional mouthrinse should be used only after sufficient time has been allowed to prove that the therapeutic effect of the previous dose requires augmentation.

Dosage Adjustments

The actual maximum dose for each patient must be individualized depending on factors such as his or her size, age, and physical status; ability to effectively rinse and expectorate; oral health; and sensitivity. Mouthrinses are not often prescribed for young pediatric patients. As patients often swallow some of the product, reduced maximum doses may be indicated for geriatric patients, patients with serious illness or disability, and patients with medical conditions who are taking drugs that alter oral responses to mouthrinses.

Special Dental Considerations

Drug Interactions of Dental Interest

Concurrent use of agents that contain either calcium hydroxide or aluminum hydroxide may form a complex with fluoride ions and reduce a rinse's effectiveness in the mouth. Concomitant use of chlorhexidine and stannous fluoride mouthrinses may reduce the efficacy of each agent. Dentifrice ingredients can decrease the antibacterial effect of chlorhexidine and cetylpyridinium chloride. Therefore, following brushing with a dentifrice, a vigorous water rinse is recommended prior to rinsing.

Cross-Sensitivity

Some patients can develop allergic reactions (eg, skin rash, hives, and facial swelling) to rinses. If this occurs, discontinue treatment immediately.

Special Patients

Problems in women who are pregnant or breastfeeding have not been documented with normal daily use of oral rinses containing fluorides.

Patient Monitoring: Aspects to Watch

- Extrinsic staining and increased calculus buildup is possible in some instances (see **Table 9.1**).
- Use caution in prescribing mouthrinses containing alcohol to patients in recovery from alcoholism.
- Avoid rinsing with water or drinking anything after using the mouthrinse for at least 30 minutes to prevent clearance of the drug from the mouth and a subsequent reduction in its effectiveness.

Adverse Effects and Precautions

The incidence of adverse reactions to mouthrinses is relatively low. Many reactions (eg, burning, taste alterations, tooth staining) are temporary. Idiosyncratic and allergic reactions account for a small minority of adverse responses. The adverse effects listed in **Table 9.1** apply to all major types of mouthrinses.

Pharmacology

Chlorhexidine

Chlorhexidine is a bisbiguanide with broad-spectrum antibacterial activity. It is a symmetrical, cationic molecule that binds strongly to hydroxylapatite, the organic pellicle of the tooth, oral mucosa, salivary proteins, and bacteria. As a result of the binding of chlorhexidine to oral structures, the drug exhibits substantivity (for example, 30% of the drug is retained after rinsing, with subsequent slow release over time). Chlorhexidine is poorly absorbed from the gastrointestinal tract, and whatever is absorbed is excreted primarily in the feces. Depending on the dose, chlorhexidine can be bacteriostatic or bactericidal. Bacteriostasis results from interference with bacterial cell wall transport systems. Bactericidal concentrations disrupt the cell wall, which leads to leakage of intracellular proteins.

Chlorhexidine can also be administered to subgingival sites in a controlled local delivery system called PerioChip. Subgingival delivery of chlorhexidine in a biodegradable hydrolyzed gelatin matrix maintains an antimicrobial concentration in the periodontal pocket for at least seven days. Clinical studies have not demonstrated staining or adverse effects using this agent in a local delivery system (see **Chapter 4, Table 4.2**, for usage information).

Delmopinol

Delmopinol hydrochloride is a morpholinoethanol compound that acts as a cationic surfactant and prevents the attachment, as well as the adherence, of plaque bacteria to the tooth surface. Although it is not yet marketed in the United States (as a 0.2% oral rinse), it is the first mouthrinse that the FDA has approved as a device. Two long-term supervised studies using delmopinol demonstrated reduced plaque, gingivitis, and bleeding sites when compared with a placebo rinse. But delmopinol was found to cause significantly higher staining of the teeth and transient anesthesia of the oral mucosa.

Essential Oils

Antibacterial activity is created by a combination of essential oils (eucalyptol [0.092%], thymol [0.062%], methyl salicylate [0.06%], and menthol [0.042%]) in an alcohol-based (21.6% to 26.9%) vehicle. Essential oils have been implicated in inhibiting bacterial enzymes and reducing pathogenicity of plaque. The substantivity of these agents, also called phenolics, is poor.

Fluorides

Fluoride has been shown to reduce carious lesions dramatically in both children and adults. Fluoride ion is assimilated into the apatite crystal of enamel and stabilizes the crystal, making teeth more resistant to decay. Fluoride also has been shown to help remineralize incipient carious lesions. The germicidal activity of these agents, which include various liquid formulations of stannous fluoride, is negligible.

Oxygenating Agents

Oxygenating agents release oxygen as an active intermediate, loosening debris in inaccessible areas. Oxygenating agents also have been reported to induce damage in bacterial cells by altering membrane permeability. The germicidal activity of these agents is negligible. The substantivity of oxygenating agents is poor.

Prebrushing Rinses

The exact mechanism that prebrushing rinses use to "loosen" plaque is not known and is questionable. However, it has been suggested that surface-active agents (sodium lauryl sulfate and sodium benzoate, for example) make plaque soluble and therefore easier to remove.

Herbal Agents

Some mouthrinses and dentifrices contain a variety of mixtures of herbal agents (such as aloe vera, sodium carrageenan, echinacea, goldenseal, bee propolis, and many others). At this time, controlled long-term studies to ascertain the efficacy of these agents in patients are lacking. A more extensive discussion of herbal agents can be found in **Chapter 25**.

Patient Advice

- The effectiveness of any mouthrinse is tied to the use of the agent as prescribed by the dentist. This means the proper dose, duration of time in the mouth, and frequency of rinsing must be carefully followed. If a patient misses a dose, he or she should apply the mouthrinse as soon as possible; however, doubling the dose will offer no benefit.
- To receive the greatest antiplaque or anticaries benefit, the patient should rinse before retiring to bed.
- After using a mouthrinse, the patient should not rinse with water or drink anything for at least 30 minutes. Immediately drinking or rinsing with water will increase the drug's clearance from the mouth and reduce its effectiveness. Furthermore, changes in taste sensation may occur if the mouth is rinsed with water immediately after mouthrinse use.
- These mouthrinses should be kept out of the reach of young children, as their ingestion of 4 or more ounces of rinses containing alcohol can cause alcohol intoxication.

DENTIFRICES

Oral hygiene is a critical aspect of all dental therapy. Proper oral hygiene reduces the buildup of dental plaque on tooth surfaces and reduces the incidence of dental caries as well as various types of periodontal diseases. Dentifrices are pastes, gels, or powders used to help remove dental plaque by enhancing the mechanical scrubbing and cleaning power of a toothbrush. Dentifrices typically contain abrasives (to remove debris and residual stain), foaming agents, or detergents (a preference of consumers), humectants (to prevent loss of water from the preparation), thickening agents or binders (to stabilize dentifrice formulations and prevent separation of liquid and solid phases), flavoring (also a preference of consumers), and therapeutic agents (see **Table 9.2**).

Depending on the dentifrice, the principal outcomes can include reduction of caries incidence by assimilation of the fluoride ion into the apatite crystal of enamel (as a result of sodium fluoride, stannous fluoride, or sodium monofluorophosphate); reduction of tooth hypersensitivity by blocking the pain caused by fluid exchange between dentinal tubules and pulp (as a result of arginine bicarbonate/calcium carbonate complex, potassium nitrate, or stabilized stannous fluoride); cosmetic whitening of teeth (as a result of hydrogen peroxide, papain/sodium citrate, or sodium tripolyphosphate and/or abrasives); reduction of calculus (as a result of pyrophosphates, zinc citrate, chloride, triclosan, or stabilized stannous fluoride); and reduction of plaque formation by reducing enzymatic activity of microorganisms and by an antibacterial effect (as a result of triclosan with vinylmethyl-ether maleic acid, zinc citrate, stannous fluoride, or a combination of essential oils). See **Table 9.2**.

It should be noted that with few exceptions, whitening toothpastes are different from agents that bleach. Bleaching involves free radicals (usually derived from hydrogen peroxide), whereas whitening or stain removal is accomplished by abrasive agents, phosphate compounds, or papain/sodium citrate (citroxain) (see **Chapter 12**).

Most dentifrices marketed to the public can be broadly classified as agents for:

- antitartar activity (reduction of calculus formation)
- caries prevention
- cosmetic effect (tooth whitening)
- gingivitis reduction
- plaque formation reduction
- reduction of tooth sensitivity

The ADA uses several guidelines to evaluate dentifrices for its Seal program. They may be viewed at *www.ada.org/ada/seal/standards/index.asp.*

Accepted Indications

Dentifrices are used in dentistry for cosmetic purposes and to provide caries prevention, reduce tooth sensitivity, reduce calculus formation, reduce plaque formation, reduce gingivitis, or provide a combination of all of these.

General Dosing Information

Depending on the patient's age and the dentifrice used (see **Table 9.3**), the usual adult dosage is approximately 1.5 mg of fluoride. The dosage for children <6 years is about 0.25 g (a pea-sized amount).

Dosage Adjustments

The actual maximum dose for each patient must be individualized depending on factors such as his or her size, age, and physical status; ability to effectively rinse and expectorate; oral health; and sensitivity. Highly fluoridated dentifrices are not often prescribed for pediatric patients, and reduced maximum doses may be indicated for certain patients, such as those with physical or mental disabilities.

Special Dental Considerations

Drug Interactions of Dental Interest

The following drug interactions and related problems involving dentifrices are potentially of clinical significance in dentistry.

Many of the ingredients of dentifrices, as well as products containing stannous fluoride, interact with chlorhexidine and reduce its efficacy. Dentifrice ingredients can also interact with cetylpyridinium chloride. Therefore, these agents should not be used concomitantly but, rather, used at least 30 minutes apart. Use of a chlorhexidine rinse followed immediately by a fluoride dentifrice may reduce the efficacy of each agent.

Cross-Sensitivity

Some patients can develop allergic reactions (eg, skin rash, hives, desquamation) to dentifrices and should discontinue use of the product immediately.

Special Patients

Patients with physical or mental disabilities may have difficulty clearing dentifrices from the mouth. These patients should receive additional help from caretakers.

Patient Monitoring: Aspects to Watch

See **Table 9.3**.

Adverse Effects and Precautions

The incidence of adverse reactions to dentifrices is relatively low. Many reactions (burning or taste alterations) are temporary. Idiosyncratic and allergic reactions account for a small minority of adverse responses.

The adverse effects listed in **Table 9.3** apply to all major types of dentifrices. Some patients cannot use tartar-control products because of the development of dentinal hypersensitivity or soft tissue irritation. For information on desensitizing agents, see **Chapter 11**. A small percentage of patients have an adverse reaction to sodium lauryl sulfate, a detergent that is added to some toothpastes. In such instances, switching to a dentifrice without sodium lauryl sulfate (such as Rembrandt, Biotene, or Sensodyne Gel) may be beneficial. Chlorhexidine and cetylpyridinium chloride have been reported to produce an extrinsic stain on teeth with the incidence being higher for chlorhexidine than for cetylpyridinium chloride.

Pharmacology

Antitartar Formulas

The precise mechanism of supragingival calculus formation is not known. However, it is assumed that most calculus-reducing formulas reduce crystal growth on tooth surfaces. One way in which they accomplish this is the chelation of cations by the dentifrices' active ingredient.

Cosmetic Formulas

Whitening of teeth can occur by two mechanisms. One method is mechanical, in which an abrasive is used to remove debris and surface stains from the tooth. The other method involves the use of phosphate compounds, such as sodium tripolyphosphate and sodium hexametaphosphate, that break down pigments that accumulate on or in tooth enamel. Sodium bicarbonate acts as both a mild abrasive and an agent for dissolving stain pigments.

Fluoride Formulas

Fluoride has been shown to reduce carious lesions dramatically in both children and adults. Fluoride ion is assimilated into the apatite crystal of enamel and stabilizes the crystal, making it more resistant to decay. Fluoride also has been shown to remineralize carious lesions.

Gingivitis- and Plaque-Reduction Formulas

Triclosan is both a bisphenol and a nonionic germicide that is effective against gram-positive and gram-negative bacteria, and it has been shown to reduce plaque accumulation and decrease the severity of gingivitis. A dentifrice containing stabilized stannous fluoride also has been shown to reduce gingivitis. The mechanism of action is thought to depend on the inhibition of bacterial metabolism and concomitant plaque acid reduction. Dentifrices containing zinc citrate have been reported to prevent the attachment of bacteria to teeth and to be antibacterial. A dentifrice containing a combination of essential oils (eucalyptol 0.738%, menthol 0.340%, methyl salicylate 0.480%, and thymol 0.511%) also has been shown to reduce plaque accumulation and gingivitis.

Herbal Agents

Some toothpastes contain a variety of mixtures of herbal agents (such as aloe vera, sodium carrageenan, echinacea, goldenseal, and bee propolis). Currently, controlled, long-term studies to ascertain the efficacy of these agents in patients are lacking. See **Chapter 25** for a more extensive discussion of herbal agents.

Amorphous Calcium Phosphate

Some fluoride dentifrices contain soluble calcium and phosphate, which are thought to enhance remineralization, prevent dental caries, reduce enamel and/or dentin erosion, and reduce dentinal hypersensitivity. It has been hypothesized that keeping calcium and phosphate in a soluble form allows it to bind to tooth surfaces and dental plaque. Laboratory and in vitro studies have demonstrated this enhanced calcium and phosphate uptake, but there is little clinical evidence to demonstrate a clinical benefit.

Sensitivity-Reduction Formulas

The mechanisms of action to reduce tooth sensitivity are not well established. It has been hypothesized that pain sensation in teeth can be reduced by blocking dentin tubule fluid exchange, by depolarizing pulpal nerves, or by both means. Currently available sensitive-teeth formulas act via the topical application of agents to root surfaces.

SUGGESTED READING

Ciancio SG. Chemical agents: plaque control, calculus reduction and treatment of dentinal hypersensitivity. *Periodontology 2000*. 1995;8:75-86.

Davies RM, Ellwood RP, Davies GM. The effectiveness of a toothpaste containing triclosan and polyvinyl-methyl ether maleic acid copolymer in improving plaque control and gingival health: a systematic review. *J Clin Periodontol*. 2004;31:1029-1033.

Gunsolley JC. A meta-analysis of six month studies of anti-plaque and antigingivitis agents *JADA*. 2006;137:1649-1657.

Mariotti A. Antiplaque/Antigingivitis Agents. In: *Pharmacology and Therapeutics for Dentistry*. 6th ed. Yagiela JA, Dowd FJ, Mariotti A, Johnson BS, Neidle EA (eds). St. Louis: Elsevier Mosby; 2009:573-582.

Panagakos FS, Volpe AR, Petrone ME, et al. Advanced oral antibacterial/anti-inflammatory technology: a comprehensive review of the clinical benefits of a triclosan/copolymer/fluoride dentifrice. *J Clin Dent*. 2005;16:S1-S19.

Paraskevas S, van der Weijden GA. A review of the effects of stannous fluoride on gingivitis. *J Clin Periodontol*. 2006;33(1):1-13.

Quirynen M, Zhao H, van Steenberghe D. Review of the treatment strategies for oral malodour. *Clin Oral Investig*. 2002;6:1-10.

Rolla G, Ogaard B, Cruz R de A. Clinical effect and mechanism of cariostatic action of fluoride-containing toothpastes: a review. *Int Dent J*. 1991;41(3):171-174.

Topping G, Assaf A. Strong evidence that daily use of fluoride toothpaste prevents caries. *Evid Based Dent*. 2005;6:32.

Twetman S, Axelsson S, Dahlgren H et al. Caries-preventive effect of fluoride toothpaste: a systematic review *Acta Odontol Scand*. 2003;6:347-355.

Yeung CA. A systematic review of the efficacy and safety of fluoridation. *Evid Based Dent*. 2008;9(2):39-43.

Table 9.1. USAGE INFORMATION FOR MOUTHRINSES

BRAND NAME/CONTENT	DOSAGE*	WARNINGS/PRECAUTIONS & CONTRAINDICATIONS	ADVERSE EFFECTS
ANESTHETIC MOUTHRINSE			
Chloraseptic Mouthwash: 1.4% phenol, 12.5% alcohol.	***Adults:*** 10mL prn (no more often than q 3 h). ***Pediatrics:*** Not recommended.	NA	NA
ANTITARTAR MOUTHRINSES			
Advanced Listerine Antiseptic with Tartar Protection (Arctic Mint, Citrus)★: 0.064% thymol, 0.092% eucalyptol, 0.060% methyl salicylate, 0.042% menthol, 0.09% zinc chloride, 21.6% alcohol, miscellaneous ingredients; **Vi-Jon Ice Mint Tartar Control Antiseptic Mouthrinse†:** miscellaneous ingredients.	***Adults:*** Rinse with 20mL for 30 sec.	NA	NA
CETYLPYRIDINIUM CHLORIDE‡			
Cepacol: 14.5% alcohol, 0.05% cetylpyridinium chloride, miscellaneous ingredients; **Crest Pro-Health Rinse (Clean Mint, Wintergreen) (alcohol-free):** 0.07% cetylpyridinium chloride, miscellaneous ingredients; **Scope Mouthwash and Gargle:** 18.9% alcohol, sodium benzoate, cetylpyridinium chloride, benzoic acid, domiphen bromide, miscellaneous ingredients; **Scope Mouthwash and Gargle with Baking Soda:** 9.9% alcohol, cetylpyridinium chloride, domiphen bromide, miscellaneous ingredients; **Viadent Advanced Care Oral Rinse:** 6.1% SD alcohol 38-B, 0.05% cetylpyridinium chloride, miscellaneous ingredients.	***Adults:*** (Crest Pro-Health) 20mL (4 tsp) swished for 30 sec bid. Do not swallow. When used after brushing, rinse mouth with water first. (All other brands) Amount, duration, and frequency depend on individual choice. ***Pediatrics:*** (Crest Pro-Health) **<6 yrs:** Do not use. **≥6 yrs to <12 yrs:** Supervise use. (All other brands) Not recommended.	**W/P:** Should be used cautiously in young children. **Contra:** Patients with known allergies to ingredients.	NA
CHLORHEXIDINE§			
G-U-M Chlorhexidine Gluconate Oral Rinse, USP (alcohol-free): 0.12% chlorhexidine; **Peridex:** 0.12% chlorhexidine, 11.6% alcohol; **PerioGard:** 0.12% chlorhexidine, 11.6% alcohol.	***Adults:*** 15mL swished for 30 sec and expectorated; use bid. Do not swallow; do not rinse with water immediately after use.	**W/P:** Permanent staining of margins of restorations or composite restorations. Should not be used as sole treatment of gingivitis. **Contra:** Patients with sensitivity to chlorhexidine. **P/N:** Category B.	Allergic reaction (skin rash, hives, swelling of face), alteration of taste, staining of teeth, staining of restorations, discoloration of tongue, increase in calculus formation, parotid duct obstruction, parotitis, desquamation of oral mucosa, irritation to lips or tongue, oral sensitivity.
COSMETIC MOUTHRINSES			
Listerine Whitening Pre-Brush Rinse: 8% alcohol, 2% hydrogen peroxide, miscellaneous agents; **Rembrandt Age Defying Mouthwash:** 0.05% sodium fluoride wt/vol, 1.5% hydrogen peroxide solution, miscellaneous agents; **Rembrandt Dazzling Fresh Mouthrinse:** methylparaben, sodium citrate, sodium lauryl sulfate, miscellaneous ingredients.	***Adults:*** Amount, duration, and frequency of use depend on individual choice. ***Pediatrics:*** Not recommended.	**W/P:** Should be used cautiously in young children and in people who have low salivary flow due to age or drugs. **Contra:** Patients with allergic reactions, oral ulcerations, and oral desquamative diseases.	NA
Targon: 15.6% alcohol, PEG-40, hydrogenated castor oil, sodium lauryl sulfate, disodium phosphate, miscellaneous ingredients.	***Adults:*** Before brushing, rinse with 20mL for 30 sec.	NA	NA

★indicates a product bearing the ADA Seal of Acceptance. There are a significant number of generic and store-brand products that carry the ADA seal. For a complete listing of ADA-accepted OTC products, visit *www.ada.org/ada/seal/index.asp.*

NA = not available.

*Pediatric safety and efficacy have not been established except with fluoride rinses in children 6 years and older.

†Private label manufacturer.

‡Depending on the formulation, products containing cetylpyridinium chloride are used for various purposes, including control of plaque, gingivitis, and halitosis.

§Pregnancy risk category B. Pregnancy risk categories have not been established for other products.

Table 9.1. USAGE INFORMATION FOR MOUTHRINSES *(cont.)*

BRAND NAME/CONTENT	DOSAGE*	WARNINGS/PRECAUTIONS & CONTRAINDICATIONS	ADVERSE EFFECTS
DELMOPINOL††			
Decapinol Oral Rinse: classified as medical device; forms a barrier by adhering to tooth surfaces.	***Adults:*** 10mL swished for 60 sec and expectorated; use bid after brushing. ***Pediatrics* <12 yrs:** Not recommended.	**W/P:** Not recommended during pregnancy due to lack of studies.	NA
ESSENTIAL OILS			
Listerine Antiseptic¶ (Original, Cool Mint, FreshBurst, Natural Citrus, and Vanilla Mint)★: 0.092% eucalyptol, 0.064% thymol, 0.06% methyl salicylate, 0.042% menthol, and alcohol ranging from 21.6% for the flavored versions and 26.9% for the original version; **Swan (Amber, Blue Mint, Spring Mint) Antiseptic Mouthrinse★†, Vi-Jon (Regular, Blue Mint, Citrus, Fresh Mint) Antiseptic Mouthrinse★†:** ingredients equivalent to Listerine.	***Adults:*** 20mL swished full strength for 30 sec and expectorated; do not swallow. Use bid or prn. ***Pediatrics:*** Do not use in children <12 yrs.	**W/P:** Should not be used as sole treatment of gingivitis. **Contra:** Children <12 yrs.	NA
FLUORIDES			
ACT Restoring Anticavity (33 oz), Fluorigard Anti-Cavity Dental Rinse, Listerine Smart Rinse for Kids, Listerine Total Care, Pro-DenRx APF Sodium Fluoride Rinse★, Tom's of Maine Natural Anticavity Fluoride Mouthwash★: 0.02% sodium fluoride; **Phos-Flur Anti-Cavity Fluoride Rinse ★:** 0.044% sodium fluoride; **ACT Anticavity★, ACT Anticavity for Kids★, Act Restoring Anticavity (18 oz), Equate Anticavity★, Fluorigard, Hannaford Anticavity★, H.E. Buddy Anticavity★, Hello! Anticavity★, Hill Country Anticavity★, Inspector Hector Tooth Protector Anticavity★, NaFrinse Acidulated Oral Rinse, NaFrinse Neutral/Daily Mouthrinse, Oral-B Rinse Therapy Anti-Cavity Treatment, Publix Anticavity★, Publix Kids Anticavity★, REACH ACT Restoring, Reach Fluoride Dental Rinse, Rite Aid Anticavity★, Sunmark Anticavity★, Swan Anticavity★†, The Natural Dentist Healthy Teeth★, Tom's of Maine Natural Anticavity★,Vi-Jon Mint Anticavity★†, Weis Anticavity★, Western Family Anticavity★:** 0.05% sodium fluoride; **ACT Anticavity Fluoride Rinse★:** 0.05% sodium fluoride, 7% alcohol; **NaFrinse Mouthrinse Powder, NaFrinse Neutral/Weekly Mouthrinse, NaFrinse Unit Dose Mouthrinse Solution, Pro-DenRx 0.2% Neutral Sodium Fluoride Rinse:** 0.2% sodium fluoride; **PreviDent Dental Rinse:** 0.2% sodium fluoride, 6% alcohol; **Dentinbloc Dentin Desensitizer:** 1.09% sodium fluoride, 0.4% stannous fluoride, 0.14% hydrogen fluoride.	***Adults:*** 10mL of sodium fluoride swished for 60 sec and expectorated qd; patient should not eat or drink for 30 min after rinsing. ***Pediatrics:* <6 yrs:** Not recommended. **≥6 yrs:** 10mL of 0.05% sodium fluoride swished for 60 sec and expectorated qd; patient should not eat or drink for 30 min after rinsing.	**W/P:** Chronic systemic overdose may induce fluorosis and changes in bone. **Contra:** Patients with dental fluorosis, fluoride toxicity from systemic ingestion, and severe renal insufficiency.	Ulcerations of oral mucosa, fluorosis, osteosclerosis, diarrhea, bloody vomit, nausea, stomach cramps, black tarry stools, drowsiness, faintness, stomach cramps or pain, unusual excitement if swallowed.

★indicates a product bearing the ADA Seal of Acceptance. There are a significant number of generic and store-brand products that carry the ADA seal. For a complete listing of ADA-accepted OTC products, visit *www.ada.org/ada/seal/index.asp.*

NA = not available.

*Pediatric safety and efficacy have not been established except with fluoride rinses in children 6 years and older.

†Private label manufacturer.

§Pregnancy risk category B. Pregnancy risk categories have not been established for other products.

¶ Although Listerine was the first antiseptic oral rinse formulated, today there are a significant number of generic compounds with similar antibacterial properties. Various mouthrinses that carry the ADA seal are generic versions of Listerine.

††Not available in the U.S. at the time of publication.

BRAND NAME/CONTENT	DOSAGE*	WARNINGS/PRECAUTIONS & CONTRAINDICATIONS	ADVERSE EFFECTS
MOUTHRINSES FOR HALITOSIS			
Astring-O-Sol (concentrate): SD alcohol 38-B, 75.6% methyl salicylate, miscellaneous ingredients; **Breath Rx:** cetylpyridinium chloride, chloride 0.075%; **Lavoris Crystal Fresh (Original, Peppermint):** alcohol, citric acid, sodium hydroxide, zinc oxide, miscellaneous ingredients; **Lavoris (Mint, Cinnamon):** alcohol, aromatic oils, zinc chloride and/or zinc oxide; **Listermint Mint (alcohol-free):** zinc chloride, sodium benzoate, sodium lauryl sulfate, miscellaneous ingredients; **Oxyfresh Natural Mouthrinse (alcohol-free):** oxygene (contains chlorine dioxide), miscellaneous ingredients; **Platinum:** monofluorophosphate, tetrapotassium pyrophosphate, miscellaneous ingredients; **Rembrandt Mouth Refreshing Rinse (alcohol-free):** sodium benzoate, methyl paraben, miscellaneous ingredients; **Retardex Oral Rinse (alcohol free):** ciosysii (contains chlorine dioxide), miscellaneous ingredients; **Tom's of Maine Natural Mouthwash:** aloe vera, ascrobic acid, menthol, spearmint, witch hazel, miscellaneous ingredients.	***Adults:*** Amount, duration, and frequency depend on individual choice. ***Pediatrics:*** Not recommended.	**W/P:** Should be used cautiously in young children. **Contra:** Patients with known allergies to ingredients.	NA
MOUTHRINSE FOR PAIN RELIEF (CANKER AND MOUTH SORES, ETC)			
Rincinol P.R.N. Soothing Oral Rinse: sodium hyaluronate, polyvinylpyrrolidone, glycyrrhetinic acid, aloe vera extract, miscellaneous ingredients.	***Adults/Pediatrics:*** Swish for 60 sec and expectorate; use prn.	NA	NA
MOUTHRINSES TO REDUCE THE DISCOMFORT OF XEROSTOMIA‡‡			
Biotene: lactoferrin, lysozyme, lactoperoxidase, glucose oxidase; **Biotene PBF:** lactoferrin, lysozyme, lactoperoxidase, glucose oxidase, mutanase, dextranase; **Oasis:** glycerin.	***Adults:*** (Biotene, Biotene PBF) 1 tbl as needed for 30 sec; (Oasis) 1 oz for 30 sec.	NA	NA
OXYGENATING AGENTS			
Gly-Oxide: 10% carbamide peroxide; **Orajel Rinse:** 4% alcohol, 1.5% hydrogen peroxide; **Peroxyl Mouthrinse:** 1.5% hydrogen peroxide, 6% alcohol.	***Adults:*** Regimens used for rinses containing oxygenating agents will vary depending on formulation: eg, recommendation for Gly-Oxide is that several drops be applied to affected areas, followed by a 2-3 min rinsing; the recommendation for Peroxyl Mouthrinse is that 10mL of it be used, followed by a 60-sec rinsing.	**W/P:** Should not be used for extended periods of time because of possible side effects mentioned at left. **Contra:** Treatment of periodontitis or gingivitis.	Chemical burns of oral mucosa, decalcification of teeth, black hairy tongue.
PREBRUSHING RINSE			
Advanced Formula Plax (Original, Mint Sensation, SoftMint): 8.7% alcohol, tetrasodium pyrophosphate, benzoic acid, sodium lauryl sulfate, sodium benzoate, miscellaneous ingredients.	***Adults:*** Efficacy has not been established for adult or geriatric population.	NA	Negligible effects on plaque make these agents of little use in the treatment of carious lesions or periodontal diseases, including gingivitis.

‡‡See Chapter 8 for more information on agents affecting salivation.

Table 9.2. COMPONENTS OF DENTIFRICES

INGREDIENTS	FUNCTION
Abrasives: Calcium carbonate, dehydrated silica gels, hydrated aluminum oxides, magnesium carbonate, phosphate salts, silicates	Remove debris and residual stain, remove surface stains on teeth
Fluoride	Reduces caries
Peroxides, sodium tripolyphosphate, sodium hexametaphosphate, papain/sodium citrate	Remove surface stains on teeth
Potassium nitrate, sodium citrate, strontium chloride	Reduce dentinal sensitivity
Pyrophosphates, triclosan, zinc citrate	Reduce supragingival calculus
Stannous fluoride, triclosan	Reduce gingival inflammation
Detergents: Sodium lauryl sulfate, sodium N-lauryl sarcosinate	Create foaming action and may help increase the solubility of plaque and accretions during brushing
Flavoring agents: Diverse and complex agents that may contain saccharin as a sweetener	Provide taste to dentifrice (consumer preference)
Humectants: Glycerol, propylene glycol, sorbitol	Prevent water loss
Thickening agents or binders: Mineral colloids, natural gums, seaweed colloids, synthetic celluloses	Stabilize formulations

Table 9.3. USAGE INFORMATION FOR DENTIFRICES

NAME/ACTIVE INGREDIENTS	WARNINGS/PRECAUTIONS	ADVERSE EFFECTS
ANTITARTAR*		
Aim Anti-Tartar Gel Formula with Fluoride, Aim Tartar Control Gel Toothpaste: Zinc citrate, 0.76% sodium monofluorophosphate **Aquafresh ALL with Tartar Control Toothpaste:** Tetrapotassium pyrophosphate, tetrasodium pyrophosphate, 0.243% sodium fluoride **Aquafresh Whitening Tartar Protection Toothpaste:** 0.243% sodium fluoride, sodium tripolyphosphate **Close-Up Tartar Control Gel:** Zinc citrate, 0.76% sodium monofluorophosphate **Colgate Tartar Control Baking Soda and Peroxide Toothpaste:** Sodium monofluorophosphate (0.15% w/v fluoride ion) **Colgate Tartar Control Toothpaste★ or Gel:** Tetrasodium pyrophosphate, 0.243% sodium fluoride **Colgate Tartar Control Plus Whitening Gel★ or Mint Paste:** 0.243% sodium fluoride, 1% tetrasodium pyrophosphate **Colgate Total Toothpaste★, Colgate Total Clean Mint Toothpaste★, Colgate Total Fresh Stripe Toothpaste, Colgate Total Mint Stripe Gel:** 0.243% sodium fluoride, 0.30% triclosan **Colgate Total Advanced Clean Toothpaste★, Colgate Total Advanced Fresh Gel, Colgate Total 2 in 1 Advanced Fresh Liquid Toothpaste:** 0.243% sodium fluoride, 0.30% triclosan **Colgate Total Plus Whitening Toothpaste★, Colgate Total Plus Whitening Gel★:** 0.243% sodium fluoride, 0.30% triclosan **Crest Extra Whitening With Tartar Protection★:** 0.243% sodium fluoride, 5.045% tetrasodium pyrophosphate **Crest Extra Whitening with Tartar Protection Toothpaste, Clean Mint (Neat Squeeze Version)★:** 0.243% sodium fluoride (0.15% w/v fluoride ion) **Crest MultiCare:** 0.243% sodium fluoride, tetrasodium pyrophosphate **Crest MultiCare Whitening★:** 0.243% sodium fluoride, 5.045% tetrasodium pyrophosphate **Crest Pro-Health Toothpaste (Clean Cinnamon, Clean Mint)★:** 0.454% stannous fluoride (active ingredient), sodium hexametaphosphate (tartar reduction and stain inhibition ingredient) **Crest Pro-Health Night Toothpaste★:** 0.454% stannous fluoride (0.16% w/v fluoride ion) **Crest Pro-Health Whitening Toothpaste★:** 0.454% stannous fluoride (0.16% w/v fluoride ion) **Crest Tartar Protection Fluoride Gel or Toothpaste:** 0.243% sodium fluoride, tetrapotassium pyrophosphate, disodium pyrophosphate, tetrasodium pyrophosphate **Crest Tartar Protection Fresh Mint Gel★:** sodium fluoride (0.15% w/v fluoride ion) **Crest Tartar Protection Regular Paste★:** 0.243% sodium fluoride (0.15% w/v fluoride ion) **Dr. Fresh Complete Fluoride Toothpaste (MFP):** 0.24% w/w sodium fluoride **Listerine Essential Care Tartar Control Powerful Mint Gel:** 0.76% sodium monofluorophosphate, 0.738% eucalyptol, 0.340% menthol, 0.480% methyl salicylates, 0.511% thymol, zinc citrate trihydrate, miscellaneous ingredients **Pepsodent Tartar Control Toothpaste:** Ingredients not available. **Viadent Advanced Care Toothpaste:** 2% zinc citrate, 0.8% sodium monofluorophosphate	See manufacturer's labeling for specific brand information.	Development of dentinal hypersensitivity and tissue irritation, but incidence is low.

★indicates a product bearing the ADA Seal of Acceptance. There are a significant number of generic and store-brand products that carry the ADA seal. For a complete listing of ADA-accepted OTC products, visit *www.ada.org/ada/seal/index.asp.*

*These dentifrices also possess caries-preventive properties.

Table 9.3. USAGE INFORMATION FOR DENTIFRICES *(cont.)*

NAME/ACTIVE INGREDIENTS	WARNINGS/PRECAUTIONS	ADVERSE EFFECTS
CARIES PREVENTION (ACTIVE INGREDIENT: FLUORIDE†)		
Aim Cavity Protection Toothpaste★ Aquafresh Anti-Cavity Toothpaste★ Aquafresh Dr. Seuss Bubble Fresh Fluoride Toothpaste★ Aquafresh Extra Fresh Toothpaste Aquafresh Fluoride Protection Toothpaste Aquafresh for Kids Toothpaste★ Aquafresh Kids Bubblemint Toothpaste Aquafresh Triple Protection Toothpaste Arm & Hammer Advance Care Toothpaste Arm & Hammer Complete Care Toothpaste Arm & Hammer Dental Care Toothpaste Arm & Hammer Dental Care Advanced Cleaning Mint Toothpaste w/ Baking Soda★ Arm & Hammer Enamel Care Toothpaste Arm & Hammer Peroxide Care Toothpaste Biotene Toothpaste Close-Up Anticavity Gel Toothpaste Close-Up Freshening Gel Toothpaste Colgate Advanced Freshness Toothpaste Colgate 2-in-1 Advanced Fresh Liquid Toothpaste Colgate 2-in-1 Kids Toothpaste Colgate Cavity Protection Gel with Baking Soda Colgate Cavity Protection Great Regular Flavor Fluoride Toothpaste★ Colgate Cavity Protection Toothpaste with Baking Soda Colgate Cavity Protection Winterfresh Gel★ Colgate Fresh Confidence Toothpaste Colgate for Kids Toothpaste★ Colgate Junior Toothpaste★ Colgate Luminous Fluoride Toothpaste★ Colgate Tartar Control Plus Whitening Gel★ or Mint Paste Colgate Tartar Control Toothpaste★ or Gel Colgate Total Toothpaste★ Colgate Total 2 in 1 Advanced Fresh Liquid Toothpaste Colgate Total Advanced Clean Toothpaste★ Colgate Total Advanced Fresh Toothpaste★ Colgate Total Advanced Whitening Toothpaste★ Colgate Total Clean Mint Toothpaste★ Colgate Total Enamel Strength Toothpaste★ Colgate Total Mint Stripe Toothpaste★ Colgate Total Plus Whitening Liquid Toothpaste★ Colgate Total Plus Whitening Toothpaste★ or Gel★ Cool Wave Fresh Mint Gel Fluoride Anticavity Toothpaste★ Crest Advanced Cleaning Toothpaste Crest Cavity Protection Cool Mint Gel★ Crest Cavity Protection Icy Mint Crest Cavity Protection Toothpaste★ Crest Extra Whitening with Tartar Protection Toothpaste, Clean Mint (Neat Squeeze Version)★ Crest Intelliclean Toothpaste Crest Kids SparkleFun Cavity Protection Gel★ Crest MultiCare Toothpaste Crest Multicare Whitening Toothpaste★ Crest Pro-Health Night Toothpaste★ Crest Pro-Health Toothpaste (Clean Cinnamon, Clean Mint)★ Crest Pro-Health Whitening Toothpaste★ Crest Rejuvenating Effects Toothpaste Crest Sensitivity Protection Soothing Whitening Mint Paste★ Crest Tartar Protection Fresh Mint Gel★ Crest Tartar Protection Regular Paste★ DTI Toothpaste and Gel (Bubble Gum, Mint)★‡ Dr. Fresh Complete Care Toothpaste Dr. Fresh Fluoride Toothpaste Enamel Care Toothpaste Equate Cavity Protection Toothpaste Gleem Sodium Fluoride Anticavity Toothpaste Goofy Grape Natural Anticavity Fluoride Toothpaste/Liquid Gel for Children★	Tell caregivers of pediatric patients to make sure a pea-sized amount is used on toothbrush to minimize amount of fluoride ingested. **Usual adult dosage:** 1.5 mg; **pediatrics <6 yrs:** ~0.25 g (pea-sized amount). See manufacturer's labeling for specific brand information.	Fluorosis.

★indicates a product bearing the ADA Seal of Acceptance. There are a significant number of generic and store-brand products that carry the ADA seal. For a complete listing of ADA-accepted OTC products, visit *www.ada.org/ada/seal/index.asp.*

*These dentifrices also possess caries-preventive properties.

†Fluoride from sodium fluoride, sodium monofluorophosphate, or stannous fluoride.

‡Private label manufacturer.

NAME/ACTIVE INGREDIENTS	WARNINGS/PRECAUTIONS	ADVERSE EFFECTS
CARIES PREVENTION (ACTIVE INGREDIENT: FLUORIDE[†]) *(cont.)*		
Mentadent Cavity Fighting Toothpaste Mentadent Fluoride Toothpaste w/Baking Soda & Peroxide Orajel Sensitive Pain Relieving Toothpaste for Adults OraLine Fluoride Mint Toothpaste★ OraLine Kids Bubblegum Toothpaste★ OraLine Secure Clear Fluoride Mint Toothpaste★ Pepsodent Original Toothpaste with Cavity Protection Pepsodent Baking Soda Toothpaste Plak Smacker Dinosaur Fluoride Gel Toothpaste (Bubblegum)★ Plak Smacker Great White Shark Fluoride Gel Toothpaste (Cool Berry)★ Quality Choice Mint Flavor Toothpaste Rembrandt Whitening Toothpaste Sensodyne Fresh Impact Toothpaste★ Shane Aloe Sense Toothpaste★ Sheffield Fluoride Toothpaste (Original, Bubble Gum, Mint)★‡ Stages Toothpaste Tom's of Maine Natural Baking Soda Toothpaste (Peppermint)★ Tom's of Maine Natural Fluoride Toothpaste for Children (Strawberry, Orange Mango)★ Tom's of Maine Natural Fluoride Toothpaste (Wintermint)★ Tom's of Maine Natural Toothpaste (Spearmint, Wintermint)★ Topol Whitening Anticavity Toothpaste Ultra Brite Advanced Whitening Fluoride Toothpaste Ultra Fresh Fluoride Toothpaste Viadent Advanced Care Toothpaste Zooth Children's Toothpaste		
COSMETIC*		
Aim Whitening Gel Toothpaste with Baking Soda: 0.8% sodium monofluorophosphate **Aquafresh Multi-Action Whitening Toothpaste:** 0.243% sodium fluoride, sodium tripolyphosphate **Aquafresh Whitening Advanced Freshness:** 0.243% sodium fluoride, sodium tripolyphosphate **Aquafresh Whitening Toothpaste:** 0.243% sodium fluoride, 10% sodium tripolyphosphate **Close-Up Whitening Gel Toothpaste:** Ingredients not available. **Colgate Baking Soda & Peroxide Whitening Toothpaste:** 0.15% w/v fluoride ion, sodium monofluorophosphate **Colgate Luminous Fluoride Toothpaste★:** 0.243% sodium fluoride, tetrasodium pyrophosphate **Colgate Platinum Tooth Whitener Toothpaste:** 2% tetrasodium phosphate, 10% aluminum oxide, 0.76% sodium monofluorophosphate **Colgate Simply White Toothpaste:** 0.24% sodium fluoride (0.13% w/v fluoride ion) **Colgate Sparkling White Toothpaste:** 0.24% sodium fluoride (0.13% w/v fluoride ion) **Colgate Total Advanced Clean Toothpaste★, Colgate Total 2-in-1 Advanced Fresh Liquid Toothpaste:** 0.243% sodium fluoride, 0.30% triclosan **Colgate Total Plus Whitening Gel★, Liquid Toothpaste★ or Toothpaste★:** 0.243% sodium fluoride, 0.30% triclosan **Crest Baking Soda Whitening Tartar Protection Toothpaste:** 0.243% sodium fluoride **Crest Dual Action Whitening Toothpaste:** 0.243% sodium fluoride (0.15% w/v fluoride ion) **Crest Extra Whitening With Tartar Protection★:** 0.243% sodium fluoride, 5.045% tetrasodium pyrophosphate **Crest MultiCare Whitening★:** 0.243% sodium fluoride, 5.045% tetrasodium pyrophosphate **Crest Pro-Health Toothpaste (Clean Cinnamon, Clean Mint)★:** 0.454% stannous fluoride (active ingredient), sodium hexametaphosphate (tartar reduction and stain inhibition ingredient) **Crest Rejuvenating Effects Toothpaste:** 0.243% sodium fluoride, silica	Not all discolorations of enamel (for example, enamel mottling, tetracycline staining, aging-extrinsic enamel) are responsive to extrinsic bleaching via dentifrices. See manufacturer's labeling for specific brand information.	Burning sensation, drying out of mucous membranes, taste alteration, gingival abrasion, enamel erosion.

Table 9.3. USAGE INFORMATION FOR DENTIFRICES *(cont.)*

NAME/ACTIVE INGREDIENTS	WARNINGS/PRECAUTIONS	ADVERSE EFFECTS
COSMETIC* *(cont.)*		
Crest Vivid White Toothpaste: 0.243% sodium fluoride, 0.15% w/v fluoride ion **Crest Whitening Expressions Toothpaste & Liquid Gel, Crest Whitening Plus Scope:** 0.243% sodium fluoride, 0.15% w/v fluoride ion **Mentadent Advanced Whitening Toothpaste, Mentadent Replenishing White Toothpaste:** 0.24% sodium fluoride **Pearl Drops Baking Soda Whitening Toothpaste:** Fluoride **Pearl Drops Extra Strength Whitening Toothpaste with Fluoride:** Fluoride **Pearl Drops Whitening Gel:** Fluoride **Pearl Drops Whitening Toothpolish with Fluoride:** Fluoride **Rembrandt Age Defying Toothpaste:** 0.76% sodium monofluorophosphate, tribon, papain/sodium citrate (citroxain), dicalcium orthophosphate, 6% carbamide peroxide **Rembrandt Dazzling White Toothpaste:** 0.76% sodium monofluorophosphate, 6% carbamide peroxide, papain/sodium citrate (citroxain) **Rembrandt Whitening Toothpaste:** 44% dicalcium phosphate dihydrate, 0.76% sodium monofluorophosphate (1,000 ppm), papain/sodium citrate (citroxain) **Sensodyne Extra Whitening:** 5% potassium nitrate, 0.243% sodium fluoride, pentasodium triphosphate		
PLAQUE AND/OR GINGIVITIS REDUCTION*		
Colgate Total Toothpaste★, Colgate Total Clean Mint Toothpaste★, Colgate Total Fresh Stripe Toothpaste, Colgate Total Mint Stripe Gel: 0.243% sodium fluoride, 0.30% triclosan **Colgate Total Advanced Clean Toothpaste★, Colgate Total Advanced Fresh Gel, Colgate Total 2 in 1 Advanced Fresh Liquid Toothpaste:** 0.243% sodium fluoride, 0.30% triclosan **Crest Pro-Health Toothpaste (Clean Cinnamon, Clean Mint)★:** 0.454% stannous fluoride (active ingredient), sodium hexametaphosphate (tartar reduction and stain inhibition ingredient) **Viadent Advanced Care Toothpaste:** 2% zinc citrate, 0.8% sodium monofluorophosphate	See manufacturer's labeling for specific brand information.	Allergic reaction, burning sensation, bitter taste. Products containing stannous fluoride may produce reversible staining of teeth.

★indicates a product bearing the ADA Seal of Acceptance. There are a significant number of generic and store-brand products that carry the ADA seal. For a complete listing of ADA-accepted OTC products, visit *www.ada.org/ada/seal/index.asp.*
*These dentifrices also posses caries-preventive properties.
§All these dentifrices also possess caries-preventive properties except for Protect Desensitizing Solution.
¶In sensitivity-reduction dentifrices, fluoride is the active agent only for caries prevention; the exception is stannous fluoride, which has both caries-preventive and sensitivity-reducing properties.

NAME/ACTIVE INGREDIENTS	WARNINGS/PRECAUTIONS	ADVERSE EFFECTS
SENSITIVITY REDUCTION§¶		
Aquafresh Sensitive Toothpaste: 5% potassium nitrate, 0.243% sodium fluoride **Butler Maximum Strength Sensitive Toothpaste:** 5% potassium nitrate, 0.22% sodium fluoride **Colgate Sensitive Maximum Strength:** 5% potassium nitrate, 0.454% stannous fluoride **Colgate Sensitive Plus Whitening Toothpaste:** 5% potassium nitrate; 0.24% sodium fluoride (0.14% w/v fluoride ion) **Crest Pro-Health Toothpaste (Clean Cinnamon, Clean Mint)★:** 0.454% stannous fluoride (active ingredient), sodium hexametaphosphate (tartar reduction and stain inhibition ingredient) **Crest Sensitivity Protection Soothing Whitening Mint Paste★:** 5% potassium nitrate, 0.243% sodium fluoride **Dr. Fresh T-Sensitive Toothpaste, Dr. Fresh T-Sensitive Tartar Control Toothpaste:** Ingredients not available. **Orajel Sensitive Pain-Relieving Toothpaste for Adults:** 5% potassium nitrate, 1.15% sodium monofluorophosphate **Oral-B Sensitive with Fluoride Paste:** 5% potassium nitrate, sodium fluoride (0.14% w/v fluoride ion) **Protect Sensitive Teeth Gel Toothpaste:** 5% potassium nitrate, 0.243% sodium fluoride **Protect Desensitizing Solution (with activating swabs):** hydroxypropyl cellulose, potassium fluoride, polyethyleneglycol dimethacrylate and other methacrylates **Rembrandt Whitening Toothpaste for Sensitive Teeth:** 5% potassium nitrate, 0.76% sodium monofluorophosphate, sodium citrate **Sensiv for Sensitive Teeth:** potassium nitrate, sodium monofluorophosphate **Sensodyne Baking Soda, Sensodyne Cool Gel, Sensodyne Fresh Impact:** 5% potassium nitrate, 0.243% sodium fluoride **Sensodyne Original, Sensodyne Fresh Mint:** 5% potassium nitrate, sodium fluoride (0.13% w/v fluoride ion) **Sensodyne ProNamel:** 5% potassium nitrate, 0.243% sodium fluoride **Sensodyne Extra Whitening:** 5% potassium nitrate, 0.243% sodium fluoride, pentasodium triphosphate **Sensodyne Tartar Control Plus Whitening:** 5% potassium nitrate, sodium fluoride (0.145% w/v fluoride ion), tetrasodium pyrophosphate **Sensodyne Toothpaste for Sensitive Teeth, Tartar Control Plus Whitening:** 5% potassium nitrate, sodium fluoride (0.145% w/v fluoride ion), tetrasodium pyrophosphate **Tom's of Maine Natural Sensitive Anticavity Toothpaste ★ & Gel Toothpaste ★:** potassium nitrate, sodium fluoride	Differential diagnosis is important to rule out other reasons for sensitivity—for example, cracked tooth or caries. Toothpastes containing 5% potassium nitrate are not recommended for children <12 yrs. See manufacturer's labeling for specific brand information.	Allergic reactions (most products contain parabens, to which some patients may be allergic).

Chapter 10

Fluorides

Kenneth H. Burrell, D.D.S., S.M.

When considering a fluoride regimen from among the many available, take into account the patient's caries risk and age.

The Patient's Caries Risk

According to the Centers for Disease Control and Prevention, populations believed to be at increased risk for dental caries are those with low socioeconomic status or low levels of parental education; those who do not seek regular dental care; and those without dental insurance or access to dental services. Individual factors that may increase risk include:

- active dental caries
- a history of high caries experience in older siblings or caregivers
- root surfaces exposed by gingival recession
- high levels of infection with cariogenic bacteria
- impaired ability to maintain oral hygiene
- malformed enamel or dentin
- reduced salivary flow because of medication, radiation treatment, or disease
- low salivary buffering capacity (ie, decreased ability of saliva to neutralize acids)
- wearing space maintainers, orthodontic appliances, or dental prostheses

The CDC further states that risk can increase if any of the factors above are combined with dietary practices conducive to dental caries (eg, frequent consumption of refined carbohydrates), and that risk decreases with adequate exposure to fluoride. For the ADA Council on Scientific Affairs' definition of caries risk, see the box on the next page.

Age of the Patient

Fluoride regimens vary according to age (see **Table 10.1**). Patients <6 years are at risk of developing enamel fluorosis from excessive amounts of fluoride in the water supply, inappropriate and injudicious use of fluoride supplements, and regular, inadvertent ingestion of fluoride-containing over-the-counter products such as toothpaste. Ingestion of fluoride in food products also contributes to a child's total daily fluoride intake.

Principles of Dosing

According to Adair (2006), "Therapeutic use of fluoride in children should focus on regimens that maximize topical contact, preferably in lower dose, higher frequency approaches. Current best practice includes recommending twice-daily use of a fluoridated dentifrice for children in optimally fluoridated and fluoride-deficient communities, coupled with professional application of topical fluoride gel, foam, or varnish. The addition of other fluoride regimens should be based on periodic risk assessments recognizing that

CARIES RISK CRITERIA AS DEFINED BY THE ADA COUNCIL ON SCIENTIFIC AFFAIRS

Patients should be evaluated using caries risk criteria such as those below.

LOW CARIES RISK

All age groups

No incipient or cavitated primary or secondary carious lesions during the last 3 years and no factors that may increase caries risk*

MODERATE CARIES RISK

Younger than 6 years

No incipient or cavitated primary or secondary carious lesions during the last 3 years but presence of at least one factor that may increase caries risk*

Older than 6 years (any of the following)

One or two incipient or cavitated primary or secondary carious lesions in the last 3 years

No incipient or cavitated primary or secondary carious lesions in the last 3 years but presence of at least one factor that may increase caries risk*

HIGH CARIES RISK

Younger than 6 years (any of the following)

Any incipient or cavitated primary or secondary carious lesion during the last 3 years

Presence of multiple factors that may increase caries risk*

Low socioeconomic status†

Suboptimal fluoride exposure

Xerostomia‡

Older than 6 years (any of the following)

Three or more incipient or cavitated primary or secondary carious lesions in the last 3 years

Presence of multiple factors that may increase caries risk*

Suboptimal fluoride exposure

Xerostomia‡

* Factors increasing the risk of developing caries also may include, but are not limited to, high titers of cariogenic bacteria, poor oral hygiene, prolonged nursing (bottle or breast), poor family dental health, developmental or acquired enamel defects, genetic abnormality of teeth, many multisurface restorations, chemotherapy or radiation therapy, eating disorders, drug or alcohol abuse, irregular dental care, cariogenic diet, active orthodontic treatment, presence of exposed root surfaces, restoration overhangs and open margins, and physical or mental disability with inability or unavailability of performing proper oral health care.

† On the basis of findings from population studies, groups with low socioeconomic status have been found to have an increased risk of developing caries. In children too young for their risk to be based on caries history, low socioeconomic status should be considered as a caries risk factor.

‡ Medication-, radiation-, or disease-induced xerostomia.

ADA Council on Scientific Affairs. Professionally applied topical fluoride. Evidence-based clinical recommendations. *JADA*. 2006;137(8):1151-1159.
Copyright © 2006 American Dental Association. All rights reserved. Reprinted by permission.

the additive effects of multiple fluoride modalities exhibit diminishing returns."

Sufficient evidence exists to apply these principles to adolescents. Although few randomized controlled clinical trials have been conducted to determine the anticaries effectiveness of fluorides in adults, it is reasonable to assume that these dosing principles apply. An application of these principles according to the patient's caries risk and age can be found in **Table 10.1**.

FLUORIDATED WATER AND FLUORIDE SUPPLEMENTS

Accepted Indications

Fluoride in community and school water supplies is responsible to a great degree for the fact that most people in the United States have a low risk of experiencing dental caries. When fluoride levels in drinking water are <0.6 ppm and when children from 6 months to 16 years are considered to be at increased risk of experiencing dental caries, a fluoride supplement should be prescribed (see **Table 10.2**). An analysis of the home drinking water may not be adequate, however. The patient's parents or guardians may need to be questioned about the child's usual source of drinking water. For example, day-care centers may have fluoridated drinking water that is at levels adequate to preclude prescribing a fluoride supplement.

General Dosing Information

The recommended concentration of fluoride in fluoridated water supply systems that offers the maximum reduction in dental caries with the minimal amount of enamel mottling or fluorosis varies with the annual average of maximum daily air temperature (people living in warmer climates tend to drink more water than those in cooler climates). It may range from 0.7 ppm in Houston to 1.2 ppm in Duluth, Minnesota.

The fluoride level in drinking water is a major factor in determining the dosage for fluoride supplements that are used for children between the ages of 6 months and 16 years. Many bottled waters do not contain optimal amounts of fluoride. **Table 10.2** shows the recommended fluoride supplement dosage schedule.

Systemic dosing of fluoride supplements is typically prescribed in the form of drops, tablets, or swish-and-swallow solutions.

General dosage forms include tablets and lozenges available in 0.25 mg, 0.50 mg, and 1 mg. Fluoride drops are available in various concentrations, which affects the number of drops per dose. Thus, it is important to specify the concentration of the drops prescribed. A combination fluoride supplement/mouthrinse is also available, with each 5 mL (1 teaspoonful) containing 1 mg of fluoride from 2.20 mg of sodium fluoride and orthophosphoric acid.

Prenatal fluoride

The efficacy of prenatal dietary fluoride supplements in preventing dental caries has been well-established in animal studies. However, well-designed clinical studies to demonstrate the safety and efficacy of prenatal fluoride in preventing caries in human subjects still are lacking. Therefore, no definitive recommendations regarding the use of prenatal fluoride can be made. Furthermore, prenatal dietary fluoride supplements will not affect the permanent dentition because permanent teeth do not begin to develop in utero.

Maximum Recommended Doses

No more than 120 mg of fluoride should be dispensed per household at one time. One tablet of the prescribed dose should be taken per day with water or juice. Taking fluoride supplements with milk and other dairy products is not recommended because they can combine with the calcium to become poorly absorbed calcium fluoride. The tablet strength is determined by the concentration of fluoride in the patient's source of drinking water and the age of the child. **Tables 10.2** and **10.3** show the maximum recommended dose: 1 mg per day.

Dosage Adjustments

The actual maximum dose for each patient must be individualized depending on the patient's weight, age, physical status, and other dietary sources of fluoride intake. Reduced doses may be indicated for patients based on changes in their water supply's fluoride content, which may result from relocation or any adverse side effects experienced.

Special Dental Considerations

Drug Interactions of Dental Interest

Calcium-containing products and food interfere with the absorption of systemic fluoride.

Cross-Sensitivity

Allergic rash and other idiosyncratic reactions have rarely been reported. Gastric distress, headache, and weakness have been reported in cases of excessive ingestion.

Special Patients

Fluoride supplements are not recommended for patients other than children with high caries risk who live in areas with fluoride levels such as those described in **Table 10.2**.

Patient Monitoring: Aspects to Watch

Fluoride supplements can cause fluorosis in children living in areas where drinking water contains fluoride levels at or above 0.6 ppm (see **Table 10.2**).

Adverse Effects and Precautions

No adverse reactions or undesirable side effects have been reported when fluoride supplements have been taken as directed. Excessive use may result in dental fluorosis, especially in areas where the fluoride level in drinking water is high. Therefore, fluoride supplements are not recommended where the water content of fluoride is at or above 0.6 ppm.

In children, acute ingestion of 10 mg to 20 mg of sodium fluoride can cause excessive salivation and gastrointestinal disturbances. Ingestion of 500 mg can be fatal. Oral or intravenous fluids containing calcium, or both, may be indicated.

Precautions

If the fluoride level is unknown, the drinking water must be tested for fluoride content before supplements are prescribed. For testing information, ask the local or state health department or dental school. Determining a proper dosage schedule can be a complex task if a patient has exposure to a number of different water supplies. Once a proper schedule is established, however, the effectiveness of the schedule requires the patient's long-term compliance.

Contraindications

The fluoride dosage schedule was designed to take into account the widespread use of fluorides that can contribute to the increased frequency and severity of fluorosis. Fluoride supplements are contraindicated for children drinking water with fluoride concentrations at or above 0.6 ppm.

Pharmacology

Mechanism of action/effect

After early studies showed that fluoride reduced the solubility of powdered enamel and dentin, investigators began trying to determine how fluoride works to reduce dental caries. However, the mechanism(s) of action is still incompletely understood. Nevertheless, fluoride is thought to work topically. It has been speculated that a combination of actions work to reduce the severity and frequency of dental caries, which is the result of excessive demineralization in the demineralization-remineralization process. This excessive demineralization occurs after repeated acid attacks that result when bacterial plaque metabolizes sugars ingested during meals and snacks. Clinical manifestations of dental caries become evident when demineralization predominates over time and upsets the demineralization-remineralization equilibrium. Fluoride reduces the demineralization of enamel and dentin by reducing the acid production of bacterial plaque and decreasing the solubility of apatite crystals. When fluoride is exposed to apatite crystals, it readily becomes incorporated to reduce the dissolution of apatite during acid attacks. The presence of fluoride, therefore, inhibits demineralization and helps to maintain the equilibrium between demineralization and remineralization during acid attacks.

Absorption

Fluoride is absorbed in the gastrointestinal tract, 90% of it in the stomach. Calcium, iron, and magnesium ions may delay absorption.

Distribution

After absorption, 50% of fluoride is deposited in bones and teeth in healthy young adults, 80% in children. Bones and teeth account for 99% of the fluoride taken up by the body.

Elimination

The major route of excretion is the kidneys. Fluoride is also excreted by the sweat glands, the tear glands, the gastrointestinal tract, and in breast milk.

Patient Advice

- Advise patients and their parents or caregivers to take systemic fluorides as directed.
- Patients or their parents or guardians should notify the prescriber when their water supply has changed as the result of a move, a change in schools, or by the addition of fluoride to the water supply.
- Fluoride products should be kept from children's reach; they are often formulated to have a pleasant taste and children therefore are more likely to consume them if they are easily accessible.

TOPICALLY APPLIED FLUORIDES

Accepted Indications

Topically applied preparations are used in the prevention and treatment of dental caries. Concentrations of ≤1,500 ppm can be sold as over-the-counter preparations for the prevention of dental caries. Preparations that are prescribed for topical home use generally consist of higher concentrations of fluoride and are indicated for both treatment and prevention. Patients who are either at high risk of developing dental caries or who experience high caries rates are candidates for daily use of these products. However, high-concentration preparations that are usually applied annually in children are applied to prevent caries.

Some kinds of fluoride compounds at certain concentrations can be used to reduce dentinal hypersensitivity. Sodium fluoride (151,000 ppm fluoride ion), in equal amounts of kaolin and glycerin, has been shown to be effective for this purpose when professionally applied and burnished into affected areas using orangewood sticks. A water-free 0.4% (1,000 ppm fluoride ion) stannous fluoride gel has also been demonstrated to reduce dentinal hypersensitivity when patients use it daily at home. A dentifrice containing 0.454% stannous fluoride and 5% potassium nitrate also has been shown to reduce dentin hypersensitivity. Further, a stabilized 0.454% stannous fluoride toothpaste has been shown to reduce plaque activity, gingivitis, and dentinal hypersensitivity (see **Chapter 11**).

General Dosing Information

Topical dosing is typically provided in the form of liquid solutions, gels, foams, varnishes, pastes, rinses, and dentifrices. Concentrations can vary depending on oral health and sensitivity, the particular indication involved, region of treatment, response to previous or existing concentrations and doses of fluoride as well as individual patient characteristics such as age, weight, physical status, and ability to effectively rinse and expectorate. See **Table 10.4**.

Doses of topically applied solutions, gels, foams, and varnishes are typically applied with a cotton swab, a toothbrush, a carrier, or as a rinse. To control the dosing of high fluoride concentrations so that excessive amounts of fluoride are not in the mouth and to control salivary contamination, use of cotton rolls, a saliva ejector, or high vacuum suction is recommended. Because varnishes are applied to adhere to teeth for prolonged periods, all residual fluoride is swallowed. Between 0.3 and 0.5 mL of varnish is used per patient, meaning about 5 mg to 11 mg is ingested. This amount is consistent with ingestion calculations for other professionally applied fluoride preparations.

With fluoride dentifrices, brushing more than twice a day may be required, but this depends on the patient's caries risk. A 0.4% stannous fluoride gel might be considered as an alternative to brushing with a dentifrice, however. In this way, the patient can receive the benefit of the same fluoride exposure as with the dentifrice without a dentifrice's cleansing properties, which may not be necessary.

Maximum Recommended Doses

The maximum recommended doses for topical fluoride formulations per procedure or appointment are listed in **Table 10.4**.

Dosage Adjustments

The actual maximum dose for each patient can be individualized depending on the patient's age and physical status, ability to effectively rinse and expectorate, and oral health and sensitivity.

Special Dental Considerations

Cross-Sensitivity

Although allergies to fluoride probably do not exist, patients may be allergic to some of the ingredients in the various formulations. Some of the 1.23% acidulated phosphate fluoride solutions and gels as well as some dentifrices contain tartrazines used as color additives. They can cause allergic reactions, especially in patients with hypersensitivity to aspirin.

Adverse Effects and Precautions

Excessive ingestion of fluoride products can produce acute and chronic effects. Ingestion of quantities of fluoride as low as 1 mg per day have been shown to produce mild fluorosis in a small percentage of the population if the ingestion takes place during tooth crown development. The severity and frequency of fluorosis can increase in a population if the recommended dose is exceeded and if the quantity of daily fluoride ingestion increases. Chronic fluoride toxicity, or skeletal fluorosis, may occur after years of daily ingestion of 20 mg to 80 mg of fluoride; however, such heavy doses are far in excess of the average intake in the United States. There is no evidence that skeletal changes are produced by ingestion of therapeutic doses of fluoride.

Accidental ingestion of fluoride, >120 mg in the form of fluoride supplements and mouthrinses or >260 mg in a toothpaste, can cause gastrointestinal disturbances such as excessive salivation, nausea, vomiting, abdominal pain, and diarrhea. Central nervous system disturbances that have been observed include irritability, paresthesia, tetany, and convulsions. Respiratory failure and cardiac failure have also been observed. See **Table 10.4**.

Therefore, as a precautionary measure, no large quantities of fluoride-containing products should be stored in the home. The ADA recommends that no more than 120 mg should be prescribed at one time in the form of mouthrinses and supplements and no individual toothpaste tube should contain more than 260 mg of fluoride. Toothpaste may contain the greater quantity of fluoride because dentifrice humectants and detergents induce vomiting.

Laboratory studies have shown that low-pH topical fluoride preparations react with glass and quartz filler particles in resin-based composites and dental ceramics (porcelains). Although this reaction is not noticeable after one application, the cumulative effect of several applications may compromise the esthetic appearance of these kinds of restorations. Therefore, it is prudent to consider using nonacidic fluoride preparations with patients who have extensive ceramic and composite restorations when daily applications are required.

Pharmacology

See the discussion earlier in this chapter.

Patient Advice

Although the gel form of 2% neutral sodium fluoride may be more easily applied, clinical evidence of its effectiveness has not been demonstrated. The original application schedule was four times per year and was for children at the specific ages of 3, 7, 10, and 13 years. Currently the caries-inhibiting properties of this solution are considered to be equivalent to the APF gels and solutions, which contain a higher concentration of fluoride (12,300 ppm).

SUGGESTED READING

Adair SM. Evidence-based use of fluoride in contemporary pediatric dental practice. *Pediatr Dent*. 2006 Mar-Apr;28(2):133-142; discussion 192-198.

American Dental Association Council on Scientific Affairs. Professionally applied topical fluoride. Evidence-based clinical recommendations. *JADA*. 2006;137(8):1151-1159.

Centers for Disease Control and Prevention, National Center for Chronic Disease Prevention and Health Promotion, Division of Oral Health. Recommendations for using fluoride to prevent and control dental caries in the United States. *MMWR Recomm Rep*. 2001 Aug 17;50(RR-14):1-42.

Ismail AI, Hasson H. Fluoride supplements, dental caries, and fluorosis: a systematic review. *JADA*. 2008;139(11):1457-1468.

Levy SM. Review of fluoride exposures and ingestion. *Community Dent Oral Epidemiol*. 1994;22(3):173-180.

Marinho VCC, Higgins JPT, Logan S, Sheiham A. Fluoride gels for preventing dental caries in children and adolescents. *Cochrane Database Systematic Rev*. 2002, Issue 1. Art. No.: CD002280. DOI: 10.1002/14651858. CD002280.

Marinho VCC, Higgins JPT, Logan S, Sheiham A. Fluoride varnishes for preventing dental caries in children and adolescents. *Cochrane Database Systematic Rev*. 2002, Issue 1. Art. No: CD002279. DOI: 10.1002/14651858. CD002279.

Marinho VCC, Higgins JPT, Logan S, Sheiham A. Fluoride toothpastes for preventing dental caries in children and adolescents. *Cochrane Database Systematic Rev*. 2003, Issue 1. Art. No.: CD002278. DOI: 10. 1002/14651858. CD002278.

Marinho VCC, Higgins JPT, Logan S, Sheiham A. Fluoride mouthrinses for preventing dental caries in children and adolescents. *Cochrane Database Systematic Rev*. 2003, Issue 3. Art. No.: CD002284. DOI: 10.1002/14651858. CD002284.

Marinho VCC, Higgins JPT, Logan S, Sheiham A. Topical fluoride (toothpastes, mouthrinses, gels or varnishes) for preventing dental caries in children and adolescents. *Cochrane Database Systematic Rev*. 2003, Issue 4. Art. No.: CD002782. DOI: 10.1002/14651858. CD002782.

Marinho VCC, Higgins JPT, Sheiham A, Logan S. Combination of topical fluoride (toothpastes, mouthrinses, gels, varnishes) versus single topical fluoride for preventing dental caries in children and adolescents. *Cochrane Database Systematic Rev*. 2004, Issue 1. Art. No.: CD002781. DOI: 10.1002/14651858. CD002781.pub2.

Newbrun E. Current regulations and recommendations concerning water fluoridation, fluoride supplements, and topical fluoride agents. *J Dent Res*. 1992;71(5):1255-1265.

Twetman S, Axelsson S, Dahlgren H, et al. Caries-preventive effect of fluoride toothpaste: a systematic review. *Acta Odontol Scand*. 2003 Dec;61(6):347-355.

Twetman S, Petersson L, Axelsson S, et al. Caries-preventive effect of sodium fluoride mouthrinses: a systematic review of controlled clinical trials. *Acta Odontol Scand*. 2004 Aug;62(4):223-230.

Warren DP, Chan JT. Topical fluorides: efficacy, administration, and safety. *J Acad Gen Dent*. 1997;45(2):134-140, 142.

Whitford GM, Allmann DW, Shaked AR. Topical fluoride: effects on physiologic and biochemical process. *J Dent Res*. 1987;66(5):1072–1078.

Table 10.1. SUGGESTED FLUORIDE REGIMENS ACCORDING TO CARIES RISK AND AGE

<6 YEARS	6 TO 18 YEARS	>18 YEARS
LOW CARIES RISK*		
Optimally fluoridated (0.7-1.2 ppm fluoride ion) water or fluoride supplement after 6 months old, twice daily fluoride toothpaste after 2 years.	Optimally fluoridated (0.7-1.2 ppm fluoride ion) water or fluoride supplement to 16 years old, twice daily fluoride toothpaste.	Optimally fluoridated (0.7-1.2 ppm fluoride ion) water, twice daily fluoride toothpaste.
MODERATE CARIES RISK		
Optimally fluoridated (0.7-1.2 ppm fluoride ion) water or fluoride supplement after 6 months old, twice daily fluoride toothpaste after 2 years, fluoride varnish applications every 6 months.	Optimally fluoridated (0.7-1.2 ppm fluoride ion) water or fluoride supplement to 16 years old; twice daily fluoride toothpaste; over-the-counter fluoride mouthrinse or gel; fluoride varnish, gel, foam, or solution every 6 months.	Optimally fluoridated (0.7-1.2 ppm fluoride ion) water; twice daily fluoride toothpaste; over-the-counter fluoride mouthrinse or gel; fluoride varnish, gel, foam, or solution every 6 months.
HIGH CARIES RISK		
Optimally fluoridated (0.7-1.2 ppm fluoride ion) water or fluoride supplements after 6 months old, twice daily fluoride toothpaste after 2 years, prescription topical fluoride product, fluoride varnish every 3 to 6 months.	Optimally fluoridated (0.7-1.2 ppm fluoride ion) water; twice daily fluoride toothpaste; over-the-counter fluoride mouthrinse or gel or prescription topical fluoride product; fluoride varnish, gel, foam, or solution every 3 to 6 months.	Optimally fluoridated (0.7-1.2 ppm fluoride ion) water; twice daily fluoride toothpaste; over-the-counter fluoride mouthrinse or gel or prescription topical fluoride product; fluoride varnish, gel, foam, or solution every 3 to 6 months.

ALL AGES: Application time for gel and foam should be 4 minutes. Evidence of foam effectiveness is not as strong as fluoride gel or varnish, but foam does offer lower fluoride dosing, which reduces the risk associated with ingestion.

* Application of professionally applied fluoride products is dependent on clinical judgment and patient preference.

ADA Council on Scientific Affairs. Professionally applied topical fluoride. Evidence-based clinical recommendations. *JADA.* 2006;137(8):1151-1159.
Copyright © 2006 American Dental Association. All rights reserved. Adapted 2009 with permission of the American Dental Association.

Table 10.2. DOSAGE FOR SYSTEMIC FLUORIDE SUPPLEMENTS*

AGE	FLOURIDE ION LEVEL DRINKING WATER (PPM) †		
	< 0.3	0.3-0.6	> 0.6
Birth-6 months	None	None	None
6 months-3 years	0.25mg/day‡	None	None
3-6 years	0.50mg/day	0.25mg/day	None
6-16 years	1.0mg/day	0.50mg/day	None

* Recommended dosage schedule of the American Dental Association, the American Academy of Pediatric Dentistry, and the American Academy of Pediatrics.
† 1.0 ppm = 1mg/liter.
‡ 2.2mg sodium fluoride contains 1mg fluoride ion.

Table 10.3. PRESCRIBING INFORMATION FOR FLUORIDE SUPPLEMENTS

NAME/STRENGTH	FORM/BRAND(S)	CHILD DOSAGE*	MAX CHILD DOSAGE
Sodium fluoride, drops—2mg/mL fluoride	**Drops:** Luride, Pediaflor	½ dropperful = 0.25mg 1 dropperful = 0.5mg 2 droppersful = 1mg	Prescribe no more than 200mL per household.
Sodium fluoride, drops—2.5mg/mL fluoride	**Drops:** Karidium	2 drops = 0.25mg 4 drops = 0.5mg 8 drops = 1mg	Prescribe no more than 30mL per household.
Sodium fluoride, drops—2.5mg/mL fluoride	**Drops:** Fluor-A-Day	2 drops = 0.25mg 4 drops = 0.5mg 8 drops = 1mg	Prescribe no more than 30mL per household.
Sodium fluoride, drops—5mg/mL flouride	**Drops:** Fluoritab, Flura-Drops	1 drop = 0.25mg 2 drops = 0.5mg 4 drops = 1mg	Prescribe no more than 23mL per household.
Sodium fluoride, tablets and lozenges—0.25mg fluoride	**Tablets:** Fluor-A-Day, Fluoritab, Luride Lozi-Tabs **Lozenges:** Fluor-A-Day	1 tablet or lozenge per day taken with water or juice and dissolved in mouth or chewed	Prescribe no more than 480 tablets or lozenges per household.
Sodium fluoride, tablets and lozenges—0.5mg fluoride	**Tablets:** Fluor-A-Day, Fluoritab, Luride Lozi-Tabs **Lozenges**: Fluor-A-Day, Fluorodex, Pharmaflur 1.1	1 tablet or lozenge per day taken with water or juice and dissolved in mouth or chewed	Prescribe no more than 240 tablets or lozenges per household.
Sodium fluoride, tablets and lozenges—1mg fluoride	**Tablets:** Fluor-A-Day, Fluoritab, Flura-Loz, Luride Lozi-Tabs **Lozenges:** Fluor-A-Day, Pharmaflur, Pharmaflur df	1 tablet or lozenge per day taken with water or juice and dissolved in mouth or chewed	Prescribe no more than 120 tablets or lozenges per household.

*These supplements are for children only. There is no dose for adult or geriatric patients.

Table 10.4. PRESCRIBING INFORMATION FOR TOPICAL FLUORIDES

NAME	DOSAGE†	WARNINGS/PRECAUTIONS & CONTRAINDICATIONS	ADVERSE EFFECTS
PROFESSIONALLY APPLIED FLUORIDE PRODUCTS			
Acidulated phosphate fluoride solutions, gels and foams (1.23% fluoride ion, 12,300 ppm fluoride ion) (AllSolutions APF Foam or Gel, Butler APF Fluoride Foam or Gel, Laclede, Oral-B Minute Foam, Care-4, Fluorident, FluoroCare Time Saver, Oral-B Minute Gel, Perfect Choice, Pro-DenRx, Puff Fluoride Foam, Topex 00:60 Second Fluoride Foam, Gel or Rinse)	***Adults:*** 5mL (approximately one-third of a tray) of solution or gel with 12,300 ppm fluoride ion per fluoride carrier; apply for 4 min once/yr or more frequently as needed. **Max:** 10mL.	**W/P:** Some preparations may contain tartrazines (FDC Yellow No. 5), which are used as color additives; tartrazine can cause allergic reactions, including bronchial asthma. Allergic response is rare, but is frequently observed in patients who also experience hypersensitivity to aspirin. **Contra:** Patients allergic to tartrazine.	(CNS) Inadvertent ingestion can produce headaches and weakness; more severe instances of excessive ingestion can cause CNS problems such as irritability, paresthesia, tetany, convulsions, respiratory failure, and cardiac failure; fluoride has direct toxic action on nerve tissue. (GI) Excessive salivation, nausea, vomiting. (Hema) Excessive amounts of fluoride can also cause electrolyte disturbances leading to hypocalcemia and hyperkalemia; hypoglycemia is a result of failure of enzyme systems. (Musc) Fluoride has a direct toxic action on muscle and nerve tissue.
2% neutral sodium fluoride solutions, gels, or foams (0.90% fluoride ion, 9,050 ppm fluoride ion) (AllSolutions Fluoride Foam or Rinse; Butler Neutral Fluoride Foam, Gel or Rinse; FluoroCare Neutral; Neutra-Foam; Oral-B Neutrafoam; Pro-DenRx Gel or Rinse; Topex Neutral pH)	***Adults:*** 5mL (approximately one-third of a tray) of solution, gel, or foam with 9,050 ppm fluoride ion per fluoride carrier; apply once/yr or more frequently as needed. **Max:** 10mL.	**W/P:** Not to be used with other professionally applied topical fluoride preparations.	(CV) Excessive amounts of fluoride can produce cardiac failure. (CNS) Excessive amounts of fluoride can produce irritability, paresthesia, tetany, convulsions; fluoride has direct toxic action on nerve tissue. (GI) Excessive amounts of fluoride can produce GI disturbances such as excess salivation, nausea, abdominal pain, vomiting, and diarrhea. (Hema) Excessive amounts of fluoride can cause electrolyte disturbances leading to hypocalcemia and hyperkalemia. Hypoglycemia is a result of enzyme systems failure. (Musc) Fluoride has direct toxic action on muscle tissue. (Resp) Excessive amounts of fluoride can produce respiratory failure.
Fluoride-containing varnishes, 5% sodium fluoride (2.26% fluoride ion, 22,600 ppm fluoride ion) (AllSolutions Varnish, CavityShield, Duraflor, Duraphat, Fluor Protector, Varnish America)	***Adults:*** 0.3-0.5mL of varnish containing 22,600 ppm fluoride ion after dental prophylaxis. **Max:** 0.5mL.	**W/P:** Not to be used in conjunction with other high-concentration topical fluoride solutions when varnish is applied to all tooth surfaces; use of some formulations can result in a temporary yellow discoloration of teeth, which patient can brush away 2-6 hrs after fluoride application.	(CNS) Inadvertent ingestion can produce headaches and weakness; more severe instances of excessive ingestion can cause CNS problems such as irritability, paresthesia, tetany, convulsions, respiratory failure, and cardiac failure; fluoride has direct toxic action on nerve tissue. (Hema) Excessive amounts of fluoride can also cause electrolyte disturbances leading to hypocalcemia and hyperkalemia; hypoglycemia is a result of failure of enzyme systems. (Musc) Fluoride has a direct toxic action on muscle and nerve tissue.
Fluoride prophylaxis pastes (0.40%-2% fluoride ion, 4,000-20,000 ppm fluoride) (Butler Fluoride Prophylaxis Paste, Butler NuCare Prophy Paste with Novamin, Glitter, Masnasil, Post Prophy, Prophy Gems, Radent, Teledyne Waterpik Prophylaxis Paste, Topex, Unipro Prophy Paste, Zircon F, Ziroxide)	***Adults:*** Use amount sufficient to polish the teeth (4,000-20,000 ppm fluoride ion). **Max:** Use no more than the amount required to polish the teeth.	**W/P:** Should be thoroughly rinsed from mouth on completion of prophylaxis.	(Oral) Excessive polishing may remove more fluoride from the enamel surface than fluoride prophylaxis paste can replace.

† Geriatric dosage is same as adult dosage.

Table 10.4. PRESCRIBING INFORMATION FOR TOPICAL FLUORIDES *(cont.)*

NAME	DOSAGE†	WARNINGS/PRECAUTIONS & CONTRAINDICATIONS	ADVERSE EFFECTS
PRESCRIPTION FLUORIDES			
1.1% neutral or acidulated sodium fluoride gel or dentifrice (0.50% fluoride ion, 5,000ppm fluoride ion) (Cavarest, ControlRx, EtheDent, Karigel-N, Luride Lozi-Tabs, Oral-B Neutracare, NeutraGard Advanced Gel, PreviDent Gel, PreviDent 5000 Booster, PreviDent 5000 Plus, Pro-DenRx 1.1% Plus, Theraflur-N)	***Adults/Pediatrics:*** 4-8 drops on inner surface of each custom-made tray per day (5,000 ppm fluoride ion). **Max:** Maximum amount prescribed is one 24-mL plastic squeeze bottle; maximum adult dose is 16 drops/day.	**W/P:** Repeated use of acidulated fluoride has been shown to etch glass filler particles in composite restorations and porcelain crowns, facings, and laminates. As with all fluoride products, children <6 yrs should be supervised to prevent their swallowing the product, which can lead to fluorosis, nausea, and vomiting.	(Oral) Patients with mucositis may report irritation to the acidulated preparation.
0.2% neutral sodium fluoride rinses (0.09% fluoride ion, 905 ppm fluoride ion solution) (CaviRinse, NaFrinse, Oral-B Fluorinse, PreviDent Dental Rinse)	***Adults/Pediatrics:* ≥6 yrs:** Recommended for use by children (905 ppm fluoride ion solution): 10mL (2mg fluoride); swish for 1 min, then spit out the solution; use once/day.	**Contra:** Should not be used in children <6 yrs because they cannot rinse without significant swallowing and this product is not for systemic use. Should not be swallowed by children of any age and should be kept from their reach.	(General) Allergic reaction could result from flavoring agent. (GI) Nausea and vomiting may result from inadvertent swallowing. (Oral) Irritation of oral tissues, especially in children with mucositis, may result from alcohol that might be part of the formulation.
0.044% sodium fluoride and acidulated phosphate fluoride rinse (0.02% fluoride ion) (OrthoWash)	***Adults:*** 10mL once daily after brushing (200 ppm fluoride ion solution).	NA	NA
OVER-THE-COUNTER FLUORIDES			
Fluoride-containing dentifrices (0.10-0.15% fluoride ion, 1,000-1,500 ppm fluoride ion)‡	***Adults/Pediatrics:*** Amount sufficient to cover toothbrush bristles: ≈1g per day (1,000-1,500 ppm fluoride ion). **Max:** Twice a day or more as recommended.	**W/P:** To prevent fluorosis, supervise children <6 yrs so that swallowing does not occur. Accidental ingestion of a single dose, which contains 1-2mg of fluoride ion, is not harmful. Intentional ingestion of large amounts of fluoride toothpaste can cause gastric irritation, nausea, and vomiting. No single container should exceed 260mg of fluoride ion (it is thought that quantity of fluoride in dentifrice can exceed the 120-mg limit ADA has established for other fluoride-containing products because dentifrices contain humectants and detergents that induce vomiting).	(General) Allergic reactions thought to be caused by flavoring agents in some formulations (mint-flavored products have been reported to cause these reactions; however, as a variety of flavoring agents is available, patient should be advised to change to another flavor until a suitable product is found).
0.4% stannous fluoride gels (0.10% fluoride ion, 1,000 ppm fluoride ion) and rinses (Alpha-Dent★, Easy-Gel, Florentine II, Gel-Kam, Gel-Kam Oral Rinse, Gel-Tin, Kids Choice★, Omnii Gel★, Omnii Just for Kids★, Oral-B Stop, Perfect Choice, Periocheck Oral Med★, PerioMed, Plak Smacker★, Pro-DenRx★, Schein Home Care, Super-Dent, Tandem Perio Rinse, Topex Take Home Care)	***Adults/Pediatrics:*** Amount sufficient to cover toothbrush bristles: ≈1g per day (1,000 ppm fluoride ion). **Max:** Once a day or more as recommended.	**W/P:** Children <6 yrs should be supervised to prevent swallowing and fluorosis; accidental ingestion of a single dose (1- to 2-mg ribbon of gel) is not harmful. Intentional ingestion of large amounts of gel can cause gastric irritation, nausea, and vomiting. No single container should exceed 120mg of fluoride.	(General) Allergic reactions thought to be caused by flavoring agents in some formulations (mint-flavored products have been reported to cause these reactions; however, as a variety of flavoring agents is available, patient should be advised to change to another flavor until a suitable product is found). Reversible black stain may occur in pits and fissures and along cervical aspect of a tooth or teeth.

NA = not available. † Geriatric dosage is same as adult dosage. ‡ See Table 9.3 in Chapter 9 for a list of products. § Private label manufacturer.

★ indicates a product bearing the ADA Seal of Acceptance. There are a significant number of generic and store-brand fluoride products that carry the ADA seal. For a complete listing of ADA-accepted OTC products, visit *www.ada.org/ada/seal/index.asp*.

NAME	DOSAGE†	WARNINGS/PRECAUTIONS & CONTRAINDICATIONS	ADVERSE EFFECTS
0.0221% sodium fluoride rinses (0.01% fluoride ion) (ACT Restoring Anticavity (33 oz), Listerine Smart Rinse for Kids, Listerine Total Care)	***Adults/Pediatrics:* ≥6 yrs:** 10mL of solution with 100 ppm fluoride ion. **Max:** Rinse for 1 min, twice daily.	**W/P:** Children <6 yrs generally should not use this product because of their inability to rinse without swallowing; otherwise, accidental ingestion of a single dose is not harmful. Intentional ingestion of several doses can cause gastric irritation, nausea, and vomiting. Some of these products contain alcohol to promote solubility of flavoring agents; these products should be kept out of children's reach and in childproof caps/packaging.	(General) Allergic reactions thought to be caused by flavoring agents in some formulations (mint-flavored products have been reported to cause these reactions; however, as a variety of flavoring agents is available, patient should be advised to change to another flavor until a suitable product is found).
0.044% sodium fluoride and acidulated phosphate fluoride rinse (0.02% fluoride ion) (Phos-Flur Anti-Cavity Fluoride Rinse★)	***Adults/Pediatrics:* ≥6 yrs:** 10mL of solution with 200 ppm fluoride ion. **Max:** Rinse for 1 min, once daily.	**W/P:** Children <6 yrs generally should not use this product because of their inability to rinse without swallowing; otherwise, accidental ingestion of a single dose is not harmful. Intentional ingestion of several doses can cause gastric irritation, nausea, and vomiting. Some product flavors contain alcohol to promote solubility of flavoring agents; these products should be kept out of children's reach and in childproof caps/packaging.	(General) Allergic reactions thought to be caused by flavoring agents in some formulations (mint-flavored products have been reported to cause these reactions; however, as a variety of flavoring agents is available, patient should be advised to change to another flavor until a suitable product is found).
0.05% sodium fluoride rinses (0.02% fluoride ion) (ACT Anticavity★, ACT Anticavity for Kids★, ACT Restoring Anticavity (18 oz), Equate Anticavity★, Fluorigard,Hannaford Anticavity★, H.E. Buddy Anticavity★, Hello! Anticavity★, Hill Country Anticavity★, NaFrinse Acidulated Oral Rinse, NaFrinse Neutral/Daily Mouthrinse, Publix Anticavity★, Publix Kids Anticavity★, REACH ACT Restoring, Rite Aid Anticavity★, Sunmark Anticavity★, Swan Anticavity★§,The Natural Dentist Healthy Teeth★, Tom's of Maine Natural Anticavity★, Vi-Jon Anticavity★§, Weis Anticavity★, Western Family Anticavity★)	***Adults/Pediatrics:* ≥6 yrs:** 10mL of solution with 230 ppm fluoride ion. **Max:** Rinse for 1 min, once daily.	**W/P:** Children <6 yrs generally should not use this product because of their inability to rinse without swallowing; otherwise, accidental ingestion of a single dose is not harmful. Intentional ingestion of several doses can cause gastric irritation, nausea, and vomiting. Some of these products contain alcohol to promote solubility of flavoring agents; these products should be kept out of children's reach and in childproof caps/packaging.	(General) Allergic reactions thought to be caused by flavoring agents in some formulations (mint-flavored products have been reported to cause these reactions; however, as a variety of flavoring agents is available, patient should be advised to change to another flavor until a suitable product is found).

Chapter 11

Desensitizing Agents

Martha Somerman, D.D.S., Ph.D.

Dentin hypersensitivity is characterized by a sharp pain produced in response to mild stimuli that usually disappears with removal of the stimulus. Root sensitivity is a significant problem for many individuals and may be a result of, or associated with, scaling and root planing, periodontal surgery, gingival recession, toothbrush abrasion, attrition, erosion, trauma, or chronic periodontal disease. It is important to rule out active pathology (eg, root fracture or root surface decay) before providing treatment for root sensitivity. In many situations, root sensitivity decreases with time. When it does not, it results in extreme discomfort or an inability to eat or drink certain foods, inability to function outdoors in cold weather and, at times, poor oral hygiene that can result in periodontal-related problems. Unfortunately, *ideal* over-the-counter and professional desensitizing agents with predictable outcomes have not been developed.

Desensitizing agents can be separated into two types: agents applied to the tooth by a practitioner and agents that are for home use. **Table 11.1** provides information about currently available products for use in the clinical setting, as well as some products available for home use. A major concern with products for home use is the abrasiveness of the paste; however, all ADA-accepted toothpastes have safe levels of abrasive materials.

The use of hydrostatic pressure to increase diffusion of agents into the dentinal tubules has been evaluated for several years with some indication that hydrostatic pressure may result in better desensitizing effects vs. topical application alone.

IN-OFFICE PRODUCTS

Accepted Indications

In-office desensitizing agents are used to provide relief from thermal and tactile sensitivity on exposed root surfaces when pathological causes for pain have been ruled out. Agents containing fluoride also provide an anticaries function. In addition, some remineralization agents have been reported to have desensitizing properties and thus are included in **Table 11.1**. Differential diagnoses for dentinal hypersensitivity are listed in **Table 11.2**.

Some of the desensitizing agents may be applied in conjunction with iontophoresis, which is the electrical transport of positively or negatively charged drugs across surface tissues. One of the uses of iontophoresis in dentistry is in the treatment of dentinal hypersensitivity with fluoride. Usually a 1% sodium fluoride solution is employed. Results are variable, and the time and cost of the treatment may limit patients' acceptance of it. Nd:YAG and CO2 lasers also have been used for treating root sensitivity; however, results are not conclusive, and long-term effects on pulp have not been investigated.

General Usage Information

Usage and Administration for Adults and Children

See **Table 11.1** for information on usage and administration. As with any agent, if pain persists or worsens, the situation should be reevaluated. Therefore, continued sensitivity, after ruling out other symptoms, can be treated by changing the product versus increasing the dose. Use of increased amounts, beyond those shown in **Table 11.1**, has not been reported to be effective in decreasing sensitivity. Additionally, before using pastes or gels containing desensitizing agents in children <12 years, consult a dentist or physician; supervision is recommended for children <6 years.

Special Dental Considerations

- Fluorides interact with calcium-containing products—for example, to form calcium fluoride, which is poorly absorbed.
- Certain agents, such as chlorhexidine, may decrease fluoride's ability to bind to root surfaces. Thus, after using fluoride agents, the patient should not rinse or eat for 1 hour.
- Because products with calcium sodium phosphosilicates do not contain fluoride, individuals may require additional agents/rinses with fluoride for caries control; fluoride products should be used at least 1 hour after the sensitivity treatment.
- Some agents are acidic and thus may cause sensitivity in patients with mucositis.
- Some acidic compounds, such as oxalate, may cause dulling of porcelain ceramics and decreased effectiveness of bonding cements. Therefore, surfaces treated with oxalate should be pumiced before a bonding agent is used.
- Home-use desensitizing agents should be stored out of reach of children.

Special Patients

Pregnant and nursing women

There is no evidence that desensitizing agents are harmful to pregnant women or when used by nursing women. While a minimal amount does cross the placental barrier if these agents are ingested and traces also are found in breast milk, no contraindications are reported when these agents are used as recommended.

Pediatric, geriatric, and other special patients

In children, ingestion of high levels of fluoride will cause fluorosis of teeth and osseous changes. In older patients, there is no evidence suggesting a need to modify existing procedures.

Patient Monitoring: Aspects to Watch

- Persistent or increased pain: may require re-evaluation of differential diagnosis as well as consideration of alternative agents, therapies, or both.

Adverse Effects and Precautions

Fluorides

Fluoride preparations should be kept out of reach of children. On rare occasions, adverse reactions to fluorides, including skin rash, GI upset, and headaches, may be noted. Such reactions are reversible upon discontinuing use. Fluoride should not be swallowed.

Patients with gingival sensitivity may be sensitive to the acidity of certain fluoride solutions.

Acidic fluoride solutions may cause dulling of porcelain and ceramic restorations.

Oxalates

Acids may decrease the effectiveness of bonding cements; thus, teeth treated with oxalates should be pumiced before application of bonding agents.

Varnishes, Sealants, and Bonding Agents

Copal-based products, such as Zarosen, cannot be used with bonding agents. No other adverse effects or precautions have been reported.

Pharmacology

The general principle guiding the development of desensitizing agents is that the number of dental tubules exposed to the mouth correlates with sensitivity; thus, many of the agents are designed to occlude tubules. The most popular theory, the "hydrodynamic theory," is that sensitivity in this situation results from the movement of fluid through the exposed tubules, which results in activation of the nerves within the pulp, subsequently registered as pain. A strategy used to decrease sensitivity, based on the hydrodynamic theory, includes the development of agents that can depolarize nerves directly.

Another theory of dentin hypersensitivity is that of the "dentinal receptor mechanism," which proposes that odontoblasts play a more receptive role; however, agents that induce pain normally fail to evoke pain when applied to exposed dentin. Yet a third theory is that certain polypeptides present within the pulp can modulate nerve impulses within the pulp. Thus, therapies have been directed at agents or procedures or both that can depolarize nerves directly.

More recent approaches for occluding dental tubules include the use of proteins, peptides, and/or amino acids that interact with calcium. It is believed that this interaction results in enhanced sealing of the tubules vs current strategies. Such agents on the market include the phosphoprotein casein (found in GC Tooth Mousse) and the amino acid arginine (found in Sensitive Pro-Relief Desensitizing Paste with Pro-Argin).

Patient Advice

- Patients should be aware that, in general, several factors must be carefully considered in treatment of tooth sensitivity: severity of the problem, physical findings, and past treatment. Proper diagnosis is required before initiation of treatment, whether in office or at home.
- Patients must realize that use of a desensitizing agent may not prove effective over a short time (for example, <2 weeks).

HOME-USE PRODUCTS

Accepted Indications

Desensitizing toothpaste agents are used to provide relief from thermal and tactile sensitivity on exposed root surfaces when pathological causes for pain have been ruled out. In addition, many of these toothpastes contain fluoride to prevent caries.

General Usage Information

Usage and Administration

See **Table 11.1** for general usage information on desensitizing toothpastes.

Special Dental Considerations

Following are special dental considerations for home use desensitizing agents, which are the same as or very similar to those for in-office products listed earlier in this chapter.

Drug Interactions of Dental Interest

There is some suggestion of interaction of fluorides with calcium-containing products, for example, formation of calcium fluoride, which is poorly absorbed.

- Certain agents, such as chlorhexidine, may decrease fluoride's ability to bind to root surfaces. Thus, after using fluoride agents, the patient should not rinse or eat for 1 hour.
- Some agents are acidic and thus may cause sensitivity in patients with mucositis.
- Some acidic compounds, such as oxalate, may cause dulling of porcelain ceramics and decreased effectiveness of bonding

cements. Therefore, pumicing the root surface before use of some desensitizing agents is recommended.

Special Patients

There is no evidence that desensitizing agents are harmful to pregnant women or during breast feeding. In children, high levels of fluoride will cause fluorosis of teeth and osseous changes. In older patients, no alteration of dose is required.

Patient Monitoring: Aspects to Watch

- Persistent or increased pain may require re-evaluation of differential diagnosis and consideration of alternative agents, therapies, or both.

Adverse Effects and Precautions

No adverse effects are reported beyond those related to high-dose fluoride. Precautions include the underlying possibility of an undiagnosed serious dental problem that may need prompt dental care. Products should not be used for more than four weeks unless recommended by the dentist. Keep out of reach of children. All patients, and especially those with severe dental erosion, should brush properly and lightly with any dentifrice to avoid further removal of tooth structure.

Pharmacology

The general principle guiding development of desensitizing agents, including toothpastes, is that the number of dental tubules exposed to the mouth correlates with sensitivity; thus, most agents are designed to occlude tubules. The most popular theory is that sensitivity in this situation is due to the movement of fluid through the exposed tubules, which results in activation of the nerves within the pulp and subsequently is registered as pain.

Patient Advice

- In general, several factors must be carefully considered in treatment of tooth sensitivity: problem severity, physical findings, and past treatment. Proper diagnosis is required before initiation of treatment, whether in office or at home.
- Use of a desensitizing agent will not prove effective over a short time unless the product is used for at least 2 weeks.

SUGGESTED READING

Azarpazhooh A, Limeback H. Clinical efficacy of casein derivatives: a systematic review of the literature. *JADA*. 2008;139:915-924.

Gaffar A. Treating hypersensitivity with fluoride varnishes. *Compend Contin Educ Dent*. 1998;19(11):1088-1090.

Hamlin D, Phelan Williams K, Delgado E, Zhang YP, DeVizio W, Mateo LR. Clinical evaluation of the efficacy of a desensitizing paste containing 8% arginine and calcium carbonate for the in-office relief of dentin hypersensitivity associated with dental prophylaxis. *Am J Dent*. 2009;22(special issue A):16A-20A.

Kleinberg I. Sensistat: A new saliva based composition for simple and effective treatment of dentinal sensitivity pain. *Dent Today*. 2002;21:42-47.

Lier BB, Rosing CK, Aass AM, et al. Treatment of dentin hypersensitivity by Nd:YAG laser. *J Clin Periodontol*. 2002;29:501-506.

Neuman L, Romano J, eds. *Dentin Hypersensitivity: Consensus-Based Recommendations for the Diagnosis & Management of Dentin Hypersensitivity*. Oct 2008;4 (#9, Special Issue). A supplement to *Inside Dentistry*.

Olusile AO, Bamise CT, Oginni AO, Dosumu OO. Short-term clinical evaluation of four densentizing agents. *J Contemp Dent Pract*. 2008;9(1):22-29.

Orchardson R, Gillam DG. Managing dentin hypersensitivity. *JADA*. 2006;137:990-998.

Poulsen S, Errboe M, Lescay Mevil Y, Glenny AM. Potassium containing toothpastes for dentin hypersensitivity. *Cochrane Database Syst Rev*. Jul 19 2006;3:CD001476.

Schiff T, Delgado E, Zhang YP, Cummins D, DeVizio W, Mateo LR. Clinical evaluation of the efficacy of an in-office desensitizing paste containing 8% arginine and calcium carbonate in providing instant and lasting relief of dentin hypersensitivity. *Am J Dent*. 2009;22(special issue A):8A-15A.

Zhang C, Matsumoto K, Kimura Y, et al. Effects of CO_2 laser in treatment of cervical dentinal hypersensitivity. *J Endod*. 1998;24(9):595-597.

SUGGESTED READING

Table 11.1. USAGE INFORMATION FOR DESENSITIZING PRODUCTS

NAME	FORM/CONTENT	USAGE AND ADMINISTRATION	WARNINGS/PRECAUTIONS & CONTRAINDICATIONS
DESENSITIZING AGENTS*†			
Arginine, Calcium Carbonate, Sodium Monofluorophosphate (Sensitive Pro-Relief Desensitizing Paste with Pro-Argin)	**Paste:** 8% arginine, calcium carbonate, sodium monofluorophosphate (60 unit-dose cups [0.07 oz], 3-oz tube)	***Adults:*** In-office treatment followed by home use as directed. In-office directions: 1. Place enough paste for one procedure in a clean dappen dish or other suitable container. 2. Fill a rotary cup with paste and run rotary cup at low to moderate speed. 3. Polish product into each tooth, on sensitive areas or areas that can become sensitive (can be applied to entire dentition). Apply product to sensitive area for 3 seconds, then repeat.	**P/N:** Effects on pregnancy and nursing are unknown.
Chlorhexidine/HEMA (HemaSeal & Cide)	**Liquid**	***Adults:*** Use as directed.	**P/N:** Effects on pregnancy and nursing are unknown.
Fluoride Ion (Butler APF Fluoride Foam, Butler Neutral Fluoride Foam, Butler APF Fluoride Gel, Butler Neutral Fluoride Rinse)	**Foam:** 1.23% (Butler APF Fluoride Foam), 0.9% (Butler Neutral Fluoride Foam); **Gel:** 1.23% (Butler APF Fluoride Gel), 0.9% (Butler Neutral Fluoride Gel); **Rinse:** 0.9% (Butler Neutral Fluoride Rinse)	***Adults:*** Use as directed.	NA
Oxalate Products (Bis-Block, dentin conditioners, D'Sense Crystal, MS-Coat, Pain-Free, Protect, Sensodyne Sealants, SuperSeal)	**Liquid** (aluminum oxalate, potassium oxalate, or potassium mono-oxalate)	***Adults:*** Dry dentin surface; dispense 10-12 drops into plastic dappen dish; apply saturated cotton pellets to sensitive area for 1 full minute; use light pressure and do not burnish; have patients expectorate after application; to overcome pain threshold, sequential 1-minute treatments may be required. Do not apply with wooden stick.	**W/P:** For chairside treatment of dentinal hypersensitivity, acidic reagents remove smear layer and demineralize root surface (and may also leave crystals of calcium oxalate on the root surfaces), which may decrease effectiveness of bond cements and adhesives' interaction with the root surface; therefore, surfaces treated with an oxalate should be pumiced before a bonding agent is used. **P/N:** Effects on pregnancy and nursing are unknown.
Potassium Nitrate (Den-Mat Desensitize)	**Kit**	***Adults:*** Use as directed.	**W/P:** Do not exceed recommended dose. **Contra:** Do not use in areas where water fluoride content is greater than 0.6 ppm; some brands of tablets contain too much fluoride for certain age groups or for use in areas of higher water fluoride content. If pain persists more than 4 weeks, patients should be re-evaluated to determine cause of sensitivity. **P/N:** Effects on pregnancy and nursing are unknown.
Potassium Nitrate (Professional Tooth Desensitizing Gel)	**Gel**	***Adults:*** Use as directed.	**W/P:** Do not exceed recommended dose. **Contra:** Do not use in areas where water fluoride content is greater than 0.6 ppm; some brands of tablets contain too much fluoride for certain age groups or for use in areas of higher water fluoride content. If pain persists more than 4 weeks, patients should be re-evaluated to determine cause of sensitivity. **P/N:** Effects on pregnancy and nursing are unknown.

NA = Not available.
*Mode of action: seals dentinal tubules and reduces fluid shifting.
†Mode of action: has been shown to form particles that block dentinal tubules, thereby providing temporary relief from pain.

Table 11.1. USAGE INFORMATION FOR DESENSITIZING PRODUCTS *(cont.)*

NAME	FORM/CONTENT	USAGE AND ADMINISTRATION	WARNINGS/PRECAUTIONS & CONTRAINDICATIONS
DESENSITIZING AGENTS*† *(cont.)*			
Potassium Nitrate, Fluoride (UltraEZ)	**Gel**	***Adults:*** Use as directed.	**W/P:** Do not exceed recommended dose. **Contra:** Do not use in areas where water fluoride content is greater than 0.6 ppm; some brands of tablets contain too much fluoride for certain age groups or for use in areas of higher water fluoride content. If pain persists more than 4 weeks, patients should be re-evaluated to determine cause of sensitivity. **P/N:** Effects on pregnancy and nursing are unknown.
Potassium Nitrate, Triclosan †† (Triclosan, triclosan with fluoride)	**Paste:** 5% potassium nitrate, 0.3% triclosan; also available with various fluoride strengths	***Adults:*** Apply at least a 1-inch strip of toothpaste onto a soft-bristle toothbrush. Brush teeth thoroughly for at least 1 minute twice a day or as recommended.	**W/P:** Do not exceed recommended dose. **Contra:** Do not use in areas where water fluoride content is greater than 0.6 ppm; some brands of tablets contain too much fluoride for certain age groups or for use in areas of higher water fluoride content. If pain persists more than 4 weeks, patients should be re-evaluated to determine cause of sensitivity. **P/N:** Effects on pregnancy and nursing are unknown.
Sodium Fluoride (Crayola Kids Fluoride Anticavity Toothpaste)	**Paste:** 0.239%	***Pediatrics:*** Use as directed.	**W/P:** Do not exceed recommended dose. **Contra:** Do not use in areas where water fluoride content is greater than 0.6 ppm; some brands of tablets contain too much fluoride for certain age groups or for use in areas of higher water fluoride content. If pain persists more than 4 weeks, patients should be re-evaluated to determine cause of sensitivity. **P/N:** Effects on pregnancy and nursing are unknown.
Sodium Fluoride, Neutral (NiteWhite NSF)	**Liquid**	***Adults:*** Apply in a tray and wear as directed for 5 min/day.	**W/P:** Caution in use of fluorides as desensitizing agents in children owing to possibility of fluorosis. **P/N:** Effects on pregnancy and nursing are unknown.
Sodium Fluoride (Sultan Sodium Fluoride Paste)	**Paste:** 33.50%	***Adults:*** Burnish onto sensitive area using an orangewood stick for 1 minute; followed by rinsing; to overcome pain threshold, sequential 1 minute treatments may be required.	**W/P:** Do not exceed recommended dose. **Contra:** Do not use in areas where water fluoride content is greater than 0.6 ppm; some brands of tablets contain too much fluoride for certain age groups or for use in areas of higher water fluoride content. If pain persists more than 4 weeks, patients should be re-evaluated to determine cause of sensitivity. **P/N:** Effects on pregnancy and nursing are unknown.

★ indicates a product bearing the ADA Seal of Acceptance. For a complete listing of ADA-accepted OTC products, visit *www.ada.org/ada/seal/index.asp.*
NA = Not available.
*Mode of action: seals dentinal tubules and reduces fluid shifting.
†Mode of action: has been shown to form particles that block dentinal tubules, thereby providing temporary relief from pain.
††Triclosan may have anti-inflammatory properties.

NAME	FORM/CONTENT	USAGE AND ADMINISTRATION	WARNINGS/PRECAUTIONS & CONTRAINDICATIONS
Sodium Fluoride, Potassium Nitrate (Aquafresh SensitiveTeeth, Arm & Hammer Dentacare, Butler Maximum Strength Sensitive Toothpaste, Crest Sensitivity Extra Whitening Toothpaste, Crest Sensitivity Protection Soothing Whitening Mint Paste★, Crest Sensitivity Whitening Plus Scope Toothpaste, Desensitize Plus, Oral-B Sensitive, Protect Sensitive Teeth, Sensodyne Cool Gel, Sensodyne ProNamel, Sensodyne Tartar Control, Sensodyne w/ Fluoride Tartar Control, Sensodyne w/ Fluoride/Baking Soda, Tom's of Maine Natural Sensitive Anticavity Toothpaste★ & Gel Toothpaste★)	**Paste:** 5% potassium nitrate	***Adults:*** Apply at least a 1-inch strip of toothpaste onto a soft bristle toothbrush. Brush teeth thoroughly for at least 1 minute twice a day or as recommended. ***Pediatrics:*** **<12 yrs:** Dentist or physician should be consulted before children use this product. **<6 yrs:** Children should be supervised when using this product; keep out of reach of children.	**W/P:** Do not exceed recommended dose. **Contra:** Do not use in areas where water fluoride content is greater than 0.6 ppm; some brands of tablets contain too much fluoride for certain age groups or for use in areas of higher water fluoride content. If pain persists more than 4 weeks, patients should be re-evaluated to determine cause of sensitivity. **P/N:** Effects on pregnancy and nursing are unknown.
Sodium Fluoride, Stannous Fluoride (Gel-Kam Dentin Block)	**Gel**	***Adults:*** Dry dentin surface; dispense 10-12 drops into plastic dappen dish; apply saturated cotton pellets to sensitive area for 1 full minute; use light pressure and do not burnish; have patients expectorate after application; to overcome pain threshold, sequential 1-minute treatments may be required. Do not apply with wooden stick.	**W/P:** Caution in use of fluorides as desensitizing agents in children owing to possibility of fluorosis. **P/N:** Effects on pregnancy and nursing are unknown.
Sodium Fluorescein (Plak-Check)	**Sol:** 0.75%	***Adults:*** Use as directed.	NA
Sodium Monofluorophosphate, Potassium Nitrate (Den-Mat Sensitive, Orajel Sensitive Pain-Relieving Toothpaste, Oral-B Sensitive, Rembrandt Whitening Sensitive, Sensodyne Fresh Mint, Sensodyne Original, Sensodyne w/Fluoride)	**Paste:** 5% potassium nitrate	***Adults:*** Apply at least a 1-inch strip of toothpaste onto a soft-bristle toothbrush. Brush teeth thoroughly for at least 1 minute twice a day or as recommended. ***Pediatrics:*** **<12 yrs:** Dentist or physician should be consulted before children use this product. **<6 yrs:** Children should be supervised when using this product; keep out of reach of children.	**W/P:** Do not exceed recommended dose. **Contra:** Do not use in areas where water fluoride content is greater than 0.6 ppm; some brands of tablets contain too much fluoride for certain age groups or for use in areas of higher water fluoride content. If pain persists more than 4 weeks, patients should be re-evaluated to determine cause of sensitivity. **P/N:** Effects on pregnancy and nursing are unknown.
Stannous Fluoride (Stani-Max Pro)	**Liq:** 3.28%	***Adults:*** Dilute 1:1 with water, preferably distilled water to provide a 1.64% SnF_2 rinse. Use in-office irrigation or rinse. Recommended rinse after scaling and root planning.	**W/P:** Caution in use of fluorides as desensititizing agents in children owing to possibility of fluorosis. **P/N:** Effects on pregnancy and nursing are unknown.
Stannous Fluoride, Potassium Nitrate (Colgate Sensitive Maximum Strength, Colgate Sensitive Maximum Strength plus Whitening)	**Paste:** 5% potassium nitrate	***Adults:*** Apply at least a 1-inch strip of toothpaste onto a soft-bristle toothbrush. Brush teeth thoroughly for at least 1 minute twice a day or as recommended. ***Pediatrics:*** **<12 yrs:** Dentist or physician should be consulted before children use this product. **<6 yrs:** Children should be supervised when using this product; keep out of reach of children.	**W/P:** Do not exceed recommended dose. **Contra:** Do not use in areas where water fluoride content is greater than 0.6 ppm; some brands of tablets contain too much fluoride for certain age groups or for use in areas of higher water fluoride content. If pain persists more than 4 weeks, patients should be re-evaluated to determine cause of sensitivity. **P/N:** Effects on pregnancy and nursing are unknown.
Stannous Fluoride, Sodium Fluoride, Hydrogen Fluoride (Gel-Kam, ProDentx Comfort Desensitizer, Dentiblock Dentin Desensitizer, ProDentx Office Fluorides)	**Paste:** 0.4% stannous fluoride, 1.09% sodium fluoride, 0.14% hydrogen fluoride	***Adults:*** Dry dentin surface; dispense 10-12 drops into plastic dappen dish; apply saturated cotton pellets to sensitive area for 1 full minute; use light pressure and do not burnish; have patients expectorate after application; to overcome pain threshold, sequential 1 minute treatments may be required.	**W/P:** Caution in use of fluorides as desensitizing agents in children owing to possibility of fluorosis. **P/N:** Effects on pregnancy and nursing are unknown.

Table 11.1. USAGE INFORMATION FOR DESENSITIZING PRODUCTS *(cont.)*

NAME	FORM/CONTENT	USAGE AND ADMINISTRATION	WARNINGS/PRECAUTIONS & CONTRAINDICATIONS
DESENSITIZING AGENTS*† *(cont.)*			
Stannous Fluoride, Sodium Hexametaphosphate (Crest Pro-Health Toothpaste, Clean Cinnamon or Clean Mint★; Crest Pro-Health Night Toothpaste★; Crest Pro-Health Whitening Toothpaste★)	**Paste:** 0.4% stannous fluoride, sodium hexametaphosphate (strength NA)	***Adults:*** Apply toothpaste onto soft-bristle toothbrush; brush teeth thoroughly for at least 1 min bid (morning and evening) or as recommended by a dentist or physician; make sure to brush all sensitive areas of the teeth. ***Pediatrics:*** **<12 yrs:** Dentist or physician should be consulted before children use this product. **<6 yrs:** Children should be supervised when using this product; keep out of reach of children.	Fluoride products are used for prevention of cavities, and potassium nitrate is considered to decrease dentinal hypersensitivity through nerve inhibition; if pain persists more than 4 weeks, patient should be re-evaluated to determine cause of sensitivity.
Strontium Chloride (Hyposen, Thermodent Toothpaste)	**Paste:** 10%; **Sol**	***Adults:*** Apply at least a 1-inch strip of toothpaste onto a soft-bristle toothbrush. Brush teeth thoroughly for at least 1 min bid or as recommended. Do not apply with wooden stick.	**W/P:** Do not exceed recommended dose. **Contra:** Do not use in areas where water fluoride content is greater than 0.6 ppm; some brands of tablets contain too much fluoride for certain age groups or for use in areas of higher water fluoride content. If pain persists more than 4 weeks, patients should be re-evaluated to determine cause of sensitivity. **P/N:** Effects on pregnancy and nursing are unknown.
Strontium Chloride, Sodium Fluoride (Health-Dent Desensitizer, Hema-Glu Desensitizer)	**Liq:** 3.9% strontium chloride, 0.42% sodium fluoride	***Adults:*** Dry dentin surface; dispense 10-12 drops into plastic dappen dish; apply saturated cotton pellets to sensitive area for 1 full minute; use light pressure and do not burnish; have patients expectorate after application; to overcome pain threshold, sequential 1 minute treatments may be required.	**W/P:** Caution in use of fluorides as desensititizing agents in children owing to possibility of fluorosis. **P/N:** Effects on pregnancy and nursing are unknown.
DEVICES‡/REMINERALIZATION AGENTS			
Calcium Phosphate Desensitizers (D/Sense 2, Quell Desensitizer)	**Paste**	***Adults:*** Use as directed by manufacturer.	**P/N:** Effects on pregnancy and nursing are unknown.
Calcium Sodium Phosphosilicates and other bioactive glass agents (NUPRO NUSolutions Prophy Paste, Oravive, SootheRx)	**Liquid**: 1% NovaMin in sterile water; liquid solution contains 45% SiO_2, 24.5% Na_2O, 24.5% CaO, 6% P_2O_5; **Paste:** 5% NovaMin (Oravive), 7.5% NovaMin (SootheRx); **Powder:** NovaMin, 2μ average particle size	***Adults:*** Use as directed. **Soothe Rx:** Use bid for 2 weeks then once per week thereafter. ***Pediatrics*** **(Soothe Rx):** Not recommended. ***Adults/ Pediatrics*** **(Oravive):** Apply toothpaste onto soft-bristle toothbrush; brush teeth thoroughly for at least 1 min bid (morning and evening) or as recommended by a dentist or physician; make sure to brush all sensitive areas of the teeth. Do not use mouthrinses or eat or drink for at least 30 min after brushing.	Calcium sodium phosphosilicates decrease dentinal hypersensitivity through tubule occlusion; if pain persists more than 4 weeks, patient should be re-evaluated to determine cause of sensitivity.

★ indicates a product bearing the ADA Seal of Acceptance. For a complete listing of ADA-accepted OTC products, visit *www.ada.org/ada/seal/index.asp.*
NA = Not available.
*Mode of action: seals dentinal tubules and reduces fluid shifting.
†Mode of action: has been shown to form particles that block dentinal tubules, thereby providing temporary relief from pain.
‡ Mode of action: Products with NovaMin occlude tubules. Rincinol P.R.N. forms a protective barrier. Protect Desensitizing Solution removes smear layer to expose tubules; calcium and protein plugs form deep in tubules, assisted by varnish.
§ Mode of action: appears to close dentinal tubules, protect pulp, and reduce sensitivity to temperature extremes; compatible with all restorative materials, dental cements, and cavity liners.
¶Mode of action: occludes dentinal tubules.

NAME	FORM/CONTENT	USAGE AND ADMINISTRATION	WARNINGS/PRECAUTIONS & CONTRAINDICATIONS
DEVICES‡/REMINERALIZATION AGENTS *(cont.)*			
Hydroxypropyl Cellulose, Potassium Fluoride, Polyethyleneglycol Dimethacrylate and other methacrylates (Protect Desensitizing Solution)	**Kit**: Bottle (4g), 45 applicator sticks, mixing pad	***Adults:*** Dry tooth and apply liquid with applicator provided. Do not apply with wooden stick.	NA
Sodium Hyaluronate, Polyvinylpyrrolidone, Glycyrrhetinic Acid, Aloe Vera Extract (Rincinol P.R.N. Soothing Oral Rinse)	**Packet:** Each single-dose packet contains bio-adherent mucosal coating	***Adults/Pediatrics:* ≥6 yrs:** Use as directed.	NA
SEALANTS§/ADHESIVES/RESINS/BONDING AGENTS			
Barrier Dental Sealant, Pain-Free Desensitizer (Dentin Protect, Health-Dent Desensitizer, Ivoclar Vivadent, Prime & Bond, Scotch bond)	NA	***Adults:*** Apply chairside according to manufacturer's recommendations.	**P/N:** Effects on pregnancy and nursing are unknown.
Casein Derivatives (GC Tooth Mousse, MI Paste, Recaldent)	**Paste:** casein phosphopeptides (CPP), amorphous calcium phosphate (CPP-ACP)	***Adults:*** Apply chairside according to manufacturer's recommendations.	**P/N:** Effects on pregnancy and nursing are unknown.
Light-cured Adhesives (Seal & Protect, Vitrebond-Lite)	**Liquid**	***Adults:*** Apply chairside according to manufacturer's recommendations.	**P/N:** Effects on pregnancy and nursing are unknown.
Methacrylate Polymer (All-Bond DS Desensitizer, MicroPrime, Confi-Dental, Gluma Desensitizer, Glu/Sense, Hema Seal G)	NA	***Adults:*** Apply chairside according to manufacturer's recommendations.	**P/N:** Effects on pregnancy and nursing are unknown.
Polyethylene Glycol Dimethacrylate and Glutaraldehyde (Systemp Densensitizer)	**Liq:** 35% polyethylene glycol dimethacrylate, 5% glutaraldehyde	***Adults:*** Apply chairside according to manufacturer's recommendations.	**P/N:** Effects on pregnancy and nursing are unknown.
VARNISHES¶			
Chlorhexidine (CHX) Dental Varnish (Cervitec Plus)	**Lig:** 1% CHX, 1% thymol	***Adults:*** After isolating the area and drying, apply topically to all tooth surfaces and instruct patient to avoid eating for 3 hrs and brushing teeth for 24 hrs, according to manufacturer's recommendations.	**W/P:** CHX is known to interact with fluoride. CHX/thymol varnish has been reported to control caries by controlling bacteria in selected individuals and to reduce root sensitivity.
Sodium Fluoride Solutions (Cavity Shield, Duraflor, Duraphat, Fluoline, Fluor Protector, Fluocal solution, Omni Varnish, PreviDent Clear, Waterpik UltraThin)	**Tubes:** 50mg/mL, 10mL	***Adults:*** Apply chairside according to manufacturer's recommendations.	**W/P:** Not to be used with other professional-applied topical fluoride preparations. **P/N:** Effects on pregnancy and nursing are unknown.
Strontium Chloride, Copal Resin (Zarosen)	**Liq:** 0.145% strontium chloride, 6.9% copal resin	***Adults:*** Apply topically to dentin, enamel, or cementum with cotton or brush; wipe dry with cotton roll or gauze pad; do not dry with air syringe.	**W/P:** Not to be used with other professional-applied topical fluoride preparations. **P/N:** Effects on pregnancy and nursing are unknown.

Table 11.2. DIFFERENTIAL DIAGNOSES FOR DENTINAL HYPERSENSITIVITY

PATHOLOGY	SIGNS AND SYMPTOMS	CLINICAL EVALUATION
Bleaching sensitivity	Thermal sensitivity	History of recent home/office bleaching procedure
Chipped tooth	Thermal sensitivity, pain from abrasion	Visual examination
Cracked tooth	Pain from pressure (biting)	Percussion, biting, application of dye to disclose fracture
Dental caries	Thermal sensitivity (cold), pain from pressure	Radiographic or clinical examination
Dentin hypersensitivity	Sharp, sudden, short pain; thermal sensitivity; pain from abrasion	Osmotic solution, thermal testing, mechanical abrasion, electrical vitality test
Fractured restoration	Thermal sensitivity, pain from pressure	Visual examination, biting on plastic or wood sticks
Marginal leakage	Thermal sensitivity, pain from pressure	Radiographic and clinical examination
Periodontal disease	Inflamed and bleeding tissues, loose teeth, pain from pressure	Radiographic and clinical examination
Postoperative sensitivity	Thermal sensitivity with moderate short pain	History of recent operative work
Pulpitis	Pain from pressure	Radiographic and clinical examination
Trauma from occlusion	Thermal sensitivity, pain from pressure, mobility, wear facets, short pain	Occlusal equilibration

Chapter 12

Bleaching Agents

B. Ellen Byrne, D.D.S., Ph.D.; Frederick McIntyre, D.D.S., M.S.

Tooth-bleaching agents can be classified as to whether they are used for external or internal bleaching and whether the procedure is performed in the office by a dentist or at home by a patient. For tooth bleaching, hydrogen peroxide (H_2O_2) is used alone at levels of 15% to 35% or at 10% to 44% levels in a stable gel of carbamide peroxide (urea peroxide) that breaks down to form hydrogen peroxide (3.35% hydrogen peroxide from 10% carbamide peroxide), urea, ammonia, and carbon dioxide.

The terms "whitening" and "bleaching," unfortunately, have been used interchangeably. While the mechanism is not completely understood, bleaching involves free radicals and breakdown of pigment, while whitening is accomplished by abrasive agents in the dentifrice (see **Chapter 9**).

INTERNAL BLEACHING

Internal bleaching produces reliable results when used to eliminate intrinsic stains in dentin caused by blood breakdown products or endodontics or for stains in receded pulp chambers. However, bleaching should be confined to the dentin; bleaching the cementum, which provides an attachment for the periodontal ligament, has been associated with external root resorption. External root resorption below the gingival attachment is associated with internal bleaching on nonvital teeth that have sustained trauma, poorly sealed canal spaces, or heating during the bleaching procedure. It is felt that the bleaching agent diffuses through the dentinal tubules and initiates an inflammatory resorptive response in the cervical area. Unfortunately, external cervical resorption is not seen for approximately five to six years after internal bleaching. The use of heat is not essential and should be avoided whenever possible.

Internal bleaching is always performed in the dental office. There are two common approaches to internal bleaching: the "office bleach" (a one-time application) and the "walking bleach" (sealed inside the tooth for two to three days). The office bleaching agent is a mixture of 30% to 35% hydrogen peroxide and perborate, to which heat has been applied by the use of a hot instrument, such as a ball burnisher or an electric heat-producing instrument, for two to five minutes to accelerate the bleaching process. However, heat also has been associated with external root resorption and should not be used (see above).

Walking bleach seals the hydrogen peroxide and perborate mixture inside the tooth for two to three days. The sodium perborate, a stable, water-soluable white powder, decomposes into sodium metaborate and hydrogen peroxide, thus releasing nascent oxygen. The sodium perborate, which is mixed with the hydrogen peroxide, also releases oxygen. This combination is thought to be synergistic and very effective in bleaching. There is evidence that sodium perborate may be safer alone than in combination with 30% to 35% hydrogen peroxide. Since sodium perborate is slower-acting than the combination, it requires a longer therapeutic period when used alone. This technique is called "walking bleach" because the bleaching process actually occurs between dental appointments, during which time the bleaching agents are sealed in the pulp chamber.

EXTERNAL BLEACHING

External bleaching is indicated for teeth that are discolored from aging, fluorosis, or staining due to the effects of tetracycline. External bleaching can be applied by the dentist or staff or can be applied by the patient in home-use bleaching. When dentist-administered and home-use bleaching are used together, it is called "dual or combination bleaching." An application in the office of a high-concentration hydrogen-peroxide agent is followed by a professionally dispensed and supervised product for at-home use for five days, often followed by an additional chairside application.

Dentist-applied external bleaching can be accomplished with periodically repeated use of an office-bleaching agent. Dentist-applied bleaching procedures can be divided into two types:

- Power bleaching with high concentrations of hydrogen peroxide (30% to 40%)
- Assisted bleaching with high concentrations of carbamide peroxide (35% to 44%)

The power bleaching systems are gels that either are premixed or can be prepared chair-side by the mixing of liquid bleach with powder. These products are caustic and, thus, can cause significant soft-tissue injury. The safest, most reliable gingival protection is a properly placed, sealed rubber dam. Assisted bleaches can be used to boost a home-bleaching program or as an easier, low-cost, in-office bleaching method. Because carbamide peroxide is not as strong as hydrogen peroxide, it cannot yield the same results. Even though these assisted bleaches are not as caustic as high concentrations of hydrogen peroxide, they do have the capability to irritate the gingiva.

An etching gel containing phosphoric acid that is applied to selected dark areas increases the penetration of the bleach. Light is used to produce heat, which reportedly accelerates the bleaching process. Current studies have produced equivocal results with some touting the benefits and others concluding there is not benefit. The light/heat source can be a visible curing light, overhead operatory light, light-emitting diode (LED), plasma arc, or argon laser. Externally bleached teeth may need touch-up treatment every six months or one year. Severely stained teeth may require more frequent retreatment (see **Table 12.1**).

Home bleaching, supervised by the dentist, is done by the patient at home using a custom-made plastic carrier that holds the bleach against the patient's teeth. After the desired result is achieved, overnight use on a periodic basis (one to four times per month) or daily use of a whitening dentifrice can maintain the lightening that has been achieved.

These products vary in their viscosity, flavor, and packing. Most of the home-use bleaches are supplied with material for bleaching trays. In addition, these products contain various concentrations of carbamide peroxide, hydrogen peroxide, or both. The concentrations of carbamide peroxide range from 10% to 22%; the hydrogen peroxide concentrations range from 4.5% to 9.5%. Bleaching agents are available for the patient to purchase over the counter. The product may contain hydrogen peroxide or carbamide peroxide. The delivery system varies with the product. Currently, hydrogen peroxide is available impregnated into a thin, flexible, textured strip made of polyethylene, or incorporated into mouthrinses. Carbamide peroxide is available as a gel to be used in bleaching trays. Fluoride, potassium nitrate, or both have been added to some products to reduce tooth sensitivity. The majority of side effects involving tooth sensitivity resolve within 24 to 48 hours after discontinuing use of the product.

External bleaching is seldom permanent, lasting approximately six months to two years, after which teeth gradually return to their original color. Usually, the younger the patient, the longer the bleaching will last. The more difficult it is to bleach a tooth, the more likely it is to discolor again. Bluish-gray stains seem to reappear more quickly than yellow stains. Because reoccurrence of staining is unpredictable, promises about longevity should not be made. Internal bleaching usually lasts longer than external bleaching. Some manufacturers offer post treatment "touch up" kits to extend the longevity of the bleaching effect.

The patient must understand that the bleaching agent will not lighten resin-based composite restorations as much as it will natural tooth structure. While there is evidence that resin-based composites will bleach, the results may not match those achieved in natural tooth structure. Patients should be informed that existing restorations will need to be replaced. There is in vitro evidence supporting the fact that bonding of resin-based composites to etched enamel after vital bleaching procedures results in a decreased bond strength. However, within hours to days, the bond strength returns to that achieved with nonbleached enamel. Restoration replacement should be delayed for about 48 hours to allow for return of bond strength and color rebound after bleaching.

Over-the-Counter Treatments

Over-the-counter treatments include whitening strips, paint-on brush applications, and dentifrices. The toothpastes marketed as whitening products typically contain mild abrasives and minimal amounts of peroxide. Whitening strips use 6.5% hydrogen peroxide; the paint-on brush kits contain 18% carbamide peroxide as the whitening agent. Due to decreased bleaching concentrations and reduced contact time, the OTC products must be used longer to obtain similar results as compared to the professionally prescribed products.

Accepted Indications

Types and causes of tooth discoloration and response to bleaching are provided in **Table 12.1**. Information on in-office bleaching techniques, dentist-supervised home bleaching, and OTC home bleaching agents is provided in **Table 12.2**. Brown, blue-gray, and gray stains are usually caused by caries, porphyria, fluorosis, dentinogenesis imperfecta, and erythroblastosis fetalis. They need microabrasion and restorative care and should not be bleached.

General Usage Information

Maximum Recommended Amounts

Average treatment time is generally two to six weeks. More difficult cases require extended treatment and may result in teeth that look chalky. In some patients, stains relapse when treatment is discontinued.

Usage Adjustments

Adults

When having bleaching done at the dental office, some patients, especially those with severe erosion, abrasion, or recession, may find the combination of heat and peroxide uncomfortable. These patients are not good candidates for office bleaching. For at-home bleaching, the recommended wearing time varies greatly; the wearing times are determined by the clinical study designs and vary considerably between products. The daily dosage is between one-half hour and 10 hours for one or two treatments per day.

Special Dental Considerations

Drug Interactions of Dental Interest

Possible interactions with bleaching agents are provided in **Table 12.3**.

Special Patients

Pregnant and nursing women

The long-term effects of using in-office or home bleaching agents on the teeth of pregnant women have not been studied; therefore, women who are pregnant or who have a reasonable expectation that they could become pregnant should not undergo treatment. Pregnancy risk category has not been determined.

Pediatric, geriatric, and other special patients

Bleaching agents have been used on the permanent teeth of children aged 10 to 14 years.

Patient Monitoring: Aspects to Watch

Long-term use can alter normal oral flora and contribute to lingual papillary hypertrophy (hairy tongue) and *Candida albicans*.

Adverse Effects and Precautions

See **Table 12.4** for adverse effects, precautions, and contraindications for in-office and home use of bleaching agents.

Pharmacology

The mechanism of tooth bleaching is not fully understood; however, it is felt that the unstable peroxide breaks down to highly unstable free radicals. These free radicals chemically break larger pigmented organic molecules in the enamel matrix into smaller, less pigmented constituents. Higher concentrations, such as 30% or higher, of hydrogen peroxide remove the enamel matrix, thereby creating microscopic voids that scatter light and increase the appearance of whiteness until remineralization occurs and the color partly relapses. When the morphology of unbleached teeth is compared to that of teeth that have been treated with lower concentrations of peroxide, such as carbamide peroxide 10%, the latter seem not to be affected; therefore, different bleaching materials and concentrations may have different modes of action.

The addition of carbopol, a carboxypolymethylene polymer, prolongs the release of hydrogen peroxide from carbamide peroxide. Carbopol, a water-soluble resin used in many household products such as shampoo and toothpaste, is used as a thickening agent. It does not break down, nor does it increase the breakdown of the bleaching agent. The carbopol binds to the peroxide and triples or quadruples the active release time of peroxide. Products without carbopol are more fluid and bleach more slowly due to the reduced activity time and greater loss of bleach from the tray. See the ADA's statement on the safety of home-use tooth whitening products below.

Patient Advice

The following advice pertains to patients who are using home bleaching agents:

- The more treatments per day, the faster the bleaching; however, this concentrated use of bleaching agents can also increase sensitivity.
- The bleaching agent should be tightly capped and refrigerated.
- Do not wear the bleaching appliance while eating.
- Discontinue treatment with the bleaching agent if the teeth, gums, or bite become uncomfortable.
- The dentist should check the patient's mouth every one to six weeks to ensure that no damage has been done to the teeth, gums, or dental restorations.
- Use of a whitening dentifrice after treatment may extend the whitening effect of the treatment.

SUGGESTED READING

Albers HF. Lightening natural teeth. *ADEPT Report*. 1991;2(1):1-24.

Dishman MV, Covey DA, Baughan LW. The effect of peroxide bleaching on composite to enamel bond strength. *Dent Mater*. 1994;9(1):33-36.

Harrington GW, Natkin F. External resorption associated with bleaching of pulpless teeth. *J Endod*. 1979;5:344-348.

Haywood VB, Leonard RH, Nelson CF, et al. Effectiveness, side effects and long-term status of nightguard vital bleaching. *JADA*. 1994;125(9):1219-1226.

Heithersay GS. Invasive cervical resorption: an analysis of potential predisposing factors. *Quintessence Int*. 1999;30(2):83-95.

Jorgensen MG, Carroll WB. Incidence of tooth sensitivity after home whitening treatment. *JADA*. 2002;133:1076-1082.

Kihn PW. Vital tooth whitening. *Dent Clin N Am*. 2007;51(2):319-331.

Monaghan P, Trowbridge T, Lautenschlager E. Composite resin color change after vital tooth bleaching. *J Prosthet Dent*. 1992;67:778-781.

Reality: The Information Source for Esthetic Dentistry. Houston: Reality Publishing Co; 1999, 2000, 2001, 2005.

Sarrett DC. The bottom line in office whitening systems. *ADA Professional Product Review*. 2008;3(2):7-12.

ADA STATEMENT ON THE SAFETY AND EFFECTIVENESS OF TOOTH WHITENING PRODUCTS

For more than a decade, the ADA Council on Scientific Affairs has monitored the development and the increasing numbers of whitening oral hygiene products. As the market for these products grew, the Association recognized a need for uniform definitions when discussing whiteners.

For example, "whitening" is any process that will make teeth appear whiter. This can be achieved in two ways. A product can bleach the tooth, which means that it actually changes the natural tooth color. Bleaching products contain peroxide(s) that help remove deep (intrinsic) and surface (extrinsic) stains. By contrast, non-bleaching whitening products contain agents that work by physical or chemical action to help remove surface stains only.

Whitening products may be administered by dentists in the dental office, dispensed by dentists for home-use, or purchased over-the-counter (OTC), and can be categorized into two major groups:

- peroxide-containing whiteners or bleaching agents; and
- whitening toothpastes (dentifrices)

Peroxide-Containing Whiteners or Bleaching Agents

Dentist-dispensed and OTC home-use products

Dentist-dispensed and OTC home-use tooth whitening bleaches are eligible for the ADA Seal of Acceptance (visit *www.ada.org/ada/seal/index.asp* for a complete listing). The products in this category that currently bear the ADA Seal contain 10% carbamide peroxide; however, participation in the program is not limited to products of this concentration or type of bleach. There are many whitening options currently available to consumers both from the dentist as well as from retail outlets. The ADA recommends that if you choose to use a bleaching product you should only do so after consultation with a dentist.

In a water-based solution, carbamide peroxide breaks down into hydrogen peroxide and urea, with hydrogen peroxide being the active bleaching agent. Other ingredients of peroxide-containing tooth whiteners may include glycerin, carbopol, sodium hydroxide and flavoring agents.

Accumulated clinical data on neutral pH, 10% carbamide peroxide continue to support both the safety and effectiveness of this kind of tooth-whitening agent. The most commonly observed side effects to hydrogen or carbamide peroxide are tooth sensitivity and occasional irritation of the soft tissues in the mouth (oral mucosa), particularly the gums. Tooth sensitivity often occurs during early stages of bleaching treatment. Tissue irritation, in most cases, results from an ill-fitting tray rather than the tooth-bleaching agents. Both of these conditions usually are temporary and stop after the treatment.

Professionally applied bleach whiteners

There are many professionally applied tooth whitening bleach products. These products use hydrogen peroxide in concentrations ranging from 15% to 35% and are sometimes used together with a light or laser, which the companies state accelerate or activate the whitening process. Prior to application of professional products, gum tissues are isolated either with a rubber dam or a protective gel. Whereas home-use products are intended for use over a 2- to 4-week period, the professional procedure is usually completed in about 1 hour.

As with the 10% home-use carbamide peroxide bleach products, the most commonly observed side effects of professionally applied hydrogen peroxide products are temporary tooth sensitivity and occasional irritation of oral tissues. On rare occasions, irreversible tooth damage has been reported. Due to the discontinuation of the professional component of the Seal Program on December 31, 2007, professionally applied bleach whiteners are not eligible for the ADA Seal.

The ADA advises patients to consult with their dentists to determine the most appropriate treatment. This is especially important for patients with many fillings, crowns, and extremely dark stains. A thorough oral examination, performed by a licensed dentist, is essential to determine if bleaching is an appropriate course of treatment. The dentist then supervises the use of bleaching agents within the context of a comprehensive, appropriately sequenced treatment plan.

Whitening Toothpastes

Whitening toothpastes (dentifrices) in the ADA Seal of Acceptance program contain polishing or chemical agents, rather than bleaches, to improve tooth appearance by removing surface stains. They do this through gentle polishing, chemical chelation, or some other non-bleaching action. Several whitening toothpastes that are available OTC have received the ADA Seal of Acceptance (visit *www.ada.org/ada/seal/index.asp* for a complete listing).

Editor's note: To check for ADA statement updates, visit *www.ada.org/prof/resources/positions/statements/index.asp*.

Table 12.1. TYPES OF TOOTH DISCOLORATION

COLOR OF STAIN/ETIOLOGY	EASE OR DIFFICULTY OF BLEACHING
White	
Fluorosis	Degree of difficulty depends on extent of fluorosis.
Blue-gray	
Dentinogenesis imperfecta, erythroblastosis fetalis, tetracycline	Deeply stained blue-gray discolorations, especially those associated with tetracycline, are more difficult to treat than yellow stains.
Gray	
Silver oxide from root canal sealers	Dark stains from root canal sealers are seldom bleachable; should be treated restoratively.
Yellow	
Fluorosis, physiological changes due to aging, obliteration of the pulp chamber	Mild uniform yellow discoloration associated with aging or mild uniform fluorosis is easiest to treat.
Brown	
Fluorosis, caries, porphyria, tetracycline, dentinogenesis imperfecta	Stains that are deeper in color are more difficult to treat.
Black	
Mercury stain (amalgam), caries, fluorosis	Very dark or black stains from silver-containing root canal sealers or from mercury are seldom bleachable; should be treated restoratively.
Pink	
Internal resorption	Bleaching is not indicated; treatment consists of endodontics and calcium hydroxide treatment.

Table 12.2. USAGE INFORMATION FOR BLEACHING AGENTS

PROFESSIONALLY APPLIED AGENTS–INTERNAL†	
Hydrogen peroxide 35%	Opalescence Endo; Superoxol (with sodium perborate)
PROFESSIONALLY APPLIED AGENTS–EXTERNAL	
Assisted Bleaches	
Carbamide peroxide 30%	VivaStyle 30%
Carbamide peroxide 35%	Opalescence Quick; Pola Zing; Quick Start; White Speed (35% equivalent; 18% hydrogen peroxide and 22% carbamide peroxide)
Carbamide peroxide 35%	Pola Zing
Carbamide peroxide 44%	Generic
Power Bleaches	
Hydrogen peroxide 15%	BriteSmile Whitening
Hydrogen peroxide 20%	GC TiON in Office Tooth Whitening System
Hydrogen peroxide 22%	Contrast AM
Hydrogen peroxide 25%	Niveous
Hydrogen peroxide 25%	Zoom! Advanced Power Plus Lamp
Hydrogen peroxide 25-27%	GC TiON Whitening In Office Kit, 25%; Niveous, 27%; Zoom Whitening Kit, 25%
Hydrogen peroxide 30-35%	ArcBrite, 30%; Hi Lite, 35%; Illuminé, 30%; Kreativ PowerGel, 35%; Laser Smile, 35%; Luma Arch Bleaching System, 35%; Opalescence Xtra, 35%; Pola Office Kit, 35%; Rembrandt Lightening Plus, 35%; Rembrandt One-Hour, 35%; Virtuoso Lightening, 32%
Hydrogen peroxide 35%	BEYOND Power Whitening System
Hydrogen peroxide 35%	In-Office Whitening System
Hydrogen peroxide 35%	LumaCool Whitening System/LumaWhite Plus Single Patient Kit
Hydrogen peroxide 35%	Perfection White
Hydrogen peroxide 35%	Pola Office
Hydrogen peroxide 36%	NUPRO White Gold
Hydrogen peroxide 37%	LaserSmile Soft Tissue Laser and In-Office Whitening System
Hydrogen peroxide 37.5%	Pola Office
Hydrogen peroxide 38%	Opalescence Boost
Hydrogen peroxide 38%	Opalescence Xtra Boost
Hydrogen peroxide 25%	Sapphire Chairside Whitening with Aftercare
Miscellaneous	
Chlorine dioxide (strength not available)	GentleBright Single Patient Kit
DENTIST-DISPENSED HOME BLEACHING AGENTS	
Carbamide Peroxide	
Carbamide peroxide 6%	VivaStyle Paint On Varnish (6% when applied; concentration is five times higher once dried)
Caramide peroxide 8%	Pola Paint
Carbamide peroxide 10%	Colgate Platinum Daytime Professional Whitening System; Colgate Platinum Overnight Professional Whitening System; Natural Elegance; Nite White Classic; Patterson Brand Toothwhitening; Rembrandt Lighten

†Indications: Yellow or black stains from endodontics or tetracycline; intrinsic stains when teeth have darkened from blood break-down products; or in receded pulp chambers. Usual adult dosage: Sealed into pulp chamber for up to 7 days.

Table 12.2. USAGE INFORMATION FOR BLEACHING AGENTS *(cont.)*

DENTIST-DISPENSED HOME BLEACHING AGENTS *(cont.)*

Carbamide Peroxide *(cont.)*	
Carbamide peroxide 10% and 15%	Nupro White Gold
Carbamide peroxide 10%, 15%, and 20%	Contrast P.M.; Opalescence (10%)★; Opalescence F; Opalescence PF
Carbamide peroxide 10%, 15%, and 22%	Rembrandt Bleaching Gel Plus
Carbamide peroxide 10% and 16%	VivaStyle
Carbamide peroxide 10%, 16%, and 22%	Nite White Excel 3; Nite White Excel 3NSF; Nite White Excel 3Z
Carbamide peroxide 10%, 16%, 22%	Pola Night
Carbamide peroxide 10% and 22%	Gel White; Zaris
Carbamide peroxide 10 to 38%	NightWhite ACP and DayWhite ACP
Carbamide peroxide 10%,16%, 22%	White & Brite
Carbamide peroxide 10%, 15%, 20%, 35%	Opalesecence PF
Carbamide peroxide 11%, 13%, 16%, and 21%	Perfecta Trio
Carbamide peroxide 12%, 16%, 22%, and 30%	Rembrandt Xtra Comfort
Carbamide peroxide 15%	GC TiON Take Home Whitening System
Carbamide peroxide 15% and 20%, with 0.11% fluoride ion	Opalescence F
Carbamide peroxide 15% or 10%	NUPRO White Gold Tooth Take-Home Whiteners
Carbamide peroxide 10%, 15% and 20%, with 0.11% fluoride ion and 3% potassium nitrate	Opalescence PF
Carbamide peroxide 16% and 10%	Star White
Carbamide Peroxide 16% and 22%	Natural Elegance Plus Teeth Whitening Kit
Carbamide Peroxide 16% and 22%	Venus White
Carbamide peroxide 22% and 32%	Sapphire Take Home
Carbamide peroxide 30%, 20%, 15%, 10%	Full-Kit, Mini-Kit, Singles or Bulk-Syringes
Cardamide peroxide 30% and 14% calcium perioxide	Forté
Hydrogen Peroxide	
Hydrogen peroxide 3%, 7.5%, and 9.5%	Poladay
Hydrogen peroxide 4% and 6%	Zoom! Take-Home
Hydrogen peroxide 4.5%	Perfecta 3/15 Extra Strength
Hydrogen peroxide 5%	Colgate Visible White Mint Touch-Up
Hydrogen peroxide 5%	Colgate Visible White Mint Full-Kit
Hydrogen peroxide 5.25%	Zoom! Whitening Pen
Hydrogen peroxide 6%	BEYOND StayWhite
Hydrogen peroxide 6%	Nite White Excel 3 Turbo
Hydrogen peroxide 6%	Zoom! Weekender
Hydrogen peroxide 6 to 9.5%	NightWhite ACP and DayWhite ACP
Hydrogen peroxide 7%	Colgate Visible White Melon Touch-Up
Hydrogen peroxide 7%	Colgate Visible White Mint Touch-Up
Hydrogen peroxide 7%	Colgate Visible White Melon Full-Kit
Hydrogen peroxide 7%	Colgate Visible White Mint Full-Kit
Hydrogen peroxide 7.5%	LumaCool Whitening Pen/Stay Bright Plus Professional Whitening Enhancer

★indicates a product bearing the ADA Seal of Acceptance. For a complete listing of ADA-accepted OTC products, visit *www.ada.org/ada/seal/index.asp.*

DENTIST-DISPENSED HOME BLEACHING AGENTS *(cont.)*

Hydrogen Peroxide *(cont.)*	
Hydrogen peroxide 7.5% and 9.5%	Day White Excel 3
Hydrogen peroxide 9%	Colgate Visible White Melon Touch -Up
Hydrogen peroxide 9%	Colgate Visible White Mint Touch -Up
Hydrogen peroxide 9%	Colgate Visible White Melon Full-Kit
Hydrogen peroxide 9%	Colgate Visible White Mint Full-Kit
Hydrogen peroxide 9%	Pectecta Bravó
Hydrogen peroxide 9%	trèswhite
Hydrogen peroxide 14%	Crest Whitestrips Supreme
Hydrogen peroxide 14%	Pectecta REV!
Hydrogen peroxide 15%	NUPRO White Gold Tooth Take-Home Whiteners

OVER-THE-COUNTER HOME BLEACHING AGENTS

Carbamide Peroxide	
Carbamide peroxide 9%	Power Brush Whitening Gel; Rembrandt Dazzling White Toothpaste; Rembrandt Plus Gel and Toothpaste
Carbamide peroxide 10%	Natural White Extreme Sensitive Toothpaste
Hydrogen Peroxide	
Hydrogen peroxide 0.75%	Mentadent Tooth Whitening System
Hydrogen peroxide 1.5%	Age Defying Whitening Mouthrinse; Rembrandt Plus Peroxide Whitening Rinse
Hydrogen peroxide 2%	Listerine Whitening Pre-Brush Rinse
Hydrogen peroxide 2.5% and 2.7%	Rembrandt 3-in-1; Rembrandt Whitening Wand
Hydrogen peroxide 3%	Age Defying Whitening Toothpaste; Natural White 5-Minute Kit; Natural White Pro; Rapid White
Hydrogen peroxide 4%	Quick White Portable Whitening System
Hydrogen peroxide 5%	Rembrandt 2 Hour White Kit
Hydrogen peroxide 6.5% and 10%	Crest Whitestrips; Crest Whitestrips Premium
Hydrogen peroxide 6% (as 30% PVP-hydrogen peroxide)	Natural White 3-in-3
Hydrogen peroxide 6.3%	Colgate Visible White Clear Whitening Gel
Hydrogen peroxide 8.7%	Colgate Visible White Night Clear Whitening Gel
Hydrogen peroxide (strength not available)	Rembrandt Whitening Pen; Rembrandt Whitening Strips

Table 12.3. POSSIBLE INTERACTIONS WITH BLEACHING AGENTS

Beverages	
Coffee and tea	May compromise treatment results. Advise patients to avoid these beverages.
Heavy use of alcohol	May possibly result in additive carcinogenicity because peroxides have mutagenic potential and may boost the effects of known carcinogens. Advise patients to avoid drinking excessive amounts of alcohol.
Wine, whiskey, and liqueurs	May compromise treatment results. Advise patients to avoid these beverages.
Tobacco	
Heavy use of tobacco	May compromise treatment results; may possibly result in additive carcinogenicity because peroxides have mutagenic potential and may boost the effects of known carcinogens. Advise patients to avoid tobacco products.

Table 12.4. PRECAUTIONS AND ADVERSE EFFECTS FOR BLEACHING AGENTS

PRECAUTIONS	ADVERSE EFFECTS
General	
Patients should not smoke or use other potential carcinogens during treatment.	Prolonged use of 30% or higher H_2O_2 can destroy cells, and for cells that are not destroyed, prolonged use may potentiate the carcinogenic effects of carcinogens.
Oral	
Patients with root sensitivity may not want to have treatment because it can aggravate sensitivity. In cases of tissue burns (see adverse effects at right), rinse affected area for 1-5 min.	Owing to the acidic nature of some of these products, patients can experience transient dentin sensitivity, especially in patients with gingival recession. High concentrations of H_2O_2 used in office bleaching may produce what appear to be tissue burns—white areas on the gingiva that are caused by oxygen gas bubbles and are not true burns, although discomfort can feel like a burn.

Chapter 13

Drugs for Medical Emergencies in the Dental Office

Barry C. Boyd, D.M.D., M.D.; Richard E. Hall, D.D.S., M.D., Ph.D., F.A.C.S.

Medical emergencies can and do occur in dental offices. Successful prevention, recognition, and prompt management of medical emergencies are critical to the safety of patients. Given advancements in medical and surgical care, life expectancy has improved overall. Those improvements mean a large proportion of our dental patient population have one or more serious disease conditions. The medical complexity of the at-risk patient population is ever increasing. All practicing dentists and dental specialists must be prepared for the ever-present possibility of life-threatening medical emergencies developing among their patient families. A three-pronged approach to medical emergencies encompasses *prevention, recognition, and treatment* as emergency situations arise. Successful prevention rests in obtaining and frequently updating a thorough medical history on each and every patient. Obtain vital signs at each visit.

Each professional staff member in every dental office should be trained to recognize and manage any emergency situation that might arise. At a minimum, the doctor and critical clinical staff members must acquire timely Basic Life Support training and certification. Training in basic life support focuses upon recognition and initial nondrug management of cardiopulmonary resuscitation, including the use of the automated external defibrillator (AED).

Those dentists treating especially complex patients, hospital dental providers, and specialists may also be required to obtain and maintain certification in Advanced Cardiac Life Support (ACLS) and Pediatric Advanced Life Support (PALS). Coursework in ACLS and PALS adds additional skills such as arrhythmia recognition and management, advanced airway management, and defibrillation for cardiac arrest victims. In the adult course, additional emphasis is placed upon management of non-arrest acute coronary syndromes (ACS) as well as upon recognition and initial management of stroke victims. As children are infrequent victims of cardiac arrest caused by cardiac disease, cardiac arrest in pediatric patients is more often the result of respiratory arrest, thus emphasis in PALS is given to management of respiratory emergencies aimed at prevention of cardiac arrest.

Although certain categories of emergency drugs are suggested for the dental office emergency kit, it must be emphasized that administering emergency drugs will always be secondary to providing Basic Life Support (BLS) during an emergency.

Because dentists' levels of training in emergency management can vary significantly, it is impossible to recommend any one list of emergency drugs or any one proprietary emergency drug kit that meets the needs and abilities of all dentists. There are several commercially available prepackaged emergency kits appropriate for use in the dental practice. In addition to emergency drugs, many include venipuncture kits, emergency airways, oxygen supply, and wound care materials. If a commercially available kit is not acquired, the practitioner must develop his or her own emergency drug and equipment kits, based on their level of expertise in managing emergencies.

Although no state dental boards have established specific recommendations as to which emergency drugs and equipment a dentist must have available, state boards of dental examiners do mandate that certain drugs and medical emergency armamentaria be available in offices where dentists employ nitrous oxide/oxygen analgesia, enteral sedation, parenteral sedation, or general anesthesia to patients of all ages. Specialty groups, such as the American Dental Society of Anesthesiology, the American Association of Oral and Maxillofacial Surgeons, and the Academy of Pediatric Dentistry, have instituted guidelines for the use of sedation and general anesthesia, which dictate the emergency drugs that must be readily available. The following drug categories are mandated by many state boards of dental examiners for doctors who have been permitted to use oral conscious sedation, parenteral conscious sedation, deep sedation, or general anesthesia:

- oxygen supply
- vasopressors
- corticosteroids
- bronchodilators
- muscle relaxants
- opioid antagonists
- benzodiazepine antagonists
- antihistamines (histamine blocker)
- anticholinergics
- cardiac medications: epinephrine, antidysrhythmic, antianginal
- antihypertensives

Dentists should not include in the emergency kit any drug or piece of emergency equipment for which they are not trained to use. For example, dentists who are not well-trained in tracheal intubation should not include a laryngoscope and endotracheal tubes in their emergency kits; likewise, dentists who are not proficient in venipuncture should not have an anticonvulsant drug, such as diazepam, in their kits because anticonvulsant drugs must be administered intravenously.

Also, dentists should not use anticonvulsants if they are unable to ventilate a patient who is unconscious and apneic, as is likely to occur when anticonvulsant drugs are administered to terminate a seizure.

Table 13.1 lists four levels of drugs and medical equipment that can help the dentist design an emergency kit that will be suitable for the level of emergency preparedness of his or her dental office:

- Level 1 drugs are those deemed most important or critical
- Level 2 drugs are those employed for ACLS
- Level 3 drugs are those employed for PALS
- Level 4 drugs are those used to reverse the clinical actions of previously administered medications

General Dosing Information

Table 13.2 provides dosing information for injectable and noninjectable drugs.

Adverse Effects and Precautions

Table 13.2 lists the adverse effects and precautions related to injectable and noninjectable emergency drugs with other drugs.

Pharmacology

Injectable Drugs

Level 1 (Basic Agents)

Antianginal agent

Morphine sulfate: Morphine exerts its primary effects on the CNS and organs containing smooth muscle. Pharmacological effects include analgesia, drowsiness, euphoria (mood alteration), reduction in body temperature (at low doses), dose-related respiratory depression, interference with adrenocortical response to stress (at high doses), and reduction of peripheral resistance.

Anticonvulsants

Diazepam: Diazepam, a benzodiazepine that acts on parts of the limbic system, thalamus, and hypothalamus, provides anticonvulsant effects reserved for use in the treatment of status epilepticus.

Phenytoin: Phenytoin is both an anticonvulsant and an antiarrhythmic. It acts via neuronal membrane stabilization and reduction of Na^+ conductance and reduction of Ca^{2+} transport limiting development of and spread of seizure foci. It is used in the treatment and prevention of tonic clonic seizures and in the treatment status epilepticus. A well-known adverse effect of its use is gingival hyperplasia.

Antihistamine

Diphenhydramine: Antihistamine blockers appear to compete with histamine for H_1 receptor sites on effector cells. These drugs also have anti-inflammatory, antiemetic, anticholinergic, and sedative properties.

Antihypertensive, antianginal, β-adrenergic blocking agents

Esmolol: This is a β_1 (cardioselective) adrenergic receptor blocking agent with rapid onset, a very short duration of action and no significant membrane-stabilizing or intrinsic sympathomimetic (partial agonist) activities at therapeutic doses. Esmolol inhibits β_1 receptors located chiefly in cardiac muscle. At higher doses, it can inhibit β_2 receptors located chiefly in the bronchial and vascular musculature. Clinical actions include a decrease in heart rate, an increase in sinus cycle length, prolongation of sinus node recovery time, prolongation of the A-H interval during normal sinus rhythm and during atrial pacing, and an increase in the antegrade Wenckebach cycle length.

Labetalol: Labetalol combines both selective competitive α_1-adrenergic blocking and nonselective competitive β-adrenergic blocking activity. Blood pressure is lowered more when the patient is in the standing rather than in the supine position, and symptoms of postural hypotension can occur. During IV dosing, the patient should not be permitted to move to an erect position unmonitored until ability to do so has been established. Labetalol is metabolized primarily through conjugation to glucuronide metabolites.

Corticosteroid

Dexamethasone: See description under Level 4

Hydrocortisone sodium succinate: Hydrocortisone sodium succinate has the same metabolic and anti-inflammatory actions as hydrocortisone. After intravenous administration of hydrocortisone sodium succinate, demonstrable effects are evident within 1 hour and persist for a variable period. The preparation also may be administered IM.

Glycemic agents

Glucagon: Glucagon, which causes an increase in blood glucose concentration, is used to treat hypoglycemia. It is effective in small doses, and no evidence of toxicity has been reported with its use. Glucagon acts only on liver glycogen by converting it to glucose.

Dextrose 50% (D_{50}): Intravenous administration of 50% dextrose also can be used to manage hypoglycemia.

Pressor

Epinephrine (1:1,000): Epinephrine, a sympathomimetic drug, acts on both α- and β-adrenergic receptors. It is the most potent α-adrenergic receptor agonist available. Clinical actions of benefit during anaphylaxis include increased systemic vascular resistance, increased arterial blood pressure, increased coronary and cerebral blood flow, and bronchodilation.

Level 2 (Advanced Cardiac Life-Support Drugs)

Antiarrhythmics

Adenosine: Adenosine is a nucleoside metabolic byproduct of adenosine monophosphate (AMP) that acts by increasing K^+ conductance, thereby promoting efflux of K^+ from cardiac pacemaker cells in the SA and AV nodes. Hyperpolarization of the atrial cells occurs, leading to reduction of the duration of the action potential and reduction of the diastolic depolarization phase of the SA node pacemaker cells. Adenosine also promotes a reduction in the upstroke of the action potential of AV nodal cells, resulting in AV nodal blockade and reduction of accessory pathway conduction.

Amiodarone: As a Class III antiarrhythmic, amiodarone slows SA automaticity and prolongs action potentials and refractoriness. The primary uses for amiodarone include treatment of ventricular fibrillation (VF), pulseless ventricular tachycardia (VT), and refractory supraventricular tachycardias.

Diltiazem: Dilitiazem is a calcium channel blocker and Class IV antiarrhythmic that exerts its primary effects by modulating the influx of ionic calcium across the cell membrane. These agents are negative inotropes that effectively increase refractoriness and slow conduction through the AV node and, as such, are used for ventricular rate control in the treatment of supraventricular tachycardia, atrial fibrillation, and atrial flutter.

Lidocaine: Lidocaine as a Class IB antiarrhythmic that suppresses ventricular dysrhythmias primarily by decreasing automaticity via fast Na+ channel blockade and reduction of the slope of Phase 4 diastolic depolarization. It suppresses automaticity of ectopic ventricular pacemakers and in Purkinje fibers with little effect on the SA or AV nodes. In myocardial ischemia, the threshold for the induction of ventricular fibrillation is reduced. Some studies have shown that lidocaine elevates the fibrillation threshold; therefore, elevation of the fibrillation threshold correlates closely with blood levels of lidocaine.

Lidocaine is indicated in the management of refractory or recurrent ventricular fibrillation, ventricular tachycardia, and suppression of ventricular ectopy.

Anticholinergic, vagolytic

Atropine: Though commonly classified as an anticholinergic drug, atropine is more precisely an antimuscarinic agent. Atropine-induced parasympathetic inhibition can be preceded by a transient phase of stimulation. This is most notable in the heart, where small doses often first slow the rate before the more characteristic tachycardia develops owing to inhibition of vagal control. Compared with scopolamine, atropine's actions on the heart, intestine, and bronchial smooth muscle are more potent and longer-lasting. Also, unlike scopolamine, atropine, in clinical doses, does not depress the CNS, but may stimulate the medulla and higher cerebral centers.

Adequate doses of atropine abolish various types of reflex vagal cardiac slowing, or asystole. It also prevents or eliminates bradycardia (asystole produced by injection of choline esters, anticholinesterase agents, or other parasympathomimetic drugs), and cardiac arrest produced by vagal stimulation. Atropine can also lessen the degree of partial heart block when vagal activity is an etiologic factor.

Systemic doses can raise systolic and diastolic pressures slightly and can produce significant postural hypotension. Such doses also slightly increase cardiac output and decrease central venous pressure. Occasionally, therapeutic doses dilate cutaneous blood vessels, particularly in the blush area, producing atropine flush, and can cause atropine fever owing to suppression of sweat gland activity in infants and small children.

Atropine disappears from the blood rapidly after administration and is metabolized primarily by enzymatic hydrolysis in the liver.

Atropine is indicated in the initial management of asystole, symptomatic bradycardias, and second- and third-degree heart blocks.

Electrolytes

Calcium chloride: Calcium ions increase the force of myocardial contraction. Calcium's positive inotropic effects are modulated by its action on systemic vascular resistance. Calcium can either increase or decrease systemic vascular resistance.

Magnesium sulfate: Magnesium is primarily indicated in the emergency management of a specific type of ventricular dysrhythmia known as torsades de pointes. It is also indicated for use as an adjunct to other agents in patients with arrhythmias and nutritional magnesium deficiency.

Sodium bicarbonate: Intravenous sodium bicarbonate therapy increases plasma bicarbonate, buffers excess hydrogen ion concentration, raises blood pH and reverses the clinical manifestations of acidosis in prolonged cardiac arrest resuscitations. Administration of sodium bicarbonate does not facilitate ventricular defibrillation or survival in patients who have had a cardiac arrest.

Pressors

Epinephrine: Epinephrine is a sympathomimetic drug with both α- and β-adrenergic activity. Clinical actions of benefit during cardiac arrest include increased systemic vascular resistance, increased arterial blood pressure, increased heart rate, increased coronary and cerebral blood flow, increased myocardial contraction and increased myocardial oxygen requirements, and increased automaticity.

Vasopressin: Vasopressin is a nonadrenergic peripheral vasoconstrictor that also produces coronary and renal vasoconstriction. It may be used in place of or after the first dose of epinephrine in the treatment of ventricular fibrillation, pulseless ventricular tachycardia, or asystole in adults. Its clinical effects are equivalent to epinephrine.

Level 3 (Pediatric Advanced Life-Support Drugs)

Antiarrhythmics

Adenosine: See description under Level 2.

Amiodarone: See description under Level 2.

Lidocaine: See description under Level 2.

Procainamide: Procainamide effectively suppresses ventricular ectopy and may be effective when lidocaine has not achieved suppression of life-threatening ventricular dysrhythmias. Procainamide suppresses Phase 4 diastolic depolarization, reducing the automaticity of ectopic pacemakers. Procainamide also slows intraventricular conduction.

Anticholinergic/vagolytic

Atropine: See description under Level 2.

Antihistamine

Diphenhydramine: Indications for diphenhydramine include the treatment of anaphylaxis in pediatric patients following epinephrine administration. The drug acts via competitive antagonism of interaction of histamine with H_1 receptors in blood vessels and mucosal surfaces. This results in reduction of release of cytokines and mediators of the inflammatory response to antigens.

Bronchodilators

Albuterol: Albuterol has mixed β_2 and β_1 stimulation with a preferential effect on β_2-adrenergic receptors. β_2-adrenergic receptors are the predominant receptors in bronchial smooth muscle. The action of albuterol is attributable, at least in part, to stimulation through β-adrenergic receptors of ATP to cyclic-AMP. Increased cyclic-AMP levels are associated with bronchial smooth muscle relaxation and the inhibition of the release of mediators of immediate hypersensitivity from cells, especially mast cells.

Albuterol has a greater effect on the respiratory tract, in the form of bronchial smooth muscle relaxation, while producing fewer cardiovascular (CV) side effects than most bronchodilators at comparable doses. However, in some patients, albuterol, like other bronchodilators, can produce significant CV effects, such as increased pulse rate, blood pressure, symptoms such as palpitation and tremor, and/or electrocardiographic changes.

Ipratropium bromide: Ipratropium bromide blocks the action of acetylcholine at parasympathetic receptors of bronchiolar smooth muscle, producing bronchodilation in asthmatics. Cardiac stimulation is minimal compared to albuterol.

Magnesium sulfate: Magnesium sulfate blocks calcium uptake by bronchiolar smooth muscle and prevents contraction resulting in bronchodilation in refractory asthma or status asthmaticus. Also used in treatment of hypomagnesemia, hypercalcemia and torsades de pointes.

Terbutaline: Terbutaline is a selective β_2 agonist that brings about bronchodilation and is used in the treatment of status asthmaticus.

Corticosteroids

Dexamethasone: Dexamethasone is a potent corticosteroid used in the emergency treatment of moderate to severe croup and mild to moderate asthma. This class of medications functions to modulate the immune response and inflammatory responses to antigenic exposure by reduction of activation, chemotaxis of lymphocytes, macrophages, and eosinophils. They also reduce production of pro-inflammatory substances and mediators of inflammation by those cell populations. Reduction of vasogenic edema and vasodilation also occurs. These agents also enhance responsiveness to sympathomimetic drugs by upregulation of cell surface β receptors.

Hydrocortisone: Hydrocortisone is indicated for prophylaxis and treatment of adrenal insufficiency and the treatment of anaphylaxis.

Methylprednisolone: Methylprednisolone is indicated in the treatment of status asthmaticus and anaphylaxis.

Diuretic

Furosemide: Furosemide is a diuretic that acts at the ascending limb of the loop of Henle by inhibition of reabsorption of sodium and chloride, resulting in excretion of water, sodium, and chloride. Loss of potassium occurs as a result of excretion in the distal tubule of the nephron. Furosemide is indicated in the treatment of pulmonary edema.

Electrolytes

Calcium chloride: See description under Level 2.

Magnesium sulfate: See description under Level 2.

Sodium bicarbonate: See description under Level 2.

Pressors

Dopamine: Dopamine is a unique agent with clinical actions which vary in dose-dependent fashion. It is considered a renal vasodilator and low doses via stimulation of renal dopaminergic receptors thus improving blood flow and renal function. At higher doses this agent stimulates α, β_1 and β_2 receptors to bring about increased peripheral vascular resistance, enhanced venous return, cardiac rate and stroke volume thus acting as a positive inotrope. It is indicated for the treatment of hypotension associated with various forms of shock.

Dobutamine: Dobutamine is an inotropic agent with sympathomimetic activity. Its primary mechanism of action is stimulation of cardiac β_1 receptors enhancing heart rate and contractility. It has less pronounced effects at β_2 and α_1 receptors and tends to produce vasodilation via β_2 stimulation and α_1 blockade.

Epinephrine: See description under Level 2. Indications include anaphylaxis, status asthmaticus, severe croup, ventricular fibrillation/pulseless ventricular tachycardia, asystole, pulseless electrical activity, shock, and antihypertensive toxicity.

Norepinephrine: Norepinephrine is an adrenergic agent with chronotropic and inotropic effects (via cardiac β_1 receptor stimulation) and pressor effects (via α_1 stimulation). Indications for its use include forms of shock with hypotension associated with low peripheral vascular resistance (vasodilation).

Reversal agent

Naloxone: See description under Level 4.

Vasodilators

Nitroglycerin: Indications for nitroglycerin in pediatric patients include treatment of congestive heart failure and cardiogenic shock. It acts via generation of nitric oxide, leading to accumulation of intracellular second messenger cyclic GMP with resulting smooth muscle relaxation and dilation of capacitance vessels, coronary arteries, and pulmonary vessels. Preload reduction and improved coronary blood flow are achieved.

Sodium nitroprusside: Indications include treatment of shock states associated with elevated peripheral vascular resistance (cardiogenic shock) and hypertensive emergencies. Smooth muscle relaxation is produced via nitric oxide release and activation of intracellular cyclic GMP with resulting vasodilation of resistance vessels. Both preload and afterload reduction are produced.

Level 4 (Reversal Agents)

Naloxone: Naloxone prevents or reverses the actions of opioids, including respiratory depression, sedation, and hypotension. It also can reverse the psychotomimetic and dysphoric effects of agonist-antagonists such as pentazocine.

As a "pure" opioid antagonist, naloxone does not produce respiratory depression, psychotomimetic effects, or pupillary constriction. In the absence of opioids or agonistic effects of other opioid antagonists, naloxone exhibits essentially no pharmacological activity.

Naloxone is a competitive antagonist for opioid receptor sites. The onset of action after IV administration is apparent within 2 minutes, with an only slightly slower onset after subcutaneous or IM administration. Duration depends on the route of administration; IM administration produces a more prolonged effect than IV administration. The need for repeated doses of naloxone depends on the dose, route of administration, and the type of opioid being antagonized.

Naloxone is rapidly distributed in the body and is metabolized in the liver.

Flumazenil: Flumazenil, which antagonizes the actions of benzodiazepines on the CNS, competitively inhibits the activity at the benzodiazepine recognition site on the GABA/benzodiazepine receptor complex. Flumazenil has little or no agonist activity in humans. Flumazenil does not antagonize the CNS effects of drugs affecting GABA-ergic neurons by means other than the benzodiazepine receptor (that is, ethanol, barbiturates, or general anesthetics) and does not reverse the effects of opioids.

Flumazenil antagonizes sedation, impairment of recall, and psychomotor impairment produced by benzodiazepines in healthy human volunteers. The duration and degree of reversal of benzodiazepine effects are related to the dose and plasma concentration of flumazenil as well as that of the sedating benzodiazepine. Onset of reversal is usually evident within 1-2 minutes after IV injection. An 80% response is reached within 3 minutes, with peak effect noted at 6-10 minutes.

Non-injectable Drugs

Level 1

Antianginal agent

Nitroglycerin: The primary action of the vasodilator nitroglycerin is to relax vascular smooth muscle. Although venous effects predominate, nitroglycerin produces, in a dose-related manner, dilation of both venous and arterial beds. It decreases venous return to the heart and reduces systemic vascular resistance and arterial pressure. These effects lead to a decrease in myocardial oxygen consumption, resulting in a more favorable supply-demand ratio and the cessation of anginal discomfort.

Antiplatelet agent

Aspirin: Aspirin, at doses of 81 mg to 325 mg, is recommended in the prehospital phase of management of the acute coronary syndromes, unstable angina, and myocardial ischemia and infarction. Its platelet aggregation inhibition may prevent thrombus formation in narrowed, atherosclerotic coronary arteries.

Bronchodilator

Albuterol: Albuterol has mixed β_2 and β_1 stimulation with a preferential effect on β_2-adrenergic receptors. β_2-adrenergic receptors are the predominant receptors in bronchial smooth muscle. The action of albuterol is attributable, at least in part, to stimulation through β-adrenergic receptors of ATP to cyclic-AMP. Increased cyclic-AMP levels are associated with bronchial smooth muscle relaxation and the inhibition of the release of mediators of immediate hypersensitivity from cells, especially mast cells.

Albuterol has a greater effect on the respiratory tract, in the form of bronchial smooth muscle relaxation, while producing fewer cardiovascular (CV) side effects than most bronchodilators at comparable doses. However, in some patients, albuterol, like other bronchodilators, can produce significant CV effects, such as increased pulse rate, blood pressure, symptoms such as palpitation and tremor, and/or electrocardiographic changes.

Antihistamine

Diphenhydramine (oral form): This drug is recommended for postoperative management of mild allergy (itching, hives, rash).

Aromatic stimulant

Aromatic ammonia, spirits of ammonia: Ammonia, which is a noxious-smelling vapor, acts by irritating the mucous membrane of the upper respiratory tract, thereby stimulating the respiratory and vasomotor centers of the medulla. This, in turn, increases respiration and blood pressure.

Glycemic agents

Insta-glucose gel or other oral glucose tablets, orange juice, regular [non-diet] soft drinks: Antihypoglycemics are rapidly absorbed sources of glucose for the management of hypoglycemia.

SUGGESTED READING

American Heart Association. *Advanced Cardiac Life Support Provider Manual.* Dallas, TX; 2006.

American Heart Association. *Pediatric Advanced Life Support Provider Manual.* Dallas, TX; 2006.

American Association of Oral and Maxillofacial Surgeons. *Office Anesthesia Evaluation Manual,* 4th ed. Rosemont, IL; 1991.

Table 13.1. DRUGS AND EQUIPMENT FOR DENTAL OFFICE EMERGENCIES

INJECTABLE DRUGS	NONINJECTABLE DRUGS	EQUIPMENT
LEVEL 1 (basic)		
Antianginal: Morphine sulfate **Anticonvulsants:** Diazepam, phenytoin **Antihistamine:** Diphenhydramine **Antihypertensives:** Esmolol, labetalol **Glycemic agents:** Dextrose (D_{50}), glucagon **Glucocorticoids:** Dexamethasone, hydrocortisone **Vasopressor:** Epinephrine	**Antianginal:** Nitroglycerin **Antihistamine:** Diphenhydramine (oral) **Antiplatelet agent:** Aspirin **Aromatic stimulant:** Spirits of ammonia **Bronchodilators:** Albuterol, ipratropium bromide **Glucose sources:** Fruit juice, non-diet soft drinks **Oxygen**	**High-volume suction** **Intravenous solutions** **Oxygen delivery systems:** Nasal cannula: 1L/min: 21%-24% O_2 2L/min: 25%-28% O_2 3L/min: 29%-32% O_2 4L/min: 33%-36% O_2 5L/min: 37%-40% O_2 6L/min: 41%-44% O_2 Face mask: up to 60% O_2 Face mask with reservoir, non-rebreather, ambu-bag: 60%-100% O_2 **Venipuncture equipment:** Tourniquets; intravenous catheters and tubing; infusion sets, tape
LEVEL 2 (advanced cardiac life-support drugs)		
Antiarrhythmics: Adenosine, amiodarone, diltiazem, lidocaine **Electrolytes:** Calcium chloride, magnesium sulfate, sodium bicarbonate **Pressors:** Epinephrine, vasopressin **Vagolytic:** Atropine		**Airway Equipment:** Laryngeal mask airways; laryngoscopes and endotracheal tubes, holders, CO_2 detectors; Magill forceps, suction catheters and tubes **Intravenous solutions:** Normal saline, lactated ringers, 5% dextrose in normal saline (D_5 normal saline), 5% dextrose in lactated ringers **Venipuncture equipment:** Tourniquets; intravenous catheters, tubing, tape, infusion sets
LEVEL 3 (pediatric advanced life-support drugs)		
Antiarrhythmics: Adenosine, amiodarone, lidocaine, procainamide **Antihistamine:** Diphenhydramine **Bronchodilator:** Magnesium sulfate, terbutaline **Corticosteroids:** Dexamethasone, hydrocortisone, methylprednisolone **Diuretic:** Furosemide **Electrolytes:** Calcium chloride, magnesium sulfate, sodium bicarbonate **Opioid antagonist:** Naloxone **Pressors:** Dobutamine, dopamine, epinephrine, norepinephrine **Vagolytic:** Atropine **Vasodilators:** Nitroglycerin, sodium nitroprusside	**Bronchodilators:** Albuterol, ipratropium bromide	
LEVEL 4 (reversal agents)		
Benzodiazepine antagonist: Flumazenil **Opioid antagonist:** Naloxone		

Table 13.2. PRESCRIBING INFORMATION FOR EMERGENCY DRUGS

NAME	FORM	DOSAGE	WARNINGS/PRECAUTIONS, CONTRAINDICATIONS & ADVERSE EFFECTS	INDICATIONS
ANTIANGINALS				
Morphine sulfate	IV	***Adults:*** 2-4mg (over 1-5 min) q3-5 min; repeat dose 2-8mg at 5-15 min intervals.	**W/P:** Have resuscitation equipment, trained personnel and narcotic antagonists available; severe respiratory depression may occur. Avoid rapid administration. May be habit-forming. Caution with head injury, increased intracranial/intraocular pressure, decreased respiratory reserve, hepatic/renal dysfunction, elderly, debilitated. High doses may cause seizures. Smooth muscle hypertonicity may cause biliary colic, urinary difficulty, or retention. Orthostatic hypotension may occur with hypovolemia or myocardial dysfunction. Acute respiratory failure reported with COPD or acute asthmatic attack. **Contra:** Allergy to opiates, acute bronchial asthma, upper airway obstruction. **P/N:** Category C, safety in nursing not known. **A/E:** Respiratory depression, hypotension, pruritus, urinary retention, N/V, constipation, anxiety, cough reflex depression, oliguria.	Angina unresponsive to nitrate, pulmonary edema.
Nitroglycerin	Sublingual, Spray	***Adults:*** Tab: 0.4mg at 5-min intervals to total of 3 doses. Spray: 1-2 sprays (0.4mg each) at 5-min intervals to 3 doses.	**W/P:** Do not swallow tabs. Severe hypotension may occur; caution with volume depletion or hypotension. May aggravate angina caused by hypertrophic cardiomyopathy. D/C if develop blurred vision or dry mouth. May interfere with cholesterol test. Monitor with acute MI or CHF. Tolerance to other nitrate forms may decrease effects. Caution in elderly. **Contra:** Early MI, severe anemia, increased ICP, concomitant phosphodiesterases. **P/N:** Category C, caution in nursing. **A/E:** Headache, vertigo, dizziness, weakness, palpitation, syncope, flushing, postural hypotension, drug rash, exfoliative dermatitis.	Angina.
Nitroglycerin	IV	***Adults:*** 12.5-25mcg bolus (if no tablet or spray given); infusion 10-20mcg/min titrate up 5-10mcg/min every 5-10 min to effect.	**W/P:** Amplification of the vasodilatory effects in combination with sildenafil can result in severe hypotension. Because of the problem of absorption by polyvinyl chloride (PVC) tubing, the injection should be used with the least absorptive infusion tubing (ie, non-PVC tubing) available. Severe hypotension and shock may occur with even small doses of nitroglycerin; use with caution in patients who may be volume depleted. Nitrate therapy may aggravate the angina caused by hypertrophic cardiomyopathy. Infusions should be administered only via a pump that can maintain a constant infusion rate. **Contra:** Pericardial tamponade, restrictive cardiomyopathy, and constrictive pericarditis. **P/N:** Category C, caution in nursing. **A/E:** Headache, lightheadedness, hypotension, syncope, crescendo angina, rebound hypertension.	Angina, acute MI, CHF, persistent/recurrent ischemia, severe HTN.

BB = black box warning; **W/P** = warnings/precautions; **Contra** = contraindications; **P/N** = pregnancy category rating and nursing considerations; **A/E** = adverse effects.

Table 13.2. PRESCRIBING INFORMATION FOR EMERGENCY DRUGS *(cont.)*

NAME	FORM	DOSAGE	WARNINGS/PRECAUTIONS, CONTRAINDICATIONS & ADVERSE EFFECTS	INDICATIONS
ANTIARRHYTHMICS				
Adenosine	IV	***Adults:*** Initially 6mg, followed by 2nd and 3rd doses of 12mg if needed. ***Pediatrics:*** 0.1mg/kg 1st, 0.2mg/kg 2nd if needed.	**W/P:** May produce short-lasting heart block. Transient or prolonged asystole, respiratory alkalosis, ventricular fibrillation reported. Caution with obstructive lung disease not associated with bronchoconstriction (eg, emphysema, bronchitis). Avoid with bronchoconstriction/bronchospasm (eg, asthma). D/C if severe respiratory difficulties develop. New arrhythmias may appear on ECG at time of conversion. Caution in elderly. **Contra:** 2nd- or 3rd-degree AV block (except with pacemaker), sinus node disease such as sick sinus syndrome, or symptomatic bradycardia (except with pacemaker). **P/N:** Category C, safety in nursing not known. **A/E:** Facial flushing, dyspnea/SOB, chest pressure, nausea.	Narrow complex SVT.
Amiodarone	IV	***Adults:*** 300mg followed by one 150mg dose if needed. ***Pediatrics:*** 5mg/kg, repeat 5mg/kg up to total 15mg/kg/24 hr if needed.	**W/P:** Bradycardia and AV block reported. Hypotension reported; do not exceed initial rate of infusion. Correct hypokalemia or hypomagnesemia before therapy to prevent exaggeration of QTc prolongation. Congenital goiter/hypothyroidism, hyperthyroidism, postoperative adult respiratory distress syndrome (ARDS) reported with oral therapy. Hyperthyroidism may result in thyrotoxicosis and/or the possibility of arrhythmia breakthrough or aggravation. Elevations of hepatic enzymes reported. May worsen or precipitate a new arrhythmia; monitor for QTc prolongation. Pulmonary toxicity reported. Contains benzyl alcohol. Caution in elderly. **Contra:** Cardiogenic shock, marked sinus bradycardia, 2nd- or 3rd-degree AV block (unless a functioning pacemaker is available). Hypersensitivity to iodine. **P/N:** Category D, not for use in nursing. **A/E:** Hypotension, fever, bradycardia, CHF, heart arrest, ventricular tachycardia, abnormal LFTs, nausea.	***Adults:*** Recurrent VF, pulseless VT; ***Pediatrics:*** VF, pulseless VT, SVT, ventricular arrhythmias.
Diltiazem	IV	***Adults:*** 15-20mg (0.25mg/kg) over 2 min; may give another 20-25mg (0.35mg/kg) in 15 min.	**W/P:** Initiate in setting with resuscitation capabilities. Caution if hemodynamically compromised, and in patients with renal, hepatic, or ventricular dysfunction. Monitor ECG continuously and BP frequently. Symptomatic hypotension, acute hepatic injury reported. D/C if high-degree AV block occurs in sinus rhythm or if persistent rash occurs. Ventricular premature beats may be present on conversion of PSVT to sinus rhythm. **Contra:** Sick sinus syndrome and 2nd- or 3rd-degree AV block (except with functioning pacemaker), severe hypotension, cardiogenic shock, concomitant IV β-blockers or within a few hrs of use, A-Fib/Flutter associated with accessory bypass tract (eg, Wolff-Parkinson-White syndrome, short PR syndrome), ventricular tachycardia. **P/N:** Category C, not for use in nursing. **A/E:** Hypotension, injection-site reactions (eg, itching, burning), vasodilation (flushing), arrhythmias.	Ventricular rate control in A-Fib/Flutter; refractory re-entry SVT.

BB = black box warning; **W/P** = warnings/precautions; **Contra** = contraindications; **P/N** = pregnancy category rating and nursing considerations; **A/E** = adverse effects.

NAME	FORM	DOSAGE	WARNINGS/PRECAUTIONS, CONTRAINDICATIONS & ADVERSE EFFECTS	INDICATIONS
Lidocaine	IV	***Adults:*** VF/VT 1-1.5mg/kg, refractory VF additional 0.5-0.75mg/kg in 5-10 min (max. 3mg/kg); infusion 1-4mg/min. ***Pediatrics:*** 1mg/kg (max. 100 mg); infusion 20-50mcg/kg/min.	**W/P:** Systemic toxicity may result in CNS depression or irritability which may progress to convulsions. Ventilatory therapy with oxygen or small increments of anticonvulsant drugs may be necessary. Constant ECG monitoring is essential to proper administration. Signs of excessive depression (sinus node dysfunction, prolongation of P-R interval and QRS complex, arrhythmias) should be followed by flow adjustment or cessation. Caution with severe liver or kidney disease, hypovolemia, CHF, shock, all heart block, and sinus bradycardia. **P/N:** Category B, caution in nursing. **A/E:** Lightheadedness, nervousness, euphoria, confusion, dizziness, drowsiness, tinnitus, blurred vision, vomiting, heat/cold sensations, twitching, tremors, convulsions, respiratory depression, bradycardia, hypotension.	VF/pulseless VT, refractory VF, stable VT, wide complex tachycardias.
Procainamide	IV	***Adults:*** 20-50mg/min (max. 17mg/kg) (endpoints=arrhythmia suppression, hypotension, QRS widening by >50% or 17mg/kg given). ***Pediatrics:*** 15mg/kg of 30-60 min.	**W/P:** Monitor for QRS widening or QT prolongation. Cardiovert or digitalize before use with A-Fib/Flutter. Caution with AV conduction disturbances and 1st-degree heart block; reduce dose. Caution with myasthenia gravis; adjust dose of anticholinesterases. Caution in digitalis intoxication, pre-existing marrow failure, cytopenia, CHF, ischemic heart disease, cardiomyopathy. May induce lupoid syndrome. Reserve for life-threatening ventricular arrhythmias. Fatal blood dyscrasias reported; obtain CBC, WBC, differential, and platelets weekly for 1st 3 months, then periodically. **Contra:** Complete heart block, SLE, torsades de pointes. **P/N:** Category C, not for use in nursing. **A/E:** GI disturbances, lupus-like symptoms, elevated LFTs, angioneurotic edema, flushing, psychosis, dizziness, depression, urticaria, pruritus, rash, agranulocytosis.	Recurrent VF/VT, stable VT, PSVT, A-Fib in Wolff-Parkinson-White syndrome.
ANTICHOLINERGIC				
Atropine	IV	***Adults:*** Asystole, pulseless electrical activity: 1mg; may repeat q3-5 min (max. 3mg) if necessary in asystole; bradycardia 0.5mg q3-5 min (max. 3mg). ***Pediatrics:*** Symptomatic bradycardia: 0.02mg/kg (max. single child dose 0.5mg, total dose 1mg) (max. single adolescent dose 1mg, total dose 2mg).	**W/P:** Avoid overdose in IV administration. Increased susceptibility to toxic effects in children. Caution in patients >40 yrs. Conventional doses may precipitate glaucoma in susceptible patients, convert partial organic pyloric stenosis into complete obstruction, lead to complete urinary retention in patients with prostatic hypertrophy, or cause inspissation of bronchial secretions and formation of dangerous viscid plugs in patients with chronic lung disease.	***Adults:*** Asystole, pulseless electrical activity, bradycardia.

Table 13.2. PRESCRIBING INFORMATION FOR EMERGENCY DRUGS *(cont.)*

NAME	FORM	DOSAGE	WARNINGS/PRECAUTIONS, CONTRAINDICATIONS & ADVERSE EFFECTS	INDICATIONS
ANTICHOLINERGIC *(cont.)*				
Atropine *(cont.)*			**Contra:** Glaucoma, pyloric stenosis, or prostatic hypertrophy except in doses used for preanesthetic medication. **P/N:** Category C, safety in nursing not known. **A/E:** Dryness of the mouth, blurred vision, photophobia, tachycardia, anhidrosis.	
ANTICONVULSANTS				
Diazepam	IV	***Adults:*** 0.15-0.25mg/kg.	**W/P:** Inject slowly and avoid small veins. Do not mix or dilute with other products in syringe or infusion flask. Extreme caution in elderly, severely ill, and those with limited pulmonary reserve. Avoid if in shock, coma, or acute alcohol intoxication with depressed vital signs. May impair mental/physical abilities. Increase in grand mal seizures reported. Caution with kidney or hepatic dysfunction. Not for obstetrical use. Withdrawal symptoms may occur. Hypotension and muscular weakness reported. Monitor blood counts and LFTs. Not for maintenance of seizures once controlled. **Contra:** Acute narrow-angle glaucoma, untreated open-angle glaucoma. **P/N:** Not for use during pregnancy, safety in nursing unknown. **A/E:** Drowsiness, fatigue, ataxia, venous thrombosis and phlebitis (injection site).	Status epilepticus.
Phenytoin	IV	***Adults:*** 15-20mg/kg, infuse at rate of 50mg/min.	**W/P:** IV administration should not exceed 50mg/min in adults. Severe cardiotoxic reactions have been reported with atrial and ventricular conduction depression and ventricular fibrillation. Use with caution in patients with hypotension and severe myocardial insufficiency. There is a suggested relationship between use and the development of lymphadenopathy (local or generalized). Patients with impaired liver function, are elderly, or are gravely ill may show early signs of toxicity. D/C use if skin rash appears. Hyperglycemia has been reported. **Contra:** Sinus bradycardia, sino-atrial block, 2nd- and 3rd-degree AV block, and patients with Adams-Stokes syndrome. Hypersensitivity to hydantoin products. **P/N:** Use with caution; a number of reports suggests an association between the use of antiepileptic drugs by women with epilepsy and a high incidence of birth defects. Not for use in nursing. **A/E:** Cardiovascular collapse (toxicity), CNS depression (toxicity), cardiotoxic reactions/fatalities, nystagmus, ataxia, slurred speech, decreased coordination, mental confusion, NV, constipation, rash.	Status epilepticus.

BB = black box warning; **W/P** = warnings/precautions; **Contra** = contraindications; **P/N** = pregnancy category rating and nursing considerations; **A/E** = adverse effects.

NAME	FORM	DOSAGE	WARNINGS/PRECAUTIONS, CONTRAINDICATIONS & ADVERSE EFFECTS	INDICATIONS
ANTIHISTAMINE				
Diphenhydramine	IV, PO	***Adults:*** 25-50mg q4-6h. Max: 300mg/24 hrs. ***Pediatrics:*** **≥12 yrs:** 25-50mg q4-6h. **Max:** 300mg/24 hrs.; **6-11 yrs:** 12.5-25mg q4-6h. **Max:** 150mg/24 hrs.	**W/P:** Caution with narrow-angle glaucoma, stenosing peptic ulcer, pyloroduodenal obstruction, symptomatic prostatic hypertrophy, or bladder-neck obstruction. May cause excitation in pediatrics. Increased risk of dizziness, sedation, and hypotension in elderly. Caution with lower respiratory diseases, bronchial asthma, increased IOP, hyperthyroidism, CV disease, or HTN. Local necrosis with SQ or intradermal use. **Contra:** Neonates, premature infants, nursing, use as a local anesthetic. **P/N:** Category B, contraindicated in nursing. **A/E:** Sedation, drowsiness, dizziness, disturbed coordination, epigastric distress, thickening of bronchial secretions.	Anaphylaxis.
ANTIHYPERTENSIVES				
Esmolol	IV	***Adults:*** 500mcg/kg over 1 min, then 50mcg/kg titrate to BP.	**W/P:** Hypotension may occur; monitor BP and reduce dose or d/c if needed. May cause cardiac failure; withdraw at 1st sign of impending cardiac failure. Caution with supraventricular arrhythmias when patient is compromised hemodynamically or is taking other drugs that decrease peripheral resistance, myocardial filling/contractility, and/or electrical impulse propagation in the myocardium. Not for HTN associated with hypothermia. Caution in bronchospastic diseases; titrate to lowest possible effective dose and terminate immediately in the event of bronchospasm. Caution in diabetics; may mask tachycardia occurring with hypoglycemia. Caution in impaired renal function. Avoid concentrations >10mg/mL and infusions into small veins or through butterfly catheters. Sloughing of skin and necrosis reported with infiltration and extravasation. Use caution when discontinuing infusion in coronary artery disease patients. **Contra:** Sinus bradycardia, heart block greater than first degree, cardiogenic shock, or overt heart failure. **P/N:** Category C, caution in nursing. **A/E:** Hypotension, dizziness, diaphoresis, somnolence, confusion, headache, agitation, bronchospasm, nausea, infusion site reactions.	Severe HTN.
Labetalol	IV	***Adults:*** 10-20mg, repeat 10-40mg q10 min. Titrate to BP (max. 300mg).	**W/P:** Severe hepatocellular injury reported; caution with hepatic dysfunction. Monitor LFTs periodically; d/c at 1st sign of hepatic injury. Caution with well-compensated HF. Can cause HF. Exacerbation of ischemic heart disease with abrupt withdrawal. Caution in nonallergic bronchospasm patients refractory to or intolerant to other antihypertensives. May mask hypoglycemia symptoms. Withdrawal before surgery is controversial. Paradoxical HTN may occur with pheochromocytoma. Death reported during surgery. Avoid injection with low cardiac indices and elevated	Severe HTN.

Table 13.2. PRESCRIBING INFORMATION FOR EMERGENCY DRUGS *(cont.)*

NAME	FORM	DOSAGE	WARNINGS/PRECAUTIONS, CONTRAINDICATIONS & ADVERSE EFFECTS	INDICATIONS
ANTIHYPERTENSIVES *(cont.)*				
Labetalol *(cont.)*			systemic vascular resistance. **Contra:** Bronchial asthma, obstructive airway disease, overt cardiac failure, >1st-degree heart block, cardiogenic shock, severe bradycardia, other conditions associated with severe and prolonged hypotension. **P/N:** Category C, caution in nursing. **A/E:** Fatigue, dizziness, dyspepsia, nausea, nasal stuffiness.	
ANTIPLATELET AGENT				
Aspirin	Oral	***Adults:*** 160-325mg.	**W/P:** Increased risk of bleeding with heavy alcohol use (≥3 drinks/day). May inhibit platelet function; can adversely affect inherited (hemophilia) or acquired (hepatic disease, vitamin K deficiency) bleeding disorders. Monitor for bleeding and ulceration. Avoid in history of active peptic ulcer, severe renal failure, severe hepatic insufficiency, and sodium restricted diets. Associated with elevated LFTs, BUN, and SrCr; hyperkalemia; proteinuria; and prolonged bleeding time. Avoid 1 week before and during labor. **Contra:** NSAID allergy, viral infections in children or teenagers, syndrome of asthma, rhinitis, and nasal polyps. **P/N:** Avoid in 3rd trimester of pregnancy and nursing. **A/E:** Fever, hypothermia, dysrhythmias, hypotension, agitation, cerebral edema, dehydration, hyperkalemia, dyspepsia, GI bleed, hearing loss, tinnitus, problems in pregnancy.	Acute coronary syndromes: angina, MI, symptoms suggestive of ischemia.
BRONCHODILATORS				
Albuterol	MDI	***Adults:*** 4-8 puffs q20 min up to 4 hrs, then q1-2 hr prn. ***Pediatrics:*** 4-8 puffs q20 min.	**W/P:** Hypersensitivity reactions reported. Monitor for worsening asthma. Fatalities reported with excessive use. Caution with cardiovascular disorders, especially coronary insufficiency, arrhythmias, and HTN. May need concomitant corticosteroids. Can produce paradoxical bronchospasm. Caution with DM, hyperthyroidism, seizures. May cause transient hypokalemia. **P/N:** Category C, not for use in nursing. **A/E:** Tachycardia, tremor, dizziness, N/V, palpitations, rhinitis, upper respiratory tract infection, fever, inhalation site and taste sensation, back pain, and nervousness.	Asthma, anaphylaxis.
Ipratropium bromide	MDI	***Adults:*** 8 puffs q20 min prn up to 3 hours. ***Pediatrics:*** 4–8 puffs q20 min prn up to 3 hrs.	**W/P:** Not for acute episodes. Immediate hypersensitivity reaction reported. Caution with narrow-angle glaucoma, prostatic hypertrophy, or bladder-neck obstruction. **Contra:** Hypersensitivity to atropine or its derivatives. **P/N:** Category B, caution in nursing. **A/E:** Back pain, bronchitis, dyspnea, dizziness, headache, nausea, blurred vision, dry mouth, exacerbation of symptoms.	Asthma.

BB = black box warning; **W/P** = warnings/precautions; **Contra** = contraindications; **P/N** = pregnancy category rating and nursing considerations; **A/E** = adverse effects.

NAME	FORM	DOSAGE	WARNINGS/PRECAUTIONS, CONTRAINDICATIONS & ADVERSE EFFECTS	INDICATIONS
Magnesium sulfate	IV	***Adults:*** 2g IV. ***Pediatrics:*** 25-50mg/kg (max. 2g) over 15-30 min.	**W/P:** Reserve IV use for immediate control of life-threatening convulsion. Use in presence of renal insufficiency may lead to magnesium intoxication. Product contains aluminum that may reach toxic levels with prolonged administration if kidney function is impaired, esp in premature neonates. Use with caution in patients with renal impairment. Clinical indications of a safe dosage regimen include the presence of the patellar reflex. Rate of administration should be slow and cautious to avoid producing hypermagnesemia. **P/N:** Category A, use with caution in nursing. **A/E:** Flushing, sweating, hypotension, depressed reflexes, flaccid paralysis, hypothermia, circulatory collapse, cardiac and CNS depression proceeding to respiratory paralysis.	Status asthmaticus.
Terbutaline	IV, SQ	***Adults:*** SQ: 0.25mg into lateral deltoid area. May repeat within 15-30 min. if no improvement. **Max:** 0.5mg/4 hrs. ***Pediatrics:*** IV: 0.1-10mcg/kg/min; SQ: 10mcg/kg q10-15 min until IV infusion started (max 0.4mg).	**W/P:** Caution with ischemic heart disease, HTN, arrhythmias, hyperthyroidism, DM, seizures. Not approved for tocolysis. Hypersensitivity and exacerbation of bronchospasm reported. Monitor for transient hypokalemia. **Contra:** Hypersensitivity to sympathomimetic amines. **P/N:** Category B, caution in nursing. **A/E:** Nervousness, tremor, headache, somnolence, palpitations, dizziness, tachycardia, nausea.	Status asthmaticus.
CORTICOSTEROIDS				
Dexamethasone	IV	***Adults:*** Give dose equivalent to prednisone 40-80mg/day in 1-2 divided doses. ***Pediatrics:*** 0.6mg/kg q24h x 2 (max. 16mg).	**W/P:** Increase dose before, during, and after stressful situations. Avoid abrupt withdrawal. May mask signs of infection, activate latent amebiasis, elevate BP, cause salt/water retention, increase excretion of K^+ and calcium. Prolonged use may produce cataracts, glaucoma, secondary ocular infections. Caution with recent MI, ocular herpes simplex, emotional instability, nonspecific ulcerative colitis, diverticulitis, peptic ulcer, renal insufficiency, HTN, osteoporosis, myasthenia gravis, threadworm infection, active TB. Enhanced effect with hypothyroidism, cirrhosis. Consider prophylactic therapy if exposed to measles or chickenpox. Risk of glaucoma, cataracts, and eye infections. **Contra:** Systemic fungal infections. **P/N:** Category C, not for use in nursing. **A/E:** Fluid/electrolyte disturbances, muscle weakness, osteoporosis, peptic ulcer, pancreatitis, ulcerative esophagitis, impaired wound healing, headache, psychic disturbances, growth suppression (pediatrics), glaucoma, hyperglycemia, weight gain, nausea, malaise.	Status asthmaticus.

Table 13.2. PRESCRIBING INFORMATION FOR EMERGENCY DRUGS *(cont.)*

NAME	FORM	DOSAGE	WARNINGS/PRECAUTIONS, CONTRAINDICATIONS & ADVERSE EFFECTS	INDICATIONS
CORTICOSTEROIDS *(cont.)*				
Hydrocortisone	IV	***Adults:*** Adrenal insufficiency: 100mg q8hr. ***Pediatrics:*** 2mg/kg (max. 100mg). ***Adults:*** Status asthmaticus: 6mg/kg/day divided in 4 doses.	**W/P:** May need to increase dose before, during, and after stressful situations. May mask signs of infection or cause new infections. Prolonged use may produce glaucoma, optic nerve damage, secondary ocular infections. Increases BP, salt/water retention, K^+ and calcium excretion. More severe/fatal course of infections reported with chickenpox, measles. Enhanced effect with hypothyroidism or cirrhosis. Caution with strongyloides, latent TB, ocular herpes simplex, HTN, diverticulitis, fresh intestinal anastomoses, ulcerative colitis, osteoporosis, myasthenia gravis, renal insufficiency, peptic ulcer disease. Kaposi's sarcoma reported. Monitor for psychic disturbances. Acute myopathy with high doses. Avoid abrupt withdrawal. Monitor growth and development of children on prolonged therapy. Hypernatremia may occur with high-dose therapy >48-72 hrs. **Contra:** Premature infants, systemic fungal infections. **P/N:** Safety in pregnancy and nursing not known. **A/E:** Fluid and electrolyte disturbances, HTN, osteoporosis, muscle weakness, cushingoid state, menstrual irregularities, vertigo, headache, impaired wound healing, DM, ulcerative esophagitis, peptic ulcer, pancreatitis, increased sweating, increased ICP, carbohydrate intolerance, glaucoma, cataracts.	Adrenal insufficiency, status asthmaticus.
Methylprednisolone	IV	***Pediatrics:*** **LD:** 2mg/kg (max. 80mg); **Maint:** 0.5mg/kg q6hr or 1mg/kg q12hr (max. 120mg/day).	**W/P:** May need to increase dose before, during, and after stressful situations. May mask signs of infection or cause new infections. Prolonged use may produce cataracts, glaucoma, secondary ocular infections. Increases BP, salt/water retention, K^+ and calcium excretion. More severe/fatal course of infections reported with chickenpox, measles. Caution with latent TB, hypothyroidism, cirrhosis, ocular herpes simplex, HTN, diverticulitis, fresh intestinal anastomoses, ulcerative colitis, osteoporosis, myasthenia gravis, renal insufficiency, peptic ulcer disease. Kaposi's sarcoma reported. Growth and development of children on prolonged therapy should be monitored. Monitor for psychic disturbances. Avoid abrupt withdrawal. Reports of cardiac arrhythmias, circulatory collapse, cardiac arrest following rapid administration of large IV doses. Effectiveness not established for the treatment of sepsis syndrome and septic shock. Bradycardia reported with high doses. **Contra:** Premature infants (due to benzyl alcohol diluent) and systemic fungal infections. **P/N:** Safety in pregnancy and nursing not known. **A/E:** Fluid and electrolyte disturbances, HTN, osteoporosis, muscle weakness, cushingoid state, menstrual irregularities, insomnia, impaired wound healing, DM, ulcerative esophagitis, excessive sweating, increased intracranial pressure, carbohydrate intolerance, glaucoma, cataracts, nausea.	Status asthmaticus, anaphylaxis.

BB = black box warning; **W/P** = warnings/precautions; **Contra** = contraindications; **P/N** = pregnancy category rating and nursing considerations; **A/E** = adverse effects.

NAME	FORM	DOSAGE	WARNINGS/PRECAUTIONS, CONTRAINDICATIONS & ADVERSE EFFECTS	INDICATIONS
DIURETIC				
Furosemide	IV	***Adults:*** 0.5-1mg/kg over 1-2 min, 2nd dose 2mg/kg prn. ***Pediatrics:*** 1mg/kg (max. 20mg).	**W/P:** Monitor for fluid/electrolyte imbalance (eg, hypokalemia), renal or hepatic dysfunction. Initiate in hospital with hepatic cirrhosis and ascites. Tinnitus, hearing impairment, hyperglycemia, hyperuricemia reported. May activate SLE. Cross-sensitivity with sulfonamide allergy. Avoid excessive diuresis, especially in elderly. **Contra:** Anuria. **P/N:** Category C, caution in nursing. **A/E:** Pancreatitis, jaundice, anorexia, paresthesias, ototoxicity, blood dyscrasias, dizziness, rash, urticaria, photosensitivity, fever, thrombophlebitis, restlessness.	Pulmonary edema, fluid overload.
ELECTROLYTES				
Calcium chloride	IV	***Adults:*** 500mg-1000mg (5-10mL of 10% sol). ***Pediatrics:*** 20mg/kg.	**W/P:** Do not inject into tissues, since severe necrosis and sloughing may occur. Caution in patients taking effective doses of digitalis. **Contra:** Existing digitalis toxicity. Cardiac resuscitation in the presence of ventricular fibrillation. **P/N:** Category C, safety in nursing not known. **A/E:** Tingling sensation, calcium taste, sense of oppression or "heat wave," peripheral vasodilation, local "burning" sensation, moderate fall in BP.	Hypocalcemia, hyperkalemia, hypermagnesemia, CCB overdose.
Magnesium sulfate	IV	***Adults:*** 1-2g in 10mL D5W over 5-20 min. ***Pediatrics:*** 25-50mg/kg bolus (pulseless VT with torsades de pointes); dose over 10-20 min for VT with pulses in torsades de points and hypomagnesemia.	**W/P:** Reserve IV use for immediate control of life-threatening convulsion. Use in the presence of renal insufficiency may lead to magnesium intoxication. Product contains aluminum that may reach toxic levels with prolonged administration if kidney function is impaired, esp in premature neonates. Use with caution in patients with renal impairment. Clinical indications of a safe dosage regimen include the presence of the patellar reflex. Rate of administration should be slow and cautious, to avoid producing hypermagnesemia. **P/N:** Category A, use with caution in nursing. **A/E:** Flushing, sweating, hypotension, depressed reflexes, flaccid paralysis, hypothermia, circulatory collapse, cardiac and CNS depression proceeding to respiratory paralysis.	Torsades de pointes, hypomagnesemia.
Sodium bicarbonate	IV	***Adults:*** 1mEq/kg bolus. ***Pediatrics:*** 1mEq/kg slow bolus.	**W/P:** Caution in patients with CHF, severe renal insufficiency, and edema with sodium retention. **Contra:** Vomiting (if losing chloride), continuous GI suction, or concomitant diuretics known to produce a hypochloremic alkalosis. **P/N:** Category C, safety in nursing not known. **A/E:** Metabolic alkalosis, hypernatremia.	Metabolic acidosis, hyperkalemia, sodium channel blocker overdose.

Table 13.2. PRESCRIBING INFORMATION FOR EMERGENCY DRUGS *(cont.)*

NAME	FORM	DOSAGE	WARNINGS/PRECAUTIONS, CONTRAINDICATIONS & ADVERSE EFFECTS	INDICATIONS
GLYCEMIC AGENTS				
Dextrose 50%	IV	***Adults:*** 20-50mL IV bolus. May repeat dose if necessary.	**W/P:** Rapid rate of administration may cause hyperglycemia or hyperosmolar syndrome esp in patients with chronic uremia or with known carbohydrate intolerance. Electrolyte deficits may occur. When a concentrated infusion is withdrawn abruptly, administer 5% or 10% dextrose to avoid rebound hypoglycemia. **Contra:** Intracranial or intraspinal hemorrhage. Delirium tremens in dehydrated patients. **P/N:** Category C, safety in nursing not known. **A/E:** Hyperosmolar syndrome, injection-site reaction, hyperglycemia, electrolyte disturbances.	Hypoglycemia.
$D_{50}W$, $D_{25}W$, $D_{10}W$, D_5W	IV	***Pediatrics:*** $D_{50}W$ 1-2mL/kg; $D_{25}W$ 2-4mL/kg; $D_{10}W$ 5-10mL/kg; D_5W 10-20mL/kg.	**W/P:** Monitor changes in fluid balance, electrolyte concentrations, and acid base balance during prolonged therapy. Avoid circulatory overload, esp if there is cardiac insufficiency. Caution with patients with overt or subclinical DM. **Contra:** Intracranial or intraspinal hemorrhage, severe dehydration, anuric, in a hepatic coma, or allergic to corn or corn products. **P/N:** Category C, caution in nursing. **A/E:** Diuresis, hyperglycemia, glycosuria, and hyperosmolar coma.	Hypoglycemia.
Fruit juice, nondiet soft drinks	Oral	***Adults/Pediatrics:*** Administer to effect only if conscious.	**W/P:** Should not be given to patients who are unconscious or unable to swallow due to risk of choking and aspiration.	Hypoglycemia.
Glucagon	IV	***Adults:*** 3mg then 3mg/hr infusion prn.	**W/P:** Caution with history suggestive of insulinoma and/or pheochromocytoma. Glucagon can cause pheochromocytoma tumor to release catecholamines, which may result in a sudden and marked increase in BP. Effective in treating hypoglycemia only if sufficient liver glycogen is present. Glucagon is not effective in states of starvation, adrenal insufficiency, or chronic hypoglycemia; use glucose to treat instead. **Contra:** Pheochromocytoma. **P/N:** Category B, caution in nursing. **A/E:** NV, allergic reactions, urticaria, respiratory distress, hypotension.	Hypoglycemia; treatment of toxicity from CCBs or β-blocker.
Insta-glucose	Oral	***Adults/Pediatrics:*** Administer to effect only if conscious.	**W/P:** Do not give if patient is unconscious or cannot swallow. Recheck glucose 15 min after ingestion, if still low, another dose may be taken. A meal or snack should be consumed to prevent reoccurrence.	Hypoglycemia.

BB = black box warning; **W/P** = warnings/precautions; **Contra** = contraindications; **P/N** = pregnancy category rating and nursing considerations; **A/E** = adverse effects.

NAME	FORM	DOSAGE	WARNINGS/PRECAUTIONS, CONTRAINDICATIONS & ADVERSE EFFECTS	INDICATIONS
PRESSORS				
Dopamine	IV	***Adults:*** 2-20mcg/kg/min; ***Pediatrics:*** 2-20mcg/kg/min titrate to effect.	**W/P:** Contains sulfites. Monitor BP, urine flow, cardiac output, and pulmonary wedge pressure. Correct hypovolemia, hypoxia, hypercapnia, and acidosis prior to use. Reduce infusion rate with increase in diastolic BP/marked decrease in pulse pressure; increase rate if hypotension occurs. D/C if hypotension persists. Reduce dose if increased ectopic beats occurs. Caution with history of occlusive vascular disease (eg, atherosclerosis, arterial embolism, Raynaud's disease, cold injury, diabetic endarteritis, and Buerger's disease); monitor for changes in skin color or temperature. Administer phentolamine if extravasation noted. Avoid abrupt withdrawal. **Contra:** Pheochromocytoma, uncorrected tachyarrhythmias or ventricular fibrillation. **P/N:** Category C, caution in nursing. **A/E:** Tachycardia, palpitation, ventricular arrhythmia (high doses), dyspnea, nausea, vomiting, headache, anxiety, bradycardia, hypotension, HTN, vasoconstriction.	***Adults:*** Hypotension, 2nd line for bradycardia; ***Pediatrics:*** Cardiogenic or distributive shock.
Dobutamine	IV	***Adults:*** 2-20mcg/kg/min. ***Pediatrics:*** 2-20mcg/kg/min titrate to effect.	**W/P:** May increase HR or BP, especially systolic pressure; caution with atrial fibrillation and HTN. May precipitate or exacerbate ventricular ectopic activity. Hypersensitivity reactions (eg, skin rash, fever, eosinophilia, bronchospasm) reported. Contains sulfites. Monitor EKG, BP, pulmonary wedge pressure, and cardiac output. Correct hypovolemia prior to infusion. Caution in elderly. May decrease serum K^+ levels. Improvement may not be observed with marked mechanical obstruction (eg, severe valvular aortic stenosis). Safety following acute MI has not been established. **Contra:** Idiopathic hypertrophic subaortic stenosis. **P/N:** Category B, not for use in nursing. **A/E:** Increased HR, BP and ventricular ectopic activity, hypotension, infusion site reactions, nausea, headache, anginal pain, palpitations, shortness of breath, decreased K^+ levels.	***Adults:*** CHF, pulmonary edema; ***Pediatrics:*** CHF, cardiogenic shock.
Epinephrine	IV, SQ	***Adults:*** Cardiac arrest: 1mg q3-5min; Bradycardia, Hypotension: 2-10mcg/min. ***Pediatrics:*** Anaphylaxis: 0.01mg/kg q3-5 min; Asthma: 0.01mg/kg SQ q15 min; Cardiac arrest: 0.01mg/kg IV q3-5 min (max 1mg); Shock: 0.1-1mcg/kg IV per min.	**W/P:** Caution in elderly, CV disease, HTN, diabetes, hyperthyroidism, and psychoneurotic individuals. Extreme caution with long-standing bronchial asthma or emphysema patients who also have degenerative heart disease. Overdosage may cause cerebrovascular hemorrhage due to sharp rise in BP. Fatalities from pulmonary edema reported. Contains sulfites. **Contra:** Narrow-angle glaucoma, shock, use during general anesthesia, organic brain damage, local anesthesia of certain areas (fingers, toes). **P/N:** Category C, safety in nursing not known. **A/E:** Palpitations, anxiety, headache, fear.	***Adults:*** Cardiac arrest, bradycardia, hypotension; ***Pediatrics:*** Anaphylaxis, asthma (severe), cardiac arrest, shock.

Table 13.2. PRESCRIBING INFORMATION FOR EMERGENCY DRUGS *(cont.)*

NAME	FORM	DOSAGE	WARNINGS/PRECAUTIONS, CONTRAINDICATIONS & ADVERSE EFFECTS	INDICATIONS
PRESSORS *(cont.)*				
Norepinephrine	IV	***Adults:*** 0.5-1 mcg/min up to 30 mcg/min titrate to effect. ***Pediatrics:*** 0.1-2 mcg/kg/min titrate to effect.	**W/P:** Use extreme caution with patients receiving MAOIs or antidepressants of the triptyline or imipramine types; may result in severe prolonged HTN. Avoid HTN; record BP every 2 min from time of administration until desired BP, then every 5 min. The rate of flow must be watched constantly; never leave patient unattended. Give infusions into a large vein. Check infusion site frequently for free flow. **Contra:** Hypotensive from blood volume deficits except when given as an emergency measure. Do not give to patients with mesenteric or peripheral vascular thrombosis. Cyclopropane and halothane anesthesia. **P/N:** Category C, caution in nursing. **A/E:** Ischemic injury, bradycardia, arrhythmias, anxiety, transient headache, respiratory difficulty, extravasation necrosis at injection site.	***Adults:*** Shock with low total peripheral resistance; ***Pediatrics:*** Hypotension due to distributive shock.
Vasopressin	IV	***Adults:*** One 40-unit dose in place of 1st or 2nd dose of epinephrine.	**W/P:** Not to be used in patients with vascular disease. May produce water intoxication; signs include drowsiness, listlessness, and headaches. Use with caution in the presence of epilepsy, migraine, asthma, or heart failure. **Contra:** Chronic nephritis with nitrogen retention until reasonable nitrogen levels are reached. **P/N:** Category C, caution in nursing. **A/E:** Anaphylaxis (cardiac arrest and/or shock), circumoral pallor, arrhythmias, abdominal cramps, nausea, vomiting, tremor, vertigo, bronchial constriction, sweating, urticaria.	Refractory VF, asystole, pulseless electrical activity.
REVERSAL AGENTS				
Flumazenil	IV	***Adults:*** 1st 0.2mg over 15 sec, 2nd 0.3mg over 30 sec, 3rd 0.5mg over 30 sec may repeat q1min to response or total 3mg given.	**W/P:** Caution in overdoses involving multiple drug combinations. Risk of seizures, especially with long-term benzodiazepine (BZD)-induced sedation, cyclic antidepressant overdose, concurrent major sedative-hypnotic drug withdrawal, recent therapy with repeated doses of parenteral BZDs, myoclonic jerking or seizure prior to flumazenil administration. Monitor for resedation, respiratory depression, or other residual BZD effects (up to 2 hrs). Avoid use in the ICU; increased risk of unrecognized BZD dependence. Caution with head injury, alcoholism, and other drug dependencies. Does not reverse respiratory depression/hypoventilation or cardiac depression. May provoke panic attacks with history of panic disorder. Adjust subsequent doses in hepatic dysfunction. Not for use as treatment for BZD dependence or for management of protracted abstinence syndromes. May trigger dose-dependent withdrawal syndromes. Extravasation may occur; administer IV into a large vein. **Contra:** Patients given BZDs for life-threatening conditions (eg, control of ICP or status epilepticus), signs of serious cyclic antidepressant overdose. **P/N:** Category C, caution in nursing. **A/E:** N/V, dizziness, injection-site pain, increased sweating, headache, abnormal or blurred vision, agitation.	Reversal of toxicity from BZD overdose.

BB = black box warning; **W/P** = warnings/precautions; **Contra** = contraindications; **P/N** = pregnancy category rating and nursing considerations; **A/E** = adverse effects.

NAME	FORM	DOSAGE	WARNINGS/PRECAUTIONS, CONTRAINDICATIONS & ADVERSE EFFECTS	INDICATIONS
Naloxone	IV, IM, SQ	***Adults:*** 0.4-2mg titrate to resolution of respiratory depression. ***Pediatrics:*** 0.1mg/kg bolus q2min; titrate to effect (max 2mg) 0.002-0.16mg/kg/hr infusion.	**W/P:** Caution in patients, including newborns of mothers known or suspected of opioid physical dependence. May precipitate acute withdrawal syndrome. Have other resuscitative measures available. Caution with cardiac, renal, or hepatic disease. Monitor patients satisfactorily responding due to extended opioid duration of action. Abrupt postoperative opioid depression reversal may result in serious adverse effects leading to death. **P/N:** Category C, caution in nursing. **A/E:** HTN, hypotension, ventricular tachycardia and fibrillation, dyspnea, pulmonary edema, cardiac arrest, NV, sweating, seizures, body aches, fever, nervousness.	Reversal of toxicity from opioid overdose.
VASODILATORS				
Nitroglycerin	Sublingual, Spray	***Adults:*** Tablet: 0.4mg at 5-min intervals to total of 3 doses. Spray: 1-2 sprays (0.4mg each) at 5-min intervals to 3 doses.	**W/P:** Do not swallow tabs. Severe hypotension may occur; caution with volume depletion or hypotension. May aggravate angina caused by hypertrophic cardiomyopathy. D/C if blurred vision or dry mouth develops. May interfere with cholesterol tests. Monitor with acute MI or CHF. Tolerance to other nitrate forms may decrease effects. Caution in elderly. **Contra:** Early MI, severe anemia, increased ICP, concomitant phosphodiesterases. **P/N:** Category C, caution in nursing. **A/E:** Headache, vertigo, dizziness, weakness, palpitation, syncope, flushing, postural hypotension, drug rash, exfoliative dermatitis.	Angina, CHF, pulmonary edema.
Sodium nitroprusside	IV	***Adults:*** 0.1mcg/kg/min, titrate up to 5-10mcg/kg/min q3-5min to effect. ***Pediatrics:*** <40kg: 1-8mcg/kg/min infusion. >40kg: 0.1-5mcg/kg/min infusion.	**W/P:** Not suitable for direct injection. May cause excessive hypotension and excessive accumulation of cyanide. Can cause increases in intracranial pressure. Use with caution in patients with hepatic insufficiency. When used for controlled hypotension during anesthesia, capacity to compensate for anemia and hypovolemia may be diminished. **Contra:** Not to be used in the treatment of compensatory HTN. Should not be used to produce hypotension during surgery in patients with known inadequate cerebral circulation. Do not use in patients with congenital (Leber's) optic atrophy or with tobacco amblyopia. **P/N:** Category C, not for use in nursing. **A/E:** Methemoglobinemia, thiocyanate toxicity, bradycardia, ECG changes, tachycardia, rash, hypothyroidism, ileus, decreased platelet aggregation, increased intracranial pressure, flushing, venous streaking, irritation at the infusion site.	***Adults:*** Hypertensive crisis, heart failure with pulmonary edema.

Section II.

Drugs Used in Medicine: Treatment and Pharmacological Considerations for Dental Patients Receiving Medical Care

Chapter 14

Cardiovascular Drugs

Steven Ganzberg, D.M.D., M.S

Cardiovascular disease affects one in six men and one in seven women aged 45 to 64 years in the United States. The incidence increases to one in three for people >65 years. Numerous medications, with considerably different mechanisms of action, are prescribed to treat these disorders. Primary mechanisms involve the renin-angiotensin system mediated via renal mechanisms and nervous-system control via adrenergic supply. Not surprisingly, medications to treat cardiovascular disease modify these systems or associated receptor systems.

This chapter will discuss the medications used for the following cardiovascular disorders: dysrhythmias, congestive heart failure, angina, hypertension, and hypercholesterolemia. The chapter is organized by drug class or therapeutic use and provides a brief explanation of each. It should be noted that drugs utilized for erectile dysfunction are included in the antihypertensive drugs section of this chapter because they are vasodilators. Sildenafil (Viagra) was originally tested as a systemic antihypertensive with poor results but is currently available for use in pulmonary hypertension (Revatio).

Special Dental Considerations

Before performing any dental procedure with a patient who has cardiovascular disease, evaluate the patient's blood pressure, heart rate, and regularity of rhythm. Review any change in medication regimen. It is important for patients to take their cardiovascular medications at their usual scheduled time, irrespective of a dental appointment, to minimize the possibility of intraoperative hypertension or tachycardia.

Noncompliance with medication regimens is not uncommon. Special precautions should be taken to minimize the stress or pain of a dental procedure so that adverse cardiovascular responses are, in turn, minimized.

Many of these drugs can cause orthostatic hypotension. Make sure the patient sits up in the dental chair for 1 to 2 minutes after being in a supine position and monitor the patient when he or she is standing. Minimize use of epinephrine in local anesthetic solutions and take extra care with aspiration to avoid intravascular injection. If local anesthetic solutions containing epinephrine are deemed necessary, it has been recommended that no more than 40 μg of epinephrine (0.04 mg or approximately two 1.7-mL cartridges of local anesthetic with 1:100,000 epinephrine) should be used for successive dental anesthetic injections in patients with cardiovascular disease. Vital sign monitoring may be of value between injections for selected patients with severe disease. Additional injections of local anesthetic with epinephrine can be given after approximately 5 to 10 minutes if vital signs are satisfactory. *The use of gingival retraction cord with epinephrine is absolutely contraindicated in all patients with cardiovascular disease; this cord should be used with extreme caution, if at all, in other patients.*

Patients with cardiovascular disease may also be taking anticoagulants. Therefore, before dental procedures involving bleeding are performed, consultation with the patient's physician may be indicated to adjust the anticoagulant dose as discussed in Chapter 19 (Hematologic Drugs).

ANTIARRHYTHMIC DRUGS

In cardiac dysrhythmia, some aspect of normal cardiac electrophysiology is disturbed. This may manifest in one or more of the following: the sinoatrial (SA) node, atrioventricular (AV) node, Bundle of His, Purkinje fibers, or in cardiac muscle itself. Antidysrhythmic drugs modify aberrant electrophysiological processes to help restore or improve an unacceptable rate, an unacceptable rhythm, or both. Some antidysrhythmic drugs, such as β-blockers and calcium channel blockers, are also used for the treatment of other cardiovascular diseases, such as hypertension.

See **Tables 14.1** and **14.2** for basic information on antidysrhythmic drugs.

Special Dental Considerations

If dental patients have been taking these drugs for long periods and their symptoms are under adequate control, the management of these patients in an outpatient dental setting without continuous cardiac monitoring is generally acceptable. Hypotension may be encountered. Quinidine is used for several dysrhythmias, but commonly for atrial fibrillation. Other Class I (Na^+ channel blockers) and Class III (K^+ channel blockers) agents are frequently administered either intravenously or orally for severe cardiac dysrhythmias such as ventricular tachycardia. Class II (β-blockers) and Class IV (Ca^{++} channel blockers) agents can be used for hypertension, dysrhythmia control, or angina. Consider ECG and continual vital-sign monitoring for patients with serious dysrhythmia. In addition, follow the recommendations listed under "Special Dental Considerations" at the beginning of this chapter for all drugs in this category.

Use of large quantities of injected local anesthetics may have additive and possibly detrimental cardiac effects. Minimize use of epinephrine in local anesthetic solutions, and take extra care with aspiration to avoid intravascular injection. A stress-reduction protocol is appropriate.

Most Class I and Class III agents may, in rare cases, cause leukopenia, thrombocytopenia, or agranulocytosis. Consider medication-induced adverse effects if gingival bleeding or infection occurs. Defer elective dental treatment if hematologic parameters are compromised.

Quinidine and amiodarone can cause bitter or altered taste. Amiodarone can cause facial flushing.

In orofacial pain management, oral analogues of lidocaine, such as mexiletine, have been reported to be of some use in certain neuropathic pain states. The dentist using these drugs as therapeutic agents is presumed to be proficient in prescribing and managing these medications.

Drug Interactions of Dental Interest

The use of local anesthetics with or without vasoconstrictors is described earlier under "Special Dental Considerations." There may be additive anticholinergic effects, such as dry mouth and constipation, with anticholinergic drugs and some sedating antihistamines. Additionally, the cardio-accelerating effect of these medications may be undesirable. Barbiturates, especially when chronically administered, may induce hepatic enzymes and decrease the plasma levels of many antidysrhythmics. Neuromuscular blockade during general anesthesia may be prolonged. Phenytoin interactions are covered in Chapter 17 (Neurological Drugs), although this agent typically is used as an antidysrhythmic only in acute cases, for digitalis overdose.

Laboratory Value Alterations

- Most Class I and Class III agents may cause leukopenia, thrombocytopenia, or agranulocytosis in rare cases. Bleeding times may be affected.
- Quinidine may cause anemia.
- Disopyramide may lower blood glucose levels.

Pharmacology

The antidysrhythmic drugs, classified in four groups from Class I to Class IV, modify the aberrant electrophysiological process to help restore more normal rate and rhythm. The classification of antidysrhythmic drugs is based on the predominant electrophysiological effect of each drug on the various components of the cardiac conduction system in regard to automaticity, refractoriness, and responsiveness. Examples of conditions in which these drugs are useful include atrial fibrillation and other atrial dysrhythmias, emergency treatment of ventricular fibrillation, ventricular dysrhythmias (including premature ventricular contractions, or PVCs), ventricular tachycardia, and drug-induced dysrhythmias.

CARDIAC GLYCOSIDES

These drugs are used mainly to treat congestive heart failure and certain cardiac dysrhythmias such as atrial fibrillation. Digoxin is the only commonly used cardiac glycoside in the U.S.

See **Tables 14.1** and **14.2** for basic information on cardiac glycosides.

Special Dental Considerations

Increased gag reflex is possible. Bright dental lights may not be tolerated. Evaluate the patient's anticoagulation status and follow the recommendations listed under "Special Dental Considerations" at the beginning of this chapter for drugs in this category.

Drug Interactions of Dental Interest

Minimize use of epinephrine in local anesthetic solutions, and take extra care with aspiration to avoid intravascular injection.

Sudden increases in potassium, such as through rapid IV administration of penicillin G potassium or succinylcholine, may precipitate digitalis-induced dysrhythmia.

Pharmacology

These drugs increase the force of cardiac contraction and decrease heart rate. By these mechanisms, an enlarged heart is allowed to function more efficiently and its size may be reduced. Because of the rate-slowing effects of these drugs, they are also used to treat specific supraventricular tachycardias. The primary mechanisms of action include inhibition of the sodium-potassium adenosinetriphosphatase (or ATPase) pump and increases in the availability of myocardial Ca^{++} ions intracellularly. This drug has a narrow therapeutic index that necessitates frequent plasma level determinations.

ANTIANGINAL AGENTS

Angina pectoris, literally "pain in the chest," usually results from a lack of adequate oxygen (ischemia) for myocardial need secondary to coronary atherosclerosis. There are three types of angina—chronic stable exertional angina, vasospastic (Prinzmetal's) angina, and unstable angina. Chronic stable exertional angina usually occurs in patients when increased activity is such that myocardial oxygen requirement exceeds supply. These patients typically carry a sublingual tablet or spray nitroglycerin, which usually aborts attacks in combination with rest. Vasospastic angina usually occurs at rest secondary to coronary vasospasm rather than atherosclerosis. Unstable angina is, as the name implies, new-onset angina or worsening angina in a patient who was previously stable. No elective dental procedures should be performed for patients with unstable angina until medically stabilized.

Immediate-acting nitrates, long-acting nitrates, β-blockers and calcium channel blockers are used in the management of angina.

See **Tables 14.1** and **14.2** for basic information on antianginal drugs.

Special Dental Considerations

Patients with angina who are taking sublingual nitroglycerin on an as-needed basis should have this medication available at all dental appointments. In the event of chest pain during a dental visit, the prompt use of nitroglycerin is indicated. Supplemental oxygen and vital-sign monitoring are appropriate. Nitroglycerin in the dentist's emergency kit should be checked regularly, as its shelf life is generally short. This is especially true of sublingual nitroglycerin tablets after the container has been opened.

In addition, follow the recommendations listed under "Special Dental Considerations" at the beginning of this chapter.

Nitroglycerin may cause flushing of the face, headache, and xerostomia.

Drug Interactions of Dental Interest

Minimize use of epinephrine in local anesthetic solutions, and take extra care with aspiration to avoid intravascular injection. Opioids may have added hypotensive effects.

Laboratory Value Alterations

- Use of nitrate-based antianginal agents may increase the risk of methemoglobinemia. Pulse oximetry may overestimate oxygen saturation.

Pharmacology

Four types of drugs are used to treat angina. The nitrates, typified by nitroglycerin, are direct-acting vasodilators. The primary effect is reduction in venous and arterial tone (former more than the latter) leading to decreased myocardial workload and less so, coronary vasodilation. Long-acting nitrates, such as isosorbide dinitrate, are also somewhat effective; however, tolerance to these agents limits their long-term value. β-blockers, which block adrenergic responses, may be helpful in treating angina by decreasing myocardial rate and workload. Calcium channel blockers cause vasodilation and slow heart rate, thus decreasing anginal attacks. Lastly, antiplatelet and anticoagulation agents, such as aspirin, may be of value in preventing myocardial infarction.

ANTIHYPERTENSIVE AGENTS

Hypertension is common in the U.S., affecting 15% to 20% of the population. The risk of hypertension increases dramatically with age. Physiological blood pressure regulation is a complex interrelationship of multiple overlapping systems. Generally, ACE inhibitors or diuretics are considered first-line agents. Other medications—such as ß-blockers, calcium channel blockers, α-blockers and direct-acting vasodilators—are then used, alone or in combination, to control blood pressure. Most patients require a multiple-medication regimen.

As dental therapeutic agents, many of these drugs are used to treat chronic orofacial pain conditions. β-blockers and calcium channel blockers are used to manage migraine and other neurovascular conditions. Verapamil is used for prevention of cluster headache. β-blockers and α-blockers are used in the management of complex regional pain syndrome (sympathetically maintained pain). Clonidine is used for a variety of painful conditions. The dentist using these drugs as therapeutic agents is presumed to be proficient in prescribing and managing these medications.

DIURETICS

Diuretic drugs generally exert an antihypertensive effect by increasing sodium and water excretion, thus decreasing blood volume. This decrease in blood volume decreases arterial tone and reduces myocardial workload. These drugs are commonly first-line agents and frequently are combined with other antihypertensives.

See **Tables 14.1** and **14.2** for basic information on diuretics.

Special Dental Considerations

Potassium-sparing diuretics may rarely cause agranulocytosis and thrombocytopenia. Consider medication-induced adverse effects if gingival bleeding or infection occurs. In addition, some patients taking diuretics may experience xerostomia, which may require special dental care.

In addition, follow the recommendations listed under "Special Dental Considerations" at the beginning of this chapter.

Drug Interactions of Dental Interest

NSAIDs may antagonize natriuresis and the antihypertensive effects of some diuretics.

Diflunisal, specifically, may increase the plasma concentration of hydrochlorothiazide. Excessive use of epinephrine in local anesthetic solutions may antagonize the antihypertensive effects of these agents. All diuretics, except potassium-sparing agents, may enhance neuromuscular blockade during general anesthesia.

Laboratory Value Alterations

- Loop diuretics and thiazide diuretics can increase blood glucose levels as well as lead to hypokalemia.
- Potassium-sparing diuretics may rarely cause agranulocytosis and thrombocytopenia.

Pharmacology

The site of action of these drugs can be any portion of the kidney from the glomerulus to the distal tubule. Modulation of electrolytes and water reabsorption are common mechanisms of action. It should be noted that patients may be taking these drugs for conditions other than essential hypertension, such as renal failure, glaucoma, or congestive heart failure. A thorough health history review should provide the necessary information.

ADRENERGIC BLOCKING AGENTS

Adrenergic blocking agents include β-blockers, α-blockers, and combined α- and β-blockers. These drugs are used to manage hypertension by decreasing sympathetic nervous system activity.

See **Tables 14.1** and **14.2** for basic information on adrenergic blocking agents.

Special Dental Considerations

Rarely, taste changes have been reported. In addition, the dentist should follow the recommendations listed under "Special Dental Considerations" at the beginning of this chapter.

A rebound hypertensive crisis may occur if a patient abruptly stops taking drugs in this category prior to a dental appointment. Instruct dental patients to take their medications at the usual time irrespective of the time of their dental appointment.

Drug Interactions of Dental Interest

Vasoconstrictors in local anesthetics

β-Blockers. Hypertension and bradycardia can occur when epinephrine or levonordefrin in local anesthetic solutions is administered to patients taking nonselective β-blockers. Monitor vital signs before and after injection of local anesthetics containing vasoconstrictors. There is generally minimal interaction of local anesthetic solutions containing epinephrine with cardioselective β-blockers.

α-Blockers. Hypotension and tachycardia can rarely occur when commonly used doses of epinephrine in local anesthetic solutions is administered to patients taking α-blockers. Monitor vital signs before and after injection of local anesthetics containing vasoconstrictors.

Combined α- and β-blockers. There is generally minimal interaction with local anesthetic solutions containing epinephrine or levonordefrin.

For patients taking medications with β-blockade, long-term NSAID use can lead to significant renal compromise. Careful laboratory monitoring is recommended.

All adrenergic blocking agents

NSAIDs may partially antagonize the antihypertensive effects of these medications. Opioids may potentiate the hypotensive effect of these medications.

β-Blockers only

These agents may decrease the clearance of injected local anesthetics from the peripheral circulation. Phenothiazines may increase the plasma concentration of both drugs.

Pharmacology

The peripheral adrenergic autonomic system principally consists of β_1, β_2, α_1, and α_2 receptors. Catecholamines, such as epinephrine and norepinephrine, act as agonists at these receptors, which have numerous physiological effects. In regard to blood pressure control:

- β_1 activity increases force and rate of cardiac contraction, thus causing tachycardia and increase in blood pressure
- β_2 activity causes vasodilation in skeletal muscles, thus decreasing blood pressure
- α_1 receptors cause peripheral vasoconstriction, thus causing an increase in blood pressure
- α_2 activity causes a decrease in the release of norepinephrine in the central nervous system, thus decreasing adrenergic tone; α_2 activity in some peripheral vascular beds can cause transient vasoconstriction

Adrenergic blocking agents work on one or more of these receptors to alter the sympathetic nervous system response.

β-Blockers

β-Blockers provide blood pressure control by decreasing the force and rate of cardiac contraction. They are also useful in tachydysrhythmias and angina pectoris. β-blockers are either nonselective or cardioselective. The nonselective β-blockers are antagonists at both the β_1 and β_2 receptors. The cardioselective β-blockers are antagonists at predominantly the β_1 receptor. Because of this difference in receptor activity, patients taking β_1 cardioselective agents experience little interaction with epinephrine in local anesthetic solutions, while those taking nonselective agents may experience unwanted hypertension and bradycardia.

α-Blockers

α-Blockers block either the α_1 receptor (making them selective) or both the α_1 and α_2 receptors (making them nonselective). These drugs control blood pressure by decreasing peripheral vascular tone. The resulting reflex tachycardia makes these agents less useful in hypertension management. Since activation of α_2 receptors decreases adrenergic tone, agents that block both α_1 and α_2 receptors may not be desirable in some patients. These drugs are more commonly used to improve urinary flow in prostatic hypertrophy. A nonselective α-blocker, phentolamine (OraVerse), has recently been marketed for use in reversal of soft tissue anesthesia associated with dental local anesthetic injection and is discussed in Chapter 1.

Combined α- and β-blockers

Labetalol and carvedilol block both α_1 and β_1/β_2 receptors with more activity at α-receptors than at β-receptors. Labetalol and carvedilol thus possess properties of a nonselective β-blocker and a vasodilator.

DIRECT-ACTING VASODILATORS

Vasodilators include hydralazine, minoxidil, diazoxide, nitroglycerin and its derivatives, as well as the calcium channel blockers, which are discussed in a separate section below. These drugs work directly on the peripheral vasculature to decrease arterial and/or venous tone.

See **Tables 14.1** and **14.2** for basic information on direct-acting vasodilators.

Special Dental Considerations

Hydralazine may, rarely, cause agranulocytosis and thrombocytopenia. Consider medication effects if gingival bleeding or infection occurs. Facial flushing may occur. Excessive facial hair growth may be seen with minoxidil.

In addition, follow the recommendations listed under "Special Dental Considerations" at the beginning of this chapter.

Drug Interactions of Dental Interest

Excessive use of epinephrine in local anesthetic solutions may antagonize the antihypertensive effects of these agents. NSAIDs may partially antagonize the antihypertensive effects of these medications. Opioids may potentiate the hypotensive effect of these medications.

Laboratory Value Alterations

- Erythrocyte concentration, hemoglobin, and hematocrit may be artificially decreased due to hemodilution.

Pharmacology

These agents provide hypertension control predominantly by various direct actions on vascular smooth muscle. The mechanism of action is believed to be mediated via nitric oxide, which alters Ca^{++} dependent muscular contractility or via vascular potassium channels and thus produces vascular muscle relaxation.

PDE5 INHIBITORS FOR ERECTILE DYSFUNCTION

Phosphodiesterase 5 (PDE5) inhibitors are used mainly to treat erectile dysfunction, which is caused by organic, psychogenic, or mixed etiologies. Diseases such as diabetes and peripheral vascular disease, as well as postsurgical sequelae such as those following prostatectomy, can cause erectile dysfunction.

See **Tables 14.1** and **14.2** for basic information on PDE5 inhibitors.

Special Dental Considerations

Glossitis, stomatitis, gingivitis, and xerostomia have been reported; however, a causal relationship to drug use is unclear.

Drug Interactions of Dental Interest

Erythromycin, ketoconazole, and itraconazole may increase plasma levels of PDE5 inhibitors. Nitroglycerin, as may be administered by the dentist for acute chest pain, is contraindicated if there has been recent use of a PDE5 inhibitor.

Pharmacology

The mechanism of erection of the penis involves release of nitric oxide (NO) in the corpus cavernosum during sexual stimulation. NO activates guanylate cyclase, which increases cGMP levels to produce smooth muscle relaxation and increase blood flow to the corpus cavernosum. The PDE5 inhibitors block the degradation of cGMP, thus increasing the effects of NO. At recommended doses, these drugs have no effect in the absence of sexual stimulation.

CALCIUM CHANNEL BLOCKERS

Calcium channel blockers are commonly prescribed antihypertensive, antianginal, and antidysrhythmic agents.

See **Tables 14.1** and **14.2** for basic information on calcium channel blockers.

Special Dental Considerations

Gingival enlargement can occur with these agents. Meticulous oral hygiene can reduce these effects. If gingival enlargement occurs, consult the patient's physician about changing the medication to a non-calcium channel blocker antihypertensive. Nimodipine may cause thrombocytopenia. Other agents rarely cause blood dyscrasias. Consider medication-induced adverse effects if gingival bleeding or infection occurs.

In addition, follow the recommendations listed under "Special Dental Considerations" at the beginning of this chapter.

Drug Interactions of Dental Interest

Excessive use of epinephrine in local anesthetic solutions may antagonize the antihypertensive effects of these agents. NSAIDs may partially antagonize the antihypertensive effects of these medications. Opioids may potentiate the hypotensive effect of these medications. There is a possible increased hypotensive effect with aspirin.

Pharmacology

These drugs decrease peripheral vascular tone by decreasing calcium influx in vascular smooth muscle. The antidysrhythmic effect is due primarily to decreasing the slow inward Ca^{++} current in the cardiac conduction system. The agents also depress force and rate of cardiac contraction to various degrees. For instance, verapamil and diltiazem control heart rate more effectively than other calcium channel blockers while most other agents act more prominently by direct vasodilation.

DRUGS ACTING ON THE RENIN-ANGIOTENSIN SYSTEM

These drugs are considered first-line agents in the control of hypertension. By blocking the effects of angiotensin II, a potent vasoconstrictor, these agents decrease high blood pressure in many patients. The angiotensin receptor blockers exert antagonist activity at the receptor on the blood vessel wall while angiotensin-converting enzyme (ACE) inhibitors block the formation of angiotensin II. A new renin inhibiting agent has more recently become available as well.

See **Tables 14.1** and **14.2** for basic information on drugs acting on the renin-angiotensin system.

Special Dental Considerations

These agents may cause neutropenia or agranulocytosis. Consider medication-induced adverse effects if gingival bleeding or infection occurs. Angioneurotic edema may occur on the face, tongue, or hypopharynx with ACE inhibitors. Coughing is a common side effect of ACE inhibitors. Loss of taste has been reported, but rarely.

In addition, follow the recommendations listed under "Special Dental Considerations" at the beginning of this chapter.

Drug Interactions of Dental Interest

Excessive use of epinephrine in local anesthetic solutions may antagonize the antihypertensive effects of these agents. NSAIDs may partially antagonize the antihypertensive effects of these medications. Long-term NSAID use can lead to significant renal compromise and careful monitoring is recommended. Opioids may potentiate the hypotensive effect of these medications. Potassium-containing medications, such as penicillin G potassium administered IV, may exacerbate medication-induced hyperkalemia.

Laboratory Value Alterations

- Agranulocytosis and neutropenia may occur.

Pharmacology

Under normal conditions, the renin-angiotensin system provides for an increase in blood pressure when hypotension occurs. Renin released from the renal glomerulus leads to the formation of angiotensin I, which is converted to angiotensin II, primarily in the lung by angiotensin converting enzyme (ACE). Angiotensin II is a potent vasoconstrictor and also stimulates aldosterone release. The antihypertensive effect of these agents occurs when angiotensin II is blocked, either at the angiotensin II receptor on the blood vessel wall or by decreased formation of angiotensin II itself. This latter effect occurs when angiotensin-converting enzyme (ACE) in the lung is inhibited, thus blocking the metabolism of angiotensin I to angiotensin II. The term "ACE inhibitor" is therefore commonly used with these medications. A newer renin-inhibiting agent blocks the release of renin early in this cascade, providing another way to modify this system.

CENTRALLY ACTING ANTIHYPERTENSIVE AGENTS

These drugs act in the central nervous system (CNS) to decrease peripheral sympathetic tone.

See **Tables 14.1** and **14.2** for basic information on centrally acting antihypertensive agents.

Special Dental Considerations

A rebound hypertensive crisis may occur if patients abruptly stop taking drugs in this category prior to a dental appointment. Instruct dental patients to take their medications at the usual time irrespective of the time of their dental appointment.

These drugs may inhibit salivary flow. Parotid pain may occur.

In addition, follow the recommendations listed under "Special Dental Considerations" at the beginning of this chapter.

Drug Interactions of Dental Interest

Excessive use of epinephrine in local anesthetic solutions may antagonize the antihypertensive effects of these agents and produce a serious hypertensive crisis. NSAIDs may partially antagonize the antihypertensive effects of these medications. Opioids may potentiate the hypotensive and sedative effects of these medications. Other oral or IV sedative agents may be potentiated by these agents. There may be a decreased antihypertensive effect with tricyclic antidepressants. Methyldopa may increase the anticoagulant effect of coumarin anticoagulants.

Pharmacology

The mechanism of action of these agents is chiefly via activation of CNS α_2 agonist action. As the α_2 receptor decreases adrenergic tone, there is a decrease in sympathetic outflow. This causes a decrease in blood pressure and heart rate.

PERIPHERAL ADRENERGIC NEURON ANTAGONISTS

This diverse group of drugs is rarely prescribed today due to numerous undesirable side effects and the availability of other more efficacious agents.

See **Tables 14.1** and **14.2** for basic information on peripheral adrenergic neuron antagonists.

Special Dental Considerations

These drugs may inhibit salivary flow.

In addition, follow the recommendations listed under "Special Dental Considerations" at the beginning of this chapter.

Drug Interactions of Dental Interest

Peripheral adrenergic neuron antagonists can cause administered epinephrine to have an exaggerated cardiovascular effect. Carefully monitor blood pressure and heart rate if local anesthetic solutions containing epinephrine are deemed essential. NSAIDs may partially antagonize the antihypertensive effects of these medications. Opioids may potentiate the hypotensive and sedative effects of these medications. Other oral or IV sedative agents may be potentiated by these agents. Phenothiazines may exhibit increased extrapyramidal reactions.

Pharmacology

These drugs act principally by depleting norepinephrine and other catecholamines from the adrenergic nerve endings. Therefore, decreases in heart rate, force of cardiac contraction, and peripheral vascular resistance result. These drugs can have complex effects when initially administered.

ANTICHOLESTEROL DRUGS

3-Hydroxy-3-methylglutaryl coenzyme A (HMG CoA) reductase inhibitors (statins) are the primary drugs used to lower cholesterol, predominantly low-density lipoproteins (LDLs), also called "bad cholesterol." Some agents increase HDLs, the "good cholesterol." Drugs that lower LDLs and raise HDLs can prevent the formation of, slow the progression of, or decrease already-formed atherosclerotic plaques. This can lead to improved coronary blood flow and a decrease in morbidity and mortality associated with coronary artery disease.

Other agents used to modify triglyceride levels and cholesterol include resins (cholestyramine and colestipol), fibrates (clofibrate, gemfibrozil, and fenofibrate), inhibitors of cholesterol absorption (ezetimibe), and niacin.

See **Tables 14.1** and **14.2** for dosage and prescribing information on anticholesterol drugs.

Special Dental Considerations

There are no specific dental considerations other than evaluating the overall cardiovascular risk in patients who are hypercholesterolemic, as this indicates at least one risk factor for coronary artery disease.

Drug Interactions of Dental Interest

Use of erythromycin with lovastatin has been associated with increased risk of rhabdomyolysis and acute renal failure. Although this has not been reported for other HMG CoA reductase inhibitors, it is recommended that erythromycin not be given to patients taking any agent in this class. It is not clear if other macrolides, such as clarithromycin, also exhibit this interaction but caution is warranted.

Laboratory Value Alterations

- Levels of serum transaminase may increase.
- Creatinine kinase levels may increase, although this usually is not associated with myositis or rhabdomyolysis.

Pharmacology

The conversion of HMG CoA to mevalonate is the rate-limiting step in the synthesis of cholesterol, primarily in the liver. The inhibition of cholesterol synthesis by HMG CoA reductase inhibitors, which block this rate-limiting step, leads to upregulation of LDL receptors and a subsequent increase in degradation of LDLs. There also is a decrease in the synthesis of LDLs.

Adverse Effects

Table 14.1 lists adverse effects of cardiovascular medications.

SUGGESTED READING

Drugs for cardiac arrhythmias. *Med Lett Drugs Ther.* 1991;33(846):55-60.

Follath F. Clinical pharmacology of antiarrhythmic drugs: variability of metabolism and dose requirements. *J Cardiovasc Pharmacol.* 1991;17(Suppl 6):S74-76.

Friedman L, Schron E, Yusuf S. Risk-benefit assessment of antiarrhythmic drugs: an epidemiological perspective. *Drug Saf.* 1991;6:323-331.

Kaplan NM, ed. *Clinical Hypertension.* 6th ed. Baltimore: Williams & Wilkins; 1994.

Laragh JH, Brenner BM, eds. *Hypertension: Pathology, Diagnosis, and Management*. New York: Raven Press; 1990.

Muzyka BC, Glick M. The hypertensive dental patient. *JADA.* 1997;128:1109-1120.

Nichols C. Dentistry and hypertension. *JADA.* 1997;128:1557-1562.

Veterans Administration Cooperative Study Group on Antihypertensive Agents. Effects of treatment on morbidity in hypertension. *JAMA.* 1967;202:1028-1034.

Table 14.1. PRESCRIBING INFORMATION FOR CARDIOVASCULAR DRUGS

NAME	FORM/ STRENGTH	DOSAGE	WARNINGS/PRECAUTIONS & CONTRAINDICATIONS	ADVERSE EFFECTS†
ANTIANGINALS				
CALCIUM CHANNEL BLOCKERS				
Diltiazem HCl (Cardizem)	**Tab:** 30mg, 60mg*, 90mg*, 120mg*	***Adults:*** **Initial:** 30mg qid (before meals and qhs). Adjust at 1-2 day intervals. **Usual:** 180-360mg/day.	**W/P:** Caution in renal, hepatic, or ventricular dysfunction. Monitor LFTs and renal function with prolonged use. D/C if persistent rash occurs. Symptomatic hypotension may occur. Acute hepatic injury reported. **Contra:** Sick sinus syndrome and 2nd- or 3rd-degree AV block (except with functioning pacemaker), hypotension (<90mmHg systolic), acute MI, pulmonary congestion. **P/N:** Category C, not for use in nursing.	Headache, dizziness, asthenia, flushing, 1st-degree AV block, edema, nausea, bradycardia, rash.
Nifedipine (Procardia)	**Cap:** 10mg, 20mg	***Adults:*** **Initial:** 10mg tid. Titrate over 7-14 days. **Usual:** 10-20mg tid. **Max:** 180mg/day. **Elderly:** Start at low end of dosing range.	**W/P:** May cause hypotension; monitor BP initially or with titration. May exacerbate angina from β-blocker withdrawal. CHF risk, especially with aortic stenosis or β-blockers. Peripheral edema reported. Not for acute reduction of BP or essential HTN. May increase angina or MI with severe obstructive CAD. Avoid with acute coronary syndrome or within 1-2 weeks of MI. Caution in elderly. **P/N:** Category C, unknown use in nursing.	Dizziness, lightheadedness, giddiness, flushing, muscle cramps, headache, weakness, nausea, peripheral edema, nervousness/mood changes.
Verapamil HCl (Calan, Covera-HS)	**Tab:** (Calan) 40mg, 80mg*, 120mg*; **Tab, Extended-Release:** (Covera-HS) 180mg, 240mg	***Adults:*** (Calan) **HTN: Initial:** 80mg tid. **Usual:** 360-480mg/day. **Elderly/Small Stature: Initial:** 40mg tid. **Angina: Usual:** 80-120mg tid. **Elderly/Small Stature: Initial:** 40mg tid. **Titrate:** Increase daily or weekly. **A-Fib (Digitalized): Usual:** 240-320mg/day given tid-qid. **PSVT Prophylaxis (Nondigitalized):** 240-480mg/day given tid-qid. **Max:** 480mg/day. **Severe Hepatic Dysfunction:** Give 30% of normal dose. (Covera-HS) **HTN/Angina: Initial:** 180mg qhs. **Titrate:** May increase to 240mg qhs, then 360mg qhs, then 480mg qhs, if needed. Swallow tab whole. **Elderly:** Start at the low end of the dosing range.	**W/P:** Avoid with moderate-to-severe cardiac failure, and ventricular dysfunction if taking a β-blocker. May cause hypotension, AV block, transient bradycardia, PR-interval prolongation. Monitor LFTs periodically; hepatocellular injury reported. Give 30% of normal dose with severe hepatic dysfunction. Caution with hypertrophic cardiomyopathy, renal or hepatic dysfunction. Decrease dose in those with decreased neuromuscular transmission. **Contra:** Severe ventricular dysfunction, hypotension, cardiogenic shock, sick sinus syndrome or 2nd- or 3rd-degree AV block (except with functioning ventricular pacemaker), A-fib/flutter with an accessory bypass tract. **P/N:** Category C, not for use in nursing.	Constipation, dizziness, nausea, hypotension, headache, peripheral edema, CHF, fatigue, pulmonary edema, elevated liver enzymes, dyspnea, bradycardia, AV block, rash, flushing, infection, flu syndrome.
NITRATE VASODILATORS				
Isosorbide Dinitrate (Dilatrate-SR, Isordil, Isordil Titradose)	**Cap, Extended-Release:** 40mg **Tab:** 5mg*, 10mg*, 20mg*, 30mg*; **Tab, Extended-Release:** 40mg; Tab, **Sublingual:** 2.5mg	***Adults:*** **(Dilatrate-SR)** 40mg bid (separate doses by 6 hrs). **Max:** 160mg/day. Should have >18 hr nitrate-free interval. **(Isordil, Isordil Titradose) Prevention: Initial:** 5-20mg bid-tid. **Maint:** 10-40mg bid-tid. Allow a dose-free interval of at least 14 hrs for both formulations. **Elderly:** Start at low end of dosing range.	**W/P:** Severe hypotension may occur; caution with volume depletion and hypotension. Hypotension may cause paradoxical bradycardia and increased angina pectoris. May aggravate angina caused by hypertrophic cardiomyopathy. Monitor for tolerance. Not for use with CHF or acute MI. **P/N:** Category C, caution in nursing.	Headache, lightheadedness, hypotension, syncope, rebound HTN.
Isosorbide Mononitrate (Imdur, Ismo, Monoket)	**Tab:** (Ismo) 20mg* (Monoket) 10mg*, 20mg* **Tab, Extended-Release:** (Imdur) 30mg*, 60mg*, 120mg	***Adults:*** **(Imdur) Initial:** 30-60mg qd in am. **Titrate:** May increase after several days to 120mg/day. Swallow whole with fluids. **Elderly:** Start at lower end of dosing range. **(Ismo)** 20mg bid (space doses 7 hours apart). **(Monoket)** 20mg bid (space doses 7 hours apart). **Small Patients: Initial:** 5mg per dose for 1 day, then increase to 10mg by 2nd or 3rd day.	**W/P:** Not for use with acute MI or CHF. Severe hypotension may occur; caution with volume depletion and hypotension. Hypotension may increase angina pectoris. May aggravate angina caused by hypertrophic cardiomyopathy. Monitor for tolerance. May interfere with cholesterol test. **P/N:** Category B, caution with nursing.	Headache, dizziness, hypotension, N/V, fatigue, GI upset.

*Scored. †Bold entries denote special dental considerations.
BB = black box warning; **W/P** = warnings/precautions; **Contra** = contraindications; **P/N** = pregnancy category rating and nursing considerations.

Table 14.1. PRESCRIBING INFORMATION FOR CARDIOVASCULAR DRUGS *(cont.)*

NAME	FORM/ STRENGTH	DOSAGE	WARNINGS/PRECAUTIONS & CONTRAINDICATIONS	ADVERSE EFFECTS†
ANTIANGINALS *(cont.)*				
NITRATE VASODILATORS *(cont.)*				
Nitroglycerin (Minitran, Nitrek, Nitro-Bid, Nitro-Dur, Nitrolingual Spray, NitroMist, Nitro-quick, Nitrostat)	**Patch:** (Minitran) 0.1mg/hr, 0.2mg/hr, 0.4mg/hr, 0.6mg/hr [30^s]; (Nitrek) 0.2mg/hr, 0.4mg/hr, 0.6mg/hr [30^s]; (Nitro-Dur) 0.1mg/hr, 0.2mg/hr, 0.3mg/hr, 0.4mg/hr, 0.6mg/hr, 0.8mg/hr [30^s] **Oint:** (Nitro-Bid) 2%(15mg/inch) [1g (48^s), 30g, 60g] **Spray:** (Nitrolingual Spray, NitroMist)	***Adults:* (Minitran, Nitrek, Nitro-Dur) Initial:** 0.2-0.4mg/hr for 12-14 hrs. Remove for 10-12 hrs. **(Nitro-Bid) Initial:** Apply 0.5 inch bid (once in the am and 6 hrs later). **Titrate:** May increase to 1 inch bid, then to 2 inches bid. Should have 10-12 hr nitrate-free period. **(Nitrolingual Spray, NitroMist) Acute:** 1-2 sprays at onset of attack onto or under tongue. **Max:** 3 sprays/15 min. **Prophylaxis:** 1-2 sprays onto or under tongue 5-10 min before activity that may cause acute attack. Do not expectorate medication or rinse mouth for 5-10 min after administration. **(Nitroquick, Nitrostat) Treatment:** 1 tab SL or in buccal pouch at onset of attack. May repeat in 5 min. **Max:** 3 tabs in 15 min. **Prophylaxis:** Take 5-10 min	**W/P:** Severe hypotension may occur; caution with volume depletion or hypotension. Vasodilatory effects with phosphodiesterase inhibitors (eg, sildenafil) can result in severe hypotension. May aggravate angina caused by hypertrophic cardiomyopathy. Tolerance to other nitrate forms may decrease effects. Monitor with acute MI or CHF. Do not discharge defibrillator/cardioverter through the patch. The ointment is only for topical use. **Contra:** Concomitant use with phosphodiesterase type 5 (PDE5) inhibitors such as sildenafil, vardenafil, and tadalafil. (Minitran, Nitrek, Nitro-Dur) Allergy to adhesives in NTG patches. (Nitroquick, Nitrostat) Early MI, severe anemia, increased ICP. **P/N:** Category C, caution in nursing.	Headache, lightheadedness, hypotension, flushing, syncope, vertigo, dizziness, weakness, palpitation, rebound HTN, drug rash, exfoliative dermatitis.
Nitroglycerin (Minitran, Nitrek, Nitro-Bid, Nitro-Dur, Nitrolingual Spray, NitroMist, Nitro-quick, Nitrostat) *(cont.)*	400mcg/spray **Tab, Sublingual:** (Nitroquick, Nitrostat) 0.3mg, 0.4mg, 0.6mg	before activity that may cause acute attack. Administer in sitting position.		
MISCELLANEOUS ANTIANGINALS				
Ranolazine (Ranexa)	**Tab, Extended-Release:** 500mg, 1000mg	***Adults:* Initial:** 500mg bid. **Titrate:** May increase to 1000mg bid. **Max:** 1000mg bid. **Concurrent With Diltiazem/Verapamil/Other Moderate CYP3A Inhibitors:** 500mg bid. **Concurrent With P-gp Inhibitors:** Down titrate dose based on clinical response. Swallow whole; do not crush, break, or chew.	**W/P:** May prolong QTc interval in a dose-related manner; avoid with known QT prolongation (including congenital long QT syndrome, uncorrected hypokalemia), known history of ventricular tachycardia, hepatic dysfunction. Monitor BP with severe renal impairment. **Contra:** Strong CYP3A inhibitors (eg, ketoconazole, clarithromycin, saquinavir), CYP3A inducers (eg, rifampin, phenobarbital, carbamazepine), and hepatic dysfunction (Child-Pugh Classes A and B). **P/N:** Category C, not for use in nursing.	Dizziness, nausea, asthenia, constipation, and headache.
ANTIARRHYTHMICS				
CLASS IA ANTIARRHYTHMICS				
Disopyramide Phosphate (Norpace, Norpace CR)	**Cap:** (Norpace) 100mg, 150mg; **Cap, Extended-Release:** (Norpace CR) 100mg, 150mg	***Adults:* Usual:** 400-800mg/day in divided dose. **Recommended:** 150mg q6h immediate-release (IR) or 300mg q12h extended-release (ER). Adjust dose with anticholinergic effects. **Weight <110lbs/Moderate Hepatic or Renal Insufficiency (CrCl >40mL/min):** 100mg q6h IR or 200mg q12h ER. **Severe Renal Insufficiency (with or without initial 150mg LD): CrCl 30-40mL/min:** 100mg q8h IR. **CrCl 30-15mL/min:** 100mg q12h IR. **CrCl <15mL/min:** 100mg q24h IR. **Rapid Control of Ventricular Arrhythmia: LD:** 300mg IR (200mg if <110lbs). Follow with maint dose. **Cardiomyopathy/Cardiac Decompensation: Initial:** 100mg q6-8h IR. Adjust gradually. See PI if no response or toxicity occurs. **Elderly:** Start at low end of dosing range.	**W/P:** Proarrhythmic; reserve for life-threatening ventricular arrhythmias. May cause or worsen CHF and produce hypotension due to negative inotropic properties. Reduce dose if 1st-degree heart block occurs. Avoid with urinary retention, glaucoma, and myasthenia gravis unless adequate overriding measures taken. Atrial flutter/fibrillation; digitalize first. Monitor closely or withdraw if QT prolongation >25% occurs and ectopy continues. D/C if QRS widening >25% occurs. Avoid LD with cardiomyopathy or cardiac decompensation. Correct K^+ abnormalities before therapy. Reduce dose with renal/hepatic dysfunction; monitor ECG. Avoid CR formulation with CrCl ≤40mL/min. Caution with sick sinus syndrome, Wolff-Parkinson-White syndrome,	**Dry mouth,** urinary retention/frequency/urgency, constipation, blurred vision, GI effects, dizziness, fatigue, headache.

†Bold entries denote special dental considerations.
BB = black box warning; **W/P** = warnings/precautions; **Contra** = contraindications; **P/N** = pregnancy category rating and nursing considerations.

NAME	FORM/ STRENGTH	DOSAGE	WARNINGS/PRECAUTIONS & CONTRAINDICATIONS	ADVERSE EFFECTS†
Disopyramide Phosphate (Norpace, Norpace CR) *(cont.)*		***Pediatrics:*** **<1 yr:** 10-30mg/kg/day. **1-4 yrs:** 10-20mg/kg/day. **4-12 yrs:** 10-15mg/kg/day. **12-18 yrs:** 6-15mg/kg/day. Give in equally divided doses q6h. Hospitalize patient during initial therapy. Start dose titration at lower end of range.	bundle branch block, or elderly. May significantly lower blood glucose. **Contra:** Cardiogenic shock, 2nd- or 3rd-degree AV block (if no pacemaker present), congenital QT prolongation. **P/N:** Category C, not for use in nursing.	
Procainamide HCl	**Inj:** 100mg/mL [10mL], 500mg/mL [2mL]	***Adults:*** (IM) **Arrhythmias Associated with Anesthesia/Surgical Operation:** 100-500mg IM. (IV) **Bolus:** 50mg/min. Doses of 100mg may be administered every 5 min at this rate until the arrhythmia is suppressed or until 500mg has been administered, after which it is advisable to wait ≥10 min to allow for more distribution into the tissue before continuing. **Max:** 1g. **Continuous Infusion: LD:** 20mg/mL administered at a constant rate of 1mL/min for 25-30 min to deliver 500-600mg. **Maint:** 2mg/mL administered at a rate of 1-3mL/minute. **Fluid Restricted:** 4mg/mL administered at a rate of 0.5-1.5mL/min. **Max:** 1g.	**BB:** Reserve for life-threatening ventricular arrhythmias. Positive ANA titer may develop with prolonged use. Agranulocytosis, bone marrow depression, neutropenia, hypoplastic anemia, and thrombocytopenia have been reported in approximately 0.5% of patients. **W/P:** Caution in digitalis intoxication; consider use only if discontinuation of digitalis, and therapy with potassium, lidocaine, or phenytoin are ineffective. Caution with AV conduction disturbances and 1st-degree heart block; reduce dose. Cardiovert or digitalize patients with A-fib/flutter before use. Monitor for QRS widening or QT prolongation. Caution in patients with CHF, acute ischemic heart disease, or cardiomyopathy. Concurrent use of additional antiarrhythmic agents enhance prolongation of conduction or depression of contractility; reserve combination therapy for serious arrhythmias unresponsive to monotherapy. Adjust dose in patients with renal insufficiency. Caution with myasthenia gravis; adjust dose of anticholinesterases. Contains sodium metabisulfite, which may induce sulfite hypersensitivity. Monitor BP with the patient supine during administration; ECG monitoring is advisable as well. **Contra:** Complete heart block, 2nd-degree AV block (without pacemaker), SLE, torsades de pointes. **P/N:** Category C, not for use in nursing.	GI disturbances, lupus-like symptoms, elevated LFTs, **bitter taste,** N/V, flushing, psychosis, dizziness, depression, urticaria, pruritus, rash, agranulocytosis.
Quinidine Gluconate	**Inj:** 80mg/mL. **Tab, Extended-Release:** 324mg	***Adults:*** **Inj: A-Fib/Flutter and Ventricular Arrhythmia:** 0.25mg/kg/min. **Max:** 5-10mg/kg. Consider alternate therapy if conversion to sinus rhythm not achieved. **Renal/Hepatic Impairment or CHF:** Reduce dose. **Elderly:** Start at low end of dosing range. **Tab: A-Fib/Flutter Conversion: Initial:** 2 tabs q8h. **Titrate:** Increase cautiously if no effect after 3-4 doses. **Alternate Regimen:** 1 tab q8h for 2 days, then 2 tabs q12h for 2 days, then 2 tabs q8h up to 4 days. **A-Fib/Flutter Relapse Reduction:** 1 tab q8-12h. **Titrate:** Increase cautiously if needed. **Ventricular Arrhythmia:** Dosing regimens not adequately studied. Generally similar to A-Fib/Flutter. **Renal/Hepatic Impairment or CHF:** Reduce dose. May break tab in half. Do not chew or crush.	**W/P:** Increases risk of mortality, especially with structural heart disease. May prolong QTc interval. Paradoxical increase in ventricular rate in A-Fib/Flutter. Caution in those at risk of complete AV block without implanted pacemakers, renal/hepatic dysfunction, and CHF. Physical/pharmacologic maneuvers to terminate paroxysmal supraventricular tachycardia may be ineffective. Exacerbated bradycardia in sick sinus syndrome. (Inj) Rapid infusion can cause peripheral vascular collapse and hypotension. **Contra:** Cardiac rhythm dependent upon a junctional or idioventricular pacemaker (absent of functioning pacemaker), thrombocytopenic purpura with previous treatment, patients adversely affected by anticholinergics. **P/N:** Category C, not for use in nursing.	GI distress, lightheadedness, fatigue, palpitations, weakness, visual problems, N/V, diarrhea, sleep disturbances, rash, headache, cinchonism, hepatotoxicity, autoimmune/inflammatory syndromes.
Quinidine Sulfate	**Tab:** 200mg, 300mg	***Adults:*** **A-Fib/Flutter Conversion: Initial:** 400mg q6h. **Titrate:** Increase cautiously if no effect after 4-5 doses. **A-Fib/Flutter Relapse Reduction:** 200mg q6h. **Titrate:** Increase cautiously if needed. **Ventricular Arrhythmia:** Dosing regimens not adequately studied. D/C and consider other means	**W/P:** Increases risk of mortality, especially with structural heart disease. May prolong QTc interval. Paradoxical increase in ventricular rate in A-fib/flutter. Adjust dose in renal/hepatic dysfunction and CHF. Caution if at risk of complete AV-block in those without implanted pacemakers or in elderly. Physical/	Diarrhea, N/V, headache, esophagitis, lightheadedness, fatigue, palpitations, angina-like pain, weakness, rash, visual problems, cinchonism, hepa-

Table 14.1. PRESCRIBING INFORMATION FOR CARDIOVASCULAR DRUGS *(cont.)*

NAME	FORM/ STRENGTH	DOSAGE	WARNINGS/PRECAUTIONS & CONTRAINDICATIONS	ADVERSE EFFECTS†
ANTIARRHYTHMICS *(cont.)*				
CLASS IA ANTIARRHYTHMICS *(cont.)*				
Quinidine Sulfate *(cont.)*		of cardioversion if the QRS complex widens to 130% of its pre-treatment duration; the QTC interval widens to 130% of its pre-treatment duration and is then longer than 500 ms; P waves disappear; or the patient develops significant tachycardia, symptomatic bradycardia, or hypotension.	pharmacologic maneuvers to terminate paroxysmal supraventricular tachycardia may be ineffective. Exacerbated bradycardia in sick sinus syndrome. Monitor blood counts, hepatic and renal function periodically with long-term therapy. D/C if blood dyscrasia or hepatic/renal dysfunction occurs. **Contra:** Cardiac rhythm dependent upon a junctional or idioventricular pacemaker (in the absence of functioning pacemaker), thrombocytopenic purpura with previous treatment, patients adversely affected by anticholinergics (eg, myasthenia gravis). **P/N:** Category C, not for use in nursing.	totoxicity, autoimmune/inflammatory syndromes.
CLASS IB ANTIARRHYTHMICS				
Lidocaine HCl	**Inj:** 10mg/mL [5mL], 20mg/mL [5mL], 100mg/mL [10mL], 200mg/mL [20mL]	***Adults:* Ventricular Arrhythmias: IV: Bolus: Usual:** 50-100mg (0.35-0.70mg/kg/min; 0.16-0.32mg/lb/min). If the initial injection does not produce the desired response, a second dose may be given after 5 min. **Max:** 200-300mg/hr. **Continuous Infusion: Initial:** 1-4mg/min (0.014-0.057mg/kg/min; 0.006-0.026mg/lb/min). Reassess infusion rate basic as soon as cardiac rhythm appears to be stable or at the earliest signs of toxicity. It should rarely be necessary to continue infusions for prolonged periods. ***Pediatrics:* Ventricular Arrhythmias:** 1mg/kg infused at a rate of 20-50µg/kg/min for prolonged therapy. **Reduced Drug Clearance (eg, Shock, CHF, Cardiac Arrest):** Infusion rate ≤20 µg/kg/min.	**W/P:** Resuscitative equipment, oxygen, and other resuscitative drugs should be immediately available. The 10% and 20% concentrated solutions must not be injected undiluted. Systemic toxicity may result in convulsions accompanied by respiratory depression and/or arrest. Should convulsions persist despite ventilatory therapy with oxygen, small increments of IV anticonvulsants may be used. Use vasopressors if circulatory depression occurs. Monitor ECG constantly; signs of excessive depression of cardiac electrical activity, such as sinus node dysfunction, prolongation of the P-R interval and QRS complex, or the appearance or aggravation of arrhythmias, should be followed by flow adjustment and, if necessary, prompt cessation of the infusion of this agent. Acceleration of ventricular rate may occur when administered to patients with atrial flutter or fibrillation. Caution in patients with severe liver or kidney disease because accumulation of the drug or metabolites may occur. Caution in the treatment of patients with hypovolemia, severe congestive heart failure, shock, the genetic predisposition of malignant hyperthermia, and all forms of heart block. Large doses of lidocaine HCl may cause malignant hyperthermia. In patients with sinus bradycardia or incomplete heart block, the IV administration of lidocaine HCl for the elimination of ventricular ectopic beats without prior acceleration in heart rate (eg, by atropine, isoproterenol, or electric pacing) may promote more frequent and serious ventricular arrhythmias or complete heart block. Reduce dose for pediatric patients and for debilitated and/or elderly patients. **Contra:** History of hypersensitivity to local anesthetics of the amide type, Stokes-Adams syndrome, Wolff-Parkinson-White syndrome, or severe degrees of sinoatrial, atrioventricular, or intraventricular block (without pacemaker). **P/N:** Category B, caution in nursing.	Light-headedness, nervousness, apprehension, euphoria, confusion, dizziness, drowsiness, tinnitus, blurred or double vision, vomiting, sensations of heat/cold/numbness, twitching, tremors, convulsions, unconsciousness, respiratory depression and arrest, bradycardia, hypotension, cardiovascular collapse (which may lead to cardiac arrest), permanent injury to extraocular muscles.

*Scored. †Bold entries denote special dental considerations.
BB = black box warning; **W/P** = warnings/precautions; **Contra** = contraindications; **P/N** = pregnancy category rating and nursing considerations.

NAME	FORM/ STRENGTH	DOSAGE	WARNINGS/PRECAUTIONS & CONTRAINDICATIONS	ADVERSE EFFECTS†
Mexiletine HCl	**Cap:** 150mg, 200mg, 250mg	***Adults:* Initial:** 200mg q8h when rapid control not essential. **Titrate:** Adjust by 50-100mg, not less than every 2-3 days. **Usual:** 200-300mg q8h. **Max:** 1200mg/day. If control with ≤300mg q8h, then may divide daily dose and give q12h. **Max:** 450mg q12h. **For Rapid Control: LD:** 400mg, then 200mg in 8 hrs. **Transfer from Other Class I Oral Agents: Initial:** 200mg and titrate as above, 6-12 hrs after last quinidine sulfate or disopyramide dose, 3-6 hrs after last procainamide dose, or 8-12 hrs after last tocainide dose. **Severe Hepatic Disease:** May need lower dose. Take with food or antacid.	**W/P:** Reserve for life-threatening arrhythmias. May treat patients with 2nd- or 3rd-degree AV block with a pacemaker; monitor continuously. Can worsen arrhythmias. Caution with hypotension, severe CHF, seizure disorder, hepatic impairment, sinus node dysfunction, or intraventricular conduction abnormalities. Leukopenia, agranulocytosis, and abnormal LFTs reported. Monitor ECG. **Contra:** Cardiogenic shock, preexisting 2nd- or 3rd-degree AV block (without pacemaker). **P/N:** Category C, not for use in nursing.	GI distress, tremor, lightheadedness, coordination difficulties, N/V, heartburn.
CLASS IC ANTIARRHYTHMICS				
Flecainide Acetate (Tambocor)	**Tab:** 50mg, 100mg*, 150mg*	***Adults:* PSVT/PAF: Initial:** 50mg q12h. **Titrate:** May increase by 50mg bid every 4 days. **Max:** 300mg/day. **Sustained VT: Initial:** 100mg q12h. **Titrate:** May increase by 50mg bid every 4 days. **Max:** 400mg/day. **CrCl ≤35mL/min: Initial:** 100mg qd or 50mg bid. Reduce dose by 50% with amiodarone. ***Pediatrics:* <6 months: Initial:** 50mg/m^2/day given bid-tid. **≥6 months: Initial:** 100mg/m^2/day given bid-tid. **Max:** 200mg/m^2/day. Reduce dose by 50% with amiodarone.	**W/P:** Avoid with non–life-threatening ventricular arrhythmias. Increased mortality and noncardiac arrests reported. Ventricular proarrhythmic effects may occur with atrial fibrillation/flutter. May cause or worsen CHF, arrhythmias. Slows cardiac conduction; dose-related increases in PR, QRS, and QT intervals reported. Conduction changes may cause sinus pause, sinus arrest, bradycardia, 2nd- or 3rd-degree AV block. Extreme caution with sick sinus syndrome. May increase endocardial pacing thresholds and suppress ventricular escape with pacemakers. Correct hypokalemia or hyperkalemia before therapy. Monitor with significant hepatic impairment. Initiate treatment of sustained VT in the hospital. **Contra:** Right bundle branch block associated with left hemiblock (without a pacemaker), preexisting 2nd- or 3rd-degree AV block, cardiogenic shock. **P/N:** Category C, safety in nursing unknown.	Arrhythmias, hepatic dysfunction, cardiac arrest, CHF, flushing, anxiety, vomiting, diarrhea, tinnitus.
Propafenone HCl (Rythmol, Rythmol SR)	**Cap, Extended-Release:** (Rythmol SR) 225mg, 325mg, 425mg **Tab:** (Rythmol) 150mg*, 225mg*, 300mg*	***Adults:* (Rythmol) *Adults:* Initial:** 150mg q8h. **Titrate:** May increase at minimum 3-4 day intervals to 225mg q8h, then to 300mg q8h if needed. **Max:** 900mg/day. **Elderly/Marked Myocardial Damage:** Increase more gradually during initial phase. **Hepatic Dysfunction:** Reduce dose by 20-30%. **(Rythmol SR) Initial:** 225mg q12h. **Titrate:** May increase at minimum 5 day intervals to 325mg q12h, then to 425mg q12h if needed. **Hepatic Impairment/QRS Widening/2nd- or 3rd-degree AV Block:** Reduce dose.	**W/P:** Avoid with non–life-threatening ventricular arrhythmias, bronchospastic disease, and AV/intraventricular conduction defects unless paced. May cause new or worsened arrhythmias, provoke overt CHF. Caution with hepatic or renal dysfunction. Slows AV conduction. 1st-degree AV block, agranulocytosis, myasthenia gravis exacerbation, positive ANA titers reported. May alter pacing and sensing thresholds of artificial pacemakers. **Contra:** CHF, cardiogenic shock, bradycardia, marked hypotension, bronchospastic disorders, electrolyte imbalance, and sinoatrial, atrioventricular (AV), and intraventricular disorders of impulse generation or conduction (eg, sick sinus node syndrome, AV block) unless paced. **P/N:** Category C, caution in nursing.	Dizziness, chest pain, palpitations, **taste disturbance,** dyspnea, N/V, constipation, anxiety, fatigue, upper respiratory tract infection, headache, influenza, 1st-degree heart block, blood dyscrasias, blurred vision.
CLASS II ANTIARRHYTHMICS (β-BLOCKERS). SEE ANTIHYPERTENSIVES/HEART FAILURE AGENTS FOR OTHER β-BLOCKERS.				
Esmolol HCl (Brevibloc)	**Inj:** 10mg/mL [10mL, 250mL], 20mg/mL [5mL, 100mL]	***Adults:* Supraventricular Tachycardia:** Titrate dose based on ventricular rate. **Load:** 0.5mg/kg over 1 min. **Maint:** 0.05mg/kg/min for next 4 min. **Titrate:** May increase by 0.05mg/kg/min at intervals of 4 min or more up to	**W/P:** Hypotension may occur; monitor BP and reduce dose or d/c if needed. May cause cardiac failure; withdraw at first sign of impending cardiac failure. Caution with supraventricular arrhythmias when patient is compromised	Hypotension, dizziness, diaphoresis, somnolence, confusion, headache, agitation, bronchospasm,

Table 14.1. PRESCRIBING INFORMATION FOR CARDIOVASCULAR DRUGS *(cont.)*

NAME	FORM/ STRENGTH	DOSAGE	WARNINGS/PRECAUTIONS & CONTRAINDICATIONS	ADVERSE EFFECTS†
ANTIARRHYTHMICS *(cont.)*				
CLASS II ANTIARRHYTHMICS (β-BLOCKERS). SEE ANTIHYPERTENSIVES/HEART FAILURE AGENTS FOR OTHER β-BLOCKERS. *(cont.)*				
Esmolol HCl (Brevibloc) *(cont.)*		0.2mg/kg/min. **Rapid Slowing of Ventricular Response:** Repeat 0.5mg/kg load over 1 min, then 0.1mg/kg/min for 4 min. If needed, another (final) load of 0.5mg/kg over 1 min, then 0.15mg/kg/min for 4 min up to 0.2mg/kg/min. May continue infusions for 24-48hrs. **Intraoperative/Postoperative Tachycardia and/or HTN: Immediate Control: Initial:** 80mg bolus over 30 sec. **Maint:** 0.15mg/kg/min. May titrate up to 0.3mg/kg/min. **Gradual Control: Initial:** 0.5mg/kg over 1 min. **Maint:** 0.05mg/kg/min for 4 min. Then, if needed, may repeat load and increase to 0.1mg/kg/min.	hemodynamically or is taking other drugs that decrease peripheral resistance, myocardial filling/contractility, and/or electrical impulse propagation in the myocardium. Not for HTN associated with hypothermia. Caution in bronchospastic diseases; titrate to lowest possible effective dose and terminate immediately in the event of bronchospasm. Caution in diabetics; may mask tachycardia occurring with hypoglycemia. Caution in impaired renal function. Avoid concentrations >10mg/mL and infusions into small veins or through butterfly catheters. Sloughing of skin and necrosis reported with infiltration and extravasation. Use caution when discontinuing infusion in CAD patients. **Contra:** Sinus bradycardia, heart block greater than first degree, cardiogenic shock, or overt heart failure. **P/N:** Category C, caution in nursing.	nausea, infusion-site reactions
Propranolol HCl (Inderal)	**Inj:** 1mg/mL; Tab: 10mg*, 20mg*, 40mg*, 60mg*, 80mg*	***Adults:*** (PO) **HTN: Initial:** 40mg bid. **Titrate:** Increase gradually. **Maint:** 120-240mg/day. **Angina:** 80-320mg/day, given bid-qid. **Arrhythmia:** 10-30mg tid-qid ac and qhs. **MI:** 180-240mg/day, given bid-tid. **Migraine: Initial:** 80mg/day in divided doses. **Usual:** 160-240mg/day in divided doses. **Tremor: Initial:** 40mg bid. **Maint:** 120mg/day. **Max:** 320mg/day. **Hypertrophic Subaortic Stenosis:** 20-40mg tid-qid, ac, and qhs. **Pheochromocytoma:** 60mg/day in divided doses for 3 days before surgery with α-blocker. **Inoperable Tumor:** 30mg/day in divided doses. (IV) **Arrhythmia:** 1-3mg IV at 1mg/min.	**W/P:** Caution with well-compensated cardiac failure, nonallergic bronchospasm, Wolff-Parkinson-White (WPW) syndrome, hepatic or renal dysfunction. Withdrawal before surgery is controversial. May mask hypoglycemia or hyperthyroidism symptoms. Avoid abrupt discontinuation. May reduce IOP. Can cause cardiac failure. Both digitalis glycosides and β-blockers slow atrioventricular conduction and decrease HR. Concomitant use can increase risk of bradycardia. Stevens-Johnson syndrome, toxic epidermal necrolysis, exfoliative dermatitis, erythema multiforme, and urticaria reported. **Contra:** Bronchial asthma, cardiogenic shock, sinus bradycardia, 2nd- and 3rd-degree AV block, CHF (unless failure is secondary to tachyarrhythmia treatable with propranolol). **P/N:** Category C, caution in nursing.	Bradycardia, CHF, hypotension, lightheadedness, mental depression, N/V, allergic reactions, agranulocytosis, dry eyes, alopecia, SLE-like reactions, male impotence, Peyronie's disease, fatigue, dizziness (except vertigo), constipation.
CLASS II/III ANTIARRHYTHMICS				
Sotalol HCl (Betapace AF)	**Tab:** 80mg*, 120mg*, 160mg*	***Adults:*** Initiate with continuous ECG monitoring. **Initial:** 80mg bid. Monitor QT 2-4 hrs after each dose. Reduce dose or d/c if QT ≥500msec. If QT <500msec after 3 days (after 5th or 6th dose if receiving qd dosing), discharge on current treatment. **Titrate:** May increase dose to 120mg during hospitalization. Monitor closely for 3 days with bid dose and for 5-6 doses with qd dose. **Max:** 160mg bid. **CrCl 40-60mL/min: Initial:** 80mg qd. Dose q24h. **CrCl <40mL/min:** Betapace AF is contraindicated. ***Pediatrics:*** **≥2 yrs: Initial:** 30mg/m^2 tid. **Titrate:** Wait at least 36 hrs between dose increases. Guide dose by response, ie heart rate and QTc. **Max:** 60mg/m^2. **<2 yrs:** See	**BB:** To minimize risk of arrhythmia, place patients initiated or reinitiated on therapy for minimum of 3 days in a facility that can provide CrCl, ECG monitoring, and cardiac resuscitation. Do not substitute Betapace for Betapace AF. **W/P:** Can cause serious ventricular arrhythmias. Avoid with hypokalemia, hypomagnesemia. Correct electrolyte imbalances before therapy. Bradycardia reported. Caution with heart failure controlled by digitalis and/or diuretics, nonallergic bronchospasm, sick sinus syndrome, left ventricular dysfunction, DM, renal dysfunction, post-MI. Avoid abrupt withdrawal. Use in surgery is controversial. May mask hypoglycemia, hyperthyroidism symptoms. **Contra:**	Bradycardia, dyspnea, fatigue, dose-related QT interval prolongation, abnormal ECG, chest pain, diarrhea, N/V, hyperhidrosis, dizziness.

*Scored. †Bold entries denote special dental considerations.
BB = black box warning; **W/P** = warnings/precautions; **Contra** = contraindications; **P/N** = pregnancy category rating and nursing considerations.

NAME	FORM/ STRENGTH	DOSAGE	WARNINGS/PRECAUTIONS & CONTRAINDICATIONS	ADVERSE EFFECTS†
Sotalol HCl (Betapace AF) *(cont.)*		dosing chart in PI. Reduce dose or d/c if QTc >550msec. **Renal Impairment:** Reduce dose or increase interval.	Sinus bradycardia (<50bpm during waking hrs), sick sinus syndrome, or 2nd- or 3rd-degree AV block (unless a functioning pacemaker is present), long QT syndromes, baseline QT interval >450msec, cardiogenic shock, uncontrolled heart failure, hypokalemia (<4meq/L), CrCl <40mL/min, bronchial asthma. **P/N:** Category B, not for use in nursing.	
Sotalol HCl (Betapace)	**Tab:** 80mg*, 120mg*, 160mg*	***Adults:*** Initiate with continuous ECG monitoring. **Initial:** 80mg bid. **Titrate:** Increase to 120-160mg bid if needed. Allow 3 days between dose increments. Reduce dose or d/c if QTC ≥550msec. **Usual:** 160-320mg/day given bid-tid. **Refractory Patients:** up to 480-640mg/day. **CrCl 30-59mL/min:** Dose q24h. **CrCl 10-29mL/min:** Dose q36-48h. **CrCl <10mL/min:** Individualize dose. May increase dose with renal impairment after at least 5-6 doses. ***Pediatrics:*** **≥2 yrs: Initial:** 30mg/m^2 tid. **Titrate:** Wait at least 36 hrs between dose increases. Guide dose by response, ie HR and QTc. **Max:** 60mg/m^2. **<2 yrs:** See dosing chart in PI. Reduce dose or d/c if QTc >550msec. **Renal Impairment:** Reduce dose or increase interval.	**BB:** To minimize risk of arrhythmia, place patients initiated or reinitiated on therapy for minimum of 3 days in a facility that can provide ECG monitoring and cardiac resuscitation. Perform CrCl before therapy. Do not substitute Betapace for Betapace AF. **W/P:** May provoke new or worsen ventricular arrhythmias. Caution with heart failure controlled by digitalis and/or diuretics, DM, left ventricular dysfunction, nonallergic bronchospasm, sick sinus syndrome, renal impairment, 2-weeks post-MI. Avoid with hypokalemia, hypomagnesemia, excessive QT interval prolongation (>550msec). Correct electrolyte imbalances before therapy. Avoid abrupt withdrawal. Use in surgery is controversial. May mask hypoglycemia, hyperthyroidism symptoms. Proarrhythmic events reported. **Contra:** Bronchial asthma, sinus bradycardia, 2nd- and 3rd-degree AV block (unless a functioning pacemaker is present), long QT syndromes, cardiogenic shock, uncontrolled CHF. **P/N:** Category B, not for use in nursing.	Dyspnea, fatigue, dizziness, bradycardia, chest pain, palpitation, asthenia, abnormal ECG, hypotension, headache, lightheadedness, edema.
CLASS III ANTIARRHYTHMICS				
Amiodarone HCl (Amiodarone IV, Cordarone, Pacerone)	**Inj:** (Amiodarone IV) 50mg/mL [3mL]. **Tab:** (Cordarone) 200mg*; (Pacerone) 100mg, 200mg*, 300mg*, 400mg*	***Adults:*** **(Amiodarone IV): LD:** 150mg over first 10 min (15mg/min), then 360mg over next 6 hrs (1mg/min), then 540mg over remaining 18 hrs (0.5mg/min). **Maint:** 0.5mg/min for 2-3 weeks. **Breakthrough Ventricular Tachycardia/ Ventricular Fibrillation:** 150mg supplement IV over 10 min. Increase rate to achieve suppression. **Elderly:** Start at low end of dosing range. Administer infusions >2 hrs in a glass or polyolefin bottle containing D5W. Amiodarone leaches out plasticizers (eg, DEHP from IV tubing) especially at higher infusion concentrations, and lower flow rates. **(Cordarone, Pacerone):** Give LD in hospital. **LD:** 800-1600mg/day in divided doses for 1-3 weeks. After control is achieved, then 600-800mg/day for 1 month. **Maint:** 400mg/day; up to 600mg/day if needed. Use lowest effective dose. Take with meals. **Elderly:** Start at low end of dosing range.	**W/P:** Only for life-threatening arrhythmias due to its substantial toxicity (eg, pulmonary toxicity including pulmonary alveolar hemorrhage, hepatic injury, arrhythmia exacerbation). Hospitalize when giving LD. May cause a clinical syndrome of cough and progressive dyspnea. D/C if LFTs are 3x ULN or if elevated baseline doubles; monitor LFTs regularly. Optic neuropathy, optic neuritis reported. Fetal harm in pregnancy. May develop reversible corneal micro deposits (eg, visual halos, blurred vision), photosensitivity, peripheral neuropathy (rare). May decrease T^3 levels, increase thyroxine levels, increase inactive reverse T^3 levels, and can cause hypo- or hyperthyroidism. Hyperthyroidism may result in thyrotoxicosis and/or the possibility of arrhythmia breakthrough or aggravation. ARDS reported with surgery. Correct K^+ or magnesium deficiency before therapy. Caution in elderly. (Cordarone IV) Hypotension reported; do not exceed initial rate of infusion. Contains benzyl alcohol. **Contra:** Cardiogenic shock. Severe sinus-node dysfunction causing marked sinus bradycardia; 2nd- and	Pulmonary toxicity (eg, inflammation, fibrosis), arrhythmia exacerbation, hepatic injury, malaise, fatigue, tremor, poor coordination, paresthesis, N/V, constipation, anorexia, ophthalmic abnormalities, photosensitivity, akinesia, bradykinesia, **taste alteration.**

Table 14.1. PRESCRIBING INFORMATION FOR CARDIOVASCULAR DRUGS *(cont.)*

NAME	FORM/ STRENGTH	DOSAGE	WARNINGS/PRECAUTIONS & CONTRAINDICATIONS	ADVERSE EFFECTS†
ANTIARRHYTHMICS *(cont.)*				
CLASS III ANTIARRHYTHMICS *(cont.)*				
Amiodarone HCl (Amiodarone IV, Cordarone, Pacerone) *(cont.)*			3rd-degree AV block; when episodes of bradycardia have caused syncope (except when used with a pacemaker). Hypersensitivity to iodine. **P/N:** Category D, not for use in nursing.	
Dofetilide (Tikosyn)	**Cap:** 125mcg, 250mcg, 500mcg	***Adults:*** **CrCl: >60mL/min:** 500mcg bid. **CrCl 40-60mL/min:** 250mcg bid. **CrCl 20** to **<40mL/min:** 125mcg bid. Determine QTc interval 2-3 hrs after 1st dose and adjust dose if QTc >500msec or if >15% increase from baseline. **QTc/Renal Dose Adjustment:** Reduce 500mcg bid to 250mcg bid. Reduce 250mcg bid to 125mcg bid. Reduce 125mcg bid to 125mcg qd. D/C anytime after 2nd dose if QTc >500 msec (550msec with ventricular conduction abnormalities).	**BB:** To minimize risk of arrhythmia, place patients initiated or reinitiated on therapy for minimum of 3 days in a facility that can provide CrCl, ECG monitoring, and cardiac resuscitation. Dofetilide is available only to hospitals and prescribers who have received appropriate dofetilide dosing and treatment initiation education. **W/P:** Can cause serious ventricular arrhythmia. Calculate CrCl before first dose; adjust dose based on CrCl. Caution in severe hepatic impairment. Maintain normal K^+ levels. **Contra:** Long QT syndromes, baseline QT interval or QTc >440msec (500msec with ventricular conduction abnormalities), severe renal impairment (CrCl <20mL/min). Concomitant verapamil, cimetidine, trimethoprim, ketoconazole, and inhibitors of renal cation transport system (eg, megestrol, prochlorperazine). **P/N:** Category C, not for use in nursing.	Headache, chest pain, dizziness, arrhythmia, conduction disturbances, dyspnea, nausea, insomnia.
Ibutilide Fumarate (Corvert)	**Inj:** 0.1mg/mL	***Adults:*** **≥60kg:** 1mg over 10 min. **<60kg:** 0.01mg/kg over 10 min. If arrhythmia still present within 10 min after the end of the initial infusion, repeat infusion 10 min after completion of 1st infusion.	**W/P:** Proarrhythmic; can cause potentially fatal arrhythmias. Administer in setting with continuous ECG monitoring and person able to treat acute ventricular arrhythmia. Adequately anticoagulate if A-Fib >2-3 days. Correct hypokalemia and hypomagnesemia before therapy. Caution in elderly. **P/N:** Category C, not for use in nursing.	Sustained and nonsustained polymorphic ventricular tachycardia, sustained and nonsustained monomorphic ventricular tachycardia, bundle branch and AV block, ventricular and supraventricular extrasystoles, hypotension, bradycardia.
CLASS IV ANTIARRYTHMICS (CALCIUM CHANNEL BLOCKERS)				
Diltiazem HCl	**Inj:** 5mg/mL	***Adults:*** **Bolus:** (Injection/Lyo-Ject) 0.25mg/kg IV over 2 min. If no response after 15 min, may give 2nd dose of 0.35mg/kg over 2 min. **Continuous Infusion:** (Injection/Lyo-Ject/Monovial) 0.25-0.35mg/kg IV bolus, then 10mg/hr. **Titrate:** Increase by 5mg/hr. **Max:** 15mg/hr and duration up to 24 hrs.	**W/P:** Initiate in setting with resuscitation capabilities. Caution if hemodynamically compromised, and renal, hepatic, or ventricular dysfunction. Monitor ECG continuously and BP frequently. Symptomatic hypotension, acute hepatic injury reported. D/C if high-degree AV block occurs in sinus rhythm or if persistent rash occurs. Ventricular premature beats may be present on conversion of PSVT to sinus rhythm. **Contra:** Sick sinus syndrome and 2nd- or 3rd-degree AV block (except with functioning pacemaker), severe hypotension, cardiogenic shock, concomitant IV β-blockers or within a few hrs of use, A-Fib/Flutter associated with accessory bypass tract (eg, Wolff-Parkinson-White syndrome, short PR syndrome), ventricular tachycardia, (Lyo-Ject) neonates due to benzyl alcohol. **P/N:** Category C, not for use in nursing	Hypotension, injection-site reactions (eg, itching, burning), vasodilation (flushing), arrhythmias.

*Scored. †Bold entries denote special dental considerations.
BB = black box warning; **W/P** = warnings/precautions; **Contra** = contraindications; **P/N** = pregnancy category rating and nursing considerations.

NAME	FORM/ STRENGTH	DOSAGE	WARNINGS/PRECAUTIONS & CONTRAINDICATIONS	ADVERSE EFFECTS†
Verapamil HCl (Calan)	**Tab:** 40mg, 80mg*, 120mg*	***Adults:*** **HTN: Initial:** 80mg tid. **Usual:** 360-480mg/day. **Elderly/Small Stature: Initial:** 40mg tid. **Angina: Usual:** 80-120mg tid. **Elderly/Small Stature: Initial:** 40mg tid. **Titrate:** Increase daily or weekly. **A-Fib (Digitalized): Usual:** 240-320mg/day given tid-qid. **PSVT Prophylaxis (Nondigitalized):** 240-480mg/day given tid-qid. **Max:** 480mg/day. **Severe Hepatic Dysfunction:** Give 30% of normal dose.	**W/P:** Avoid with moderate-to-severe cardiac failure, and ventricular dysfunction if taking a β-blocker. May cause hypotension, AV block, transient bradycardia, PR-interval prolongation. Monitor LFTs periodically; hepatocellular injury reported. Give 30% of normal dose with severe hepatic dysfunction. Caution with hypertrophic cardiomyopathy, renal or hepatic dysfunction. Decrease dose in those with decreased neuromuscular transmission. **Contra:** Severe ventricular dysfunction, hypotension, cardiogenic shock, sick sinus syndrome, or 2nd- or 3rd-degree AV block (except with functioning ventricular pacemaker), A-fib/flutter with an accessory bypass tract. **P/N:** Category C, not for use in nursing.	Constipation, dizziness, nausea, hypotension, headache, peripheral edema, CHF, fatigue, pulmonary edema, elevated liver enzymes, dyspnea, bradycardia, AV block, rash, flushing, infection, flu syndrome.
MISCELLANEOUS ANTIARRHYTHMICS				
Adenosine (Adenocard)	**Inj:** 3mg/mL [2mL, 4mL]	***Adults:*** 6mg rapid IV bolus infusion over 1-2 sec. If not converted to SR within 1-2 min, give 12mg rapid IV bolus; may give 2nd 12mg dose if needed. **Max:** 12mg/dose. ***Pediatrics:*** **<50kg:** 0.05-0.1mg/kg rapid IV bolus. If not converted to SR within 1-2 min, give additional bolus doses, incrementally increasing amount by 0.05-0.1mg/kg. Follow each bolus with a saline flush. Continue process until SR or a maximum single dose of 0.3mg/kg is used. **≥50kg:** 6mg rapid IV bolus infusion over 1-2 sec. If not converted to SR within 1-2 min, give 12mg rapid IV bolus; may give 2nd 12mg dose if needed. **Max:** 12mg/dose.	**W/P:** May produce short-lasting heart block. Transient or prolonged asystole, respiratory alkalosis, ventricular fibrillation reported. Caution with obstructive lung disease not associated with bronchoconstriction (eg, emphysema, bronchitis). Avoid with bronchoconstriction/bronchospasm (eg, asthma). D/C if severe respiratory difficulties develop. New arrhythmias may appear on ECG at time of conversion. Caution in elderly. **Contra:** 2nd- or 3rd-degree AV block (except with pacemaker), sinus node disease such as sick sinus syndrome or symptomatic bradycardia (except with pacemaker). **P/N:** Category C, safety in nursing not known.	Facial flushing, dyspnea/SOB, chest pressure, nausea.
ANTIHYPERTENSIVES/HEART FAILURE AGENTS				
ACE INHIBITORS				
Benazepril HCl (Lotensin)	**Tab:** 5mg, 10mg, 20mg, 40mg	***Adults:*** If possible, d/c diuretic 2-3 days prior to initiation of therapy. **Initial:** 10mg qd or 5mg with concomitant diuretic. **Maint:** 20-40mg/day given qd-bid. Resume diuretic if BP not controlled. **Max:** 80mg/day. **CrCl <30mL/min/1.73m²: Initial:** 5mg qd. **Max:** 40mg/day. ***Pediatrics:*** **≥6 yrs: Initial:** 0.2mg/kg qd. **Max:** 0.6mg/kg.	**BB:** ACE inhibitors can cause death/injury to developing fetus during 2nd and 3rd trimesters. Stop therapy if pregnancy detected. **W/P:** D/C if angioedema, jaundice, or if marked LFT elevation occurs. Risk of hyperkalemia with DM, renal dysfunction. Persistent nonproductive cough reported. Monitor WBCs in renal and collagen vascular disease. Anaphylactoid reactions reported. Fetal/neonatal morbidity and death reported. Monitor for hypotension in high risk patients (eg, surgery/anesthesia, prolonged diuretic therapy, heart failure, volume and/or salt depletion, etc). Caution with CHF, renal dysfunction, and renal artery stenosis. Less effective on BP in blacks and more reports of angioedema than nonblacks. **P/N:** Category D, not for use in nursing.	Cough, dizziness, headache, fatigue, somnolence, postural dizziness, nausea.
Captopril (Capoten)	**Tab:** 12.5mg*, 25mg*, 50mg*, 100mg*	***Adults:*** Take 1 hour before meals. **HTN:** If possible, d/c recent antihypertensive drug for 1 week prior to therapy. **Initial:** 25mg bid-tid. **Titrate:** May increase to 50mg bid-tid after 1-2 weeks. **Usual:** 25-150mg bid-tid. **Max:** 450mg/day. **CHF: Initial:** 25mg tid; 6.25-12.5mg tid with risk of hypotension or salt/volume depletion. **Usual:** 50-100mg tid.	**BB:** ACE inhibitors can cause death/injury to developing fetus during 2nd and 3rd trimesters. Stop therapy if pregnancy detected. **W/P:** D/C if jaundice or marked LFT elevation occurs. Risk of hyperkalemia with DM, renal dysfunction. Persistent nonproductive cough, anaphylactoid reactions, neutropenia with myeloid hypoplasia reported. Fetal/	Proteinuria, rash, hypotension, **dysgeusia,** cough, MI, CHF.

Table 14.1. PRESCRIBING INFORMATION FOR CARDIOVASCULAR DRUGS *(cont.)*

NAME	FORM/ STRENGTH	DOSAGE	WARNINGS/PRECAUTIONS & CONTRAINDICATIONS	ADVERSE EFFECTS†
ANTIHYPERTENSIVES/HEART FAILURE AGENTS *(cont.)*				
ACE INHIBITORS *(cont.)*				
Captopril (Capoten) *(cont.)*		**Max:** 450mg/day. **Left Ventricular Dysfunction Post-MI: Initial:** 6.25mg single dose, then 12.5mg tid. **Titrate:** Increase to 25mg tid over next several days, then to 50mg tid over next several weeks. **Usual:** 50mg tid. **Diabetic Nephropathy:** 25mg tid. **Significant Renal Dysfunction:** Decrease initial dose and titrate slowly.	neonatal morbidity and death reported. Monitor for hypotension in high-risk patients (surgery/anesthesia, dialysis, heart failure, volume/salt depletion, etc). Caution with CHF, renal dysfunction, renal artery stenosis, collagen vascular disease (especially with renal dysfunction). Monitor WBC before therapy, then every 2 weeks for 3 months, then periodically. Less effective on BP in blacks and more reports of angioedema than nonblacks. **P/N:** Category C (1st trimester) and D (2nd and 3rd trimesters), not for use in nursing.	
Enalapril Maleate (Vasotec), **Enalaprilat** (Vasotec I.V.)	**Inj:** 1.25mg/mL **Tab:** 2.5mg*, 5mg*, 10mg*, 20mg*	***Adults:*** **(IV)** Administer IV over 5 min. **Usual:** 1.25mg q6h for no longer than 48 hrs. **Max:** 20mg/day. **Concomitant Diuretic/CrCl ≤30mL/min: Initial:** 0.625mg, may repeat after 1 hr. **Maint:** 1.25mg q6h. **Risk of Excessive Hypotension: Initial:** 0.625mg over 5 min to 1 hr. **PO/IV Conversion:** Give 5mg/day PO for 1.25mg IV q6h and 2.5mg/day PO for 0.625mg q6h IV. **(Tab) HTN:** If possible, d/c diuretic 2-3 days prior to therapy. **Initial:** 5mg qd, 2.5mg qd with concomitant diuretic. **Usual:** 10-40mg/day given qd or bid. Resume diuretic if BP not controlled. **CrCl ≤30mL/min: Initial:** 2.5mg/day. **Dialysis:** 2.5mg/day on dialysis days. **Heart Failure: Initial:** 2.5mg/day. **Usual:** 2.5-20mg given bid. **Max:** 40mg/day. **Left Ventricular Dysfunction: Initial:** 2.5mg bid. **Titrate:** Increase to 20mg/day. **Hyponatremia or SrCr 1.6mg/dL with Heart Failure: Initial:** 2.5mg qd. **Titrate:** Increase to 2.5mg bid, then 5mg bid. **Max:** 40mg/day. ***Pediatrics:*** **HTN: 1 month-16 yrs: Initial:** 0.08mg/kg (up to 5mg) qd. **Titrate:** Adjust according to response. **Max:** 0.58mg/kg/dose (or 40mg/dose). Avoid if GFR <30mL/min/1.73m^2.	**BB:** ACE inhibitors can cause death/injury to developing fetus during 2nd and 3rd trimesters. Stop therapy if pregnancy detected. **W/P:** D/C if angioedema, jaundice, or if marked LFT elevation occurs. Risk of hyperkalemia with DM, renal dysfunction. Persistent nonproductive cough reported. Monitor WBCs in renal or collagen vascular disease. Anaphylactoid reactions reported. Fetal/neonatal morbidity and death reported. Monitor for hypotension in high-risk patients (heart failure, surgery/anesthesia, hyponatremia, high-dose diuretic therapy, severe volume and/or salt depletion, etc). Caution with CHF, obstruction to left ventricle outflow tract, renal dysfunction, and renal artery stenosis. Less effective on BP in blacks and more reports of angioedema than nonblacks. Intestinal angioedema reported. **Contra:** Hereditary or idiopathic angioedema. **P/N:** Category C (1st trimester) and D (2nd and 3rd trimesters), not for use in nursing.	Fatigue, orthostatic effects, asthenia, diarrhea, N/V, headache, dizziness, cough, rash, hypotension, angioedema, fever, constipation.
Fosinopril Sodium (Monopril)	**Tab:** 10mg*, 20mg, 40mg	***Adults:*** If possible, d/c diuretic 2-3 days before therapy. **Initial:** 10mg qd, monitor carefully; if cannot d/c diuretic. **Maint:** 20-40mg/day. Resume diuretic if BP not controlled. **Max:** 80mg/day. **Heart Failure: Initial:** 10mg qd, 5mg with moderate-to-severe renal failure or vigorous diuresis. **Titrate:** Increase over several weeks. **Maint:** 20-40mg qd. **Max:** 40mg qd. **Elderly:** Start at low end of dosing range.	**BB:** ACE inhibitors can cause death/injury to developing fetus during 2nd and 3rd trimesters. Stop therapy if pregnancy detected. **W/P:** D/C if angioedema, jaundice, or if marked LFT elevation occur. Risk of hyperkalemia with DM, renal dysfunction. Persistent nonproductive cough reported. Monitor WBCs in renal and collagen vascular disease. Anaphylactoid reactions reported. Fetal/neonatal morbidity and death reported. Monitor for hypotension in high-risk patients (heart failure, volume and/or salt depletion, surgery/anesthesia, etc.). Less effective on BP in blacks and more reports of angioedema than nonblacks. Caution with CHF, renal or hepatic dysfunction, renal artery stenosis. May cause false low measurement of serum digoxin level. **P/N:** Category C (1st trimester) and D (2nd and 3rd trimesters), not for use in nursing.	Dizziness, cough, hypotension, musculoskeletal pain.

*Scored. †Bold entries denote special dental considerations.
BB = black box warning; **W/P** = warnings/precautions; **Contra** = contraindications; **P/N** = pregnancy category rating and nursing considerations.

NAME	FORM/ STRENGTH	DOSAGE	WARNINGS/PRECAUTIONS & CONTRAINDICATIONS	ADVERSE EFFECTS†
Lisinopril (Prinivil)	**Tab:** (Prinvil) 5mg*, 10mg*, 20mg*	***Adults:*** **(Prinvil) HTN:** If possible, d/c diuretic 2-3 days prior to therapy. **Initial:** 10mg qd; 5mg qd with diuretic. **Usual:** 20-40mg qd. Resume diuretic if BP not controlled. **Max:** 80mg/day. **CrCl 10-30mL/min: Initial:** 5mg/day. **Max:** 40mg/day. **CrCl <10mL/min: Initial:** 2.5mg/day. **Max:** 40mg/day. **Heart Failure: Initial:** 5mg qd. **Usual:** 5-20mg qd. **Hyponatremia or CrCl ≤30mL/min: Initial:** 2.5mg qd. **AMI: Initial:** 5mg within 24 hrs, then 5mg after 24 hrs, then 10mg after 48 hrs, then daily. Use 2.5mg during first 3 days with low SBP. **Maint:** 10mg qd for 6 weeks, 2.5-5mg with hypotension. D/C with prolonged hypotension. **Elderly:** Caution with dose adjustment. ***Pediatrics:*** **≥6 yrs: (Prinvil, Zestril) HTN: Initial:** 0.07mg/kg qd (up to 5mg total). Adjust dose based on BP response. **Max:** 0.61mg/kg qd (40mg/day).	**BB:** ACE inhibitors can cause death/injury to developing fetus during 2nd and 3rd trimesters. Stop therapy if pregnancy detected. **W/P:** D/C if angioedema, jaundice, or marked LFT elevation occur. Risk of hyperkalemia, hypoglycemia with DM, renal dysfunction. Persistent nonproductive cough reported. Monitor WBCs in renal and collagen vascular disease. Anaphylactoid reactions during membrane exposure reported. Fetal/neonatal morbidity and death reported. Monitor for hypotension in high-risk patients (heart failure with SBP <100mmHg, surgery/anesthesia, hyponatremia, high-dose diuretic therapy, severe volume and/or salt depletion, etc). Caution with CHF, aortic stenosis/hypertrophic cardiomyopathy, renal dysfunction, and renal artery stenosis. Less effective on BP in blacks and more reports of angioedema than nonblacks. Caution in hypoglycemia and leukopenia/neutropenia. Patients should report any indication of infection which may be sign of leukopenia/neutropenia. **Contra:** Hereditary or idiopathic angioedema. **P/N:** Category C (1st trimester) and D (2nd and 3rd trimesters), not for use in nursing.	Hypotension, diarrhea, headache, dizziness, hyperkalemia, chest pain, cough, cutaneous pseudolymphoma.
Lisinopril (Zestril)	**Tab:** 2.5mg, 5mg, 10mg, 20mg, 30mg, 40mg	***Adults:*** **HTN:** If possible, d/c diuretic 2-3 days prior to therapy. **Initial:** 10mg qd, 5mg qd with diuretic. **Usual:** 20-40mg qd. Resume diuretic if BP not controlled. **Max:** 80mg/day. **CrCl 10-30mL/min: Initial:** 5mg/day. **Max:** 40mg/day. **CrCl <10mL/min: Initial:** 2.5mg/day. **Max:** 40mg/day. **Heart Failure: Initial:** 5mg qd. **Usual:** 5-40mg qd. May increase by 10mg every 2 weeks. **Max:** 40mg/day. **Hyponatremia or CrCl ≤30mL/min or SrCr >3mg/dL: Initial:** 2.5mg qd. **AMI: Initial:** 5mg within 24 hrs, then 5mg after 24 hrs, then 10mg after 48 hrs, then 10mg qd. Use 2.5mg during first 3 days with low SBP. **Maint:** 10mg qd for 6 weeks, 2.5-5mg with hypotension. D/C with prolonged hypotension. **Elderly:** Caution with dose adjustment. ***Pediatrics:*** **≥6 yrs: HTN: Initial:** 0.07mg/kg qd up to 5mg total. Dose adjust according to response. **Max:** 0.61mg/kg qd or 40mg/day.	**BB:** ACE inhibitors can cause death/injury to developing fetus during 2nd and 3rd trimesters. Stop therapy if pregnancy detected. **W/P:** D/C if angioedema, jaundice, or marked LFT elevation occur. Risk of hyperkalemia, hypoglycemia with DM, renal dysfunction. Persistent nonproductive cough reported. Monitor WBCs in renal and collagen vascular disease. Anaphylactoid reactions during membrane exposure reported. Fetal/neonatal morbidity and death reported. Monitor for hypotension in high-risk patients (heart failure with SBP <100mmHg, surgery/anesthesia, hyponatremia, high-dose diuretic therapy, severe volume and/or salt depletion, etc). Caution with CHF, aortic stenosis/hypertrophic cardiomyopathy, renal dysfunction, and renal artery stenosis. Less effective on BP in blacks and more reports of angioedema than nonblacks. Caution in hypoglycemia and leukopenia/neutropenia. Patients should report any indication of infection which may be sign of leukopenia/neutropenia. **Contra:** Hereditary or idiopathic angioedema. **P/N:** Category C (1st trimester) and D (2nd and 3rd trimesters), not for use in nursing.	Hypotension, diarrhea, headache, dizziness, hyperkalemia, chest pain, cough, cutaneous pseudolymphoma.

Table 14.1. PRESCRIBING INFORMATION FOR CARDIOVASCULAR DRUGS *(cont.)*

NAME	FORM/ STRENGTH	DOSAGE	WARNINGS/PRECAUTIONS & CONTRAINDICATIONS	ADVERSE EFFECTS†
ANTIHYPERTENSIVES/HEART FAILURE AGENTS *(cont.)*				
ACE INHIBITORS *(cont.)*				
Moexipril HCl (Univasc)	**Tab:** 7.5mg*, 15mg*	***Adults:*** If possible, d/c diuretic 2-3 days prior to therapy. Take 1 hr before meals. **Initial:** 7.5mg qd, 3.75mg with concomitant diuretic therapy. **Maint:** 7.5-30mg/day given qd-bid. Resume diuretic if BP not controlled. **Max:** 60mg/day. **CrCl ≤40mL/min: Initial:** 3.75mg qd. **Max:** 15mg/day.	**BB:** ACE inhibitors can cause death/ injury to developing fetus during 2nd and 3rd trimesters. Stop therapy if pregnancy detected. **W/P:** D/C if angioedema, jaundice, or if marked LFT elevation occurs. Intestinal angioedema reported. Risk of hyperkalemia with DM, renal dysfunction. Persistent nonproductive cough reported. Monitor WBCs in renal and collagen vascular disease. Anaphylactoid reactions reported. Fetal/neonatal morbidity and death reported. Monitor for hypotension in high-risk patients (heart failure, surgery/anesthesia, prolonged diuretic therapy, volume and/ or salt depletion, etc.). Caution with CHF, renal dysfunction, and renal artery stenosis. Less effective on BP in blacks and more reports of angioedema than nonblacks. **P/N:** Category C (1st trimester) and D (2nd and 3rd trimesters), not for use in nursing.	Cough, dizziness, diarrhea, flu syndrome, fatigue, pharyngitis, flushing, rash, myalgia.
Perindopril Erbumine (Aceon)	**Tab:** 2mg*, 4mg*, 8mg*	***Adults:*** **HTN:** If possible, d/c diuretic 2-3 days prior to therapy. **Initial:** 4mg qd; 2-4mg/day given qd-bid with concomitant diuretic. **Maint:** 4-8mg/ day given qd-bid. Resume diuretic if BP not controlled. **Max:** 16mg/day. **Elderly (>65 yrs): Initial:** 4mg/day given qd-bid. **Max (usual):** 8mg/day. **Renal Impairment: CrCl >30mL/min: Initial:** 2mg/day. **Max:** 8mg/day. **CAD: Initial:** 4mg qd for 2 weeks. **Maint:** 8mg qd. **Elderly (>70 yrs): Initial:** 2mg qd for 1 week. **Titrate:** 4mg qd for Week 2. **Maint:** 8mg qd.	**BB:** ACE inhibitors can cause death/ injury to developing fetus during 2nd and 3rd trimesters. Stop therapy if pregnancy detected. **W/P:** D/C if angioedema, jaundice, or if marked LFT elevation occurs. Risk of hyperkalemia with DM, renal dysfunction. Persistent nonproductive cough reported. Monitor WBCs in renal and collagen vascular disease. Anaphylactoid reactions reported. Fetal/neonatal morbidity and death reported. Monitor for hypotension in high-risk patients (heart failure, surgery/ anesthesia, hyponatremia, prolonged diuretic therapy, or volume and/or salt depletion). Caution with CHF, renal dysfunction, and renal artery stenosis. Less effective on BP in blacks and more reports of angioedema than nonblacks. Avoid if CrCl <30mL/min. **P/N:** Category D, caution in nursing.	Cough, headache, asthenia, dizziness, diarrhea, edema, respiratory infection, lower extremity pain.
Quinapril HCl (Accupril)	**Tab:** 5mg*, 10mg, 20mg, 40mg	***Adults:*** **HTN:** If possible, d/c diuretic 2-3 days prior to therapy. **Initial:** 10-20mg qd; 5mg qd with concomitant diuretic. Titrate at intervals of at least 2 weeks. **Usual:** 20-80mg/day given qd-bid. **CrCl >60mL/min: Initial:** 10mg/ day. **CrCl 30-60mL/min: Initial:** 5mg/ day. **CrCl 10-30mL/min: Initial:** 2.5mg/ day. **Heart Failure: Initial:** 5mg bid. Titrate at weekly intervals. **Usual:** 10-20mg bid. **CrCl >30mL/min: Initial:** 5mg/day. **CrCl 10-30mL/min: Initial:** 2.5mg/day.	**BB:** ACE inhibitors can cause death/ injury to developing fetus during 2nd and 3rd trimesters. Stop therapy if pregnancy detected. **W/P:** D/C if angioedema, jaundice, or if marked LFT elevation occurs. Risk of hyperkalemia with DM, renal dysfunction. Persistent nonproductive cough reported. Monitor WBCs in renal or collagen vascular disease. Anaphylactoid reactions reported. Fetal/neonatal morbidity and death reported. Monitor for hypotension in high risk patients (heart failure, surgery/ anesthesia, hyponatremia, high-dose diuretic therapy, recent intensive diuresis, dialysis, or severe volume and/or salt depletion, etc). Caution with CHF, renal dysfunction, and renal artery stenosis. Less effective on BP in blacks and more reports of angioedema than nonblacks. **P/N:** Category C (1st trimester) and D (2nd and 3rd trimesters), not for use in nursing.	Fatigue, headache, dizziness, cough, N/V, hypotension, chest pain.

*Scored. †Bold entries denote special dental considerations.
BB = black box warning; **W/P** = warnings/precautions; **Contra** = contraindications; **P/N** = pregnancy category rating and nursing considerations.

NAME	FORM/ STRENGTH	DOSAGE	WARNINGS/PRECAUTIONS & CONTRAINDICATIONS	ADVERSE EFFECTS†
Ramipril (Altace)	**Cap:** 1.25mg, 2.5mg, 5mg, 10mg	***Adults:*** **HTN: Initial:** 2.5mg qd. **Maint:** 2.5-20mg/day given qd or bid. Add diuretic if BP not controlled. **CrCl <40mL/ min: Initial:** 1.25mg qd. **Titrate/Max:** 5mg/day. **CHF Post-MI: Initial:** 2.5mg bid, 1.25mg bid if hypotensive. **Titrate:** increase to 5mg bid. **CrCl <40mL/ min: Initial:** 1.25mg qd. **Titrate:** May increase to 1.25mg bid. **Max:** 2.5mg bid. **Risk Reduction of MI, Stroke, Death (≥55 yrs): Initial:** 2.5mg qd for 1 week. Increase to 5mg qd for next 3 weeks. **Maint:** 10mg qd. Reduce or d/c diuretic if possible. **With Volume Depletion/Renal Artery Stenosis: Initial:** 1.25mg qd.	**BB:** ACE inhibitors can cause death/ injury to developing fetus during 2nd and 3rd trimesters. Stop therapy if pregnancy detected. **W/P:** D/C if angioedema, jaundice, or if marked LFT elevation occurs. Risk of hyperkalemia with DM, renal dysfunction. Persistent nonproductive cough and anaphylactoid reactions reported. Monitor WBCs in renal and collagen vascular disease. Fetal/neonatal morbidity and death reported. Monitor for hypotension in high-risk patients (heart failure, surgery/ anesthesia, hyponatremia, high-dose diuretic therapy, recent intensive diuresis, dialysis, or severe volume and/ or salt depletion, etc). Caution with CHF, renal dysfunction, severe liver cirrhosis and/or ascites, and renal artery stenosis. Less effective on BP in blacks and more reports of angioedema than nonblacks. May reduce RBCs, Hgb, WBCs, or platelets. May cause agranulocytosis, pancytopenia, and bone marrow depression. **P/N:** Category C (1st trimester) and D (2nd and 3rd trimesters), not for use in nursing.	Hypotension, cough, dizziness, fatigue, angina, impotence, Stevens-Johnson syndrome.
Trandolapril (Mavik)	**Tab:** 1mg*, 2mg, 4mg	***Adults:*** **HTN:** If possible, d/c diuretic 2-3 days before therapy. **Initial:** 1mg qd in nonblack patients; 2mg qd in black patients; 0.5mg with concomitant diuretic. **Titrate:** Adjust at 1-week intervals. **Usual:** 2-4mg qd. Resume diuretic if not controlled. **Max:** 8mg/day. **Post-MI: Initial:** 1mg qd. **Titrate:** Increase to target dose of 4mg qd as tolerated. **CrCl <30mL/min/Hepatic Cirrhosis for HTN or Post-MI: Initial:** 0.5mg qd.	**BB:** ACE inhibitors can cause death/ injury to developing fetus during 2nd and 3rd trimesters. Stop therapy if pregnancy detected. **W/P:** D/C if angioedema or jaundice occurs. Risk of hyperkalemia with DM, renal dysfunction. Persistent nonproductive cough reported. Monitor WBCs in renal impairment and/or collagen vascular disease. Anaphylactoid reactions reported. Fetal/neonatal morbidity and death reported. Monitor for hypotension in high-risk patients (heart failure, surgery/anesthesia, prolonged diuretic therapy, volume and/ or salt depletion, etc). Caution with CHF, renal dysfunction, and renal artery stenosis. More reports of angioedema in blacks than nonblacks. **P/N:** Category C (1st trimester) and D (2nd and 3rd trimesters), not for use in nursing.	Cough, dizziness, hypotension, elevated serum uric acid, elevated BUN, elevated creatinine, asthenia, syncope, myalgia, gastritis, hypocalcemia, hyperkalemia, dyspepsia.
ACE INHIBITORS/CALCIUM CHANNEL BLOCKERS				
Benazepril HCl/ Amlodipine Besylate (Lotrel)	**Cap:** (Amlodipine-Benazepril) 2.5mg-10mg, 5mg-10mg, 5mg-20mg, 5mg-40mg, 10mg-20mg, 10mg-40mg	***Adults:*** **Usual:** 2.5-10mg amlodipine and 10-80mg benazepril per day. **Small/Elderly/Frail/Hepatic Impairment: Initial:** 2.5mg amlodipine.	**BB:** When used in pregnancy, ACE inhibitors can cause injury and even death to the developing fetus. D/C therapy when pregnancy detected. **W/P:** D/C if angioedema, jaundice, or if marked LFT elevation occurs. Risk of hyperkalemia with DM, renal dysfunction. Persistent nonproductive cough reported. Monitor WBCs in collagen vascular disease. Anaphylactoid reactions reported. Fetal/ neonatal morbidity and death reported. Monitor for hypotension in high-risk patients (heart failure, surgery/ anesthesia, volume and/or salt depletion, etc). Caution with CHF, severe hepatic or renal dysfunction, and renal artery stenosis. Avoid if GFR ≤30mL/ min/1.73m^2. **P/N:** Category D, not for use in nursing.	Cough, headache, dizziness, edema.

Table 14.1. PRESCRIBING INFORMATION FOR CARDIOVASCULAR DRUGS *(cont.)*

NAME	FORM/ STRENGTH	DOSAGE	WARNINGS/PRECAUTIONS & CONTRAINDICATIONS	ADVERSE EFFECTS†
ANTIHYPERTENSIVES/HEART FAILURE AGENTS *(cont.)*				
ACE INHIBITORS/CALCIUM CHANNEL BLOCKERS *(cont.)*				
Trandolapril/ Verapamil HCl (Tarka)	**Tab:** (Trandolapril Verapamil) 2mg-180mg, 1mg-240mg, 2mg-240mg, 4mg-240mg	***Adults:*** **Replacement Therapy:** 1 tab qd with food. **Severe Hepatic Dysfunction:** Give 30% of normal dose.	**BB:** ACE inhibitors can cause death/ injury to developing fetus during 2nd and 3rd trimesters. Stop therapy if pregnancy detected. **W/P:** Monitor for hypotension with surgery or anesthesia. Risk of hyperkalemia with renal insufficiency, DM. D/C if jaundice develops. Avoid with moderate to severe cardiac failure and ventricular dysfunction if taking a β-blocker. May cause angioedema, cough, fetal/neonatal morbidity, hypotension, AV block, anaphylactoid reactions, transient bradycardia, PR-interval prolongation. Monitor LFTs periodically. Give 30% of normal dose with severe hepatic dysfunction. Caution with CHF, hypertrophic cardiomyopathy, renal or hepatic dysfunction. Decrease dose in those with decreased neuromuscular transmission. Monitor WBC with collagen-vascular disease and/or renal disease. **Contra:** Severe ventricular dysfunction, hypotension, cardiogenic shock, sick sinus syndrome or 2nd- or 3rd-degree AV block (except with functioning ventricular pacemaker), A-Fib/Flutter with an accessory bypass tract. **P/N:** Category C (1st trimester) and D (2nd and 3rd trimesters), not for use in nursing.	AV block, constipation, cough, dizziness, fatigue, headache, increased hepatic enzymes, chest pain, upper respiratory tract infection/ congestion.
ACE INHIBITORS/DIURETICS				
Benazepril HCl/Hydrochlorothiazide (Lotensin HCT)	**Tab:** (Benazepril-HCTZ) 5mg-6.25mg*, 10mg-12.5mg*, 20mg-12.5mg*, 20mg-25mg*	***Adults:*** **Initial (if not controlled on benazepril monotherapy):** 10mg-12.5mg or 20mg-12.5mg. **Titrate:** May increase after 2-3 weeks. **Initial (if controlled on 25mg HCTZ/day with hypokalemia):** 5mg-6.25mg. **Replacement Therapy:** Substitute combination for titrated components.	**BB:** ACE inhibitors can cause death/ injury to developing fetus during 2nd and 3rd trimesters. Stop therapy if pregnancy detected. **W/P:** Avoid if GFR ≤30mL/min/1.73m^2. D/C if angioedema, jaundice, or marked LFT elevation occur. Risk of hyperkalemia with DM, renal dysfunction. May cause persistent nonproductive cough, hypokalemia, hyperuricemia, hypomagnesemia, hypercalcemia, hypophosphatemia. Monitor WBCs in renal and collagen vascular disease. Anaphylactoid reactions reported. Fetal/neonatal morbidity and death reported. Monitor for hypotension in high-risk patients (eg, surgery/ anesthesia, prolonged diuretic therapy, heart failure, volume and/or salt depletion, etc). Caution with CHF, renal dysfunction, and renal artery stenosis. More reports of angioedema in blacks than nonblacks. Monitor for fluid/electrolyte imbalance. May increase cholesterol and TG levels. May exacerbate/activate SLE. **Contra:** Anuria, sulfonamide hypersensitivity. **P/N:** Category D, not for use in nursing.	Cough, dizziness/ postural dizziness, headache, fatigue.
Captopril/Hydrochlorothiazide (Capozide)	**Tab:** (Captopril-HCTZ) 25mg-15mg*, 25mg-25mg*, 50mg-15mg*, 50mg-25mg*	***Adults:*** **Initial:** 25mg-15mg tab qd. **Titrate:** Adjust dose at 6-week intervals. **Max:** 150mg captopril/50mg HCTZ per day. **Replacement Therapy:** Substitute combination for titrated components. **Renal Impairment:** Decrease dose	**BB:** ACE inhibitors can cause death/ injury to developing fetus during 2nd and 3rd trimesters. Stop therapy if pregnancy detected. **W/P:** D/C if angioedema, jaundice, or if marked LFT elevation occurs. Risk of hyperkalemia with DM,	Cough, hypotension, rash, pruritus, fever, arthralgia, eosinophilia, dysgeusia, neutropenia/ thrombocytopenia.

*Scored. †Bold entries denote special dental considerations.
BB = black box warning; **W/P** = warnings/precautions; **Contra** = contraindications; **P/N** = pregnancy category rating and nursing considerations.

NAME	FORM/ STRENGTH	DOSAGE	WARNINGS/PRECAUTIONS & CONTRAINDICATIONS	ADVERSE EFFECTS†
Captopril/Hydro-chlorothiazide (Capozide) *(cont.)*		or increase interval. Take 1 hr before meals.	renal dysfunction. Monitor WBCs in renal and collagen vascular disease. Fetal/neonatal morbidity and death reported. Monitor for hypotension in high-risk patients (eg, surgery/anesthesia, volume/salt depletion). Caution with renal or hepatic dysfunction. More reports of angioedema in blacks than nonblacks. May exacerbate or activate systemic lupus erythematosus. Monitor electrolytes. Hypercalcemia, hypomagnesemia, hyperuricemia may occur. With renal impairment, monitor WBCs and differential before therapy, every 2 weeks for 3 months, then periodically. Neutropenia with myeloid hypoplasia, persistent nonproductive cough, anaphylactoid reactions, proteinuria reported. **Contra:** Anuria, sulfonamide hypersensitivity. **P/N:** Category C (1st trimester) and D (2nd and 3rd trimesters), not for use in nursing.	
Enalapril Maleate/Hydro-chlorothiazide (Vaseretic)	**Tab:**(Enalapril-HCTZ) 5mg-12.5mg, 10mg-25mg	***Adults:* Initial (if not controlled with enalapril/HCTZ monotherapy):** 5mg-12.5mg tab or 10mg-25mg tab qd. **Titrate:** May increase after 2-3 weeks. **Max:** 20mg enalapril/50mg HCTZ per day. **Replacement Therapy:** Substitute combination for titrated components	**BB:** ACE inhibitors can cause death/injury to developing fetus during 2nd and 3rd trimesters. Stop therapy if pregnancy detected. **W/P:** D/C if angioedema, jaundice, or if marked LFT elevation occurs. Risk of hyperkalemia with DM, renal dysfunction. Persistent nonproductive cough reported. Monitor WBCs in renal and collagen vascular disease. Anaphylactoid reactions reported. Fetal/neonatal morbidity and death reported. Monitor for hypotension in high-risk patients (surgery/anesthesia, hyponatremia, severe volume/salt depletion, etc). Caution with CHF, renal or hepatic dysfunction, obstruction to left ventricle outflow tract, elderly, renal artery stenosis. More reports of angioedema in blacks than nonblacks. May exacerbate or activate SLE. Monitor serum electrolytes. Avoid if GFR ≤30mL/min/1.73m^2. May increase cholesterol, TG, uric acid levels, and blood glucose. Intestinal angioedema reported. **Contra:** Hereditary or idiopathic angioedema, anuria, sulfonamide hypersensitivity. **P/N:** Category C (1st trimester) and D (2nd and 3rd trimesters), not for use in nursing.	Dizziness, cough, fatigue, orthostatic effects, diarrhea, nausea, muscle cramps, asthenia, impotence.
Fosinopril Sodium/Hydro-chlorothiazide (Monopril HCT)	**Tab:** (Fosinopril-HCTZ) 10mg-12.5mg, 20mg-12.5mg	***Adults:* Initial (if not controlled with fosinopril/HCTZ monotherapy):** 12.5mg-10mg tab or 12.5mg-20mg tab qd.	**BB:** ACE inhibitors can cause death/injury to developing fetus during 2nd and 3rd trimesters. Stop therapy if pregnancy detected. **W/P:** D/C if angioedema, jaundice, or marked LFT elevation occur. Risk of hyperkalemia with DM, renal dysfunction. Persistent nonproductive cough reported. Monitor WBCs in renal and collagen vascular disease. Anaphylactoid reactions reported. Fetal/neonatal morbidity and death reported. Monitor for hypotension in high-risk patients (eg, surgery/anesthesia, volume/salt depletion). Caution with CHF, renal or hepatic dysfunction. More reports of angioedema in blacks than nonblacks. May exacerbate or activate SLE. Monitor	Headache, cough, fatigue, dizziness, upper respiratory infection, musculo-skeletal pain.

Table 14.1. PRESCRIBING INFORMATION FOR CARDIOVASCULAR DRUGS *(cont.)*

NAME	FORM/ STRENGTH	DOSAGE	WARNINGS/PRECAUTIONS & CONTRAINDICATIONS	ADVERSE EFFECTS†
ANTIHYPERTENSIVES/HEART FAILURE AGENTS *(cont.)*				
ACE INHIBITORS/DIURETICS *(cont.)*				
Fosinopril Sodium/Hydro-chlorothiazide (Monopril HCT) *(cont.)*			electrolytes. Avoid if GFR ≤30mL/min/1.73m². May increase cholesterol, TG. Hypercalcemia, hypomagnesemia, hyperuricemia may occur. **Contra:** Anuria, sulfonamide hypersensitivity. **P/N:** Category C (1st trimester) and D (2nd and 3rd trimesters), not for use in nursing.	
Lisinopril/Hydro-chlorothiazide (Prinzide, Zestoretic)	**Tab:** [Prinzide, Zestoretic] (Lisinopril-HCTZ) 10mg-12.5mg, 20mg-12.5mg, 20mg-25mg	***Adults:* Initial (if not controlled with lisinopril/HCTZ monotherapy):** 10mg-12.5mg tab or 20mg-12.5mg tab daily. **Titrate:** May increase after 2-3 weeks. **Initial (if controlled on 25mg HCTZ/day with hypokalemia):** 10mg-12.5mg tab. **Replacement Therapy:** Substitute combination for titrated components.	**BB:** ACE inhibitors can cause death/injury to developing fetus during 2nd and 3rd trimesters. Stop therapy if pregnancy detected. **W/P:** D/C if angioedema, jaundice, or if marked LFT elevation occurs. Risk of hyperkalemia with DM, renal dysfunction. Persistent nonproductive cough reported. Agranulocytosis and bone marrow depression in renal impairment, especially with collagen vascular disease; monitor WBCs in renal disease and collagen vascular disease. Anaphylactoid reactions reported. Fetal/neonatal morbidity and death reported. Monitor for hypotension in high-risk patients (eg, surgery/anesthesia,volume/salt depletion). Caution with CHF, renal or hepatic dysfunction, obstruction to left ventricle outflow tract, renal artery stenosis, elderly. More reports of angioedema in blacks than nonblacks. May exacerbate or activate SLE. Monitor electrolytes. Avoid if GFR ≤30mL/min/1.73m². May increase cholesterol, TG. Hypercalcemia, hyperglycemia, hypomagnesemia, hyperuricemia may occur. Caution with left ventricle outflow obstruction. **Contra:** Hereditary or idiopathic angioedema, anuria, sulfonamide hypersensitivity. **P/N:** Category C (1st trimester) and D (2nd and 3rd trimesters), not for use in nursing.	Dizziness, headache, cough, fatigue, orthostatic effects, diarrhea, nausea, muscle cramps, angioedema, cutaneous pseudo-lymphoma.
Moexipril HCl/Hydro-chlorothiazide (Uniretic)	**Tab:** (Moexipril-HCTZ) 7.5mg-12.5mg*, 15mg-12.5mg*, 15mg-25mg*	***Adults:* Initial (if not controlled on moexipril/HCTZ monotherapy):** Switch to 7.5mg-12.5mg tab, 15mg-12.5mg tab, or 15mg-25mg tab qd. **Titrate:** May increase after 2-3 weeks. **Initial (if controlled on 25mg HCTZ/day with hypokalemia):** 3.75mg-6.25mg (1/2 of 7.5mg-12.5mg tab). If excessive reduction with 7.5mg-12.5mg tab, may switch to 3.75mg-6.25mg. **Replacement Therapy:** Substitute combination for titrated components. Take 1 hr before meals.	**BB:** ACE inhibitors can cause death/injury to developing fetus during 2nd and 3rd trimesters. Stop therapy if pregnancy detected. **W/P:** D/C if angioedema, jaundice, or if marked LFT elevation occurs. Intestinal angioedema reported. Risk of hyperkalemia with DM, renal dysfunction. Persistent nonproductive cough reported. Monitor WBCs in renal and collagen vascular disease. Anaphylactoid reactions reported. Fetal/neonatal morbidity and death reported. Monitor for hypotension in high-risk patients (eg, surgery/anesthesia, volume/salt depletion). Caution in elderly, CHF, renal or hepatic dysfunction. More reports of angioedema in blacks than nonblacks. May exacerbate or activate SLE. Monitor electrolytes. Avoid if GFR ≤40mL/min/1.73m². May increase cholesterol, TG. Hypercalcemia, hypomagnesemia, hyperuricemia may occur. **Contra:** Anuria, sulfonamide hypersensitivity. **P/N:** Category C (1st trimester) and D (2nd and 3rd trimesters), not for use in nursing.	Cough, dizziness, fatigue.

*Scored. †Bold entries denote special dental considerations.
BB = black box warning; **W/P** = warnings/precautions; **Contra** = contraindications; **P/N** = pregnancy category rating and nursing considerations.

NAME	FORM/ STRENGTH	DOSAGE	WARNINGS/PRECAUTIONS & CONTRAINDICATIONS	ADVERSE EFFECTS†
Quinapril HCl/Hydro-chlorothiazide (Accuretic)	**Tab:** (Quinapril-HCTZ) 10mg-12.5mg*, 20mg-12.5mg*, 20mg-25mg*	***Adults:* Initial (if not controlled on quinapril monotherapy):** 10mg-12.5mg or 20mg-12.5mg tab qd. **Titrate:** May increase after 2-3 weeks. **Initial (if controlled on HCTZ 25mg/day but significant K^+ loss):** 10mg-12.5mg or 20mg-12.5mg tab qd. If previously treated with 20mg quinapril and 25mg HCTZ, may switch to 20mg-25mg tab qd.	**BB:** ACE inhibitors can cause death/injury to developing fetus during 2nd and 3rd trimesters. Stop therapy if pregnancy detected. **W/P:** D/C if angioedema, jaundice, or marked LFT elevation occurs. Risk of hyperkalemia with DM, renal dysfunction. Persistent nonproductive cough reported. Monitor WBCs in renal or collagen vascular disease. Anaphylactoid reactions reported. Fetal/neonatal morbidity and death reported. Monitor for hypotension in high-risk patients (heart failure, surgery/anesthesia, hyponatremia, severe volume/salt depletion, etc). Caution with CHF, renal or hepatic dysfunction, and renal artery stenosis. Less effective on BP in blacks and more reports of angioedema than nonblacks. May exacerbate or activate SLE. Monitor serum electrolytes. Avoid if GFR ≤30mL/min/1.73m². May increase cholesterol, TGs, and uric acid levels and decrease glucose tolerance. **Contra:** History of ACE inhibitor–associated angioedema, anuria, sulfonamide hypersensitivity. **P/N:** Category C (1st trimester) and D (2nd and 3rd trimesters), not for use in nursing.	Dizziness, headache, cough, myalgia.
α-ADRENERGIC BLOCKERS				
Doxazosin Mesylate (Cardura)	**Tab:** 1mg*, 2mg*, 4mg*, 8mg*	***Adults:* HTN: Initial:** 1mg qd (am or pm). Monitor BP 2-6 hrs and 24 hrs after 1st dose. **Titrate:** Increase to 2mg qd then upwards as needed. **Max:** 16mg/day. **BPH: Initial:** 1mg qd (am or pm). **Titrate:** May double the dose every 1-2 weeks. **Max:** 8mg/day.	**W/P:** Monitor for orthostatic hypotension and syncope with first dose and dose increase. Caution with hepatic dysfunction. Rule out prostate cancer. Priapism (rare), leukopenia/neutropenia reported. **P/N:** Category C, caution with nursing.	Fatigue/malaise, hypotension, edema, dizziness, dyspnea, weight gain.
Phenoxybenzamine HCl (Dibenzyline)	**Cap:** 10mg	***Adults:* Pheocromocytoma induced HTN/Diaphoresis: Initial:** 10mg bid. **Titrate:** Increase every other day to 20-40mg bid-tid, until BP is controlled.	**W/P:** Caution with marked cerebral or coronary arteriosclerosis, or renal damage. May aggravate symptoms of respiratory infections. **Contra:** Conditions where fall in BP may be undesirable. **P/N:** Category C, not for use in nursing.	Postural hypotension, tachycardia, ejaculation inhibition, nasal congestion, miosis, GI irritation, drowsiness, fatigue.
Prazosin HCl (Minipress)	**Cap:** 1mg, 2mg, 5mg	***Adults:* Initial:** 1mg bid-tid. **Maint:** 6-15mg/day in divided doses. **Max:** 40mg/day. **Concomitant Diuretic/Antihypertensive:** Reduce to 1-2mg tid, then retitrate.	**W/P:** Syncope may occur, usually after initial dose or dose increase. Excessive postural hypotensive effects. Avoid driving for 24 hrs after first dose or dose increase. Always start on 1mg cap. False (+) for pheochromocytoma. **P/N:** Category C, caution in nursing.	Dizziness, headache, drowsiness, lack of energy, weakness, palpitations, nausea.
Terazosin HCl (Hytrin)	**Cap:** 1mg, 2mg, 5mg, 10mg	***Adults:* HTN: Initial:** 1mg hs, then slowly increase dose. **Usual:** 1-5mg/day. **Max:** 20mg/day. If response is substantially diminished at 24 hrs, may increase dose or give in 2 divided doses. **BPH: Initial:** 1mg qhs. **Titrate:** Increase stepwise as needed. **Usual:** 10mg/day. May increase to 20mg/day after 4-6 weeks. **Max:** 20mg/day. If discontinued for several days, restart at initial dose.	**W/P:** Monitor for orthostatic hypotension and syncope initially and with dose increase. Rule out prostate cancer. Priapism (rare) reported. Possibility of hemodilution. **P/N:** Category C, caution with nursing.	Asthenia, postural hypotension, headache, dizziness, dyspnea, nasal congestion/rhinitis, somnolence, impotence, blurred vision, palpitations, nausea, peripheral edema, priapism, thrombocytopenia, atrial fibrillation.

Table 14.1. PRESCRIBING INFORMATION FOR CARDIOVASCULAR DRUGS *(cont.)*

NAME	FORM/ STRENGTH	DOSAGE	WARNINGS/PRECAUTIONS & CONTRAINDICATIONS	ADVERSE EFFECTS†
ANTIHYPERTENSIVES/HEART FAILURE AGENTS *(cont.)*				
α-ADRENERGIC AGONISTS, CENTRALLY ACTING				
Clonidine (Catapres, Catapres-TTS)	**Patch, Extended-Release (TTS):** 0.1mg/24 hr [4[s]], 0.2mg/ 24 hr [4[s]], 0.3mg/ 24 hr [4[s]]; **Tab:** 0.1mg*, 0.2mg*, 0.3mg*	***Adults:* (Patch)** Apply to hairless, intact area of upper arm or chest weekly. Taper withdrawal of previous antihypertensive. **Initial:** 0.1mg/24 hr patch weekly. **Titrate:** May increase after 1-2 weeks. **Max:** 0.6mg/24 hr. **(Tab) Initial:** 0.1mg bid. **Titrate:** May increase by 0.1mg weekly. **Usual:** 0.2-0.6mg/day in divided doses. **Max:** 2.4mg/day. **(Patch, Tab) Renal Impairment:** Adjust according to degree of impairment.	**W/P:** Avoid abrupt discontinuation. Tabs may cause rash if have allergic reaction to patch. Continue tabs within 4 hrs of surgery and resume as soon as possible thereafter. Do not remove patch for surgery. Caution with severe coronary insufficiency, conduction disturbances, recent MI, cerebrovascular disease or chronic renal failure. Remove patch before defibrillation or cardioversion due to the potential risk of altered electrical conductivity or MRI due to the ocurrence of burns. **P/N:** Category C, caution in nursing.	**Dry mouth,** drowsiness, dizziness, constipation, sedation, impotence/sexual dysfunction, N/V, alopecia, weakness, orthostatic symptoms, nervousness, localized skin reactions (patch).
Guanfacine HCl (Tenex)	**Tab:** 1mg, 2mg	***Adults:*** 1mg qhs. **Titrate:** May increase to 2mg qhs after 3-4 weeks. **Max:** 3mg/day.	**W/P:** Caution with severe coronary insufficiency, recent MI, cerebrovascular disease, chronic renal or hepatic failure. Avoid abrupt discontinuation. Dose-related drowsiness and sedation. **P/N:** Category B, caution with nursing.	**Dry mouth,** somnolence, asthenia, dizziness, constipation, impotence, headache.
Methyldopa, Methyldopate HCl	**Inj:** (Methyldopate HCl) 50mg/mL **Tab:** (Methyldopa) 125mg, 250mg, 500mg	***Adults:* (Tab) Initial:** 250mg bid-tid for 48 hrs. Adjust dose at intervals of not less than 2 days. **Maint:** 500mg-2g/day given bid-qid. **Max:** 3g/day. **Concomitant Antihypertensives (other than thiazides): Initial:** Limit to 500mg/day. **Renal Impairment:** May respond to lower doses. **(Inj)** 250-500mg IV q6h as needed. **Max:** 1gm q6h. **Elderly/Renal Dysfunction:** May reduce dose. Switch to oral therapy once BP is controlled. ***Pediatrics:* (Tab) Initial:** 10mg/kg/day given bid-qid. **Max:** 65mg/kg/day or 3g/day, whichever is less. **(Inj)** 20-40mg/kg/day IV given q6h. **Max:** 65mg/kg/day or 3 g/day, whichever is less. Switch to oral therapy once BP is controlled.	**W/P:** Positive Coombs' test, hemolytic anemia, and liver disorders may occur. Fever reported within the first 3 weeks of therapy. HTN has recurred after dialysis. Caution with liver disease or dysfunction. D/C if signs of heart failure or involuntary choreoathetotic movements develop. Edema and wt gain reported. Blood count, Coombs' test and LFTs prior to therapy and periodically thereafter. Caution with cerebrovascular disease. **Contra:** Active hepatic disease, concomitant MAOIs. **P/N:** Category B, caution in nursing.	Sedation, headache, asthenia, weakness, edema, weight gain, hepatic disorders, N/V, diarrhea, **sore or "black" tongue,** blood dyscrasias, BUN increase, gynecomastia, impotence.
α-ADRENERGIC AGONISTS, CENTRALLY ACTING/DIURETICS				
Clonidine HCl/ Chlorthalidone (Clorpres)	**Tab:** (Clonidine-Chlorthalidone) 0.1mg-15mg*, 0.2mg-15mg*, 0.3mg-15mg*	***Adults:*** Determine dose by individual titration. 0.1mg clonidine-15mg chlorthalidone tab qd-bid. **Max:** 0.6mg clonidine-30mg chlorthalidone/day.	**W/P:** Caution with severe renal disease, hepatic dysfunction, asthma, severe coronary insufficiency, recent MI, cerebrovascular disease. May develop allergic reaction to oral clonidine if sensitive to clonidine patch. Avoid abrupt withdrawal. Continue therapy to within 4 hrs of surgery and resume after. Monitor for fluid/electrolyte imbalance. Hyperuricemia, hypokalemia, hyponatremia, hypochloremic alkalosis, and hyperglycemia may occur. **Contra:** Anuria, sulfonamide hypersensitivity. **P/N:** (Clonidine) Category C, caution in nursing. (Chlorthalidone) Category B, not for use in nursing.	Drowsiness, dizziness, constipation, sedation, N/V, blood dyscrasias, hypersensitivity reactions, orthostatic symptoms, impotence.
Methyldopa/Hydrochlorothiazide	**Tab:** (Methyldopa-HCTZ) 250mg-15mg, 250mg-25mg	***Adults:* Initial:** 250mg-15mg tab bid-tid, 250mg-25mg tab bid, or 500mg-30mg qd. **Max:** 50mg HCTZ/day or 3g methyldopa/day.	**BB:** Not for initial therapy of HTN. **W/P:** Positive Coombs' test, hemolytic anemia, liver disorders, sensitivity reactions, hypokalemia, hyperuricemia, hyperglycemia, hypomagnesemia, hypercalcemia may occur. Fever reported within first 3 weeks of therapy. HTN has recurred after dialysis. Caution with liver disease or dysfunction, severe renal disease. D/C if signs of heart	Weakness, asthenia, headache, pancreatitis, diarrhea, N/V, constipation, blood dyscrasias, rash, electrolyte imbalance, renal failure, impotence, vertigo.

*Scored. †Bold entries denote special dental considerations.

BB = black box warning; **W/P** = warnings/precautions; **Contra** = contraindications; **P/N** = pregnancy category rating and nursing considerations.

NAME	FORM/ STRENGTH	DOSAGE	WARNINGS/PRECAUTIONS & CONTRAINDICATIONS	ADVERSE EFFECTS†
Methyldopa/Hydrochlorothiazide *(cont.)*			failure, progressive renal dysfunction, or involuntary choreoathetotic movements develop. Edema and weight gain reported. Blood count, Coombs' test, and LFTs before therapy and periodically thereafter. Monitor electrolytes. May exacerbate or activate SLE. May increase cholesterol and TG levels. Enhanced effects in postsympathectomy patient. **Contra:** Active hepatic disease, anuria, sulfonamide allergy, concomitant MAOIs. **P/N:** Category C, not for use in nursing.	
ANGIOTENSIN II RECEPTOR BLOCKERS				
Candesartan Cilexetil (Atacand)	**Tab:** 4mg, 8mg, 16mg, 32mg	***Adults:*** **HTN: Monotherapy Without Volume Depletion: Initial:** 16mg qd. **Usual:** 8-32mg/day given qd-bid. May add diuretic if BP not controlled. **Intravascular Volume Depletion/ Moderate Hepatic Impairment:** Lower initial dose. **Heart Failure: Initial:** 4mg qd. **Usual:** 32mg qd. **Titrate:** Double dose every 2 weeks, as tolerated.	**BB:** Can cause death/injury to developing fetus during 2nd and 3rd trimesters. Stop therapy if pregnancy detected. **W/P:** Can cause fetal injury/death. Correct volume or salt depletion before therapy or monitor closely. Changes in renal function may occur; caution with renal artery stenosis, CHF. Risk of hypotension; caution in major surgery and anesthesia, or when initiating therapy in heart failure. May cause hyperkalemia in heart failure patients; monitor serum potassium. **P/N:** Category C (1st trimester) and D (2nd and 3rd trimesters), not for use in nursing.	Back pain, dizziness, upper respiratory infection, pharyngitis, rhinitis, headache.
Eprosartan Mesylate (Teveten)	**Tab:** 400mg, 600mg	***Adults:*** **Initial:** 600mg qd. **Usual:** 400-800mg/day, given qd-bid. **Moderate-to-Severe Renal Impairment: Max:** 600mg/day.	**BB:** Can cause death/injury to developing fetus during 2nd and 3rd trimesters. Stop therapy if pregnancy detected. **W/P:** Can cause fetal injury/death. Correct volume or salt depletion before therapy. Changes in renal function may occur; caution with renal artery stenosis, severe CHF. **P/N:** Category C (1st trimester) and D (2nd and 3rd trimesters), not for use in nursing.	Upper respiratory infection, rhinitis, pharyngitis, cough.
Irbesartan (Avapro)	**Tab:** 75mg, 150mg, 300mg	***Adults:*** **HTN: Initial:** 150mg qd. **Titrate:** May increase to 300mg qd. **Intravascular Volume/Salt Depletion: Initial:** 75mg qd. **Nephropathy: Maint:** 300mg qd. ***Pediatrics:*** **HTN: ≥17 yrs: Initial:** 150mg qd. **Titrate:** May increase to 300mg qd. **Intravascular Volume/Salt Depletion: Initial:** 75mg qd.	**BB:** Can cause death/injury to developing fetus during 2nd and 3rd trimesters. Stop therapy if pregnancy detected. **W/P:** Can cause fetal injury/death. Correct volume or salt depletion before therapy. Changes in renal function may occur; caution with renal artery stenosis, severe CHF. Angioedema reported. **P/N:** Category C (1st trimester) and D (2nd and 3rd trimesters), not for use in nursing.	Diarrhea, dyspepsia/ heartburn, musculoskeletal trauma, fatigue, upper respiratory infection.
Losartan Potassium (Cozaar)	**Tab:** 25mg, 50mg, 100mg	***Adults:*** **HTN: Initial:** 50mg qd. **Usual:** 25-100mg/day given qd-bid. **Intravascular Volume Depletion/ Hepatic Impairment: Initial:** 25mg qd. **HTN with LVH: Initial:** 50mg qd. Add hydrochlorothiazide (HCTZ) 12.5mg qd and/or increase losartan to 100mg qd, followed by an increase in HCTZ to 25mg qd based on BP response. **Nephropathy: Initial:** 50 mg qd. **Titrate:** Increase to 100mg qd based on BP response. ***Pediatrics:*** **≥6 yrs: HTN: Initial:** 0.7mg/kg qd (up to 50mg/day). **Max:** 1.4mg/kg/day (100mg/day).	**BB:** Can cause death/injury to developing fetus during 2nd and 3rd trimesters. Stop therapy if pregnancy detected. **W/P:** Can cause fetal injury/death. Correct volume or salt depletion before therapy. Changes in renal function may occur; caution with renal artery stenosis, severe CHF. Angioedema reported. Consider dose adjustment with hepatic dysfunction. **P/N:** Category C (1st trimester) and D (2nd and 3rd trimesters), not for use in nursing.	Dizziness, cough, upper respiratory infection, diarrhea.

Table 14.1. PRESCRIBING INFORMATION FOR CARDIOVASCULAR DRUGS *(cont.)*

NAME	FORM/ STRENGTH	DOSAGE	WARNINGS/PRECAUTIONS & CONTRAINDICATIONS	ADVERSE EFFECTS†
ANTIHYPERTENSIVES/HEART FAILURE AGENTS *(cont.)*				
ANGIOTENSIN II RECEPTOR BLOCKERS *(cont.)*				
Olmesartan Medoxomil (Benicar)	**Tab:** 5mg, 20mg, 40mg	***Adults:* Monotherapy Without Volume Depletion: Initial:** 20mg qd. **Titrate:** May increase to 40mg qd after 2 weeks if needed. May add diuretic if BP not controlled. **Intravascular Volume Depletion (eg, with diuretics, impaired renal function):** Lower initial dose; monitor closely.	**BB:** Can cause death/injury to developing fetus during 2nd and 3rd trimesters. Stop therapy if pregnancy detected. **W/P:** Can cause fetal injury/death. Symptomatic hypotension may occur in volume- and/or salt-depleted patients; monitor closely. Changes in renal function may occur; caution with severe CHF. Increases in SrCr or BUN reported with renal artery stenosis. **P/N:** Category C (1st trimester) and D (2nd and 3rd trimesters), not for use in nursing.	Dizziness, transient hypotension, hyperkalemia.
Telmisartan (Micardis)	**Tab:** 20mg, 40mg*, 80mg*	***Adults:* Initial:** 40mg qd. **Usual:** 20-80mg/day. May add diuretic if need additional BP reduction after 80mg/day.	**BB:** Can cause death/injury to developing fetus during 2nd and 3rd trimesters. Stop therapy if pregancy detected. **W/P:** Can cause fetal injury/death. Correct volume or salt depletion before therapy. Changes in renal function may occur; caution with renal artery stenosis, severe CHF. Closely monitor with biliary obstructive disorders or hepatic dysfunction. **P/N:** Category C (1st trimester) and D (2nd and 3rd trimesters), not for use in nursing.	Upper respiratory infection, back pain, sinusitis, diarrhea, bradycardia, eosinophilia, thrombocytopenia, increased uric acid, increased CPK, increased sweating, abnormal hepatic function/ liver disorder, renal impairment including acute renal failure, anemia, edema, and cough.
Valsartan (Diovan)	**Tab:** 40mg*, 80mg, 160mg, 320mg	***Adults:* HTN: Monotherapy Without Volume Depletion: Initial:** 80mg or 160mg qd. **Titrate:** May increase to 320mg qd or add diuretic (greater effect than increasing dose >80mg). **Hepatic/ Severe Renal Dysfunction:** Use with caution. **Heart Failure: Initial:** 40mg bid. **Titrate:** May increase to 80mg or 160mg bid (use highest dose tolerated). **Max:** 320mg/day in divided doses. **Post-MI: Initial:** 20mg bid. **Titrate:** May increase to 40mg bid within 7 days, with subsequent titrations up to 160mg bid. ***Pediatrics:* 6-16 yrs: HTN: Initial:** 1.3mg/kg qd (up to 40mg total). Adjust dose according to BP response. **Max:** 2.7mg/kg (up to 160mg) qd. Use of a sus recommended for children who cannot swallow tabs, or children for whom calculated dosage (mg/kg) does not correspond to available tab strengths. Adjust dose accordingly when switching dosage forms. **Hepatic/ Severe Renal Impairment:** Use with caution. Avoid use in pediatrics with GFR <30mL/min/1.73m^2.	**BB:** Can cause death/injury to developing fetus during 2nd and 3rd trimesters. Stop therapy if pregnancy detected. **W/P:** Changes in renal function may occur; caution with renal artery stenosis, severe CHF. Caution with hepatic dysfunction, renal dysfunction, and obstructive biliary disorder. Risk of hypotension; caution when initiating therapy in heart failure or post-MI. Correct volume or salt depletion before therapy. Avoid use in pediatric patients with GFR <30mL/ min/1.73m^2. May cause fetal harm when administered to pregnant women. **P/N:** Category D, not for use in nursing.	(HTN) Headache, dizziness, viral infection, fatigue, abdominal pain. (Heart Failure) Dizziness, hypotension, diarrhea, arthralgia, fatigue, back pain, hyperkalemia. (Post-MI) Hypotension, cough, increased blood creatinine.
ANGIOTENSIN II RECEPTOR BLOCKERS/CALCIUM CHANNEL BLOCKERS				
Olmesartan Medoxomil/ Amlodipine Besylate (Azor)	**Tab:** (Amlodipine-Olmesartan) 5mg-20mg, 10mg-20mg, 5mg-40mg, 10mg-40mg	***Adults:* Replacement Therapy:** May substitute for individually titrated components for patients on amlodipine and olmesartan. When substituting for individual components, the dose of 1 or both components may be increased if needed. **Add-On Therapy:** May use	**BB:** Can cause death/injury to developing fetus during 2nd and 3rd trimesters. Stop therapy if pregnancy detected. **W/P:** Hypotension, especially in volume- or salt-depleted patients, may occur with treatment initiation; monitor closely. Caution with severe aortic stenosis,	Edema.

*Scored. †Bold entries denote special dental considerations.
BB = black box warning; **W/P** = warnings/precautions; **Contra** = contraindications; **P/N** = pregnancy category rating and nursing considerations.

NAME	FORM/ STRENGTH	DOSAGE	WARNINGS/PRECAUTIONS & CONTRAINDICATIONS	ADVERSE EFFECTS†
Olmesartan Medoxomil/ Amlodipine Besylate (Azor) *(cont.)*		as add-on therapy when not adequately controlled on amlodipine or olmesartan. May increase dose after 2 weeks to maximum dose of 10mg-40mg qd.	heart failure, or severe hepatic impairment. Increased angina or MI with CCBs may occur with dosage initiation or increase. Changes in renal function, oliguria, progressive azotemia, or acute renal failure may occur. **P/N:** Category C (1st trimester) and D (2nd and 3rd trimester), not for use in nursing.	
Valsartan/ Amlodipine Besylate (Exforge)	**Tab:** (Amlodipine-Valsartan) 5mg-160mg, 10mg-160mg, 5mg-320mg, 10mg-320mg	***Adults:*** **Initial Therapy:** 5mg-160mg qd. **Add-On/Replacement Therapy:** May be substituted for titrated components. **Titrate:** If inadequate control, may increase after 1-2 weeks of therapy. **Max:** 10mg-320mg qd. **Elderly: Initial:** 2.5mg amlodipine.	**BB:** When used in pregnancy, drugs that act directly on the renin-angiotensin system can cause injury and even death to the developing fetus. D/C therapy when pregnancy is detected. **W/P:** May cause excessive hypotension. May increase risk of angina and MI in patients with severe obstructive CAD. Caution with CHF, severe hepatic impairment, renal dysfunction, or renal artery stenosis. **P/N:** Category D, not for use in nursing.	Peripheral edema, vertigo, nasopharyngitis, upper respiratory tract infection, dizziness.
ANGIOTENSIN II RECEPTOR BLOCKERS/DIURETICS				
Candesartan Cilexetil/Hydrochlorothiazide (Atacand HCT)	**Tab:** (Candesartan-HCTZ) 16mg-12.5mg, 32mg-12.5mg, 32mg-25mg	***Adults:*** **Initial: If BP not controlled on HCTZ 25mg/day or controlled but serum K⁺ decreased:** 16mg-12.5mg tab qd. If BP not controlled on 32mg candesartan/day, give 32mg-12.5mg qd; may increase to 32mg-25mg qd.	**BB:** Can cause death/injury to developing fetus during 2nd and 3rd trimesters. Stop therapy if pregnancy detected. **W/P:** Can cause fetal injury/death. Correct volume or salt depletion before therapy. Caution with hepatic or renal dysfunction, renal artery stenosis, severe CHF, history of allergies, and asthma. May exacerbate or activate SLE. Monitor serum electrolytes. Avoid if CrCl ≤30mL/min. Hyperuricemia, hyperglycemia, hypokalemia, hypomagnesemia, hyponatremia, hypercalcemia may occur. Enhanced effects in postsympathectomy patient. May increase cholesterol and triglyceride levels. Risk of hypotension; caution in major surgery or anesthesia. **Contra:** Anuria, sulfonamide hypersensitivity. **P/N:** Category C (1st trimester) and D (2nd and 3rd trimesters), not for use in nursing.	Upper respiratory infection, back pain, influenza-like symptoms, dizziness, headache.
Eprosartan Mesylate/Hydrochlorothiazide (Teveten HCT)	**Tab:** (Eprosartan-HCTZ) 600mg-12.5mg, 600mg-25mg	***Adults:*** **Usual (Not Volume Depleted):** 600mg-12.5mg qd. **Titrate:** May increase to 600mg-25mg qd if needed. **Renal Impairment: Max:** 600mg/day (eprosartan).	**BB:** Can cause death/injury to developing fetus during 2nd and 3rd trimesters. Stop therapy if pregnancy detected. **W/P:** Hypersensitivity reactions reported. Fetal/neonatal morbidity and death reported. Monitor for hypotension in volume/salt depletion. Caution with CHF, renal or hepatic dysfunction. May exacerbate or activate SLE. Monitor electrolytes periodically. Hypercalcemia, hypomagnesemia, hyperuricemia, hyperglycemia may occur. Enhanced effects in postsympathectomy patient. **Contra:** Anuria, sulfonamide hypersensitivity. **P/N:** Category C (1st trimester) and D (2nd and 3rd trimesters), not for use in nursing.	Dizziness, headache, back pain, fatigue, myalgia, upper respiratory tract infection, sinusitis, viral infection.
Irbesartan/Hydrochlorothiazide (Avalide)	**Tab:** (Irbesartan-HCTZ) 150mg-12.5mg, 300mg-12.5mg, 300mg-25mg	***Adults:*** **Not Controlled on Monotherapy:** 150mg/12.5mg qd. **Titrate:** May increase to 300mg/12.5mg, then 300mg/25mg qd if needed. **Intial Therapy:** Initiate with 150mg/12.5mg qd for 1 to 2 weeks. **Titrate:** As needed to maximum 300mg/25mg qd. **Replacement Therapy:** May substitute for titrated components. **Elderly:** Start at low end of dosing range. Avoid with CrCl ≤30mL/min.	**BB:** Can cause death/injury to developing fetus during 2nd and 3rd trimesters. Stop therapy if pregnancy detected. **W/P:** Can cause fetal injury/death when administered to pregnant women. Correct volume or salt depletion before therapy. Caution with hepatic or renal dysfunction, renal artery stenosis, severe CHF, history of allergies, elderly, and asthma. May exacerbate or activate SLE. Monitor serum electrolytes. Avoid	Dizziness, fatigue, musculoskeletal pain, influenza, edema, N/V, fever, chills, flushing, HTN, pruritus, sexual dysfunction, diarrhea, anxiety, vision disturbance, pancreatitis, aplastic anemia.

Table 14.1. PRESCRIBING INFORMATION FOR CARDIOVASCULAR DRUGS *(cont.)*

NAME	FORM/ STRENGTH	DOSAGE	WARNINGS/PRECAUTIONS & CONTRAINDICATIONS	ADVERSE EFFECTS†
ANTIHYPERTENSIVES/HEART FAILURE AGENTS *(cont.)*				
ANGIOTENSIN II RECEPTOR BLOCKERS/DIURETICS *(cont.)*				
Irbesartan/Hydro-chlorothiazide (Avalide) *(cont.)*			if CrCl ≤30mL/min. Hyperuricemia, hyperglycemia, hypokalemia, hypomagnesemia, and hypercalcemia may occur. Enhanced effects in postsympathectomy patient. May increase cholesterol and triglyceride levels. Caution in elderly. **Contra:** Anuria, sulfonamide hypersensitivity. **P/N:** Category D, not for use in nursing.	
Losartan Potassium/Hydro-chlorothiazide (Hyzaar)	**Tab:** (Losartan-HCTZ) 50mg-12.5mg, 100mg-12.5mg, 100mg-25mg	***Adults:* HTN:** If BP uncontrolled on losartan monotherapy, HCTZ alone or controlled with HCTZ 25mg/day but hypokalemic, 50mg-12.5mg tab qd. **Titrate/Max:** If uncontrolled after 3 weeks, increase to 2 tabs of 50mg-12.5mg qd or 1 tab of 100mg-25mg qd. If uncontrolled on losartan 100mg monotherapy, may switch to 100mg-12.5mg qd. **Severe HTN: Initial:** 50mg-12.5mg qd. **Titrate/Max:** If inadequate response after 2-4 weeks, increase to 1 tab of 100mg-25mg qd. **HTN With Left Ventricular Hypertrophy: Initial:** Losartan 50mg qd. If BP reduction inadequate, add HCTZ 12.5mg or substitute losartan/HCTZ 50mg-12.5mg. If additional BP reduction is needed, losartan 100mg and HCTZ 12.5mg or losartan/HCTZ 100mg-12.5mg may be substituted, followed by losartan 100mg and HCTZ 25mg or losartan/HCTZ 100mg-25mg.	**BB:** Can cause death/injury to developing fetus during 2nd and 3rd trimesters. Stop therapy if pregnancy detected. **W/P:** Can cause fetal injury/death. Correct volume or salt depletion before therapy. Caution with hepatic or renal dysfunction, renal artery stenosis, severe CHF, history of allergies, asthma. May exacerbate or activate SLE. Monitor serum electrolytes. Avoid if CrCl ≤30mL/min. Observe for signs of fluid or electrolyte imbalance. May precipitate hyperuricemia or gout. Enhanced effects in postsympathectomy patient. May increase cholesterol, TG levels. Angioedema reported. Not recommended with hepatic dysfunction requiring losartan titration. **Contra:** Anuria, sulfonamide hypersensitivity. **P/N:** Category C (1st trimester) and D (2nd and 3rd trimesters), not for use in nursing.	Dizziness, upper respiratory infection, back pain, cough.
Olmesartan Medoxomil/Hydro-chlorothiazide (Benicar HCT)	**Tab:** (Olmesartan-HCTZ) 20mg-12.5mg, 40mg-12.5mg, 40mg-25mg	***Adults:*** If BP not controlled with olmesartan alone, add HCTZ 12.5mg qd. May titrate to 25mg qd if BP uncontrolled after 2-4 weeks. If BP not controlled with HCTZ alone, add olmesartan 20mg qd. May titrate to 40mg qd if BP uncontrolled after 2-4 weeks. **Intravascular Volume Depletion (eg, with diuretics, impaired renal function):** Lower initial dose; monitor closely. **Elderly:** Start at lower end of dosing range.	**BB:** Can cause death/injury to developing fetus during 2nd and 3rd trimesters. Stop therapy if pregnancy detected. **W/P:** Can cause fetal injury/death. Correct volume or salt depletion before therapy or monitor closely. Caution with hepatic or severe renal dysfunction, progressive liver disease, history of allergies or asthma, renal artery stenosis, severe CHF. Avoid if CrCl ≤30mL/min. May exacerbate or activate SLE. Monitor serum electrolytes. Hyperuricemia, hyperglycemia, hypercalcemia, hypomagnesemia may occur. May increase cholesterol and triglyceride levels. **Contra:** Anuria, sulfonamide hypersensitivity. **P/N:** Category C (1st trimester) and D (2nd and 3rd trimesters), not for use in nursing.	Dizziness, upper respiratory tract infection, hyperuricemia, N/V, asthenia, angioedema, hyperkalemia, rhabdomyolysis, ARF, alopecia, urticaria.
Telmisartan/Hydro-chlorothiazide (Micardis HCT)	**Tab:** (Telmisartan-HCTZ) 40mg-12.5mg, 80mg-12.5mg, 80mg-25mg	***Adults:*** If BP not controlled on 80mg telmisartan, or 25mg HCTZ/day, or controlled on 25mg HCTZ/day but serum K^+ decreased, 80mg-12.5mg tab qd. **Titrate/Max:** If uncontrolled after 2-4 weeks, increase to 160mg-25mg. **Biliary Obstruction/Hepatic Dysfunction: Initial:** 40mg-12.5mg tab qd; monitor closely.	**BB:** Can cause death/injury to developing fetus during 2nd and 3rd trimesters. Stop therapy if pregnancy detected. **W/P:** Can cause fetal injury/death. Correct volume or salt depletion before therapy. Caution with hepatic or renal dysfunction, biliary obstructive disorders, renal artery stenosis, severe CHF, history of allergies, and asthma. May exacerbate or activate SLE. Monitor serum electrolytes. Avoid if CrCl ≤30mL/min. Hyperuricemia, hyperglycemia, hypokalemia, hypomagnesemia, hypercalcemia may occur. Enhanced effects in postsympathectomy patient. May increase cholesterol and triglyceride	Dizziness, fatigue, sinusitis, upper respiratory infection, diarrhea, bradycardia, eosinophilia, thrombocytopenia, uric acid increased, abnormal hepatic function/liver disorder, renal impairment including acute renal failure, anemia, and increased CPK.

*Scored. †Bold entries denote special dental considerations.
BB = black box warning; **W/P** = warnings/precautions; **Contra** = contraindications; **P/N** = pregnancy category rating and nursing considerations.

NAME	FORM/ STRENGTH	DOSAGE	WARNINGS/PRECAUTIONS & CONTRAINDICATIONS	ADVERSE EFFECTS†
Telmisartan/Hydrochlorothiazide (Micardis HCT) *(cont.)*			levels. **Contra:** Anuria, sulfonamide hypersensitivity. **P/N:** Category C (1st trimester) and D (2nd and 3rd trimesters), not for use in nursing.	
Valsartan/Hydrochlorothiazide (Diovan HCT)	**Tab:** (Valsartan-HCTZ) 80mg-12.5mg, 160mg-12.5mg, 160mg-25mg, 320mg-12.5mg, 320mg-25mg	***Adults:*** **Add-On/Initial Therapy:** 160mg-12.5mg qd. **Titrate:** May increase after 1-2 weeks of therapy. **Max:** 320mg-25mg. **Replacement Therapy:** May be substituted for titrated components. **CrCl ≤30mL/min:** Use not recommended.	**BB:** Can cause death/injury to developing fetus during 2nd and 3rd trimesters. Stop therapy if pregnancy detected. **W/P:** Correct volume or salt depletion before therapy. Caution with hepatic or renal dysfunction, biliary obstructive disorders, renal artery stenosis, severe CHF, history of allergies, and asthma. May exacerbate or activate SLE. Monitor serum electrolytes. Avoid if CrCl ≤30mL/min. Hyperuricemia, hyperglycemia, hypokalemia, hypomagnesemia, hypercalcemia may occur. Enhanced effects in postsympathectomy patient. May increase cholesterol and triglyceride levels. May cause fetal and neonatal morbidity and death when given to pregnant women. **Contra:** Anuria, sulfonamide hypersensitivity. **P/N:** Category D, not for use in nursing.	Cough, headache, dizziness, fatigue, viral infection, pharyngitis, diarrhea.
β_1-BLOCKERS, CARDIOSELECTIVE				
Acebutolol HCl (Sectral)	**Cap:** 200mg, 400mg	***Adults:*** **HTN: Initial:** 400mg/day, given qd-bid. **Usual:** 200-800mg/day. **Max:** 1200mg/day. **Ventricular Arrhythmia: Initial:** 200mg bid. **Maint:** Increase gradually to 600-1200mg/day. **Elderly:** Lower daily doses. **Max:** 800mg/day. **CrCl <50mL/min:** Decrease daily dose by 50%. **CrCl <25mL/min:** Decrease daily dose by 75%.	**W/P:** Withdrawal before surgery is controversial. Caution with bronchospastic disease, peripheral or mesenteric vascular disease, aortic or mitral valve disease, left ventricular dysfunction, heart failure controlled by digitalis and/or diuretics, hepatic or renal dysfunction. May mask hypoglycemia or hyperthyroidism symptoms. Avoid abrupt discontinuation. May develop antinuclear antibodies (ANA). **Contra:** Cardiogenic shock, persistently severe bradycardia, 2nd- and 3rd-degree AV block, overt cardiac failure. **P/N:** Category B, not for use in nursing.	Fatigue, dizziness, headache, constipation, diarrhea, dyspepsia, flatulence, nausea, dyspnea, urinary frequency, insomnia.
Atenolol (Tenormin)	**Tab:** 25mg, 50mg*, 100mg	***Adults:*** **HTN: Initial:** 50mg qd. **Titrate:** May increase after 1-2 weeks. **Max:** 100mg qd. **Angina: Initial:** 50mg qd. **Titrate:** May increase to 100mg after 1 week. **Max:** 200mg qd. **AMI: Initial:** 5mg IV over 5 min, repeat 10 min later. If tolerated, give 50mg PO 10 min after the last IV dose, followed by another 50mg PO 12 hrs later. **Maint:** 100mg qd or 50mg bid for 6-9 days. **Renal Impairment/Elderly: HTN: Initial:** 25mg qd. **HTN/Angina/AMI: Max: CrCl 15-35mL/min:** 50mg/day. **CrCl <15mL/min:** 25mg/day. **Hemodialysis:** 25-50mg after each dialysis.	**BB:** Avoid abrupt discontinuation of therapy in coronary artery disease. Severe exacerbation of angina and occurrence of MI and ventricular arrhythmias reported in angina patients following abrupt discontinuation of therapy with β-blockers. **W/P:** Withdrawal before surgery is not recommended. Caution with bronchospastic disease, conduction abnormalities, left ventricular dysfunction, heart failure controlled by digitalis and/or diuretics, renal or hepatic dysfunction. Can cause heart failure with prolonged use, hyperuricemia, hypercalcemia, hypokalemia, hypophosphatemia. May mask hypoglycemia or hyperthyroidism symptoms. Avoid abrupt discontinuation. Avoid with untreated pheochromocytoma. Possible fetal harm in pregnancy. May aggravate peripheral arterial circulatory disorders. May manifest latent DM. Monitor for fluid or electrolyte imbalance. May develop antinuclear antibodies (ANA). Neonates born to mothers receiving atenolol may be at risk of hypoglycemia and bradycardia. **Contra:** Cardiogenic shock, sinus bradycardia, 2nd- and 3rd-degree AV block, overt cardiac failure. **P/N:** Category D, caution in nursing.	Bradycardia, hypotension, dizziness, fatigue, nausea, depression, dyspnea.

Table 14.1. PRESCRIBING INFORMATION FOR CARDIOVASCULAR DRUGS *(cont.)*

NAME	FORM/ STRENGTH	DOSAGE	WARNINGS/PRECAUTIONS & CONTRAINDICATIONS	ADVERSE EFFECTS†
ANTIHYPERTENSIVES/HEART FAILURE AGENTS *(cont.)*				
β_1-BLOCKERS, CARDIOSELECTIVE *(cont.)*				
Betaxolol HCl (Kerlone)	**Tab:** 10mg*, 20mg	***Adults:*** **Initial:** 10mg qd. **Titrate:** May increase to 20mg qd after 7-14 days. **Max (usual):** 20mg/day. **Severe Renal Impairment/Dialysis: Initial:** 5mg qd. **Titrate:** May increase by 5mg/day every 2 weeks. **Max:** 20mg/day. **Elderly: Initial:** 5mg qd.	**W/P:** Caution in CHF controlled by digitalis and diuretics, bronchospastic disease, renal or hepatic dysfunction. Can cause cardiac failure. Avoid abrupt withdrawal. Withdrawal before surgery is controversial. May mask hypoglycemia and hyperthyroidism symptoms. May decrease IOP and interfere with glaucoma-screening test. Bradycardia may occur more often in elderly. May develop antinuclear antibodies (ANA). **Contra:** Sinus bradycardia, >1st-degree heart block, cardiogenic shock, overt cardiac failure. **P/N:** Category C, caution in nursing.	Bradycardia, fatigue, dyspnea, lethargy, impotence, dyspepsia, arthralgia, headache, dizziness, insomnia.
Bisoprolol Fumarate (Zebeta)	**Tab:** 5mg*, 10mg	***Adults:*** **Initial:** 2.5-5mg qd. **Max:** 20mg/day. **Hepatic Dysfunction or CrCl <40mL/min: Initial:** 2.5mg qd; caution with dose titration.	**W/P:** Avoid abrupt withdrawal. May mask hypoglycemia or hyperthyroidism symptoms. Caution with compensated cardiac failure, DM, bronchospastic disease, hepatic/renal impairment, or peripheral vascular disease. May precipitate cardiac failure. Both digitalis glycosides and β-blockers slow atrioventricular conduction and decrease HR. Concomitant use can increase risk of bradycardia. **Contra:** Cardiogenic shock, sinus bradycardia, 2nd- and 3rd-degree AV block, overt cardiac failure. **P/N:** Category C, caution in nursing.	Diarrhea, URI, fatigue.
Metoprolol Succinate (Toprol-XL)	**Tab, Extended-Release:** 25mg*, 50mg*, 100mg*, 200mg*	***Adults:*** **HTN: Initial:** 25-100mg qd. **Titrate:** May increase weekly or at longer intervals. **Max:** 400mg/day. **Angina: Initial:** 100mg qd. **Titrate:** May increase weekly. **Max:** 400mg/day. **Heart Failure: Initial:** (NYHA Class II) 25mg qd for 2 weeks. **Severe Heart Failure:** 12.5mg qd for 2 weeks. **Titrate:** Double dose every 2 weeks as tolerated. **Max:** 200mg/day. ***Pediatrics:*** **≥6 yrs: HTN:** 1mg/kg qd. **Max:** 50mg/day. Dose adjust according to BP response. Doses above 2mg/kg have not been studied.	**W/P:** Exacerbation of angina pectoris and MI reported following abrupt withdrawal; taper over 1-2 weeks. Caution with heart failure, bronchospastic disease, DM, hepatic dysfunction, hyperthyroidism, or peripheral vascular disease. May mask symptoms of hyperthyroidism and hypoglycemia. Withdrawal prior to surgery is controversial. Worsening cardiac failure may occur during up titration; lower dose or temporarily d/c. **Contra:** Cardiogenic shock, severe bradycardia, 2nd- and 3rd-degree AV block, overt cardiac failure, sick sinus syndrome (unless a pacemaker is present), decompensated cardiac failure. **P/N:** Category C, caution with nursing.	Bradycardia, SOB, fatigue, dizziness, depression, diarrhea, pruritus, rash, hepatitis, arthralgia.
Metoprolol Tartrate (Lopressor)	**Inj:** 1mg/mL; **Tab:** 50mg*, 100mg*	***Adults:*** **HTN: Initial:** 100mg/day in single or divided doses. **Titrate:** May increase at weekly (or longer) intervals. **Usual:** 100-450mg/day. **Max:** 450mg/day. **Angina: Initial:** 50mg bid. **Titrate:** May increase weekly. **Usual:** 100-400mg/day. **Max:** 400mg/day. **MI (Early Phase):** 5mg IV every 2 min for 3 doses (monitor BP, HR, and ECG). If tolerated, give 50mg PO q6h for 48 hrs. If not tolerated, give 25-50mg PO q6h. Initiate PO dose 15 min after last IV dose. **MI (Late Phase):** 100mg bid for at least 3 months. Take PO with or immediately following meals.	**W/P:** Caution with ischemic heart disease, avoid abrupt withdrawal; taper over 1-2 weeks. Withdrawal before surgery is controversial. May mask hyperthyroidism and hypoglycemia symptoms. May exacerbate cardiac failure. Caution with hepatic dysfunction, CHF controlled by digitalis. Avoid in bronchospastic disease. May decrease sinus HR and/or slow AV conduction. D/C if heart block or hypotension occurs. **Contra:** (HTN, Angina) Cardiogenic shock, sinus bradycardia, 2nd- and 3rd-degree AV block, overt cardiac failure, sick-sinus syndrome, severe peripheral	Bradycardia, SOB, fatigue, dizziness, depression, diarrhea, pruritus, rash, heart block, hypotension.

*Scored. †Bold entries denote special dental considerations.
BB = black box warning; **W/P** = warnings/precautions; **Contra** = contraindications; **P/N** = pregnancy category rating and nursing considerations.

NAME	FORM/ STRENGTH	DOSAGE	WARNINGS/PRECAUTIONS & CONTRAINDICATIONS	ADVERSE EFFECTS†
Metoprolol Tartrate (Lopressor) *(cont.)*			arterial circulatory disorders, pheochromocytoma. (MI) HR <45 beats/min, 2nd- and 3rd-degree AV block, significant 1st-degree AV block, SBP <100mmHg, moderate-to-severe cardiac failure. **P/N:** Category C, caution in nursing.	
Nebivolol (Bystolic)	**Tab:** 2.5mg, 5mg, 10mg, 20mg	***Adults:*** **Monotherapy/Combination Therapy: Initial:** 5mg qd. **Titrate:** May increase dose if needed at 2-week intervals. **Max:** 40mg. **Hepatic Impairment/ CrCl <30mL/min:** 2.5mg qd; upward titration may be performed cautiously.	**W/P:** Exacerbation of angina, and occurrence of MI and ventricular arrhythmias reported in patients with CAD following abrupt withdrawal; taper over 1-2 weeks when possible. Avoid with bronchospastic disease. Caution with compensated CHF; consider d/c if heart failure worsens. Caution with PVD, severe renal/moderate hepatic impairment. May mask signs/symptoms of hypoglycemia or hyperthyroidism. Abrupt withdrawal may also exacerbate symptoms of hyperthyroidism or precipitate a thyroid storm. Caution with history of severe anaphylactic reactions. Patients with known/suspected pheochromocytoma should initially receive an α-blocker prior to use of any β-blocker. No studies done in patients with angina pectoris, recent MI, or severe hepatic impairment. **Contra:** Cardiogenic shock, severe bradycardia, 2nd- and 3rd-degree AV block, decompensated cardiac failure, sick sinus syndrome (unless permanent pacemaker in place), severe hepatic impairment (Child-Pugh >B). **P/N:** Category C, not for use in nursing.	Headache, fatigue, dizziness, diarrhea, nausea.
β_1-BLOCKERS, CARDIOSELECTIVE/DIURETICS				
Atenolol/ Chlorthalidone (Tenoretic)	**Tab:** (Atenolol-Chlorthalidone) 50mg-25mg*, 100mg-25mg	***Adults:*** **Initial:** 50mg-25mg tab qd. May increase to 100mg-25mg tab qd. **CrCl 15-35mL/min: Max:** 50mg atenolol/day. **CrCl <15mL/min: Max:** 50mg atenolol qod.	**W/P:** Withdrawal before surgery is not recommended. Caution with bronchospastic disease, conduction abnormalities, left ventricular dysfunction. Caution in patients with impaired renal and hepatic function. Can cause heart failure with prolonged use. May mask hypoglycemia or hyperthyroidism symptoms. Avoid abrupt discontinuation. Avoid with untreated pheochromocytoma. Possible fetal harm in pregnancy. May aggravate peripheral arterial circulatory disorders. Enhanced effects in postsympathectomy patient. Neonates born to mothers receiving atenolol may be at risk of hypoglycemia and bradycardia. **Contra:** Cardiogenic shock, sinus bradycardia, 2nd- and 3rd-degree AV block, overt cardiac failure, anuria, sulfonamide hypersensitivity. **P/N:** Category D, caution in nursing.	Bradycardia, hypotension, dizziness, fatigue, nausea, depression, dyspnea, blood dyscrasias.
Bisoprolol Fumarate/Hydrochlorothiazide (Ziac)	**Tab:** (Bisoprolol-HCTZ) 2.5mg-6.25mg, 5mg-6.25mg, 10mg-6.25mg	***Adults:*** **Initial:** 2.5mg-6.25mg tab qd. **Maint:** May increase every 14 days. **Max:** 20mg bisoprolol-12.5mg HCTZ/ day. **Renal/Hepatic Dysfunction:** Caution in dosing/titrating.	**W/P:** Caution with compensated cardiac failure, DM, bronchospastic disease, hepatic/renal impairment, or peripheral vascular disease. Avoid abrupt withdrawal. Photosensitivity reactions, hypokalemia, hypercalcemia, hypophosphatemia reported. May activate/exacerbate SLE. Enhanced effects in postsympathectomy patients. May mask hyperthyroidism or hypoglycemia symptoms. Monitor for fluid/	Cough, diarrhea, myalgia, headache, dizziness, fatigue, upper respiratory infection.

Table 14.1. PRESCRIBING INFORMATION FOR CARDIOVASCULAR DRUGS *(cont.)*

NAME	FORM/ STRENGTH	DOSAGE	WARNINGS/PRECAUTIONS & CONTRAINDICATIONS	ADVERSE EFFECTS†
ANTIHYPERTENSIVES/HEART FAILURE AGENTS *(cont.)*				
β_1-BLOCKERS, CARDIOSELECTIVE/DIURETICS *(cont.)*				
Bisoprolol Fumarate/Hydrochlorothiazide (Ziac) *(cont.)*			electrolyte imbalance. May precipitate hyperuricemia, acute gout, cardiac failure. **Contra:** Cardiogenic shock, marked sinus bradycardia, 2nd- and 3rd-degree AV block, overt cardiac failure, anuria, sulfonamide hypersensitivity. **P/N:** Category C, not for use in nursing.	
Metoprolol Tartrate/Hydrochlorothiazide (Lopressor HCT)	**Tab:** (Metoprolol-HCTZ) 50mg-25mg*, 100-25mg*, 100mg-50mg*	***Adults:*** **Usual:** 100-450mg metoprolol/day and 12.5-50mg HCTZ/day. **Max:** 50mg HCTZ/day.	**W/P:** Avoid abrupt withdrawal; taper over 1-2 weeks. Withdrawal before surgery is controversial. May mask hyperthyroidism and hypoglycemia symptoms. May cause cardiac failure. Caution with hepatic dysfunction, CHF controlled by digitalis, severe renal disease, allergy or asthma history. Avoid in bronchospastic disease. Monitor for fluid/electrolyte imbalance. May manifest latent DM. Hypokalemia, hyperuricemia, hypercalcemia, hypophosphatemia, and hypomagnesemia may occur. May exacerbate SLE. Enhanced effects in postsympathectomy patient. **Contra:** Cardiogenic shock, sinus bradycardia, 2nd- and 3rd-degree AV block, overt cardiac failure, sick-sinus syndrome, severe peripheral arterial circulatory disorders, pheochromocytoma, anuria, sulfonamide hypersensitivity. **P/N:** Category C, not for use in nursing.	Fatigue, dizziness, flu syndrome, drowsiness, hypokalemia, headache, bradycardia.
β-BLOCKERS, NONSELECTIVE				
Nadolol (Corgard)	**Tab:** 20mg*, 40mg*, 80mg*, 120mg*, 160mg*	***Adults:*** **Angina Pectoris: Initial:** 40mg qd. **Titrate:** Increase by 40-80mg every 3-7 days. **Usual:** 40-80mg qd. **Max:** 240mg/day. **HTN: Initial:** 40mg qd. **Titrate:** Increase by 40-80mg. **Max:** 320mg/day. **CrCl 31-50mL/min:** Dose q24-36h. **CrCl 10-30mL/min:** Dose q24-48h. **CrCl <10mL/min:** Dose q40-60h.	**W/P:** Caution in well-compensated cardiac failure, nonallergic bronchospasm, renal dysfunction. Exacerbation of ischemic heart disease with abrupt withdrawal. Withdrawal before surgery is controversial. May mask hyperthyroidism or hypoglycemia symptoms. Can cause cardiac failure. **Contra:** Bronchial asthma, cardiogenic shock, sinus bradycardia, 2nd- and 3rd-degree AV block, overt cardiac failure. **P/N:** Category C, not for use in nursing.	Bradycardia, peripheral vascular insufficiency, dizziness, fatigue.
Penbutolol Sulfate (Levatol)	**Tab:** 20mg*	***Adults:*** 20mg qd.	**W/P:** Caution with well-compensated heart failure, elderly, nonallergic bronchospasm, renal impairment. Can cause cardiac failure. Avoid abrupt withdrawal. Withdrawal before surgery is controversial. May mask hypoglycemia or hyperthyroidism symptoms. **Contra:** Bronchial asthma, cardiogenic shock, sinus bradycardia, 2nd- and 3rd-degree AV block. **P/N:** Category C, caution in nursing.	Diarrhea, nausea, dyspepsia, dizziness, fatigue, headache, insomnia, cough.
Pindolol	**Tab:** 5mg, 10mg	***Adults:*** **Initial:** 5mg bid. **Titrate:** May increase by 10mg/day after 3-4 weeks. **Max:** 60mg/day.	**W/P:** Caution with well-compensated heart failure, nonallergic bronchospasm, renal or hepatic impairment. Can cause cardiac failure. Avoid abrupt withdrawal. Withdrawal before surgery is controversial. May mask hypoglycemia or hyperthyroidism symptoms. **Contra:** Bronchial asthma, cardiogenic shock, severe bradycardia, 2nd- and 3rd-degree AV block, overt cardiac failure. **P/N:** Category B, not for use in nursing.	Dizziness, fatigue, insomnia, nervousness, dyspnea, edema, joint pain, muscle cramps/pain.

*Scored. †Bold entries denote special dental considerations.
BB = black box warning; **W/P** = warnings/precautions; **Contra** = contraindications; **P/N** = pregnancy category rating and nursing considerations.

NAME	FORM/ STRENGTH	DOSAGE	WARNINGS/PRECAUTIONS & CONTRAINDICATIONS	ADVERSE EFFECTS†
Propranolol HCl (Inderal, Inderal IV, Inderal LA, InnoPran XL)	**Cap, Extended-Release:** (Inderal LA) 60mg, 80mg, 120mg, 160mg (InnoPran XL) 80mg, 120mg; **Inj:** 1mg/mL; **Tab:** (Inderal) 10mg*, 20mg*, 40mg*, 60mg*, 80mg*	***Adults:*** **(Inderal) HTN: Initial:** 40mg bid. **Titrate:** Increase gradually. **Maint:** 120-240mg/day. **Angina:** 80-320mg/day, given bid-qid. **Arrhythmia:** 10-30mg tid-qid ac and qhs. **MI:** 180-240mg/day, given bid-tid. **Migraine: Initial:** 80mg/day in divided doses. **Usual:** 160-240mg/day in divided doses. **Tremor: Initial:** 40mg bid. **Maint:** 120mg/day. **Max:** 320mg/day. **Hypertrophic Subaortic Stenosis:** 20-40mg tid-qid, ac, and qhs. **Pheochromocytoma:** 60mg/day in divided doses for 3 days before surgery with α-blocker. **Inoperable Tumor:** 30mg/day in divided doses. **(Inderal IV) Arrhythmia:** 1-3mg IV at 1 mg/min. **(Inderal LA) HTN: Initial:** 80mg qd. **Maint:** 120-160mg qd. **Angina: Initial:** 80mg qd. **Titrate:** Increase gradually every 3-7 days. **Maint:** 160mg qd. **Max:** 320mg/day. **Migraine: Initial:** 80mg qd. **Maint:** 160-240mg qd. Discontinue gradually if no response within 4-6 weeks. **Hypertrophic Subaortic Stenosis:** 80-160mg qd. **(InnoPran XL): HTN: Initial:** 80mg qhs (approximately 10 pm) consistently either on empty stomach or with food. **Titrate:** Based on response may titrate to dose of 120mg. ***Pediatrics:*** **HTN: Initial:** 1mg/kg/day PO. **Usual:** 1-2mg/kg bid. **Max:** 16mg/kg/day.	**BB (InnoPran XL only):** Avoid abrupt discontinuation of therapy in coronary artery disease. Severe exacerbation of angina and occurrence of MI and ventricular arrhythmias reported in angina patients following abrupt discontinuation of therapy with β-blockers. **W/P:** Caution with well-compensated cardiac failure, nonallergic bronchospasm, Wolff-Parkinson-White (WPW) syndrome, hepatic or renal dysfunction. Withdrawal before surgery is controversial. May mask hypoglycemia or hyperthyroidism symptoms. Avoid abrupt discontinuation. May reduce IOP. Can cause cardiac failure. Both digitalis glycosides and β-blockers slow atrioventricular conduction and decrease HR. Concomitant use can increase risk of bradycardia. Stevens-Johnson syndrome, toxic epidermal necrolysis, exfoliative dermatitis, erythema multiforme, and urticaria reported. **Contra:** Bronchial asthma, cardiogenic shock, sinus bradycardia, 2nd- and 3rd-degree AV block, CHF (unless failure is secondary to tachyarrhythmia treatable with propranolol). **P/N:** Category C, caution in nursing.	Bradycardia, CHF, hypotension, lightheadedness, mental depression, N/V, allergic reactions, agranulocytosis, dry eyes, alopecia, SLE-like reactions, male impotence, Peyronie's disease, fatigue, dizziness (except vertigo), constipation.
Timolol Maleate	**Tab:** 5mg, 10mg*, 20mg*	***Adults:*** **HTN: Initial:** 10mg bid. **Maint:** 20-40mg/day. Wait at least 7 days between dose increases. **Max:** 60mg/day given bid. **MI:** 10mg bid. **Migraine: Initial:** 10mg bid. **Maint:** 20mg qd. **Max:** 30mg/day in divided doses. May decrease to 10mg qd. D/C if inadequate response after 6-8 weeks with max dose.	**W/P:** Caution with well-compensated cardiac failure, DM, mild-to-moderate COPD, bronchospastic disease, dialysis, hepatic/renal impairment, or cerebrovascular insufficiency. Exacerbation of ischemic heart disease with abrupt cessation. May mask hyperthyroidism or hypoglycemia symptoms. Withdrawal before surgery is controversial. May potentiate weakness with myasthenia gravis. Can cause cardiac failure. Caution and consider monitoring renal function in elderly. **Contra:** Bronchial asthma, severe COPD, cardiogenic shock, sinus bradycardia, 2nd- and 3rd-degree AV block, overt cardiac failure. **P/N:** Category C, not for use in nursing.	Fatigue, headache, nausea, arrhythmia, pruritus, dizziness, dyspnea, asthenia, bradycardia.
β-BLOCKERS, NONSELECTIVE/α_1-BLOCKERS				
Carvedilol (Coreg, Coreg CR)	**Tab:** 3.125mg, 6.25mg, 12.5mg, 25mg; **Cap, Extended-Release:** 10mg, 20mg, 40mg, 80mg	***Adults:*** Individualize dose. Take with food. Monitor dose increases. Take extended-release capsules in am and swallow whole. **CHF: Tab: Initial:** 3.125mg bid for 2 weeks. **Titrate:** May double dose every 2 weeks as tolerated. **Max:** 50mg bid if >85kg. Reduce dose if HR <55 beats/min. **Cap, Extended-Release: Initial:** 10mg qd for 2 weeks. **Titrate:** May double dose every 2 weeks as tolerated. **Max:** 80mg/day. Reduce dose if HR <55 beats/min. **HTN: Tab: Initial:** 6.25mg bid for 7-14 days. **Titrate:** May double dose at 7-14 day intervals. **Max:** 50mg/day. **Cap, Extended-Release: Initial:** 20mg qd for 7-14 days. **Titrate:** May double dose every 7-14 days as tolerated. **Max:** 80mg/day. **LVD Post-MI: Tab: Initial:** 6.25mg bid for 3-10 days. **Titrate:**	**W/P:** Avoid abrupt discontinuation; taper over 1-2 weeks. Hepatic injury reported; d/c and do not restart if develop hepatic injury. Hypotension and syncope reported, most commonly during up-titration period; avoid driving or hazardous tasks during initiation period. May mask hypoglycemia and hyperthyroidism. May potentiate insulin-induced hypoglycemia and delay recovery of serum glucose levels. Decrease dose if pulse <55 beats/min. Monitor renal function during up-titration with low BP (SBP <100mmHg), ischemic heart disease, diffuse vascular disease and/or renal insufficiency. Worsening heart failure or fluid retention may occur with up-titration. Caution in pheochromocytoma, peripheral vascular disease, major surgery with anesthesia, Prinzmetal's variant angina, and	Bradycardia, fatigue, edema, hypotension, dizziness, headache, diarrhea, N/V, hyperglycemia, weight increase, dyspnea, anemia, increased cough, arthralgia.

Table 14.1. PRESCRIBING INFORMATION FOR CARDIOVASCULAR DRUGS *(cont.)*

NAME	FORM/ STRENGTH	DOSAGE	WARNINGS/PRECAUTIONS & CONTRAINDICATIONS	ADVERSE EFFECTS†
ANTIHYPERTENSIVES/HEART FAILURE AGENTS *(cont.)*				
β-BLOCKERS, NONSELECTIVE/α_1-BLOCKERS *(cont.)*				
Carvedilol (Coreg, Coreg CR) *(cont.)*		May double dose every 3-10 days to target of 25mg bid. May begin with 3.125mg bid and slow up-titration rate if clinically indicated. **Cap, Extended-Release: Initial:** 20mg qd for 3-10 days. **Titrate:** May double dose every 3-10 days to target of 80mg qd.	bronchospastic disease. Effectiveness of carvedilol in patients younger than 18 years of age has not been established. **Contra:** Bronchial asthma or related bronchospastic conditions, 2nd- or 3rd-degree AV block, sick sinus syndrome, severe bradycardia (without permanent pacemaker), cardiogenic shock, decompensated heart failure requiring IV inotropic therapy, severe hepatic impairment. **P/N:** Category C, not for use in nursing.	
Labetalol HCl (Trandate)	**Inj:** 5mg/mL; **Tab:** (Trandate) 100mg*, 200mg*, 300mg*	***Adults:*** **(Tab) HTN: Initial:** 100mg bid. **Titrate:** May increase by 100mg bid every 2-3 days. **Maint:** 200-400mg bid. **Severe HTN:** 1200-2400mg/day given bid-tid. **Titrate:** Do not increase by more than 200mg bid. **Elderly: Initial:** 100mg bid. **Titrate:** May increase by 100mg bid. **Maint:** 100-200mg bid. **(Inj) Severe HTN:** Administer in supine position. **Repeated IV Infusion: Initial:** 20mg over 2 min. **Titrate:** Give additional 40-80mg at 10 min intervals if needed. **Max:** 300mg. **Slow Continuous Infusion:** 200mg at rate of 2mg/min. May adjust dose according to BP. Switch to tabs when BP is stable while in hospital. **Initial:** 200mg, then 200-400mg 6-12 hrs later on Day 1. **Titrate:** May increase at 1-day interval.	**W/P:** Severe hepatocellular injury reported; caution with hepatic dysfunction. Monitor LFTs periodically; d/c at first sign of hepatic injury. Caution with well-compensated heart failure. Caution with latent cardiac insufficiency, may exacerbate cardiac failure, reduce sinus HR, and slow AV conduction. Exacerbation of ischemic heart disease with abrupt withdrawal. Caution in nonallergic bronchospasm patients refractory to or intolerant to other antihypertensives. May mask hypoglycemia symptoms. Caution with DM; may mask symptoms of hypoglycemia. Withdrawal before surgery is controversial. Paradoxical HTN may occur with pheochromocytoma. Death reported during surgery. Avoid injection with low cardiac indices and elevated systemic vascular resistance. **Contra:** Bronchial asthma, severe COPD, cardiogenic shock, severe bradycardia, 2nd- and 3rd-degree AV block, overt cardiac failure, other conditions associated with severe and prolonged hypotension. **P/N:** Category C, caution in nursing.	Dizziness, fatigue, N/V, dyspepsia, paresthesia, nasal stuffiness, ejaculation failure, impotence, edema, dyspnea, headache, vertigo, postural hypotension, increased sweating.
β-BLOCKERS, NONSELECTIVE/DIURETICS				
Nadolol/Bendroflumethiazide (Corzide)	**Tab:** (Nadolol-Bendroflumethiazide) 40mg-5mg*, 80mg-5mg*	***Adults:*** **Initial:** 40mg-5mg tab qd. **Max:** 80mg-5mg tab qd. **CrCl >50mL/min:** Dose q24h. **CrCl 31-50mL/min:** Dose q24-36h. **CrCl 10-30mL/min:** Dose q24-48h. **CrCl <10mL/min:** Dose q40-60h.	**W/P:** Caution in well-compensated cardiac failure, nonallergic bronchospasm, progressive hepatic disease, and renal or hepatic dysfunction. Exacerbation of ischemic heart disease with abrupt withdrawal. Withdrawal before surgery is controversial. May mask hyperthyroidism or hypoglycemia symptoms. Can cause cardiac failure, sensitivity reactions, hypokalemia, hyperuricemia, hypomagnesemia, hypophosphatemia. May activate or exacerbate SLE. Monitor for fluid/electrolyte imbalance. Enhanced effects in postsympathectomy patient. May manifest latent DM. May decrease PBI levels. **Contra:** Bronchial asthma, severe COPD, cardiogenic shock, sinus bradycardia, 2nd- and 3rd-degree AV block, overt cardiac failure, anuria, sulfonamide hypersensitivity. **P/N:** Category C, not for use in nursing.	Bradycardia, peripheral vascular insufficiency, dizziness, fatigue, N/V, blood dyscrasias, hypersensitivity reactions.

*Scored. †Bold entries denote special dental considerations.
BB = black box warning; **W/P** = warnings/precautions; **Contra** = contraindications; **P/N** = pregnancy category rating and nursing considerations.

NAME	FORM/ STRENGTH	DOSAGE	WARNINGS/PRECAUTIONS & CONTRAINDICATIONS	ADVERSE EFFECTS†
Propranolol HCl/Hydrochlorothiazide (Inderide)	**Tab:** (Propranolol-HCTZ) (Inderide) 40mg-25mg*, 80mg-25mg*	***Adults:*** **Initial:** 80-160mg propranolol/day; 25-50mg HCTZ/day. **Max:** (propranolol-HCTZ) 160mg-50mg/day. **Elderly:** Start at low end of dosing range. Do not substitute mg-for-mg of extended-release cap for immediate-release tab plus HCTZ. Dose tab bid and extended-release cap qd.	**W/P:** Caution with well-compensated cardiac failure, nonallergic bronchospasm, Wolff-Parkinson-White syndrome, hepatic or renal dysfunction. Withdrawal before surgery is controversial. May mask hypoglycemia or hyperthyroidism symptoms. Avoid abrupt discontinuation. May reduce IOP. Can cause cardiac failure, hypokalemia, hyperuricemia, hypercalcemia, hypophosphatemia. May exacerbate or activate SLE. Monitor for fluid/electrolyte imbalance. May manifest latent DM. Enhanced effect in postsympathectomy patient. Concomitant use with alcohol may increase plasma levels of propranolol **Contra:** Bronchial asthma, cardiogenic shock, sinus bradycardia, 2nd- and 3rd-degree AV block, CHF (unless failure is secondary to tachyarrhythmia treatable with propranolol), anuria, sulfonamide hypersensitivity. **P/N:** Category C, not for use in nursing.	Bradycardia, CHF, hypotension, lightheadedness, mental depression, N/V, allergic reactions, blood dyscrasias, pancreatitis.
CALCIUM CHANNEL BLOCKERS				
Amlodipine Besylate (Norvasc)	**Tab:** 2.5mg, 5mg, 10mg	***Adults:*** **HTN: Initial:** 5mg qd. Titrate over 7-14 days. **Max:** 10mg qd. **Small, Fragile, or Elderly/Hepatic Dysfunction/Concomitant Antihypertensive: Initial:** 2.5mg qd. **Angina:** 5-10mg qd. **Elderly/Hepatic Dysfunction:** 5mg qd. **CAD:** 5-10mg qd. ***Pediatrics:*** **6-17 yrs: HTN:** 2.5-5mg qd.	**W/P:** May increase angina or MI with severe obstructive CAD. Caution with severe aortic stenosis, CHF, severe hepatic impairment, and in elderly. **P/N:** Category C, not for use in nursing.	Edema, flushing, palpitation, dizziness, headache, fatigue.
Diltiazem HCl (Cardizem CD, Cardizem LA, Cartia XT, Dilacor XR, Diltia XT, Taztia XT, Tiazac)	**Cap, Extended-Release:** (Cartia XT) 120mg, 180mg, 240mg, 300mg; (Cardizem CD, Taztia XT) 120mg, 180mg, 240mg, 300mg, 360mg; (Dilacor XR, Diltia XT) 120mg, 180mg, 240mg; (Tiazac) 120mg, 180mg, 240mg, 300mg, 360mg, 420mg; **Tab, Extended-Release:** (Cardizem LA) 120mg, 180mg, 240mg, 300mg, 360mg, 420mg	***Adults:*** **(Cardizem CD, Cartia XT): HTN: Initial (monotherapy):** 180-240mg qd. **Titrate:** Adjust at 2-week intervals. **Usual:** 240-360mg qd. **Max:** 480mg qd. **Angina: Initial:** 120-180mg qd. Adjust at 1-2 week intervals. **Max:** 480mg/day. **(Cardizem LA) HTN: Initial:** 180-240mg qd. Adjust at 2-week intervals. **Max:** 540mg qd. **Angina: Initial:** 180mg qd. Adjust at 1-2 week intervals. **(Dilacor XR, Diltia XT): HTN: Initial:** 180-240mg qd. **Usual:** 180-480mg qd. **Max:** 540mg qd. **≥60 yrs: Initial:** 120mg qd. **Angina: Initial:** 120mg qd. **Titrate:** Adjust at 1-2 week intervals. **Max:** 480mg/day. Swallow whole on an empty stomach in the am. **(Taztia XT, Tiazac) HTN: Initial:** 120-240mg qd. **Titrate:** Adjust at 2-week intervals. **Usual:** 120-540mg qd. **Max:** 540mg qd. **Angina: Initial:** 120-180mg qd. **Titrate:** Increase over 7-14 days. **Max:** 540mg qd.	**W/P:** Caution in renal, hepatic, or ventricular dysfunction. Monitor LFTs and renal function with prolonged use. D/C if persistent rash occurs. Symptomatic hypotension may occur. Acute hepatic injury reported. **Contra:** Sick sinus syndrome and 2nd- or 3rd-degree AV block (except with functioning pacemaker), hypotension (<90mmHg systolic), acute MI, pulmonary congestion. **P/N:** Category C, not for use in nursing.	Headache, dizziness, asthenia, flushing, 1st-degree AV block, peripheral edema, bradycardia, rash, vasodilation, dyspepsia, rhinitis, pharyngitis, cough, flu syndrome, myalgia, N/V, sinusitis, constipation, diarrhea.
Felodipine (Plendil)	**Tab, Extended-Release:** 2.5mg, 5mg, 10mg	***Adults:*** **Initial:** 5mg qd. **Titrate:** Adjust at no less than 2-week intervals. **Maint:** 2.5-10mg qd. **Elderly: Initial:** 2.5mg qd. Take without food or with a light meal. Swallow tab whole.	**W/P:** May cause hypotension and lead to reflex tachycardia with precipitation of angina. Caution with heart failure or ventricular dysfunction, especially with concomitant β-blockers. Monitor dose adjustment with hepatic dysfunction or elderly. Peripheral edema reported. Maintain good dental hygiene; gingival hyperplasia reported. **P/N:** Category C, not for use in nursing.	Peripheral edema, headache, flushing, dizziness.

Table 14.1. PRESCRIBING INFORMATION FOR CARDIOVASCULAR DRUGS *(cont.)*

NAME	FORM/ STRENGTH	DOSAGE	WARNINGS/PRECAUTIONS & CONTRAINDICATIONS	ADVERSE EFFECTS†
ANTIHYPERTENSIVES/HEART FAILURE AGENTS *(cont.)*				
CALCIUM CHANNEL BLOCKERS *(cont.)*				
Isradipine (DynaCirc CR)	**Cap:** (Isradipine) 2.5mg, 5mg **Tab, Controlled-Release:** (DynaCirc CR) 5mg, 10mg	***Adults:*** **(DynaCirc CR) Initial:** 5mg qd alone or with a thiazide diuretic. **Titrate:** May adjust by 5mg/day at 2-4 week intervals. **Max:** 20mg/day. Swallow whole. **(Isradipine) Initial:** 2.5mg bid alone or with a thiazide diuretic. **Titrate:** May adjust by 5mg/day at 2-4 week intervals. **Max:** 20mg/day.	**W/P:** May produce symptomatic hypotension. Caution in CHF, especially with concomitant β-blockers. Caution with preexisting severe GI narrowing. Peripheral edema reported. Increased bioavailability in elderly, patients with hepatic functional impairment, and mild renal impairment. **P/N:** Category C, not for use in nursing.	Headache, edema, dizziness, palpitations, chest pain, constipation, fatigue, flushing, abdominal discomfort, tachycardia, rash, pollakiura, weakness, vomiting.
Nicardipine HCl (Cardene SR, Cardene IV)	**Cap:** (Nicardipine HCl) 20mg, 30mg **Cap, Extended-Release:** (Cardene SR) 30mg, 45mg, 60mg **Inj:** (Cardene IV) 2.5mg/mL	***Adults:*** **(Cardene IV)** Individualized dose; Administer by slow continuous infusion at a concentration of 0.1mg/mL. **Gradual Reduction: Initial:** 50mL/hr (5mg/hr). **Titrate:** May increase by 25mL/hr (2.5mg/hr) q15 min. **Max:** 150mL/hr (15mg/hr). **Rapid BP Reduction: Initial:** 50mL/hr (5mg/hr). **Titrate:** 25mL/hr(2.5mg/hr) q5 min. Max 150mL/hr (15mg/hr). Decrease rate to 30mL/hr (3mg/hr) after BP reduction is achieved. Equiv. **PO/IV Dose:** 20mg q8h=0.5mg/hr, 30mg q8h=1.2mg/hr, 40mg q8h=2.2mg/hr. **(Cardene SR) Initial:** 30mg bid. **Usual:** 30-60mg bid. **(Nicardipine HCl) ≥18 yrs: Initial:** 20mg tid. **Titrate:** Increase dose every 3 days if needed. **Usual:** 20-40mg tid. **Hepatic Dysfunction: Initial:** 20mg bid.	**W/P:** May induce or exacerbate angina. Caution with CHF, significant left ventricular dysfunction, or pheochromocytoma. Change IV site every 12 hrs to minimize risk of peripheral venous irritation. Monitor BP during administration. Measure BP 2-4 hrs after 1st dose or dose increase of extended release caps. Measure BP 1-2 hrs and 8 hrs after dosing of capsules. May cause symptomatic hypotension. Caution in hepatic/renal impairment or reduced hepatic blood flow. **Contra:** Advanced aortic stenosis. **P/N:** Category C, not for use in nursing.	Headache, pedal edema, vasodilation, palpitations, nausea, dizziness, asthenia, flushing, increased angina, hypotension, tachycardia, N/V.
Nifedipine (Adalat CC, Afeditab CR, Procardia XL)	**Tab, Extended-Release:** (Adalat CC, Procardia XL) 30mg, 60mg, 90mg (Afeditab CR) 30mg, 60mg	***Adults:*** **(Adalat CC, Afeditab CR) Initial:** 30mg qd. Titrate over 7-14 days. **Usual:** 30-60mg qd. **Max:** 90mg/day. Take on empty stomach. Swallow tab whole. **(Procardia XL) Angina/HTN: Initial:** 30-60mg qd. Titrate over 7-14 days. **Max:** 120mg/day. Caution if dose >90mg with angina.	**W/P:** May cause hypotension; monitor BP initially or with titration. May exacerbate angina from β-blocker withdrawal. CHF risk, especially with aortic stenosis or β-blockers. Peripheral edema reported. May increase angina or MI with severe obstructive CAD. Caution in elderly. **P/N:** Category C, not for use in nursing.	Dizziness, lightheadedness, giddiness, flushing, muscle cramps, headache, weakness, nausea, peripheral edema, nervousness/mood changes.
Nisoldipine (Sular)	**Tab, Extended-Release:** 10mg, 20mg, 30mg, 40mg	***Adults:*** **Initial:** 20mg qd. **Titrate:** Increase by 10mg weekly or longer. **Maint:** 20-40mg qd. **Max:** 60mg/day. **Elderly (>65 yrs)/Hepatic Dysfunction: Initial:** Do not exceed 10mg/day. Do not chew, divide, or crush tabs.	**W/P:** May increase angina or MI with severe obstructive CAD. May cause hypotension; monitor BP initially or with titration. Caution with heart failure or compromised ventricular function, especially with concomitant β-blockers. Caution with severe hepatic dysfunction or in elderly. **P/N:** Category C, not for use in nursing.	Peripheral edema, headache, dizziness, pharyngitis, vasodilation, sinusitis, palpitations.
Verapamil HCl (Calan, Covera-HS, Isoptin SR, Verelan, Verelan PM)	**Cap, Extended-Release:** (Verelan) 120mg, 180mg, 240mg, 360mg; (Verelan PM) 100mg, 200mg, 300mg; **Tab:** (Calan) 40mg, 80mg*, 120mg*; **Tab, Extended-Release:** (Covera-HS) 180mg, 240mg; (Calan SR, Isoptin SR) 120mg, 180mg*, 240mg	***Adults:*** **(Calan): HTN: Initial:** 80mg tid. **Usual:** 360-480mg/day. **Elderly/Small Stature: Initial:** 40mg tid. **Angina: Usual:** 80-120mg tid. **Elderly/Small Stature: Initial:** 40mg tid. **Titrate:** Increase daily or weekly. **A-Fib (Digitalized): Usual:** 240-320mg/day given tid-qid. **PSVT Prophylaxis (Nondigitalized):** 240-480mg/day given tid-qid. **Max:** 480mg/day. **Severe Hepatic Dysfunction:** Give 30% of normal dose. **(Calan SR, Isoptin SR): ≥18 yrs: Essential HTN: Initial:** 180mg qam. **Titrate:** If inadequate response, increase to 240mg qam, then 180mg bid; or 240mg qam plus 120mg qpm, then 240mg q12h. **Elderly/Small Stature: Initial:** 120mg qam. Take with food. **(Covera-HS): HTN/Angina: Initial:**	**W/P:** Avoid with moderate-to-severe cardiac failure, and ventricular dysfunction if taking a β-blocker. May cause hypotension, AV block, transient bradycardia, PR-interval prolongation. Monitor LFTs periodically; hepatocellular injury reported. Give 30% of normal dose with severe hepatic dysfunction. Caution with hypertrophic cardiomyopathy, renal or hepatic dysfunction. Decrease dose in those with decreased neuromuscular transmission. **Contra:** Severe ventricular dysfunction, hypotension, cardiogenic shock, sick sinus syndrome or 2nd- or 3rd-degree AV block (except with functioning ventricular pacemaker), A-Fib/Flutter with an accessory bypass tract. **P/N:** Category C, not for use in nursing.	Constipation, dizziness, nausea, hypotension, headache, peripheral edema, CHF, fatigue, pulmonary edema, elevated liver enzymes, dyspnea, bradycardia, AV block, rash, flushing, infection, flu syndrome.

*Scored. †Bold entries denote special dental considerations.
BB = black box warning; **W/P** = warnings/precautions; **Contra** = contraindications; **P/N** = pregnancy category rating and nursing considerations.

NAME	FORM/ STRENGTH	DOSAGE	WARNINGS/PRECAUTIONS & CONTRAINDICATIONS	ADVERSE EFFECTS†
Verapamil HCl (Calan, Covera-HS, Isoptin SR, Verelan, Verelan PM) *(cont.)*		180mg qhs. **Titrate:** May increase to 240mg qhs, then 360mg qhs, then 480mg qhs, if needed. Swallow tab whole. **Elderly:** Start at the low end of the dosing range. **(Verelan): Usual:** 240mg qam. **Titrate:** May increase by 120mg qam. **Max:** 480mg qam. **Elderly/Small People: Initial:** 120mg qam. **Titrate:** May increase to 180mg qam, then 240mg qam, then 360mg qam, then 480mg qam. May sprinkle on applesauce; do not crush or chew. **(Verelan PM) Usual:** 200mg qhs. **Titrate:** May increase to 300mg qhs, then 400mg qhs. **Renal or Hepatic Dysfunction/Elderly/Small People: Initial:** 100mg qhs. **Max:** 400mg qhs. May sprinkle on applesauce; do not crush or chew.		
CALCIUM CHANNEL BLOCKER/HMG-CoA REDUCTASE INHIBITOR				
Amlodipine Besylate/ Atorvastatin Calcium (Caduet)	**Tab:** (Amlodipine-Atorvastatin) 2.5mg-10mg, 2.5mg-20mg, 2.5mg-40mg, 5mg-10mg, 5mg-20mg, 5mg-40mg, 5mg-80mg, 10mg-10mg, 10mg-20mg, 10mg-40mg, 10mg-80mg	***Adults:*** Dosing should be individualized and based on the appropriate combination of recommendations for the monotherapies. **(Amlodipine): HTN: Initial:** 5mg qd. Titrate over 7-14 days. **Max:** 10mg qd. **Small, Fragile, or Elderly/ Hepatic Dysfunction/Concomitant Antihypertensive: Initial:** 2.5mg qd. **Angina:** 5-10mg qd. **Elderly Hepatic Dysfunction:** 5mg qd. **(Atorvastatin): Hypercholesterolemia/Mixed Dyslipidemia: Initial:** 10-20mg qd (or 40mg qd for LDL-C reduction >45%). **Titrate:** Adjust dose if needed at 2-4 week intervals. **Usual:** 10-80mg qd. **Homozygous Familial Hypercholesterolemia:** 10-80mg qd. ***Pediatrics:*** **≥10 yrs (postmenarchal): (Amlodipine): HTN:** 2.5-5mg qd. **10-17 yrs (postmenarchal): (Atorvastatin): Heterozygous Familial Hypercholesterolemia: Initial:** 10mg/day. **Titrate:** Adjust dose if needed at intervals of ≥4 weeks. **Max:** 20mg/day.	**W/P:** May rarely increase angina or MI with severe obstructive CAD. Monitor LFTs prior to therapy, at 12 weeks after initiation, with dose elevation, and periodically thereafter. Reduce dose or withdraw if AST or ALT >3x ULN persist. Caution with heavy alcohol use and/or history of hepatic disease, severe aortic stenosis, CHF. D/C if markedly elevated CPK levels occur, if myopathy is diagnosed or suspected, or if predisposition to renal failure secondary to rhabdomyolysis. Increased risk of hemorrhagic stroke in patients with recent stroke or TIA. **Contra:** Active liver disease, unexplained persistent elevations of serum transaminases, pregnancy, nursing mothers. **P/N:** Category X, not for use in nursing.	Headache, edema, palpitation, dizziness, fatigue, constipation, flatulence, dyspepsia, abdominal pain.
CARDIAC GLYCOSIDES				
Digoxin (Digitek, Lanoxicaps, Lanoxin)	**Cap:** (Lanoxicaps) 0.1mg, 0.2mg; **Inj:** (Pediatric Inj) 0.1mg/mL, 0.25mg/mL; **Sol:** (Pediatric Sol) 0.05mg/ mL [60mL]; **Tab:** 0.125mg*, 0.25mg*	***Adults:*** **Rapid Digitalization: LD:** (Cap/Inj) 0.4-0.6mg PO/IV or (Tab) 0.5-0.75mg PO, may give additional (Cap/Inj) 0.1-0.3mg or (Tab) 0.125-0.375mg at 6-8 hr intervals until clinical effect. **Maint:** (Tab) 0.125-0.5mg qd. **Elderly (>70 yrs)/Renal Dysfunction: Initial:** 0.125mg qd. **Marked Renal Dysfunction: Initial:** 0.0625mg qd. **Titrate:** Increase every 2 weeks based on response. **A-Fib:** Titrate to minimum effective dose for desired response. ***Pediatrics:*** (Ped Sol) **Oral Digitalizing Dose: Premature Infants:** 20-30mcg/ kg. **Full-Term Infants:** 25-35mcg/kg. **1-24 months:** 35-60mcg/kg. **2-5 yrs:** 30-40mcg/kg. **5-10 yrs:** 20-35mcg/kg. **>10 yrs:** 10-15mcg/kg. **Maint: Premature Infants:** 20-30% of PO digitalizing dose/day. **Full-Term Infants to >10 yrs:** 25-35% of PO digitalizing dose. (Ped Inj) **IV Digitalizing Dose: Premature Infants:** 15-25mcg/kg. **Full-Term Infants:** 20-30mcg/kg. **1-24 months:** 30-50mcg/kg.	**W/P:** May cause severe sinus bradycardia or sinoatrial block with preexisting sinus node disease. May cause advanced or complete heart block with preexisting incomplete AV block. May cause very rapid ventricular response or ventricular fibrillation. Caution with thyroid disorders, AMI, hypermetabolic states, restrictive cardiomyopathy, constrictive pericarditis, amyloid heart disease, elderly, acute cor pulmonale, and idiopathic hypertrophic subaortic stenosis. Caution with renal dysfunction; high risk for toxicity. Caution with hypokalemia, hypomagnesemia, or hypercalcemia; toxicity may occur. Hypocalcemia can nullify effects of digoxin. Monitor electrolytes and renal function periodically. Risk of ventricular arrhythmia with electrical cardioversion. Bioavailability is different between dosage forms. **Contra:** Ventricular fibrillation, digitalis hypersensitivity. **P/N:** Category C, caution in nursing.	Heart block, rhythm disturbances, anorexia, N/V, diarrhea, visual disturbances, headache, weakness, dizziness, mental disturbances.

Table 14.1. PRESCRIBING INFORMATION FOR CARDIOVASCULAR DRUGS *(cont.)*

NAME	FORM/ STRENGTH	DOSAGE	WARNINGS/PRECAUTIONS & CONTRAINDICATIONS	ADVERSE EFFECTS†
ANTIHYPERTENSIVES/HEART FAILURE AGENTS *(cont.)*				
CARDIAC GLYCOSIDES *(cont.)*				
Digoxin (Digitek, Lanoxicaps, Lanoxin) *(cont.)*		**2-5 yrs:** 25-35mcg/kg. **5-10 yrs:** 15-30mcg/kg. **>10 yrs:** 8-12mcg/kg. **Maint: Premature Infants:** 20-30% of IV digitalizing dose. Full-Term Infants to **>10 yrs:** 25-35% of IV digitalizing dose/day. (Cap) **Oral Digitalizing Dose: 2-5 yrs:** 25-35mcg/kg. **5-10 yrs:** 15-30mcg/kg. **>10 yrs:** 8-12mcg/kg. **Maint: ≥2 yrs:** 25-25% of PO or IV digitalizing dose. (Tab) **Maint: 2-5 yrs:** 10-15mcg/kg. **5-10 yrs:** 7-10mcg/kg. **>10 yrs:** 3-5mcg/kg. **A-Fib:** Titrate to minimum effective dose for desired response.		
DIURETIC, INDOLINE				
Indapamide	**Tab:** 1.25mg, 2.5mg	***Adults:*** **HTN:** 1.25mg qam. **Titrate:** May increase to 2.5mg qd after 4 weeks, then to 5mg qd after another 4 weeks. **Max:** 5mg/day. **CHF:** 2.5mg qam. **Titrate:** May increase to 5mg qd after 1 week. **Max:** 5mg/day.	**W/P:** Caution in severe renal disease, liver dysfunction. May exacerbate or activate SLE. Monitor for fluid/electrolyte imbalance. Hyperuricemia, hypercalcemia, hypokalemia, hypophosphatemia, and hyperglycemia may occur. Monitor renal function, serum uric acid levels periodically. May precipitate gout. May manifest latent DM. Enhanced effects in postsympathectomy patient. **Contra:** Anuria, sulfonamide hypersensitivity. **P/N:** Category B, not for use in nursing.	Headache, infection, pain, back pain, dizziness, rhinitis, fatigue, muscle cramps, nervousness, numbness of extremities, electrolyte imbalance, anxiety, agitation.
DIURETICS, K^+-SPARING				
Amiloride HCl	**Tab:** 5mg	***Adults:*** **Initial:** 5mg qd. **Titrate:** Increase to 10mg/day. If hyperkalemia persists, may increase to 15mg/day then to 20mg/day with careful monitoring. Take with food.	**W/P:** Risk of hyperkalemia (>5.5mEq/L) especially with renal impairment, elderly, DM; monitor levels frequently. D/C if hyperkalemia occurs. Caution in severely ill in whom respiratory or metabolic acidosis may occur; monitor acid-base balance frequently. Hepatic encephalopathy reported with severe hepatic disease. Increased BUN reported. D/C at least 3 days before glucose tolerance test. Monitor electrolytes and renal function in DM. **Contra:** Hyperkalemia, anuria, acute or chronic renal insufficiency, diabetic neuropathy, K^+-sparing agents (eg, diuretics), and K^+ supplements, K^+-salt substitutes, K^+-rich diet (except with severe hypokalemia). **P/N:** Category B, not for use in nursing.	Headache, N/V, anorexia, elevated serum potassium, diarrhea, muscle cramps, impotence.
Eplerenone (Inspra)	**Tab:** 25mg, 50mg	***Adults:*** **CHF Post-MI: Initial:** 25mg qd. **Titrate:** To 50mg qd within 4 weeks. **Maint:** 50mg qd. Adjust dose based on K^+ level (see PI). **HTN: Initial:** 50mg qd. May increase to 50mg bid if inadequate effect on BP. **Max:** 100mg/day. **With Weak CYP3A4 Inhibitors: Initial:** 25mg qd.	**W/P:** Risk of hyperkalemia (>5.5mEq/L); monitor periodically. With CHF post-MI use caution with SCr >2mg/dL (males) or >1.8mg/dL (females), CrCl ≤50mL/min, and in diabetics (also with proteinuria). **Contra: All:** Serum K^+ >5.5mgEq/L at initiation, CrCl ≤30mL/min, with potent CYP3A4 inhibitors (eg, ketoconazole, itraconazole, nefazodone, troleandomycin, clarithromycin, ritonavir, nelfinavir). **When treating HTN:** Type 2 diabetes with microalbuminuria, SCr >2mg/dL (males) or >1.8mg/dL (females), CrCl <50mg/min, with K^+ supplements or K^+-sparing diuretics (eg, amiloride, spironolactone, triamterene). **P/N:** Category B, not for use in nursing.	Headache, dizziness, hyperkalemia, increased SCr/triglycerides/GGT, angina/MI.

*Scored. †Bold entries denote special dental considerations.
BB = black box warning; **W/P** = warnings/precautions; **Contra** = contraindications; **P/N** = pregnancy category rating and nursing considerations.

NAME	FORM/ STRENGTH	DOSAGE	WARNINGS/PRECAUTIONS & CONTRAINDICATIONS	ADVERSE EFFECTS†
Spironolactone (Aldactone)	**Tab:** 25mg, 50mg*, 100mg*	***Adults:*** **Hyperaldosteronism: Diagnostic:** 400mg/day for 3-4 weeks or 400mg/day for 4 days. **Preoperative:** 100-400mg/day. **Maint:** Lowest effective dose. **Edema: Initial:** 100mg/day given qd or in divided doses for at least 5 days. **Maint:** 25-200mg/day given qd-bid. **HTN: Initial:** 50-100mg/day given qd or in divided doses. **Titrate:** Adjust at 2-week intervals. **Hypokalemia:** 25-100mg/day.	**BB:** Tumorigenic in chronic toxicity animal studies; avoid unnecessary use. **W/P:** Monitor for fluid/electrolyte imbalance. Caution with renal and hepatic dysfunction. Hyperchloremic metabolic acidosis reported with decompensated hepatic cirrhosis. Mild acidosis, gynecomastia, transient BUN elevation may occur. D/C and monitor ECG if hyperkalemia occurs. Risk of dilutional hyponatremia. **Contra:** Anuria, acute renal insufficiency, significantly impaired renal excretory function, hyperkalemia. **P/N:** Category C, not for use in nursing.	Gastric bleeding, ulceration, gynecomastia, impotence, agranulocytosis, fever, urticaria, confusion, ataxia, renal dysfunction, irregular menses, amenorrhea.
Triamterene (Dyrenium)	**Cap:** 50mg, 100mg	***Adults:*** **Initial:** 100mg bid pc. **Max:** 300mg/day.	**BB:** Abnormal elevation of serum K^+ levels (≥5.5mEq/L) can occur with all K^+-sparing agents, including triamterene. Hyperkalemia is more likely to occur with renal impairment and diabetes (even without evidence of renal impairment), and in the elderly, or severely ill. Monitor serum K^+ at frequent intervals. **W/P:** Check ECG if hyperkalemia occurs. May cause decreased alkali reserve with possibility of metabolic acidosis, mild nitrogen retention. Monitor BUN periodically. May contribute to megaloblastosis in folic acid deficiency. Caution with gouty arthritis; may elevate uric acid levels. May aggravate or cause electrolyte imbalances in CHF, renal disease, or cirrhosis. Caution with history of renal stones. **Contra:** Anuria, severe or progressive kidney disease or dysfunction (except with nephrosis), severe hepatic disease, hyperkalemia, K^+ supplements, K^+-salt substitutes, K^+-sparing agents (eg, diuretics). **P/N:** Category C, not for use in nursing.	Hypersensitivity reactions, hyper- or hypokalemia, azotemia, renal stones, jaundice, N/V, diarrhea, weakness, dizziness.
DIURETICS, K^+-SPARING/DIURETICS, THIAZIDE				
Amiloride HCl/Hydrochlorothiazide	**Tab:** (Amiloride-HCTZ) 5mg-50mg* *scored	***Adults:*** **Initial:** 1 tab qd. **Titrate:** May increase to 2 tabs qd or in divided doses. **Max:** 2 tabs/day. May give intermittently once diuresis is achieved. Take with food.	**W/P:** Risk of hyperkalemia (≥5.5mEq/L), especially with renal impairment or DM; d/c if hyperkalemia occurs. Monitor for fluid/electrolyte imbalance; hyponatremia and hypochloremia may occur. Caution in severely ill (risk of respiratory or metabolic acidosis). Increases BUN, cholesterol, and TG levels. D/C at least 3 days before glucose tolerance test. May precipitate gout or exacerbate SLE. May precipitate azotemia with renal disease. **Contra:** Hyperkalemia, anuria, sulfonamide hypersensitivity, acute or chronic renal insufficiency, diabetic neuropathy. Concomitant K^+-sparing agents (eg, spironolactone, triamterene), K^+ supplements, salt substitutes, K^+-rich diet (except with severe hypokalemia). **P/N:** Category B, not for use in nursing.	Nausea, anorexia, rash, headache, weakness, hyperkalemia, dizziness.
Spironolactone/ Hydrochlorothiazide (Aldactazide)	**Tab:** (Spironolactone-HCTZ) 25mg-25mg, 50mg-50mg*	***Adults:*** **Edema:** 100mg/day per component qd or in divided doses. **Maint:** 25-200mg/day per component. **HTN:** 50-100mg/day per component qd or in divided doses.	**BB:** Tumorigenic in chronic toxicity animal studies; avoid unnecessary use. Not for initial therapy. **W/P:** Monitor for fluid/electrolyte imbalance. Caution with renal and hepatic dysfunction. Hyperchloremic metabolic acidosis reported with decompensated hepatic cirrhosis. Mild acidosis, gynecomastia, transient	Gastric bleeding, ulceration, gynecomastia, impotence, agranulocytosis, fever, urticaria, confusion, ataxia, renal dysfunction, blood dyscrasias,

Table 14.1. PRESCRIBING INFORMATION FOR CARDIOVASCULAR DRUGS *(cont.)*

NAME	FORM/ STRENGTH	DOSAGE	WARNINGS/PRECAUTIONS & CONTRAINDICATIONS	ADVERSE EFFECTS†
ANTIHYPERTENSIVES/HEART FAILURE AGENTS *(cont.)*				
DIURETICS, K⁺-SPARING/DIURETICS, THIAZIDE *(cont.)*				
Spironolactone/ Hydrochlorothiazide (Aldactazide) *(cont.)*			BUN elevation, hypercalcemia, hyperglycemia, hyperuricemia, hypomagnesemia, and sensitivity reactions may occur. D/C if hyperkalemia occurs. Risk of dilutional hyponatremia. Enhanced effects in postsympathetectomy patient. May increase cholesterol and TG levels. May manifest latent DM. **Contra:** Acute renal impairment, significantly impaired renal excretory function, hyperkalemia, acute or severe hepatic dysfunction, anuria, sulfonamide hypersensitivity. **P/N:** Category C, not for use in nursing	electrolyte disturbances, weakness, irregular menses, amenorrhea.
Triamterene/ Hydrochlorothiazide (Dyazide, Maxzide, Maxzide-25)	(Triamterene HCTZ) **Cap:** (Dyazide) 37.5mg-25mg **Tab:** (Maxzide) 75mg-50mg*, (Maxzide-25) 37.5mg-25mg*	***Adults:*** (37.5mg-25mg) 1-2 caps/tabs qd. (75mg-50mg) 1 tab qd.	**W/P:** Risk of hyperkalemia (≥5.5mEq/L) especially with renal impairment, elderly, DM or severely ill; monitor levels frequently. Check ECG if hyperkalemia occurs. Caution with history of renal lithiasis, hepatic dysfunction. Monitor BUN and creatinine periodically. D/C if azotemia increases. May contribute to megaloblastosis in folic acid deficiency. Hyperuricemia, hypercalcemia, hypophosphatemia, hypokalemia may occur. May manifest latent DM. May decrease serum PBI levels. Monitor for fluid/electrolyte imbalance. **Contra:** Hyperkalemia, anuria, acute or chronic renal insufficiency, sulfonamide hypersensitivity, diabetic neuropathy, K^+-sparing agents (eg, diuretics), K^+ supplements (except with severe hypokalemia), K^+-salt substitutes, K^+-rich diet. **P/N:** Category C, not for use in nursing.	Muscle cramps, GI effects, arrhythmia, impotence, paresthesia, renal stones, hypersensitivity reactions, weakness, jaundice, pancreatitis, N/V, taste alteration, drowsiness, dry mouth, depression, anxiety, tachycardia, blood dyscrasias, electrolyte disturbances.
DIURETICS, LOOP				
Bumetanide (Bumex)	**Inj:** 0.25mg/mL; **Tab:** 0.5mg*, 1mg*, 2mg*	***Adults:*** **≥18 yrs: PO: Usual:** 0.5-2mg qd. **Maint:** May give every other day or every 3-4 days. **Max:** 10mg/day. **IV/ IM: Initial:** 0.5-1mg over 1-2 min, may repeat every 2-3 hrs for 2-3 doses. **Max:** 10mg/day. **Elderly:** Start at low end of dosing range.	**BB:** Can lead to profound water and electrolyte depletion with excessive use. **W/P:** Monitor for volume/electrolyte depletion, hypokalemia, blood dyscrasias, hepatic damage. Elderly are prone to volume/electrolyte depletion. Caution in elderly, hepatic cirrhosis and ascites. Associated with ototoxicity, hypocalcemia, thrombocytopenia, hypomagnesemia, hypokalemia, and hyperuricemia. Hypersensitivity with sulfonamide allergy. D/C if marked increase in BUN or creatinine or if develop oliguria with progressive renal disease. **Contra:** Anuria, hepatic coma, severe electrolyte depletion. **P/N:** Category C, not for use in nursing.	Muscle cramps, dizziness, hypotension, headache, nausea, hyperuricemia, hypokalemia, hyponatremia, hyperglycemia, azotemia, increase serum creatinine.
Ethacrynate Sodium, Ethacrynic Acid (Edecrin)	**Inj:** (Ethacrynate Sodium) 50mg **Tab:** (Ethacrynic Acid) 25mg*	***Adults:*** (Inj) 50mg or 0.5-1mg/kg IV single dose. May give 2nd dose if necessary. **(Tab) Initial:** 50-100mg qd. **Titrate:** 25-50mg increments. **Usual:** 50-200mg/day. After diuresis achieved, give smallest effective dose continuously or intermittently. ***Pediatrics:*** **Initial:** 25mg. **Titrate:** Increase by 25mg increments. **Maint:** Reduce dose and frequency once dry wt achieved; may give intermittently.	**W/P:** Caution in advanced liver cirrhosis. Monitor serum electrolytes, CO^2, BUN early in therapy and periodically during active diuresis. Vigorous diuresis may induce acute hypotensive episode and in elderly cardiac patients, hemoconcentration resulting in thromboembolic disorders. Ototoxicity reported with severe renal dysfunction. Hypomagnesemia and transient increase in serum urea nitrogen may occur. Reduce dose or	Anorexia, malaise, abdominal discomfort, gout, deafness, tinnitus, vertigo, headache, fatigue, rash, chills.

*Scored. †Bold entries denote special dental considerations.
BB = black box warning; **W/P** = warnings/precautions; **Contra** = contraindications; **P/N** = pregnancy category rating and nursing considerations.

NAME	FORM/ STRENGTH	DOSAGE	WARNINGS/PRECAUTIONS & CONTRAINDICATIONS	ADVERSE EFFECTS†
Ethacrynate Sodium, Ethacrynic Acid (Edecrin) *(cont.)*			withdraw if excessive electrolyte loss occurs. Initiate therapy in the hospital for cirrhotic patients with ascites. Liberalize salt intake and supplement with K^+ if needed. Reduced responsiveness in renal edema with hypoproteinemia; use salt-poor albumin. **Contra:** Anuria, infants. D/C if increasing electrolyte imbalance, azotemia, or oliguria develops during treatment of severe, progressive renal disease. D/C if severe, watery diarrhea occurs. **P/N:** Category B, not for use in nursing.	
Furosemide (Lasix)	**Inj:** 10mg/mL; **Sol:** 10mg/mL, 40mg/5mL; **Tab:** 20mg, 40mg*, 80mg	***Adults:*** (PO) **HTN: Initial:** 40mg bid. **Edema: Initial:** 20-80mg PO. May repeat or increase by 20-40mg after 6-8 hrs. **Max:** 600mg/day. **Alternative Regimen:** Dose on 2-4 consecutive days each week. Closely monitor if on >80mg/day. (Inj) **Edema: Initial:** 20-40mg IV/IM. May repeat or increase by 20mg after 2 hrs. **Acute Pulmonary Edema: Initial:** 40mg IV. May increase to 80mg IV after 1 hr. ***Pediatrics:*** **Edema:** (PO) **Initial:** 2mg/kg single dose. May increase by 1-2mg/kg after 6-8 hrs. **Max:** 6mg/kg. (Inj) **Initial:** 1mg/kg IV/IM single dose. May increase by 1mg/kg IV/IM after 2 hrs. **Max:** 6mg/kg.	**BB:** Can lead to profound water and electrolyte depletion with excessive use. **W/P:** Monitor for fluid/electrolyte imbalance (eg, hypokalemia), renal or hepatic dysfunction. Initiate in hospital with hepatic cirrhosis and ascites. Tinnitus, hearing impairment, hyperglycemia, hyperuricemia reported. May activate SLE. Cross-sensitivity with sulfonamide allergy. Avoid excessive diuresis, especially in elderly. **Contra:** Anuria. **P/N:** Category C, caution in nursing.	Pancreatitis, jaundice, anorexia, paresthesias, ototoxicity, blood dyscrasias, dizziness, rash, urticaria, photosensitivity, fever, thrombophlebitis, restlessness.
Torsemide (Demadex)	**Inj:** 10mg/mL; **Tab:** 5mg*, 10mg*, 20mg*, 100mg*	***Adults:*** PO/IV (bolus over 2 min or continuous): **CHF: Initial:** 10-20mg qd. **Max:** 200mg single dose. **Chronic Renal Failure: Initial:** 20mg qd. **Max:** 200mg single dose. **Hepatic Cirrhosis: Initial:** 5-10mg qd with aldosterone antagonist or K^+-sparing diuretic. **Titrate:** Double dose. **Max:** 40mg single dose. **HTN: Initial:** 5mg qd. **Titrate:** May increase to 10mg qd in 4-6 weeks, then may add additional antihypertensive agent.	**W/P:** Caution with cirrhosis and ascites in hepatic disease. Tinnitus and hearing loss (usually reversible) reported. Avoid excessive diuresis, especially in elderly. Caution with brisk diuresis, inadequate oral intake of electrolytes, and cardiovascular disease, especially with digitalis glycosides. Monitor for electrolyte/volume depletion. Hyperglycemia, hypokalemia, hypermagnesemia, hypercalcemia, gout reported. May increase cholesterol and TG. **Contra:** Anuria, sulfonamide hypersensitivity. **P/N:** Category B, caution in nursing.	Headache, excessive urination, dizziness, cough, ECG abnormality, asthenia, rhinitis, diarrhea.
DIURETICS, MONOSULFAMYL				
Chlorthalidone (Thalitone)	**Tab:** 15mg	***Adults:*** **HTN: Initial:** 15mg qd. **Titrate:** May increase to 30mg qd, then to 45-50mg qd. **Edema: Initial:** 30-60mg/day or 60mg every other day, up to 90-120mg/day. **Maint:** May be lower than initial; adjust to patient. Take in the morning with food.	**W/P:** Caution in severe renal disease, liver dysfunction, allergy history, asthma. May exacerbate or activate SLE. Monitor for fluid and electrolyte imbalance. Hyperuricemia, hypomagnesemia, hypokalemia, hypercalcemia, hypophosphatemia, and hyperglycemia may occur. May manifest latent DM. **Contra:** Anuria, sulfonamide hypersensitivity. **P/N:** Category B, not for use in nursing.	Pancreatitis, jaundice, diarrhea, N/V, constipation, blood dyscrasias, rash, photosensitivity, dizziness, headache, electrolyte disturbance, impotence.
DIURETICS, QUINAZOLINE				
Metolazone (Zaroxolyn)	**Tab:** 2.5mg, 5mg, 10mg	***Adults:*** **Edema:** 5-20mg qd. **HTN:** 2.5-5mg qd. **Elderly:** Start at low end of dosing range.	**BB:** Do not interchange rapid and complete bioavailability metolazone formulations for other slow and incomplete bioavailability metolazone formulations; they are not therapeutically equivalent. **W/P:** Risk of hypokalemia, orthostatic hypotension, hypercalcemia, hyperuricemia, azotemia and rapid onset hyponatremia. Cross-allergy with	Chest pain/discomfort, orthostatic hypotension, syncope, neuropathy, necrotizing angiitis, hepatitis, jaundice, pancreatitis, blood dyscrasias, joint pain.

Table 14.1. PRESCRIBING INFORMATION FOR CARDIOVASCULAR DRUGS *(cont.)*

NAME	FORM/ STRENGTH	DOSAGE	WARNINGS/PRECAUTIONS & CONTRAINDICATIONS	ADVERSE EFFECTS†
ANTIHYPERTENSIVES/HEART FAILURE AGENTS *(cont.)*				
DIURETICS, QUINAZOLINE *(cont.)*				
Metolazone (Zaroxolyn) *(cont.)*			sulfonamide-derived drugs, thiazides, or quinethazone. Sensitivity reactions may occur with first dose. Monitor electrolytes. May cause hyperglycemia and glycosuria in diabetics. Caution in elderly or severe renal impairment. May exacerbate or activate SLE. **Contra:** Anuria, hepatic coma or precoma. **P/N:** Category B, not for use in nursing	
DIURETICS, THIAZIDE				
Chlorothiazide (Diuril, Intravenous Sodium Diuril)	**Inj:** 0.5g; **Sus:** 250mg/ 5mL [237mL]	***Adults:*** (PO/IV) **Edema:** 0.5-1g qd-bid. May give every other day or 3-5 days/ week. Substitute IV for oral using same dosage. (PO) **HTN:** 0.5-1g qd or in divided doses. **Max:** 2g/day. ***Pediatrics:*** (PO) **Diuresis/HTN: Usual:** 10-20mg/ kg/day given qd-bid. **Max: <6 months:** Up to 15mg/kg bid may be required. **Infants up to 2 yrs:** 375mg/day. **2-12 yrs:** 1g/day.	**W/P:** Caution in severe renal disease, liver dysfunction, electrolyte/fluid imbalance. Monitor electrolytes. Hyperuricemia, hyperglycemia, hypokalemia, hyponatremia, hypomagnesemia, hypercalcemia may occur. Increases in cholesterol and triglyceride levels reported. May exacerbate SLE. Sensitivity reactions reported. D/C prior to parathyroid test. Enhanced effects in postsympathectomy patient. IV use not recommended in infants or children. **Contra:** Anuria, sulfonamide hypersensitivity. **P/N:** Category C, not for use in nursing.	Weakness, hypotension, pancreatitis, jaundice, diarrhea, vomiting, blood dyscrasias, rash, photosensitivity, electrolyte imbalance, impotence
Hydro-chlorothiazide (Microzide)	**Cap:** (Microzide) 12.5mg **Tab:** 12.5mg, 25mg*, 50mg*	***Adults:*** (Cap) **Initial:** 12.5mg qd. **Max:** 50mg/day. (Tab) **Edema:** 25-100mg qd or in divided doses. May give every other day or 3-5 days/week. **HTN: Initial:** 25mg qd. **Titrate:** May increase to 50mg/day. ***Pediatrics:*** **Diuresis/HTN:** 1-2mg/kg/day given qd-bid. **Max: <6 months:** Up to 1.5mg/kg bid may be required. **Infants up to 2 yrs:** 37.5mg/ day. **2-12 yrs:** 100mg/day.	**W/P:** Caution in severe renal disease, liver dysfunction, electrolyte/fluid imbalance. Monitor electrolytes. Hyperuricemia, hyperglycemia, hypokalemia, hyponatremia, hypomagnesemia, hypercalcemia may occur. Increases in cholesterol and triglyceride levels reported. May exacerbate SLE. Sensitivity reactions reported. D/C prior to parathyroid test. Enhanced effects in postsympathectomy patients. **Contra:** Anuria, sulfonamide hypersensitivity. **P/N:** Category B, not for use in nursing.	Weakness, hypotension, pancreatitis, jaundice, diarrhea, vomiting, blood dyscrasias, rash, photosensitivity, electrolyte imbalance, impotence.
Methyclothiazide (Enduron)	**Tab:** 5mg*	***Adults:*** **Edema:** 2.5-10mg qd. **Max:** 10mg/dose. **HTN:** 2.5-5mg qd.	**W/P:** Caution in severe renal disease, liver dysfunction, electrolyte/fluid imbalance. Monitor electrolytes. Hyperuricemia, hyperglycemia, hypokalemia, hyponatremia, hypomagnesemia, hypercalcemia may occur. Increases in cholesterol and triglyceride levels reported. May exacerbate SLE. Sensitivity reactions reported. D/C prior to parathyroid test. Enhanced effects in postsympathectomy patient. **Contra:** Anuria, sulfonamide hypersensitivity. **P/N:** Category B, not for use in nursing.	Headache, cramping, weakness, orthostatic hypotension, pancreatitis, hyperglycemia, hyperuricemia, electrolyte imbalance, blood dyscrasias, hypersensitivity reactions.
GANGLIONIC BLOCKER				
Mecamylamine HCl (Inversine)	**Tab:** 2.5mg	***Adults:*** **Initial:** 2.5mg bid after meals. **Titrate:** Increase by 2.5mg/day at intervals of not less than 2 days. **Usual:** 25mg/day given tid. Give larger doses at noontime and evening. Reduce dose by 50% with thiazides.	**W/P:** Caution with renal, cerebral, or cardiovascular dysfunction, marked cerebral or coronary insufficiency, prostatic hypertrophy, bladder neck obstruction, urethral stricture. Large doses in cerebral or renal insufficiency may produce CNS effects. Withdraw gradually and add other antihypertensives. May be potentiated by excessive heat, fever, infection, hemorrhage,	Ileus, constipation, N/V, anorexia, **dryness of mouth,** syncope, postural hypotension, convulsions, tremor, interstitial pulmonary edema, urinary retention, impotence, blurred vision.

†Bold entries denote special dental considerations.
BB = black box warning; **W/P** = warnings/precautions; **Contra** = contraindications; **P/N** = pregnancy category rating and nursing considerations.

NAME	FORM/ STRENGTH	DOSAGE	WARNINGS/PRECAUTIONS & CONTRAINDICATIONS	ADVERSE EFFECTS†
Mecamylamine HCl (Inversine) *(cont.)*			pregnancy, anesthesia, surgery, vigorous exercise, other antihypertensive drugs, alcohol, salt depletion. D/C if paralytic ileus occurs. **Contra:** Coronary insufficiency, recent MI, uremia, glaucoma, organic pyloric stenosis, uncooperative patients, mild to moderate or labile HTN, with antibiotics or sulfonamides. Administer with great discretion in renal insufficiency. **P/N:** Category C, not for use in nursing.	
PHOSPHODIESTERASE 5 INHIBITORS				
Sildenafil Citrate (Revatio, Viagra)	**Tab:** (Revatio) 20mg; (Viagra) 25mg, 50mg, 100mg.	***Adults:*** **(Revatio) Pulmonary Arterial HTN:** 20mg tid 4-6 hours apart. **(Viagra) Usual:** 50mg 1 hr (range 0.5-4 hrs) prior to sexual activity at frequency of up to once daily. **Titrate:** May decrease to 25mg qd or increase to 100mg qd. **Max:** 100mg qd. **Elderly/ Hepatic Impairment/CrCl <30mL/min/ Concomitant CYP450 3A4 Inhibitors (eg, ketoconazole, itraconazole, erythromycin, saquinavir): Initial:** 25mg qd. **Concomitant Ritonavir: Max:** 25mg q48h. **Concomitant α-blocker:** Avoid doses >25mg sildenafil within 4 hours of an α-blocker.	**W/P:** Caution with MI, stroke, or life-threatening arrhythmia within last 6 months; with resting hypotension (BP <90/50mmHg), fluid depletion, severe left ventricular outflow obstruction, autonomic dysfunction, or HTN (BP >170/110mmHg); unstable angina due to cardiac failure or CAD; anatomical penile deformation; predisposition to priapism; and retinitis pigmentosa. Avoid in patients with veno-occlusive disease. Decrease in supine BP reported. Rare reports of non-arteritic anterior ischemic optic neuropathy (NAION) with PDE5 inhibitors. Patients may experience a sudden decrease or loss of hearing while PDE5 inhibitors. If erection persists >4 hrs, seek immediate medical assistance; penile tissue damage and permanent loss of potency could result if priapism not treated immediately. (Viagra) Avoid in men where sexual activity is inadvisable due to underlying CV status. **Contra:** Organic nitrates taken regularly and/or intermittently. **P/N:** Category B, caution in nursing.	Epistaxis, headache, flushing, dyspepsia, insomnia, erythema, dyspnea, rhinitis, diarrhea, myalgia, pyrexia, gastritis, sinusitis, paresthesia.
Tadalafil (Cialis)	**Tab:** 2.5mg, 5mg, 10mg, 20mg	***Adults:*** **Prn Use:** Take prior to sexual activity. **Initial:** 10mg. **Range:** 5-20mg. **Renal Impairment: CrCl 31-50mL/ min: Initial:** 5mg. **Max:** 10mg/48 hrs. **CrCl <30mL/min/Hemodialysis: Max:** 5mg/72 hrs. **Mild/Moderate Hepatic Impairment: Max:** 10mg. **Severe Hepatic Impairment:** Avoid use. **With Potent CYP3A4 Inhibitors (eg, ketoconazole, itraconazole, ritonavir): Max:** 10mg/72 hrs. **Once-Daily Use: Initial:** 2.5mg qd without regard to timing of sexual activity. **Titrate:** May increase to 5mg qd based on efficacy and tolerability. **CrCl <30mL/ min/Hemodialysis/Severe Hepatic Impairment:** Avoid use. **Mild/Moderate Hepatic Impairment:** Use with caution. **With Potent CYP3A4 Inhibitors (eg, ketoconazole, itraconazole, ritonavir): Max:** 2.5mg. Take with or without food.	**W/P:** Increased sensitivity to vasodilatory effect with left ventricular outflow obstruction. Avoid with MI (within last 90 days); unstable angina or angina occurring during sexual intercourse; NYHA Class 2 or greater heart failure (in the last 6 months); uncontrolled arrhythmias, hypotension (<90/50mmHg); or uncontrolled HTN (>170/100mmHg); stroke within the last 6 months; severe hepatic impairment (Child-Pugh Class C); degenerative retinal disorders, including retinitis pigmentosa. Prolonged erection reported. Substantial consumption of alcohol with tadalafil can increase HR, decrease BP, cause dizziness and headache. Caution with predisposition to priapism (eg, sickle cell anemia, multiple myeloma, leukemia), anatomical deformation of the penis, bleeding disorders, or active peptic ulceration. May cause transient decrease in BP. Caution with coadministration of PDE5 inhibitors and β-blockers. May cause additive hypotensive effect. Initiate at lowest dose once patient is stable on either therapy. Rare reports of nonarteritic anterior ischemic optic neuropathy (NAION) with PDE5 inhibitors. Sudden decrease or loss of	Headache, dyspepsia, back pain, myalgia, nasal congestion, flushing, limb pain, urticaria, Stevens-Johnson syndrome, exfoliative dermatitis, migraine, visual field defect, retinal vein occlusion, retinal artery occlusion, sudden decrease or loss of hearing, tinnitus.

Table 14.1. PRESCRIBING INFORMATION FOR CARDIOVASCULAR DRUGS *(cont.)*

NAME	FORM/ STRENGTH	DOSAGE	WARNINGS/PRECAUTIONS & CONTRAINDICATIONS	ADVERSE EFFECTS†
ANTIHYPERTENSIVES/HEART FAILURE AGENTS *(cont.)*				
PHOSPHODIESTERASE 5 INHIBITORS *(cont.)*				
Tadalafil (Cialis) *(cont.)*			hearing, tinnitus, and dizziness reported. D/C if experienced these symptoms. **Contra:** Organic nitrates taken regularly and/or intermittently. **P/N:** Category B, not for use in women	
Vardenafil HCl (Levitra)	**Tab:** 2.5mg, 5mg, 10mg, 20mg	***Adults:*** **Initial:** 10mg one hour prior to sexual activity at frequency of up to once daily. **Titrate:** May decrease to 5mg or increase to max of 20mg based on response. **Elderly: ≥65 yrs: Initial:** 5mg. **Moderate Hepatic Impairment: Initial:** 5mg; **Max:** 10mg. **Concomitant Ritonavir: Max:** 2.5mg/72 hrs. **Concomitant Indinavir/Saquinavir/ Atazanavir/Clarithromycin/Ketoconazole 400mg daily/Itraconazole 400mg daily: Max:** 2.5mg/24 hrs. **Concomitant Ketoconazole 200mg daily/Itraconazole 200mg daily/Erythromycin: Max:** 5mg/24 hrs.	**W/P:** Avoid when sexual activity is inadvisable due to underlying CV status. Increased sensitivity to vasodilation effects with left ventricular outflow obstruction. Decrease in supine BP reported. Avoid with unstable angina, hypotension (SBP<90 mmHg), uncontrolled HTN (>170/100 mmHg), recent history of stroke, life-threatening arrhythmia, MI (within last 6 months), severe cardiac failure, severe hepatic impairment (Child-Pugh C), end-stage renal disease requiring dialysis, hereditary degenerative retinal disorders including retinitis pigmentosa, congenital QT prolongation. Caution with bleeding disorders, peptic ulcers, anatomical deformation of the penis, or predisposition to priapism. Rare reports of non-arteritic anterior ischemic optic neuropathy (NAION) with PDE5 inhibitors. Sudden decrease or loss of hearing accompanied by tinnitus and dizziness reported. **Contra:** Organic nitrates taken regularly and/or intermittently. **P/N:** Category B, not for use in women	Headache, flushing, rhinitis, dyspepsia, sinusitis, flu syndrome, sudden decrease or loss of hearing, tinnitus.
RAUWOLFIA ALKALOID				
Reserpine	**Tab:** 0.1mg, 0.25mg	***Adults:*** **HTN: Initial:** 0.5mg/day for 1-2 weeks. **Maint:** reduce to 0.1-0.25mg/ day. **Psychotic Disorders: Initial:** 0.5mg/day. **Range:** 0.1-1mg/day.	**W/P:** Caution with renal insufficiency. May cause depression; d/c at first sign. Caution with history of peptic ulcer, ulcerative colitis, or gallstones. **Contra:** Active or history of mental depression, active peptic ulcer, ulcerative colitis, current electroconvulsive therapy. **P/N:** Category C, not for use in nursing.	GI effects, **dry mouth,** hypersecretion, arrhythmia, syncope, edema, dyspnea, muscle aches, dizziness, depression, nervousness, impotence, gynecomastia, rash.
RENIN INHIBITOR				
Aliskiren (Tekturna)	**Tab:** 150mg, 300mg	***Adults:*** **Usual:** 150mg qd. **Titrate:** May increase to 300mg/day if needed. High-fat meals decrease absorption.	**BB:** When used in pregnancy, drugs that act directly on the renin-angiotensin system can cause injury and even death to the developing fetus. D/C therapy when pregnancy is detected. **W/P:** Caution with greater than moderate renal dysfunction (SCr >1.7mg/dL (women) or >2mg/dL (men) and/or GFR <30mL/ min), history of dialysis, nephrotic syndrome, or renovascular hypertension. May increase serum K^+, especially when used in combination with ACE inhibitors in diabetics. Angioedema of face, extremities, lips, tongue, glottis, and/or larynx reported; d/c and monitor until complete resolution of signs and symptoms. Hypotension rarely seen. **P/N:** Category C (1st trimester) and D (2nd and 3rd trimesters); not for use in nursing.	Diarrhea, headache, nasopharyngitis, dizziness, fatigue, upper respiratory tract infection, back pain, cough.

*Scored. †Bold entries denote special dental considerations.
BB = black box warning; **W/P** = warnings/precautions; **Contra** = contraindications; **P/N** = pregnancy category rating and nursing considerations.

NAME	FORM/ STRENGTH	DOSAGE	WARNINGS/PRECAUTIONS & CONTRAINDICATIONS	ADVERSE EFFECTS†
RENIN INHIBITORS/DIURETIC				
Aliskiren/ Hydrochlor-othiazide (Tekturna HCT)	**Tab:** (Aliskiren-HCTZ) 150mg-12.5mg, 150mg-25mg, 300mg-12.5mg, 300mg-25mg	***Adults:*** **Initial: Not Controlled on Monotherapy:** 150mg-12.5mg qd. **Titrate:** May increase to 150mg-25mg, 300mg-12.5mg qd if uncontrolled after 2-4 weeks. **Max:** 300mg-25mg. Avoid with CrCl ≤30mL/min.	**BB:** Drugs that act directly on the renin-angiotensin system can cause injury and even death to the developing fetus. D/C therapy when pregnancy is detected. **W/P:** Angioedema of head and neck may occur; d/c therapy and monitor until signs and symptoms resolve. May cause symptomatic hypotension in volume- and/or salt-depleted patients; correct condition prior to therapy. Avoid with CrCl <30mL/min. Caution with hepatic impairment, or history of allergy or bronchial asthma. May exacerbate or activate SLE. Monitor serum electrolytes periodically to detect possible electrolyte imbalance. **Contra:** Anuria, sulfonamide hypersensitivity. **P/N:** Category D, not for use in nursing.	Dizziness, influenza, diarrhea, cough, vertigo, asthenia, arthralgia.
TYROSINE HYDROXYLASE INHIBITOR				
Metyrosine (Demser)	**Cap:** 250mg	***Adults:*** **Initial:** 250mg qid. **Titrate:** May increase by 250-500mg/day. **Max:** 4g/day. Titrate based on clinical symptoms and catecholamine excretion. **Usual:** 2-3g/day. **Preoperative Preparation:** Take 5-7 days before surgery. ***Pediatrics:*** **≥12 yrs: Initial:** 250mg qid. **Titrate:** May increase by 250-500mg/day. **Max:** 4g/day. Titrate based on clinical symptoms and catecholamine excretion. **Usual:** 2-3g/day. **Preoperative Preparation:** Take 5-7 days before surgery.	**W/P:** When used preoperatively or with β-adrenergic blockers, maintain intravascular volume intra- and post-operatively to avoid hypotension and decreased perfusion. Maintain adequate water intake to achieve urine volume of ≥2000mL to prevent crystalluria. Risk of hypertensive crisis or arrhythmias during tumor manipulation. Monitor BP and ECG continuously during surgery. **P/N:** Category C, caution in nursing.	Sedation, EPS, anxiety, depression, hallucinations, disorientation, confusion, diarrhea.
VASODILATORS				
Diazoxide (Hyperstat)	**Inj:** 300mg/ 20mL	***Adults:*** **Minibolus:** 1-3mg/kg IV q5-10min until a satisfactory reduction in BP (DBP <100mmHg) is achieved. **Max:** 150mg/dose. The dose should be administered in 30sec or less in recumbent patients. It is preferable that a patient remain supine for 1 hr after the injection. **Controlled HTN:** q4-24h will maintain the blood pressure below pretreatment levels until oral antihypertensive medication can be instituted. It is usually unnecessary to continue treatment for more than 4-5 days.	**W/P:** May cause a rapid reduction BP which has been observed to cause angina, MI, cerebral infarction and one case of optic nerve infarction. The desired BP lowering should be achieved over as long a period of time as is compatible with the patient's status; at least 1-2 hours and preferably 1-2 days. Hypotension may occur so it is recommended that diazoxide only be used in a setting where the proper response can be made; diazoxide induced hypotension is usually responsive to the Trendelenberg maneuver and if necessary administer sympathomimetics. Use of diazoxide may lead to a retention of sodium and water, warrenting the use of concomitant diuretics. Caution in patients in whom water/sodium retention will be problematic, those in whom abrupt reduction in BP might be detrimental or those in whom mild tachycardia or decreased blood perfusion may be deleterious, and in patients with diabetes mellitus. Do not administer IM or SC. If diazoxide leaks into the subcutaneous tissue treat with a warm compress. **Contra:** Compensatory HTN (eg HTN associated with aortic coarctation or arteriovenous shunt), hypersensitivity to sulfonamides. **P/N:** Category C, safety in nursing not known.	Hypotension, N/V, dizziness, weakness, **alteration in taste,** parotid swelling, **salivation, dry mouth.**

Table 14.1. PRESCRIBING INFORMATION FOR CARDIOVASCULAR DRUGS *(cont.)*

NAME	FORM/ STRENGTH	DOSAGE	WARNINGS/PRECAUTIONS & CONTRAINDICATIONS	ADVERSE EFFECTS†
ANTIHYPERTENSIVES/HEART FAILURE AGENTS *(cont.)*				
VASODILATORS *(cont.)*				
Hydralazine HCl	**Inj:** 20mg/mL; **Tab:** 10mg, 25mg, 50mg, 100mg	***Adults:*** **Initial:** 10mg qid for 2-4 days. **Titrate:** Increase to 25mg qid for the rest of the week, then increase to 50mg qid. **Maint:** Use lowest effective dose. **Resistant Patients:** 300mg/day or titrate to lower dose combined with thiazide diuretic and/or reserpine, or β-blocker. ***Pediatrics:*** **Initial:** 0.75mg/kg/day given qid. **Titrate:** Increase gradually over 3-4 weeks to a max of 7.5mg/kg/day or 200mg/day.	**W/P:** D/C if SLE symptoms occur. May cause angina and ECG changes of MI. Caution with suspected CAD, CVA, advanced renal impairment. May increase pulmonary artery pressure in mitral valvular disease. Postural hypotension reported. Add pyridoxine if peripheral neuritis develops. Monitor CBC and ANA titer before and periodically during therapy. **Contra:** CAD and mitral valvular rheumatic heart disease. **P/N:** Category C, safety in nursing not known.	Headache, anorexia, N/V, diarrhea, tachycardia, angina.
Minoxidil	**Tab:** 2.5mg*, 10mg*	***Adults:*** **Initial:** 5mg qd. **Titrate:** Increase by no less than 3 days; may increase every 6 hrs if closely monitored. **Usual:** 10-40mg/day. **Max:** 100mg/day. **Frequency:** Give qd if diastolic BP is reduced to <30mmHg and if reduced to >30mmHg give bid. Give with a diuretic (eg, HCTZ 50mg bid, furosemide 40mg bid) and a β-blocker (equivalent to propranolol 80-160mg/day) or methyldopa (250-750mg bid starting 24 hrs before therapy). **Renal Failure/Dialysis:** Reduce dose. ***Pediatrics:*** **>12 yrs: Initial:** 5mg qd. **Titrate:** Increase by no less than 3 days; may increase every 6 hrs if closely monitored. **Usual:** 10-40mg/day. **Max:** 100mg/day. **Frequency:** Give qd if diastolic BP is reduced to <30mmHg and if reduced to >30mmHg give bid. Give with a diuretic (eg, HCTZ 50mg bid, furosemide 40mg bid) and a β-blocker (equivalent to propranolol 80-160mg/day) or methyldopa (250-750mg bid starting 24 hrs before therapy). **<12 yrs:** 0.2mg/kg qd. **Titrate:** May increase by 50-100% increments. **Usual:** 0.25-1mg/kg/day. **Max:** 50mg/day. **Renal Failure/Dialysis:** Reduce dose.	**BB:** May cause pericardial effusion, occasionally progressing to tamponade, and angina pectoris may be exacerbated. Only for nonresponders to maximum therapeutic doses of two other antihypertensives and a diuretic. Administer under supervision with a β-blocker and diuretic. Monitor in hospital for a decrease in BP in those receiving guanethidine with malignant hypertension. **W/P:** Administer with a diuretic and β-blocker. Pericarditis, pericardial effusion and tamponade reported. With renal failure or dialysis, reduce dose to prevent renal failure exacerbation and precipitation of cardiac failure. Avoid rapid control with severe HTN. Monitor body wt, fluid and electrolyte balance. Extreme caution with post-MI. Hypersensitivity reactions reported. **Contra:** Pheochromocytoma. **P/N:** Category C, not for use in nursing.	Salt and water retention, pericarditis, pericardial effusion, tamponade, hypertrichosis, N/V, rash, ECG changes, hemodilution effects.
VASODILATOR COMBINATION				
Hydralazine HCl/ Isosorbide Dinitrate (BiDil)	**Tab:** (Hydralazine-Isosorbide) 37.5mg-20mg	***Adults:*** **Initial:** 1 tab tid. **Max:** 2 tabs tid.	**W/P:** May produce a clinical picture simulating SLE including glomerulonephritis. May cause symptomatic hypotension, tachycardia, peripheral neuritis. Caution in patients with acute MI, hemodynamic and clinical monitoring recommended. May aggravate angina associated with hypertrophic cardiomyopathy. **Contra:** Allergies to organic nitrates. **P/N:** Category C, caution in nursing.	Headache, dizziness, chest pain, asthenia, N/V, bronchitis, hypotension, sinusitis, ventricular tachycardia, palpitations, hyperglycemia, rhinitis, paresthesia, amblyopia, hyperlipidemia.
ANTILIPIDEMIC AGENTS				
BILE ACID SEQUESTRANTS				
Cholestyramine (Questran, Questran Light)	**Powder:** 4g/pkt [60s, 378g], (Light) 4g/scoopful [60s, 268g]	***Adults:*** **Initial:** 1 pkt or scoopful qd or bid. **Maint:** 2-4 pkts or scoopfuls/day, given bid. **Titrate:** Adjust at no less than 4 week intervals. **Max:** 6 pkts/day or 6 scoopfuls/day. May also give as 1-6 doses/day. Mix with fluid or highly fluid food. ***Pediatrics:*** **Usual:** 240mg/kg/day of anhydrous cholestyramine resin in 2-3 divided doses. **Max:** 8g/day.	**W/P:** May produce hyperchloremic acidosis with prolonged use. Caution in renal insufficiency, volume depletion, and with concomitant spironolactone. Chronic use may produce or worsen constipation. Avoid constipation with symptomatic CAD. May increase bleeding tendency due to vitamin K deficiency. Serum or red cell folate	Constipation, heartburn, N/V, abdominal pain, flatulence, diarrhea, anorexia, osteoporosis, rash, hyperchloremic

*Scored. †Bold entries denote special dental considerations.
BB = black box warning; **W/P** = warnings/precautions; **Contra** = contraindications; **P/N** = pregnancy category rating and nursing considerations.

NAME	FORM/ STRENGTH	DOSAGE	WARNINGS/PRECAUTIONS & CONTRAINDICATIONS	ADVERSE EFFECTS†
Cholestyramine (Questran, Questran Light) *(cont.)*			reduced with chronic use. Constipation may aggravate hemorrhoids. Light formulation contains phenylalanine. Measure cholesterol during first few months; periodically thereafter. Measure TG periodically. **Contra:** Complete biliary obstruction. **P/N:** Category C, caution in nursing.	acidosis (children), vitamin A and D deficiency, steatorrhea, hypoprothrombinemia (vitamin K deficiency).
Colesevelam HCl (WelChol)	**Tab:** 625mg	***Adults:*** **Hyperlipidemia/Type 2 DM:** 3 tabs bid or 6 tabs qd. Take with liquids and a meal.	**W/P:** Monitor lipids, including TG and non–HDL-cholesterol levels prior to initiation of treatment and periodically thereafter. Caution in TG levels >300mg/dL, dysphagia or swallowing disorders, gastroparesis, GI motility disorders, major GI tract surgery, bowel obstruction, and those susceptible to vitamin K or fat-soluble vitamin deficiencies. Coadministered drugs should be given at least 4 hrs prior to treatment; monitor drug levels. Not for use in treatment of Type 1 DM or for diabetic ketoacidosis. **Contra:** Bowel obstruction, hypertriglyceridemia-induced pancreatitis, serum TG concentrations >500mg/dL. **P/N:** Category B, caution in nursing.	Asthenia, constipation, dyspepsia, pharyngitis, myalgia, nausea, hypoglycemia, bowel obstruction, **dysphagia,** esophageal obstruction, fecal impaction, hypertriglyceridemia, pancreatitis, increased transaminases.
Colestipol HCl (Colestid)	**Granules:** 5g/pkt [30^{s} 90^{s}], 5g/scoopful [300g, 500g]; **Tab:** 1g	***Adults:*** **Initial:** 2g, 1 pkt or 1 scoopful qd-bid. **Titrate:** Increase by 2g qd or bid at 1-2 month intervals. **Usual:** 2-16g/day (tab) or 1-6 pkts or scoopfuls qd or in divided doses. Always mix granules with liquid. Swallow tabs whole with plenty of liquid.	**W/P:** Exclude secondary causes of hypercholesterolemia and perform a lipid profile. May produce hyperchloremic acidosis with prolonged use. Monitor cholesterol and TG based on NCEP guidelines. May cause hypothyroidism. May interfere with normal fat absorption. Chronic use may produce or worsen constipation. Avoid constipation with symptomatic CAD. May increase bleeding tendency due to vitamin K deficiency. **P/N:** Safety in pregnancy not known, caution in nursing.	Constipation, musculoskeletal pain, headache, migraine or sinus headache.
CHOLESTEROL ABSORPTION INHIBITOR				
Ezetimibe (Zetia)	**Tab:** 10mg	***Adults:*** 10mg qd. May give with HMG-CoA reductase inhibitor (with primary hypercholesterolemia) or fenofibrate (with mixed hyperlipidemia) for incremental effect. **Concomitant Bile Sequestrant:** Give either ≥2 hrs before or ≥4 hrs after bile-acid sequestrant.	**W/P:** Monitor LFTs with concurrent statin therapy. Not recommended with moderate or severe hepatic insufficiency. **Contra:** When used with a statin, refer to the statin graphs. **P/N:** Category C, contraindicated in nursing.	Back pain, arthralgia, diarrhea, sinusitis, abdominal pain, myalgia.
FIBRIC ACID DERIVATIVES				
Fenofibrate (Antara, Lofibra, Tricor, Triglide)	**Cap:** (Antara) 43mg, 130mg (Lofibra)67mg, 134mg, 200mg; **Tab:** (Lofibra) 54mg, 160mg (Tricor) 48mg, 145mg (Triglide) 50mg, 160mg	***Adults:*** **(Antara): Hypercholesterolemia/Mixed Dyslipidemia: Initial:** 130mg qd. **Hypertriglyceridemia: Initial:** 43-130mg/day. **Titrate:** Adjust if needed after repeat lipid levels at 4-8 week intervals. **Max:** 130mg/day. **Renal Dysfunction/Elderly: Initial:** 43mg/day. Take with meals. **(Lofibra): Hypercholesterolemia/Mixed Dyslipidemia: Initial: Cap:** 200mg qd. **Hypercholesterolemia/Mixed Hyperlipidemia: Tab:** 160mg qd. **Hypertriglyceridemia: Initial: Cap:** 67-200mg/day. **Tab:** 54-160mg qd. **Titrate:** Adjust if needed after repeat lipid levels at 4-8 week intervals. **Max: Cap:** 200mg/day. **Tab:** 160mg/day. **Renal Dysfunction/Elderly: Initial: Cap:** 67mg/day. **Tab:** 54mg/day. Take with meals. **(Tricor): Hypercholesterolemia/Mixed Dyslipidemia: Initial:** 145mg qd.	**W/P:** Monitor LFTs regularly; d/c if >3x ULN. May cause cholelithiasis; d/c if gallstones found. D/C if myopathy or marked CPK elevation occurs. Decreased Hgb, Hct, WBCs, thrombocytopenia, and agranulocytosis reported; monitor CBCs during first 12 months of therapy. Acute hypersensitivity reactions (rare) and pancreatitis reported. Rare cases of rhabdomyolysis. Evaluate for myopathy. Monitor lipids periodically initially, d/c if inadequate response after 2 months on 130mg/day. Minimize dose in severe renal impairment. Caution in elderly. **Contra:** Hepatic or severe renal dysfunction (including primary biliary cirrhosis), unexplained persistent hepatic function abnormality, preexisting gallbladder disease. **P/N:** Category C, not for use in nursing.	Abdominal pain, back pain, headache, abnormal LFTs, respiratory disorder, increased creatinine phosphokinase.

Table 14.1. PRESCRIBING INFORMATION FOR CARDIOVASCULAR DRUGS *(cont.)*

NAME	FORM/ STRENGTH	DOSAGE	WARNINGS/PRECAUTIONS & CONTRAINDICATIONS	ADVERSE EFFECTS†
ANTILIPIDEMIC AGENTS *(cont.)*				
FIBRIC ACID DERIVATIVES *(cont.)*				
Fenofibrate (Antara, Lofibra, Tricor. Triglide) *(cont.)*		**Hypertriglyceridemia: Initial:** 48-145mg/day. **Titrate:** Adjust if needed after repeat lipid levels at 4-8 week intervals. **Max:** 145mg/day. **Renal Dysfunction/Elderly: Initial:** 48mg/day. Take without regards to meals. **(Triglide): Hypercholesterolemia/ Mixed Hyperlipidemia:** 160mg qd. **Hypertriglyceridemia: Initial:** 50-160mg/day. **Titrate:** Adjust if needed after repeat lipid levels at 4-8 week intervals. **Max:** 160mg/day. Renal Dysfunction/**Elderly: Initial:** 50mg/day. Take without regards to meals.		
Gemfibrozil (Lopid)	**Tab:** 600mg*	***Adults:*** 600mg bid. Give 30 min before morning and evening meals.	**W/P:** Abnormal LFTs reported; monitor periodically. Only use if indicated and d/c if significant lipid response not obtained. Associated with myositis. Cholelithiasis reported. D/C if suspect or diagnose myositis, if abnormal LFTs persist, or gallstones develop. Monitor blood counts periodically during first 12 months. May worsen renal insufficiency. **Contra:** Hepatic or severe renal dysfunction, including primary biliary cirrhosis; preexisting gallbladder disease, concomitant cerivastatin. **P/N:** Category C, not for use in nursing.	Dyspepsia, abdominal pain, diarrhea, fatigue, bacterial and viral infections, musculoskeletal symptoms, abnormal LFTs, hematologic changes, hypesthesia, paresthesia, **taste alteration.**
HMG-CoA REDUCTASE INHIBITORS (STATINS)				
Atorvastatin Calcium (Lipitor)	**Tab:** 10mg, 20mg, 40mg, 80mg	***Adults:*** **Hypercholesterolemia/Mixed Dyslipidemia: Initial:** 10-20mg qd (or 40mg qd for LDL-C reduction >45%). **Titrate:** Adjust dose if needed at 2-4 week intervals. **Usual:** 10-80mg qd. **Homozygous Familial Hypercholesterolemia:** 10-80mg qd. ***Pediatrics:*** **Heterozygous Familial Hypercholesterolemia: 10-17 yrs (postmenarchal): Initial:** 10mg/day. **Titrate:** Adjust dose if needed at intervals of ≥4 weeks. **Max:** 20mg/day.	**W/P:** Monitor LFTs prior to therapy, at 12 weeks or with dose elevation, and periodically thereafter. Reduce dose or withdraw if AST or ALT ≥3x ULN persist. Caution with heavy alcohol use and/ or history of hepatic disease. D/C if markedly elevated CPK levels occur, if myopathy is diagnosed or suspected, or if predisposition to renal failure secondary to rhabdomyolysis. Caution in patients with recent stroke or TIA. Rare cases of rhabdomyolysis reported. **Contra:** Active liver disease, unexplained persistent elevations of serum transaminases, pregnancy, nursing mothers. **P/N:** Category X, not for use in nursing.	Constipation, flatulence, dyspepsia, abdominal pain, transaminase and CK elevation in higher doses.
Fluvastatin Sodium (Lescol, Lescol XL)	**Cap:** (Lescol) 20mg, 40mg; **Tab, Extended-Release:** (Lescol XL) 80mg	***Adults:*** **≥18 yrs: (For LDL-C reduction of ≥25%) Initial:** 40mg cap qpm or 80mg XL tab at any time of day or 40mg cap bid. **(For LDL-C Reduction of <25%) Initial:** 20mg cap qpm. **Range:** 20-80mg/day. **Severe Renal Impairment:** Caution with dose >40mg/day. Take 2 hrs after bile-acid resins qhs. ***Pediatrics:*** **Heterozygous Familial Hypercholesterolemia: 10-16 yrs (≥1 yr postmenarche): Individualize dose: Initial:** One 20mg cap. **Titrate:** Adjust dose at 6-week intervals. **Max:** 40mg cap bid or 80mg XL tab qd.	**W/P:** Monitor LFTs prior to therapy, at 12 weeks, or with dose elevation. D/C if AST or ALT ≥3x ULN on 2 consecutive occasions. Risk of myopathy and/ or rhabdomyolysis reported. D/C if markedly elevated CPK levels occur, if myopathy is diagnosed or suspected, or if predisposition to renal failure secondary to rhabdomyolysis. Less effective with homozygous familial hypercholesterolemia. Caution with heavy alcohol use and/or history of hepatic disease. Evaluate if endocrine dysfunction develops. **Contra:** Active liver disease or unexplained, persistent elevations of serum transaminases, pregnancy, nursing mothers. **P/N:** Category X, not for use in nursing.	Dyspepsia, abdominal pain, headache, nausea, diarrhea, abnormal LFTs, myalgia, flu-like symptoms.

*Scored. †Bold entries denote special dental considerations.
BB = black box warning; **W/P** = warnings/precautions; **Contra** = contraindications; **P/N** = pregnancy category rating and nursing considerations.

NAME	FORM/ STRENGTH	DOSAGE	WARNINGS/PRECAUTIONS & CONTRAINDICATIONS	ADVERSE EFFECTS†
Lovastatin (Altoprev, Mevacor)	**Tab:** (Mevacor) 20mg, 40mg; **Tab, Extended-Release:** (Altoprev) 20mg, 40mg, 60mg	***Adults:* (Altoprev): Initial:** 20, 40, or 60mg qhs. Consider immediate-release lovastatin in patients requiring smaller reductions. May adjust at intervals of ≥4 weeks. **Concomitant Fibrates/Niacin (≥1g/day):** Try to avoid. **Max:** 20mg/day. **Concomitant Amiodarone/Verapamil: Max:** 20mg/day. **CrCl <30mL/min:** Consider dose increase of >20mg/day carefully and implement cautiously. Swallow whole; do not chew or crush. **(Mevacor): Initial:** 20mg qd at dinner (10mg/day if need LDL-C reduction <20%). **Usual:** 10-80mg/day given qd or bid. May adjust every 4 weeks. **Max:** 80mg/day. **Concomitant Cyclosporine: Initial:** 10mg/day. **Max:** 20mg/day. **Fibrates/Niacin (≥1g/day): Max:** 20mg/day. **Concomitant Amiodarone/Verapamil: Max:** 40mg/day. **CrCl <30mL/min:** Consider dose increase of >20mg/day carefully and implement cautiously. ***Pediatrics:* (Mevacor): Heterozygous Familial Hypercholesterolemia: 10-17 yrs (at least 1-yr postmenarchal): Initial: If <20% LDL-C Reduction Needed:** 10mg qd. If ≥20% **LDL-C Reduction Needed:** 20mg qd. May adjust every 4 weeks. **Max:** 40mg/day. **Concomitant Cyclosporine: Initial:** 10mg/day. **Max:** 20mg/day. **Fibrates/Niacin (≥1g/day): Max:** 20mg/day. **Concomitant Amiodarone/Verapamil: Max:** 40mg/day. **CrCl <30mL/min:** Consider dose increase of >20mg/day carefully and implement cautiously.	**W/P:** May increase serum transaminases and CPK levels; consider in differential diagnosis of chest pain. D/C if AST or ALT ≥3x ULN persist, if myopathy diagnosed or suspected, and a few days before major surgery. Monitor LFTs prior to therapy, at 6 weeks, 12 weeks, then periodically or with dose elevation. Caution with heavy alcohol use and/or history of hepatic disease. Caution with dose escalation in renal insufficiency. Lovastatin immediate-release found to be less effective with homozygous familial hypercholesterolemia. Rhabdomyolysis (rare), myopathy reported. **Contra:** Active liver disease, unexplained persistent elevations of serum transaminases, pregnancy, nursing mothers. **P/N:** Category X, not for use in nursing.	Nausea, abdominal pain, constipation, flatulence, dizziness, rash, elevated transaminases or CK levels, blurred vision, insomnia, dyspepsia, headache, asthenia, myalgia.
Pravastatin Sodium (Pravachol)	**Tab:** 10mg, 20mg, 40mg, 80mg	***Adults:* ≥18 yrs: Initial:** 40mg qd. Perform lipid tests within 4 weeks and adjust according to response and guidelines. **Titrate:** May increase to 80mg qd if needed. Significant **Renal/Hepatic Dysfunction: Initial:** 10mg qd. **Concomitant Immunosuppressives (eg, cyclosporine): Initial:**10mg qhs. **Max:** 20mg/day. ***Pediatrics:* Heterozygous Familial Hypercholesterolemia:** 14-18 yrs: **Initial:** 40mg qd. **8-13 yrs:** 20mg qd. **Concomitant Immunosuppressives (eg, cyclosporine): Initial:** 10mg qhs. **Max:** 20mg/day.	**W/P:** Perform LFTs before therapy, before dose increases, and if clinically indicated. Risk of myopathy, myalgia, and rhabdomyolysis. D/C if AST or ALT ≥3x ULN persists, if elevated CPK levels occur, or if myopathy diagnosed or suspected. Less effective with homozygous familial hypercholesterolemia. Monitor for endocrine dysfunction. Closely monitor with heavy alcohol use, recent history or signs of hepatic disease, or renal dysfunction. **Contra:** Active liver disease, unexplained persistent elevations of LFTs, pregnancy, nursing mothers. **P/N:** Category X, not for use in nursing.	Rash, N/V, diarrhea, headache, chest pain, influenza, abdominal pain, dizziness, increases ALT, AST, CPK.
Rosuvastatin Calcium (Crestor)	**Tab:** 5mg, 10mg, 20mg, 40mg	***Adults:* Hypercholesterolemia/Mixed Dyslipidemia/Hypertriglyceridemia/Primary Dysbetalipoproteinemia/Slowing Progression of Atherosclerosis: Initial:** 10mg qd. (20mg qd with LDL-C >190mg/dL). **Titrate:** Adjust dose if needed at 2-4 week intervals. **Range:** 5-40mg qd. **Homozygous Familial Hypercholesterolemia:** 20mg qd. **Max:** 40mg qd. **Asian Patients:** 5mg qd. **Concomitant Cyclosporine: Max:** 5mg qd. **Concomitant Lopinavir/Ritonavir:** Max 10mg qd. **Concomitant Gemfibrozil: Max:** 10mg qd. **Severe Renal Impairment: CrCl <30mL/min/1.73m² (not on hemodialysis): Initial:** 5mg qd. **Max:** 10mg qd.	**W/P:** Increased risk of myopathy with other lipid-lowering therapies, cyclosporine, or lopinavir/ritonavir. Rare cases of rhabdomyolysis with acute renal failure secondary to myoglobinuria reported. Monitor LFTs prior to therapy, at 12 weeks or with dose elevation, and periodically thereafter. Reduce dose or d/c if AST/ALT ≥3x ULN persist. Caution with heavy alcohol use, history of hepatic disease, renal impairment, hypothyroidism, elderly. D/C if markedly elevated CPK levels occur, if myopathy is diagnosed or suspected, or if predisposition to renal failure secondary to rhabdomyolysis. Approximately twofold elevation in median exposure in Asian subjects. Persistent elevations in hepatic transaminase occurred. Monitor liver enzymes. **Contra:** Active liver disease, unexplained, persistent elevations	Headache, myalgia, abdominal pain, asthenia, constipation, nausea, rhabdomyolysis with myoglobinuria, acute renal failure, myopathy, liver enzyme abnormalities.

Table 14.1. PRESCRIBING INFORMATION FOR CARDIOVASCULAR DRUGS *(cont.)*

NAME	FORM/ STRENGTH	DOSAGE	WARNINGS/PRECAUTIONS & CONTRAINDICATIONS	ADVERSE EFFECTS†
ANTILIPIDEMIC AGENTS *(cont.)*				
HMG-CoA REDUCTASE INHIBITORS *(cont.)*				
Rosuvastatin Calcium (Crestor) *(cont.)*			of hepatic transaminase levels, pregnancy, nursing mothers. **P/N:** Category X, not for use in nursing.	
Simvastatin (Zocor)	**Tab:** 5mg, 10mg, 20mg, 40mg, 80mg	***Adults:*** **Initial:** 20-40mg qpm. **Usual:** 5-80mg/day. **Titrate:** Adjust at ≥4-week intervals. **High Risk for CHD Events: Initial:** 40mg/day. **Homozygous Familial Hypercholesterolemia:** 40mg qpm or 80mg/day given as 20mg bid plus 40mg qpm. **Concomitant Cyclosporine: Initial:** 5mg/day. **Max:** 10mg/day. **Concomitant Gemfibrozil (try to avoid): Max:** 10mg/day. **Concomitant Amiodarone/Verapamil: Max:** 20mg/day. **Severe Renal Insufficiency:** 5mg/day; monitor closely. ***Pediatrics:*** **Heterozygous Familial Hypercholesterolemia: 10-17 yrs (at least 1 yr postmenarchal): Initial:** 10mg qpm. **Usual:** 10-40mg/day. **Titrate:** Adjust at ≥4-week intervals. **Max:** 40mg/day.	**W/P:** Caution with heavy alcohol use, severe renal insufficiency or history of hepatic disease. Monitor LFTs prior to therapy, periodically thereafter for first yr, or until 1 yr after last dose elevation (additional test at 3 months for 80mg dose). D/C if AST or ALT ≥3x ULN persist, if myopathy is suspected or diagnosed, a few days prior to major surgery. Rhabomyolysis (rare), myopathy reported. **Contra:** Active liver disease, unexplained persistent elevations of serum transaminases, pregnancy, nursing mothers. **P/N:** Category X, not for use in nursing.	Abdominal pain, headache, CK and transaminase elevations, constipation, upper respiratory infection, hepatic failure.
HMG-CoA REDUCTASE INHIBITOR/CHOLESTEROL ABSORPTION INHIBITOR				
Simvastatin/ Ezetimibe (Vytorin)	**Tab:** (ezetimibe-simvastatin) 10mg-10mg, 10mg-20mg, 10mg-40mg, 10mg-80mg	***Adults:*** Take once daily in the evening. **Initial:** 10mg-20mg qd. **Less Aggressive LDL-C Reductions: Initial:** 10mg-10mg qd. **LDL-C Reduction >55%: Initial:** 10mg-40mg qd. **Titrate:** Adjust at ≥2 weeks. **Homozygous Familial Hypercholesterolemia:** 10mg-40mg or 10mg-80mg qd. **Severe Renal Insufficiency:** Avoid unless tolerant of ≥5mg of simvastatin; monitor closely. **Concomitant Bile-Acid Sequestrant:** Take either ≥2 hrs before or ≥4 hrs after bile-acid sequestrant. **Concomitant Cyclosporine:** Avoid unless tolerant of ≥5mg of simvastatin. **Max:** 10mg-10mg/day. **Concomitant Amiodarone/ Verapamil: Max:** 10mg-20mg/day.	**W/P:** Rhabdomyolysis (rare), myopathy reported. D/C therapy if myopathy is suspected or diagnosed, if AST or ALT ≥3x ULN persist, a few days prior to major surgery or when any major medical or surgical condition supervenes. Monitor LFTs prior to therapy and thereafter when clinically indicated. With 10mg-80mg dose, monitor LFTs prior to titration, 3 months after titration and periodically thereafter for first yr. Caution with heavy alcohol use, severe renal insufficiency, or history of hepatic disease. Avoid use in moderate or severe hepatic insufficiency. **Contra:** Active liver disease, unexplained persistent elevations in serum transaminases, pregnancy, lactation. **P/N:** Category X, not for use in nursing.	Headache, upper respiratory tract infection, myalgia, CK and transaminase elevations, urticaria, arthralgia
HMG-CoA REDUCTASE INHIBITORS/NICOTINIC ACID				
Lovastatin/Niacin (Advicor)	**Tab:** (Extended-Release Niacin-Lovastatin) 500mg-20mg, 750mg-20mg, 1000mg-20mg, 1000mg-40mg	***Adults:*** **≥18 yrs: Initial:** 500mg-20mg qhs. **Titrate:** Increase by no more than 500mg of niacin every 4 weeks. **Max:** 2000mg-40mg. **Concomitant Cyclosporine/Danazol: Max Lovastatin:** 20mg/day. **Concomitant Amiodarone/ Verapamil: Max Lovastatin:** 40mg/day. Swallow tab whole. Take with low-fat snack. Pretreat 30 min prior with ASA to reduce flushing.	**W/P:** Do not substitute for equivalent dose of immediate-release niacin. Myopathy, rhabdomyolysis, severe hepatotoxicity reported. Caution with history of liver disease or jaundice, heavy alcohol use, hepatobiliary disease, peptic ulcer, diabetes, unstable angina, acute phase of MI, gout, renal dysfunction. Monitor LFTs prior to therapy, every 6-12 weeks for first 6 months, and periodically thereafter. May elevate PT, uric acid levels. D/C if AST or ALT ≥3x ULN persist, if myopathy diagnosed or suspected, and a few days before surgery. May reduce phosphorous levels. May disrupt therapy during a course of treatment with systemic antifungal azole, a macrolide antibiotic or ketolide antibiotic. **Contra:** Active liver disease, unexplained persistent elevations in serum	Flushing, asthenia, flu syndrome, headache, infection, pain, GI effects, hyperglycemia, myalgia, pruritus, rash.

*Scored. †Bold entries denote special dental considerations.
BB = black box warning; **W/P** = warnings/precautions; **Contra** = contraindications; **P/N** = pregnancy category rating and nursing considerations.

NAME	FORM/ STRENGTH	DOSAGE	WARNINGS/PRECAUTIONS & CONTRAINDICATIONS	ADVERSE EFFECTS†
Lovastatin/Niacin (Advicor) *(cont.)*			transaminases, active PUD, arterial bleeding, pregnancy, nursing mothers. **P/N:** Category X, not for use in nursing.	
Simvastatin/ Niacin (Simcor)	**Tab, Extended-Release:** (Niacin-Simvastatin) 500mg/20mg, 750mg/20mg, 1000mg/20mg	***Adults:*** Patients not currently on niacin extended-release or switching from immediate-release niacin: **Initial:** 500mg/20mg qd hs, with a low fat snack. **Titrate:** Adjust dose at ≥4 weeks. After Week 8, titrate to response and tolerance. **Maint:** 1000mg/20mg to 2000mg/40mg qd. **Max:** 2000mg/40mg qd. Do not break, crush or chew before swallowing.	**W/P:** Do not substitute for equivalent dose of immediate-release niacin. Myopathy and rhabdomyolysis reported; monitor serum creatine kinase (CK) periodically. D/C therapy if myopathy is suspected or diagnosed, if transaminase levels increase ≥3 ULN persist, or a few days prior to major surgery or when any major medical or surgical condition supervenes. Increased risk with higher doses, advanced age (≥65 yrs), hypothyroidism, renal impairment. Caution with heavy alcohol use, or history of liver disease; monitor LFTs prior to therapy, every 12 weeks for the first 6 months and periodically thereafter. Severe hepatic toxicity may occur in patients substituting sustained-release niacin for immediate-release niacin at equivalent doses. May increase serum glucose levels in diabetic or potentially diabetic patients, particularly the first few months of therapy; adjust diet and/or hypoglycemic therapy or d/c if necessary. May reduce platelet count. Caution with those predisposed to gout. **Contra:** Active liver disease (unexplained persistent elevations of serum transaminases), active peptic ulcer disease, arterial bleeding, pregnancy/nursing. **P/N:** Category X, not for use in nursing.	Flushing, headache, backpain, diarrhea, nausea, pruritus.
LIPID-REGULATING AGENT				
Omega-3-Acid Ethyl Esters (Lovaza)	**Cap:** 1g	***Adults:*** 4g qd. Given as single 4g dose (4 caps) or as two 2g doses (2 caps bid).	**W/P:** Caution in patients with diabetes, hypothyroidism, hepatic or pancreatic problems, or known sensitivity or allergy to fish. Lower alcohol use. Excess body weight may be a contributing factor to elevated cholesterol and should be addressed before initiating therapy. Possible increases in alanine aminotransferase levels without a concurrent increase in aspartate aminotransferase levels. Possible increase in LDL-C levels. **P/N:** Category C, caution in nursing.	Eructation, infection, flu-syndrome, dyspepsia.
NICOTINIC ACID				
Niacin (Niaspan)	**Tab, Extended-Release:** 500mg, 750mg, 1000mg	***Adults:*** Take qhs after low-fat snack. **Initial:** 500mg qhs. **Titrate:** Increase by 500mg every 4 weeks. **Maint:** 1-2g qhs. **Max:** 2g/day. Take ASA or NSAIDs 30 min before to reduce flushing. Do not chew, crush, or break; swallow whole. Women may respond to lower doses than men.	**W/P:** Do not substitute with equivalent doses of immediate-release niacin (severe hepatic toxicity may occur). Associated with abnormal LFTs; monitor LFTs before therapy, every 6-12 weeks during first yr, then periodically thereafter. D/C if LFTs ≥3x ULN persist or develop signs of hepatotoxicity. Monitor for rhabdomyolysis. Observe closely with history of jaundice, hepatobiliary disease, and peptic ulcer; monitor LFTs and blood glucose frequently. Dose-related rise in glucose tolerance in diabetics. Caution with history of hepatic disease, heavy alcohol use, renal dysfunction, unstable angina, and acute phase of MI. Elevated uric acid levels reported. May reduce platelet and phosphorous levels. **Contra:** Unexplained or significant hepatic dysfunction, active peptic ulcer disease, arterial bleeding. **P/N:** Category C, not for use in nursing.	Flushing episodes (eg, warmth, redness, itching, tingling), dizziness, tachycardia, SOB, sweating, chills, edema, headache, diarrhea.

Table 14.2. DRUG INTERACTIONS FOR CARDIOVASCULAR DRUGS

ANTIANGINALS

Calcium Channel Blockers

Diltiazem HCl (Cardizem)	
Anesthetics	Potentiates depression of cardiac contractility, conductivity, automaticity, and vascular dilation.
Benzodiazepines	Increases AUC of midazolam, triazolam; may require dose adjustment due to increased clinical effects or increased adverse events.
β-Blockers, IV	Avoid IV β-blockers.
β-Blockers, oral	Possible bradycardia, AV block, and contractility depression with oral β-blockers.
Buspirone	Increases AUC of buspirone; may require dose adjustment due to increased clinical effects or increased adverse events.
Carbamazepine	Elevates carbamazepine levels, which may result in toxicity; monitor closely.
Cardiac function, drugs affecting	Caution with drugs that decrease peripheral resistance, intravascular volume, myocardial contractility or conduction.
Cimetidine	Increases levels of diltiazem.
Cyclosporine	Increases levels of cyclosporine; may need dose adjustment; monitor closely.
CYP3A4 inducers	Avoid concurrent use with CYP3A4 inducers (eg, rifampin).
CYP3A4 substrates	May require dose adjustment with concomitant CYP3A4 substrates.
CYP450 substrates	Possible competitive inhibition of metabolism with drugs metabolized by CYP450.
Digoxin	Monitor for excessive slowing of HR and/or AV block.
Lovastatin	Increases AUC of lovastatin; may require dose adjustment due to increased clinical effects or increased adverse events.
Propranolol	Increases levels of propranolol; monitor closely.
Quinidine	Increases AUC of quinidine; may require dose adjustment due to increased clinical effects or increased adverse events; monitor closely.
Nifedipine (Procardia)	
β-Blockers	β-Blockers may increase risk of CHF, severe hypotension, or angina exacerbation.
Cimetidine	Increases levels of nifedipine.
Coumarin	Increases prothrombin time.
Digoxin	Increases levels of digoxin.
Fentanyl	Possible hypotension with fentanyl.
Grapefruit juice	Potentiated by grapefruit juice; avoid grapefruit juice.
Quinidine	Decreased plasma levels of quinidine.

Nitrate Vasodilators

Isosorbide Dinitrate (Dilatrate-SR, Isordil, Isordil Titradose, Isosorbide Dinitrate)	
Sildenafil	Severe hypotension.

Table 14.2. DRUG INTERACTIONS FOR CARDIOVASCULAR DRUGS *(cont.)*

ANTIANGINALS *(cont.)*

Nitrate Vasodilators

Isosorbide Dinitrate (Dilatrate-SR, Isordil, Isordil Titradose, Isosorbide Dinitrate) *(cont.)*	
Vasodilators	Additive vasodilating effects with other vasodilators (eg, alcohol).
Isosorbide Mononitrate (Imdur, Ismo, Monoket)	
Calcium channel blockers (CCBs)	Orthostatic hypotension reported with CCBs.
Sildenafil	Severe hypotension.
Vasodilators	Additive vasodilating effects with other vasodilators (eg, alcohol).
Nitroglycerin (Minitran, Nitrek, Nitro-Bid, Nitro-Dur, Nitrolingual Spray, NitroMist, Nitroquick, Nitrostat)	
Alcohol	Additive hypotension.
Alteplase	Caution with alteplase.
Anticholinergics	Anticholinergics may make sublingual dissolution difficult. (Nitroquick, Nitrostat)
Antihypertensives	Additive hypotension with β-blockers, calcium channel blockers, and other antihypertensives.
Aspirin (ASA)	Vasodilatory and hemodynamic effects potentiated by ASA.
β-Blockers	(NitroMist) Increases hypotensive effects with β-adrenergic blockers (eg, labetolol).
Calcium channel blockers (CCBs)	Orthostatic hypotension reported with CCBs.
Ergotamine	Avoid ergotamine.
Heparin	May decrease anticoagulant effect of heparin.
Nitrates, long-acting	Long-acting nitrates may decrease effects.
PDE5 inhibitors	Avoid PDE5 inhibitors (eg, sildenafil, vardenafil, tadalafil); severe hypotension may occur.
Phenothiazines	Additive hypotension.
Plasminogen activator, tissue type	Caution with tissue-type plasminogen activator.
Tricyclic antidepressants (TCAs)	TCAs may make sublingual dissolution difficult. (Nitroquick, Nitrostat)
Vasodilators	Additive vasodilating effects with other vasodilators (eg, alcohol).

Miscellaneous Antianginal

Ranolazine (Ranexa)	
Antiarrhythmics	Avoid with drugs that may prolong the QTc interval, such as Class Ia (eg, quinidine) and Class III (eg, dofetilide, sotalol) antiarrhythmics.
Antipsychotics	Avoid with drugs that may prolong the QTc interval, such as antipsychotics (eg, thioridazine, ziprasidone).
CYP2D6 substrates	May increase levels of drugs metabolized by CYP2D6 such as TCAs and some antipsychotics; consider dosage reduction of these drugs.
CYP3A inducers	Avoid coadministration with CYP3A inducers, eg, rifampin, rifabutin, rifapentin, phenobarbital, phenytoin, carbamazepine, and St. John's wort.

ANTIANGINALS *(cont.)*

Miscellaneous Antianginal

Ranolazine (Ranexa) *(cont.)*	
CYP3A inhibitors	Avoid coadministration with moderately CYP3A inhibitors, eg, fluconazole, diltiazem, verapamil, macrolide antibiotics, HIV protease inhibitors, grapefruit juice, or grapefruit-containing products. Do not use with strong CYP3A inhibitors, eg, ketoconazole.
Digoxin	May increase levels of digoxin; consider dose reduction of digoxin.
Simvastatin	May increase levels of simvastatin; consider dose reduction of simvastatin.

ANTIARRHYTHMICS

Class IA Antiarrhythmics

Disopyramide Phosphate (Norpace, Norpace CR)	
Alcohol	Monitor blood glucose.
Antiarrhythmics	Avoid Class 1a and 1c antiarrhythmics and propranolol except in unresponsive, life-threatening arrhythmias.
β-Blockers	Monitor blood glucose.
CYP3A4 inhibitors	Possible fatal interactions.
Hepatic enzyme inducers	Hepatic enzyme inducers may lower levels.
Verapamil	Avoid within 48 hrs before or 24 hrs after verapamil.
Procainamide HCl	
Antiarrhythmics	Concomitant antiarrhythmics potentiate effects; dose reduction may be necessary.
Anticholinergics	Concomitant anticholinergics may produce additive antivagal effects on A-V nodal conduction.
Neuromuscular blocking agents	Patients requiring neuromuscular blocking agents (eg, succinylcholine) may require lower doses due to procainamide reducing the release of acetylcholine.
Quinidine Gluconate	
Amiodarone	Amiodarone increases quinidine levels.
Anticholinergics	Additive effects with anticholinergics.
β-blockers	β-Blockers decrease clearance.
Cholinergics	Antagonistic effects with cholinergics.
Cimetidine	Cimetidine increases quinidine levels.
CYP3A4 inducers	CYP3A4 inducers (eg, phenobarbital, phenytoin, rifampin) may accelerate hepatic elimination.
CYP450 3A4/2D6 substrates	Caution with drugs metabolized by CYP450 3A4 (eg, nifedipine, felodipine, nicardipine, nimodipine) and 2D6 (eg, mexiletine, phenothiazines, polycyclic antidepressants, codeine, hydrocodone).
Digoxin	Increases levels of digoxin; digoxin may require dose reduction.

Table 14.2. DRUG INTERACTIONS FOR CARDIOVASCULAR DRUGS *(cont.)*

ANTIARRHYTHMICS *(cont.)*

Class IA Antiarrhythmics

Quinidine Gluconate *(cont.)*	
Diltiazem	Diltiazem decreases clearance.
Grapefruit juice	Avoid grapefruit juice with oral formulation.
Haloperidol	Increases levels of haloperidol.
Inotropes, positive	Antagonistic effects with positive inotropes.
Inotropics, negative	Additive effects with negative inotropics.
Ketoconazole	Ketoconzaole increases quinidine levels.
Neuromuscular blockers	Potentiates depolarizing (eg, succinylcholine, decamethonium) and nondepolarizing (eg, d-tubocurarine, pancuronium) neuromuscular blockers.
Procainamide	Increases levels of procainamide.
Salt	Dietary salt may affect absorption with oral formulation.
Urine alkalinizers	Urine alkalinizers (eg, carbonic anhydrase inhibitors, sodium bicarbonate, thiazide diuretics) reduce renal elimination.
Vasoconstrictors	Antagonistic effects with vasoconstrictors.
Vasodilators	Additive effects with vasodilators.
Verapamil	Verapamil decreases clearance.
Warfarin	Potentiates the effects of warfarin.
Quinidine Sulfate	
Amiodarone	Amiodarone increases quinidine levels.
Anticholinergics	Additive effects with anticholinergics.
β-Blockers	β-Blockers decrease clearance.
Cimetidine	Cimetidine increases quinidine levels.
CYP3A4 inducers	CYP3A4 inducers (eg, phenobarbital, phenytoin, rifampin) may accelerate hepatic elimination.
CYP3A4/2D6 substrates	Caution with drugs metabolized by CYP450 3A4 (eg, nifedipine, felodipine, nicardipine, nimodipine) and 2D6 (eg, mexiletine, phenothiazines, polycyclic antidepressants, codeine, hydrocodone).
Digoxin	Increases levels of digoxin; may require dose reduction of digoxin.
Diltiazem	Diltiazem decreases clearance.
Grapefruit juice	Avoid grapefruit juice.
Haloperidol	Increases levels of haloperidol.
Inotropes, positive	Antagonistic effects with positive inotropes.
Inotropics, negative	Additive effects with negative inotropics.
Ketoconazole	Ketoconazole increases quinidine levels.
Neuromuscular blockers	Potentiates depolarizing (eg, succinylcholine, decamethonium) and non-depolarizing (eg, d-tubocurarine, pancuronium) neuromuscular blockers.

ANTIARRHYTHMICS *(cont.)*

CLASS IA ANTIARRHYTHMICS

Quinidine Sulfate *(cont.)*	
Procainamide	Increases levels of procainamide.
Salt	Dietary salt may affect absorption.
Urine alkalinizers	Urine alkalinizers (eg, carbonic anhydrase inhibitors, sodium bicarbonate, thiazide diuretics) reduce renal elimination.
Vasodilators	Additive effects with vasodilators.
Verapamil	Verapamil decreases clearance.
Warfarin	Potentiates the effects of warfarin.

CLASS IB ANTIARRHYTHMICS

Lidocaine HCl	
β-Blockers	β-Blockers may reduce hepatic blood flow and thereby reduce lidocaine clearance.
Cimetidine	Cimetidine may reduce hepatic blood flow and thereby reduce lidocaine clearance.
Digoxin	Caution with digoxin toxicity accompanied by atrioventricular block.
Mexiletine HCl	
Caffeine	Decreases caffeine clearance.
Cimetidine	Cimetidine may alter plasma levels.
CYP2D6/CYP1A2 inhibitors/inducers	Inhibition or induction of CYP2D6 and CYP1A2 enzymes may alter plasma levels.
Enzyme inducers	Hepatic enzyme inducers (eg, rifampin, phenobarbital, phenytoin) lower plasma levels.
Fluvoxamine	Slowly titrate dose of mexiletine to desired effect with concomitant fluvoxamine.
Propafenone	Slowly titrate dose of mexiletine to desired effect with concomitant propafenone.
Theophylline	May increase theophylline levels.
Urinary pH, drugs altering	Avoid drugs or diet regimens that may alter urinary pH.

CLASS IC ANTIARRHYTHMICS

Flecainide Acetate (Tambocor)	
Amiodarone	The effects of flecainide are potentiated by amiodarone.
Anticonvulsants	Increases elimination with phenytoin, phenobarbital, carbamazepine.
β-Blockers	Additive negative inotropic effects with β-blockers (eg, propranolol).
Calcium channel blockers	Diltiazem, nifedipine, verapamil are not recommended.
Cimetidine	Effects are potentiated by cimetidine.
CYP2D6 inhibitors	Inhibitors of CYP2D6 (eg, desipramine, paroxetine, quinidine, ritonavir, sertraline) may increase levels; monitor closely.

Table 14.2. DRUG INTERACTIONS FOR CARDIOVASCULAR DRUGS *(cont.)*

ANTIARRHYTHMICS *(cont.)*

Class IC Antiarrhythmics

Flecainide Acetate (Tambocor) *(cont.)*	
Digoxin	Increases digoxin levels.
Disopyramide	Disopyramide not recommended.
Propafenone HCl (Rythmol, Rythmol SR)	
Cimetidine	Cimetidine may increase plasma levels.
CYP1A2 inhibitors	Inhibitors of CYP1A2 (eg, amiodarone) may increase levels; monitor closely.
CYP2D6 inhibitors	Inhibitors of CYP2D6 (eg, desipramine, paroxetine, quinidine ritonavir, sertraline) may increase levels; monitor closely.
CYP2D6 substrates	May increase levels of drugs metabolized by CYP2D6 (eg, desipramine, imipramine, haloperidol, venlafaxine).
CYP3A4 inhibitors	Inhibitors of CYP3A4 (eg, ketoconazole, ritonavir, saquinavir, erythromycin, grapefruit juice) may increase levels; monitor closely.
Digoxin	May increase levels of digoxin; monitor closely.
Lidocaine	May increase CNS side effects of lidocaine.
Orlistat	Orlistat may decrease plasma levels.
Propranolol	May increase levels of propranolol; monitor closely.
Rifampin	Rifampin may decrease plasma levels.
Warfarin	May increase levels of warfarin; monitor closely.

Class II Antiarrhythmics (β-blockers). See Antihypertensives/Heart Failure Agents for other β-blockers.

Esmolol HCl (Brevibloc)	
Catecholamine-depleting agents	Additive effects with catecholamine-depleting agents (eg, reserpine); monitor for hypotension or bradycardia.
Digoxin	May increase digoxin levels; titrate with caution.
Epinephrine	Patients with history of severe anaphylactic reaction may be more reactive to repeated challenge and unresponsive to the usual doses of epinephrine.
Inotropic drugs	Do not use to control supraventricular tachycardia with vasoconstrictive and inotropic agents (eg, dopamine, epinephrine, norepinephrine); high risk of blocking cardiac contractility when systemic vascular resistance is high.
Morphine	Levels increased by morphine; titrate with caution.
Succinylcholine	May prolong effects of succinylcholine; titrate with caution.
Vasoconstrictive/ inotropic agents	Do not use to control supraventricular tachycardia with vasoconstrictive and inotropic agents (eg, dopamine, epinephrine, norepinephrine); high risk of blocking cardiac contractility when systemic vascular resistance is high.
Verapamil	Caution when using with verapamil in depressed myocardial function; fatal cardiac arrest may occur.
Warfarin	Levels increased by warfarin; titrate with caution.

ANTIARRHYTHMICS *(cont.)*

CLASS II/III ANTIARRHYTHMIC

Sotalol HCl (Betapace, Betapace AF)	
Antacids	Avoid within 2 hrs of aluminum- or magnesium-containing antacids.
Antiarrhythmics	Avoid Class 1A and Class III antiarrhythmics; potential to prolong refractoriness.
Antidiabetic agents	Antidiabetic agents may need adjustment.
β_2-Agonist	β_2-agonists (eg, terbutaline) may need dose increase.
β-Blockers	Additive Class II effects with β-blockers.
Calcium channel blockers (CCBs)	Additive conduction abnormalities with CCBs.
Catecholamine-depleting drugs	May potentiate bradycardia or hypotension with catecholamine-depleting drugs (eg, reserpine).
Clonidine	Potentiates rebound HTN with clonidine withdrawal.
Digoxin	Additive conduction abnormalities with digoxin.
Diuretics	Caution with diuretics.
Epinephrine	May block epinephrine effects.
QT interval, drugs prolonging	Avoid with drugs that prolong the QT interval (eg, Class I and III antiarrhythmics, phenothiazines, TCAs, bepridil, certain quinolones and oral macrolides, astemizole).

CLASS III ANTIARRHYTHMICS

Amiodarone HCl* (Amiodarone IV, Cordarone, Pacerone)	
Anesthetics	May increase sensitivity to myocardial depressant and conduction defects of halogenated inhalational anesthetics.
Antiarrhythmics	Initiate additional antiarrhythmic drug at lower than usual dose.
Antidepressants	QT prolongation and torsades de pointes with antidepressants (eg, trazodone) reported.
Azoles	QTc prolongation reported.
β-blockers	Risk of bradycardia, hypotension with β-blockers.
Calcium channel blockers (CCBs)	Increases risk of AV block with verapamil or diltiazem and hypotension with CCBs. Concomitant administration with diltiazem and verapamil may result in hemodynamic and electrophysiologic interactions.
Cholestyramine	Cholestyramine may decrease levels and half-life.
Clopidogrel	Concomitant use may result in ineffective inhibition of platelet aggregation.
Cyclosporine	May elevate plasma levels of cyclosporine.
CYP1A2 substrates	Increased levels of CYP1A2 substrates reported.
CYP2C8 inhibitors	CYP2C8 inhibitors may increase amiodarone levels.
CYP2C9 substrates	Increased levels of CYP2C9 substrates reported.

*Risk of interactions may persist after discontinuation due to long half-life.

Table 14.2. DRUG INTERACTIONS FOR CARDIOVASCULAR DRUGS *(cont.)*

ANTIARRHYTHMICS *(cont.)*

Class III Antiarrhythmics

Amiodarone HCl* (Amiodarone IV, Cordarone, Pacerone) *(cont.)*	
CYP2D6 substrates	Increased levels of CYP2D6 substrates reported.
CYP3A4 inducers	CYP3A4 inducers (eg, rifampin, St. John's wort) may decrease levels.
CYP3A4 inhibitors	CYP3A4 inhibitors (eg, protease inhibitors, cimetidine, grapefruit juice) may increase amiodarone levels.
CYP3A4 substrates	Increased levels of CYP3A4 substrates reported.
Digoxin	May elevate plasma levels of digoxin; d/c or reduce digoxin dose by 50%.
Disopyramide	May elevate plasma levels of disopyramide. Caution with disopyramide; QT prolongation reported.
Fentanyl	Concomitant use may cause hypotension, bradycardia, and decreased cardiac output.
Flecainide	May increase levels of flecainide.
Fluoroquinolones	Caution with fluoroquinolones; QTc prolongation reported.
H_1 antagonists	QT prolongation and torsades de pointes with H_1 antagonists (eg, loratadine) reported.
HMG-CoA reductase inhibitors (statins)	May elevate plasma levels of statins; rhabdomyolysis/myopathy reported with simvastatin and atorvastatin.
Loratadine	Caution with loratadine; QT prolongation reported.
Macrolides	Caution with macrolides; QTc prolongation reported with macrolides.
Methotrexate	Caution with methotrexate.
Phenytoin	May elevate plasma levels of phenytoin. Phenytoin may decrease levels of amiodarone.
Procainamide	May increase levels of procainamide; d/c or decrease procainamide dose by 1/3.
Propranolol	Concomitant administration with propranolol may result in hemodynamic and electrophysiologic interactions.
Protease inhibitors	Increases levels with protease inhibitors; monitor for toxicity.
Quinidine	May increase levels of quinidine; d/c or decrease quinidine dose by 1/3 to 1/2.
Trazadone	Caution with trazadone; QT prolongation reported.
Warfarin	May increase PT with warfarin; d/c or decrease warfarin dose by 1/3 to 1/2.
Dofetilide (Tikosyn)	
Amiodarone	Reduce amiodarone to <3mcg/mL or withdraw at least 3 months before initiating dofetilide.
Antiarrhythmics	Hold Class I and III antiarrhythmics for at least 3 half-lives before initiating dofetilide.
Cationic secreters	Caution with actively secreting cation drugs (eg, amiloride, triamterene, metformin).

*Risk of interactions may persist after discontinuation due to long half-life.

ANTIARRHYTHMICS *(cont.)*

Class III Antiarrhythmics

Dofetilide (Tikosyn) *(cont.)*	
Cimetidine	Contraindicated.
CYP3A4 inhibitors	CYP3A4 inhibitors (eg, macrolides, protease inhibitors, grapefruit juice, etc) may potentiate dofetilide.
Diuretics	Hypokalemia or hypomagnesemia may occur with K^+-depleting diuretics.
Hydrochlorothiazide (HCTZ)	HCTZ (alone or in combinations such as with triamterene) is contraindicated; concomitant use can significantly increase dofetilide plasma concentrations and QT interval prolongation.
Ketoconazole	Contraindicated.
QT interval, drugs prolonging	Not recommended.
Renal cationic secretion, inhibitors of	Contraindicated.
Trimethoprim	Contraindicated (alone or in combination with sulfamethoxazole).
Verapamil	Contraindicated.
Ibutilide Fumarate (Corvert)	
Antiarrhythmics	Avoid Class IA (eg, disopyramide, quinidine, procainamide) and other Class III (eg, amiodarone, sotalol) antiarrhythmics with or within 4 hrs postinfusion of ibutilide.
Digoxin	Supraventricular arrhythmias may mask cardiotoxicity associated with excessive digoxin levels.
QT interval, drugs prolonging	Increased proarrhythmia potential with drugs that prolong the QT interval (eg, phenothiazines, TCAs).

Class IV Antiarrhythmic (Calcium Channel Blockers)

Diltiazem HCl Injection	
Anesthetics	Potentiates depression of cardiac contractility, conductivity, automaticity, and vascular dilation with anesthetics.
Benzodiazepines	Increases AUC of midazolam, triazolam; may require dose adjustment due to increased clinical effects or increased adverse events.
β-Blockers, IV	Avoid IV β-blockers.
β-Blockers, oral	Possible bradycardia, AV block, and contractility depression with oral β-blockers.
Buspirone	Increases AUC of buspirone; which may require a dose adjustment due to increased clinical effects or increased adverse events.
Carbamazepine	Elevates carbamazepine levels, which may result in toxicity; monitor closely.
Cardiac function, drugs affecting	Caution with drugs that decrease peripheral resistance, intravascular volume, myocardial contractility, or conduction.
Cimetidine	Increases levels of diltiazem with cimetidine.

Table 14.2. DRUG INTERACTIONS FOR CARDIOVASCULAR DRUGS *(cont.)*

ANTIARRHYTHMICS *(cont.)*

Class IV Antiarrhythmic (Calcium Channel Blockers)

Diltiazem HCl Injection *(cont.)*	
Cyclosporine	Increases levels of cyclosporine; may need dose adjustment, monitor closely.
CYP3A4 inducers	Avoid with CYP3A4 inducers (eg, rifampin).
CYP450 substrates	Possible competitive inhibition of metabolism with drugs metabolized by CYP450.
Digoxin	Monitor for excessive slowing of HR and/or AV block with digoxin.
Lovastatin	Increases AUC of lovastatin; may require dose adjustment due to increased clinical effects or increased adverse events.
Propranolol	Increases levels of propranolol; monitor closely.
Quinidine	Increases AUC of quinidine; may require dose adjustment due to increased clinical effects or increased adverse events; monitor closely.
Rifampin, IV	Avoid IV rifampin.

Miscellaneous Antiarrhythmic

Adenosine (Adenocard)	
Carbamazepine	Possible higher degrees of heart block with carbamazepine.
Digoxin	Caution with digoxin; ventricular fibrillation reported and potential for additive synergistic depressant effects on SA and AV nodes.
Dipyridamole	Potentiated by dipyridamole; use lower adenosine dose.
Methylxanthines	Antagonized by methylxanthines (eg, theophylline, caffeine); may need larger adenosine dose.
Verapamil	Caution with verapamil; ventricular fibrillation reported and potential for additive/synergistic depressant effects on SA and AV nodes.

ANTIHYPERTENSIVES/HEART FAILURE AGENTS

ACE Inhibitors

Benazepril HCl (Lotensin)	
Diuretics	Risk of hypotension.
Lithium	May reduce excretion of lithium; monitor lithium levels.
Potassium	Increases risk of hyperkalemia with K^+ supplements, K^+-sparing diuretics, or K^+-containing salt substitutes.
Captopril (Capoten)	
Antihypertensives	Augmented effect by antihypertensives that cause renin release (eg, thiazides).
Diuretics	Risk of hypotension.
Lithium	May reduce excretion of lithium; monitor lithium levels.
NSAIDs	May further decrease renal dysfunction with NSAIDs. NSAIDs may diminish antihypertensive effect.

ANTIHYPERTENSIVES/HEART FAILURE AGENTS *(cont.)*

ACE Inhibitors

Captopril (Capoten) *(cont.)*	
Potassium	Increases risk of hyperkalemia with K^+ supplements, K^+-sparing diuretics, or K^+-containing salt substitutes.
Vasodilators	Caution with vasodilators or agents affecting sympathetic activity.
Enalapril Maleate (Vasotec), **Enalaprilat** (Vasotec IV)	
Antihypertensives	Augmented effect by antihypertensives that cause renin release (eg, thiazides).
Diuretics	Risk of hypotension.
Lithium	May reduce excretion of lithium; monitor lithium levels.
NSAIDs	May further decrease renal dysfunction with NSAIDs. NSAIDs may diminish antihypertensive effect.
Potassium	Increases risk of hyperkalemia with K^+ supplements, K^+-sparing diuretics, or K^+-containing salt substitutes.
Fosinopril Sodium (Monopril)	
Antacids	Decreased absorption with antacids; space dosing by 2 hrs.
Diuretics	Risk of hypotension.
Lithium	May reduce excretion of lithium; monitor lithium levels.
Potassium	Increases risk of hyperkalemia with K^+ supplements, K^+-sparing diuretics, or K^+-containing salt substitutes.
Lisinopril (Prinivil)	
Antidiabetic medications	Concomitant use with antidiabetic medications may increase risk of hypoglycemia.
Diuretics	Risk of hypotension.
Gold, injectable	Nitritoid reactions have been reported rarely in patients on therapy with injectable gold and concomitant ACE inhibitor therapy.
Lithium	May reduce excretion of lithium; monitor lithium levels.
NSAIDs	Coadministration with NSAIDs (eg, indomethacin) in patients with compromised renal function may further deteriorate renal function. NSAIDs may diminish antihypertensive effects.
Potassium	Increases risk of hyperkalemia with K^+ supplements, K^+-sparing diuretics, or K^+-containing salt substitutes.
Moexipril HCl (Univasc)	
Diuretics	Risk of hypotension with diuretics.
Lithium	May reduce excretion of lithium; monitor lithium levels.
Potassium	Increases risk of hyperkalemia with K^+ supplements, K^+-sparing diuretics, or K^+-containing salt substitutes.
Perindopril Erbumine (Aceon)	
Diuretics	Risk of hypotension.
Gentamicin	Caution with gentamicin.

Table 14.2. DRUG INTERACTIONS FOR CARDIOVASCULAR DRUGS *(cont.)*

ANTIHYPERTENSIVES/HEART FAILURE AGENTS *(cont.)*

ACE Inhibitors

Perindopril Erbumine (Aceon) *(cont.)*	
Lithium	May reduce excretion of lithium; monitor lithium levels.
Potassium	Increases risk of hyperkalemia with K^+ supplements, K^+-sparing diuretics, or K^+-containing salt substitutes.
Quinapril HCl (Accupril)	
Diuretics	Risk of hypotension.
Lithium	May reduce excretion of lithium; monitor lithium levels.
Magnesium	Consider interaction with drugs that interact with magnesium.
Potassium	Increases risk of hyperkalemia with K^+ supplements, K^+-sparing diuretics, K^+-containing salt substitutes.
Tetracycline	Decreases tetracycline absorption (possibly due to magnesium content in quinapril).
Ramipril (Altace)	
Diuretics	Risk of hypotension with diuretics.
Lithium	May reduce excretion of lithium; monitor lithium levels.
NSAIDs	May further decrease renal dysfunction with NSAIDs. NSAIDs may diminish antihypertensive effect.
Potassium	Increases risk of hyperkalemia with K^+ supplements, K^+-sparing diuretics, or K^+-containing salt substitutes.
Trandolapril (Mavik)	
Diuretics	Risk of hypotension.
Lithium	May reduce excretion of lithium; monitor lithium levels.
Potassium	Increases risk of hyperkalemia with K^+-sparing diuretics, K^+ supplements, or K^+-containing salt substitutes.

ACE Inhibitors/Calcium Channel Blockers

Benazepril HCl/Amlodipine Besylate (Lotrel)	
Diuretics	Risk of hypotension.
Lithium	May reduce excretion of lithium; monitor lithium levels.
Potassium	Increases risk of hyperkalemia with K^+ supplements, K^+-sparing diuretics, or K^+-containing salt substitutes.
Vasodilators, peripheral	Caution with other peripheral vasodilators.
Trandolapril/Verapamil HCl (Tarka)	
Alcohol	May increase alcohol blood levels and prolong effects.
Anesthetics, inhaled	Caution with inhalation anesthetics.
Antihypertensives	Potentiates other antihypertensives.
β-Blockers	Additive effects on HR, AV conduction, and contractility with β-blockers.
Carbamazepine	May increase carbamazepine levels.

ANTIHYPERTENSIVES/HEART FAILURE AGENTS *(cont.)*

ACE INHIBITORS/CALCIUM CHANNEL BLOCKERS

Trandolapril/Verapamil HCl (Tarka) *(cont.)*	
Cyclosporine	May increase cyclosporine levels.
Digoxin	May increase digoxin levels.
Disopyramide	Avoid disopyramide within 48 hrs before or 24 hrs after verapamil.
Flecainide	Additive negative inotropic effects and AV conduction prolongation with flecainide.
Lithium	Monitor lithium.
Neuromuscular blockers	May potentiate neuromuscular blockers; both agents may need dose reduction.
Phenobarbital	Increases clearance with phenobarbital.
Potassium	Increases risk of hyperkalemia with K^+ supplements, K^+-sparing diuretics, or K^+-containing salt substitutes.
Quinidine	Avoid quinidine with hypertrophic cardiomyopathy.
Rifampin	Rifampin may reduce oral bioavailability.
Theophylline	May increase theophylline levels.

ACE INHIBITORS/DIURETICS

Benazepril HCl/Hydrochlorothiazide (Lotensin HCT)	
ACTH	ACTH depletes electrolytes.
Cholestyramine	Reduced absorption with cholestyramine.
Colestipol	Reduced absorption with colestipol.
Corticosteroids	Corticosteroids deplete electrolytes.
Insulin	Insulin may need adjustment.
Lithium	May reduce excretion of lithium; monitor lithium levels.
Norepinephrine	May decrease arterial responsiveness to norepinephrine.
NSAIDs	NSAIDs reduce effects.
Potassium	Increases risk of hyperkalemia with K^+ supplements, K^+-sparing diuretics, or K^+-containing salt substitutes.
Tubocurarine	May increase responsiveness to tubocurarine.

Captopril/Hydrochlorothiazide (Capozide)	
ACTH	ACTH depletes electrolytes.
Alcohol	Potentiates orthostatic hypotension.
Amphotericin B	Amphotericin B, corticosteroids, ACTH deplete electrolytes.
Anesthetics	May potentiate anesthetics.
Anticoagulants	Adjust anticoagulants.
Antidiabetic drugs	Adjust antidiabetic drugs.
Antigout drugs	Adjust antigout drugs.

Table 14.2. DRUG INTERACTIONS FOR CARDIOVASCULAR DRUGS *(cont.)*

ANTIHYPERTENSIVES/HEART FAILURE AGENTS *(cont.)*

ACE Inhibitors/Diuretics

Captopril/Hydrochlorothiazide (Capozide) *(cont.)*	
Antihypertensives	Adjust other antihypertensives.
Barbiturates	Potentiates orthostatic hypotension.
Calcium salts	Monitor serum calcium levels.
Cardiac glycosides	Monitor potassium levels.
Cholestyramine	Reduced absorption with cholestyramine.
Colestipol	Reduced absorption with colestipol.
Corticosteroids	Corticosteroids deplete electrolytes.
Diazoxide	Diazoxide enhances hyperglycemic, hyperuricemic, and antihypertensive effects.
Lithium	May reduce excretion of lithium; monitor lithium levels.
Methenamine	May decrease methenamine effects.
MAOIs	Enhanced hypotensive effects with MAOIs.
Narcotics	Potentiates orthostatic hypotension with narcotics.
NSAIDs	NSAIDs (eg, indomethacin) reduce effects.
Potassium	Increases risk of hyperkalemia with K^+ supplements, K^+-sparing diuretics, or K^+-containing salt substitutes.
Pressor amines	May decrease response to pressor amines.
Probenecid	Probenecid may need dose increase.
Skeletal muscle relaxants, non-depolarizing	May potentiate non-depolarizing skeletal muscle relaxants.
Sulfinpyrazone	Sulfinpyrazone may need dose increase.
Sympathetic activity, agents affecting	Caution with agents affecting sympathetic activity.
Vasodilators	D/C vasodilators before therapy. Caution and decrease vasodilator dose if resumed during therapy.
Enalapril Maleate/Hydrochlorothiazide (Vaseretic)	
ACTH	ACTH depletes electrolytes.
Alcohol	Potentiates orthostatic hypotension with alcohol.
Antidiabetic drugs	Adjust insulin and antidiabetic drugs.
Antihypertensives	Potentiates other antihypertensives.
Barbiturates	Potentiates orthostatic hypotension with barbiturates.
Cholestyramine	Reduced absorption with cholestyramine.
Colestipol	Reduced absorption with colestipol.
Corticosteroids	Corticosteroids deplete electrolytes.

ANTIHYPERTENSIVES/HEART FAILURE AGENTS *(cont.)*

ACE Inhibitors/Diuretics

Enalapril Maleate/Hydrochlorothiazide (Vaseretic) *(cont.)*	
Lithium	May reduce excretion of lithium; monitor lithium levels.
Narcotics	Potentiates orthostatic hypotension with narcotics.
NSAIDs	NSAIDs may reduce antihypertensive effect and worsen renal dysfunction.
Potassium	Increases risk of hyperkalemia with K^+ supplements, K^+-sparing diuretics, or K^+-containing salt substitutes.
Pressor amines	May decrease response to pressor amines.
Skeletal muscle relaxants	May increase responsiveness to skeletal muscle relaxants.
Fosinopril Sodium/Hydrochlorothiazide (Monopril HCT)	
ACTH	ACTH depletes electrolytes.
Antacids	Antacids may impair absorption; space dose by 2 hrs.
Antihypertensives	Caution with other antihypertensives.
Cholestyramine	Reduced absorption with cholestyramine.
Colestipol	Reduced absorption with colestipol.
Insulin	May alter insulin requirements.
Lithium	May reduce excretion of lithium; monitor lithium levels.
Methenamine	May decrease effects of methenamine.
Norepinephrine	May decrease response to norepinephrine.
NSAIDs	NSAIDs reduce effects.
Potassium	Increases risk of hyperkalemia with K^+ supplements, K^+-sparing diuretics, or K^+-containing salt substitutes.
Tubocurarine	May increase responsiveness to tubocurarine.
Lisinopril/Hydrochlorothiazide (Prinzide, Zestoretic)	
ACTH	ACTH depletes electrolytes.
Alcohol	Potentiates orthostatic hypotension.
Antidiabetic drugs	Adjust antidiabetic drugs.
Antihypertensives	Potentiates other antihypertensives.
Barbiturates	Potentiates orthostatic hypotension with barbiturates.
Cholestyramine	Reduced absorption with cholestyramine.
Colestipol	Reduced absorption with colestipol.
Corticosteroids	Corticosteroids deplete electrolytes.
Diuretics	Patients on diuretics may experience an excessive reduction of blood pressure.
Gold, injectable	Nitritoid reactions have been reported rarely in patients on therapy with injectable gold and concomitant ACE inhibitor therapy.
Lithium	May reduce excretion of lithium; monitor lithium levels.

Table 14.2. DRUG INTERACTIONS FOR CARDIOVASCULAR DRUGS *(cont.)*

ANTIHYPERTENSIVES/HEART FAILURE AGENTS *(cont.)*

ACE Inhibitors/Diuretics

Lisinopril/Hydrochlorothiazide (Prinzide, Zestoretic) *(cont.)*	
Narcotics	Potentiates orthostatic hypotension.
NSAIDs	NSAIDs reduce effects and worsen renal dysfunction.
Potassium	Increases risk of hyperkalemia with K^+ supplements, K^+-sparing diuretics, or K^+-containing salt substitutes.
Pressor amines	May decrease response to pressor amines.
Skeletal muscle relaxants	May increase responsiveness to skeletal muscle relaxants.
Moexipril HCl/Hydrochlorothiazide (Uniretic)	
ACTH	ACTH depletes electrolytes.
Alcohol	Potentiates orthostatic hypotension.
Antidiabetic drugs	Adjust antidiabetic drugs.
Antihypertensives	Potentiates other antihypertensives.
Barbiturates	Potentiates orthostatic hypotension.
Cholestyramine	Reduced absorption with cholestyramine.
Colestipol	Reduced absorption with colestipol.
Corticosteroids	Corticosteroids deplete electrolytes.
Guanabenz	Increases absorption of HCTZ with guanabenz.
Lithium	May reduce excretion of lithium; monitor lithium levels.
Narcotics	Potentiates orthostatic hypotension.
NSAIDs	NSAIDs reduce effects.
Potassium	Increases risk of hyperkalemia with K^+ supplements, K^+-sparing diuretics, or K^+-containing salt substitutes.
Pressor amines	May decrease response to pressor amines.
Propantheline	Increases absorption of HCTZ with propantheline.
Skeletal muscle relaxants	May increase responsiveness to skeletal muscle relaxants.
Quinapril HCl/Hydrochlorothiazide (Accuretic)	
ACTH	ACTH depletes electrolytes.
Alcohol	Potentiates orthostatic hypotension.
Antidiabetic drugs	Adjust insulin and antidiabetic drugs.
Antihypertensives	Potentiates other antihypertensives.
Barbiturates	Potentiates orthostatic hypotension with barbiturates.
Cholestyramine	Impaired absorption with cholestyramine.
Colestipol	Impaired absorption with colestipol.
Corticosteroids	Corticosteroids deplete electrolytes.
Lithium	May reduce excretion of lithium; monitor lithium levels.
Narcotics	Potentiates orthostatic hypotension.
NSAIDs	NSAIDs decrease diuretic effects.

ANTIHYPERTENSIVES/HEART FAILURE AGENTS *(cont.)*

ACE Inhibitors/Diuretics

Quinapril HCl/Hydrochlorothiazide (Accuretic) *(cont.)*	
Potassium	Increases risk of hyperkalemia with K^+ supplements, K^+-sparing diuretics, or K^+-containing salt substitutes.
Pressor amines	May decrease response to pressor amines.
Skeletal muscle relaxants	May increase responsiveness to skeletal muscle relaxants.
Tetracycline	Decreases tetracycline absorption (possibly due to magnesium content in quinapril); consider interaction with drugs that interact with magnesium.

α-Adrenergic Blockers

Doxazosin Mesylate (Cardura)	
Antihypertensives	Additive antihypertensive effects with other antihypertensive agents.
PDE-5 inhibitors	Concomitant use may result in additive BP lowering effects and symptomatic hypotension.
Phenoxybenzamine HCl (Dibenzyline)	
Adrenergic receptors, α and β stimulators	Exaggerated hypotensive response and tachycardia with agents that stimulate both α- and β-adrenergic receptors (eg, epinephrine).
Levarterenol	Blocks hyperthermia production by levarterenol.
Reserpine	Blocks hypothermia production by reserpine.
Prazosin HCl (Minipress)	
Alcohol	Dizziness or syncope may occur.
Antihypertensives	Additive hypotensive effects with diuretics, β-blockers, or other antihypertensives.
Terazosin HCl (Hytrin)	
Antihypertensives	Additive hypotensive effects with other antihypertensives; may need dose reduction or retitration of either agent.
Verapamil	Increases levels with verapamil.

α-Adrenergic agonists, Centrally Acting

Clonidine (Catapres, Catapres-TTS)	
Sedatives	May potentiate CNS depression with alcohol, barbiturates, or other sedatives.
Sinus/AV node function, agents affecting	Additive bradycardia and AV block with agents that affect sinus node function or AV nodal conduction (eg, digitalis, CCBs, and β-blockers).
Tricyclic antidepressants (TCAs)	Hypotensive effect reduced by TCAs.
Guanfacine HCl (Tenex)	
CNS depressants	Additive sedation with other CNS depressants.
CYP450 inducers	Caution with CYP450 inducers (eg, phenobarbital, phenytoin) in renal dysfunction.
Methyldopa, Methyldopate HCl	
Anesthetics	Anesthetics may need dose reduction.
Antihypertensives	May potentiate other antihypertensives.
Ferrous products	Ferrous sulfate and ferrous gluconate may decrease bioavailability; avoid coadministration.

Table 14.2. DRUG INTERACTIONS FOR CARDIOVASCULAR DRUGS *(cont.)*

ANTIHYPERTENSIVES/HEART FAILURE AGENTS *(cont.)*

α-Adrenergic agonists, Centrally Acting

Methyldopa, Methyldopate HCl *(cont.)*	
Lithium	Monitor for lithium toxicity.
MAOIs	Contraindicated for patients on therapy with MAOIs.

α-Adrenergic Agonists, Centrally Acting/Diuretics

Clonidine HCl/Chlorthalidone (Clorpres)	
Alcohol	Orthostatic hypotension aggravated by alcohol.
Amitriptyline	Amitriptyline may enhance ocular toxicity.
Antidiabetic agents	Antidiabetic agents may need adjustment.
Antihypertensives	Potentiates other antihypertensives.
Barbiturates	Orthostatic hypotension aggravated by barbiturates.
Lithium	May reduce excretion of lithium; monitor lithium levels.
Narcotics	Orthostatic hypotension aggravated by narcotics.
Norepinephrine	May decrease arterial response to norepinephrine.
Sedatives	Enhanced CNS-depressive effects of alcohol, barbiturates, or other sedatives.
Tricyclic antidepressants (TCAs)	TCAs may reduce effects of clonidine.
Tubocurarine	May increase response to tubocurarine.
Methyldopa/Hydrochlorothiazide	
ACTH	ACTH intensifies electrolyte depletion.
Alcohol	Potentiates orthostatic hypotension.
Anesthetics	Reduce dose of anesthetics.
Antidiabetic drugs	Adjust antidiabetic drugs.
Antihypertensives	May potentiate antihypertensives.
Barbiturates	Potentiates orthostatic hypotension.
Cholestyramine	Impaired absorption with cholestyramine.
Colestipol	Impaired absorption with colestipol.
Corticosteroids	Corticosteroids intensify electrolyte depletion.
Ferrous products	Ferrous sulfate and ferrous gluconate may decrease bioavailability; avoid coadministration.
Lithium	Lithium toxicity.
MAOIs	Contraindicated for patients on therapy with MAOIs.
Narcotics	Potentiates orthostatic hypotension.
NSAIDs	NSAIDs decrease diuretic effects.
Pressor amines	May decrease response to pressor amines.
Skeletal muscle relaxants, nondepolarizing	May potentiate nondepolarizing skeletal muscle relaxants.

ANTIHYPERTENSIVES/HEART FAILURE AGENTS *(cont.)*

Angiotensin II Receptor Blockers (ARBs)

Candesartan Cilexetil (Atacand)	
Lithium	Increases lithium levels.
Eprosartan Mesylate (Teveten)	
Diuretics	Risk of hypotension.
Irbesartan (Avapro)	
Nifedipine	Nifedipine may inhibit the formation of an oxidized metabolite.
Sulphenazole	Sulphenazole may inhibit the formation of an oxidized metabolite.
Tolbutamide	Tolbutamide may inhibit the formation of an oxidized metabolite.
Losartan Potassium (Cozaar)	
Lithium	May reduce excretion of lithium; monitor lithium levels.
NSAIDs	Combination with NSAIDs, including COX-2 inhibitors, may lead to further deterioration of renal function and diminish antihypertensive effect.
Potassium	Concomitant use of K^+ supplements, K^+-sparing diuretics, or K^+-containing salt substitutes may increase serum K^+ levels; may increase SrCr in heart failure patients.
Olmesartan Medoxomil (Benicar)	
Diuretics	Risk of hypotension with high-dose diuretics.
Telmisartan (Micardis)	
Digoxin	Increases digoxin levels.
Warfarin	May alter warfarin levels.
Valsartan (Diovan)	
Potassium	Concomitant use of K^+ supplements, K^+-sparing diuretics, or K^+-containing salt substitutes may increase serum K^+ levels; may increase SrCr in heart failure patients.

Angiotensin II Receptor Blockers/Calcium Channel Blockers

Valsartan/Amlodipine Besylate (Exforge)	
Potassium	Concomitant use of K^+ supplements, K^+-sparing diuretics, or K^+-containing salt substitutes may increase serum K^+ levels; may increase SrCr in heart failure patients.

Angiotensin II Receptor Blockers/Diuretics

Candesartan Cilexetil/Hydrochlorothiazide (Atacand HCT)	
ACTH	ACTH depletes electrolytes.
Alcohol	Potentiates orthostatic hypotension.
Antidiabetic drugs	Insulin and antidiabetic agents may require dosage adjustment.
Antihypertensives	Potentiates other antihypertensives.
Barbiturates	Potentiates orthostatic hypotension.
Cholestyramine	Impaired absorption with cholestyramine.
Colestipol	Impaired absorption with colestipol.

Table 14.2. DRUG INTERACTIONS FOR CARDIOVASCULAR DRUGS *(cont.)*

ANTIHYPERTENSIVES/HEART FAILURE AGENTS *(cont.)*

ANGIOTENSIN II RECEPTOR BLOCKERS/DIURETICS

Candesartan Cilexetil/Hydrochlorothiazide (Atacand HCT) *(cont.)*	
Corticosteroids	Corticosteroids deplete electrolytes.
Lithium	Risk of lithium toxicity; monitor lithium levels during concomitant use.
Narcotics	Potentiates orthostatic hypotension.
NSAIDs	NSAIDs decrease diuretic effects.
Pressor amines	May decrease response to pressor amines.
Skeletal muscle relaxants	May increase responsiveness to skeletal muscle relaxants.
Eprosartan Mesylate/Hydrochlorothiazide (Teveten HCT)	
ACTH	ACTH depletes electrolytes.
Alcohol	Potentiates orthostatic hypotension with alcohol.
Antidiabetic drugs	Insulin and antidiabetic agents may require dosage adjustment.
Antihypertensives	Potentiates other antihypertensives.
Barbiturates	Potentiates orthostatic hypotension.
Cholestyramine	Impaired absorption with cholestyramine.
Colestipol	Impaired absorption with colestipol.
Corticosteroids	Corticosteroids deplete electrolytes.
Lithium	Risk of lithium toxicity; avoid use.
Narcotics	Potentiates orthostatic hypotension with narcotics.
NSAIDs	NSAIDs may decrease diuretic/antihypertensive effects.
Potassium	Increases risk of hyperkalemia with K^+ supplements, K^+-sparing diuretics, or K^+-containing salt substitutes.
Pressor amines	May decrease response to pressor amines (eg, norepinephrine).
Skeletal muscle relaxants, non-depolarizing	May increase responsiveness to non-depolarizing skeletal muscle relaxants (eg, tubocurarine).
Irbesartan/Hydrochlorothiazide (Avalide)	
ACTH	ACTH depletes electrolytes.
Alcohol	Potentiates orthostatic hypotension.
Antidiabetic agents	Insulin and oral antidiabetic agents may require dosage adjustment.
Antihypertensives	Potentiates other antihypertensives.
Barbiturates	Potentiates orthostatic hypotension.
Cholestyramine	Impaired absorption with cholestyramine.
Colestipol	Impaired absorption with colestipol.
Corticosteroids	Corticosteroids deplete electrolytes.
Lithium	May reduce excretion of lithium; monitor lithium levels.
Narcotics	Potentiates orthostatic hypotension.

ANTIHYPERTENSIVES/HEART FAILURE AGENTS *(cont.)*

Angiotensin II Receptor Blockers/Diuretics

Irbesartan/Hydrochlorothiazide (Avalide) *(cont.)*	
NSAIDs	NSAIDs may decrease diuretic effects.
Pressor amines	May decrease response to pressor amines.
Skeletal muscle relaxants	May increase responsiveness to skeletal muscle relaxants.
Losartan Potassium/Hydrochlorothiazide (Hyzaar)	
ACTH	ACTH depletes electrolytes.
Alcohol	Potentiates orthostatic hypotension.
Antidiabetic drugs	Insulin and antidiabetic agents may require dosage adjustment.
Antihypertensives	Potentiates other antihypertensives.
Barbiturates	Potentiates orthostatic hypotension.
Cholestyramine	Impaired absorption with cholestyramine.
Colestipol	Impaired absorption with colestipol.
Corticosteroids	Corticosteroids deplete electrolytes.
Fluconazole	Increases levels with fluconazole.
Lithium	May reduce excretion of lithium; monitor lithium levels.
Narcotics	Potentiates orthostatic hypotension with narcotics.
NSAIDs	NSAIDs, including COX-2 inhibitors, may decrease effects and may result in a further deterioration of renal function in the renally impaired.
Potassium	Increases risk of hyperkalemia with K^+ supplements, K^+-sparing diuretics, or K^+-containing salt substitutes.
Pressor amines	May decrease response to pressor amines (eg, norepinephrine).
Rifampin	Decreased levels with rifampin.
Skeletal muscle relaxants	May increase responsiveness to skeletal muscle relaxants (eg, tubocurarine).
Olmesartan Medoxomil/Hydrochlorothiazide (Benicar HCT)	
ACTH	ACTH depletes electrolytes.
Alcohol	Potentiates orthostatic hypotension.
Antidiabetic drugs	Antidiabetic agents may require dosage adjustment.
Antihypertensives	Potentiates other antihypertensives.
Barbiturates	Potentiates orthostatic hypotension.
Cholestyramine	Impaired absorption with cholestyramine.
Colestipol	Impaired absorption with colestipol.
Corticosteroids	Corticosteroids deplete electrolytes.
Lithium	May reduce excretion of lithium; monitor lithium levels.
Narcotics	Potentiates orthostatic hypotension.
NSAIDs	NSAIDs decrease diuretic effects.

Table 14.2. DRUG INTERACTIONS FOR CARDIOVASCULAR DRUGS *(cont.)*

ANTIHYPERTENSIVES/HEART FAILURE AGENTS *(cont.)*

Angiotensin II Receptor Blockers/Diuretics

Olmesartan Medoxomil/Hydrochlorothiazide (Benicar HCT) *(cont.)*	
Pressor amines	May decrease response to pressor amines.
Skeletal muscle relaxants, non-depolarizing	May increase responsiveness to non-depolarizing skeletal muscle relaxants.
Telmisartan/Hydrochlorothiazide (Micardis HCT)	
ACTH	ACTH depletes electrolytes.
Alcohol	Potentiates orthostatic hypotension.
Antidiabetic drugs	Insulin and antidiabetic agents may require dosage adjustment.
Antihypertensives	Potentiates other antihypertensives.
Barbiturates	Potentiates orthostatic hypotension.
Cholestyramine	Impaired absorption with cholestyramine.
Colestipol	Impaired absorption with colestipol.
Corticosteroids	Corticosteroids deplete electrolytes.
Digoxin	Increases digoxin levels.
Lithium	May reduce excretion of lithium; monitor lithium levels.
Narcotics	Potentiates orthostatic hypotension.
NSAIDs	NSAIDs decrease diuretic effects.
Pressor amines	May decrease response to pressor amines.
Skeletal muscle relaxants	May increase responsiveness to skeletal muscle relaxants.
Warfarin	May alter warfarin levels.
Valsartan/Hydrochlorothiazide (Diovan HCT)	
ACTH	ACTH depletes electrolytes.
Alcohol	Potentiates orthostatic hypotension.
Antidiabetic agents	Insulin and oral antidiabetic agents may require dosage adjustment.
Antihypertensives	Potentiates other antihypertensives.
Barbiturates	Potentiates orthostatic hypotension.
Cholestyramine	Impaired absorption with cholestyramine.
Colestipol	Impaired absorption with colestipol.
Corticosteroids	Corticosteroids deplete electrolytes.
Lithium	Risk of lithium toxicity; avoid concurrent use.
Narcotics	Potentiates orthostatic hypotension.
NSAIDs	NSAIDs may decrease diuretic effects; monitor closely.
Pressor amines	May decrease response to pressor amines.
Skeletal muscle relaxants	May increase responsiveness to skeletal muscle relaxants.

ANTIHYPERTENSIVES/HEART FAILURE AGENTS *(cont.)*

β_1-BLOCKERS, CARDIOSELECTIVE

Acebutolol HCl (Sectral)	
α Stimulants	Exaggerated hypertensive responses with α stimulants.
Catecholamine-depleting drugs	Possible additive effects.
Epinephrine	May antagonize epinephrine.
Insulin	May potentiate insulin-induced hypoglycemia.
NSAIDs	NSAIDs may reduce effects.
Atenolol (Tenormin)	
Amiodarone	Additive effects.
Calcium channel blockers (CCBs)	Additive effects. Bradycardia, heart block, and LVEDP can rise with verapamil or diltiazem.
Catecholamine-depleting drugs	Additive effects with catecholamine-depleting drugs (eg, reserpine).
Clonidine	Exacerbates rebound HTN with clonidine withdrawal.
Digitalis	Additive effects. Concomitant use with digitalis glycosides may increase risk of bradycardia.
Disopyramide	Use with disopyramide may be associated with severe bradycardia, asystole, and heart failure.
Epinephrine	May block epinephrine effects.
Myocardium, drugs depressing	Caution with drugs that depress myocardium (eg, anesthesia).
Prostaglandin synthase inhibitors	Prostaglandin synthase inhibitors (eg, indomethacin) may decrease hypotensive effects.
Betaxolol HCl (Kerlone)	
Calcium channel blockers (CCBs), oral	Avoid oral CCBs with cardiac dysfunction; may increase cardiac adverse effects.
Catecholamine-depleting drugs	Possible additive effects with catecholamine-depleting drugs (eg, reserpine).
Clonidine	D/C gradually before clonidine withdrawal.
Epinephrine	May block epinephrine effects.
Bisoprolol Fumarate (Zebeta)	
Anesthetics	Caution with anesthetics that depress myocardial function.
Antiarrhythmics	Caution with antiarrhythmic agents (eg, disopyramide).
Antidiabetic agents	Antidiabetic agents may need adjustment.
β-Blockers	Avoid other β-blockers.
Calcium channel blockers (CCBs)	Caution when used with CCBs (eg, verapamil, diltiazem).
Catecholamine-depleting drugs	Excessive reduction of sympathetic activity.
Clonidine	Caution with clonidine withdrawal.

Table 14.2. DRUG INTERACTIONS FOR CARDIOVASCULAR DRUGS *(cont.)*

ANTIHYPERTENSIVES/HEART FAILURE AGENTS *(cont.)*

β1-BLOCKERS, CARDIOSELECTIVE

Bisoprolol Fumarate (Zebeta) *(cont.)*	
Epinephrine	May block epinephrine effects.
Rifampin	Rifampin increases clearance.
Metoprolol Succinate (Toprol-XL), **Metoprolol Tartrate** (Lopressor)	
Calcium channel blockers (CCBs)	Caution when used with CCBs of the verapamil and diltiazem type.
Catecholamine-depleting drugs	Additive effects with catecholamine-depleting drugs (eg, reserpine, MAOIs).
Clonidine	May exacerbate rebound HTN following clonidine withdrawal.
CYP2D6 inhibitors	CYP2D6 inhibitors (eg, quinidine, fluoxetine, paroxetine, propafenone) may increase levels.
Digitalis glycosides	Concomitant use of digitalis glycosides and β-blockers can increase the risk of bradycardia.
Epinephrine	May block epinephrine effects.
Nebivolol (Bystolic)	
Anesthetics	May depress myocardial function with anesthetic agents (eg, ether, cyclopropane, trichloroethylene); monitor closely.
Antiarrhythmics	Caution with antiarrhythmic agents (eg, disopyramide).
Calcium antagonists	Caution with calcium antagonists (particularly verapamil and diltiazem type).
Catecholamine-depleting drugs	Excessive reduction of sympathetic activity may occur with catecholamine-depleting drugs (eg, reserpine, guanethidine); monitor closely.
Clonidine	D/C for several days before gradually tapering clonidine.
CYP2D6 inhibitors	CYP2D6 inhibitors (eg, fluoxetine, quinidine, propafenone, paroxetine) may increase nebivolol levels; monitor and consider dosage adjustment.
Diabetic agents	May potentiate hypoglycemic effect of glucose-lowering agents (eg, insulin, oral hypoglycemic agents); use with caution.
Sildenafil	Sildenafil may decrease nebivolol levels.

β1-BLOCKERS, CARDIOSELECTIVE/DIURETICS

Atenolol/Chlorthalidone (Tenoretic)	
ACTH	Possible hypokalemia with ACTH.
Amiodarone	Additive negative chronotropic effects.
Anesthetics	Caution with anesthetic agents.
Calcium channel blockers	Bradycardia, heart block, and LVEDP can rise with verapamil or diltiazem.
Catecholamine-depleting drugs	Additive effects with catecholamine-depleting drugs (eg, reserpine), CCBs, and digitalis.
Clonidine	Exacerbates rebound HTN with clonidine withdrawal.
Corticosteroids	Possible hypokalemia.

ANTIHYPERTENSIVES/HEART FAILURE AGENTS *(cont.)*

β_1-Blockers, Cardioselective/Diuretics

Atenolol/Chlorthalidone (Tenoretic) *(cont.)*	
Disopyramide	Coadministration with disopyramide has been associated with severe bradycardia, asystole, and heart failure.
Epinephrine	May block epinephrine effects.
Insulin	May alter insulin requirements.
Lithium	May reduce excretion of lithium; monitor lithium levels.
Norepinephrine	May decrease arterial response to norepinephrine.
Prostaglandin synthase inhibitors	Prostaglandin synthase inhibitors (eg, indomethacin) may decrease hypotensive effects.
Bisoprolol Fumarate/Hydrochlorothiazide (Ziac)	
ACTH	ACTH intensifies electrolyte depletion.
Alcohol	Alcohol may potentiate orthostatic hypotension.
Anesthesia	Caution with anesthesia.
Antiarrhythmics	Caution with antiarrhythmics.
Antidiabetic drugs	Adjust dose of antidiabetic drugs.
Antihypertensives	Potentiates other antihypertensives.
Barbiturates	Barbiturates may potentiate orthostatic hypotension.
β-Blockers	Avoid other β-blockers. β-blockers slow atrioventricular conduction and decrease HR; concomitant use can increase the risk of bradycardia.
Calcium channel blockers (CCBs)	Caution with CCBs.
Catecholamine-depleting drugs	Excessive reduction of sympathetic activity with catecholamine-depleting drugs.
Cholestyramine	Impaired absorption with cholestyramine.
Clonidine	Caution with clonidine withdrawal.
Colestipol	Impaired absorption with colestipol.
Corticosteroids	Corticosteroids intensify electrolyte depletion.
Digitalis glycosides	Digitalis glycosides and β-blockers slow atrioventricular conduction and decrease HR; concomitant use can increase the risk of bradycardia.
Epinephrine	May block epinephrine effects.
Lithium	May reduce excretion of lithium; monitor lithium levels.
Myocardial depressants	Caution with myocardial depressants.
Narcotics	Narcotics may potentiate orthostatic hypotension.
NSAIDs	NSAIDs may reduce effects.
Pressor amines	May decrease response to pressor amines.
Skeletal muscle relaxants, non-depolarizing	May increase response to non-depolarizing muscle relaxants.
Rifampin	Increases clearance with rifampin.

Table 14.2. DRUG INTERACTIONS FOR CARDIOVASCULAR DRUGS *(cont.)*

ANTIHYPERTENSIVES/HEART FAILURE AGENTS *(cont.)*	
β_1-Blockers, Cardioselective/Diuretics	
Metoprolol Tartrate/Hydrochlorothiazide (Lopressor HCT)	
ACTH	ACTH may increase risk of hypokalemia.
Alcohol	Alcohol may potentiate orthostatic hypotension.
Antihypertensives	Potentiates other antihypertensives.
Barbiturates	Barbiturates may potentiate orthostatic hypotension.
Catecholamine-depleting drugs	Additive effects with catecholamine-depleting drugs (eg, reserpine).
Cholestyramine	Impaired absorption with cholestyramine.
Clonidine	Stop metoprolol several days before clonidine; d/c when agents given concurrently.
Colestipol	Impaired absorption with colestipol.
Corticosteroids	Corticosteroids may increase risk of hypokalemia.
CYP2D6 inhibitors	Potent CYP2D6 inhibitors may increase levels.
Digitalis	Caution with digitalis; both agents slow AV conduction.
Epinephrine	May block epinephrine effects.
Insulin	Insulin may need adjustment.
Lithium	May reduce excretion of lithium; monitor lithium levels.
Narcotics	Narcotics may potentiate orthostatic hypotension.
Norepinephrine	May decrease arterial responsiveness to norepinephrine.
NSAIDs	NSAIDs may reduce diuretic effects.
Tubocurarine	May increase responsiveness to tubocurarine.
β-Blockers, Nonselective	
Nadolol (Corgard)	
Anesthetics, general	General anesthetics may exaggerate hypotension.
Antidiabetic agents	Antidiabetic agents may need adjustment.
Catecholamine-depleting drugs	Additive hypotension and/or bradycardia with catecholamine-depleting drugs.
Epinephrine	May block epinephrine effects.
Penbutolol Sulfate (Levatol)	
Alcohol	Caution with alcohol; may depress the myocardium.
Anesthetics	Caution with anesthetics that depress the myocardium.
Calcium channel blockers (CCBs)	Synergistic hypotensive effects, bradycardia, and arrhythmias with oral CCBs.
Catecholamine-depleting drugs	Avoid catecholamine-depleting drugs.
Epinephrine	May antagonize epinephrine.
Lidocaine	Increases volume of distribution of lidocaine; may need larger LD.

ANTIHYPERTENSIVES/HEART FAILURE AGENTS *(cont.)*

β-Blockers, Nonselective

Pindolol (Pindolol)	
Catecholamine-depleting drugs	Additive hypotension and/or bradycardia with catecholamine-depleting drugs.
Thioridazine	Both thioridazine and pindolol levels may increase when used concomitantly.
Propranolol HCl (Inderal, Inderal LA, InnoPran XL)	
ACE inhibitors	ACE inhibitors can cause hypotension and certain ACE inhibitors may increase bronchial hyperactivity.
Aluminum hydroxide	Aluminum hydroxide gel may decrease plasma concentrations.
Anesthetics	Anesthetics (eg, methoxyflurane, trichloroethylene) may depress myocardial contractility.
AV conduction, drugs affecting	Caution with drugs that slow down AV conduction.
β-Agonists	Effects may be reversed by β-agonists (eg, dobutamine, isoproterenol).
Calcium channel blockers (CCBs)	Increases levels with concurrent nisoldipine and nicardipine.
Chlorpromazine	Coadministration with chlorpromazine may increase levels of both drugs.
Cholestyramine	Decreased levels with cholestyramine.
Cigarettes	Decreased levels with cigarette smoking.
Clonidine	May antagonize clonidine effects; caution when withdrawing from clonidine.
Colestipol	Decreased levels with colestipol.
CYP1A2 substrates or inhibitors	Increases propranolol levels/toxicity with CYP1A2 inhibitors (eg, imipramine, cimetidine, ciprofloxacin, fluvoxamine, isoniazid, ritonavir, theophylline, zileuton, zolmitriptan, rizatriptan).
CYP2C19 substrates or inhibitors	Increases propranolol levels/toxicity with CYP2C19 inhibitors (eg, fluconazole, cimetidine, fluoxetine, fluvoxamine, teniposide, tolbutamide).
CYP2D6 substrates or inhibitors	Increases propranolol levels/toxicity with CYP2D6 inhibitors (eg, amiodarone, cimetidine, fluoxetine, paroxetine, quinidine, ritonavir).
Diazepam	Increases concentrations of diazepam and its metabolites with coadministration.
Digitalis glycosides	Increases risk of bradycardia with concomitant digitalis glycosides.
Disopyramide	Severe bradycardia, asystole, and heart failure associated with concomitant disopyramide.
Doxazosin	Coadministration with doxazosin may lead to postural hypotension.
Epinephrine	Uncontrolled HTN may develop with concurrent epinephrine.
Ethanol	Decreased levels with ethanol.
Haloperidol	Hypotension and cardiac arrest reported with haloperidol.
Hepatic enzyme inducers	Decreased blood levels with hepatic enzyme inducers (eg, rifampin, ethanol, phenytoin, phenobarbital, cigarette smoking).
HMG-CoA reductase inhibitors (statins)	Decreases levels of lovastatin and pravastatin.

Table 14.2. DRUG INTERACTIONS FOR CARDIOVASCULAR DRUGS *(cont.)*

ANTIHYPERTENSIVES/HEART FAILURE AGENTS *(cont.)*

β-Blockers, Nonselective

Propranolol HCl (Inderal, Inderal LA, InnoPran XL) *(cont.)*	
Lidocaine	Lidocaine metabolism is inhibited with coadministration.
MAOIs	May exacerbate hypotensive effects of MAOIs.
Nifedipine	Increases levels of nifedipine.
NSAIDs	Antagonized by NSAIDs.
Phenobarbital	Decreased levels with phenobarbital.
Phenytoin	Decreased levels with phenytoin.
Prazosin	Prolonged first-dose hypotension.
Propafenone	Propafenone levels increase with concurrent administration.
Quinidine	Increases levels of propranolol.
Reserpine	Closely monitor for excessive reduction of resting sympathetic nervous activity (eg, hypotension, bradycardia, vertigo, orthostatic hypotension, syncope) with concurrent reserpine; reserpine may also potentiate depression.
Rifampin	Decreased levels with rifampin.
Terazosin	Coadministration with terazosin may lead to postural hypotension.
Theophylline	Decreased theophylline clearance with concurrent administration.
Thioridazine	Increases thioridazine plasma concentrations with concurrent administration of doses ≥160 mg/day.
Thyroxine	May result in lower than expected T_3 level with concomitant thyroxine.
Tricyclic antidepressants (TCAs)	May exacerbate hypotensive effects of TCAs.
Triptans	Zolmitriptan and rizatriptan concentrations increase with concurrent administration.
Warfarin	Concurrent administration increases warfarin levels and PT.
Timolol Maleate	
Calcium antagonists	Hypotension, AV conduction disturbances, left ventricular failure reported with oral calcium antagonists. Caution with IV calcium antagonists. Avoid calcium antagonists with cardiac dysfunction.
Calcium channel blockers (CCBs)	AV conduction time prolonged with either diltiazem or verapamil.
Catecholamine-depleting drugs	Possible additive effects and hypotension and/or marked bradycardia with catecholamine-depleting drugs.
Clonidine	May exacerbate rebound HTN following clonidine withdrawal.
Digitalis	AV conduction time prolonged.
Epinephrine	May block effects of epinephrine.
Hypoglycemics	Caution with insulin, oral hypoglycemics.
NSAIDs	NSAIDs may reduce antihypertensive effects.
Quinidine	Quinidine may potentiate β-blockade.

ANTIHYPERTENSIVES/HEART FAILURE AGENTS *(cont.)*

β-Blockers, Nonselective/α_1-Blockers

Carvedilol (Coreg, Coreg CR)	
Alcohol	Alcohol may affect release properties of extended-release caps; space administration by ≥2 hrs.
Amiodarone	Amiodarone may increase plasma levels, resulting in further slowing of the HR or cardiac conduction.
Anesthetics	Caution with anesthetic agents that may depress myocardial function (eg, cyclopropane, trichloroethylene).
β-Blockers	β-Blockers slow atrioventricular conduction and decrease heart rate. Concomitant use can increase risk of bradycardia.
Calcium channel blockers (CCBs)	Monitor ECG and BP with CCBs (eg, verapamil, diltiazem).
Catecholamine-depleting agents	Monitor for hypotension and bradycardia with catecholamine-depleting agents (eg, reserpine, MAOIs).
Cimetidine	Cimetidine may increase AUC.
Clonidine	Clonidine may potentiate BP- and HR-lowering effects.
Cyclosporine	Monitor with cyclosporine.
CYP2D6 inhibitors	CYP2D6 inhibitors (eg, quinidine, fluoxetine, paroxetine, and propafenone) may increase levels.
Digitalis glycoside	Digitalis glycosides slow atrioventricular conduction and decrease heart rate. Concomitant use can increase the risk of bradycardia.
Digoxin	Monitor with digoxin.
Hypoglycemics, oral	Monitor with oral hypoglycemics.
Insulin	Monitor with insulin.
Rifampin	Rifampin may reduce plasma levels.
Labetalol HCl (Trandate)	
Antidiabetic agents	Antidiabetic agents may need dose adjustment.
β-Agonists	Antagonizes bronchodilator effect of β-agonists.
Calcium antagonists	Caution with calcium antagonists.
Cimetidine	Potentiated by cimetidine; may need to reduce dose.
Epinephrine	May block epinephrine effects.
Halothane	(Inj) Synergistic with halothane; do not use ≥3% halothane.
Nitroglycerin	Synergistic antihypertensive effects blunts the reflex tachycardia with nitroglycerin.
Tricyclic antidepressants (TCAs)	Increases tremors with TCAs.

β-blockers, Nonselective/Diuretics

Nadolol/Bendroflumethiazide (Corzide)	
ACTH	ACTH intensifies electrolyte imbalance.
Alcohol	Alcohol potentiates orthostatic hypotension.

Table 14.2. DRUG INTERACTIONS FOR CARDIOVASCULAR DRUGS *(cont.)*

ANTIHYPERTENSIVES/HEART FAILURE AGENTS *(cont.)*

β-Blockers, Nonselective/Diuretics

Nadolol/Bendroflumethiazide (Corzide) *(cont.)*	
Amphotericin B	Amphotericin B intensifies electrolyte imbalance.
Anesthetics	General anesthetics may exaggerate hypotension. May potentiate preanesthetics and anesthetics.
Anticoagulants	Anticoagulants may need adjustment.
Antidiabetic agents	Antidiabetic agents may need adjustment.
Antigout agents	Antigout agents may need adjustment.
Antihypertensives	Other antihypertensives may need adjustment.
Barbiturates	Barbiturates potentiate orthostatic hypotension.
Calcium salts	Monitor calcium levels with calcium salts.
Catecholamine-depleting drugs	Additive hypotension and/or bradycardia with catecholamine-depleting drugs.
Cholestyramine	Cholestyramine may delay or decrease absorption.
Colestipol	Colestipol may delay or decrease absorption.
Corticosteroids	Corticosteroids intensify electrolyte imbalance.
Diazoxide	Enhanced hyperglycemic, hyperuricemic, and antihypertensive effects with diazoxide.
Digoxin	Monitor digoxin.
Epinephrine	May block epinephrine effects.
Lithium	Lithium toxicity.
Methenamine	Possible decreased effectiveness with methenamine.
MAOIs	Enhanced hypotensive effects with MAOIs.
Narcotics	Narcotics potentiate orthostatic hypotension.
NSAIDs	NSAIDs may decrease effects.
Pressor amines	Decreased arterial responsiveness with pressor amines.
Probenedcid	Probenecid may need dose increase.
Skeletal muscle relaxants, non-depolarizing	May potentiate non-depolarizing muscle relaxants.
Sulfinpyrazone	Sulfinpyrazone may need dose increase.
Propranolol HCl/Hydrochlorothiazide (Inderide)	
ACTH	Risk of hypokalemia with ACTH.
Adrenergic blockers	Potentiation with ganglionic or peripheral adrenergic-blockers.
Alcohol	Alcohol decreases absorption rate and may potentiate orthostatic hypotension. Concomitant use may increase plasma levels of propranolol.
Aluminum hydroxide	Aluminum hydroxide gel reduces intestinal absorption.
Antipyrine	Reduces clearance of antipyrine.

ANTIHYPERTENSIVES/HEART FAILURE AGENTS *(cont.)*

β-Blockers, Nonselective/Diuretics

Propranolol HCl/Hydrochlorothiazide (Inderide) *(cont.)*	
Barbiturates	Barbiturates potentiate orthostatic hypotension.
Calcium channel blockers (CCBs)	May increase cardiac effects of CCBs.
Catecholamine-depleting drugs	Bradycardia/hypotension.
Chlorpromazine	Potentiated by chlorpromazine.
Cimetidine	Potentiated by cimetidine.
Corticosteroids	Risk of hypokalemia.
Digoxin	Monitor digoxin.
Epinephrine	May block epinephrine effects.
Haloperidol	Hypotension and cardiac arrest reported with haloperidol.
Insulin	Insulin dose may need adjustment.
Lidocaine	Reduces clearance of lidocaine.
Narcotics	Narcotics potentiate orthostatic hypotension.
Norepinephrine	May decrease arterial response to norepinephrine.
NSAIDs	Antagonized by NSAIDs.
Phenobarbital	Antagonized by phenobarbital.
Phenytoin	Antagonized by phenytoin.
Rifampin	Antagonized by rifampin.
Theophylline	Reduces clearance of theophylline.
Thyroxine	May block thyroxine effects.
Tubocurarine	May increase response to tubocurarine.

Calcium Channel Blockers

Diltiazem HCl (Cardizem, Cardizem CD, Cardizem LA, Cartia XT, Dilacor XR, Diltia XT, Taztia XT, Tiazac)	
Anesthetics	Potentiates the depression of cardiac contractility, conductivity, automaticity, and vascular dilation with anesthetics.
Benzodiazepines	Increases AUC of midazolam, triazolam; may require a dose adjustment due to increased clinical effects or increased adverse events.
β-Blockers, IV	Avoid IV β-blockers.
β-Blockers, oral	Possible bradycardia, AV block, and contractility depression with oral β-blockers.
Buspirone	Increases AUC of buspirone; may require dose adjustment due to increased clinical effects or increased adverse events.
Carbamazepine	Elevates carbamazepine levels, which may result in toxicity; monitor closely.
Cardiac function, drugs affecting	Caution with drugs that decrease peripheral resistance, intravascular volume, myocardial contractility, or conduction.

Table 14.2. DRUG INTERACTIONS FOR CARDIOVASCULAR DRUGS *(cont.)*

ANTIHYPERTENSIVES/HEART FAILURE AGENTS *(cont.)*

Calcium Channel Blockers

Diltiazem HCl (Cardizem, Cardizem CD, Cardizem LA, Cartia XT, Dilacor XR, Diltia XT, Taztia XT, Tiazac) *(cont.)*	
Cimetidine	Increases levels of diltiazem with cimetidine.
Cyclosporine	Increases levels of cyclosporine; may need dose adjustment, monitor closely.
CYP3A4 inducers	Avoid concurrent use with CYP3A4 inducers (eg, rifampin).
CYP3A4 substrates	May require dosage adjustment with concomitant CYP3A4 substrates.
CYP450 substrates	Possible competitive inhibition of metabolism with drugs metabolized by CYP450.
Digoxin	Monitor for excessive slowing of HR and/or AV block with digoxin.
Lovastatin	Increases AUC of lovastatin; may require dose adjustment due to increased clinical effects or increased adverse events.
Propranolol	Increases levels of propranolol; monitor closely.
Quinidine	Increases AUC of quinidine; may require dose adjustment due to increased clinical effects or increased adverse events; monitor closely.
Felodipine (Plendil)	
Anticonvulsants	Levels decreased with long-term anticonvulsant therapy.
CYP3A4 inhibitors	CYP3A4 inhibitors (eg, itraconazole, ketoconazole, erythromycin, grapefruit juice, cimetidine) may increase plasma levels.
Metoprolol	May increase metoprolol levels.
Tacrolimus	May increase tacrolimus levels.
Isradipine (DynaCirc, DynaCirc CR)	
Antihypertensives	Severe hypotension possible with β-blockers or CCBs.
Cimetidine	Increases mean peak plasma concentration with cimetidine.
Fentanyl	Severe hypotension possible with fentanyl.
Hydrochlorothiazide (HCTZ)	Additive effects with HCTZ.
Propranolol	Increases AUC and C_{max} of propranolol.
Rifampicin	Decreased levels with rifampicin.
Nicardipine HCl (Cardene IV, Cardene SR, Nicardipine)	
Anesthesia, fentanyl	May cause hypotension. Caution with fentanyl anesthesia.
Antihypertensives	Monitor with other antihypertensive agents.
β-Blockers	With β-blocker withdrawal, gradually reduce over 8 to 10 days.
Cimetidine	Increases levels with cimetidine.
Cyclosporine	Elevates cyclosporine levels.
Digoxin	Monitor digoxin levels.
Nifedipine (Adalat CC, Afeditab CR, Procardia XL)	
β-Blockers	β-Blockers may increase risk of CHF, severe hypotension, or angina exacerbation.

ANTIHYPERTENSIVES/HEART FAILURE AGENTS *(cont.)*

CALCIUM CHANNEL BLOCKERS

Nifedipine (Adalat CC, Afeditab CR, Procardia XL) *(cont.)*	
Cimetidine	Cimetidine may increase levels.
Coumarin	Reports of increased prothrombin time (rare). Monitor coumarin levels.
CYP3A4 inducers	CYP3A4 inducers (eg, phenytoin, St. John's wort) may decrease levels.
CYP3A4 inhibitors	CYP3A4 inhibitors (eg, ketoconazole, erythromycin, protease inhibitors) may increase levels.
Digoxin	Reports of elevated digoxin levels (rare). Monitor digoxin levels.
Fentanyl	Severe hypotension possible with fentanyl.
Grapefruit juice	Increases AUC and C_{max}. Avoid grapefruit juice.
Quinidine	May increase heart rate. Monitor quinidine levels.
Nisoldipine (Sular)	
Cimetidine	Increases AUC and C_{max} with cimetidine.
CYP3A4 inducers	Avoid CYP3A4 inducers.
Grapefruit juice	Avoid grapefruit juice; increases AUC and C_{max}.
High-fat meals	Avoid high-fat meals; increase peak drug levels.
Phenytoin	Avoid phenytoin; decreased levels of nisoldipine.
Quinidine	Decreased bioavailability with quinidine.
Verapamil HCl (Calan, Calan SR, Covera-HS, Isoptin SR, Verelan, Verelan PM)	
Alcohol	May increase alcohol levels.
Anesthetic, inhalation	Caution with inhalation anesthetics.
Antihypertensives	Potentiates other antihypertensives.
Aspirin (ASA)	Increases bleeding time with ASA.
β-Blockers	Additive effects on HR, AV conduction, and contractility with β-blockers.
Carbamazepine	May increase carbamazepine levels.
Cyclosporine	May increase cyclosporine levels.
CYP3A4 inducers	CYP3A4 inducers (eg, rifampin, phenobarbital) may decrease levels.
CYP3A4 inhibitors	CYP3A4 inhibitors (eg, erythromycin, ritonavir) and grapefruit juice may increase levels.
Cytotoxic drugs	Reduced absorption with COPP and VAC cytotoxic drug regimens.
Digoxin	May increase digoxin levels.
Disopyramide	Avoid disopyramide within 48 hrs before or 24 hrs after verapamil.
Doxorubicin	Increases efficacy of doxorubicin.
Flecainide	Additive negative inotropic effects and AV conduction prolongation with flecainide.
Lithium	May decrease levels of lithium; may increase sensitivity to effects of lithium. Monitor levels and effects of lithium.

Table 14.2. DRUG INTERACTIONS FOR CARDIOVASCULAR DRUGS *(cont.)*

ANTIHYPERTENSIVES/HEART FAILURE AGENTS *(cont.)*

Calcium Channel Blockers

Verapamil HCl (Calan, Calan SR, Covera-HS, Isoptin SR, Verelan, Verelan PM) *(cont.)*	
Neuromuscular blockers	May potentiate neuromuscular blockers; both agents may need dose reduction.
Paclitaxel	May decrease clearance of paclitaxel.
Quinidine	Avoid quinidine with hypertrophic cardiomyopathy.
Theophylline	May increase theophylline.

Calcium Channel Blockers/HMG-CoA Reductase Inhibitors (Statins)

Amlodipine Besylate/Atorvastatin Calcium (Caduet)	
Azoles	Azole antifungals may increase risk of myopathy.
Colestipol	Colestipol decreases levels when coadministered, but greater LDL-C reduction than when each drug given alone.
Contraceptives, oral	Increases levels of oral contraceptives (norethindrone, ethinyl estradiol).
Cyclosporine	Cyclosporine may increase risk of myopathy.
Digoxin	May increase levels of digoxin. Monitor digoxin levels.
Erythromycin	Increases levels with erythromycin. Erythromycin may increase risk of myopathy.
Fibrates	Avoid fibrates.
Fibric acid derivatives	Fibric acid derivatives may increase risk of myopathy.
Maalox	Decreased levels with Maalox TC, but LDL-C reduction not altered.
Niacin	Niacin may increase risk of myopathy.
Steroid hormones, drugs decreasing	Caution with drugs that decrease levels or activity of endogenous steroid hormones (eg, ketoconazole, spironolactone, cimetidine).

Cardiac Glycoside

Digoxin (Digitek, Lanoxicaps, Lanoxin)	
Alprazolam	Alprazolam increases serum levels of digoxin.
Amiodarone	Amiodarone increases serum levels of digoxin.
Antacids	Decreased intestinal absorption with antacids.
Anticancer drugs	Decreased intestinal absorption with anticancer drugs.
Antihypertensives	Additive effects on AV node conduction with β-blockers or CCBs.
Calcium	Increases risk of arrhythmias.
Cholestyramine	Decreased intestinal absorption.
Diphenoxylate	Increases absorption with diphenoxylate; monitor for toxicity.
Diuretics	Risk of toxicity with K^+-depleting diuretics.
Indomethacin	Indomethacin increases serum levels of digoxin.
Itraconazole	Itraconazole increases serum levels of digoxin.
Kaolin-pectin	Decreased intestinal absorption with kaolin-pectin.

ANTIHYPERTENSIVES/HEART FAILURE AGENTS *(cont.)*

Cardiac Glycoside

Digoxin (Digitek, Lanoxicaps, Lanoxin) *(cont.)*	
Macrolides	Increases absorption with macrolides; monitor for toxicity.
Metoclopramide	Decreased intestinal absorption with metoclopromide.
Neomycin	Decreased intestinal absorption with neomycin.
Propafenone	Propafenone increases serum levels of digoxin.
Propantheline	Increases absorption with propantheline; monitor for toxicity.
Quinidine	Quinidine increases serum levels of digoxin.
Renal function, drugs affecting	Caution with drugs that deteriorate renal function.
Rifampin	Decreased serum levels with rifampin.
Spironolactone	Spironolactone increases serum levels of digoxin.
Succinylcholine	Increases risk of arrhythmias.
Sulfasalazine	Decreased intestinal absorption with sulfasalazine.
Sympathomimetics	Increases risk of arrhythmias with sympathomimetics.
Tetracycline	Increases absorption with tetracycline; monitor for toxicity.
Thyroid supplements	Increases digoxin dose requirement with thyroid supplements.
Verapamil	Verapamil increases serum levels of digoxin.

Diuretic, Indoline

Indapamide	
ACTH	Increases risk of hypokalemia.
Antidiabetic agents	Antidiabetic agents may need adjustment.
Antihypertensives	May potentiate other antihypertensives.
Corticosteroids	Increases risk of hypokalemia with corticosteroids.
Lithium	May reduce excretion of lithium; monitor lithium levels.
Norepinephrine	May decrease arterial responsiveness to norepinephrine.

Diuretics, K^+-sparing

Amiloride HCl (Midamor)	
ACE inhibitors	Increases risk of hyperkalemia.
Angiotensin II receptor antagonists	Increases risk of hyperkalemia.
Cyclosporine	Increases risk of hyperkalemia.
Diuretics	Hyponatremia and hypochloremia with other diuretics.
Indomethacin	Increases risk of hyperkalemia.
Lithium	May reduce excretion of lithium; monitor lithium levels.
NSAIDs	Decreased effects with NSAIDs.
Tacrolimus	Increases risk of hyperkalemia.

Table 14.2. DRUG INTERACTIONS FOR CARDIOVASCULAR DRUGS ***(cont.)***

ANTIHYPERTENSIVES/HEART FAILURE AGENTS *(cont.)*

Diuretics, K⁺-sparing

Eplerenone (Inspra)	
ACE inhibitors	In HTN, use caution with ACE inhibitors; increases risk of hyperkalemia, especially with diabetics with microalbuminuria.
Angiotensin II receptor antagonists	In HTN, use caution, with angiotensin II receptor antagonists; increases risk of hyperkalemia, especially with diabetics with microalbuminuria.
CYP3A4 inhibitors	Avoid with potent CYP3A4 inhibitors (eg, ketoconazole, itraconazole, nefazodone, troleandomycin, clarithromycin, ritonavir, nelfinavir). Increases levels with other CYP3A4 inhibitors (eg, erythromycin, verapamil, saquinavir, fluconazole).
Lithium	Monitor lithium levels.
NSAIDs	Monitor antihypertensive effect with NSAIDs.
Spironolactone (Aldactone)	
ACE inhibitors	Risk of hyperkalemia.
ACTH	ACTH may intensify electrolyte depletion.
Alcohol	Alcohol potentiates orthostatic hypotension.
Barbiturates	Barbiturates potentiate orthostatic hypotension.
Corticosteroids	Corticosteroids may intensify electrolyte depletion.
Digoxin	Risk of digoxin toxicity.
Diuretics, potassium-sparing	Risk of hyperkalemia with K^+-sparing diuretics.
Lithium	May reduce excretion of lithium; monitor lithium levels.
Narcotics	Narcotics potentiate orthostatic hypotension.
Norepinephrine	Reduced vascular response to norepinephrine.
NSAIDs	Risk of hyperkalemia with NSAIDs. NSAIDs may reduce effects.
Potassium supplements	Risk of hyperkalemia with K^+ supplements.
Skeletal muscle relaxants, non-depolarizing	Increases response to non-depolarizing skeletal muscle relaxants.
Triamterene (Dyrenium)	
ACE inhibitors	Increases risk of hyperkalemia.
Anesthetics	May potentiate preanesthetics and anesthetics.
Antidiabetic agents	May cause hyperglycemia; adjust antidiabetic agents.
Antihypertensives	May potentiate antihypertensives.
Chlorpropamide	Chlorpropamide may increase risk of severe hyponatremia.
Diuretics	May potentiate other diuretics.
Lithium	May reduce excretion of lithium; monitor lithium levels.
NSAIDs	Indomethacin may cause renal failure; caution with NSAIDs.

ANTIHYPERTENSIVES/HEART FAILURE AGENTS *(cont.)*

DIURETICS, K^+-SPARING

Triamterene (Dyrenium) *(cont.)*	
Potassium	Avoid K^+-sparing diuretics, K^+ supplements, K^+-containing agents or salt substitutes, low-salt milk, and blood from blood bank; may potentiate serum K^+ levels.
Skeletal muscle relaxants, non-depolarizing	May potentiate nondepolarizing muscle relaxants.

DIURETICS, K^+-SPARING/DIURETICS, THIAZIDE

Amiloride HCl/Hydrochlorothiazide	
ACE inhibitors	Increases risk of hyperkalemia.
ACTH	ACTH intensifies electrolyte depletion.
Alcohol	Alcohol may potentiate orthostatic hypotension.
Angiotensin II receptor antagonists	Increases risk of hyperkalemia.
Antidiabetic agents	Antidiabetic agents may need adjustment.
Antihypertensives	May potentiate other antihypertensives.
Barbiturates	Barbiturates may potentiate orthostatic hypotension.
Cholestyramine	Cholestyramine impairs absorption.
Colestipol	Colestipol impairs absorption.
Corticosteroids	Corticosteroids intensify electrolyte depletion.
Cyclosporine	Increases risk of hyperkalemia.
Indomethacin	Increases risk of hyperkalemia.
Lithium	May reduce excretion of lithium; monitor lithium levels.
Narcotics	Narcotics may potentiate orthostatic hypotension.
Norepinephrine	May decrease response to norepinephrine.
NSAIDs	NSAIDs may decrease effects.
Skeletal muscle relaxants, non-depolarizing	May increase responsiveness to non-depolarizing muscle relaxants.
Tacrolimus	Increases risk of hyperkalemia.
Spironolactone/Hydrochlorothiazide (Aldactazide)	
ACE inhibitors	Risk of hyperkalemia with ACE inhibitors.
ACTH	ACTH intensifies electrolyte depletion.
Alcohol	Alcohol may potentiate orthostatic hypotension.
Antidiabetic agents	Antidiabetic agents may need adjustment.
Barbiturates	Barbiturates may potentiate orthostatic hypotension.
Corticosteroids	Corticosteroids intensify electrolyte depletion.
Digoxin	Risk of digoxin toxicity.

Table 14.2. DRUG INTERACTIONS FOR CARDIOVASCULAR DRUGS *(cont.)*

ANTIHYPERTENSIVES/HEART FAILURE AGENTS *(cont.)*

DIURETICS, K⁺-SPARING/DIURETICS, THIAZIDE

Sprironolactone/Hydrochlorothiazide (Aldactazide) *(cont.)*	
Diuretics, potassium-sparing	Risk of hyperkalemia with K^+-sparing diuretics.
Lithium	May reduce excretion of lithium; monitor lithium levels.
Narcotics	Narcotics may potentiate orthostatic hypotension.
Norepinephrine	Reduced vascular response to norepinephrine.
NSAIDs	Risk of hyperkalemia with NSAIDs. NSAIDs may decrease effects.
Potassium supplements	Risk of hyperkalemia with K^+ supplements.
Skeletal muscle relaxants, non-depolarizing	Increases response to non-depolarizing skeletal muscle relaxants.
Triamterene/Hydrochlorothiazide (Dyazide, Maxzide, Maxzide-25)	
ACE inhibitors	Increases risk of hyperkalemia.
ACTH	ACTH intensifies electrolyte depletion.
Alcohol	Alcohol may potentiate orthostatic hypotension.
Amphotericin B	Amphotericin B may intensify electrolyte depletion.
Anticoagulants	May decrease levels of oral anticoagulants. Adjust oral anticoagulants.
Antidiabetic	Adjust antidiabetic drugs.
Antigout	Dyazide may increase level of blood uric acid; adjust antigout drugs.
Antihypertensives	May potentiate other antihypertensives.
Barbiturates	Barbiturates may potentiate orthostatic hypotension.
Chlorpropamide	Increases risk of hyponatremia.
Corticosteroids	Corticosteroids intensify electrolyte depletion.
Insulin	May alter insulin requirements.
Laxatives	Overuse of laxatives reduces K^+ levels.
Lithium	May reduce excretion of lithium; monitor lithium levels.
Methanamine	Reduces methenamine effects.
Narcotics	Narcotics may potentiate orthostatic hypotension.
Norepinephrine	Decreases arterial responsiveness to norepinephrine.
NSAIDs	Possible renal dysfunction with NSAIDs.
Potassium-containing agents	Hyperkalemia risk with K^+-containing agents (eg, parenteral penicillin G potassium).
Salt	Hyperkalemia risk with low-salt milk, salt substitutes.
Skeletal muscle relaxants, nondepolarizing	Increases effects of nondepolarizing muscle relaxants.
Sodium polystyrene sulfonate	Overuse of sodium polystyrene sulfonate reduces K^+ levels.
Tubocurarine	May increase responsiveness to tubocurarine.

ANTIHYPERTENSIVES/HEART FAILURE AGENTS *(cont.)*

Diuretics, Loop

Bumetanide (Bumex)	
Aminoglycosides	Avoid aminoglycosides.
Antihypertensives	Potentiates antihypertensives.
Indomethacin	Avoid indomethacin.
Lithium	Lithium toxicity.
Nephrotoxic drugs	Avoid nephrotoxic drugs.
Ototoxic drugs	Avoid ototoxic drugs.
Probenecid	Probenecid reduces effects.
Ethacrynate Sodium, Ethacrynic Acid (Edecrin)	
Antibiotics	May increase ototoxic potential of aminoglycosides and some cephalosporins.
Antihypertensives	Orthostatic hypotension may occur with antihypertensives.
Digitalis	Excessive K^+ loss may precipitate digitalis toxicity.
Lithium	May reduce excretion of lithium; monitor lithium levels.
NSAIDs	NSAIDs may decrease effects.
Steroids	Increases risk of gastric hemorrhage with corticosteroids. Caution with K^+-depleting steroids.
Warfarin	Displaces warfarin from plasma protein; may need dose reduction.
Furosemide (Lasix)	
ACTH	Risk of hypokalemia with ACTH.
Adrenergic blockers	Potentiates ganglionic or peripheral adrenergic blockers.
Alcohol	Orthostatic hypotension may be aggravated by alcohol.
Aminoglycosides	Ototoxicity with aminoglycosides.
Antihypertensives	Potentiates antihypertensives.
Barbiturates	Orthostatic hypotension may be aggravated by barbiturates.
Corticosteroids	Risk of hypokalemia with corticosteroids.
Ethacrynic acid	Ototoxicity with ethacrynic acid.
Indomethacin	Indomethacin may decrease effects.
Lithium	Lithium toxicity.
Narcotics	Orthostatic hypotension may be aggravated by narcotics.
Norepinephrine	Decreases arterial response to norepinephrine.
NSAIDs	Possible renal dysfunction with NSAIDs.
Salicylates	Caution with high dose salicylates.
Succinylcholine	Potentiates succinylcholine.
Sucralfate	Separate sucralfate dose by 2 hrs.
Tubocurarine	Antagonizes tubocurarine.

Table 14.2. DRUG INTERACTIONS FOR CARDIOVASCULAR DRUGS *(cont.)*

ANTIHYPERTENSIVES/HEART FAILURE AGENTS *(cont.)*

DIURETICS, LOOP	
Torsemide (Demadex)	
ACTH	Risk of hypokalemia with ACTH.
Aminoglycosides	Caution with aminoglycosides.
Cholestyramine	Avoid simultaneous cholestyramine administration.
Corticosteroids	Risk of hypokalemia with corticosteroids.
Indomethacin	Indomethacin partially inhibits natriuretic effect.
Lithium	Lithium toxicity.
NSAIDs	Possible renal dysfunction with NSAIDs.
Probenecid	Probenecid decreases effects.
Salicylates	Caution with high-dose salicylates.
Spironolactone	Reduces spironolactone clearance.
DIURETIC, MONOSULFAMYL	
Chlorthalidone (Thalitone)	
Alcohol	Orthostatic hypotension aggravated by alcohol.
Antidiabetic agents	Antidiabetic agents may need adjustment.
Antihypertensives	Potentiates action of other antihypertensive drugs.
Barbiturates	Orthostatic hypotension aggravated by barbiturates.
Lithium	May reduce excretion of lithium; monitor lithium levels.
Narcotics	Orthostatic hypotension aggravated by narcotics.
Norepinephrine	May decrease arterial effectiveness of norepinephrine.
Tubocurarine	May increase responsiveness to tubocurarine.
DIURETIC, QUINAZOLINE	
Metolazone (Zaroxolyn)	
ACTH	ACTH increases hypokalemia and salt and water retention.
Alcohol	Potentiates hypotensive effects of alcohol.
Anticoagulants	Adjust anticoagulants.
Antidiabetic agents	Adjust antidiabetic agents.
Antihypertensives	Adjust dose of other antihypertensives.
Barbiturates	Potentiates hypotensive effects of barbiturates.
Corticosteroids	Corticosteroids increase hypokalemia and salt and water retention.
Curariform drugs	Enhanced neuromuscular blocking effects of curariform drugs.
Digitalis	Digitalis toxicity.
Diuretics, loop	Furosemide and other loop diuretics prolong fluid and electrolyte loss.
Lithium	Lithium toxicity.
Methenamine	Decrease in methenamine efficacy.

ANTIHYPERTENSIVES/HEART FAILURE AGENTS *(cont.)*

DIURETIC, QUINAZOLINE

Metolazone (Zaroxolyn) *(cont.)*	
Narcotics	Potentiates hypotensive effects of narcotics.
Norepinephrine	Decreased arterial response to norepinephrine.
Salicylates	Salicylates and NSAIDs decrease effects.

DIURETICS, THIAZIDE

Chlorothiazide (Diuril, Intravenous Sodium Diuril)	
ACTH	ACTH increases electrolyte depletion.
Alcohol	May potentiate orthostatic hypotension with alcohol.
Antidiabetic drugs	Adjust antidiabetic drugs.
Antihypertensives	May potentiate antihypertensives.
Barbiturates	May potentiate orthostatic hypotension with barbiturates.
Cholestyramine	Decreased PO absorption with cholestyramine.
Colestipol	Decreased PO absorption with colestipol.
Corticosteroids	Corticosteroids increase electrolyte depletion.
Lithium	Lithium toxicity.
Narcotics	May potentiate orthostatic hypotension with narcotics.
NSAIDs	NSAIDs, including COX-2 inhibitors, decrease effects.
Pressor amines	Possible decreased response to pressor amines.
Skeletal muscle relaxants, non-depolarizing	May potentiate non-depolarizing skeletal muscle relaxants.

Hydrochlorothiazide (Microzide)	
ACTH	ACTH increases electrolyte depletion.
Alcohol	May potentiate orthostatic hypotension with alcohol.
Antidiabetic drugs	Adjust antidiabetic drugs.
Antihypertensives	May potentiate antihypertensives.
Barbiturates	May potentiate orthostatic hypotension with barbiturates.
Cholestyramine	Decreased PO absorption with cholestyramine.
Colestipol	Decreased PO absorption with colestipol.
Corticosteroids	Corticosteroids increase electrolyte depletion.
Lithium	Lithium toxicity.
Narcotics	May potentiate orthostatic hypotension with narcotics.
NSAIDs	NSAIDs, including COX-2 inhibitors, decrease effects.
Pressor amines	Possible decreased response to pressor amines.
Skeletal muscle relaxants, non-depolarizing	May potentiate non-depolarizing skeletal muscle relaxants.

Table 14.2. DRUG INTERACTIONS FOR CARDIOVASCULAR DRUGS *(cont.)*

ANTIHYPERTENSIVES/HEART FAILURE AGENTS *(cont.)*

Diuretics, Thiazide

Methyclothiazide (Enduron)	
ACTH	Hypokalemia may develop with ACTH.
Antihypertensives	May potentiate other antihypertensives.
Insulin	May affect insulin requirements.
Lithium	May reduce excretion of lithium; monitor lithium levels.
Norepinephrine	May decrease arterial responsiveness to norepinephrine.
Steroids	Hypokalemia may develop with steroids.
Tubocurarine	May increase responsiveness to tubocurarine.

Ganglionic Blocker

Mecamylamine HCl (Inversine)	
Alcohol	Alcohol may potentiate effects.
Anesthesia	Anesthesia may potentiate effects.
Antibiotics	Avoid with antibiotics.
Antihypertensives	Other antihypertensives may potentiate effects.
Sulfonamides	Avoid with sulfonamides.

Phosphodiesterase 5 Inhibitors

Sildenafil Citrate (Revatio, Viagra)	
Amlodipine	Additional supine BP reduction with amlodipine reported.
β-Blockers	Simultaneous administration with β-blockers may lead to symptomatic hypotension.
Bosentan	Coadministration with bosentan resulted in decrease in AUC of sildenafil and increase in AUC of bosentan.
CYP2C9 inhibitors	CYP2C9 inhibitors may decrease sildenafil clearance.
CYP3A4 inducers	Decreased levels with CYP3A4 inducers (eg, bosentan; more potent inducers such as barbiturates, carbamazepine, phenytoin, efavirenz, nevirapine, rifampin, rifabutin).
CYP3A4 inhibitors	CYP3A4 inhibitors (eg, cimetidine, ketoconazole, itraconazole, erythromycin, saquinavir) increase levels of sildenafil.
Protease inhibitors	CYP3A4 inhibitors (eg, cimetidine, ketoconazole, itraconazole, erythromycin, saquinavir) and protease inhibitors (eg, ritonavir) increase levels of sildenafil.
Vitamin antagonists	Reports of bleeding (epistaxis) with vitamin K antagonists.
Tadalafil (Cialis)	
Alcohol	Caution with alcohol; causes additive hypotensive effects.
α-blockers	Caution with α-blockers; may cause additive hypotensive effects.
Antacids	Antacids reduce the rate of absorption.
Antihypertensives	Caution with antihypertensives (eg, amlodipine, metoprolol, bendrofluazide, enalapril, ARBs); causes additive hypotensive effects.

ANTIHYPERTENSIVES/HEART FAILURE AGENTS *(cont.)*

Phosphodiesterase 5 Inhibitors

Tadalafil (Cialis) *(cont.)*	
CYP3A4 inducers	Decreased levels with CYP3A4 inducers (eg, bosentan; more potent inducers such as barbiturates, carbamazepine, phenytoin, efavirenz, nevirapine, rifampin, rifabutin).
CYP3A4 inhibitors	CYP3A4 inhibitors (eg, cimetidine, ketoconazole, itraconazole, erythromycin, saquinavir) increase levels of tadalafil.
Nitrates	Potentiates the hypotensive effects of nitrates. Use is contraindicated.
Ritonavir	Ritonavir significantly increases the levels of tadalafil.
Vardenafil HCl (Levitra)	
α-blockers	Caution with α-blockers; may cause additive hypotensive effects.
Antiarrhythmics	Avoid use with Class IA (eg, quinidine, procainamide) or Class III (eg, amiodarone, sotalol) antiarrhythmics.
Antihypertensives	Caution with antihypertensives (eg, amlodipine, metoprolol, bendrofluazide, enalapril, ARBs); causes additive hypotensive effects.
CYP3A4 inhibitors	CYP3A4 inhibitors (eg, ketoconazole, erythromycin, indinavir, ritonavir, grapefruit juice) increase levels of vardenafil.
Nifedipine	Caution with nifedipine; causes additive hypotensive effects.
Nitrates	Potentiates the hypotensive effects of nitrates. Use is contraindicated.

Rauwolfia Alkaloid

Reserpine	
Antihypertensives	Titrate carefully with other antihypertensives.
Digoxin	Risk of arrhythmia with digoxin.
MAOIs	Avoid MAOIs or use extreme caution.
Quinidine	Risk of arrhythmia with quinidine.
Sympathomimetics, direct-acting	Prolonged effect of direct-acting sympathomimetics (eg, epinephrine, isoproterenol).
Sympathomimetics, indirect-acting	May inhibit effects of indirect-acting sympathomimetics (eg, ephedrine, tyramine).
Tricyclic antidepressants (TCAs)	Decreased effect with TCAs.

Renin Inhibitor

Aliskiren (Tekturna)	
Atorvastatin	Coadministration with atorvastatin may increase C_{max} up to 50% after multiple dosing.
Cyclosporine	Concomitant use with cyclosporine is not recommended.
Furosemide	Coadministration with furosemide may reduce AUC and C_{max} by 30% and 50%, respectively.
Irbesartan	Coadministration of irbesartan may reduce C_{max} up to 50% after multiple dosing.

Table 14.2. DRUG INTERACTIONS FOR CARDIOVASCULAR DRUGS *(cont.)*

ANTIHYPERTENSIVES/HEART FAILURE AGENTS *(cont.)*

Renin Inhibitor	
Aliskiren (Tekturna) *(cont.)*	
Ketoconazole	Coadministration of ketoconazole 200 mg bid may result in an approximate 80% increase in plasma level.
Potassium	Caution with concomitant use of K^+-sparing diuretics, K^+ supplements, K^+-containing salt substitutes, or other drugs that increase K^+ levels; may lead to increases in serum K^+.
Renin Inhibitor/Diuretic, Thiazide	
Aliskiren/Hydrochlorothiazide (Tekturna HCT)	
ACTH	ACTH depletes electrolytes.
Alcohol	Potentiation of orthostatic hypotension with HCTZ may occur with alcohol.
Antihypertensives	Potentiates effects of other antihypertensives.
Atorvastatin	Atorvastatin may increase plasma levels of aliskiren.
Barbiturates	Potentiation of orthostatic hypotension with HCTZ may occur with barbiturates.
Cholestyramine	Cholestyramine resins may impair absorption.
Colestipol	Colestipol resins may impair absorption.
Corticosteroids	Corticosteroids deplete electrolytes.
Furosemide	Coadministration may diminish furosemide levels.
Hypoglycemics	Dosage adjustment of insulin or oral hypoglycemic agents may be required.
Irbesartan	Irbesartan may reduce levels.
Ketoconazole	Ketoconazole may increase plasma levels of aliskiren.
Lithium	Increases risk of lithium toxicity; avoid concurrent use.
Narcotic	Potentiation of orthostatic hypotension with HCTZ may occur with narcotics.
NSAIDs	NSAIDs may reduce diuretic effects; monitor closely.
Pressor amines	May decrease response to pressor amines (eg, norepinephrine).
Skeletal muscle relaxants	May increase responsiveness to skeletal muscle relaxants (eg, tubocurarine).
Tyrosine Hydroxylase Inhibitor	
Metyrosine (Demser)	
CNS depressants	Additive sedative effects with alcohol and other CNS depressants (eg, hypnotics, sedatives, tranquilizers).
Haloperidol	May potentiate EPS with haloperidol.
Phenothiazines	May potentiate EPS with phenothiazines.
Vasodilators	
Diazoxide (Hyperstat)	
Alphaprodine	Diazoxide injection should not be administered within 6 hrs of alphaprodine.
Antihypertensives	Potentiates effects of other antihypertensives.
β-Blockers	Diazoxide injection should not be administered within 6 hrs of β-blockers.

ANTIHYPERTENSIVES/HEART FAILURE AGENTS *(cont.)*

Vasodilators

Diazoxide (Hyperstat) *(cont.)*	
Diuretics	Concomitant administration with diuretics (eg, thiazides) may be expected to potentiate the hyperuricemic and antihypertensive effects.
Hydralazine	Diazoxide injection should not be administered within 6 hrs of hydralazine.
Methyldopa	Diazoxide injection should not be administered within 6 hrs of methyldopa.
Minoxidil	Diazoxide injection should not be administered within 6 hrs of minoxidil.
Nitrites	Diazoxide injection should not be administered within 6 hrs of nitrites.
Papaverine-like compounds	Diazoxide injection should not be administered within 6 hrs of other papaverine-like compounds.
Prazosin	Diazoxide injection should not be administered within 6 hrs of prazosin.
Protein-bound drugs	Diazoxide is a protein-bound drug and can displace other highly protein-bound substances (ie, bilirubin, coumarin).
Reserpine	Diazoxide injection should not be administered within 6 hrs of reserpine.
Hydralazine HCl	
Antihypertensives, parenteral	Profound hypotension with potent parenteral antihypertensives (eg, diazoxide).
Epinephrine	May reduce pressor response to epinephrine.
MAOIs	Caution with MAOIs.
Minoxidil	
Guanethidine	Severe orthostatic hypotension.

Vasodilator Combination

Hydralazine HCl/Isosorbide Dinitrate (BiDil)	
Antihypertensives, parenteral	Increases risk of hypotension with potent parenteral antihypertensive agents.
MAOIs	Caution with MAOIs.
Phosphodiesterase inhibitors	Increases vasodilatory effects with phosphodiesterase inhibitors (eg, sildenafil, vardenafil, tadalafil).

ANTILIPIDEMIC AGENTS

Bile Acid Sequestrants

Cholestyramine (Questran, Questran Light)	
Digitalis	May reduce or delay absorption of digitalis.
Diuretics, thiazide	May reduce or delay absorption of thiazide diuretics.
Drugs, concomitant	Take concomitant drugs 1 hr before or 4-6 hrs after.
Enterohepatic circulation, drugs undergoing	May interfere with absorption of drugs that undergo enterohepatic circulation.
Estrogens	May reduce or delay absorption of estrogens.
HMG-CoA reductase inhibitors (statins)	Additive effects with statins.

Table 14.2. DRUG INTERACTIONS FOR CARDIOVASCULAR DRUGS *(cont.)*

ANTILIPIDEMIC AGENTS *(cont.)*

Bile Acid Sequestrants

Cholestyramine (Questran, Questran Light) *(cont.)*	
Nicotinic acid	Additive effects with nicotinic acid.
Penicillin G	May reduce or delay absorption of penicillin G.
Phenobarbital	May reduce or delay absorption of phenobarbital.
Phenylbutazone	May reduce or delay absorption of phenylbutazone.
Phosphate supplements, oral	May interfere with absorption of oral phosphate supplements.
Progestins	May reduce or delay absorption of progestins.
Propranolol	May reduce or delay absorption of propranolol.
Spironolactone	Caution with spironolactone.
Tetracycline	May reduce or delay absorption of tetracyclines.
Thyroid/thyroxine agents	May reduce or delay absorption of thyroid and thyroxine agents.
Vitamins, fat-soluable	May interfere with absorption of fat-soluble vitamins (eg, A, D, E, K).
Warfarin	May reduce or delay absorption of warfarin.
Colesevelam HCl (WelChol)	
Contraceptives, oral	May decrease level of oral contraceptives containing ethinyl estradiol and norethindrone.
Diabetic agents	May increase TG levels when used with insulin or sulfonylureas.
Glyburide	May decrease level of glyburide.
Levothyroxine	May decrease level of levothyroxine.
Phenytoin	May decrease phenytoin levels.
Thyroid hormone	May elevate TSH in patients receiving thyroid hormone replacement therapy.
Warfarin	Concomitant use with warfarin decreases INR; monitor INR.
Colestipol HCl (Colestid)	
Chlorothiazide	Reduces absorption of chlorothiazide, tetracycline, furosemide, penicillin G, HCTZ, and gemfibrozil.
Digitalis	Caution with digitalis agents.
Folic acid	May interfere with absorption of folic acid.
Furosemide	Reduces absorption of furosemide.
Gemfibrozil	Reduces absorption of gemfibrozil.
Hydrochlorothiazide (HCTZ)	Reduces absorption of HCTZ.
Hydrocortisone	May interfere with absorption of hydrocortisone.
Medication, concomitant	May delay or reduce absorption of concomitant oral medication; take other drugs 1 hr before or 4 hrs after colestipol.
Penicillin G	Reduces absorption of penicillin G.
Phosphate supplements, oral	May interfere with absorption of oral phosphate supplements.

ANTILIPIDEMIC AGENTS *(cont.)*

BILE ACID SEQUESTRANTS

Colestipol HCl (Colestid) *(cont.)*	
Propranolol	Caution with propranolol.
Tetracycline	Reduces absorption of tetracycline.
Vitamins, fat-soluble	May interfere with absorption of fat-soluble vitamins (eg, A, D,E,K).

CHOLESTEROL ABSORPTION INHIBITOR

Ezetimibe (Zetia)	
Cholestyramine	Incremental LDL-C reduction may be reduced with concomitant cholestyramine.
Cyclosporine	Monitor cyclosporine levels with concomitant use.
Fibrates	Fibrates may increase cholesterol excretion into the bile; concurrent use is not recommended.
Gemfibrozil	Increases levels with gemfibrozil.
Warfarin	Monitor INR when administered with warfarin.

FIBRIC ACID DERIVATIVES

Fenofibrate (Antara, Lofibra, Tricor, Triglide)	
Bile acid sequestrants	Bile acid sequestrants may impede absorption; take at least 1 hr before or 4-6 hrs after the resin.
Coumarin anticoagulants	May potentiate coumarin anticoagulants; reduce anticoagulant dose and monitor PT/INR.
HMG-CoA reductase inhibitors (statins)	Avoid statins unless benefits outweigh risks.
Immunosuppressants	Evaluate benefits/risks with immunosuppressants (eg, cyclosporine) and other nephrotoxic agents.
Gemfibrozil (Lopid)	
Anticoagulants	Caution with anticoagulants; reduce dose and monitor PT.
HMG-CoA reductase inhibitors (statins)	Increases risk of myopathy and rhabdomyolysis with statins. Benefit with concomitant statins does not outweigh risks.
Itraconazole	Avoid itraconazole in patients taking gemfibrozil and repaglinide.
Repaglinide	Avoid initiating therapy with repaglinide. If already on repaglinide therapy, monitor levels and adjust repaglinide dose.

HMG-COA REDUCTASE INHIBITORS (STATINS)

Atorvastatin Calcium (Lipitor)	
Azole antifungals	Azole antifungals may increase risk of myopathy.
Colestipol	Colestipol decreases levels when coadministered, but greater LDL-C reduction than when each drug given alone.
Contraceptives, oral	Increases levels of oral contraceptives (norethindrone, ethinyl estradiol).
Cyclosporine	Cyclosporine may increase risk of myopathy.

Table 14.2. DRUG INTERACTIONS FOR CARDIOVASCULAR DRUGS *(cont.)*

ANTILIPIDEMIC AGENTS *(cont.)*

HMG-CoA Reductase Inhibitors (Statins)

Atorvastatin Calcium (Lipitor) *(cont.)*	
Digoxin	Monitor digoxin.
Erythromycin	Increases levels with erythromycin. Erythromycin may increase risk of myopathy.
Fibrates	Fibrates may increase risk of myopathy. Avoid fibrates unless benefit outweighs risk.
Maalox	Decreases levels with Maalox TC, but LDL-C reduction not altered.
Niacin	Niacin may increase risk of myopathy/rhabdomyolysis.
Steroid hormone suppressors	Caution with drugs that decrease levels or activity of endogenous steroid hormones (eg, ketoconazole, spironolactone, cimetidine).
Fluvastatin Sodium (Lescol, Lescol XL)	
Anticoagulants	Monitor anticoagulants.
Cholestyramine	Cholestyramine given within 4 hrs decreases serum levels but has additive effects when given 4 hrs after fluvastatin (immediate-release).
Cimetidine	Cimetidine increases fluvastatin levels.
Colchicine	Colchicine may increase risk of myopathy/rhabdomyolysis.
Cyclosporine	Cyclosporine may increase risk of myopathy/rhabdomyolysis.
Diclofenac	Increases levels of diclofenac.
Digoxin	Monitor digoxin.
Erythromycin	May increase risk of myopathy/rhabdomyolysis.
Fibrates	Fibrates may increase risk of myopathy. Avoid fibrates unless benefit outweighs risk.
Gemfibrozil	Gemfibrozil may increase risk of myopathy/rhabdomyolysis.
Glyburide	Increases levels of glyburide. Glyburide increases fluvastatin levels.
Niacin	Niacin may increase risk of myopathy/rhabdomyolysis.
Omeprazole	Increases fluvastatin levels.
Phenytoin	Increases levels of phenytoin. Phenytoin increases fluvastatin levels.
Ranitidine	Increases fluvastatin levels.
Rifampicin	Rifampicin significantly decreases serum levels.
Steroid hormone suppressors	Caution with drugs that decrease levels or activity of endogenous steroid hormones (eg, ketoconazole, spironolactone, cimetidine).
Lovastatin (Altoprev, Mevacor)	
Amiodarone	Amiodarone may increase risk of myopathy.
Anticoagulants	Monitor anticoagulants
CYP3A4 inhibitors	CYP3A4 inhibitors (eg, cyclosporine, itraconazole, ketoconazole, erythromycin, clarithromycin, telithromycin, protease inhibitors, nefazodone, >1 qt/day of grapefruit juice) may increase risk of myopathy.

ANTILIPIDEMIC AGENTS *(cont.)*

HMG-CoA Reductase Inhibitors (Statins)

Lovastatin (Altoprev, Mevacor) *(cont.)*	
Danazol	Danazol may increase risk of myopathy.
Fibrates	Fibrates may increase risk of myopathy. Avoid fibrates unless benefit outweighs risk.
Niacin	Niacin ≥1 g/day may increase risk of myopathy.
Steroid hormone suppressors	May blunt adrenal and/or gonadal steroid production; caution with steroid hormone suppressive drugs (eg, ketoconazole, spironolactone, cimetidine).
Verapamil	May increase risk of myopathy.
Pravastatin Sodium (Pravachol)	
Cholestyramine/colestipol	Decreased levels with concomitant cholestyramine/colestipol; take 1 hr before or 4 hrs after resins.
Cyclosporine	May increase risk of myopathy.
Erythromycin	May increase risk of myopathy.
Fibrates	Fibrates may increase risk of myopathy. Avoid fibrates unless benefit outweighs risk.
Gemfibrozil	Increases levels with gemfibrozil.
Itraconazole	Increases levels with itraconazole.
Niacin	Niacin may increase risk of myopathy/rhabdomyolysis.
Steroid hormone suppressors	Caution with drugs that decrease levels or activity of endogenous steroid hormones (eg, ketoconazole, spironolactone, cimetidine).
Rosuvastatin Calcium (Crestor)	
Antacids	Space antacid dosing by 2 hrs.
Contraceptives, oral	Increases levels of oral contraceptives (norgestrel, ethinyl estradiol).
Cyclosporine	Increases levels and risk of myopathy.
Fibrates	Fibrates may increase risk of myopathy. Avoid fibrates unless benefit outweighs risk.
Lopinavir/ritonavir	Increases levels and risk of myopathy with lopinavir/ritonavir.
Niacin	Niacin may increase risk of myopathy/rhabdomyolysis.
Steroid hormone suppressors	Caution with drugs that decrease levels or activity of endogenous steroid hormones (eg, ketoconazole, spironolactone, cimetidine).
Warfarin	Increases INR with warfarin. Monitor warfarin.
Simvastatin (Zocor)	
Amiodarone	Max 20 mg/day with amiodarone.
Cyclosporine	Max 10 mg/day with cyclosporine.
CYP3A4 inhibitors	Avoid use with concomitant itraconazole, ketoconazole, erythromycin, clarithromycin, telithromycin, HIV protease inhibitors, nefazodone, grapefruit juice (>1 qt/day); increases risk of myopathy/rhabdomyolysis.

Table 14.2. DRUG INTERACTIONS FOR CARDIOVASCULAR DRUGS *(cont.)*

ANTILIPIDEMIC AGENTS *(cont.)*

HMG-CoA Reductase Inhibitors (Statins)

Simvastatin (Zocor) *(cont.)*	
Danazol	Max 10 mg/day with danazol.
Digoxin	Monitor digoxin.
Fibrates	Fibrates may increase risk of myopathy. Avoid fibrates unless benefit outweighs risk.
Gemfibrozil	Max 10 mg/day with gemfibrozil.
Niacin	Caution with ≥1 g/day of niacin; may increase risk of myopathy/ rhabdomyolysis.
Verapamil	Max 20 mg/day with verapamil.
Warfarin	Increases INR with warfarin. Monitor warfarin.

HMG-CoA Reductase Inhibitors (Statins)/Cholesterol Absorption Inhibitor

Simvastatin/Ezetimibe (Vytorin)	
Amiodarone	Max 10 mg-20 mg daily with amiodarone.
Azoles	Avoid use with concomitant itraconazole, ketoconazole; increases risk of myopathy/rhabdomyolysis.
Cholestyramine	Incremental LDL-C reductions with concomitant cholestyramine.
Cyclosporine	Max 10 mg-10 mg daily with cyclosporine.
Danazol	Max 10 mg-10 mg daily with danazol.
Digoxin	Monitor digoxin.
Fibrates	Caution with other fibrates.
Gemfibrozil	Max 10 mg-10 mg daily with gemfibrozil.
Grapefruit juice	Avoid use with concomitant grapefruit juice (>1 qt/day); increases risk of myopathy/rhabdomyolysis.
Macrolides	Avoid use with concomitant erythromycin, clarithromycin, telithromycin; increases risk of myopathy/rhabdomyolysis.
Nefazadone	Avoid use with concomitant nefazodone; increases risk of myopathy/ rhabdomyolysis.
Niacin	Caution with ≥1 g/day of niacin; may increase risk of myopathy/ rhabdomyolysis.
Protease inhibitors	Avoid use with concomitant HIV protease inhibitors; increases risk of myopathy/rhabdomyolysis.
Verapamil	Max 10 mg-20 mg daily with verapamil.
Wafarin	Monitor with warfarin.

HMG-CoA Reductase Inhibitors (Statins)/Nicotinic Acid

Lovastatin/Niacin (Advicor)	
Adrenergic blockers	Caution with adrenergic blockers.

ANTILIPIDEMIC AGENTS *(cont.)*

HMG-CoA Reductase Inhibitors (Statins)/Nicotinic Acid

Lovastatin/Niacin (Advicor) *(cont.)*	
Alcohol	Avoid concomitant alcohol and hot drinks; may increase flushing and pruritus.
Antidiabetic agents	Antidiabetic agents may need adjustment.
Aspirin (ASA)	Decreased niacin clearance with ASA.
Bile acid sequestrants	Separate bile acid sequestrants by 4 to 6 hrs.
Calcium channel blockers (CCBs)	Caution with CCBs.
CYP3A4 inhibitors	Increases risk of skeletal muscle disorders with CYP3A4 inhibitors (eg, cyclosporine, itraconazole, ketoconazole, erythromycin, clarithromycin, telithromycin, protease inhibitors, nefazodone, >1 qt/day of grapefruit juice, verapamil, fibrates [eg, gemfibrozil].
Ganglionic blockers	May potentiate ganglionic blockers.
Nitrates	Caution with acute MI and nitrates.
Steroid hormone suppressors	Caution with drugs that decrease levels or activity of endogenous steroid hormones (eg, ketoconazole, spironolactone, cimetidine).
Supplements	Caution with niacin-containing nutritional supplements.
Vasoactive drugs	May potentiate vasoactive drugs.
Warfarin	Monitor warfarin.
Simvastatin/Niacin (Simcor)	
Amiodarone	Max 20 mg/day with amiodarone.
Aspirin (ASA)	Concomitant use with ASA decreases niacin levels.
Cholestyramine	Cholestyramine may increase niacin-binding capacity.
Colestipol	Colestipol may increase niacin-binding capacity.
Coumarin anticoagulants	Potentiates effects of coumarin anticoagulants; monitor PT/INR.
CYP3A4 inhibitors	Avoid use with concomitant CYP3A4 inhibitors including itraconazole, ketoconazole, and other antifungal azoles, erythromycin, clarithromycin, telithromycin, HIV protease inhibitors, nefazodone, grapefruit juice (>1 qt/day), cyclosporine, danazol, and fibrates; increases risk of myopathy/rhabdomyolysis.
Digoxin	May increase digoxin levels; monitor appropriately.
Propranolol	Concurrent use with propranolol decreases simvastatin levels.
Supplements, nutritional	Potentiates adverse effects with nutritional supplements containing large doses of niacin or related compounds.
Verapamil	Max 20 mg/day with verapamil.

Lipid-Regulating Agent

Omega-3-Acid Ethyl Esters (Lovaza)	
Anticoagulants	Possible prolongation of bleeding time with concomitant anticoagulants (eg, aspirin, warfarin, coumarin, clopidogrel).

Table 14.2. DRUG INTERACTIONS FOR CARDIOVASCULAR DRUGS *(cont.)*

ANTILIPIDEMIC AGENTS *(cont.)*

NICOTINIC ACID

Niacin (Niaspan)	
Alcohol	Avoid concomitant alcohol or hot drinks; may increase flushing and pruritus.
Anticoagulants	Caution with anticoagulants.
Antidiabetic agents	Antidiabetic agents may need adjustment.
Antihypertensives	May potentiate antihypertensives (eg, ganglionic blockers, vasoactive drugs).
Bile acid resins	Separate dosing from bile acid resins by at least 4-6 hrs.
HMG-CoA reductase inhibitors (statins)	Rhabdomyolysis may occur with statins.
Nicotinamide	High-dose niacin or nicotinamide may potentiate adverse effects.

Chapter 15

Respiratory Drugs

Martha Somerman, D.D.S., Ph.D.

A significant number of people in the general population have respiratory disorders that require the use of medications. Bronchial asthma is the most common respiratory disease the dentist encounters; therefore, he or she should be particularly familiar with drugs taken by patients with such conditions.

Asthma is characterized physiologically by reversible airway obstruction that results from constriction of the bronchial and bronchiolar muscles and hypersecretion of viscous mucus. Factors that can precipitate an asthmatic attack include respiratory infection, physical exertion, and exposure to cold air or irritating gases, allergies, and stress.

There are three major approaches to the treatment of asthma:

- use of anti-inflammatory drugs (and more recently, diet-related products) to reduce symptoms and bronchial hyperactivity
- use of agents that reverse or inhibit bronchoconstriction
- avoidance of causative factors

Causative factors include indoor allergens and stress; thus, the dentist must be sensitive to the possibility of these factors provoking an asthmatic attack in a susceptible person while he or she is in the dental office. If a patient is using metered-dose inhalants, these inhalants should be readily accessible at his or her dental appointment.

The information in this chapter will provide summary data on special dental considerations for, use of, interactions of, adverse effects of, and contraindications for drugs taken by and potentially given to people who have respiratory conditions.

When treating a patient with a respiratory condition, the dentist must determine the nature of the condition and which, if any, drugs the patient is taking for these conditions. The American Society of Anesthesiologists classification of asthma is provided in **Table 15.1**.

Corticosteroids are covered in more detail in **Chapter 5**, while β-blockers are covered in **Chapter 14**.

Tables 15.2 and **15.3** provide general information on drugs used for respiratory diseases, including typical dosage ranges and interactions with other drugs, except for corticosteroids, which can be found in **Chapter 5**.

Special Dental Considerations

When it comes to treating patients with respiratory conditions, practitioners should keep the following important points in mind.

First, chronic obstructive pulmonary disease (COPD) is a respiratory disease of major medical concern; bronchial obstruction in this disease is irreversible, resulting in severe infections, heart disease, and respiratory failure. Respiratory conditions and the use of inhalants can result in decreased salivary flow and associated problems, including caries and candidiasis. Therefore, patients should use fluoride rinses and should be observed for the need to use antifungal agents.

Reduction of stress may require the use of sedatives, especially when complex procedures are being performed. Stress-reduction methods, including medications, may be required to prevent an asthmatic attack.

NSAIDs and aspirin are contraindicated in patients with respiratory conditions, as they may prompt an asthmatic attack.

Use a semisupine chair position for patients with respiratory diseases, especially for patients with COPD. To prevent orthostatic hypotension, patients should sit upright for a few minutes before being dismissed.

Keep inhalants that patients are using easily accessible during the dental appointment.

With patients receiving chronic steroid therapy, there is an enhanced concern about stress situations—such as the possibility of adrenal crisis—as well as increased susceptibility to infections.

With patients using β-adrenergic agonists, there is a concern about cardiovascular side effects. Most of the drugs in this category used to treat asthma are selective β_2-adrenergic agonists and thus act as bronchodilators. However, they do have some β_1 side effects, so there is a need to be aware of possible cardiovascular side effects (for example, tachycardia and hypertension).

In addition to the concerns above, patients with cystic fibrosis may be using inhalants containing pancreatic enzymes and tobramycin (or tablets/capsules with similar formulas). Beyond high risk of respiratory infections in individuals with cystic fibrosis, caution must be taken in administration of other antibiotics in patients receiving the aminoglycoside antibiotic tobramycin (see **Table 15.3**).

Drug Interactions of Dental Interest

Avoid drugs that may precipitate an asthmatic attack: aspirin, NSAIDs, and narcotics.

Special Patients

As a rule, inhalants are not recommended for use in children <5 years. Also, these drugs may have hepatic and renal side effects that often are of more concern with children and older adults.

Adverse Effects, Precautions, and Contraindications

Table 15.2 describes adverse effects, precautions, and contraindications associated with steroids and β_2-adrenergic blockers (whether taken orally or inhaled).

Pharmacology

Inhibitors of Chemical Mediators/ Anti-Inflammatory Drugs

Cromolyn sulfate

Cromolyn sulfate is thought to act by stabilizing mast cells. In addition, cromolyn also may inhibit mast cell release of histamine, leukotrienes, and other inflammatory mediators and inhibit calcium influx into mast cells. The result is decreased stimuli for bronchospasm. However, as it has no bronchodilating activity, cromolyn is useful only for prophylactic treatment and not for acute situations.

Leukotriene antagonists and inhibitors

These drugs act by blocking the synthesis of leukotriene from arachidonic acid (eg, zileuton [Zyflo]) or by acting as leukotriene receptor antagonists (eg, montelukast [Singulair], zafirlukast [Accolate]), thereby decreasing leukotriene levels and the associated increased inflammatory activity. Antileukotriene approaches are recommended as maintenance therapies for persistent asthma requiring daily bronchodilator treatment.

Corticosteroids

See **Chapter 5** for details.

Bronchodilators

β-Adrenergic agonists

β-Adrenergic agonists are used for treatment of acute bronchospasm. Ideal drugs act predominantly on β_2-adrenergic receptors and stimulate dilation of bronchial smooth muscles. This relaxes the airway's smooth muscle. β-Adrenergic agents also inhibit release of substances from mast cells and thus prevent bronchoconstriction. Most adrenergic drugs have some β_1 activity; therefore, there is a need to monitor patients for cardiovascular effects, including increased force and rate of cardiac contraction. This is especially true of epinephrine. Note: Epinephrine usually is used for emergency situations such as rapid/acute asthmatic attack, in which case 0.2 mL to 0.5 mL of 1:1,000 solution is administered subcutaneously or intramuscularly.

Intramuscular injection of epinephrine into the buttocks should be avoided, because it could cause gas gangrene. The subcutaneous route is recommended for bronchodilatory purposes; for anaphylactic reactions, either the subcutaneous or the intramuscular route could be used.

Xanthines

Xanthines relax bronchial smooth muscle (in both acute and chronic situations, and often in combination with other drugs). Several mechanisms for this activity have been proposed, but none have been definitively proven. These mechanisms include inhibition of phosphodiesterase, mobilization of calcium pools, inhibition of prostaglandin activity, and decreased uptake of catecholamines. Due to a narrow therapeutic window, high side-effect profile, and potential for drug interactions, theophylline has been largely replaced with β_2 agonists and corticosteroids.

Anticholinergic agents

Anticholinergic agents act on receptors to prevent smooth muscle contraction. They are marketed for inhalant treatment of COPD, but this use is still under investigation.

Additional Drugs for Seasonal Allergies and Coughing

The drugs noted above are used primarily to treat asthma and COPD. Another class of drugs, antihistamines, is used to treat seasonal allergic rhinitis. These H_1-receptor antagonists include cetirizine (Zyrtec, Xyzal, et al) and loratadine (Claritin et al), both second-generation H_1-antihistamines that are available OTC. They have fewer sedative effects than the first-generation H_1-antihistamines, eg, diphenhydramine (Benadryl et al) and chlorpheniramine (Chlor-Trimetron et al). Side effects include xerostomia, dose-dependent somnolence, nasopharyngitis, and pharyngitis.

In addition, there are numerous agents used (often in combination) for cough suppression, including codeine, dextromethorphan, and guaifenesin.

EVOLVING RESPIRATORY THERAPIES

New therapies continue to be targeted at decreasing inflammation. DNase inhibitors are thought to act by breaking up long extracellular DNA into smaller fragments. DNA is considered to contribute to thick sputum, especially in patients with cystic fibrosis. Omalizumab (Xolair injection) is a recombinant DNA-derived monoclonal antibody that selectively binds to human IgE, resulting in decreased IgE binding to receptors on mast cells and basophils. Reports of serious and life-threatening hypersensitivity reactions have resulted in the limiting of clinical use of Xolair to patients with severe asthma that is not adequately controlled by other drugs. In recent years, nutritional/dietary control for many diseases, including cardiovascular, gastrointestinal, and pulmonary diseases, has received much attention. There is some indication that the inflammatory state in the airways, often associated with increased oxygen species and free radical–mediated reactions, can be controlled by foods or supplements that are able to control oxidant insult, eg, antioxidants. In the area of allergen avoidance, there have been efforts to develop products that can control dust-mite allergens or denature allergens.

Note: Effective January 1, 2009, albuterol MDIs using chlorofluorocarbons (CFCs) have been discontinued, with an FDA announcement for discontinuation dates for other CFC-containing products in the near future. The CFC propellants in metered-dose inhalers (MDIs) are being replaced by hydrofluoroalkane (HFA) propellants for environmental reasons. (CFCs contribute to depletion of the ozone layer.)

SUGGESTED READING

Drugs for allergic disorders. *Treat Guideline Med Lett.* 2007;5:71.

Fanta CH. Asthma. (Review article. Drug therapy). *N Engl J Med.* Mar 5, 2009;360(10):1002-1014.

Kips JC, Pauwels RA. Long-acting inhaled β_2-agonist therapy in asthma. *Am J Respir Crit Care Med.* 2001;164:923-932.

Laube BL. The expanding role of aerosols in systemic drug delivery, gene therapy and vaccination. *Respir Care.* 2005;50(9):1161-1176.

Lukacs NW. Role of chemokines in the pathogenesis of asthma. *Nat Rev Immunol.* 2001;1(2):108-116.

Malamed SF. *Medical Emergencies in the Dental Office.* 6th ed. St. Louis: Elsevier Mosby; 2007.

Peebles RS, Hartert TV. Highlights from the annual scientific assembly: patient-centered approaches to asthma management—strategies for the treatment and management of asthma. *South Med J.* 2002;95:775-779.

Riccioni G, Di Ilio C, D'Orazio N. Review: An update of the leukotriene modulators for treatment of asthma. *Expert Opin Investig Drugs.* 2004;13(7):763-776.

Riccioni G, D'Orazio N. The role of selenium, zinc and antioxidant vitamin supplementation in the treatment of bronchial asthma: adjuvant therapy or not? *Expert Opin Investig Drugs.* 2005;14(9):1145-1155.

Table 15.1. AMERICAN SOCIETY OF ANESTHESIOLOGISTS CLASSIFICATION: ASTHMA

ASA CLASS*	DESCRIPTION	DENTAL TREATMENT MODIFICATIONS
II	**Typical extrinsic or intrinsic asthma** • Easily managed • Characterized by infrequent episodes • Does not require emergency care or hospitalization	Reduce stress as needed Determine triggering factors Avoid triggering factors Have bronchodilators available during dental treatment
III	**Exercise-induced asthma** • Often accompanied by fear • Patient with Class III asthma usually has history of emergency care or hospitalization	Follow ASA II modifications Administer sedation-inhalation with nitrous oxide, oxygen, or oral benzodiazepines, if indicated
IV	**Chronic asthma** • Signs and symptoms of asthma present at rest	Obtain medical consultation before beginning treatment Provide only emergency care in office Defer elective care until respiratory status improves or until patient can be treated in controlled environment

*Class I represents a healthy person with no asthma.

Malamed SF. *Medical Emergencies in the Dental Office.* 6th ed. St. Louis: Elsevier Mosby; 2007. Copyright © 2007 Elsevier Mosby.

Table 15.2. PRESCRIBING INFORMATION FOR RESPIRATORY DRUGS
(For all inhaled, intranasal, or systemic corticosteroids, refer to Table 5.1 starting on page 163)

NAME	FORM/ STRENGTH	DOSAGE	WARNINGS/PRECAUTIONS & CONTRAINDICATIONS	ADVERSE EFFECTS†
ASTHMA/COPD PREPARATIONS				
ANTICHOLINERGIC BRONCHODILATORS				
Ipratropium Bromide (Atrovent HFA)	**MDI:** 0.017mg/ inh [12.9g]	***Adults:*** **Initial:** 2 inh qid. **Max:** 12 inh/24hrs.	**W/P:** Not for acute episodes. Immediate hypersensitivity reaction reported. Caution with narrow-angle glaucoma, prostatic hypertrophy, or bladder-neck obstruction. **Contra:** Hypersensitivity to atropine or its derivatives. **P/N:** Category B, caution in nursing.	Back pain, bronchitis, dyspnea, dizziness, headache, nausea, blurred vision, **dry mouth,** exacerbation of symptoms.
Tiotropium Bromide (Spiriva)	**Cap, Inhalation:** 18mcg	***Adults:*** Inhale contents of one capsule (18mcg) qd, with HandiHaler device.	**W/P:** Not for initial treatment of acute episodes. D/C if hypersensitivity (eg, angioedema) or paradoxical bronchospasm occurs. Caution with narrow-angle glaucoma, prostatic hyperplasia, bladder-neck obstruction. Monitor with moderate to severe renal impairment (CrCl ≤50mL/min). Contents of caps are for oral inhalation only and must not be swallowed. **Contra:** Hypersensitivity to atropine or its derivatives (eg, ipratropium). **P/N:** Category C, caution in nursing.	**Dry mouth,** arthritis, cough, flu-like symptoms, sinusitis, constipation, abdominal pain, UTI, moniliasis, rash, dizziness, dysphagia, **hoarseness,** intestinal obstruction-ileus paralytic, increased IOP, **oral candidiasis,** tachycardia, **throat irritation.**
β_2-AGONISTS				
Albuterol Sulfate	**Sol (neb):** 0.083% [3mL, 25[s]], 0.5% [20mL]; **Syrup:** 2mg/5mL; **Tab:** 2mg*, 4mg*; **Tab, Extended-Release:** (Vospire ER) 4mg, 8mg	***Adults/Pediatrics:*** **Bronchospasm: ≥12 yrs: (Sol)** 2.5mg tid-qid by nebulizer. **>12 yrs: (Tab, Extended-Release) Usual:** 4-8mg q12h. **Low Body Weight: Initial:** 4 mg q12h. **Titrate:** May increase to 8mg q12h. **Max:** 32mg/day in divided doses. Swallow whole with liquids; do not chew or crush. **>12 yrs: (Tabs)** 2-4mg tid-qid. **Max:** 32mg/day (8mg qid). **>14yrs: (Syrup)** 2-4mg tid-qid. **Max:** 32mg/day (8mg qid). **Elderly/β-Adrenergic Sensitivity: (Syrup, Tabs) Initial:** 2mg tid-qid. **Max: (Tabs)** 8mg tid-qid. ***Pediatrics:*** **Bronchospasm: 6-14 yrs: (Syrup) Initial:** 2mg tid-qid. **Max:** 24mg/day. **6-12 yrs: (Tab, Extended-Release) Usual:** 4mg q12h. **Max:** 24mg/day in divided doses. Swallow whole with liquids; do not chew or crush. **(Tabs) Initial:** 2mg tid-qid. **Max:** 24mg/day. **2-6 yrs: (Syrup) Initial:** 0.1mg/kg tid (not to exceed 2mg tid). **Titrate:** May increase to 0.2mg/kg/day. **Max:** 4mg tid.	**W/P:** Hypersensitivity reactions reported. Monitor for worsening asthma. Fatalities reported with excessive use. Caution with cardiovascular disorders, especially coronary insufficiency, arrhythmias, and HTN. May need concomitant corticosteroids. Can produce paradoxical bronchospasm. Caution with DM, hyperthyroidism, seizures. May cause transient hypokalemia. Erythema multiforme and Stevens-Johnson (rare) reported in children. **P/N:** Category C, not for use in nursing.	Tachycardia, increased BP, headache, tremor, nervousness, dizziness, N/V, palpitations, paradoxical bronchospasm, muscle spasms, heartburn, rhinitis, respiratory tract infection.
Albuterol Sulfate (AccuNeb)	**Sol, Inhalation:** 1.25mg/3mL, 0.63mg/3mL [3mL, 25[s]]	***Pediatrics:*** **2-12 yrs: Initial:** 0.63mg or 1.25mg tid-qid via nebulizer. **6-12 yrs with Severe Asthma, >40kg or 11-12 yrs: Initial:** 1.25mg tid-qid.	**W/P:** Hypersensitivity reactions reported. Fatalities reported with excessive use. Caution with cardiovascular disorders, especially coronary insufficiency, arrhythmias, and HTN. May need concomitant anti-inflammatory agents. Can produce paradoxical bronchospasm. Caution with DM. May cause hypokalemia. **P/N:** Category C, not for use in nursing.	Asthma exacerbation, otitis media, allergic reaction, gastroenteritis, cold symptoms.
Albuterol Sulfate (ProAir HFA, Proventil HFA, Ventolin HFA)	**MDI:** 90mcg/ inh, ProAir HFA [8.5g], Proventil HFA [6.7g], Ventolin HFA [18g]	***Adults/Pediatrics:*** **≥4 yrs: Treatment/ Prevention of Bronchospasm:** 2 inh q4-6h or 1 inh q4h. **EIB:** 2 inh 15-30 min before activity.	**W/P:** Can produce paradoxical bronchospasm. Monitor for worsening asthma. May produce clinically significant cardiovascular effects; caution with cardiovascular disorders, especially coronary insufficiency, cardiac arrhythmias, and HTN. Fatalities reported with excessive use. Immediate hypersensitivity	**Pharyngitis,** headache, **throat irritation,** rhinitis, **cough,** dizziness, N/V, palpitations, pain, back pain, tachycardia, tremor,

*Scored. †Bold entries denote special dental considerations.
BB = black box warning; **W/P** = warnings/precautions; **Contra** = contraindications; **P/N** = pregnancy category rating and nursing considerations.

Table 15.2. PRESCRIBING INFORMATION FOR RESPIRATORY DRUGS *(cont.)*
(For all inhaled, intranasal, or systemic corticosteroids, refer to Table 5.1 starting on page 163)

NAME	FORM/ STRENGTH	DOSAGE	WARNINGS/PRECAUTIONS & CONTRAINDICATIONS	ADVERSE EFFECTS†
ASTHMA/COPD PREPARATIONS *(cont.)*				
β_2-AGONISTS *(cont.)*				
Albuterol Sulfate (ProAir HFA, Proventil HFA, Ventolin HFA) *(cont.)*			reactions may occur. May need concomitant corticosteroids. Caution with convulsive disorders, hyperthyroidism, DM, and in patients unusually responsive to sympathomimetic amines. May cause significant hypokalemia. **P/N:** Category C, not for use in nursing.	upper respiratory tract infection, fever, inhalation site and **taste sensations,** nervousness.
Albuterol Sulfate/ Ipratropium Bromide (Combivent)	**MDI:** 0.09mg-0.018mg/inh [14.7g]	***Adults:*** 2 inh qid. **Max:** 12 inh/24 hrs.	**W/P:** Paradoxical bronchospasm reported. Hypersensitivity reactions reported. Caution with coronary insufficiency, arrhythmias, narrow-angle glaucoma, prostatic hypertrophy, bladder-neck obstruction, HTN, DM, hyperthyroidism, seizures, renal or hepatic dysfunction, and in those unusually responsive to sympathomimetic amines. May produce transient hypokalemia. Fatalities reported with excessive use. **Contra:** History of hypersensitivity to soya lecithin or related food products (eg, soybeans, peanuts). **P/N:** Category C, not for use in nursing.	Headache, cough, respiratory disorders, pain, dyspnea, bronchitis.
Albuterol Sulfate/ Ipratropium Bromide (Duoneb)	**Sol, Inhalation:** 3mg-0.5mg/3mL [3mL, 30[s] 60[s]]	***Adults:*** 3mL qid via nebulizer. May give 2 additional doses/day.	**W/P:** Paradoxical bronchospasm and hypersensitivity reactions reported. Caution with cardiovascular disorders, convulsive disorders, hyperthyroidism, DM, narrow-angle glaucoma, prostatic hypertrophy, and bladder-neck obstruction. **Contra:** Hypersensitivity to atropine and its derivatives. **P/N:** Category C (albuterol) and B (ipratropium), not for use in nursing.	Pain, chest pain, diarrhea, dyspepsia, nausea, leg cramps, bronchitis, lung disease, **pharyngitis,** pneumonia, UTI.
Arformoterol Tartrate (Brovana)	**Sol, Inhalation:** 15mcg/2mL [30[s], 60[s]]	***Adults:*** **Usual:** 15mcg bid (am and pm). **Max:** 30mcg/day. Administer via nebulizer.	**BB:** Long-acting β_2-adrenergic agonists may increase the risk of asthma-related death. **W/P:** Not indicated for treatment of acute episodes of bronchospasm. Should not be initiated or used in children or patients with acutely deteriorating COPD. Fatalities reported with excessive use of inhaled sympathomimetics; avoid use with other long-acting β_2-agonists. D/C regular use of short acting β_2-agonists (eg, qid) before initiating therapy. May produce life-threatening paradoxical bronchospasm. Caution in patients with convulsive disorders, thyrotoxicosis, cardiovascular disorders especially coronary insufficiency, cardiac arrhythmias, and HTN. Immediate hypersensitivity reactions may occur. **Contra:** Hypersensitivity to racemic formoterol. **P/N:** Category C, caution in nursing.	Pain, chest pain, back pain , diarrhea, sinusitis, leg cramps, dyspnea, rash, flu syndrome, peripheral edema.

†Bold entries denote special dental considerations.
BB = black box warning; **W/P** = warnings/precautions; **Contra** = contraindications; **P/N** = pregnancy category rating and nursing considerations.

NAME	FORM/ STRENGTH	DOSAGE	WARNINGS/PRECAUTIONS & CONTRAINDICATIONS	ADVERSE EFFECTS†
Formoterol Fumarate (Foradil)	**Cap (Inhalation):** 12mcg [12[s], 60[s]]	***Adults/Pediatrics:*** **≥5 yrs:** Do not swallow cap; give only by inhalation with Aerolizer™ Inhaler. **Asthma/COPD:** 12mcg q12h. **Max:** 24mcg/day. **≥12yrs: EIB:** 12mcg 15 min before exercise (do not give added dose if already on q12h dose).	**BB:** Long-acting β_2-agonists may increase the risk of asthma-related death. **W/P:** Do not d/c inhaled corticosteroids. Only use short-acting β_2-agonist inhaler for acute symptoms. D/C if paradoxical bronchospasm occurs. D/C if ECG changes, QT interval increases, or ST depression occurs. Caution with cardiovascular disorders (eg, HTN, arrhythmias), thyrotoxicosis, and convulsive disorders. Anaphylactic and other allergic reactions reported. Not for use in acute asthmatic conditions. Should not be used with other long-acting β_2-agonist medications. May cause hypokalemia. **P/N:** Category C, caution in nursing.	Viral infection, dyspnea, chest pain, tremor, HTN, hypotension, tachycardia, arrhythmias, headache, N/V, fatigue, hypokalemia, hyperglycemia, exacerbation of asthma.
Formoterol Fumarate (Perforomist)	**Sol, Inhalation:** 20mcg/2mL [2.5mL, 60[s]]	***Adults:*** 20mcg bid q12h. Administer by nebulizer.	**BB:** Long-acting β_2-agonists may increase risk of asthma-related death. **W/P:** Only use short-acting β_2-agonist inhaler for acute symptoms. Should not be used with other long-acting β_2-agonist medications. D/C if paradoxical bronchospasm occurs. D/C if ECG changes, QT interval increases, or ST depression occurs. Caution with cardiovascular disorders (eg, coronary insufficiency, arrythmias, and HTN), convulsive disorders, thyrotoxicosis, and DM. May cause hypokalemia and hyperglycemia. **P/N:** Category C, caution in nursing.	Diarrhea, nausea, **nasopharyngitis, dry mouth,** angina, HTN, hypotension, tachycardia, arrythmias, nervousness, headache, tremor, muscle cramps, palpitations, dizziness.
Levalbuterol HCl (Xopenex)	**Sol, Inhalation:** 0.31mg/3mL, 0.63mg/3mL, 1.25mg/3mL [3mL, 24[s]]	***Adults/Pediatrics:*** **≥12 yrs: Initial:** 0.63mg tid, q6-8h. **Severe Asthma:** 1.25mg tid, q6-8h. Administer by nebulizer. ***Pediatrics:*** **6-11 yrs:** 0.31mg tid. **Max:** 0.63mg tid. Administer by nebulizer.	**W/P:** Hypersensitivity reactions reported. D/C immediately if paradoxical bronchospasm occurs. May produce ECG changes; caution with cardiovascular disorders, coronary insufficiency, arrhythmias, and HTN. Caution with convulsive disorders, hyperthyroidism, and diabetes. May produce transient hypokalemia. **P/N:** Category C, not for use in nursing.	Tachycardia, migraine, dyspepsia, leg cramps, nervousness, dizziness, tremor, rhinitis, increased cough, chest pain, HTN, hypotension, diarrhea, **dry mouth,** anxiety, insomnia, paresthesia, wheezing.
Levalbuterol Tartrate (Xopenex HFA)	**MDI:** 45mcg/inh [15g]	***Adults/Pediatrics:*** **≥4 yrs:** 2 inh (90mcg) q4-6h or 1 inh (45mcg) q4h may be sufficient.	**W/P:** D/C immediately if paradoxical bronchospasm occurs. May produce ECG changes; caution with cardiovascular disorders, coronary insufficiency, arrhythmias, and HTN. Caution with convulsive disorders, hyperthyroidism, and diabetes. May produce transient hypokalemia. **P/N:** Category C, not for use in nursing.	Asthma, **pharyngitis,** rhinitis, pain, vomiting.
Metaproterenol Sulfate	**MDI:** 0.65mg/inh [14g]; **Sol, Inhalation:** 0.4% [2.5mL], 0.6% [2.5mL]; **Syrup:** 10mg/5mL [480mL]; **Tab:** 10mg, 20mg	***Adults/Pediatrics:*** **≥12 yrs:** (MDI) 2-3 inh q3-4h. **Max:** 12 inh/day. (Sol 0.4%, 0.6%) 2.5mL by IPPB tid-qid, up to q4h. (Syr, Tab) 20mg tid-qid. ***Pediatrics:*** (Syr, Tab) **>9 yrs or >60 lbs:** 20mg tid-qid. **6-9 yrs or <60 lbs:** 10mg tid-qid.	**W/P:** Caution with cardiovascular disorders, (eg, ischemic heart disease, HTN, arrhythmias), hyperthyroidism, diabetes, convulsive disorders. Fatalities reported with excessive use. Can produce paradoxical bronchospasm. Monitor BP. Nebulized solution single dose may not abort an asthma attack. **Contra:** Cardiac arrhythmias associated with tachycardia. **P/N:** Category C, caution in nursing.	Headache, dizziness, HTN, GI distress, **throat irritation,** cough, asthma exacerbation, nervousness, tremor, N/V.
Pirbuterol Acetate (Maxair, Maxair Autohaler)	**Autohaler:** 0.2mg/inh [14g, 25.6g]; **MDI:** 0.2mg/inh [14g]	***Adults/Pediatrics:*** **≥12 yrs:** 1-2 inh q4-6h. **Max:** 12 inh/day.	**W/P:** Caution with cardiovascular disorders, (eg, ischemic heart disease, HTN, arrhythmias), hyperthyroidism, diabetes, convulsive disorders. Fatalities reported with excessive use. Can produce paradoxical bronchospasm. Monitor BP. **P/N:** Category C, caution in nursing.	Nervousness, tremor, headache, dizziness, palpitations, tachycardia, cough, nausea.

Table 15.2. PRESCRIBING INFORMATION FOR RESPIRATORY DRUGS *(cont.)*
(For all inhaled, intranasal, or systemic corticosteroids, refer to Table 5.1 starting on page 163)

NAME	FORM/ STRENGTH	DOSAGE	WARNINGS/PRECAUTIONS & CONTRAINDICATIONS	ADVERSE EFFECTS†
ASTHMA/COPD PREPARATIONS *(cont.)*				
β_2-AGONISTS *(cont.)*				
Salmeterol Xinafoate (Serevent)	**Disk:** 50mcg [28, 60 blisters]	***Adults/Pediatrics:* ≥4 yrs: Asthma/ COPD:** 1 inh bid, am and pm (12 hrs apart). **EIB Prevention:** 1 inh 30 min before exercise (do not give preventive doses if already on bid dose).	**BB:** Long-acting β_2-adrenergic agonists, such as salmeterol, may increase the risk of asthma-related deaths. **W/P:** Avoid with significantly worsening or acutely deteriorating asthma. Not for acute treatment or substitute for oral/ inhaled corticosteroids. Monitor for increasing use of inhaled β_2-agonists. QTc interval prolongation reported when recommended dose exceeded. D/C if paradoxical bronchospasm occurs. Immediate hypersensitivity and upper airway symptom reactions reported. Caution with cardiovascular disorder (eg, coronary insufficiency, arrhythmia, HTN), convulsive disorders, thyrotoxicosis, if usually unresponsive to sympathomimetic amines. May cause hypokalemia. **P/N:** Category C, not for use in nursing.	Nasal/sinus congestion, pallor, rhinitis, headache, **tracheitis/**bronchitis, influenza, **throat irritation.**
Terbutaline Sulfate	**Inj:** 1mg/mL [1mL]; **Tab:** 2.5mg*, 5mg*	***Adults/Pediatrics:* ≥12 yrs:** (Inj) **Usual:** 0.25mg SQ into lateral deltoid area. May repeat within 15-30 min if no improvement. **Max:** 0.5mg/4hrs. ***Adults:*** (PO) **Usual:** 5mg tid. May reduce to 2.5mg tid. **Max:** 15mg/24hrs. ***Pediatrics:* 12-15 yrs:** (PO) **Usual:** 2.5mg tid. **Max:** 7.5mg/24hrs.	**W/P:** Caution with ischemic heart disease, HTN, arrhythmias, hyperthyroidism, DM, seizures. Not approved for tocolysis. Hypersensitivity and exacerbation of bronchospasm reported. Monitor for transient hypokalemia. **Contra:** Hypersensitivity to sympathomimetic amines. **P/N:** Category B, caution in nursing.	Nervousness, tremor, headache, somnolence, palpitations, dizziness, tachycardia, nausea.
LEUKOTRIENE-RECEPTOR ANTAGONISTS				
Montelukast Sodium (Singulair)	**Granules:** 4mg/ pkt; **Tab, Chewable:** 4mg, 5mg; **Tab:** 10mg	***Adults/Pediatrics:* ≥15 yrs: Asthma:** 10mg qpm. **Allergic Rhinitis:** 10mg qd. **EIB:** 10mg 2 hrs before exercise. Do not take additional dose within 24 hrs of previous dose. ***Pediatrics:* Asthma: 6-14 yrs:** 5mg qpm. **2-5 yrs:** 4mg qpm. **6-23 months:** 4mg qpm. **Seasonal/ Perennial Allergic Rhinitis: 6-14 yrs:** 5mg qd. **2-5 yrs:** 4mg qd. **Perennial Allergic Rhinitis: 6-23 months:** 4mg qd. Do not take additional dose within 24 hrs of previous dose. Granules may be mixed with applesauce, carrots, rice, or ice cream; give within 15 min of opening pkt.	**W/P:** Not for treatment of acute asthma attacks. Do not abruptly substitute for inhaled or oral corticosteroids. Eosinophilic conditions reported (rare). **P/N:** Category B, caution in nursing.	(Adults, Pediatrics) Headache, abdominal pain, dyspepsia, cough, flu. (Pediatrics) **Pharyngitis**, flu, fever, sinusitis, nausea, diarrhea, dyspepsia, otitis, viral infection, laryngitis.
Zafirlukast (Accolate)	**Tab:** 10mg, 20mg	***Adults:*** 20mg bid. Administer 1 hr ac or 2 hrs pc. ***Pediatrics:* ≥12 yrs:** 20mg bid. **5-11 yrs:** 10mg bid. Administer 1 hr ac or 2 hrs pc.	**W/P:** Cases of life-threatening hepatic failure reported; if suspected, d/c therapy. Not for treatment of acute asthma attacks. Bioavailability decreases with food. Hepatic dysfunction and systemic eosinophilia reported. **P/N:** Category B, not for use in nursing.	Headache, infection, nausea, diarrhea, hypersensitivity reactions including angioedema.
Zileuton (Zyflo CR)	**Tab, Extended-Release:** 600mg	***Adults/Pediatrics:* ≥12 yrs:** 1200mg bid within 1 hr after am and pm meals. **Max:** 2400mg/day.	**W/P:** Not for treatment of acute attacks. Evaluate liver function prior to therapy and periodically thereafter. D/C if signs of liver disease occur. **Contra:** Active liver disease or transaminase elevations (≥3x ULN). **P/N:** Category C, not for use in nursing.	Headache, ALT elevation, dyspepsia, pain, nausea, asthenia, myalgia, sinusitis, **pharyngolaryngeal pain**.
MAST CELL STABILIZER				
Cromolyn Sodium (Intal)	**MDI:** (Intal) 0.8mg/inh [8.1g, 14.2g];	***Adults/Pediatrics:* ≥5 yrs: Acute Bronchospasm Prevention:** (Inhaler) **Usual:** 2 inh 10-60 min before exposure	**W/P:** Not for treatment of acute attack. Severe anaphylaxis may occur. D/C if eosinophilic pneumonia or pulmonary	**Throat irritation/ dryness, bad taste,** cough, nausea,

*Scored. †Bold entries denote special dental considerations.
BB = black box warning; **W/P** = warnings/precautions; **Contra** = contraindications; **P/N** = pregnancy category rating and nursing considerations.

NAME	FORM/ STRENGTH	DOSAGE	WARNINGS/PRECAUTIONS & CONTRAINDICATIONS	ADVERSE EFFECTS†
Cromolyn Sodium (Intal) *(cont.)*	**Sol**: 10mg/mL [2mL, 10^{s} 60^{s}]	to precipitant. **Asthma:** (Inhaler) **Usual/Max:** 2 inh qid. **≥2 yrs: Acute Bronchospasm Prevention:** (Sol) 20mg nebulized shortly before exposure to precipitant. **Asthma:** (Sol) 20mg qid via nebulizer. **Renal/Hepatic Dysfunction:** Decrease inhaler dose.	infiltrates with eosinophilia develop. May experience cough and/or bronchospasm. Caution with inhaler in CAD or history of cardiac arrhythmias. Decrease dose or d/c with renal/hepatic dysfunction. **P/N:** Category B, caution in nursing.	bronchospasm, sneezing, wheezing.
MONOCLONAL ANTIBODY/IgE-BLOCKER				
Omalizumab (Xolair)	**Inj:** 150mg [5mL]	***Adults/Pediatrics:*** **≥12 yrs:** 150-375mg SQ every 2 or 4 weeks based on body weight and pretreatment serum total IgE level. **Max:** 150mg/site. **30-90kg & IgE ≥30-100 IU/mL:** 150mg every 4 weeks. **>90-150kg & IgE ≥30-100 IU/mL OR 30-90kg & IgE >100-200 IU/mL OR 30-60kg & IgE >200-300 IU/mL:** 300mg every 4 weeks. **>90-150kg & IgE >100-200 IU/mL OR >60-90kg & IgE >200-300 IU/mL OR 30-70kg & IgE >300-400 IU/mL:** 225mg every 2 weeks. **>90-150kg & IgE >200-300 IU/mL OR >70-90kg & IgE >300-400 IU/mL OR 30-70kg & IgE >400-500 IU/mL OR 30-60kg & IgE >500-600 IU/mL:** 300mg every 2 weeks. **>70-90kg & IgE >400-500 IU/mL OR >60-70kg & IgE >500-600 IU/mL OR 30-60kg & IgE >600-700 IU/mL:** 375mg every 2 weeks.	**BB:** Anaphylaxis, presenting as bronchospasm, hypotension, syncope, urticaria, and/or angioedema of the throat or tongue has been reported. Monitor patients closely for an appropriate time period after administration. **W/P:** Malignant neoplasms reported. Not for use in treatment of acute bronchospasm or status asthmaticus. Systemic or inhaled corticosteroids should not be abruptly discontinued when initiating therapy. **P/N:** Category B, caution in nursing.	Anaphylaxis, malignancies, injection-site reactions, viral infections, upper respiratory infection, sinusitis, headache, **pharyngitis,** pain, arthralgia.
XANTHINE BRONCHODILATOR				
Theophylline (Theo-24, Uniphyl)	**Cap, Extended-Release:** 100mg, 200mg, 300mg, 400mg; **Tab, Extended-Release:** 400mg*, 600mg*	***Adults:*** **Initial:** 300-400mg/day. **Titrate:** After 3 days increase to 400-600mg/day if tolerated. May increase to >600mg/day if needed and tolerated after 3 more days. **Renal/Liver Dysfunction/Elderly > 60 yrs/CHF: Max:** 400mg/day. May give in divided doses q12h in fast metabolizers. Swallow tab whole with full glass of water, do not crush. Dose should be titrated based on serum levels. ***Pediatrics:*** **12-15 yrs: <45kg: Initial:** 12-14mg/kg/day. **Max:** 300mg/day. **Titrate:** After 3 days increase to 16mg/kg/day. **Max:** 400mg/day. May increase to 20mg/kg/day if tolerated and needed after 3 more days. **Max:** 600mg/day. **12-15 yrs: >45kg:** Follow adult dose schedule. **Renal/Liver Dysfunction/CHF: Max:** 16mg/kg/day or 400mg/day. May give in divided doses q12h in fast metabolizers. Swallow tab whole with full glass of water, do not crush. Dose should be titrated based on serum levels.	**W/P:** Extreme caution in PUD, seizure disorders, and/or cardiac arrhythmias (except bradycardia). Caution in neonates, children <1 yr, and the elderly. Caution in pulmonary edema, CHF, fever ≥102°F for 24 hrs, cor pulmonale, hypothyroidism, liver disease, reduced renal function, sepsis, shock, and HTN. If toxicity develops (eg, repetitive vomiting) monitor serum levels and adjust dosage. **P/N:** Category C, caution in nursing.	Diarrhea, N/V, abdominal pain, nervousness, headache, insomnia, seizures, dizziness, tachycardia, arrhythmias, restlessness, tremor, transient diuresis.
COUGH & COLD COMBINATIONS				
ANTIHISTAMINES				
Acrivastine/ Pseudoephedrine HCl (Semprex-D)	**Cap:** 8mg-60mg	***Adults/Pediatrics:*** **≥12 yrs:** 1 cap q4-6h, qid.	**W/P:** Not for use >14 days. Caution with HTN, DM, increased IOP, ischemic heart disease, hyperthyroidism, BPH, renal impairment, peptic ulcer, pyloroduodenal obstruction, and elderly. Sedation reported. Avoid with CrCl ≤48mL/min. **Contra:** Severe HTN, CAD, MAOIs during or within 14 days of use. Hypersensitivity to alkylamine antihistamines. **P/N:** Category B, caution in nursing.	Somnolence, headache, **dry mouth,** insomnia, dizziness, nervousness, **pharyngitis.**

Table 15.2. PRESCRIBING INFORMATION FOR RESPIRATORY DRUGS *(cont.)*
(For all inhaled, intranasal, or systemic corticosteroids, refer to Table 5.1 starting on page 163)

NAME	FORM/ STRENGTH	DOSAGE	WARNINGS/PRECAUTIONS & CONTRAINDICATIONS	ADVERSE EFFECTS†
COUGH & COLD COMBINATIONS *(cont.)*				
ANTIHISTAMINES *(cont.)*				
Brompheniramine Maleate/Dextromethorphan HBr/Phenylephrine HCl (Alacol DM)	**Syrup:** 2mg-10mg-5mg/5mL	***Adults:*** 10mL q4h. **Max:** 6 doses/24 hrs. ***Pediatrics:*** **>12 yrs:** 10mL q4h. **6-12 yrs:** 5mL q4h. **2-6 yrs:** 2.5mL q4h. **Max:** 6 doses/24 hrs.	**W/P:** Caution with persistent or chronic cough (eg, associated with asthma, emphysema, smoking, excessive phlegm). Persistent cough may be a sign of a serious condition. May diminish mental alertness. May produce excitation in children. Caution with asthma, narrow-angle glaucoma, GI obstruction, urinary bladder neck obstruction, DM, HTN, heart and thyroid disease. **Contra:** Newborns, premature infants, nursing, severe HTN or CAD, with MAOIs, lower respiratory tract conditions including asthma. **P/N:** Category C, contraindicated in nursing.	Sedation, thickening of bronchial secretions, dizziness, **dryness of mouth,** nose**, and throat.**
Brompheniramine Maleate/Pseudoephedrine HCl (Bromfed, Bromfed-PD, Bromfenex, Bromfenex-PD)	**Cap, Extended-Release:** (PD) 6mg- 60mg, (Bromfed, Bromfenex) 12mg-120mg	***Adults/Pediatrics:*** **≥12 yrs:** (12mg-120mg) 1 cap q12h. (6mg-60mg) 1-2 caps q12h. ***Pediatrics:*** **6-11 yrs:** (6mg-60mg) 1 cap q12h.	**W/P:** Caution with HTN, DM, ischemic heart disease, hyperthyroidism, increased IOP, prostatic hypertrophy, and elderly. Caution while operating machinery. **Contra:** Severe HTN, CAD, narrow-angle glaucoma, MAOI therapy, urinary retention, peptic ulcer, during an asthmatic attack. **P/N:** Safety in pregnancy and nursing not known.	Drowsiness, lassitude, nausea, giddiness, **dryness of the mouth,** blurred vision, palpitations, flushing, increased irritability or excitement.
Carbetapentane Tannate/Chlorpheniramine Tannate (Tussi-12)	**Sus:** 30mg-4mg/5mL [118mL]; **Tab:** 60mg-5mg*	***Adults:*** 1-2 tabs q12h. ***Pediatrics:*** **>6 yrs:** 5-10mL q12h. **2-6 yrs:** 2.5-5mL q12h.	**W/P:** Caution with HTN, CVD, hyperthyroidism, DM, elderly, narrow-angle glaucoma, or prostatic hypertrophy. Excitation in children may occur. Suspension contains tartrazine. **Contra:** Newborns, nursing mothers. **P/N:** Category C, not for use in nursing.	Drowsiness, sedation, **dryness of mucous membranes,** GI effects.
Carbetapentane Tannate/Chlorpheniramine Tannate/ Ephedrine Tannate/ Phenylephrine Tannate (Rynatuss)	**Tab:** 60mg-5mg-10mg-10mg*	***Adults:*** 1-2 tabs q12h.	**W/P:** Caution with HTN, cardiovascular disease, hyperthyroidism, DM, narrow-angle glaucoma, elderly, or prostatic hypertrophy. Suspension contains FD&C Yellow No. 5, which may cause allergic-type reactions. **Contra:** Newborns, nursing mothers. **P/N:** Category C, not for use in nursing.	Drowsiness, sedation, **dryness of mucous membranes,** GI effects.
Cetirizine HCl/ Pseudoephedrine HCl (Zyrtec-D)	**Tab, Extended-Release:** 5mg-120mg	***Adults/Pediatrics:*** **≥12 yrs:** 1 tab bid. **Hepatic Impairment/Renal Dysfunction (CrCl <31mL/min):** 1 tab qd. Swallow whole.	**W/P:** Caution with HTN, DM, ischemic heart disease, increased IOP, hyperthyroidism, renal impairment, or prostatic hypertrophy. May produce CNS stimulation with convulsions or cardiovascular collapse. May impair mental/ physical abilities. **Contra:** Narrow-angle glaucoma, urinary retention, MAOIs during or within 14 days of use, severe HTN, severe CAD, hypersensitivity to adrenergics. **P/N:** Category C, not for use in nursing.	Insomnia, **dry mouth,** fatigue, somnolence.
Chlorpheniramine Maleate/Dextromethorphan HBr/Phenylephrine HCl (Rondec-DM Oral Drops, Rondec-DM Syrup)	**Sol**: 1mg-3mg-3.5mg/mL [30mL]; **Syrup:** 4mg-15mg-12.5mg/5mL [20mL, 118mL, 473mL]	(Sol) ***Pediatrics:*** Give qid. **12-24 months:** 1mL. **6-12 months:** 3/4mL. (Syrup) ***Adults/Pediatrics:*** **≥12 yrs:** 5mL q4-6h. **Max:** 30mL/24 hrs. **Pediatrics: 6 to <12 yrs:** 2.5mL q4-6h. **Max:** 15mL/24 hrs. **2 to <6 yrs:** 1.25mL q4-6h. **Max:** 7.5mL/24 hrs.	**W/P:** Caution with HTN, DM, heart disease, asthma, hyperthyroidism, increased IOP, prostatic hypertrophy, and in atopic children, elderly, sedated, debilitated, or confined to supine positions. May cause excitability, especially in children. Do not exceed recommended doses. **Contra:** Severe HTN or CAD, narrow-angle glaucoma, urinary retention, peptic ulcer, acute asthma attack, with, or for 2 weeks after stopping, MAOI therapy. **P/N:** Category C, not for use in nursing.	Sedation, drowsiness, dizziness, diplopia, N/V, diarrhea, **dry mouth,** headache, nervousness, convulsions, CNS stimulation, arrhythmias, increased HR or BP, tremors.

*Scored. †Bold entries denote special dental considerations.
BB = black box warning; **W/P** = warnings/precautions; **Contra** = contraindications; **P/N** = pregnancy category rating and nursing considerations.

NAME	FORM/ STRENGTH	DOSAGE	WARNINGS/PRECAUTIONS & CONTRAINDICATIONS	ADVERSE EFFECTS†
Chlorpheniramine Maleate/Methscopolamine Nitrate/ Phenylephrine HCl (Dallergy)	**Syrup:** 2mg-0.625mg-10mg/5mL; **Tab:** 4mg-1.25mg-10mg*; **Tab, Extended-Release:** 12mg-2.5mg-20mg	***Adults:*** 1 tab or 10mL q4-6h. **Max:** 4 doses/24hrs. ***Pediatrics:*** **≥12 yrs:** 1 tab or 10mL q4-6h. **6-12 yrs:** 1/2 tab or 5mL q4-6h. **Max:** 4 doses/24hrs.	**W/P:** Caution in HTN, DM, ischemic heart disease, hyperthyroidism, increased IOP, prostatic hypertrophy. Adverse events more common in elderly. May cause excitability in children. **Contra:** Severe HTN, severe CAD, MAOI therapy, narrow-angle glaucoma, urinary retention, PUD, during asthma attack. **P/N:** Category C, caution in nursing.	Drowsiness, lassitude, nausea, giddiness, **dry mouth,** blurred vision, cardiac palpitations, flushing, increased irritability or excitement.
Chlorpheniramine Maleate/Methscopolamine Nitrate/ Pseudoephedrine HCl (AlleRx)	**Tab, Extended-Release, AM Dose:** (Methscopolamine-Pseudoephedrine) 2.5mg-120mg; **PM Dose:** (Chlorpheniramine-Methscopolamine) 8mg-2.5mg	***Adults/Pediatrics:*** **≥12 yrs:** 1 AM Dose tab in morning and 1 PM Dose tab in evening.	**W/P:** Caution with elderly, HTN, DM, ischemic heart disease, hyperthyroidism, prostatic hypertrophy, CVD, increased IOP. May produce CNS stimulation with convulsions or cardiovascular collapse with hypotension. Excitability reported, especially in children. **Contra:** Severe HTN or CAD, MAOI use or within 14 days of discontinuation, nursing mothers taking MAOIs, narrow-angle glaucoma, urinary retention, peptic ulcer, during asthma attack. **P/N:** Category C, not for use in nursing.	Drowsiness, lassitude, nausea, giddiness, **dry mouth,** blurred vision, cardiac palpitations, flushing, increased irritability.
Chlorpheniramine Maleate/Phenylephrine HCl (Dallergy Jr, Rondec Oral Drops, Rondec Syrup)	**Cap:** (Dallergy Jr) 4mg-20mg; **Sol**: 1mg-3.5mg/ mL [30mL]; **Syrup:** 4mg-12.5mg/5mL [20mL, 118mL, 473mL]	(Caps) ***Adults/Pediatrics:*** **>12 yrs:** 2 caps q12h. **Max:** 2 doses/24h. **6-12 yrs:** 1 cap q12h. **Max:** 2 doses/24h. (Sol) ***Pediatrics:*** Give qid. **12-24 months:** 1mL. **6-12 months:** 3/4mL. (Syrup) ***Adults/Pediatrics:*** **≥12 yrs:** 5mL q4-6h. **Max:** 30mL/24 hrs. ***Pediatrics:*** **6 to <12 yrs:** 2.5mL q4-6h. **Max:** 15mL/24 hrs. **2 to <6 yrs:** 1.25mL q4-6h. **Max:** 7.5mL/24 hrs.	**W/P:** Caution with HTN, DM, ischemic heart disease, hyperthyroidism, increased IOP, prostatic hypertrophy, the elderly. May cause excitability, especially in children. **Contra:** Severe HTN, severe CAD, MAOI therapy, narrow-angle glaucoma, urinary retention, PUD, during asthma attack. **P/N:** Category C, caution in nursing.	Drowsiness, lassitude, nausea, giddiness, **dry mouth,** blurred vision, cardiac palpitations, flushing, increased irritability or excitement.
Chlorpheniramine Maleate/Pseudoephedrine HCl (Deconamine SR)	**Cap, Sustained-Release:** (Chlorpheniramine-Pseudoephedrine) 8mg-120mg	***Adults/Pediatrics:*** **≥12 yrs:** 1 cap q12h.	**W/P:** Extreme caution in narrow-angle glaucoma, stenosing peptic ulcer, pyloroduodenal obstruction, symptomatic prostatic hypertrophy, bladder neck obstruction. Caution in bronchial asthma, emphysema, chronic pulmonary disease, HTN, ischemic heart disease, DM, increased IOP, hyperthyroidism. May cause excitability in children. May produce CNS stimulation with convulsions or cardiovascular collapse with hypotension. **Contra:** Severe HTN, severe CAD, concomitant MAOIs. **P/N:** Category C, not for use in nursing.	Drowsiness, urticaria, drug rash, hypotension, hemolytic anemia, sedation, epigastric distress, urinary frequency, nervousness, dizziness.
Chlorpheniramine Tannate/Phenylephrine Tannate (Rynatan Pediatric, Rynatan)	**Sus:** (Pediatric) 4.5mg-5mg/ 5mL; **Tab:** 9mg-25mg; **Tab, Chewable:** (Pediatric) 4.5mg-5mg	(Sus) ***Pediatrics:*** **>6 yrs:** 5-10mL q12h. **2-6 yrs:** 2.5-5mL q12h. **<2 yrs:** Titrate individually. (Tab/Tab, Chew) ***Adults/ Pediatrics:*** **>6 yrs:** 1-2 tabs q12h. **2-6 yrs:** 1/2-1 tab q12h.	**W/P:** Caution with HTN, cardiovascular disease, hyperthyroidism, DM, narrow-angle glaucoma, prostatic hypertrophy, and elderly. May impair mental alertness. Contains tartrazine. **Contra:** Newborns and nursing mothers. **P/N:** Category C, not for use in nursing.	Drowsiness, sedation, **dryness of mucous membranes,** GI effects.

Table 15.2. PRESCRIBING INFORMATION FOR RESPIRATORY DRUGS *(cont.)*
(For all inhaled, intranasal, or systemic corticosteroids, refer to Table 5.1 starting on page 163)

NAME	FORM/ STRENGTH	DOSAGE	WARNINGS/PRECAUTIONS & CONTRAINDICATIONS	ADVERSE EFFECTS†
COUGH & COLD COMBINATIONS *(cont.)*				
ANTIHISTAMINES *(cont.)*				
Desloratadine/ Pseudoephedrine Sulfate (Clarinex-D)	**Tab, Extended-Release:** (12-Hr) 2.5mg-120mg, (24-Hr) 5mg-240mg	***Adults/Pediatrics:* ≥12 yrs:** 2.5mg-120mg tab bid or 5mg-240mg tab qd w/ or w/o food. **Hepatic Impairment: 12-Hour/24-Hour:** Avoid use. **Renal Impairment: 12-Hour:** Avoid use. **24-Hour:** 1 tab qod.	**W/P:** Caution with HTN, DM, ischemic heart disease, increased IOP, hyperthyroidism, renal impairment, or prostatic hypertrophy. CNS stimulation with convulsions or cardiovascular collapse with accompanying hypotension may be produced by sympathomimetic amines. Avoid with hepatic insufficiency. **Contra:** Narrow-angle glaucoma, urinary retention, MAOI therapy or within 14 days of discontinuation, severe HTN, severe CAD, hypersensitivity or idiosyncrasy to adrenergic agents or to other drugs of similar chemical structures. **P/N:** Category C, not for use in nursing.	**Dry mouth,** headache, insomnia, fatigue, **pharyngitis,** somnolence.
Fexofenadine HCl/ Pseudoephedrine HCl (Allegra-D)	**Tab, Extended-Release:** (12-Hour) 60mg-120mg, (24-Hour) 180mg-240mg	***Adults/Pediatrics:* ≥12 yrs:** 60mg-120mg tab bid or 180mg-240mg tab qd without food. **Renal Dysfunction: Initial:** 60mg-120mg tab qd; avoid 180mg-240mg tab. Do not crush or chew.	**W/P:** Caution with HTN, DM, ischemic heart disease, increased IOP, hyperthyroidism, renal impairment, or prostatic hypertrophy. May produce CNS stimulation with convulsions or cardiovascular collapse with hypotension. **Contra:** Narrow-angle glaucoma, urinary retention, severe HTN, severe CAD, within 14 days of MAOI therapy. **P/N:** Category C, caution with nursing.	Headache, insomnia, nausea, **dry mouth,** dyspepsia, **throat irritation.**
Loratadine/ Pseudoephedrine Sulfate (Claritin-D OTC)	**Tab, Extended-Release:** (12-Hour) 5mg-120mg, (24-Hour) 10mg-240mg	***Adults/Pediatrics:* ≥12 yrs:** 5-120mg tab q12h or 10-240mg tab qd (with full glass of water). **Max:** 10-240mg/24 hrs. **Hepatic/Renal Impairment:** May need to adjust dose. Do not divide, crush, chew, or dissolve tabs.	**W/P:** Caution with hepatic or renal impairment, heart disease, thyroid disease, high BP, diabetes, enlarged prostate. **P/N:** Safety in pregnancy and nursing is not known.	Dizziness, insomnia, nervousness.
Phenylephrine HCl/ Promethazine HCl (Promethazine VC)	**Syrup:** 5mg/5mL-6.25mg	***Adults/Pediatrics:* ≥12 yrs:** 5mL q4-6h. **Max:** 30mL/24 hr. ***Pediatrics:* 6-11 yrs:** 2.5-5mL q4-6h. **Max:** 30mL/24 hr. **2-5 yrs:** 1.25-2.5mL q4-6h.	**W/P:** Caution in pediatrics ≥2 yrs. Avoid in pediatric patients whose signs and symptoms may suggest Reye's syndrome or other hepatic diseases. May impair mental/physical abilities. May lower seizure threshold; caution with seizure disorders. May lead to potentially fatal respiratory depression; avoid with compromised respiratory function (eg, COPD, sleep apnea). Caution with bone marrow depression; leukopenia and agranulocytosis reported. Neuroleptic malignant syndrome reported. Caution with narrow-angle glaucoma, prostatic hypertrophy, stenosing peptic ulcer, bladder neck or pyloroduodenal obstruction, cardiovascular disease, and elderly patients. Cholestatic jaundice reported. May alter HCG pregnancy test reading. May increase blood glucose. Avoid prolonged exposure to sunlight. **Contra:** Concomitant MAOIs, comatose states, treatment of lower respiratory tract symptoms (eg, asthma), HTN, peripheral vascular insufficiency, pediatric patients <2 yrs. **P/N:** Category C, caution in nursing.	Drowsiness, dizziness, anxiety, tremor, sedation, blurred vision, **dry mouth,** increased or decreased blood pressure, rash, N/V.

†Bold entries denote special dental considerations.
BB = black box warning; **W/P** = warnings/precautions; **Contra** = contraindications; **P/N** = pregnancy category rating and nursing considerations.

NAME	FORM/ STRENGTH	DOSAGE	WARNINGS/PRECAUTIONS & CONTRAINDICATIONS	ADVERSE EFFECTS†
COUGH SUPPRESSANTS				
Benzonatate (Tessalon)	**Cap:** 100mg, 200mg	***Adults/Pediatrics:*** **>10 yrs: Usual:** 100-200mg tid as needed. **Max:** 600mg/day.	**W/P:** Severe hypersensitivity reactions; confusion and hallucinations reported in combination with other prescribed drugs. Swallow capsules without sucking/chewing to avoid local anesthesia adverse effects. **P/N:** Category C, caution in nursing.	Sedation, headache, dizziness, confusion, hallucinations, constipation, nausea, GI upset, pruritus.
Chlorpheniramine Polistirex/Hydrocodone Polistirex (Tussionex Pennkinetic)	**Sus, Extended-Release:** 8mg-10mg/5mL	***Adults/Pediatrics:*** **≥12 yrs:** 5mL q12h. **Max:** 10mL/24 hrs. ***Pediatrics:*** **6-11 yrs:** 2.5mL q12h. **Max:** 5mL/24 hrs.	**W/P:** May produce dose-related respiratory depression. Caution with pulmonary disease, postsurgery, head injury, intracranial lesions or preexisting increase in ICP, narrow-angle glaucoma, asthma, BPH, elderly, debilitated, impaired hepatic/renal functions, hypothyroidosis, Addison's disease, or urethral stricture. May mask acute abdominal conditions and the clinical course of head injuries. May cause obstructive bowel disease. Consider risk/benefit ratio in pediatrics, especially with croup. Impairment of mental and physical performance. **Contra:** Should not be used in children less than 6 years of age due to risk of fatal respiratory depression. **P/N:** Category C, not for use in nursing.	Sedation, drowsiness, lethargy, anxiety, dysphoria, euphoria, dizziness, psychotic dependence, rash, pruritus, N/V, ureteral spasm, urinary retention, respiratory depression, **dryness of the pharynx,** tightness of the chest.
Codeine Phosphate/Guaifenesin (Cheratussin AC, Halotussin AC)	**Syrup:** 10mg-100mg/ 5mL [120mL]	***Adults/Pediatrics:*** **≥12 yrs:** 10mL q4h. **Max:** 60mL/24 hrs. ***Pediatrics:*** **6 to <12 yrs:** 5mL q4h. **Max:** 30mL/24 hrs.	**W/P:** Use caution with persistent/chronic cough, cough with excessive phlegm, chronic pulmonary disease, or shortness of breath. May cause or aggravate constipation. **P/N:** Safety in pregnancy and nursing not known.	Constipation, sedation.
Codeine Phosphate/Phenylephrine HCl/ Promethazine HCl (Promethazine VC/ Codeine)	**Syrup:** 10mg-5mg/ 5mL-6.25mg	***Adults/Pediatrics:*** **≥16 yrs:** 5mL q4-6h. **Max:** 30mL/24hr.	**W/P:** May cause or aggravate constipation. May lead to potentially fatal respiratory depression; avoid with compromised respiratory function (eg, COPD, sleep apnea). Caution in atopic children. May elevate CSF pressure; caution with head injury, intracranial lesions, or preexisting increase in ICP. Avoid with asthma, acute febrile illness with chronic cough, or with chronic respiratory disease where interference with ability to clear tracheobronchial tree of secretions would have a deleterious effect on patient's respiratory function. May cause orthostatic hypotension. May impair mental/physical abilities. May lower seizure threshold; caution with seizure disorders. Caution with bone marrow depression; leukopenia and agranulocytosis reported. Neuroleptic malignant syndrome reported. Hallucinations and convulsions have occurred in pediatrics. Cholestatic jaundice reported. Caution with acute abdominal conditions, convulsive disorders, significant hepatic/renal impairment, fever, hypothyroidism, Addison's disease, ulcerative colitis, prostatic hypertrophy, recent GI or urinary tract surgery, elderly, debilitated, narrow-angle glaucoma, stenosing peptic ulcer, pyloroduodenal or bladder-neck obstruction, cardiovascular disease, thyroid disease, DM, heart disease. Urinary retention may occur with BPH. May decrease cardiac	Drowsiness, dizziness, sedation, tremor, anxiety, blurred vision, **dry mouth,** increased or decreased blood pressure, rash, N/V, constipation, urinary retention.

Table 15.2. PRESCRIBING INFORMATION FOR RESPIRATORY DRUGS *(cont.)*
(For all inhaled, intranasal, or systemic corticosteroids, refer to Table 5.1 starting on page 163)

NAME	FORM/ STRENGTH	DOSAGE	WARNINGS/PRECAUTIONS & CONTRAINDICATIONS	ADVERSE EFFECTS†
COUGH & COLD COMBINATIONS *(cont.)*				
COUGH SUPPRESSANTS *(cont.)*				
Codeine Phosphate/Phenylephrine HCl/ Promethazine HCl (Promethazine VC/ Codeine) *(cont.)*			output; use extreme caution with arteriosclerosis, elderly, and patients with initially poor cerebral or coronary circulation. May alter HCG pregnancy test reading. May increase blood glucose. Avoid prolonged exposure to sunlight. **Contra:** Concomitant MAOIs, comatose states, treatment of lower respiratory tract symptoms (eg, asthma), HTN, peripheral vascular insufficiency, pediatric patients <16 yrs. **P/N:** Category C, caution in nursing.	
Codeine Phosphate/ Promethazine HCl (Promethazine w/ Codeine)	**Syrup:** 10mg/5mL-6.25mg	***Adults/Pediatrics:*** **≥16 yrs:** 5mL q4-6h. **Max:** 30mL/24 hr.	**W/P:** May cause or aggravate constipation. May lead to potentially fatal respiratory depression; avoid with compromised respiratory function (eg, COPD, sleep apnea). Caution in atopic children. May elevate CSF pressure; caution with head injury, intracranial lesions, or preexisting increase in ICP. Avoid with asthma, acute febrile illness with chronic cough, or with chronic respiratory disease where interference with ability to clear tracheobronchial tree of secretions would have a deleterious effect on patient's respiratory function. May cause orthostatic hypotension. May impair mental/physical abilities. May lower seizure threshold; caution with seizure disorders. Caution with bone marrow depression; leukopenia and agranulocytosis reported. Neuroleptic malignant syndrome reported. Hallucinations and convulsions have occurred in pediatrics. Cholestatic jaundice reported. Caution with acute abdominal conditions, convulsive disorders, significant hepatic/renal impairment, fever, hypothyroidism, Addison's disease, ulcerative colitis, prostatic hypertrophy, recent GI or urinary tract surgery, elderly, debilitated, narrow-angle glaucoma, stenosing peptic ulcer, pyloroduodenal or bladder-neck obstruction, or cardiovascular disease. May alter HCG pregnancy test reading. May increase blood glucose. Avoid prolonged exposure to sunlight. **Contra:** Comatose states, treatment of lower respiratory tract symptoms (eg, asthma), pediatric patients <16 yrs. **P/N:** Category C, caution in nursing.	Drowsiness, dizziness, sedation, blurred vision, **dry mouth,** increased or decreased blood pressure, rash, N/V, constipation, urinary retention.
Codeine Phosphate/Pseudoephedrine HCl (Nucofed)	**Cap:** 20mg-60mg	***Adults/Pediatrics:*** **≥12 yrs:** 1 cap q6h. **Max:** 4 caps/24 hrs.	**W/P:** Not for cough associated with smoking, emphysema, asthma, or excessive secretions. May cause constipation. Caution with pulmonary disease, shortness of breath, HTN, heart disease, DM, thyroid disease, prostatic hypertrophy, Addison's disease, children, ulcerative colitis, drug dependence, liver or kidney dysfunction. May impair alertness. **P/N:** Category C, caution in nursing.	Nervousness, restlessness, insomnia, drowsiness, dysuria, dizziness, headache, N/V, constipation, trembling, dyspnea, sweating, paleness, weakness, heart rate changes.

†Bold entries denote special dental considerations.
BB = black box warning; **W/P** = warnings/precautions; **Contra** = contraindications; **P/N** = pregnancy category rating and nursing considerations.

NAME	FORM/ STRENGTH	DOSAGE	WARNINGS/PRECAUTIONS & CONTRAINDICATIONS	ADVERSE EFFECTS†
Dextromethorphan HBr/Promethazine HCl (Promethazine DM)	**Syrup:** 15mg/5mL-6.25mg	***Adults/Pediatrics:* ≥12 yrs:** 5mL q4-6h. **Max:** 30mL/24 hr. ***Pediatrics:* 6-11 yrs:** 2.5-5mL q4-6h. **Max:** 20mL/24hr. **2-5 yrs:** 1.25-2.5mL q4-6h. **Max:** 10mL/24hr.	**W/P:** Caution in pediatrics ≥2 yrs. Avoid in pediatric patients whose signs and symptoms may suggest Reye's syndrome or other hepatic diseases. May impair mental/physical abilities. May lower seizure threshold; caution with seizure disorders. May lead to potentially fatal respiratory depression; avoid with compromised respiratory function (eg, COPD, sleep apnea). Caution with bone marrow depression; leukopenia and agranulocytosis reported. Neuroleptic malignant syndrome reported. Caution with narrow-angle glaucoma, prostatic hypertrophy, stenosing peptic ulcer, bladder neck or pyloroduodenal obstruction, cardiovascular disease, hepatic impairment, atopic children, sedated, elderly, or debilitated patients, and patients confined to supine position. Cholestatic jaundice reported. May alter HCG pregnancy test reading. May increase blood glucose. Avoid prolonged exposure to sunlight. **Contra:** Concomitant MAOIs, comatose states, treatment of lower respiratory tract symptoms (eg, asthma), pediatric patients <2 yrs. **P/N:** Category C, caution in nursing.	Drowsiness, dizziness, sedation, GI disturbance, blurred vision, dry mouth, increased or decreased BP, rash, N/V.
Dextromethorphan Hydrobromide/ Guaifenesin (Duratuss DM, Gani-Tuss-DM NR, Mucinex DM, Tussi-Organidin DM NR, Tussi-Organidin DM S NR)	**Elixir:** (Duratuss DM) 25mg-225mg/5mL; **Liq:** (Gani-Tuss-DM NR, Tussi-Organidin DM NR, Tussi-Organidin DM S NR) 10mg/5mL-100mg/5mL; **Tab:** (Mucinex DM) 30mg-600mg	***Adults/Pediatrics:* ≥12 yrs:** (Elixir) 5mL q4h. **Max:** 30mL/24 hrs. (Liq) 10mL q4h. **Max:** 60mL/24hrs. (Tab) 1-2 tabs q12hrs. **Max:** 4 tabs/24hrs. Take with full glass of water. Do not crush, chew, or break. ***Pediatrics:* 6-12 yrs:** (Elixir) 2.5mL q4h. **Max:** 15mL/24 hrs. (Liq) 5mL q4h. **Max:** 30mL/24hrs. **2-6 yrs:** (Elixir) 1.25mL q4h. **Max:** 7.5mL/24 hrs. (Liq) 2.5mL q4h. **Max:** 15mL/24hrs. **6 months to <2 yrs:** (Liq) 0.6-1.25mL q4h or 2.5mL q6-8h. **Max:** 7.5mL/24hrs.	**W/P:** Re-evaluate if cough persists >7 days, recurs, or occurs with fever, rash, or persistent headache. **Contra:** Within 14 days of MAOI therapy. **P/N:** Category C, caution in nursing.	Nausea, GI disturbances, dizziness, drowsiness, vomiting, headache, rash.
Guaifenesin (Mucinex)	**Tab, Extended-Release:** 600mg	***Adults/Pediatrics:* ≥12 yrs:** 1-2 tabs every 12hrs. **Max:** 4 tabs/24hrs. Take with full glass of water. Do not crush, chew, or break.	**W/P:** D/C if cough lasts >7 days, recurs, or occurs with fever, rash, or persistent headache. **P/N:** Safety in pregnancy or nursing not known.	
Guaifenesin/ Hydrocodone Bitartrate (CodiCLEAR DH, Hycotuss)	**Syrup:** (CodiCLEAR DH) 300mg/5mL-3.5mg; (Hycotuss) 100mg/5mL-5mg	***Adults/Pediatrics:* >12 yrs:** (CodiCLEAR) 5mL q4-6h. **Max:** 30mL/24hrs. (Hycotuss) **Initial:** 5mL after meals and hs, not less than 4 hrs apart. **Titrate:** May increase up to 15mL after meals and hs. **Max:** 30mL/24 hrs. **Max Single Dose:** 10mL. ***Pediatrics:* 6-12 yrs:** (CodiCLEAR) 2.5mL q4-6h. **Max:** 15mL/24 hrs. (Hycotuss) **Initial:** 2.5mL after meals and hs, not less than 4 hrs apart. **Max Single Dose:** 5mL.	**W/P:** Hydrocodone is potentially habit-forming. Extreme caution with severe respiratory impairment or impaired respiratory drive. May cause respiratory depression; caution with COPD. Caution with renal, hepatic, or gall bladder disease, asthma, glaucoma, urinary retention, prostatic hypertrophy, hypothyroidism, seizures or epilepsy, head injury, or Addison's disease. May cause drowsiness or dizziness; caution when operating heavy machinery or other hazardous activities. **Contra:** (Hydrocodone) Increased ICP and whenever ventilatory function is depressed. **P/N:** Category C, not for use in nursing.	Drowsiness, N/V, giddiness, constipation, respiratory depression, dizziness, restlessness, irritability, blurred vision, **dry mouth,** decreased appetite, sweating, itching, decreased urination.

Table 15.2. PRESCRIBING INFORMATION FOR RESPIRATORY DRUGS *(cont.)*
(For all inhaled, intranasal, or systemic corticosteroids, refer to Table 5.1 starting on page 163)

NAME	FORM/ STRENGTH	DOSAGE	WARNINGS/PRECAUTIONS & CONTRAINDICATIONS	ADVERSE EFFECTS†
COUGH & COLD COMBINATIONS *(cont.)*				
COUGH SUPPRESSANTS *(cont.)*				
Guaifenesin/ Hydrocodone Bitartrate/ Phenylephrine HCl (Entex HC)	**Liq:** 100mg-5mg-7.5mg/5mL [473mL]	***Adults/Pediatrics:* ≥12 yrs:** 5-10mL q4-6h. **Max:** 40mL/24 hrs. ***Pediatrics:* 6-12 yrs:** 5mL q4-6h. **Max:** 20mL/24 hrs. **2-6 yrs:** 2.5mL q4-6h. **Max:** 10mL/24 hrs.	**W/P:** May be habit-forming. May cause respiratory depression or increase CSF pressure in the presence of other intracranial pathology. May obscure head injuries or acute abdominal conditions. Caution in elderly, debilitated, hepatic/renal dysfunction, Addison's disease, hypothyroidism, postoperative use, prostatic hypertrophy, pulmonary disease, and urethral stricture. Suppresses cough reflex. **Contra:** Infants, newborns, severe HTN or CAD, hyperthyroidism, or MAOI therapy. **P/N:** Category C, not for use in nursing.	CNS stimulation, constipation, drowsiness, dizziness, excitability, headache, insomnia, lightheadedness, N/V, nervousness, respiratory depression, restlessness, tachycardia, tremors, urinary retention, weakness, arrhythmias, and cardiovascular.
Guaifenesin/ Phenylephrine HCl (Entex LA)	**Tab, Extended-Release:** 400mg-30mg*	***Adults/Pediatrics:* ≥12 yrs:** 1 tab q12h. **Max:** 2 tabs/24hrs. ***Pediatrics:* 6-12 yrs:** 1/2 tab q12h. **Max:** 1 tab/24hrs.	**W/P:** Caution in HTN, DM, ischemic heart disease, increased IOP, hyperthyroidism, or prostatic hypertrophy. May produce CNS stimulation with convulsions or cardiovascular collapse with hypotension. Adverse effects occur more often in elderly. **Contra:** HTN, ventricular tachycardia, MAOI use within 14 days. Extreme caution in elderly, hyperthyroidism, bradycardia, partial heart block, myocardial disease, severe arteriosclerosis. **P/N:** Category C, not for use in nursing.	Palpitations, headache, dizziness, nausea, anxiety, restlessness, tremor, weakness, pallor, dysuria, respiratory difficulty.
Guaifenesin/ Phenylephrine HCl (Guaifed-PD)	**Cap:** 200mg-7.5mg	***Adults/Pediatrics:* ≥12 yrs:** 1-2 caps q12h. ***Pediatrics:* 6 to <12 yrs:** 1 cap q12h.	**W/P:** Caution with HTN, DM, ischemic heart disease, hyperthyroidism, increased IOP, prostatic hypertrophy, and the elderly. Not for persistent or chronic cough such as occurs with smoking, asthma, emphysema, or where cough is accompanied by excessive secretions. **Contra:** Severe HTN, severe CAD, concomitant MAOIs, pregnancy, nursing mothers. **P/N:** Category B, not for use in nursing.	Nausea, cardiac palpitations, increased irritability, headache, dizziness, tachycardia, diarrhea, drowsiness, stomach pain, seizures, slowed heart rate, shortness of breath.
Guaifenesin/ Pseudoephedrine HCl (Ami-Tex PSE, Duratuss, Entex PSE, Guaifenex PSE 120, Mucinex D)	**Tab, Extended-Release:** (Ami-Tex PSE, Entex PSE, Guaifenex PSE) 400mg-120mg*; (Duratuss) 600mg-120mg*; 600mg-60mg; (Mucinex D) 600mg-60mg	***Adults/Pediatrics:* ≥12 yrs:** (400mg-120mg) 1 tab q12h. (600mg-120mg) 1 tab q12h. (600mg-60mg) 2 tabs q12h. **Max:** 4 tabs/24hrs. Take with full glass of water. Do not crush, chew, or break. ***Pediatrics:* 6 to <12 yrs:** (400mg-120mg) 1/2 tab q12h. (600mg-120mg) 1/2 tab q12h.	**W/P:** Caution in HTN, DM, heart disease, peripheral vascular disease, increased IOP, hyperthyroidism, or prostatic hypertrophy. **Contra:** Nursing, severe HTN, severe CAD, prostatic hypertrophy, concomitant MAOIs. **P/N:** Category C, contraindicated in nursing.	N/V, nervousness, dizziness, restlessness, sleeplessness, lightheadedness, headache, tremor, palpitations, tachycardia, weakness, respiratory difficulties.
Hydrocodone Bitartrate/ Homatropine Methylbromide (Hycodan, Hydromet)	**Syrup:** 5mg-1.5mg/5mL; **Tab:** 5mg-1.5mg*	***Adults/Pediatrics:* >12 yrs:** 1 tab or 5mL q4-6h prn. **Max:** 6 tabs/24hrs or 30mL/24hrs. ***Pediatrics:* 6-12 yrs:** 1/2 tab or 2.5mL q4-6h prn. **Max:** 3 tabs/24hrs or 15mL/24 hrs.	**W/P:** May be habit-forming. May cause respiratory depression. May obscure diagnosis or clinical course of acute abdominal conditions. Caution in elderly, debilitated, severe hepatic or renal impairment, hypothyroidism, Addison's disease, prostatic hypertrophy, urethral stricture, asthma, head injury, increased ICP, and narrow-angle glaucoma. **P/N:** Category C, not for use in nursing.	Sedation, drowsiness, lethargy, mental/physical impairment, dizziness, psychic dependence, constipation, ureteral spasm, respiratory depression, rash.

*Scored. †Bold entries denote special dental considerations.
BB = black box warning; **W/P** = warnings/precautions; **Contra** = contraindications; **P/N** = pregnancy category rating and nursing considerations.

NAME	FORM/ STRENGTH	DOSAGE	WARNINGS/PRECAUTIONS & CONTRAINDICATIONS	ADVERSE EFFECTS†
Potassium Iodide (SSKI)	**Sol**: 1g/mL [30mL]	***Adults:*** 0.3-0.6mL (300-600mg) tid-qid. Dilute in glassful of water, juice, or milk. Take with food or milk.	**W/P:** Caution with Addison's disease, cardiac disease, hyperthyroidism, myotonia congenita, tuberculosis, acute bronchitis, renal impairment. May cause fetal harm, abnormal thyroid function, and goiter in pregnant women. Prolonged use may lead to hypothyroidism or iodism; d/c if iodism occurs. May alter thyroid function tests. **Contra:** Iodide sensitivity. **P/N:** Category D, caution in nursing.	Stomach upset/ pain, diarrhea, N/V, skin rash, **salivary gland swelling/ tenderness,** thyroid adenoma, goiter, myxedema.
DECONGESTANT				
Pseudoephedrine HCl (Sudafed)	**Liq:** 15mg/5mL; **Tab:** 30mg, 60mg; **Tab, Chewable:** 15mg; **Tab, Extended-Release:** 120mg, 240mg	***Adults:*** (Tab, ER) 120mg q12h or 240mg q24h. **Max:** 240mg/24h. ***Pediatrics:*** **>12 yrs:** (Liquid/Tab/ Tab, Chew) 60mg q4-6h. **Max:** 240mg/24hrs. Tab, ER: 120mg q12h or 240mg q24h. **Max:** 240mg/24hrs. **6 to <12 yrs:** (Liquid/Tab/Tab, Chew) 30mg q4-6h. **Max:** 4 doses/24hrs. **2 to <6 yrs:** (Liquid/Tab/Tab, Chew) 15mg q4-6h. **Max:** 4 doses/24hrs.	**W/P:** Do not exceed recommended dosage. If nervousness, dizziness, or sleeplessness occurs, d/c use. Avoid with heart disease, high BP, thyroid disease, diabetes, or difficulty in urination due to prostate enlargement. **P/N:** Not rated in pregnancy or nursing.	—
NASAL PREPARATIONS				
Azelastine HCl (Astelin, Astepro)	**Spray:** 137mcg/ spray [30mL]	(Astelin) ***Adults/Pediatrics:*** **≥12 yrs: Seasonal Allergic/Vasomotor Rhinitis:** 2 sprays per nostril bid. **5-11 yrs: Seasonal Allergic Rhinitis:** 1 spray per nostril bid. (Astepro) ***Adults/Pediatrics:*** **≥12 yrs:** 1 or 2 sprays per nostril bid.	**W/P:** Somnolence reported. May impair physical/mental abilities. **P/N:** Category C, caution in nursing.	**Bitter taste,** somnolence, weight increase, headache, nasal burning, **pharyngitis,** paroxysmal sneezing, **dry mouth,** nausea, atrial fibrillation, palpitations.
Ipratropium Bromide (Atrovent Nasal)	**Spray:** (0.03%) 21mcg/spray [31g], (0.06%) 42mcg/spray [16.6g]	***Adults/Pediatrics:*** **≥6 yrs: Rhinorrhea w/Allergic/Nonallergic Perennial Rhinitis:** (0.03%) 2 sprays per nostril bid-tid. **≥12 yrs: Rhinorrhea w/Common Cold:** (0.06%) 2 sprays per nostril tid-qid. **5-11 yrs:** (0.06%) 2 sprays per nostril tid. **≥5 yrs: Rhinorrhea w/ Seasonal Allergic Rhinitis:** (0.06%) 2 sprays per nostril qid.	**W/P:** Immediate hypersensitivity reaction reported. Caution with narrow-angle glaucoma, prostatic hyperplasia or bladder-neck obstruction. **Contra:** Hypersensitivity to atropine or its derivatives. **P/N:** Category B, caution in nursing.	Epistaxis, nasal dryness, **dry mouth, dry throat,** headache, upper respiratory infection, **pharyngitis.**
MISCELLANEOUS PULMONARY AGENTS				
Alpha1-Proteinase Inhibitor (Human) (Aralast, Prolastin, Zemaira)	**Inj:** 500mg, 1000mg	***Adults:*** 60mg/kg IV once weekly. Administer at a rate not exceeding 0.08mL/kg/min. If adverse events occur, reduce rate or interrupt infusion until symptoms subside. Infusion may then be resumed at a tolerable rate.	**W/P:** For IV use only. Risk of transmitting infectious agents (eg, viruses, and theoretically, the Creutzfeldt-Jakob disease agent). Monitor VS and carefully observe during infusion. D/C immediately if anaphylactic or severe anaphylactoid reactions occur. Administer alone without mixing with other agents. **Contra:** Selective IgA deficiencies (IgA levels <15mg/dL) with known antibody against IgA. **P/N:** Category C, caution in nursing.	**Pharyngitis,** headache, increased **cough,** bronchitis, sinusitis, rash, back pain, viral infection, peripheral edema, bloating, dizziness, somnolence, asthma, rhinitis, AST/ALT elevations, injection-site pain.
Dornase Alfa (Pulmozyme)	**Sol:** 2.5mg/2.5mL [2.5mL: 1^s, 30^s]	***Adults/Pediatrics:*** **≥5 yrs: Cystic Fibrosis:** 2.5mg qd-bid via nebulizer.	**W/P:** Use with standard therapies for cystic fibrosis. **Contra:** Hypersensitivity to Chinese hamster ovary cell products. **P/N:** Category B, caution in nursing.	Voice alteration, **pharyngitis,** rash, laryngitis, chest pain, conjunctivitis, rhinitis, fever, dyspnea.

Table 15.2. PRESCRIBING INFORMATION FOR RESPIRATORY DRUGS *(cont.)*
(For all inhaled, intranasal, or systemic corticosteroids, refer to Table 5.1 starting on page 163)

NAME	FORM/ STRENGTH	DOSAGE	WARNINGS/PRECAUTIONS & CONTRAINDICATIONS	ADVERSE EFFECTS†
MISCELLANEOUS PULMONARY AGENTS *(cont.)*				
Tobramycin (TOBI)	**Sol**: 60mg/mL (300mg/amp)	***Adults/Pediatrics:* ≥6 yrs: Cystic Fibrosis with *P. aeruginosa:*** Inhale via nebulizer 300mg q12h for 28 days, then stop for 28 days. Resume therapy for next 28-day on/28-day off cycle.	**W/P:** Caution with muscular disorders (eg, myasthenia gravis, Parkinson's disease), and renal, auditory, vestibular, or neuromuscular dysfunction. May cause hearing loss, bronchospasm. Can cause fetal harm in pregnancy. D/C if nephrotoxicity occurs until serum level <2mcg/mL. **P/N:** Category D, not for use in nursing.	Voice alteration, **taste perversion,** tinnitus.

†Bold entries denote special dental considerations.
BB = black box warning; **W/P** = warnings/precautions; **Contra** = contraindications; **P/N** = pregnancy category rating and nursing considerations.

Table 15.3. DRUG INTERACTIONS FOR RESPIRATORY DRUGS
(For all inhaled, intranasal, or systemic corticosteroids, refer to Table 5.2 starting on page 183)

ASTHMA/COPD PREPARATIONS	
ANTICHOLINERGIC BRONCHODILATOR	
Ipratropium Bromide (Atrovent HFA)	
Anticholinergic-containing drugs	Caution with other anticholinergic-containing drugs.
Tiotropium Bromide (Spiriva)	
Anticholinergics	Avoid with other anticholinergics (eg, ipratropium).
β_2-AGONIST	
Albuterol Sulfate (AccuNeb, ProAir HFA, Proventil HFA, Ventolin HFA, VoSpire ER)	
Antidepressants	Avoid MAOI or TCA use within 2 weeks.
β-Blockers	β-Blockers and albuterol inhibit the effects of each other.
Digoxin	May decrease serum digoxin levels. Monitor digoxin.
Diuretics, non-K^+-sparing	ECG changes and/or hypokalemia with non-K^+-sparing diuretics may worsen.
Epinephrine	Avoid epinephrine.
Sympathomimetics	Avoid other short-acting sympathomimetic bronchodilators.
Albuterol Sulfate/Ipratropium Bromide (Combivent, Duoneb)	
Anticholinergics	Potential additive interactions with other anticholinergic drugs.
Antidepressants	Avoid MAOI or TCA use within 2 weeks.
β-Blockers	β-Blockers and albuterol inhibit the effects of each other.
Diuretics, non-K^+-sparing	ECG changes and/or hypokalemia may occur with non-K^+-sparing diuretics.
Sympathomimetics	Increased risk of cardiovascular effects with other sympathomimetics.
Arformoterol Tartrate (Brovana)	
Adrenergic agonists	Sympathetic effects may be potentiated with concomitant use of additional adrenergic agonists.
β-Blockers	Antagonized effect with β-blockers. Use with caution.
Diuretics, non-K^+-sparing	ECG changes and/or hypokalemia may occur with non-K^+-sparing diuretics.
Methylxanthines	Concomitant use with methylxanthines may potentiate hypokalemia.
QTc interval, drugs prolonging	Extreme caution with MAOIs, TCAs, and drugs known to prolong QT interval.
Steroids	Concomitant use with steroids may potentiate hypokalemia.
Formoterol Fumarate (Foradil, Perforomist)	
Adrenergic drugs	Adrenergic drugs may potentiate effects.
β-Blockers	Antagonized effect with β-blockers. Use with caution.
Diuretics, non-K^+-sparing	Concomitant use with non-K^+-sparing diuretics may potentiate hypokalemia and/or ECG changes.
Methylxanthines	Concomitant use with methylxanthines may potentiate hypokalemia.
QTc interval, drugs prolonging	Extreme caution with MAOIs, TCAs, and drugs known to prolong QT interval.
Steroids	Concomitant use with steroids may potentiate hypokalemia.
Sympathomimetics	Potentiates the effects of other sympathomimetics.

Table 15.3. DRUG INTERACTIONS FOR RESPIRATORY DRUGS *(cont.)*
(For all inhaled, intranasal, or systemic corticosteroids, refer to Table 5.2 starting on page 183)

ASTHMA/COPD PREPARATIONS *(cont.)*	
β_2-AGONIST	
Levalbuterol HCl (Xopenex, Xopenex HFA)	
Antidepressants	Extreme caution with MAOIs and TCAs.
β-Blockers	Antagonized effect with β-blockers.
Digoxin	Decreases levels of digoxin. Monitor digoxin.
Diuretics, non-K^+-sparing	ECG changes and/or hypokalemia may occur with non-K^+-sparing diuretics.
Sympathomimetics	Avoid other sympathomimetic agents.
Metaproterenol Sulfate	
Antidepressants	Vascular effects may be potentiated by MAOIs and TCAs.
β_2-Agonists	Avoid other aerosol β_2-agonists.
Sympathomimetics	Vascular effects may be potentiated by other sympathomimetics.
Pirbuterol Acetate (Maxair Autohaler)	
Antidepressants	Vascular effects may be potentiated by MAOIs and TCAs.
β-Blockers	Decreased effect with β-blockers.
β_2-Agonists	Avoid other aerosol β_2-agonists.
Diuretics, non-K^+-sparing	ECG changes and/or hypokalemia may occur with non-K^+-sparing diuretics.
Sympathomimetics	Vascular effects may be potentiated with other sympathomimetics.
Salmeterol Xinafoate (Serevent)	
Antidepressants	Extreme caution with MAOI or TCA use within 2 weeks.
β-Blockers	Avoid with β-blockers.
β_2-Agonists	Caution with >8 inhalations of short-acting β_2-agonists.
Diuretics, non-K^+-sparing	ECG changes and/or hypokalemia may occur with non-K^+-sparing diuretics. Use with caution.
Terbutaline Sulfate	
Antidepressants	Extreme caution with MAOI or TCA use within 2 weeks.
β-Blockers	Decreased effects with β-blockers.
Diuretics	ECG changes and hypokalemia may occur with loop or thiazide diuretics.
Sympathomimetics	Avoid other sympathomimetic agents (except aerosol bronchodilators).
LEUKOTRIENE RECEPTOR ANTAGONIST	
Montelukast Sodium (Singulair)	
CYP450 inducers	Monitor with potent CYP450 inducers (eg, phenobarbital, rifampin).
Zafirlukast (Accolate)	
ASA	Increased levels with ASA.
CYP2C9 substrates	Caution with drugs metabolized by CYP2C9 (eg, tolbutamide, phenytoin, carbamazepine).
CYP3A4 substrates	Caution with drugs metabolized by CYP3A4 (eg, dihydropyridine CCBs, cyclosporine, cisapride, astemizole).

ASTHMA/COPD PREPARATIONS *(cont.)*

Leukotriene receptor antagonist

Zafirlukast (Accolate) *(cont.)*	
Erythromycin	Erythromycin decreases levels of zafirlukast.
Theophylline	Theophylline decreases levels of zafirlukast and rarely increases theophylline levels.
Warfarin	Coadministration with warfarin increases PT time; monitor closely.
Zileuton (Zyflo, Zyflo CR)	
CYP3A4 substrates	Monitor drugs metabolized by CYP3A4.
Propranolol	Potentiates the effects of propranolol.
Theophylline	Increases theophylline levels; reduce theophylline by 50% and monitor levels.
Warfarin	Potentiates the effects of warfarin.

Mast cell stabilizer

Cromolyn Sodium (Intal)	
Isopreterenol	Avoid with isoproterenol during pregnancy.

Xanthine bronchodilator

Theophylline (Theo-24, Uniphyl)	
Adenosine	May need higher doses of adenosine to achieve an effect.
Alcohol	Effects are potentiated with alcohol.
Allopurinol	Effects are potentiated by allopurinol.
Aminoglutethimide	Diminished effects with aminoglutethimide.
Barbiturates	Diminished effects with barbiturates.
Benzodiazepines	Higher levels of diazepam, flurazepam, lorazepam, diazepam may be needed to cause sedation.
Carbamazepine	Diminished effects with carbamazepine.
Cimetidine	Effects are potentiated by cimetidine.
Ciprofloxacin	Effects are potentiated by ciprofloxacin.
Contraceptives, oral	Effects are potentiated by estrogen-containing oral contraceptives.
Corticosteroids	Effects are potentiated by corticosteroids.
Diet	Increased levels of theophylline with high fat content meal.
Disulfiram	Effects are potentiated by disulfiram.
Erythromycin	Effects are potentiated by erythromycin.
Fluvoxamine	Effects are potentiated by fluvoxamine.
Food	Diminished effects with charcoal-broiled food.
Interferon, human recombinant alpha-A	Effects are potentiated by interferon.
Isoproterenol	Diminished effects with isoproterenol.

Table 15.3. DRUG INTERACTIONS FOR RESPIRATORY DRUGS *(cont.)*
(For all inhaled, intranasal, or systemic corticosteroids, refer to Table 5.2 starting on page 183)

ASTHMA/COPD PREPARATIONS *(cont.)*

XANTHINE BRONCHODILATOR

Theophylline (Theo-24, Uniphyl) *(cont.)*	
Ketamine	May lower theophylline seizure threshold.
Ketoconazole	Diminished effects with ketoconazole.
Lithium	Higher levels of lithium required to reach therapeutic serum concentrations.
Methotrexate	Effects are potentiated by methoxtrexate.
Mexiletine	Effects are potentiated by mexiletine.
Pancuronium	May need higher doses of pancuronium to achieve neuromuscular blockade.
Phenobarbital	Diminished effects with phenobarbital.
Phenytoin	Diminished effects of theophylline and phenytoin.
Propafenone	Effects are potentiated by propafenone.
Propranolol	Effects are potentiated by propranolol.
Rifampin	Diminished effects with rifampin.
St. John's wort	Diminished effects with St. Johns wort.
Sulfinpyrazone	Diminished effects with sulfinpyrazone.
Thiabendazole	Effects are potentiated by thiabendazole.
Ticlopidine	Effects are potentiated by ticlopidine.
Troleandomycin	Effects are potentiated by troleandomycin.
Verapamil	Effects are potentiated by verapamil.

COUGH & COLD COMBINATIONS

ANTIHISTAMINES

Acrivastine/Pseudoephedrine HCl (Semprex-D)	
β-Agonists	β-Agonists increase effects of sympathomimetics.
CNS depressants	Increased sedation with CNS depressants, including alcohol.
MAOIs	MAOIs increase effects of sympathomimetics; avoid MAOI use during or within 2 weeks.
Brompheniramine Maleate/Dextromethorphan HBr/Phenylephrine HCl (Alacol DM)	
Antihypertensives	May reduce effects of antihypertensives.
Anxiolytics	Additive effects with anxiolytics.
CNS depressants	Additive effects with CNS depressants, including alcohol.
MAOIs	MAOIs may prolong/intensify anticholinergic effects of antihistamines and phenylephrine.
Sedatives	Additive effects with sedatives.
Tranquilizers	Additive effects with tranquilizers.
Brompheniramine Maleate/Pseudoephedrine HCl (Bromfed, Bromfed-PD, Bromfenex, Bromfenex-PD)	
Antihypertensives	Reduced antihypertensive effects of methyldopa, mecamylamine, reserpine, and veratrum alkaloids.

COUGH & COLD COMBINATIONS *(cont.)*

Antihistamines

Brompheniramine Maleate/Pseudoephedrine HCl (Bromfed, Bromfed-PD, Bromfenex, Bromfenex-PD) *(cont.)*	
β-Blockers	Effects are potentiated by β-blockers.
CNS depressants	Additive effects with alcohol and other CNS depressants.
MAOIs	Effects are potentiated by MAOIs.
Carbetapentane Tannate/Chlorpheniramine Tannate (Tussi-12)	
CNS depressants	Additive CNS effects with CNS depressants, including alcohol.
MAOIs	Avoid with or within 14 days of discontinuation of MAOIs.
Carbetapentane Tannate/Chlorpheniramine Tannate/Ephedrine Tannate/Phenylephrine Tannate (Rynatuss)	
CNS depressants	Additive CNS effects with CNS depressants, including alcohol.
MAOIs	Avoid MAOI use within 14 days.
Cetirizine HCl/Pseudoephedrine HCl (Zyrtec-D)	
MAOIs	Avoid MAOIs during or within 14 days of use.
Chlorpheniramine Maleate/Dextromethorphan HBr/Phenylephrine HCl (Rondec-DM Oral Drops, Rondec-DM Syrup)	
Antihypertensives	May reduce antihypertensive effects of reserpine, veratrum alkaloids, methyldopa, and mecamylamine.
Barbiturates	The effects of barbiturates may be enhanced.
β-Blockers	Increased sympathomimetic effect with β-blockers.
CNS depressants	Additive CNS effects with CNS depressants, including alcohol.
MAOIs	Increased sympathomimetic effect with MAOIs.
Narcotic antitussives	Additive cough-suppressant effect with narcotic antitussives.
TCAs	The effects of TCAs may be enhanced.
Chlorpheniramine Maleate/Methscopolamine Nitrate/Phenylephrine HCl (Dallergy)	
Antihypertensives	May reduce antihypertensive effect of methyldopa, mecamylamine, reserpine, and veratrum alkaloids.
β-Blockers	Increased sympathomimetic effect with β-blockers.
CNS depressants	Additive CNS effects with CNS depressants, including alcohol.
MAOIs	Increased sympathomimetic effect with MAOIs.
Chlorpheniramine Maleate/Methscopolamine Nitrate/Pseudoephedrine HCl (AlleRx)	
Antihypertensives	May diminish antihypertensive effects of reserpine, veratrum alkaloids, methyldopa, and mecamylamine.
Barbiturates	The effects of barbiturates may be enhanced.
β-Blockers	Increased sympathomimetic effect with β-blockers.
CNS depressants	Additive CNS effects with CNS depressants, including alcohol.
MAOIs	Increased sympathomimetic effect with MAOIs. Avoid MAOI use with or within 2 weeks.
Nitrates, organic	Hypotension potentiated with sildenafil or other organic nitrates; avoid concomitant use.

Table 15.3. DRUG INTERACTIONS FOR RESPIRATORY DRUGS *(cont.)*
(For all inhaled, intranasal, or systemic corticosteroids, refer to Table 5.2 starting on page 183)

COUGH & COLD COMBINATIONS *(cont.)*

ANTIHISTAMINES

Chlorpheniramine Maleate/Methscopolamine Nitrate/Pseudoephedrine HCl (AlleRx) *(cont.)*	
Sympathomimetics	Caution with hyperactivity to sympathomimetics.
TCAs	The effects of TCAs may be enhanced.
Chlorpheniramine Maleate/Phenylephrine HCl (Dallergy Jr, Rondec Oral Drops, Rondec Syrup)	
Antihypertensives	May reduce antihypertensive effects of reserpine, veratrum alkaloids, methyldopa, and mecamylamine.
Barbiturates	The effects of barbiturates may be enhanced.
Benzodiazepines	The effects of benzodiazpines may be enhanced.
β-Blockers	Increased sympathomimetic effect with β-blockers.
CNS depressants	Additive CNS effects with CNS depressants, including alcohol.
MAOIs	Increased sympathomimetic effect with MAOIs.
TCAs	The effects of TCAs may be enhanced.
Chlorpheniramine Maleate/Pseudoephedrine HCl (Deconamine SR)	
Antihypertensives	May reduce antihypertensive effect of methyldopa, reserpine, veratrum alkaloids, mecamylamine.
CNS depressants	Additive CNS effects with CNS depressants, including alcohol.
MAOIs	Hypertensive crisis may occur with MAOIs.
Chlorpheniramine Tannate/Phenylephrine Tannate (Rynatan, Rynatan Pediatric)	
CNS depressants	Additive CNS effects with CNS depressants, including alcohol (eg, sedative-hypnotics, tranquilizers).
MAOIs	Increased anticholinergic and sympathomimetic effects with MAOIs; avoid during or within 14 days of use.
Tranquilizers	Additive CNS effects with tranquilizers.
Desloratadine/Pseudoephedrine Sulfate (Clarinex-D)	
Antihypertensives	May reduce the antihypertensive effects of methyldopa, mecamylamine, reserpine.
Digitalis	Increased ectopic pacemaker activity with digitalis.
MAOIs	Avoid with MAOIs or within 14 days of discontinuation.
Fexofenadine HCl/Pseudoephedrine HCl (Allegra-D)	
Antihypertensives	May reduce the antihypertensive effects of methyldopa, mecamylamine, reserpine.
Digitalis	Increased ectopic pacemaker activity can occur with digitalis.
Erythromycin	Plasma levels of fexofenadine/pseudoephedrine are increased with erythromycin.
Ketoconazole	Plasma levels of fexofenadine/pseudoephedrine are increased with ketoconazole.
MAOIs	Avoid concomitant use or within 14 days of MAOIs.
Sympathomimetics	Caution with other sympathomimetics.

COUGH & COLD COMBINATIONS *(cont.)*

Antihistamines

Loratadine/Pseudoephedrine Sulfate (Claritin-D OTC)	
MAOIs	Avoid concomitant use or within 14 days of MAOIs.
Phenylephrine HCl/Promethazine HCl (Promethazine VC)	
Amphetamines	Synergistic adrenergic response with amphetamines.
Anesthetics, general	May increase the sedative effects of general anesthetics.
Atropine	Reflex bradycardia blocked and pressor response enhanced with atropine.
Barbiturates	May increase the sedative effects of barbiturates. Reduce barbiturate dose by at least 1/2.
β-Blockers	Cardiostimulating effects blocked with β-blockers. Pressor response decreased with β-adrenergic blockers.
Cardiac pressors	Cardiac pressor response potentiated.
CNS depressants	May increase the sedative effects of other CNS depressants, including alcohol.
Diet preparations	Synergistic adrenergic response with diet preparations (eg, amphetamines or phenylpropanolamine).
Ergot alkaloids	Excessive rise in BP with ergot alkaloids.
MAOIs	Contraindicated; possible hypertensive crisis.
Opioid analgesics	May increase the sedative effects of opioid analgesics. Reduce the dose of opioid analgesics by 1/4 to 1/2.
Phenylpropanolamine	Synergistic adrenergic response with phenylpropanolamine.
Respiratory agents	Avoid concomitant administration with other respiratory agents in pediatrics.
Seizure threshold, drugs affecting	May lower seizure threshold; caution with drugs which lower seizure threshold (eg, opioids, local anesthetics).
Sympathomimetics	Tachycardia or other arrhythmias may occur with sympathomimetics.
TCAs	Pressor response increased with TCAs. May increase the sedative effects of TCAs.
Tranquilizers	May increase the sedative effects of tranquilizers.

COUGH SUPPRESSANTS

Chlorpheniramine Polistirex/Hydrocodone Polistirex (Tussionex Pennkinetic)	
Alcohol	Additive CNS depression with alcohol.
Antianxiety agents	Additive CNS depression with antianxiety agents.
Anticholinergics	Concurrent anticholinergics may cause paralytic ileus.
Antidepressants	Concurrent MAOIs or TCAs with hydrocodone may increase the effect of the antidepressant or hydrocodone.
Antipsychotics	Additive CNS depression with antipsychotics.
Narcotics	Additive CNS depression with narcotics.

Table 15.3. DRUG INTERACTIONS FOR RESPIRATORY DRUGS *(cont.)*
(For all inhaled, intranasal, or systemic corticosteroids, refer to Table 5.2 starting on page 183)

COUGH SUPPRESSANTS *(cont.)*	
Codeine Phosphate/Guaifenesin (Cheratussin AC, Halotussin AC)	
Antidepressants	Increased sedation with antidepressants, especially MAOIs.
Sedatives	Increased sedation with sedatives.
Tranquilizers	Increased sedation with tranquilizers.
Codeine Phosphate/Phenylephrine HCl/Promethazine HCl (Promethazine VC/Codeine)	
Anesthetics, general	May increase the sedative effects of general anesthetics.
Anticholinergics	Caution with concomitant use of other agents with anticholinergic properties.
Atropine	Reflex bradycardia blocked and pressor response enhanced with atropine.
Barbiturates	May increase the sedative effects of barbiturates. Reduce barbiturate dose by at least 1/2.
β-Blockers	Cardiostimulating effects blocked with β-blockers.
CNS depressants	May increase the sedative effects of other CNS depressants, including alcohol.
Epinephrine	May reverse epinephrine's vasopressor effect.
Ergot alkaloids	Excessive rise in BP with ergot alkaloids.
MAOIs	Contraindicated; cardiac pressor response potentiated and acute hypertensive crisis may occur.
Opioids	May increase the sedative effects of opioid analgesics. Reduce the dose of opioid analgesics by 1/4 to 1/2.
Sympathomimetics	Tachycardia or other arrhythmias may occur with other sympathomimetics.
TCAs	Pressor response increased with TCAs. May increase the sedative effects of TCAs.
Tranquilizers	May increase the sedative effects of tranquilizers.
Codeine Phosphate/Promethazine HCl (Promethazine w/Codeine)	
Anesthetics, general	May potentiate the sedative effects of general anesthetics; avoid such agents or administer in reduced dosages.
Anticholinergics	Caution with concomitant use of other agents with anticholinergic properties.
Barbiturates	May potentiate the sedative effects of barbiturates; reduce barbiturate dose by at least 1/2.
CNS depressants	May potentiate the sedative effects of other CNS depressants, including alcohol. Avoid such agents or administer in reduced dosages.
Epinephrine	May reverse epinephrine's vasopressor effect.
MAOIs	Possible interaction with MAOIs; consider small test dose.
Opioid analgesics	May potentiate the sedative effects of opioid analgesics; reduce opioid dose by at least 1/4 to 1/2.
Respiratory depressants	Avoid concomitant administration with other respiratory depressants in pediatrics.

COUGH SUPPRESSANTS *(cont.)*

Codeine Phosphate/Promethazine HCl (Promethazine w/Codeine) *(cont.)*	
Sedative-hypnotics	May potentiate the sedative effects of sedative-hypnotics; avoid such agents or administer in reduced dosages.
Seizure threshold, drugs lowering	May lower seizure threshold; caution with drugs which lower seizure threshold (eg, opioids, local anesthetics).
TCAs	May potentiate the sedative effects of TCAs; avoid such agents or administer in reduced dosages.
Tranquilizers	May potentiate the sedative effects of tranquilizers; avoid such agents or administer in reduced dosages.
Codeine Phosphate/Pseudoephedrine HCl (Nucofed)	
Anticholinergics	Anticholinergics may cause paralytic ileus.
Antihypertensives	May reduce the effects of antihypertensive agents.
β-Blockers	β-Blockers may increase the effects of pseudoephedrine.
CNS depressants	Caution with CNS depressants, general anesthetics, alcohol.
Digitalis glycosides	Digitalis glycosides may cause cardiac arrhythmias.
MAOIs	MAOIs may increase the effects of pseudoephedrine. Avoid MAOI use within 2 weeks.
Sympathomimetics	Sympathomimetics may increase the effects of pseudoephedrine.
TCAs	TCAs may antagonize effects of pseudoephedrine.
Dextromethorphan Hydrobromide/Promethazine HCl (Promethazine DM)	
Anesthetics, general	May potentiate the sedative effects of general anesthetics; avoid such agents or administer in reduced dosages.
Anticholinergics	Caution with concomitant use of other agents with anticholinergic properties.
Barbiturates	May potentiate the sedative effects of barbiturates; reduce barbiturate dose by at least 1/2.
CNS depressants	May potentiate the sedative effects of other CNS depressants, including alcohol. Avoid such agents or administer in reduced dosages.
Epinephrine	May reverse epinephrine's vasopressor effect.
MAOIs	Contraindicated; hyperpyrexia, hypotension, and death associated.
Opioid analgesics	May potentiate the sedative effects of opioid analgesics; reduce opioid dose by at least 1/4 to 1/2.
Respiratory depressants	Avoid concomitant administration with other respiratory depressants in pediatrics.
Sedative-hypnotics	May potentiate the sedative effects of sedative-hypnotics; avoid such agents or administer in reduced dosages.
Seizure threshold, drugs lowering	May lower seizure threshold; caution with drugs which lower seizure threshold (eg, opioids, local anesthetics).

Table 15.3. DRUG INTERACTIONS FOR RESPIRATORY DRUGS *(cont.)*
(For all inhaled, intranasal, or systemic corticosteroids, refer to Table 5.2 starting on page 183)

COUGH SUPPRESSANTS *(cont.)*	
Dextromethorphan Hydrobromide/Promethazine HCl (Promethazine DM) *(cont.)*	
TCAs	May potentiate the sedative effects of TCAs; avoid such agents or administer in reduced dosages.
Tranquilizers	May potentiate the sedative effects of tranquilizers; avoid such agents or administer in reduced dosages.
Dextromethorphan Hydrobromide/Guaifenesin (Duratuss DM, Gani-Tuss-DM NR, Mucinex DM, Tussi-Organidin DM NR, Tussi-Organidin DM S NR)	
Antihistamines	Additive CNS depressant effcts with antihistamines.
CNS depressants	Additive CNS depression with other CNS depressants, including alcohol.
MAOIs	Avoid MAOI use within 2 weeks of discontinuation.
Psychotropics	Additive CNS depressant effects with psychotropics.
Guaifenesin/Hydrocodone Bitartrate (CodiCLEAR DH, Hycotuss)	
Anesthetics, general	Additive CNS depressant effects with general anesthetics.
CNS depressants	Additive CNS depressant effects with other CNS depressants, including alcohol.
Opioid analgesics	Additive CNS depressant effects with opioid analgesics.
Phenothiazines	Additive CNS depressant effects with phenothiazines.
Sedative-hypnotics	Additive CNS depressant effects with sedative-hypnotics.
Tranquilizers	Additive CNS depressant effects with tranquilizers.
Guaifenesin/Hydrocodone Bitartrate/Phenylephrine HCl (Entex HC)	
Antianxiety agents	Additive CNS effects with antianxiety agents.
Antihistamines	Additive CNS effects with antihistamines.
Antihypertensives	May reduce antihypertensive effects of methyldopa, mecamylamine, reserpine, and veratrum alkaloids.
Barbiturates	May enhance the effects of barbiturates.
β-Blockers	Increased sympathomimetic effects with β-blockers.
CNS depressants	Additive CNS effects with other CNS depressants, including alcohol.
MAOIs	Increased sympathomimetic effects with MAOIs.
Opioid analgesics	Additive CNS effects with opioid analgesics.
Psychotropics	Additive CNS effects with psychotropics.
TCAs	May enhance the effects of TCAs.
Tranquilizers	Additive CNS effects with tranquilizers.
Guaifenesin/Phenylephrine HCl (Entex LA)	
Anesthetics	Increased risk of arrhythmias with halothane anesthesia.
Antihypertensives	May reduce hypotensive effects of guanethidine, mecamylamine, methyldopa, and reserpine.
β-Blockers	β-Blockers may potentiate pressor response.
Digitalis glycosides	Increased risk of arrhythmias with digitalis glycosides.

COUGH SUPPRESSANTS *(cont.)*

Guaifenesin/Phenylephrine HCl (Entex LA) *(cont.)*	
MAOIs	MAOIs may potentiate pressor response.
TCAs	TCAs may antagonize effects.
Guaifenesin/Phenylephrine HCl (Guaifed-PD)	
Antihypertensives	May reduce the antihypertensive effects of methyldopa, mecamylamine, and reserpine.
β-Blockers	Increased sympathomimetic effects with β-blockers.
Digitalis glycosides	Increased risk of arrhythmias with digitalis glycosides.
MAOIs	Increased sympathomimetic effects with MAOIs.
Guaifenesin/Pseudoephedrine HCl (Ami-Tex PSE, Duratuss, Entex PSE, Guaifenex PSE 120, Mucinex D)	
Antihypertensives	May reduce antihypertensive effects of methyldopa, guanethidine, mecamylamine, and reserpine.
β-Blockers	Increased sympathomimetic effects with β-blockers.
MAOIs	Increased sympathomimetic effects with MAOIs.
Sympathomimetics	Caution with concomitant sympathomimetic amines.
Homatropine Methylbromide/Hydrocodone Bitartrate (Hycodan, Hydromet)	
Antihistamines	May increase the CNS depressant effects of antihistamines.
Antipsychotics	May increase the CNS depressant effects of antipsychotics.
Anxiolytics	May increase the CNS depressant effects of anxiolytics.
Atropine	Reflex bradycardia blocked; pressor response enhanced with atropine.
CNS depressants	May increase the CNS depressant effects of other CNS depressants, including alcholol.
MAOIs	Concomitant use may increase the effect of MAOIs or hydrocodone.
Opioids	May increase the CNS depressant effects of opioids.
Respiratory depressants	Avoid concomitant administration with other respiratory depressants in pediatrics.
Seizure threshold, drugs lowering	May lower seizure threshold; caution with drugs which lower seizure threshold (eg, opioids, local anesthetics).
TCAs	Concomitant use may increase the effect of TCAs or hydrocodone. May increase CNS depressant effects of TCAs.
Potassium Iodide (SSKI)	
ACE inhibitors	ACE inhibitors may cause hyperkalemia, cardiac arrhythmias, or cardiac arrest.
Antithyroid drugs	May potentiate the hypothyroid and goitrogenic effects of lithium and other antithyroid drugs.
Diuretics, K^+-sparing	K^+-sparing diuretics may cause hyperkalemia, cardiac arrhythmias, or cardiac arrest.
K^+-containing medications	K^+-containing medications may cause hyperkalemia, cardiac arrhythmias, or cardiac arrest.

Table 15.3. DRUG INTERACTIONS FOR RESPIRATORY DRUGS *(cont.)*
(For all inhaled, intranasal, or systemic corticosteroids, refer to Table 5.2 starting on page 183)

COUGH SUPPRESSANTS *(cont.)*

DECONGESTANT

Pseudoephedrine HCl (Sudafed)	
MAOIs	Avoid MAOI use within 2 weeks of discontinuation.

NASAL PREPARATIONS

Azelastine HCl (Astelin, Astepro)	
Cimetidine	Increased azelastine levels with cimetidine.
CNS depressants	Avoid alcohol or other CNS depressants; additive CNS impairment may occur.
Ipratropium Bromide (Atrovent Nasal)	
Anticholinergic agents	May produce additive effects with other anticholinergic agents.

MISCELLANEOUS PULMONARY AGENT

Tobramycin (TOBI)	
Aminoglycosides	Avoid with other aminoglycosides; potential for additive nephrotoxicity and neurotoxicity.
Diuretics	Avoid with diuretics (eg, ethacrynic acid, furosemide, urea, mannitol); may enhance aminoglycoside toxicity, including neurotoxicity.
Nephrotoxic drugs	Avoid with nephrotoxic drugs; potential for additive nephrotoxicity.
Neurotoxic drugs	Avoid with neurotoxic drugs; potential for additive neurotoxicity.

Chapter 16

Gastrointestinal Drugs

B. Ellen Byrne, D.D.S., Ph.D.

"Heartburn" occurs daily in approximately 7% of the population. It is a symptom of reflux esophagitis, an irritation and inflammation of the esophageal mucosa caused by the reflux of acidic stomach or duodenal contents retrograde into the esophagus. Reflux esophagitis is commonly seen in gastroesophageal reflux disease (GERD) and peptic ulcer disease (PUD), which are considered together in this chapter because the same drugs are used to treat them. Other symptoms associated with GERD include regurgitation, dysphagia, bleeding, and chest pain. Regurgitation is the most specific symptom of GERD and may result in morning hoarseness, laryngitis, and pulmonary aspiration.

PUD is a heterogeneous group of disorders characterized by ulceration of the upper gastrointestinal tract. Peptic ulcer disease can occur at any place in the gastrointestinal (GI) tract that is exposed to the erosive action of pepsin and acid. It can be exacerbated by stress, alcohol, cigarette smoking, some foods, aspirin, and aspirin-like drugs. Medical therapy for GERD and PUD consists mainly of neutralizing the stomach contents or reducing gastric acid secretions and using promotility agents to enhance peristalsis. Infections with a bacterium, *Helicobacter pylori*, also have been implicated in the pathogenesis of PUD, and eradication of this organism with antibiotics, bismuth compounds, and an antisecretory agent has been shown to alter the natural course of peptic ulcer disease. Although the optimal regimen to eradicate *H. pylori* and cure PUD has not been established, a number of combinations are effective. An antisecretory drug often is added to achieve more rapid relief from ulcer symptoms as well as ulcer healing. Antibiotics used in PUD therapy include amoxicillin, clarithromycin, metronidazole, and tetracycline. The antisecretory drugs include H_2 receptor antagonists such as cimetidine and proton pump inhibitors such as omeprazole. Bismuth subsalicylate, the third drug in this triad, is found in Pepto-Bismol.

Diarrhea is usually caused by infection, toxins, or drugs. Antidiarrheal agents can be sold over the counter or by prescription only. Virally or bacterially induced diarrhea is usually transient and requires only a clear liquid diet and increased fluid intake. Antimicrobial therapy may be indicated. Intravenous fluids may be required if dehydration occurs.

Drug- or toxin-induced diarrhea is best treated by discontinuing the causative agent when possible. Chronic diarrhea may be caused by laxative abuse, lactose intolerance, inflammatory bowel disease, malabsorption syndromes, endocrine disorders, or irritable bowel syndrome. Treatment of chronic diarrhea should be aimed at correcting the cause of diarrhea rather than alleviating the symptoms.

"Gastroparesis" is the term for disorders causing gastric stasis. Nausea, vomiting, bloating, fullness, and early satiety are signs of gastroparesis. Treatment is aimed at accelerating gastric emptying. This condition is often associated with diabetes.

Crohn's disease and ulcerative colitis are considered together because the same drugs are used to treat these disorders. Crohn's disease is a chronic inflammatory disease that can affect any part of the gastrointestinal system, from mouth to anus. The etiology is unknown. The most common symptoms are abdominal pain and diarrhea. Perirectal fissure with sinus formation and strictures is common.

Ulcerative colitis is an inflammatory disease of the gastrointestinal tract that is limited to the colon and rectum. Typically, patients with ulcerative colitis present with bloody diarrhea. The disease primarily affects young adults. The etiology is unknown. Management of both Crohn's disease and ulcerative colitis is aimed at decreasing the inflammation and providing symptomatic relief.

Nausea and vomiting usually are self-limiting events without serious sequelae. Protracted vomiting may result in dehydration, malnutrition, metabolic alkalosis, hyponatremia, hypokalemia, and hypochloremia. Infants and children are at greatest risk.

Nausea and vomiting may occur in patients with inferior myocardial infarction or diabetic ketoacidosis, Addisonian crisis, acute pancreatitis, or acute appendicitis.

Drug-induced nausea and vomiting are common in cancer chemotherapy. However, numerous other drugs—such as narcotics, antibiotics (erythromycin, quinolones, flucytosine, nitrofurantoin, and tetracyclines), digoxin, and theophylline—also may cause nausea and vomiting.

Viral gastroenteritis is the most common cause of nausea and vomiting. Bacterial infections, motion sickness, and pregnancy are other frequently encountered etiologies of nausea and vomiting.

Treatment of nausea and vomiting can include removal or treatment of the underlying cause. Antiemetic therapy is indicated in patients with electrolyte disturbances secondary to vomiting, severe anorexia, or weight loss. Antiemetic drugs are available over the counter and by prescription. If a patient is unable to retain oral medication, rectal and injectable routes of administration may be preferable. Many classes of drugs have been used to treat nausea and vomiting, including antihistamines, anticholinergics, seratonin antagonists, dopamine antagonists, phenothiazines, cannabinoids, and butyrophenones.

ANTIDIARRHEAL AGENTS

Special Dental Considerations

There are no contraindications to the dental treatment of patients with diarrhea.

Most acute diarrhea is self-limiting. The opiate-related drugs and anticholinergics used to treat diarrhea produce xerostomia; therefore, meticulous oral hygiene should be stressed. These drugs also produce drowsiness and this effect is additive with other CNS depressants, thereby producing greater drowsiness. For general prescribing information on antidiarrheal agents, see **Table 16.1**.

Drug Interactions of Dental Interest

Drugs used to treat diarrhea include antimotility opioids and derivatives (including loperamide and diphenoxylate) and adsorbents. Drug interactions of concern with opioids would occur if the patient took another CNS depressant drug, such as alcohol, antidepressants, antianxiety agents, anticholinergics, antihistamines, or barbiturates. This combination of drugs may seriously increase the side effects of either drug.

Adsorbent drugs such as bismuth salts can bind with various drugs, resulting in decreased absorption of the coadministered drug and a decreased therapeutic response. If these drugs must be taken together it is best to space dosing by 6 hours.

For information on drug interactions with antidiarrheal agents, see **Table 16.2**.

Pharmacology

Antidiarrheal agents can be divided into antibiotic and nonantibiotic drugs. Antibiotics are the mainstay of treatment of acute bacterial diarrhea. Whenever possible, antibiotics should be directed toward specific microorganisms either identified by culture or clinically suspected.

There are many commercial preparations sold for symptomatic relief of diarrhea. Controlled clinical trials have not proven the safety and effectiveness of most of them.

Adsorbents have been shown to increase stool consistency but do not decrease stool water content.

Anticholinergics relieve cramps by reducing contractile activity but have no effect on diarrhea.

Bismuth subsalicylate binds toxins and prevents bacteria from attaching to intestinal epithelium.

Loperamide and diphenoxylate have a profound effect on motility. These agents are generally contraindicated in dysentery.

In general, these nonspecific antidiarrheal agents should not be used as a substitute for oral rehydration and directed antibiotics.

CROHN'S DISEASE AND ULCERATIVE COLITIS DRUGS

Special Dental Considerations

There are no contraindications to the dental treatment of patients with Crohn's disease. The leukopenic and thrombocytopenic effects of sulfasalazine may increase the incidence of certain microbial infections, delay healing, and increase gingival bleeding. If a patient has leukopenia or thrombocytopenia, dental treatment should be deferred until laboratory counts have returned to normal. Patients treated with glucocorticoids are likely to have a decreased resistance to infection and a poor wound healing response. Actual and potential sources of infection in the mouth should be treated promptly. If surgical procedures are necessary, they should be as atraumatic, conservative, and aseptic as possible. Prophylactic antibiotic coverage should be considered in most cases. Adrenal suppression owing to the administration of glucocorticoids is also a consideration. Depending on the dose and length of treatment, the patient may require an increased dose of glucocorticoids before undergoing stressful dental treatment.

For patients with ulcerative colitis, use of antibiotics may aggravate the problem. Antibiotics most often associated with ulcerative colitis are broad-spectrum penicillins.

See **Table 16.1** for general prescribing information on Crohn's disease and ulcerative colitis drugs.

Drug Interactions of Dental Interest

See **Table 16.2** for drug interaction information on Crohn's disease and ulcerative colitis drugs.

Pharmacology

Crohn's disease is a chronic inflammatory condition of the gastrointestinal tract. Current therapy is directed at reducing inflammation and providing systematic relief. Initial treatment includes the aminosalicylates such as sulfasalazine or mesalamine. Sulfasalazine (through its active component 5-aminosalicylic acid [5ASA]) exerts an anti-inflammatory effect on the colon. Antibiotics such as ciprofloxacin and metronidazole are most commonly used and likely function by reducing bacterial endotoxin and granuloma formation. Antibiotics are also used to treat fistulas.

Corticosteroids such as budesonide, hydrocortisone, and prednisone are given to reduce inflammation. Due to serious side effects such as increased blood pressure, osteoporosis, and increased risk of infection, steroids are only indicated for short-term use.

Medications that suppress the immune system, called immunomodulators, such as azathioprine (AZA), 6-mercaptopurine (6-MP), or methotrexate may be used. Tumor necrosis factor (TNF) antagonists, such as infliximab and adalimumab may be used as maintenance medications.

GASTRIC MOTILITY DISORDER (GASTROPARESIS) DRUG

Special Dental Considerations

There are no contraindications to the dental treatment of patients with gastroparesis. See **Table 16.1** for general prescribing information on the gastric motility drug metoclopramide.

Drug Interactions of Dental Interest

Metocloptamide treats gastroparesis by increasing gastrointestinal mobility and decreasing gastric emptying time. Oral absorption from the stomach may be decreased while absorption from the small intestine may be enhanced. See **Table 16.2** for drug interaction information on metoclopramide.

Pharmacology

Diabetic gastroparesis is a common GI complication of diabetes mellitus. Caused by delayed gastric emptying, the symptoms range from early satiety and bloating to severe gastric retention with nausea, vomiting, and abdominal pain. Impaired gastric emptying is caused by abnormal motility of the stomach or a reduction in motor activity in the intestine. Metoclopramide affects gut motility through indirect cholinergic stimulation of the gut muscle.

GASTROESOPHAGEAL REFLUX DISEASE AND PEPTIC ULCER DISEASE DRUGS

Special Dental Considerations

There are no contraindications to the dental treatment of patients with GERD or PUD; however, drugs that cause gastrointestinal injury should be avoided in patients with GERD or PUD. These drugs include erythromycin, aspirin, corticosteroids, and nonsteroidal anti-inflammatory agents.

Dental patients with GERD should be kept in a semi-supine chair position for patient comfort because of the reflux effects of this disease. Xerostomia is a common side effect of the anticholinergic agents and meticulous oral hygiene must be emphasized. Many anticholinergic agents also induce orthostatic or postural hypotension. Therefore, dental patients treated with one of these agents should remain in the dental chair in an upright position for several minutes before being dismissed.

For general prescribing information on GERD and PUD drugs, see **Table 16.1**.

Drug Interactions of Dental Interest

Drugs used to treat GERD and PUD include antacids, H_2 histamine receptor antagonists, anticholinergics, and promotility agents.

Antacids potentially interfere with the absorption of many drugs by forming a complex with these drugs or by altering gastric pH. Antacids containing metal cations (Mg^{2+}, Ca^{2+}, Al^{3+}) have a strong affinity for tetracycline, and response to the antibiotic can vary according to the extent of the complex.

Antacids increase the gastric pH, and this can decrease the absorption of drugs that require an acidic environment for dissolution and absorption. Conversely, enteric-coated drugs such as erythromycin may be released prematurely.

Most of these drug-antacid interactions can be minimized by administering each drug 2 hours from the other.

The H_2 histamine receptor antagonist cimetidine can bind to the cytochrome P450 mixed-function oxidase system and can inhibit the biotransformation of drugs by the liver. This results in inhibition of metabolism and increased serum drug concentrations of the drug not metabolized. Serum levels of some benzodiazepines (diazepam, alprazolam, chlorodiazepoxide, midazolam, triazolam) have been shown to increase, resulting in enhanced sedation.

Anticholinergics can decrease gastric emptying time, which can increase the amount of drug absorbed or increase the degradation of a drug in the stomach, thus decreasing the amount of drug absorbed. Overall, this interaction appears to have minor significance.

For drug interaction information on GERD and PUD drugs, see **Table 16.2**.

Pharmacology

Histamine H_2-receptor antagonists are effective for short-term treatment of GERD and PUD. These agents prevent histamine-induced acid release by competing with histamine for H_2-receptors.

Proton pump inhibitors (such as omeprazole) act by irreversibly blocking the H^+/K^+-ATPase pump. These agents markedly inhibit both basal and stimulated gastric acid secretion.

Antacids act by neutralizing gastric acid and thus raising the gastric pH. This has the effect of inhibiting peptic activity, which practically ceases at pH 5. The antacids in common use are salts of magnesium and aluminum. Magnesium salts cause diarrhea and aluminum salts cause constipation, so mixtures of the two are used to maintain bowel function.

Drugs that protect the mucosa can do so by either forming a protective physical barrier over the surface of the ulcer (sucralfate) or enhancing or augmenting endogenous prostaglandins (misoprostol) to promote bicarbonate and mucin release, and inhibit acid secretion.

Anticholinergic agents (such as propantheline bromide) have played a limited role in the treatment of PUD by inhibiting vagally stimulated gastric acid secretion. These agents are not considered first-line agents for treatment of PUD.

ANTIEMETIC DRUGS

Special Dental Considerations

Be aware of why the patient is taking a drug for nausea and vomiting. If the patient is receiving the drug for cancer chemotherapy, he or she may require palliative therapy for stomatitis. Patients with cancer may be taking chronic opioids for pain. Additional drugs for pain should not be prescribed without reviewing the patient's medication profile. Also, procedures or drugs that could promote nausea and vomiting should be avoided. An increased gag reflex makes it difficult for the patient to undergo dental procedures such as obtaining radiographs or impressions. Many antiemetic drugs cause xerostomia, so these patients should avoid mouthrinses containing alcohol because of its drying effects. They also should use sugarless gum or saliva substitutes or take sips of water.

For general prescribing information on antiemetic drugs, see **Table 16.1**.

Drug Interactions of Dental Interest

Antacids can decrease the absorption of many drugs, including tetracycline, digoxin, benzodiazepines, iron salts, and indomethacin. Antihistamines, phenothiazines, and butyrophenones cause drowsiness. This drowsiness may be additive with that caused by other CNS depressants.

For drug interaction information on antiemetic drugs, see **Table 16.2**.

Pharmacology

Numerous pathways are capable of stimulating the vomiting center and chemoreceptor trigger zone in the brain, so it is not surprising that a wide variety of drugs can be used in treating nausea and vomiting. Phenothiazines and butyrophenones block dopamine receptors and are believed to act at the chemoreceptor trigger zone. Antihistamines and anticholinergics are effective in managing vomiting associated with vestibular disturbances by blocking acetylcholine receptors in the vestibular center. Metoclopramide is a dopamine antagonist that has both peripheral and central antiemetic actions. This drug accelerates gastric emptying, inhibits gastric relaxation, and appears to block the chemoreceptor trigger zone. Ondansetron is a highly selective and potent antagonist of 5-HT_3 (serotonin) receptors. Cannabinoids such as dronabinol are believed to inhibit emesis by blocking descending impulses from the cerebral cortex. Glucocorticoids have demonstrated antiemetic activity in patients receiving cancer chemotherapy. Their mechanism of action is unknown.

LAXATIVES

Constipation generally is defined as a decrease in the frequency of fecal elimination and is characterized by the difficult passage of hard, dry stools. By definition, laxatives facilitate the passage and elimination of feces from the large intestine (colon) and rectum. Laxatives can be divided into bulk products, lubricants, osmotics, saline laxatives, stimulants, and stool softeners.

Bulk laxatives work by absorbing water and expanding to increase moisture content and bulk in the stool. Lubricants increase water retention in the stool, causing reabsorption of water in the bowel. Stimulants act by increasing peristalsis by direct effect on the intestines. Saline draws water into the intestinal lumen. Osmotics increase distension and promote peristalsis. Stool softeners, also known as emollients, reduce surface tension of liquids in the bowel.

For general prescribing information on laxatives, see **Table 16.1**. For information on drug interactions, see **Table 16.2**.

SUGGESTED READING

Anderson PO, Knoben JE, eds. *Handbook of Clinical Drug Data*. 8th ed. Stamford, Conn: Appleton & Lange; 1997.

Berardi RR. GI disorders. In: Allen LV, ed. *Handbook of Nonprescription Drugs.* 12th ed. Washington: American Pharmaceutical Association; 2000:241-737.

Tatro DS, ed. *Drug Interactions Facts: Facts and Comparisons*. St. Louis: Facts and Comparisons; 1995.

Wells BG, DiPiro JT, Schwinghammer TL, et al. *Pharmacotherapy Handbook*. Stamford, Conn: Appleton & Lange; 1998.

Young LY, Koda-Kimble MA, eds. *Applied Therapeutics: The Clinical Use of Drugs.* 6th ed. Vancouver, Wash: Applied Therapeutics; 1995.

Table 16.1. PRESCRIBING INFORMATION FOR GASTROINTESTINAL DRUGS

NAME	FORM/ STRENGTH	DOSAGE	WARNINGS/PRECAUTIONS & CONTRAINDICATIONS	ADVERSE EFFECTS†
ANTIDIARRHEALS				
Atropine Sulfate/ Diphenoxylate HCl (Lomotil, Lonox) CV	(Diphenoxylate-Atropine) **Sol:** 2.5mg-0.025/ 5mL [60mL]; **Tab:** 2.5mg-0.025mg	***Adults:*** **Initial:** 2 tabs or 10mL qid. **Titrate:** Reduce dose after symptoms are controlled. **Maint:** 2 tabs or 10mL qd. **Max:** 20mg/day diphenoxylate. D/C if symptoms not controlled after 10 days at max dose of 20mg/day (diphenoxylate). ***Pediatrics:*** **2-12 yrs: Initial:** 0.3-0.4mg/kg/day of solution given qid. **13-16 yrs: Initial:** 2 tabs or 10mL tid. **Titrate:** Reduce dose after symptoms are controlled. **Maint:** 25% of initial dose. D/C if no improvement within 48 hrs.	**W/P:** May induce toxic megacolon in ulcerative colitis; d/c if abdominal distention occurs. May cause intestinal fluid retention. Avoid with diarrhea associated with organisms that penetrate the intestinal mucosa, and with pseudomembranous enterocolitis. Caution in pediatrics, especially with Down's syndrome. Extreme caution with advanced hepatorenal disease and liver dysfunction. Do not use with severe dehydration or electrolyte imbalance until corrective therapy is initiated. **Contra:** Obstructive jaundice, diarrhea associated with pseudomembranous enterocolitis or enterotoxin-producing bacteria. **P/N:** Category C, caution in nursing.	Numbness of extremities, dizziness, anaphylaxis, hyperthermia, tachycardia, urinary retention, flushing, drowsiness, toxic megacolon, N/V.
Bismuth Subsalicylate (Pepto-Bismol, Pepto-Bismol Maximum Strength) OTC	**Sus:** 262mg/ 15mL; **Sus, Maximum Strength:** 525mg/15mL; **Tab:** 262mg; **Tab, Chewable:** 262mg	***Adults:*** (Sus) 30mL every 0.5-1 hr prn. **Max:** 8 doses/24hrs. (Sus, Max Strength) 30mL hourly prn. **Max:** 4 doses/24 hrs. (Tab; Tab, Chewable) 2 tabs every 0.5-1 hr prn. **Max:** 8 doses/24hrs. Drink plenty of clear fluids. ***Pediatrics:*** **9-12 yrs:** (Sus) 15mL every 0.5-1 hr prn. (Sus, Max Strength) 15mL hourly prn. (Tab; Tab, Chewable) 1 tab every 0.5-1 hr prn. **6-9 yrs:** (Sus) 10mL every 0.5-1 hr prn. (Sus, Max Strength) 10mL hourly prn. (Tab; Tab, Chewable) 2/3 tab every 0.5-1 hr prn. **3-6 yrs:** (Sus) 5mL every 0.5-1 hr. **Max:** 8 doses/24hrs. (Sus, Max Strength) 5mL hourly prn. **Max:** 4 doses/24hrs. (Tab; Tab, Chewable) 1/3 tab every 0.5-1 hr prn. **Max:** 8 doses/24 hrs. Drink plenty of clear fluids.	**W/P:** Avoid in children and teenagers with or recovering from chickenpox or flu. Do not give with ASA or non–ASA salicylate allergy. May cause temporary darkening of tongue or stool. Product may contain small amounts of naturally occurring lead. **P/N:** Safety in pregnancy and nursing not known.	—
Loperamide HCl (Imodium A-D) OTC	**Sol:** 1mg/7.5mL [120mL]; **Tab:** 2mg	***Adults/Pediatrics:*** **≥12 yrs:** (Tab) **Initial:** 4mg after the first loose stool then 2mg after each additional loose stool, take with plenty of liquid. **Max:** 8mg/day for no more than 2 days. (Sol) 30mL after first loose stool then 15mL after each additional loose stool. **Max:** 60mL/day for no more than 2 days. ***Pediatrics:*** **9-11 yrs (60-95 lbs):** (Tab) 2mg after the first loose stool then 1mg after each additional loose stool, take with plenty of liquid. **Max:** 6mg/day for no more than 2 days. (Sol) 15mL after first loose stool then 7.5mL after each additional loose stool. **Max:** 45mL/day for no more than 2 days. **6-8 yrs (48-59 lbs):** (Tab) 2mg after the first loose stool then 1mg after each additional loose stool. **Max:** 4mg/day for no more than 2 days. (Sol) 15mL after first loose stool then 7.5mL after each additional loose stool. **Max:** 30mL/day for no more than 2 days.	**W/P:** Do not use if diarrhea is accompanied with high fever, blood, or mucus in stool. Caution with history of liver disease. D/C if diarrhea worsens, lasts more than 2 days, or abdominal swelling or bulging occurs. **P/N:** Safety in pregnancy and nursing is not known.	—
Nitazoxanide (Alinia)	**Sus:** 100mg/ 5mL [60mL]; **Tab:** 500mg [60[s], 3-Day Therapy Packs, 6[s]]	***Adults/Pediatrics:*** **≥12 yrs:** ***G.lamblia*** **Diarrhea:** 500mg (25mL) q12h for 3 days. Take with food. ***Pediatrics: C.parvum/G.lamblia*** **Diarrhea: 4-11yrs:** 200mg (10mL) q12h for 3 days. **1-3 yrs:** 100mg (5mL) q12h for 3 days.	**W/P:** Caution with hepatic and biliary disease, renal disease. Contains 1.48g sucrose/5mL. Safety and effectiveness have not been established in HIV positive or immunodeficient patients. **P/N:** Category B, caution in nursing.	Abdominal pain, diarrhea, headache, nausea.

†Bold entries denote special dental considerations.
BB = black box warning; **W/P** = warnings/precautions; **Contra** = contraindications; **P/N** = pregnancy category rating and nursing considerations.

Table 16.1. PRESCRIBING INFORMATION FOR GASTROINTESTINAL DRUGS *(cont.)*

NAME	FORM/ STRENGTH	DOSAGE	WARNINGS/PRECAUTIONS & CONTRAINDICATIONS	ADVERSE EFFECTS†
ANTIDIARRHEALS *(cont.)*				
Rifaximin (Xifaxan)	**Tab:** 200mg	***Adults/Pediatrics:* ≥12 yrs:** 1 tab tid for 3 days.	**W/P:** Avoid in diarrhea complicated by fever or blood in the stool or diarrhea due to pathogens other than *E.coli.* D/C if diarrhea symptoms worsen or persist >24-48 hrs; consider alternative antibiotic therapy. Pseudomembranous colitis reported. **P/N:** Category C; not for use in nursing.	Flatulence, headache, abdominal pain, rectal tenesmus, defecation urgency, nausea, constipation, pyrexia.
ANTIEMETICS				
Aprepitant (Emend)	**Cap:** 40mg, 80mg, 125mg; **Tri-Pak:** (one 125mg & two 80mg caps)	***Adults:* Prevention of CINV: Day 1:** 125mg 1 hr prior to chemotherapy. **Days 2 and 3:** 80mg qam. Regimen should include a corticosteroid and a 5-HT_3 antagonist. **Concomitant Corticosteroid:** Reduce dexamethasone PO or methylprednisolone PO by 50% and methylprednisolone IV by 25%. **Prevention of PONV:** 40mg within 3 hrs prior to induction of anesthesia.	**W/P:** Chronic continuous use is not recommended. Caution with severe hepatic insufficiency. **Contra:** Concurrent treatment with pimozide, terfenadine, astemizole, or cisapride. **P/N:** Category B, not for use in nursing.	Asthenia/fatigue, N/V, constipation, diarrhea, hiccups, anorexia, headache, dizziness, dehydration, heartburn, abdominal pain, epigastric discomfort, gastritis, tinnitis, neutropenia.
Dolasetron Mesylate (Anzemet)	**Inj:** 20mg/mL; **Tab:** 50mg, 100mg	***Adults:* Prevention of CINV:** (IV) 1.8mg/kg IV single dose or 100mg IV 30 min before chemotherapy. (PO) 100mg PO within 1 hr before chemotherapy. **Prevention/Treatment of PONV:** (IV)12.5mg IV single dose 15 min before cessation of anesthesia or as soon as N/V presents. (PO) 100mg PO within 2 hrs before surgery. ***Pediatrics:* 2-16 yrs: Prevention of CINV:** (IV)1.8mg/kg IV single dose 30 min before chemotherapy. **Max:** 100mg. May mix injection solution in apple or grape juice and take orally within 1 hr before chemotherapy. (PO) 1.8mg/kg PO within 1 hr before chemotherapy. **Max:** 100mg. **Prevention/Treatment of PONV:** (IV) 0.35mg/kg IV single dose 15 min before cessation of anesthesia or as soon as N/V presents. **Max:** 12.5mg single dose. May mix 1.2mg/kg injection solution in apple or grape juice and take orally within 2 hrs before surgery. **Max:** 100mg/dose. (PO) 1.2mg/kg PO within 2 hrs before surgery. **Max:** 100mg.	**W/P:** Caution in patients with or who may develop cardiac conduction interval prolongation, especially those with congenital QT syndrome, hypokalemia, and hypomagnesemia. Cross-sensitivity may occur with other 5-HT_3 antagonists. Can cause ECG interval changes. **P/N:** Category B, caution in nursing.	Headache, diarrhea, fever, fatigue, dizziness, abnormal hepatic function, chills/shivering, urinary retention, abdominal pain, HTN, wide complex tachycardia or ventricular tachycardia, ventricular fibrillation.
Dronabinol (Marinol) CIII	**Cap:** 2.5mg, 5mg, 10mg	***Adults:* Appetite Stimulation: Initial:** 2.5mg bid before lunch and supper or 2.5mg qpm or qhs if 5mg/day is intolerable. **Max:** 20mg/day in divided doses. **Antiemetic: Initial:** 5mg/m^2 given 1-3 hrs before chemotherapy, then q2-4h after chemotherapy, up to 4-6 doses/day. **Titrate:** May increase by 2.5mg/m^2 increments. **Max:** 15mg/m^2/dose.	**W/P:** Do not engage in any hazardous activity until ability to tolerate drug is established. Caution with cardiac disorders due to possible HTN/hypotension, syncope, tachycardia. Caution with history of substance abuse. Monitor with mania, depression, schizophrenia; may exacerbate illness. Caution in elderly due to increased sensitivity to the psychoactive, neurological, and postural hypotensive effects. Initial dose and adjustments should be supervised by responsible adult. Caution with history of seizure disorders, may lower seizure threshold. **Contra:** Hypersensitivity to sesame oil and cannabinoids. **P/N:** Category C, not for use in nursing.	Euphoria, dizziness, paranoid reaction, somnolence, abnormal thinking, abdominal pain, N/V, diarrhea, conjunctivitis, hypotension, flushing.

†Bold entries denote special dental considerations.
BB = black box warning; **W/P** = warnings/precautions; **Contra** = contraindications; **P/N** = pregnancy category rating and nursing considerations.

NAME	FORM/ STRENGTH	DOSAGE	WARNINGS/PRECAUTIONS & CONTRAINDICATIONS	ADVERSE EFFECTS†
Droperidol (Inapsine)	**Inj:** 2.5mg/mL	***Adults:*** Individualize dose. **Initial (Max):** 2.5mg IM/IV. May give additional 1.25mg cautiously to achieve desired effect. Lower initial doses in elderly, debilitated, poor-risk patients. ***Pediatrics:*** **2-12 yrs: Initial (Max):** 0.1 mg/kg IM/IV. May give additional doses cautiously. Lower initial doses in debilitated, poor-risk patients.	**BB:** QT prolongation, torsade de pointes, arrhythmias reported. Use in patients resistant or intolerant to other therapies. Monitor ECG before and 2-3 hrs after treatment. Extreme caution if at risk for developing prolonged QT syndrome. **W/P:** Caution with renal/hepatic impairment. HTN, tachycardia reported with pheochromocytoma. Risk of prolonged QT syndrome with CHF, cardiac disease, bradycardia, cardiac hypertrophy, electrolyte imbalances (eg, hypokalemia, hypomagnesemia), >65 yrs, alcohol abuse. NMS reported; give dantrolene with increased temperature, HR, or carbon dioxide production. May decrease pulmonary arterial pressure. **Contra:** Known or suspected QT prolongation, including congenital long QT syndrome. **P/N:** Category C, caution in nursing.	QT-interval prolongation, torsade de pointes, cardiac arrest, hypotension, tachycardia, dysphoria, post-op drowsiness, restlessness, hyperactivity, anxiety, depression, syncope, irregular cardiac rhythm.
Fosaprepitant Dimeglumine (Emend for Injection)	**Inj:** 115mg/ 10mL	***Adults:*** **3-Day CINV Regimen: Day 1 only:** 115mg IV may be substituted for aprepitant 125mg PO 30 min prior to chemotherapy, as an infusion over 15 min. **Days 2-3:** 80mg aprepitant PO. Give with a corticosteroid and 5-HT_3 antagonist.	**W/P:** Use caution with concomitant medications primarily metabolized through CYP3A4. Inhibition of CYP3A4 by aprepitant could result in elevated plasma concentrations of these concomitant medications. When fosaprepitant is used concomitantly with another CYP3A4 inhibitor, aprepitant plasma concentrations could be elevated. Chronic continuous use is not recommended. Caution with severe hepatic insufficiency. **Contra:** Concurrent treatment with astemizole, cisapride, pimozide, or terfenadine. **P/N:** Category B, not for use in nursing.	Infusion site pain, infusion site induration, headache, asthenia, abdominal pain, dehydration, dizziness, constipation, pruritus, rash, urticaria, anaphylactic reactions.
Granisetron (Sancuso)	**Patch:** 3.1mg/ 24 hrs	***Adults:*** Apply single patch to upper outer arm a minimum of 24 hrs before chemotherapy. May be applied up to a maximum of 48 hrs before chemotherapy. Remove patch a minimum of 24 hrs after completion of chemotherapy. Patch can be worn for up to 7 days depending on duration of chemotherapy regimen.	**W/P:** May mask progressive ileus and/or gastric distention. Avoid placing on red, irritated, or damaged skin. Generalized skin reaction (eg, allergic rash, including erythematous, macular, papular rash, pruritis) may occur; d/c and remove patch immediately. Avoid direct natural or artificial sunlight. Cover application site in case of risk of exposure to sunlight throughout the period of wear and for 10 days following removal. **P/N:** Category B, caution in nursing.	Constipation, abdominal pain, diarrhea, HTN, hypotension, dizziness, insomnia, fever.
Granisetron HCl (Kytril)	**Inj:** 0.1mg/ mL, 1mg/mL; **Sol:** 2mg/10mL [30mL]; **Tab:** 1mg	***Adults:*** **Prevention of CINV:** (IV) 10mcg/kg within 30 min before chemotherapy. (PO) 2mg qd up to 1 hr before chemotherapy or 1mg bid (up to 1 hr before chemotherapy and 12 hrs later). **Prevention of Radiation-Induced N/V:** (PO) 2mg within 1 hr of radiation. **Prevention/Treatment of PONV:** (IV) Administer 1mg over 30 sec before induction of anesthesia or immediately before anesthesia reversal. ***Pediatrics:*** **2-16 yrs: Prevention of CINV:** (IV)10mcg/kg IV within 30 min before chemotherapy.	**W/P:** Does not stimulate gastric or intestinal peristalsis. Do not use instead of nasogastric suction. May mask progressive ileus or gastric distension. **P/N:** Category B, caution in nursing.	Headache, asthenia, somnolence, diarrhea, constipation, abdominal pain, dizziness, insomnia, increased hepatic enzymes.
Meclizine HCl (Antivert)	**Tab:** 12.5mg, 25mg, 50mg*	***Adults/Pediatrics:*** **≥12 yrs: Motion Sickness:** 25-50mg 1 hr prior to trip/ departure, repeat q24h prn. **Vertigo:** 25-100mg/day in divided doses.	**W/P:** Caution with asthma, glaucoma, prostatic hypertrophy. **P/N:** Category B, safety in nursing is not known.	Drowsiness, **dry mouth,** blurred vision (rare).

Table 16.1. PRESCRIBING INFORMATION FOR GASTROINTESTINAL DRUGS *(cont.)*

NAME	FORM/ STRENGTH	DOSAGE	WARNINGS/PRECAUTIONS & CONTRAINDICATIONS	ADVERSE EFFECTS†
ANTIEMETICS *(cont.)*				
Metoclopramide HCl (Reglan)	**Inj:** 5mg/mL; **Syr:** 5mg/5mL; **Tab:** 5mg, 10mg*	***Adults:*** **GERD:** 10-15mg PO qid 30 min ac and hs. **Elderly:** 5 mg qid. **Max:** 12 weeks of therapy. **Intermittent Symptoms:** Up to 20mg PO as single dose prior to provoking situation. **Gastroparesis:** 10mg PO 30 min ac and hs for 2-8 weeks. **Severe Gastroparesis:** May give same doses IV/IM for up to 10 days if needed. **Antiemetic: (PONV)** 10-20mg IM near end of surgery. **(CINV)** 1-2mg/kg 30 min before chemotherapy then q2h for 2 doses, then q3h for 3 doses. **For Highly Emetogenic Chemotherapy:** Give 2mg/kg as initial 2 doses. **Small-Bowel Intubation/ Radiological Exam:** 10mg IV as single dose. **CrCl <40mL/min:** 50% of normal dose. ***Pediatrics:*** **Small-Bowel Intubation: 6-14 yrs:** 2.5-5mg IV single dose. **<6 yrs:** 0.1mg/kg IV single dose. **CrCl <40mL/min:** 50% of normal dose.	**BB:** D/C if signs/symptoms of tardive dyskinesia develop; avoid ≥12 weeks of therapy. **W/P:** Caution with HTN, Parkinson's disease, depression. EPS, tardive dyskinesia, Parkinsonian-like symptoms, neuroleptic malignant syndrome reported. Administer IV injection slowly. Risk of developing fluid retention and volume overload especially with cirrhosis or CHF; d/c if these occur. May increase pressure of suture lines. **Contra:** Where GI mobility stimulation is dangerous (eg, perforation, obstruction, hemorrhage), pheochromocytoma, seizure disorder, concomitant drugs that cause EPS effects. **P/N:** Category B, caution with nursing.	Restlessness, drowsiness, fatigue, EPS effects (acute dystonic reactions), galactorrhea, hyperprolactinemia, hypotension, arrhythmia, diarrhea, dizziness, urinary frequency.
Nabilone (Cesamet) CII	**Cap:** 1mg	***Adults:*** **Initial:** 1 or 2mg bid; given 1-3 hrs before chemotherapy. A dose of 1 or 2mg the night before may be useful. **Max:** 6mg/day given in divided doses tid.	**W/P:** Patients should remain under the supervision of a responsible adult during treatment, especially during initial use and dose adjustments. Caution when initiating therapy with HTN, heart disease, current or previous psychiatric disorders, and with history of substance abuse. Avoid driving, operating heavy machinery, or engaging in any hazardous activity during treatment. May cause dizziness, euphoria, ataxia, anxiety, disorientation, depression, hallucinations, and psychosis. Adverse psychiatric reactions can persist for 48-72 hrs following cessation of treatment. Avoid with alcohol, sedatives, hypnotics, or other psychoactive substances. May cause tachycardia and orthostatic hypotension. **P/N:** Category C, not for use in nursing.	Drowsiness, vertigo, **dry mouth,** euphoria, ataxia, headache, concentration difficulties, nausea, dysphoria, sleep/ visual disturbance, asthenia, anorexia.
Ondansetron (Zofran)	**Inj:** 2mg/mL, 32mg/50mL; **Sol:** 4mg/5mL [50mL]; **Tab:** 4mg, 8mg, 24mg; **Tab, Disintegrating:** 4mg, 8mg	***Adults:*** **Prevention of CINV:** (Inj) 32mg single dose or three 0.15mg/kg doses, 1st dose 30 min before chemotherapy, then 4 and 8 hrs after first dose. **With Highly Emetogenic Chemotherapy:** (Tab) 24mg given as three 8-mg tabs 30 min before chemotherapy. **With Moderately Emetogenic Chemotherapy:** (Sol/Tab) 8mg bid, first dose 30 min before chemotherapy, then 8 hrs later, then bid for 1-2 days after chemotherapy. **Prevention of PONV:** (Inj) 4mg IM/IV immediately before anesthesia or after surgery if nausea or vomiting occurs. (Sol/Tab) 16mg 1 hr before anesthesia. **Prevention of Radiation-Induced N/V:** (Sol/Tab) **Usual:** 8mg tid. **Total Body Irradiation:** 8mg 1-2 hrs before therapy daily. **Single High-Dose Therapy to Abdomen:** 8mg 1-2 hrs before therapy then q8h after first dose for 1-2 days after completion of therapy. **Daily Fractionated Therapy To Abdomen:** 8mg 1-2 hrs before therapy then q8h after first dose. **Severe Hepatic Dysfunction (Child-Pugh ≥10): Max:** 8mg/day IV single dose infused over 15 min,	**W/P:** Hypersensitivity reactions reported in those hypersensitive to other 5-HT_3 receptor antagonists. Transient ECG changes including QT interval prolongation reported with IV administration. May mask progressive ileus or gastric distension. Orally disintegrating tabs contain phenylalanine; caution in phenylketonurics. **P/N:** Category B, caution in nursing.	Headache, diarrhea, dizziness, drowsiness, malaise/ fatigue, constipation, LFT abnormalities.

*Scored. †Bold entries denote special dental considerations.
BB = black box warning; **W/P** = warnings/precautions; **Contra** = contraindications; **P/N** = pregnancy category rating and nursing considerations.

NAME	FORM/ STRENGTH	DOSAGE	WARNINGS/PRECAUTIONS & CONTRAINDICATIONS	ADVERSE EFFECTS†
Ondansetron (Zofran) *(cont.)*		start 30 min before chemotherapy or 8mg/day PO. ***Pediatrics:* Prevention of CINV:** (Inj) **6 months-18 yrs:** Three 0.15mg/kg doses, first dose 30 min before chemotherapy, then 4 and 8 hrs after the first dose. **With Moderately Emetogenic Chemotherapy:** (Sol/Tab) **≥12 yrs:** 8mg bid, first dose 30 min before chemotherapy, then 8mg 8 hrs later, then bid for 1-2 days. **4-11 yrs:** 4mg tid, first dose 30 min before chemotherapy, then 4 and 8 hrs after first dose, then tid for 1-2 days. **Prevention of PONV:** (Inj) **>12 yrs:** 4mg IM/IV immediately before anesthesia or post-op after surgery if nausea or vomiting occurs. **1 month-12 yrs: ≤40kg:** 0.1mg/kg single dose. **>40kg:** 4mg single dose. **Severe Hepatic Dysfunction: Max:** 8mg/day IV single dose infused over 15 min, start 30 min before chemotherapy or 8mg/day PO.		
Palonosetron HCl (Aloxi)	**Cap:** 0.5mg; **Inj:** 0.25mg/ 5mL, 0.075mg/ 1.5mL	***Adults:* CINV:** (Cap) 0.5mg 1 hr prior to chemotherapy with or without food. (Inj) 0.25mg IV single dose 30 min before start of chemo. Repeated dosing within 7-day interval not recommended. **PONV:** 0.075mg IV single dose 10 sec before induction of anesthesia.	**W/P:** Hypersensitivity reaction may occur. **P/N:** Category B, not for use in nursing.	(Cap/Inj) Headache, constipation; (Inj) diarrhea, dizziness.
Prochlorperazine	**Inj:** (Edisylate) 5mg/mL; **Supp:** 5mg, 25mg; **Tab:** (Maleate) 5mg, 10mg	***Adults:* N/V:** (Tab) **Usual:** 5-10mg tid-qid. **Max:** 40mg/day. (IM) 5-10mg IM q3-4h prn. **Max:** 40mg/day. (IV) 2.5-10mg IV (not bolus). **Max:** 10mg single dose and 40mg/day. **PONV:** 5-10mg IM 1-2 hrs or 5-10mg IV 15-30 min before anesthesia, or during or after surgery; repeat once if needed. **Non-Psychotic Anxiety:** (Tab) 5mg tid-qid; **Max:** 20mg/ day and/or ≤12 weeks.**Psychosis: Mild/Outpatient:** 5-10mg PO tid-qid. **Moderate-Severe/Hospitalized: Initial:**10mg PO tid-qid. May increase in small increments every 2-3 days. **Severe:** (PO) 100-150mg/day. (IM) 10-20mg, may repeat q2-4 hrs if needed. Switch to oral after obtain control or if needed, 10-20mg IM q4-6h. **Elderly:** Use lower dosing range and titrate more gradually. ***Pediatrics:* N/V: >2 yrs and >20 lbs:** (PO/PR) **20-29 lbs: Usual:** 2.5mg qd-bid. **Max:** 7.5mg/day. **30-39 lbs:** 2.5mg bid-tid. **Max:** 10mg/day. **40-85 lbs:** 2.5mg tid or 5mg bid. **Max:** 15mg/day. (IM) 0.06mg/lb, usually single dose for control. **Psychosis:** (PO/ PR) **2-12 yrs: Initial:** 2.5mg bid-tid, up to 10mg/day on first day. **Max: 2-5 yrs:** 20mg/day. **6-12 yrs:** 25mg/day. (IM) **<12 yrs:** 0.06mg/lb single dose. Switch to oral after obtain control.	**W/P:** Secondary extrapyramidal symptoms can occur. Tardive dyskinesia and neuroleptic malignant syndrome (NMS) may develop. Caution with activities requiring alertness. May mask symptoms of overdose of other drugs. May obscure diagnosis of intestinal obstruction, brain tumor, and Reye's syndrome. May interfere with thermoregulation. Caution with glaucoma, cardiac disorders. Caution in children with dehydration or acute illness and the elderly. D/C 48 hrs before myelography and may resume after 24 hrs post-procedure. **Contra:** Comatose states, concomitant large dose CNS depressants (alcohol, barbiturates, narcotics), pediatric surgery, pediatrics <2 yrs or <20lbs. **P/N:** Safety in pregnancy is not known; caution in nursing.	Drowsiness, dizziness, amenorrhea, blurred vision, skin reactions, hypotension, NMS, cholestatic jaundice.
Promethazine Injection	**Inj:** 25mg/mL, 50mg/mL	***Adults:*** (IM/IV) IM is preferred. **Allergy: Initial:** 25mg, may repeat within 2 hrs. **Sedation:** 25-50mg qhs. **Nausea/Vomiting:** 12.5-25mg q4h. **Pre-Op/Post-Op:** 25-50mg. **Obstetrics:** 50mg in early labor, 25-75mg in established labor, may repeat once or twice q4h. **Max:** 100mg/24 hrs of labor. Do not give IV administration >25mg/mL and at a rate >25mg/min. ***Pediatrics:* ≥2 yrs:** Dose	**W/P:** Caution in patients ≥2 yrs. Not recommended for uncomplicated vomiting in pediatrics. May cause marked drowsiness; caution with operating machinery. Fatal respiratory depression reported; avoid with respiratory dysfunction (eg, COPD, sleep apnea). Avoid prolonged sun exposure. May lower seizure threshold. Caution with bone marrow depression. NMS reported. Caution in	Drowsiness, dizziness, tinnitus, blurred vision, **dry mouth,** increased or decreased blood pressure, urticaria, N/V, blood dyscrasia.

Table 16.1. PRESCRIBING INFORMATION FOR GASTROINTESTINAL DRUGS *(cont.)*

NAME	FORM/ STRENGTH	DOSAGE	WARNINGS/PRECAUTIONS & CONTRAINDICATIONS	ADVERSE EFFECTS†
ANTIEMETICS *(cont.)*				
Promethazine Injection *(cont.)*		should not exceed half of adult dose. **Premedication: Usual:** 0.5mg/lb. Do not give IV administration >25mg/mL and at a rate >25mg/min.	acutely ill pediatric patients. Avoid in pediatrics with Reye's syndrome or hepatic disease. Avoid perivascular extravasation or inadvertent intraarterial injection. Caution with narrow-angle glaucoma, prostatic hypertrophy, stenosing peptic ulcer, bladder-neck or pyloroduodenal obstruction, cardiovascular disease, hepatic dysfunction. Cholestatic jaundice reported. Alters HCG pregnancy test reading. May increase blood glucose. **Contra:** Comatose states, intraarterial or subcutaneous injection. Hypersensitivity to other phenothiazines. **P/N:** Category C, caution in nursing.	
Scopolamine (Transderm Scop)	**Patch:** 0.33mg/ 24 hrs [4[s]]	***Adults:* Motion Sickness:** Apply 1 patch 4 hrs before travel. Replace after 3 days. **PONV:** Apply 1 patch the evening before surgery or 1 hr prior to cesarean section. Keep in place for 24 hrs. Apply patch to a hairless area behind the ear. Do not cut patch in half.	**W/P:** Monitor IOP with open-angle glaucoma. Not for use in children. Caution with pyloric obstruction, urinary bladder neck or intestinal obstruction, elderly. Increased CNS effects with liver or kidney dysfunction. May aggravate seizures or psychosis. Idiosyncratic reactions reported (rare). Remove patch before MRI. **Contra:** Angle-closure (narrow-angle) glaucoma, hypersensitivity to belladonna alkaloids. **P/N:** Category C, caution in nursing.	**Dry mouth,** drowsiness, blurred vision, dilation of pupils, dizziness, disorientation, confusion.
Trimethobenzamide HCl (Tigan)	**Cap:** 300mg; **Inj:** 100mg/mL	***Adults:*** (Cap) 300mg tid-qid. (Inj) 200mg IM tid-qid.	**W/P:** Caution in children; may cause EPS, which may be confused with CNS signs of undiagnosed primary disease (eg, Reye's syndrome) and may unfavorably alter the course of Reye's syndrome due to hepatotoxic potential. Caution with acute febrile illness, encephalitides, gastroenteritis, dehydration, electrolyte imbalance, and in elderly; CNS reactions reported. May produce drowsiness. **Contra:** Injection in children. **P/N:** Safety in pregnancy and nursing not known.	Hypersensitivity reactions, Parkinson-like symptoms, hypotension (inj), blood dyscrasias, blurred vision, coma, convulsions, mood depression, diarrhea, disorientation, dizziness, drowsiness, headache, jaundice, muscle cramps, opisthotonos.
ANTISPASMODICS/IBS AGENTS				
Alosetron HCl (Lotronex)	**Tab:** 0.5mg, 1mg	***Adults:* Initial:** 0.5mg bid. If constipation occurs, d/c until constipation resolves. May restart at 0.5mg qd. **Titrate:** If tolerated and IBS symptoms not controlled at 0.5mg qd or bid, may increase to 1mg bid. D/C after 4 weeks if symptoms not controlled on 1mg bid.	**BB:** Serious GI adverse events, some fatal, reported (eg, ischemic colitis, serious constipation complications). Physicians must enroll in the Prescribing Program for Lotronex and patients must sign the Patient-Physician Agreement. Discontinue immediately if constipation or symptoms of ischemic colitis develop (rectal bleeding, bloody diarrhea, abdominal pain); do not resume therapy. **W/P:** Increased risk of constipation and ischemic colitis. Caution with mild or moderate hepatic impairment. **Contra:** Current constipation. History of chronic/ severe constipation or sequelae of constipation, intestinal obstruction/stricture, toxic megacolon, GI perforation/ adhesions, ischemic colitis, impaired intestinal circulation, thrombophlebitis, hypercoagulable state, Crohn's disease, ulcerative colitis, diverticulitis, severe hepatic impairment. Inability to understand/comply with Patient-Physician Agreement. **P/N:** Category B, caution in nursing.	Constipation, abdominal discomfort/pain, nausea, GI discomfort/pain.

†Bold entries denote special dental considerations.
BB = black box warning; **W/P** = warnings/precautions; **Contra** = contraindications; **P/N** = pregnancy category rating and nursing considerations.

NAME	FORM/ STRENGTH	DOSAGE	WARNINGS/PRECAUTIONS & CONTRAINDICATIONS	ADVERSE EFFECTS†
Atropine Sulfate/ Hyoscyamine Sulfate/Phenobarbital/Scopolamine Hydrobromide (Donnatal, Donnatal Extentabs)	**(Atropine-Hyoscyamine-Phenobarbital-Scopolamine) Elixir:** 0.0194mg-0.1037mg-16.2mg-0.0065mg/5mL; **Tab:** 0.0194mg-0.1037mg-16.2mg-0.0065mg; **Tab, Extended-Release (Extentabs):** 0.0582mg-0.3111mg-48.6mg-0.0195mg	***Adults:*** (Elixir/Tab) 1-2 tabs or 5-10mL tid-qid. (Extentabs) 1 tab q8-12h. **Hepatic Disease:** Use lower doses. ***Pediatrics:*** (Elixir) **4.5kg:** 0.5mL q4h or 0.75mL q6h. 9.1kg: 1mL q4h or 1.5mL q6h. **13.6kg:** 1.5mL q4h or 2mL q6h. **22.7kg:** 2.5mL q4h or 3.75mL q6h. **34kg:** 3.75mL q4h or 5mL q6h. **45.4kg:** 5mL q4h or 7.5mL q6h. **Hepatic Disease:** Use lower doses.	**W/P:** Inconclusive whether anti-cholinergic/antispasmodic drugs aid in duodenal ulcer healing, decrease recurrence rate, or prevent complications. Heat prostration can occur with high environmental temperatures. Avoid with intestinal obstruction. May be habit-forming; caution with history of physical and/or psychological drug dependence. Caution with hepatic disease, renal disease, autonomic neuropathy, hyperthyroidism, coronary heart disease, CHF, arrhythmias, tachycardia, HTN. May delay gastric emptying. Diarrhea may be an early symptom of incomplete intestinal obstruction, especially with ileostomy or colostomy; treatment would be inappropriate. **Contra:** Glaucoma, obstructive uropathy, obstructive GI disease, paralytic ileus, intestinal atony in elderly or debilitated, unstable cardiovascular status in acute hemorrhage, severe ulcerative colitis, myasthenia gravis, hiatal hernia with reflux esophagitis, intermittent porphyria, and for patients in whom phenobarbital produces restlessness and/or excitement. **P/N:** Category C, caution in nursing.	**Xerostomia,** urinary hesitancy/retention, blurred vision, tachycardia/palpitation, mydriasis, cycloplegia, increased ocular tension, **loss of taste,** headache, nervousness, drowsiness, weakness, dizziness, insomnia, N/V, impotence, suppression of lactation, constipation, bloated feeling, musculoskeletal pain, allergic reaction/drug idiosyncrasies, decreased sweating.
Chlordiazepoxide HCl/Clidinium Bromide (Librax) CIV	**Cap:** (Chlordiazepoxide-Clidinium) 5mg-2.5mg	***Adults:*** **Usual/Maint:** 1-2 caps tid-qid ac and hs. **Elderly/Debilitated: Initial:** 2 caps/day and increase gradually, if needed.	**W/P:** Risk of congenital malformations during first trimester of pregnancy; avoid use. Avoid abrubt withdrawal. Paradoxical reactions reported in psychiatric patients. Caution with depression, renal or hepatic dysfunction, the elderly. Inhibition of lactation may occur. **Contra:** Glaucoma, prostatic hypertrophy, benign bladder neck obstruction. **P/N:** Not for use in pregnancy; safety in nursing is not known.	Drowsiness, ataxia, confusion, skin eruptions, extrapyramidal symptoms, **dry mouth,** nausea, constipation, altered libido, blood dyscrasias, jaundice, hepatic dysfunction.
Dicyclomine HCl (Bentyl)	**Cap:** 10mg; **Inj:** 10mg/mL; **Syrup:** 10mg/5mL; **Tab:** 20mg	***Adults:*** (Tab/Syrup) **Initial:** 20mg qid. **Usual:** 40mg qid if tolerated. D/C if no improvement after 2 weeks or if doses ≥80mg/day are not tolerated. (Inj) 20mg IM qid for 1-2 days, followed by oral dicyclomine. Not for IV use.	**W/P:** Caution in autonomic neuropathy, hepatic/renal impairment, ulcerative colitis, hyperthyroidism, HTN, CHF, cardiac tachyarrhythmia, coronary heart disease, hiatal hernia, and prostatic hypertrophy. Heat prostration may occur in high environmental temperature. Monitor for diarrhea, may be the early symptom of intestinal obstruction. Psychosis reported. Serious respiratory symptoms, seizures, syncope, and death reported in infants. **Contra:** GI tract obstruction, obstructive uropathy, severe ulcerative colitis, reflux esophagitis, glaucoma, myasthenia gravis, unstable cardiovascular status, and in acute hemorrhage, nursing mothers, infants <6 months of age. **P/N:** Category B, contraindicated in nursing.	**Dry mouth,** N/V, blurred vision, dizziness, drowsiness, nervousness, mental confusion/excitement (especially in the elderly), mydriasis, increased ocular tension, urinary retention, dyspnea, apnea, tachycardia, decreased sweating, lactation suppression, impotence.
Hyoscyamine Sulfate	**Sol:** (IB-Stat) 0.125mg/mL [30mL]; **Tab, Disintegrating:** 0.125mg	***Adults/Pediatrics:*** **≥12 yrs:** (Sol) 1-2 sprays q4h or prn. **Max:** 12 sprays/24hrs. (Tab, Disintegrating) 0.125-0.25mg q4h or prn. **Max:** 1.5mg/24hrs. Take with or without water. **2 to <12 yrs:** (Tab, Disintegrating) 0.0625-0.125mg q4h or prn. **Max:** 0.75mg/24hrs. Take with or without water.	**W/P:** Risk of heat prostration with high environmental temperature. Avoid activities requiring mental alertness. Psychosis has been reported in sensitive patients. Caution with diarrhea, autonomic neuropathy, hyperthyroidism, coronary heart disease, CHF, arrhythmias/tachycardia, HTN, renal disease, and hiatal hernia associated with reflux	Anticholinergic effects, drowsiness, headache, nervousness, dizziness, blurred vision, **dry mouth,** urinary hesitancy/retention, tachycardia, palpitations.

Table 16.1. PRESCRIBING INFORMATION FOR GASTROINTESTINAL DRUGS *(cont.)*

NAME	FORM/ STRENGTH	DOSAGE	WARNINGS/PRECAUTIONS & CONTRAINDICATIONS	ADVERSE EFFECTS†
ANTISPASMODICS/IBS AGENTS *(cont.)*				
Hyoscyamine Sulfate *(cont.)*			esophagitis. Contains phenylalanine. **Contra:** Glaucoma, obstructive uropathy, GI tract obstruction, paralytic ileus; intestinal atony of elderly/debilitated, unstable cardiovascular status in acute hemorrhage, toxic megacolon complicating ulcerative colitis, myasthenia gravis. **P/N:** Category C, caution in nursing.	
Hyoscyamine Sulfate (Levbid, Levsin, Levsinex)	**(Levbid) Tab, Extended-Release:** 0.375mg. **(Levsin) Drops:** 0.125mg/mL [15mL]; **Elixir:** 0.125mg/5mL [473mL]; **Inj:** 0.5mg/mL; **Tab:** 0.125mg*; **Tab, SL:** 0.125mg*. **(Levsinex) Cap, Extended-Release:** 0.375mg	***Adults:*** May also chew or swallow SL tab. (Drops/Elixir/Tab/Tab, SL) 0.125-0.25mg q4h or prn. **Max:** 1.5mg/24 hrs. (Cap/Tab, ER) 0.375-0.75mg q12h; or 1 cap q8h. **Max:** 1.5mg/24 hrs. Do not crush or chew. (Inj) **Anesthesia:** 5mcg/kg IM/IV/SQ 30-60 min before anesthesia or with narcotic/sedative administration. **GI Disorders:** 0.25-0.5mg IM/IV/SQ as single dose; may require bid-qid administration at 4-hr intervals. **Diagnostic Procedures:** 0.25-0.5mg IV 5-10 min prior. **Drug-Induced Bradycardia (Surgery):** Increments of 0.25mL IV; repeat prn. **Neuromuscular Blockade Reversal:** 0.2mg for every 1mg neostigmine or equal dose of physostigmine or pyridostigmine. ***Pediatrics:*** May also chew or swallow SL tab. **≥12 yrs:** (Drops, Elixir, Tab, and Tab, SL) 0.125-0.25mg q4h or prn. **Max:** 1.5mg/24 hrs. (Cap/Tab, ER) 0.375-0.75mg q12h; or 1 cap may be given q8h. **Max:** 1.5mg/24 hrs. Do not crush or chew. **2 to <12 yrs:** (Tab/Tab, SL) 0.0625-0.125mg q4h or prn. **Max:** 0.75mg/24 hrs. (Elixir) Give q4h or prn. **10kg:** 1.25mL. **20kg:** 2.5mL. **40kg:** 3.75mL. **50kg:** 5mL. **Max:** 30mL/24 hrs. (Drops) 0.25-1mL q4h or prn. **Max:** 6mL/24 hrs. **<2 yrs:** (Drops) Give q4h or prn. **3.4kg:** 4 drops. **Max:** 24 drops/24 hrs. **5kg:** 5 drops. **Max:** 30 drops/24 hrs. **7kg:** 6 drops. **Max:** 36 drops/24 hrs. **10kg:** 8 drops. **Max:** 48 drops/24 hrs. **>2 yrs: Anesthesia:** (Inj) 5mcg/kg IM/IV/SQ 30-60 min before anesthesia or with narcotic/sedative administration.	**W/P:** Risk of heat prostration with high environmental temperature. Avoid activities requiring mental alertness. Psychosis has been reported. Caution with diarrhea, autonomic neuropathy, hyperthyroidism, coronary heart disease, CHF, arrhythmias/tachycardia, HTN, renal disease, and hiatal hernia associated with reflux esophagitis. D/C if diarrhea occurs. **Contra:** Glaucoma, obstructive uropathy, GI tract obstruction, paralytic ileus; intestinal atony of elderly/debilitated, unstable CV status in acute hemorrhage, toxic megacolon complicating ulcerative colitis, myasthenia gravis. **P/N:** Category C, caution in nursing.	Anticholinergic effects, drowsiness, headache, nervousness.
ANTIULCER/GERD AGENTS				
Aluminum Hydroxide OTC	**Sus:** 320mg/5mL	***Adults:*** 10mL 5-6 times daily, between meals and qhs. **Max:** 60mL/24hrs.	**W/P:** Extreme caution with renal failure and dialysis. Prolonged use of aluminum-containing antacids with renal failure may result in or worsen dialysis osteomalacia. Elevated tissue aluminum levels contribute to development of dialysis encephalopathy and osteomalacia syndromes. **P/N:** Safety in pregnancy and nursing not known.	Constipation.

*Scored. †Bold entries denote special dental considerations.
BB = black box warning; **W/P** = warnings/precautions; **Contra** = contraindications; **P/N** = pregnancy category rating and nursing considerations.

NAME	FORM/ STRENGTH	DOSAGE	WARNINGS/PRECAUTIONS & CONTRAINDICATIONS	ADVERSE EFFECTS†
Aluminum Hydroxide/Magnesium Hydroxide/Simethicone (Mylanta Maximum Strength Liquid, Mylanta Regular Strength Liquid) OTC	**Liq: (Aluminum Hydroxide-Magnesium Hydroxide-Simethicone) Maximum Strength:** 400mg/5mL-400mg/5mL-40mg/5mL. **Regular Strength:** 200mg/5mL-200mg/5mL-20mg/5mL	***Adults/Pediatrics:*** **≥12 yrs:** 2-4 tsp between meals or at bedtime. **Max:** 24 tsp/day for 2 weeks. Shake well.	—	—
Amoxicillin/Clarithromycin/Lansoprazole (Prevpac)	**Cap: (Amoxicillin)** 500mg, **Tab: (Clarithromycin)** 500mg, **Cap, Delayed-Release: (Lansoprazole)** 30mg	***Adults:*** 1g amoxicillin, 500mg clarithromycin, and 30mg lansoprazole, all bid (am and pm) before meals for 10 or 14 days. Swallow each pill whole. **Renal Impairment (with or without hepatic impairment):** Decrease clarithromycin dose or prolong intervals. Avoid with CrCl <30mL/min.	**W/P:** Avoid if CrCl <30mL/min. Caution with cephalosporin/PCN allergy; anaphylactic reactions have been reported. Pseudomembranous colitis reported. Possibility of superinfections. Caution in elderly. Clarithromycin may increase colchicine; monitor for toxicity. Do not use clarithromycin during pregnancy. Symptomatic response to lansoprazole does not preclude the presence of gastric malignancy. *Clostridium difficile*–associated diarrhea (CDAD) reported. D/C if confirmed. **Contra:** Concomitant cisapride, pimozide, astemizole, terfenadine, ergotamine, or dihydroergotamine. Hypersensitivity to prevacid, macrolide or penicillin antibiotics. **P/N:** Category C, not for use in nursing.	Diarrhea, **taste perversion,** headache.
Bismuth Subsalicylate/Metronidazole/Tetracycline HCl (Helidac)	**Cap (Tetracycline):** 500mg; **Tab (Metronidazole):** 250mg; **Tab, Chewable (Bismuth Subsalicylate):** 262.4mg	***Adults:*** **(Bismuth)** 2 tabs (525mg) qid + **(Metronidazole)** 250mg qid + **(Tetracycline)** 500mg qid, all for 14 days with an H_2-antagonist. Take with meals and hs. Take metronidazole and tetracycline with a full glass of water; swallow whole.	**W/P:** Do not use to treat nausea and vomiting in children or teenagers who have or are recovering from chickenpox or flu. Rare reports of neurotoxicity with excessive bismuth doses. Seizures and peripheral neuropathy reported with metronidazole; caution with CNS disease; d/c with abnormal neurological signs. Caution with blood dyscrasias. Unrecognized candidiasis may be unmasked. Avoid exposure to sunlight/UV light. Caution in elderly. **Contra:** Pregnancy, nursing, pediatrics, nitroimidazole hypersensitivity, ASA or salicylate hypersensitivity, renal/hepatic impairment. **P/N:** Category D, not for use in nursing.	N/V, diarrhea, abdominal pain, melena, constipation, anorexia, asthenia, **discolored tongue,** headache, dyspepsia, dizziness. **Temporary, harmless darkening of tongue** and black stool with bismuth. **Tetracycline may cause permanent discoloration of teeth during tooth development, enamel hypoplasia,** photosensitivity reactions, BUN increase, breakthrough bleeding, pseudotumor cerebri.
Calcium Carbonate (Children's Mylanta) OTC	**Tab, Chewable:** 400mg	***Pediatrics:*** **24-47 lbs or 2-5 yrs:** 1 tab; **48-95 lbs or 6-11 yrs:** 2 tabs. **Max: 2-5 yrs:** 3 tabs/24hrs; **6-11 yrs:** 6 tabs/24hrs. Repeat as needed. Do not use for >2 weeks unless under supervision of a doctor.	—	—
Calcium Carbonate/Famotidine/Magnesium Hydroxide (Pepcid Complete) OTC	**Tab, Chewable:** (Famotidine-Calcium Carbonate-Magnesium Hydroxide) 10mg-800mg-165mg	***Adults/Pediatrics:*** **≥12 yrs:** Chew 1 tab to relieve symptoms. **Max:** 2 tabs/24hrs.	**W/P:** Not for use in those with trouble swallowing. Avoid use with other acid reducers. **P/N:** Safety in pregnancy and nursing not known.	

Table 16.1. PRESCRIBING INFORMATION FOR GASTROINTESTINAL DRUGS *(cont.)*

NAME	FORM/ STRENGTH	DOSAGE	WARNINGS/PRECAUTIONS & CONTRAINDICATIONS	ADVERSE EFFECTS†
ANTIULCER/GERD AGENTS *(cont.)*				
Calcium Carbonate/ Magnesium Hydroxide (Mylanta Gelcaps Antacid, Mylanta Supreme, Mylanta Ultra Tabs) OTC	**Cap (Calcium Carbonate-Magnesium Hydroxide):** 550mg-125mg. **Tab:** 700mg-300mg. **Liq:** 400mg/5mL-135mg/5mL	***Adults:*** (Gelcaps) 2-4 caps prn. **Max:** 12 caps/24hrs. (Ultra Tabs) Chew 2-4 tabs between meals or at bedtime. **Max:** 10 tabs/24hrs. (Supreme Liquid) 2-4 tsp between meals or at bedtime. **Max:** 18 tsp/24hrs. Shake well.	**W/P:** Caution with kidney disease.	—
Cimetidine (Tagamet)	**Inj (HCl):** 150mg/mL, 300mg/5mL; **Sol (HCl):** 300mg/5mL; **Tab:** 200mg, 300mg, 400mg*, 800mg*	***Adults/Pediatrics:*** **≥16 yrs:** (PO) **Active DU:** 800mg qhs or 300mg qid or 400mg bid for 4-8 weeks. **Maint:** 400mg qhs. **Active Benign GU:** 800mg qhs or 300mg qid for 6 weeks. **GERD:** 800mg bid or 400mg qid for 12 weeks. **Hypersecretory Conditions:** 300mg qid. **Max:** 2400mg/day. (Inj) 300mg IM/IV q6-8h. **Max:** 2400mg/day. **Rapid Gastric pH Elevation: LD:** 150mg IV, then 37.5mg/hr IV. **Upper GI Bleed Prevention:** Continuous IV infusion of 50mg/hr for 7 days. **CrCl <30mL/min:** Give half the recommended dose.	**W/P:** Cardiac arrhythmias and hypotension reported following rapid IV administration (rare). Symptomatic response does not preclude the presence of gastric malignancy. Reversible confusional states reported, especially in severely ill patients. Elderly, renal, and/or hepatic impairment are risk factors for confusional states. Risk of hyperinfection of strongyloidiasis in immunocompromised patients. **P/N:** Category B, not for use in nursing.	Diarrhea, headache, dizziness, somnolence, reversible confusional states, impotence, increased serum transaminases, rash, gynecomastia, blood dyscrasias.
Esomeprazole Magnesium (Nexium)	**Cap, Delayed-Release:** 20mg, 40mg; **Sus, Delayed-Release:** 10mg, 20mg, 40mg (granules/pkt).	***Adults:*** **Erosive Esophagitis: Healing:** 20mg or 40mg qd for 4-8 weeks; may extend treatment for 4-8 weeks if not healed. **Maint:** 20mg qd for up to 6 months. **Risk Reduction of NSAID-Associated Gastric Ulcer:** 20mg or 40mg qd for up to 6 months. **Symptomatic GERD:** 20mg qd for 4 weeks; may extend treatment for 4 weeks if symptoms do not resolve. ***H.pylori:*** **Triple Therapy:** 40mg qd + amoxicillin 1000mg bid + clarithromycin 500mg bid, all for 10 days. **Zollinger-Ellison Syndrome:** 40mg bid. **Severe Hepatic Dysfunction: Max:** 20mg/day. Take 1 hr before meals. Swallow capsule whole. Contents may be mixed with soft food (eg, applesauce, yogurt) that does not require chewing. ***Pediatrics:*** **GERD: 12-17 yrs:** 20mg or 40mg qd for up to 8 weeks. **1-11 yrs:** 10mg qd for up to 8 weeks. **Erosive Esophagitis: 1-11 yrs: ≥20kg:** 10mg or 20mg qd for 8 weeks. **<20kg:** 10mg qd for 8 weeks. **Severe Hepatic Dysfunction: Max:** 20mg/day. Take 1 hr before meals. Swallow capsule whole. Contents may be mixed with soft food (eg, applesauce, yogurt) that does not require chewing.	**W/P:** Atrophic gastritis may occur. Symptomatic response does not preclude gastric malignancy. **Contra:** Hypersensitivity to substituted benzimidazoles. **P/N:** Category B, not for use in nursing.	Headache, diarrhea, abdominal pain, constipation, nausea, flatulence, **dry mouth.**
Esomeprazole Sodium (Nexium IV)	**Inj:** 20mg, 40mg	***Adults:*** 20mg or 40mg qd IV injection (no less than 3 min) or infusion (10-30 min). D/C as soon as patient able to resume oral therapy. **Severe Hepatic Dysfunction: Max:** 20mg/day.	**W/P:** Atrophic gastritis may occur. Symptomatic response does not preclude gastric malignancy. D/C and convert to oral therapy as soon as possible. **Contra:** Hypersensitivity to substituted benzimidazoles. **P/N:** Category B, not for use in nursing.	Headache, flatulence, dyspepsia, nausea, abdominal pain, diarrhea, **dry mouth.**
Famotidine (Pepcid AC) OTC	**Cap:** 10mg; **Tab:** 10mg, 20mg; **Tab, Chewable:** 10mg	***Adults/Pediatrics:*** **≥12yrs: Relief:** 1 tab/cap prn. **Max:** 2 doses/24 hrs. **Prevention:** 1 tab/cap 15-60 min before food or beverages that cause heartburn. **Max:** 2 doses/24 hrs.	—	—

*Scored. †Bold entries denote special dental considerations.
BB = black box warning; **W/P** = warnings/precautions; **Contra** = contraindications; **P/N** = pregnancy category rating and nursing considerations.

NAME	FORM/ STRENGTH	DOSAGE	WARNINGS/PRECAUTIONS & CONTRAINDICATIONS	ADVERSE EFFECTS†
Famotidine (Pepcid, Pepcid RPD)	**Inj:** 0.4mg/mL, 10mg/mL; **Sus:** 40mg/5mL [50mL]; **Tab:** 20mg, 40mg; **Tab, Disintegrating:** (RPD) 20mg, 40mg	***Adults:*** (PO) **Acute DU:** 40mg qhs or 20mg bid for 4-8 weeks. **Maint DU:** 20mg qhs. **GU:** 40mg qhs. **GERD:** 20mg bid up to 6 weeks. **GERD with Esophagitis:** 20-40mg bid up to 12 weeks. **Hypersecretory Conditions: Initial:** 20mg q6h. **Max:** 160mg q6h. (Inj) 20mg IV q12h, hypersecretory conditions may require higher doses. **CrCl <50mL/min:** Reduce to 1/2 dose, or increase interval to q36-48h. ***Pediatrics:*** **1-16 yrs:** (PO) **DU/GU: Usual:** 0.5mg/kg/day qhs or divided bid. **Max:** 40mg/day. **GERD With or Without Esophagitis:** 0.5mg/kg PO bid. **Max:** 40mg bid. (Inj) 0.25mg/kg IV q12h up to 40mg/day. Base duration of therapy on clinical response, and/or pH, and endoscopy. (PO) **GERD: 3 months-1 yr:** 0.5mg/kg bid for up to 8 weeks. **<3 months:** 0.5mg/kg qd for up to 8 weeks. **CrCl <50mL/min:** Reduce to 1/2 dose, or increase interval to q36-48h.	**W/P:** CNS adverse effects reported with moderate to severe renal insufficiency; adjust dose. Disintegrating tabs contain phenylalanine; caution in phenylketonurics. Symptomatic response does not preclude the presence of gastric malignancy. May be given with antacids if needed. **Contra:** Hypersensitivity to other H_2-antagonists. **P/N:** Category B, not for use in nursing.	Headache, dizziness, constipation, diarrhea, convulsions, interstitial pneumonia, Stevens-Johnson syndrome.
Glycopyrrolate (Robinul Injection)	**Inj:** 0.2mg/mL	***Adults:*** **Preanesthesia:** 0.004mg/kg IM 30-60 min before anesthesia induction or at time of preanesthetic narcotic/sedative. **Intraoperatively:** 0.1mg IV, repeat prn every 2-3 min. **Reverse Neuromuscular Blockade:** 0.2mg IV for each 1mg neostigmine or 5mg pyridostigmine. **Peptic Ulcer:** 0.1mg IV/IM q4h, tid-qid. May use 0.2mg if needed. ***Pediatrics:*** **Preanesthesia:** 0.004mg/kg IM 30-60 min before anesthesia induction or at time of preanesthetic narcotic/sedative. **1 month-2 yrs:** May require up to 0.009mg/kg. **Intraoperatively:** 0.004mg/kg IV. **Max:** 0.1mg single dose. May repeat prn every 2-3 min. **Reverse Neuromuscular Blockade:** 0.2mg IV for each 1mg neostigmine or 5mg pyridostigmine.	**W/P:** Caution with CAD, CHF, arrhythmias, HTN, hyperthyroidism, elderly, autonomic neuropathy, hepatic or renal disease, ulcerative colitis, or hiatal hernia. May produce drowsiness and blurred vision; caution when operating machinery. Risk of fever and heat stroke due to decreased sweating in high environmental temperature. Diarrhea may be early symptom of incomplete intestinal obstruction. **Contra:** Newborns (<1 month) due to benzyl alcohol content. For long treatment duration: Glaucoma, obstructive uropathy, obstructive disease of GI tract, paralytic ileus, intestinal atony of elderly or debilitated, unstable cardiovascular status in acute hemorrhage, severe ulcerative colitis, toxic megacolon complicating ulcerative colitis, myasthenia gravis. **P/N:** Category B, caution in nursing.	Drowsiness, blurred vision, **dry mouth,** urinary retention and hesitancy, increased ocular tension, tachycardia, palpation, decreased sweating, **loss of taste.**
Glycopyrrolate (Robinul, Robinul Forte)	**Tab:** 1mg*, (Forte) 2mg*	***Adults/Pediatrics:*** **≥12 yrs: Peptic Ulcer: Usual:** (Tab) 1mg tid (am, pm and hs); may increase to 2mg qhs if needed. **Maint:** 1mg bid. (Forte) 2mg bid-tid. **Max:** 8mg/day.	**W/P:** May produce drowsiness and blurred vision; avoid operating machinery. Risk of heat prostration with high environmental temperature. Diarrhea may be early symptom of incomplete intestinal obstruction especially with ileostomy or colostomy. Caution in elderly, autonomic neuropathy, hepatic/renal disease, ulcerative colitis, hyperthyroidism, coronary heart disease, CHF, tachyarrhythmias, tachycardia, HTN, prostatic hypertrophy, hiatal hernia associated with reflux esophagitis. **Contra:** Glaucoma, obstructive uropathy, GI tract obstruction, paralytic ileus, intestinal atony of elderly or debilitated, unstable cardiovascular status in acute hemorrhage, severe ulcerative colitis, toxic megacolon complicating ulcerative colitis, myasthenia gravis. **P/N:** Safety in pregnancy is not known; not for use in nursing.	Blurred vision, **dry mouth,** urinary retention and hesitancy, increased ocular tension, tachycardia, decreased sweating, **loss of taste,** headache.

Table 16.1. PRESCRIBING INFORMATION FOR GASTROINTESTINAL DRUGS *(cont.)*

NAME	FORM/ STRENGTH	DOSAGE	WARNINGS/PRECAUTIONS & CONTRAINDICATIONS	ADVERSE EFFECTS†
ANTIULCER/GERD AGENTS *(cont.)*				
Lansoprazole (Prevacid, Prevacid IV, Prevacid So-lutab)	**Cap, Delayed-Release:** 15mg, 30mg; **Inj:** 30mg; **Sus, Delayed-Release:** 15mg, 30mg (granules/pkt); **Tab, Disintegrating (SoluTab):** 15mg, 30mg.	***Adults:*** **>17 yrs:** (PO) **DU:** 15mg qd for 4 weeks. **Maint:** 15mg qd. **GU:** 30mg qd up to 8 weeks. **GERD:** 15mg qd up to 8 weeks. **Erosive Esophagitis:** 30mg qd up to 8 weeks. May repeat for 8 weeks if needed. **Maint:** 15mg qd. **NSAID-Induced GU:** 30mg qd for 8 weeks. **Reduce Risk of NSAID-Induced GU:** 15mg qd for 12 weeks. **Hypersecretory Conditions: Initial:** 60mg qd, then adjust. **Max:** 90mg bid. Divide dose if >120mg/day. ***H.pylori:*** **Triple Therapy:** 30mg + clarithromycin 500mg + amoxicillin 1000mg, all bid (q12h) for 10-14 days. **Dual Therapy:** 30mg + amoxicillin 1000mg both tid (q8h) for 14 days. Take before eating. **Caps:** Swallow whole or sprinkle cap contents on 1 tbsp of applesauce, ENSURE pudding, cottage cheese, yogurt, strained pears, or in 60mL orange juice or tomato juice; swallow immediately. **Sus:** Do not chew or crush. Mix pkt with 30mL of water; stir well and drink immediately; not for use with NG tube. **SoluTab:** Place on tongue with or without water. **Oral Syringe (SoluTab):** Place 15mg tab in oral syringe and draw up 4mL of water, or 30mg tab in oral syringe and draw up 10mL of water. Shake contents and administer after tablet has dispersed within 15 mins. Refill syringe with 2mL (5mL for 30mg tab) of water, shake, and give any remaining contents. **NG Tube (Cap):** Mix cap contents with 40mL apple juice and inject into NG tube; flush with additional juice to clear tube. **(SoluTab)** Place 15mg tab and draw up 4mL of water, or 30mg tab and draw up 10mL of water. Shake contents and after tablet has dispersed, inject through NG tube into stomach within 15 mins. Refill syringe with 5mL of water, shake, and flush NG tube. (Inj) **Erosive Esophagitis:** 30mg IV qd over 30 mins for 7 days. May switch to PO formulation for total of 6 to 8 weeks of therapy once patient is able to take oral medications. **Severe Hepatic Impairment:** Adjust dose. ***Pediatrics:*** **12-17 yrs: Short-Term Symptomatic GERD:** 15mg qd for up to 8 weeks. **Erosive Esophagitis:** 30mg qd for up to 8 weeks. **1-11 yrs: Short-Term Symptomatic GERD/Erosive Esophagitis: ≤30kg:** 15mg qd for up to 12 weeks. **>30kg:** 30mg qd for up to 12 weeks. **Titrate:** May increase up to 30mg bid after 2 weeks if symptomatic. **Severe Hepatic Impairment:** Adjust dose. Take before eating. **Caps:** Swallow whole or sprinkle contents on 1 tbsp of applesauce, ENSURE pudding, cottage cheese, yogurt, strained pears, or in 60mL orange juice or tomato juice; swallow	**W/P:** Symptomatic response does not preclude the presence of gastric malignancy. Adjust dose with hepatic impairment. **P/N:** Category B, not for use in nursing.	Abdominal pain, constipation, diarrhea, nausea, myositis, interstitial nephritis.

*Scored. †Bold entries denote special dental considerations.
BB = black box warning; **W/P** = warnings/precautions; **Contra** = contraindications; **P/N** = pregnancy category rating and nursing considerations.

NAME	FORM/ STRENGTH	DOSAGE	WARNINGS/PRECAUTIONS & CONTRAINDICATIONS	ADVERSE EFFECTS†
Lansoprazole (Prevacid, Prevacid IV, Prevacid So-lutab) *(cont.)*		immediately. **Sus:** Do not chew or crush granules. Mix pkt with 30mL water; stir well and drink immediately; not for use with NG tube. **SoluTab:** Place on tongue with or without water. **Oral Syringe: (SoluTab)** Place 15mg tab in oral syringe and draw up 4mL of water, or 30mg tab in oral syringe and draw up 10mL of water. Shake contents and administer after tablet has dispersed within 15 mins. Refill syringe with 2mL (5mL for 30mg tab) of water, shake, and give any remaining contents. **NG Tube: (Cap)** Mix cap contents with 40mL apple juice and inject into NG tube; flush with additional juice to clear tube. **(SoluTab)** Place 15mg tab and draw up 4mL of water, or 30mg tab and draw up 10mL of water. Shake contents and after tablet has dispersed, inject through NG tube into stomach within 15 mins. Refill syringe with 5mL of water, shake, and flush NG tube.		
Methscopolamine Bromide (Pamine, Pamine Forte)	**Tab:** 2.5mg; (Forte) 5mg	***Adults:*** 2.5mg tid 30 min ac and 2.5-5mg qhs. **Severe Symptoms:** 5mg 30 min ac and qhs. **Max:** 30mg/day.	**W/P:** Heat prostration may occur with high environmental temperatures. Avoid or d/c use if diarrhea develops, especially with ileostomy or colostomy. Caution in elderly, autonomic neuropathy, hepatic/renal disease, ulcerative colitis, hyperthyroidism, coronary heart disease, CHF, tachyrhythmia, tachycardia, HTN, or prostatic hypertrophy. May impair mental/physical abilities. **Contra:** Glaucoma, obstructive uropathy, obstructive GI disease, paralytic ileus, intestinal atony of the elderly or debilitated, unstable cardiovascular status in acute hemorrhage, severe ulcerative colitis, toxic megacolon, myasthenia gravis. **P/N:** Category C, caution in nursing.	Constipation, decreased sweating, headache, drowsiness, dizziness.
Misoprostol (Cytotec)	**Tab:** 100mcg, 200mcg*	***Adults:*** 200mcg qid, or if not tolerated, 100mcg qid. Take for the duration of NSAID therapy. Take with meals; last dose at bedtime.	**BB:** Can cause abortion, premature birth, or birth defects. Uterine rupture reported when used to induce labor or induce abortion beyond 8th week of pregnancy. Not for use by pregnant women to reduce risk of NSAID-induced ulcers. Only use in women of childbearing age if at high risk of GI ulcers or complications with NSAID therapy; patient must then have negative serum pregnancy test within 2 weeks before therapy, maintain contraceptive measures, and begin therapy on 2nd or 3rd day of menstrual period. **Contra:** Pregnant women to reduce risk of NSAID-induced ulcers, prostaglandin allergy. **P/N:** Category X, not for use in nursing.	Diarrhea, abdominal pain, nausea, flatulence, headache, dyspepsia.
Nizatidine (Axid, Axid Oral Solution)	**Cap:** 150mg, 300mg; **Sol:** 15mg/mL	***Adults:*** **Active DU/Active Benign GU: Usual:** 300mg qhs or 150mg bid up to 8 weeks. **Healed DU: Maint:** 150mg qhs, up to 1 year. **GERD:** 150mg bid up to 12 weeks. **Renal Impairment: Treatment: CrCl 20-50mL/min:** 150mg/day. **CrCl <20mL/min:** 150mg every other day. **Maint: CrCl 20-50mL/min:** 150mg every other day. **CrCl <20mL/min:** 150mg every 3 days. ***Pediatrics:*** **≥12 yrs: Erosive Esophagitis/GERD:** 150mg bid up to 8 weeks. **Max:** 300mg/day.	**W/P:** Caution with renal dysfunction; reduce dose. Symptomatic response does not preclude the presence of gastric malignancy. False positive tests for urobilinogen with Multistix. **P/N:** Category B, not for use in nursing.	Headache, abdominal pain, pain, asthenia, diarrhea, N/V, flatulence, dyspepsia, rhinitis, **pharyngitis,** dizziness, headache.

Table 16.1. PRESCRIBING INFORMATION FOR GASTROINTESTINAL DRUGS *(cont.)*

NAME	FORM/ STRENGTH	DOSAGE	WARNINGS/PRECAUTIONS & CONTRAINDICATIONS	ADVERSE EFFECTS†
ANTIULCER/GERD AGENTS *(cont.)*				
Nizatidine (Axid, Axid Oral Solution) *(cont.)*		**Renal Impairment: Treatment: CrCl 20-50mL/min:** 150mg/day. **CrCl <20mL/min:** 150mg every other day. **Maint: CrCl 20-50mL/min:** 150mg every other day. **CrCl <20mL/min:** 150mg every 3 days		
Omeprazole (Prilosec)	**Cap, Delayed-Release:** 10mg, 20mg, 40mg; **Sus, Delayed-Release:** 2.5mg, 10mg granules/pkt	***Adults:* DU:** 20mg qd for 4-8 weeks. **GU:** 40mg qd for 4-8 weeks. **GERD:** 20mg qd up to 4 weeks without esophageal lesions. **Treatment Erosive Esophagitis with GERD:** 20mg qd for 4-8 weeks. **Maint:** 20mg qd. **Hypersecretory Conditions: Initial:** 60mg qd, then adjust if needed. Divide dose if >80mg/day. Doses up to 120mg tid have been given. ***H.pylori* Triple Therapy:** 20mg + clarithromycin 500mg + amoxicillin 1g, all bid for 10 days. Give additional 18 days of omeprazole 20mg every morning if ulcer present initially. **Dual Therapy:** 40mg qd + clarithromycin 500mg tid for 14 days. Give additional 14 days of omeprazole 20mg every morning if ulcer present initially. Do not crush or chew. Take before eating. Can add contents of caps to applesauce if difficulty swallowing; swallow immediately without chewing. ***Pediatrics:* 1-16 yrs: GERD/Erosive Esophagitis: ≥20kg:** 20mg qd. **10 to <20kg:** 10mg qd. **5 to <10kg:** 5mg qd. Do not crush or chew. Take before eating. Can add contents of caps to applesauce if difficulty swallowing; swallow immediately without chewing.	**W/P:** Atrophic gastritis reported with long-term use. Symptomatic response does not preclude the presence of gastric malignancy. **P/N:** Category C, not for use in nursing.	Headache, diarrhea, abdominal pain, flatulence, N/V.
Omeprazole Magnesium (Prilosec OTC) OTC	**Tab, Delayed-Release:** 20mg	***Adults:*** 20mg qd for 14 days. Take with water in morning before food. May repeat q 4 months.	**Contra:** Trouble or pain swallowing food, vomiting with blood, or bloody or black stools. **P/N:** Safety in pregnancy and nursing not known.	
Omeprazole/ Sodium Bicarbonate (Zegerid)	(Omeprazole-Sodium Bicarbonate) **Cap:** 20mg-1100mg, 40mg-1100mg; **Powder:** 20mg-1680mg/pkt [30^s], 40mg-1680mg/pkt [30^s]	***Adults:* DU:** 20mg qd for 4-8 weeks. **GU:** 40mg qd for 4-8 weeks. **GERD:** 20mg qd up to 4 weeks without esophageal lesions and for 4-8 weeks with erosive esophagitis. **Maintenance of Healing Erosive Esophagitis:** 20mg qd. **Powder (40mg-1680mg): Risk Reduction of Upper GI Bleeding in Critically Ill Patients: Initial:** 40mg, followed by 40mg after 6-8 hrs. **Maint:** 40mg qd for 14 days. Take 1 hr before a meal. Add pkt contents to 2 tablespoons of water; do not use other liquids or foods. Stir powder well and drink immediately. Swallow caps whole with water.	**W/P:** Atrophic gastritis reported with long-term use. Symptomatic response does not preclude the presence of gastric malignancy. Due to sodium bicarbonate content, avoid with metabolic alkalosis, hypocalcemia, and use caution with a sodium-restricted diet, Bartter's syndrome, hypokalemia, respiratory alkalosis. Long-term use of bicarbonate with calcium or milk may cause milk-alkali syndrome. **P/N:** Category C, not for use in nursing.	Abdominal pain, headache, N/V.
Pantoprazole Sodium (Protonix, Protonix IV)	**Inj:** 40mg; **Sus, Delayed-Release:** 40mg (granules/pkt); **Tab, Delayed-Release:** 20mg, 40mg	***Adults:*** (PO) **Erosive Esophagitis Treatment:** 40mg qd for up to 8 weeks. May repeat for 8 weeks if needed. **Maint:** 40mg qd. **Hypersecretory Conditions: Initial:** 40mg bid. Adjust to patient's needs. **Max:** 240mg/day. (Inj) **GERD:** 40mg IV qd for 7-10 days. **Pathological Hypersecretory Conditions:** 80mg IV q12h. May adjust up to 80mg IV q8h	**W/P:** Symptomatic response does not preclude the presence of gastric malignancy. Atrophic gastritis has been noted occasionally in gastric corpus biopsies from patients treated for long-term. False (+) urine screening test for THC reported. Vitamin B_{12} deficiency reported with long-term use (>3 yrs). (Inj) Immediate hypersensitivity	(Inj) Abdominal pain, headache, constipation, dyspepsia, nausea, injection-site reactions. (PO) Headache, flatulence, diarrhea, abdominal pain.

*Scored. †Bold entries denote special dental considerations.
BB = black box warning; **W/P** = warnings/precautions; **Contra** = contraindications; **P/N** = pregnancy category rating and nursing considerations.

NAME	FORM/ STRENGTH	DOSAGE	WARNINGS/PRECAUTIONS & CONTRAINDICATIONS	ADVERSE EFFECTS†
Pantoprazole Sodium (Protonix, Protonix IV) *(cont.)*		based on acid output. **Max:** 240mg/day. Duration >6 days not studied. Do not split, crush, or chew tabs.	reactions reported (eg, thrombophlebitis, LFT elevation). **P/N:** Category B, not for use in nursing.	
Rabeprazole Sodium (Aciphex)	**Tab, Delayed-Release:** 20mg	***Adults:* Erosive/Ulcerative GERD: Healing:** 20mg qd for 4-8 weeks. May repeat for 8 weeks if needed. **Maint:** 20mg qd. **Symptomatic GERD:** 20mg qd for 4 weeks. May repeat for 4 weeks if needed. **DU:** 20mg qd after morning meal for up to 4 weeks. May need additional therapy. ***H.pylori* Triple Therapy:** 20mg + clarithromycin 500mg + amoxicillin 1g, all bid (qam and qpm) with food for 7 days. **Pathological Hypersecretory Conditions: Initial:** 60mg qd. **Titrate:** Adjust according to need. **Maint:** Up to 100mg qd or 60mg bid. May treat up to 1 yr. Swallow tabs whole; do not chew, crush, or split. ***Pediatrics:* ≥12 yrs: Symptomatic GERD:** 20mg qd for up to 8 weeks.	**W/P:** Symptomatic response does not preclude the presence of gastric malignancy. Caution with severe hepatic impairment. **P/N:** Category B, not for use in nursing.	Headache, diarrhea, N/V, abdominal pain, and **taste perversion with triple therapy**.
Ranitidine HCl (Zantac 150, Zantac 75, Zantac OTC) OTC	**Tab:** 75mg, 150mg	***Adults/Pediatrics:* ≥12 yrs: Treatment/ Relief of Heartburn:** 75-150mg with water. **Heartburn Prevention:** 75-150mg 30-60 min before eating food or drinking beverages that cause heartburn. **Max:** 300mg/24 hrs.	**W/P:** Do not use if trouble or pain swallowing food, vomiting with blood, or bloody or black stools; with other acid reducers; or in patients with kidney disease. D/C if heartburn continues/worsens or use for >14 days. **P/N:** Safety in pregnancy and nursing not known.	
Ranitidine HCl (Zantac)	**Inj:** 1mg/mL, 25mg/mL; **Syrup:** 15mg/mL; **Tab:** 150mg, 300mg; **Tab, Effervescent:** 25mg	***Adults:* DU/GU:** PO: **Usual:** 150mg bid or 300mg after evening meal or qhs for DU. **Maint:** 150mg qhs. **GERD:** PO: **Usual:** 150mg bid. **Erosive Esophagitis:** PO: 150mg qid. **Maint:** 150mg bid. **Hypersecretory Conditions:** PO: **Usual:** 150mg bid. May give up to 6g/day with severe disease. IM/IV: **Usual:** 50mg IM/ IV q6-8 hrs or 6.25mg/hr continuous IV. **Max:** 400mg/day. **Zollinger-Ellison:** IV: **Initial:** 1mg/kg/hr. **Titrate:** May increase after 4 hrs by 0.5mg/kg/hr increments. **Max:** 2.5mg/kg/hr or 220mg/ hr. **CrCl <50mL/min:** 50mg IV q18-24 hrs or 150mg PO q24h. Give more frequent (q12h) if necessary. **Hemodialysis:** Give dose at end of treatment. Dissolve each 150mg effervescent tab in 6-8oz of water before administration. ***Pediatrics:* 1 month-16 yrs: DU/GU:** PO: **Usual:** 2-4mg/kg bid. **Max:** 300mg/ day. **Maint:** 2-4mg/kg qd or ≤150mg/ day. **GERD/Erosive Esophagitis:** PO: 2.5-5mg/kg bid. **DU:** IV: 2-4mg/kg/day IV given q6-8 hrs. **Max:** 50mg q6-8 hrs. **CrCl <50mL/min:** 50mg IV q18-24 hrs or 150mg PO q24h. Give more frequent (q12h) if necessary. **Hemodialysis:** Give dose at end of treatment. Dissolve each 25mg effervescent tab in 5mL of water before administration.	**W/P:** Do not exceed recommended infusion rates; bradycardia reported with rapid infusion. Caution with liver and renal dysfunction. Monitor SGPT if on IV therapy for ≥5 days at dose >100mg qid. Avoid use with history of acute porphyria. Symptomatic response does not preclude the presence of gastric malignancy. May cause false (+) urine protein test. Granules and effervescent tablets contain phenylalanine. **P/N:** Category B, caution with nursing.	Headache, constipation, diarrhea, N/V, abdominal discomfort, hepatitis, blood dyscrasias, rash, injection site reactions (IV/IM).
Sucralfate (Carafate)	**Sus:** 1g/10mL [414mL]; **Tab:** 1g*	***Adults:* Active Ulcer:** (Sus/Tab) 1g qid for 4-8 weeks. **Maint:** (Tab) 1g bid. Take on empty stomach.	**W/P:** Caution with chronic renal failure and dialysis. **P/N:** Category B, caution with nursing.	Constipation, diarrhea, N/V, pruritus, rash, dizziness, insomnia, back pain, headache.

Table 16.1. PRESCRIBING INFORMATION FOR GASTROINTESTINAL DRUGS *(cont.)*

NAME	FORM/ STRENGTH	DOSAGE	WARNINGS/PRECAUTIONS & CONTRAINDICATIONS	ADVERSE EFFECTS†
COLORECTAL AGENTS				
Balsalazide Disodium (Colazal)	**Cap:** 750mg	***Adults:*** 3 caps tid for up to 8 weeks (or 12 weeks if needed). May open cap and sprinkle on applesauce. ***Pediatrics:*** **5-17 yrs:** 1 or 3 caps tid for 8 weeks. May open cap and sprinkle on applesauce.	**W/P:** May exacerbate symptoms of colitis. Prolonged gastric retention with pyloric stenosis. Caution with renal dysfunction or history of renal disease. **Contra:** Hypersensitivity to salicylates. **P/N:** Category B, caution in nursing.	Headache, abdominal pain, diarrhea, N/V, respiratory problems, arthralgia, rhinitis, insomnia, fatigue, rectal bleeding, flatulence, fever, dyspepsia.
Budesonide (Entocort EC)	**Cap, Delayed-Release:** 3mg	***Adults:*** **Usual:** 9mg qd, in the am for up to 8 weeks. **Recurring Episodes:** Repeat therapy for 8 weeks. **Maint:** 6mg qd for 3 months, then taper to complete cessation. **Moderate-to-Severe Hepatic Insufficiency/Concomitant CYP3A4 Inhibitors:** Reduce dose. Swallow whole; do not chew or break.	**W/P:** May reduce response of HPA axis to stress. Supplement with systemic glucocorticosteroids if undergoing surgery or other stressful situations. Increased risk of infection; avoid exposure to chickenpox and measles. Caution with TB, HTN, DM, osteoporosis, peptic ulcer, glaucoma, cirrhosis, cataracts, family history of DM or glaucoma. Replacement of systemic glucocorticosteroids may unmask allergies. Chronic use may cause hypercorticism and adrenal suppression. **P/N:** Category C, not for use in nursing.	Headache, respiratory infection, N/V, back pain, dyspepsia, dizziness, abdominal pain, diarrhea, flatulence, sinusitis, viral infection, arthralgia.
Hydrocortisone (Anusol-HC Cream, Proctocream HC, Proctosol HC, Proctozone-HC)	**Cre:** 2.5% [30g]	***Adults/Pediatrics:*** Apply bid-qid. May use occlusive dressings for psoriasis or recalcitrant conditions; d/c dressings if infection develops.	**W/P:** May cause reversible adrenal suppression, manifestations of Cushing's syndrome, hyperglycemia, glucosuria. Caution when applied to large surface areas or under occlusive dressings. Use appropriate therapy with infections. Pediatrics may be more susceptible to systemic toxicity. D/C if irritation occurs. Avoid eyes. **P/N:** Category C, caution in nursing.	Burning, itching, irritation, dryness, folliculitis, hypertrichosis, acneiform eruptions, hypopigmentation, **perioral dermatitis,** allergic contact dermatitis, maceration skin, secondary infection, skin atrophy, striae, miliaria.
Hydrocortisone (Colocort)	**Enema:** 100mg/ 60mL	***Adults:*** 1 enema qhs for 21 days or until remission. After 21 days, decrease to every other night for 2-3 weeks. D/C if no clinical improvement after 2-3 weeks. Difficult cases may require 2-3 months of therapy. Retain for 1 hr minimum, preferably all night.	**W/P:** Rectal wall damage with improper insertion. May mask signs of infection and cause new infections; avoid exposure to chickenpox and measles. Prolonged use may cause adrenocortical insufficiency, cataracts, glaucoma, optic nerve damage, and may enhance secondary ocular infections. May cause elevated BP, salt and water retention, increased potassium and calcium excretion, and reactivation of TB. Caution with perforation, abscess, obstruction, fistulas, sinus tracts, peptic ulcer, diverticulitis, renal impairment, HTN, osteoporosis, ocular herpes simplex, and myasthenia gravis. Enhanced effects in hypothyroidism and cirrhosis. May need increased dose in stressful situation. Do not vaccinate against smallpox or perform other immunization procedure; risk of neurological complications and lack of antibody response. Observe growth in pediatrics. Psychic derangement may appear; caution with emotional instability or psychotic tendencies. **Contra:** Systemic fungal infections, ileocolostomy during the immediate or early postoperative. **P/N:** Safety in pregnancy and nursing is not known.	Local pain/burning/bleeding, fluid retention, HTN, muscle weakness, osteoporosis, peptic ulcer, abdominal distention, impaired wound healing, ecchymosis, facial erythema, sweating, menstrual disorders, Cushingoid state, decreased glucose tolerance.

†Bold entries denote special dental considerations.
BB = black box warning; **W/P** = warnings/precautions; **Contra** = contraindications; **P/N** = pregnancy category rating and nursing considerations.

NAME	FORM/ STRENGTH	DOSAGE	WARNINGS/PRECAUTIONS & CONTRAINDICATIONS	ADVERSE EFFECTS†
Hydrocortisone (Proctocort Cream)	**Cre:** 1% [30g]	***Adults:*** Apply bid-qid. May use occlusive dressings for psoriasis or recalcitrant conditions; d/c dressings if infection develops. ***Pediatrics:*** Use least amount necessary for effective regimen.	**W/P:** May produce reversible HPA axis suppression, manifestations of Cushing's syndrome, hyperglycemia, and glucosuria. Caution when applied to large surface areas or under occlusive dressings. Use appropriate therapy with infections. Pediatrics may be more susceptible to systemic toxicity. D/C if irritation occurs. Avoid eyes. **P/N:** Category C, caution in nursing.	Burning, itching, irritation, dryness, folliculitis, hypertrichosis, acneiform eruptions, hypopigmentation, **perioral dermatitis,** allergic contact dermatitis, maceration skin, secondary infection, skin atrophy, striae, miliaria.
Hydrocortisone Acetate (Anucort HC, Anusol-HC Suppository, Hemorrhoidal HC)	**Sup:** (Anusol-HC) 25mg [12[s], 24[s]]	***Adults:*** **Nonspecific Proctitis:** 1 sup rectally bid for 2 weeks. **More Severe Cases:** 1 sup rectally tid or 2 sup rectally bid. **Factitial Proctitis:** Use up to 6-8 weeks.	**W/P:** D/C if irritation develops. D/C if infection develops that does not respond to appropriate therapy. May stain fabric. Only use after adequate proctologic exam. **P/N:** Category C, not for use in nursing.	Burning, itching, irritation, dryness, folliculitis, hypopigmentation, allergic contact dermatitis, secondary infection.
Hydrocortisone Acetate (Cortifoam)	**Foam:** 10% [15g]	***Adults:*** 1 applicatorful rectally qd-bid for 2-3 weeks, and every 2nd day thereafter. **Maint:** Decrease in small amounts to lowest effective dose. D/C if no improvement within 2-3 weeks.	**W/P:** Absorption may be greater than from other corticosteroid enemas. May elevate BP, cause salt and water retention, IOP, or increase potassium and calcium excretion. Caution with recent MI, hypo- or hyperthyroidism, Strongyloides infestation, TB, CHF, HTN, renal insufficiency, peptic ulcers, diverticulitis, nonspecific ulcerative colitis, cirrhosis, risk of osteoporosis. May produce reversible HPA axis suppression, posterior subcapsular cataracts, glaucoma with possible optic nerve damage. May mask signs of infection or cause new infections. Kaposi's sarcoma reported with chronic use. Avoid with cerebral malaria, systemic fungal infections, active ocular herpes simplex, postoperative ileorectostomy. Rule out latent or active amebiasis. Avoid exposure to chickenpox and/or measles. Observe growth in pediatrics. Withdraw gradually. Acute myopathy observed with high steroid doses. May aggravate existing emotional instability or psychosis. D/C if severe reaction occurs. **Contra:** Obstruction, abscess, perforation, peritonitis, fresh intestinal anastomoses, extensive fistulas, and sinus tracts. **P/N:** Category C, caution in nursing.	Bradycardia, acne, abdominal distention, convulsions, depression, abnormal fat deposits, fluid/electrolyte disturbances, muscle weakness, osteoporosis, peptic ulcer, pancreatitis, impaired wound healing, headache, psychic disturbances, suppression of growth in children, glaucoma, hyperglycemia, weight gain, thromboembolism, malaise, hypersensitivity reactions.
Hydrocortisone Acetate (Proctocort Suppository)	**Sup:** 30mg [12[s], 24[s]]	***Adults:*** **Nonspecific Proctitis:** 1 sup rectally bid for 2 weeks. **More Severe Cases:** 1 sup rectally tid or 2 sup rectally bid. **Factitial Proctitis:** Use up to 6-8 weeks.	**W/P:** D/C if irritation develops. D/C if infection that does not respond to appropriate therapy develops. May stain fabric. Only use after adequate proctologic exam. **P/N:** Category C, not for use in nursing.	Burning, itching, irritation, dryness, folliculitis, hypopigmentation, allergic contact dermatitis, secondary infection.
Hydrocortisone Acetate/ Lidocaine HCl (AnaMantle HC)	**Cre:** (Hydrocortisone-Lidocaine): 0.5%-3% [7g]	***Adults:*** Apply rectally bid.	**W/P:** Caution with impaired liver function, debilitated, elderly. D/C if irritation occurs. Not for prolonged use. May cause adrenal suppression with systemic absorption. **Contra:** Tuberculosis, fungal lesions, skin vaccinia, varicella, acute herpes simplex. **P/N:** Category B, caution in nursing.	Transient stinging or burning, transient blanching, erythema.

Table 16.1. PRESCRIBING INFORMATION FOR GASTROINTESTINAL DRUGS *(cont.)*

NAME	FORM/ STRENGTH	DOSAGE	WARNINGS/PRECAUTIONS & CONTRAINDICATIONS	ADVERSE EFFECTS†
COLORECTAL AGENTS *(cont.)*				
Hydrocortisone Acetate/ Pramoxine HCl (Analpram-HC)	**Cre:** (Hydrocortisone-Pramoxine) 1%-1%, 2.5%-1% [30g]; **Lot:** 2.5%-1% [60mL]	***Adults:*** Apply tid-qid. May use occlusive dressings in psoriasis or recalcitrant conditions. For cleansing anogenital area, spread lotion on cotton or tissue and wipe affected area. ***Pediatrics:*** Use least amount necessary for effective regimen.	**W/P:** May produce reversible HPA axis suppression, manifestations of Cushing's syndrome, hyperglycemia, and glucosuria. D/C use if irritation occurs. Avoid eyes. Peds may be more susceptible to systemic toxicity. Use appropriate therapy with infections. **P/N:** Category C, caution in nursing.	Burning, itching, irritation, dryness, folliculitis, hypertrichosis, acneiform eruptions, hypopigmentation, perioral dermatitis, allergic contact dermatitis, secondary infection, skin maceration, skin atrophy, striae, miliaria.
Hydrocortisone Acetate/ Pramoxine HCl (ProctoFoam-HC)	**Foam:** (Hydrocortisone-Pramoxine) 1%-1% [10g]	***Adults:*** Apply to anal/perianal area tid-qid. ***Pediatrics:*** Use least amount necessary for effective regimen.	**W/P:** D/C if no improvement in 2-3 weeks. May produce reversible HPA axis suppression, manifestations of Cushing's syndrome, hyperglycemia, and glucosuria. Caution when applied to large surface areas or under occlusive dressings. Use appropriate therapy if infections develop; d/c if favorable response does not occur promptly. D/C if irritation develops. Pediatrics may be more susceptible to systemic toxicity. Avoid eyes. **P/N:** Category C, caution in nursing.	Burning, itching, irritation, dryness, folliculitis, hypertrichosis, acneiform eruptions, hypopigmentation, **perioral dermatitis,** allergic contact dermatitis, skin maceration, secondary infection, skin atrophy, striae, miliaria.
Mesalamine (Asacol)	**Tab, Delayed-Release:** 400mg	***Adults:*** **Mild-Moderate Active Ulcerative Colitis: Usual:** 800mg tid for 6 weeks. **Maintenance of Remission:** 1.6g/day in divided doses.	**W/P:** Exacerbation of colitis reported upon initiation of therapy; symptoms abate with discontinuation. Caution with sulfasalazine hypersensitivity. Caution with renal dysfunction or history of renal disease. Monitor renal function prior to therapy and periodically after. Pyloric stenosis could delay mesalamine release in the colon. **Contra:** Hypersensitivity to salicylates. **P/N:** Category B, caution in nursing.	Diarrhea, headache, N/V, **pharyngitis,** abdominal pain, pain, eructation, dizziness, asthenia, fever, dysmenorrhea, arthralgia, dyspepsia.
Mesalamine (Canasa)	**Sup:** 1000mg	***Adults:*** 1000mg rectally qhs. Retain suppository for at least 1-3 hrs.	**W/P:** D/C if acute intolerance syndrome develops (eg, cramping, bloody diarrhea, abdominal pain, headache); consider sulfasalazine hypersensitivity. If rechallenge is considered, perform under careful observation. Caution with sulfasalazine hypersensitivity. Carefully monitor with renal dysfunction. Pancolitis, pericarditis (rare) reported. **Contra:** Hypersensitivity to suppository vehicle (eg, saturated vegetable fatty acid esters) or salicylates. **P/N:** Category B, caution in nursing.	Dizziness, rectal pain, fever, acne, colitis, rash, hair loss.
Mesalamine (Lialda)	**Tab, Delayed-Release:** 1.2g	***Adults:*** 2-4 tabs qd with meals for up to 8 weeks. **Max:** 2.4g or 4.8g per day.	**W/P:** Prolonged gastric retention with pyloric stenosis, delaying mesalamine release in the colon. Caution with sulfasalazine allergy. May cause acute intolerance syndrome; if suspected, prompt withdrawal is required. Caution with cardiac hypersensitivity reactions, myocarditis and pericarditis reported. Renal impairment, including minimal change nephropathy, and acute or chronic interstitial nephritis reported; caution with known renal dysfunction. Monitor renal function prior to therapy and periodically after. **P/N:** Category B, caution in nursing.	Headache, flatulence.

*Scored. †Bold entries denote special dental considerations.
BB = black box warning; **W/P** = warnings/precautions; **Contra** = contraindications; **P/N** = pregnancy category rating and nursing considerations.

NAME	FORM/ STRENGTH	DOSAGE	WARNINGS/PRECAUTIONS & CONTRAINDICATIONS	ADVERSE EFFECTS†
Mesalamine (Pentasa)	**Cap, Extended-Release:** 250mg, 500mg	***Adults:*** 1g qid. Can be given up to 8 weeks.	**W/P:** Caution with hepatic and renal dysfunction; monitor closely. D/C if acute intolerance syndrome develops (eg, cramping, bloody diarrhea, abdominal pain, headache). If rechallenge is considered, perform under careful observation. **Contra:** Hypersensitivity to salicylates. **P/N:** Category B, caution in nursing.	Diarrhea, headache, nausea, abdominal pain.
Mesalamine (Rowasa)	**Enema:** 4g/ 60mL	***Adults:*** Use 1 enema rectally qhs for 3-6 weeks. Retain for 8 hrs. Empty bowel prior to administration.	**W/P:** D/C if acute intolerance syndrome develops (eg, cramping, bloody diarrhea, abdominal pain, headache); consider sulfasalazine hypersensitivity. If rechallenge is considered, perform under careful observation. Caution with sulfasalazine hypersensitivity. Carefully monitor with renal dysfunction. Contains potassium metabisulfite; caution with sulfite sensitivity, especially in asthmatics. Pancolitis, pericarditis (rare) reported. **P/N:** Category B, not for use in nursing.	Abdominal problems, headache, flatulence, flu, fever, nausea, malaise/ fatigue.
Mineral Oil/ Pramoxine HCl/ Zinc Oxide (Tucks Ointment) OTC	**Oint:** (Mineral Oil-Pramoxine-Zinc Oxide) 46.6%-1%-12.5% [30g]	***Adults/Pediatrics:*** **≥12 yrs:** Cleanse area with soap and water, then rinse and dry. Apply externally to the affected area. **Max:** 5 times/day for 7 days. To use dispensing cap, attach it to tube, lubricate well, then gently insert part into anal canal. Squeeze tube to deliver medication.	**W/P:** Allergic reactions may develop. D/C if redness, irritation, swelling, pain, other symptoms develop or increase, or if condition worsens within 7 days. Do not administer into rectum by using fingers or any mechanical device or applicator. **P/N:** Safety in pregnancy and nursing not known.	—
Olsalazine Sodium (Dipentum)	**Cap:** 250mg	***Adults:*** 500mg bid with food.	**W/P:** May exacerbate colitis symptoms. Diarrhea may be dose related, or an underlying symptom of the disease. Caution with renal dysfunction; monitor urinalysis, BUN, creatinine levels. Monitor patients with severe allergies or asthma and impaired hepatic function. **Contra:** Salicylate hypersensitivity. **P/N:** Category C, caution with nursing.	Diarrhea, abdominal pain, nausea, dyspepsia, headache, rash/itching, arthralgia.
Starch (Tucks Suppositories) OTC	**Sup:** 51% [12[s], 24[s]]	***Adults/Pediatrics:*** **≥12 yrs:** Cleanse area with soap and water, then rinse and dry. Insert 1 sup rectally. **Max:** 6 times/day for 7 days.	**W/P:** D/C if rectal bleeding occurs or if condition worsens or does not improve within 7 days. **P/N:** Safety in pregnancy and nursing not known.	—
Sulfasalazine (Azulfidine EN)	**Tab, Delayed-Release:** 500mg	***Adults:*** **Ulcerative Colitis: Initial:** 1-4g/day in divided doses at intervals not exceeding 8 hrs. **Maint:** 2g/day. **Rheumatoid Arthritis: Initial:** 0.5-1g/day. **Maint:** 2g/day given bid. Swallow tabs whole after meals. ***Pediatrics:*** **≥6 yrs: Ulcerative Colitis: Initial:** 40-60mg/kg/24 hrs in 3-6 divided doses. **Maint:** 7.5mg/kg qid. **Juvenile Rheumatoid Arthritis:** 30-50mg/kg/day given bid. To reduce GI effects give 1/4 to 1/3 initial dose; increase weekly for 1 month. **Max:** 2g/day. Swallow tabs whole after meals.	**W/P:** Caution with hepatic or renal impairment, blood dyscrasias, severe allergy, bronchial asthma or G6PD deficiency. Monitor CBC, WBC, and LFTs prior to therapy and every other week for the first 3 months, once monthly for next 3 months, then every 3 months. Monitor renal function periodically. Maintain adequate fluid intake. Fatal hypersensitivity reactions reported. D/C if tabs pass undisintegrated or if hypersensitivity reactions occur. **Contra:** Intestinal or urinary obstruction, porphyria, hypersensitivity to sulfonamides or salicylates. **P/N:** Category B, caution in nursing.	Anorexia, headache, N/V, gastric distress, oligospermia, rash, pruritus, urticaria, fever, orange-yellow urine or skin.
Sulfasalazine (Azulfidine)	**Tab:** 500mg*	***Adults:*** **Initial:** 3-4g/day in divided doses. May initiate at 1-2g/day to reduce GI intolerance. **Maint:** 2g/day. ***Pediatrics:*** **≥2 yrs:** 40-60mg/kg/day divided into 3-6 doses. **Maint:** 7.5mg/kg qid.	**W/P:** Caution with hepatic/renal impairment, blood dyscrasias, severe allergy, bronchial asthma, G6PD deficiency. Monitor CBC, WBC, LFTs, at baseline, every 2nd week for first 3 months, monthly for next 3 months, and every 3 months thereafter. Monitor renal function periodically. Maintain adequate	Anorexia, headache, N/V, gastric distress, reversible oligospermia.

Table 16.1. PRESCRIBING INFORMATION FOR GASTROINTESTINAL DRUGS *(cont.)*

NAME	FORM/ STRENGTH	DOSAGE	WARNINGS/PRECAUTIONS & CONTRAINDICATIONS	ADVERSE EFFECTS†
COLORECTAL AGENTS *(cont.)*				
Sulfasalazine (Azulfidine) *(cont.)*			fluid intake to prevent crystalluria and stone formation. D/C if hypersensitivity or toxic reaction occurs. **Contra:** <2 yrs, intestinal or urinary obstruction, porphyria, hypersensitivity to sulfonamides, salicylates. **P/N:** Category B, caution in nursing.	
DIGESTIVE ENZYMES/BILE ACIDS				
Amylase/Lipase/ Protease (Creon)	**Cap, Delayed-Release:** (Amylase-Lipase-Protease) **(Creon 5)** 30,000 U-6,000 U-19,000 U, **(Creon 10)** 60,000 U-12,000 U-38,000 U, **(Creon 20)** 120,000 U-24,000 U-76,000 U	***Adults/Pediatrics:* >4 yrs:** Individualize dose. **Initial:** 500 U lipase/kg/meal. **Titrate:** May increase dose based on clinical symptoms, degree of steatorrhea present, and fat content of diet. **Max:** 2500 U lipase/kg/meal. Swallow whole; do not crush or chew. ***Pediatrics:*** Individualize dose. **12 mos-4 yrs: Initial:** 1000 U lipase/kg/meal. **Titrate:** May increase dose based on clinical symptoms, degree of steatorrhea present, and fat content of diet. **Max:** 2500 U lipase/kg/meal. **Infants-12 mos:** 2000-4000 U lipase/120 mL of formula or breast milk.	**W/P:** Fibrosing colonopathy reported; monitor closely. Increased risk of progressing to stricture formation. Caution in doses >2500 U lipase/kg/meal. Caution with gout, renal impairment, or hyperuricemia. May increase serum uric acid levels. Risk for transmission of viral disease, including diseases caused by novel or unidentified viruses reported. Caution with a known allergy to porcine protein. Do not interchange with any other pancrealipase products. Not recommended to mix with milk formula or breast milk. **P/N:** Category C, safety not known in nursing.	Abnormal feces, flatulence, abdominal pain, weight loss, diarrhea, constipation, nausea, skin disorders (eg, pruritus, urticaria, and rash) headache, dizziness, cough.
Amylase/Lipase/ Protease (Viokase)	(Amylase-Lipase-Protease) **Powder:** 70,000 U-16,800 U-70,000 U/0.7g [240g]; **Tab: (Viokase 8)** 30,000 U-8,000 U-30,000 U; **(Viokase 16)** 60,000 U-16,000 U-60,000 U	***Adults:*** (Powder) **CF:** 0.7g (1/4 tsp) with meals. (Tab) **CF/Pancreatitis:** 8,000-32,000 U Lipase with meals. **Pancreatectomy/Pancreatic Duct Obstruction:** 8,000-16,000 U Lipase q2h. ***Pediatrics:*** (Powder) **CF:** 0.7g (1/4 tsp) with meals. (Tab) **CF/ Pancreatitis:** 8,000-32,000 U Lipase with meals. **Pancreatectomy/Pancreatic Duct Obstruction:** 8,000-16,000 U Lipase q2h.	**W/P:** May have allergic reactions if previously sensitized to trypsin, pancreatin, or pancrelipase. Irritating to oral mucosa if held in mouth. Inhalation of powder can cause an asthma attack. High doses can cause hyperuricemia and hyperuricosuria. **Contra:** Pork protein hypersensitivity. **P/N:** Category C, caution in nursing.	Irritation to nasal mucosa and respiratory tract with inhaled powder.
Ursodiol (Actigall)	**Cap:** 300mg	***Adults:* Gall Stones: Treatment:** 8-10mg/kg/day given bid-tid. Obtain ultrasound at 6 month intervals for 1 yr. Continue therapy after stones have dissolved and confirm with repeat ultrasound within 1-3 months. **Prevention:** 300mg bid.	**W/P:** Therapy is not associated with liver damage. Monitor LFTs at the initiation of therapy and periodically thereafter. Caution in elderly. **Contra:** Calcified cholesterol stones, radiopaque stones, radiolucent bile pigment stones, unremitting acute cholecystitis, cholangitis, biliary obstruction, gallstone pancreatitis, biliary-gastrointestinal fistula, bile-acid hypersensitivity. **P/N:** Category B, caution in nursing.	Abdominal pain, constipation, diarrhea, dyspepsia, flatulence, N/V, arthralgia, coughing, viral infection, bronchitis, **pharyngitis,** back pain, myalgia, headache, sinusitis, upper respiratory tract infection.
Ursodiol (Urso 250, Urso Forte)	**Tab: (Urso 250)** 250mg, **(Urso Forte)** 500mg*	***Adults:* Primary Biliary Cirrhosis: Usual:** 13-15mg/kg/day given bid-qid with food.	**W/P:** Administer appropriate specific treatment with variceal bleeding, hepatic encephalopathy, ascites, or when in need of urgent liver transplant. **P/N:** Category B, caution in nursing.	Diarrhea, leukopenia, peptic ulcer, hyperglycemia, skin rash, increased creatinine.
LAXATIVES/EVACUANTS				
Ascorbic Acid/Polyethylene Glycol 3350/Potassium Chloride/Sodium Ascorbate/Sodium Chloride/Sodium Sulfate (MoviPrep)	**Pow:** (PEG 3350-Sodium Sulfate-Sodium Chloride-Potassium Chloride-Ascorbic Acid-Sodium Ascorbate) 100g-7.5g-2.69g-1.015g-4.7g-5.9g	***Adults:* ≥18 yrs: Split-Dose Regimen:** 8oz every 15 min (first liter) followed by 0.5 liters of clear liquid the evening prior, then another liter over 1 hr followed by 0.5 liters of clear liquid in the morning at least 1 hr prior to colonoscopy. **Evening-Only Regimen:** Around 6 pm take 8oz every 15 min (first liter), then 1.5 hrs later take second liter over 1 hour, additionally take 1 liter of clear liquid.	**W/P:** Rare reports of generalized tonic-clonic seizures with use of PEG colon preparations. Caution with concomitant medications that increase risk of electrolyte abnormalities (eg, diuretics, ACEIs) or in patients with hyponatremia; consider baseline and postcolonoscopy lab tests (eg, sodium, potassium, calcium, creatinine, BUN). **P/N:** Category C, caution in nursing.	Abdominal distension, anal discomfort, thirst, N/V, abdominal pain, sleep disorder, rigors, hunger, malaise, dizziness.

*Scored. †Bold entries denote special dental considerations.
BB = black box warning; **W/P** = warnings/precautions; **Contra** = contraindications; **P/N** = pregnancy category rating and nursing considerations.

NAME	FORM/ STRENGTH	DOSAGE	WARNINGS/PRECAUTIONS & CONTRAINDICATIONS	ADVERSE EFFECTS†
Bisacodyl (Dulcolax) OTC	**Sup:** 10mg; **Tab, Delayed-Release:** 5mg	***Adults/Pediatrics:*** **≥12 yrs:** (Tab) Take 1-3 tabs qd. (Sup) Insert 1 sup rectally; retain for 15-20 min. **6-12 yrs:** (Tab) 1 tab qd. Do not crush/chew. (Sup) Insert 1/2 sup rectally qd. May coat tip with petroleum jelly with anal fissures or hemorrhoids. **≥6 yrs: X-Ray Endoscopy For Barium Enema:** Avoid food after tab administration. Insert 1 sup rectally 1-2 hrs before exam. **<6 yrs: X-Ray Endoscopy For Barium Enema:** Avoid tab. Insert 1/2 sup rectally 1-2 hrs before exam.	**W/P:** Avoid with abdominal pain, nausea, or vomiting. Not for long-term use (>7 days). D/C with rectal bleeding or fail to have bowel movement. **Contra:** Acute abdominal surgery, appendicitis, rectal bleeding, gastroenteritis, intestinal obstruction. **P/N:** Safety in pregnancy and nursing not known.	Abdominal discomfort.
Bisacodyl (Fleet Bisacodyl) OTC	**Enema:** 10mg; **Sup:** 10mg; **Tab, Delayed-Release:** 5mg	***Adults/Pediatrics:*** **≥12yrs:** (Enema) Use 1 rectally single dose qd. (Sup) Insert 1 rectally qd. (Tab) 2-3 tabs single dose qd. **6-11 yrs:** (Sup) Insert 1/2 sup rectally qd. Retain for 15-20 min. (Tab) 1 tab qd. Swallow tabs whole; do not chew or crush.	**W/P:** Do not use with nausea, vomiting, or abdominal pain. Rectal bleeding or failure to have a bowel movement after use may indicate a serious condition. Should not be used longer than 1 week. **P/N:** Safety in pregnancy and nursing is not known.	Abdominal discomfort, faintness, cramps.
Bisacodyl/ Polyethylene Glycol 3350/ Potassium Chloride/Sodium Bicarbonate/ Sodium Chloride (HalfLytely)	**Kit: Tab, Delayed-Release:** (Bisacodyl) 5mg [4[s]]. **Sol:** (Polyethylene Glycol 3350-Potassium Chloride-Sodium Bicarbonate-Sodium Chloride) 210g-0.74g-2.86g-5.60g [2000mL]	***Adults:*** Consume only clear liquids on day of preparation. Swallow all 4 bisacodyl tabs at noon (do not chew or crush). After first bowel movement (or max of 6 hrs) begin drinking sol, 240mL every 10 min (approx. 8 glasses). Drink all sol.	**W/P:** Do not add additional ingredients (eg, flavorings). Caution with severe ulcerative colitis, ileus or gastric retention. Monitor with impaired gag reflex, prone to regurgitation or aspiration. Slow administration or temporarily d/c if severe bloating, distention, or abdominal pain develops. Avoid large quantities of water during or after preparation or colonoscopy. Monitor closely with impaired water handling. Generalized tonic-clonic seizures, hives, and skin rashes reported. **Contra:** Ileus, GI obstruction, gastric retention, bowel perforation, toxic colitis, toxic megacolon. **P/N:** Category C, caution in nursing.	N/V, abdominal fullness, cramping, overall discomfort.
Docusate Sodium (Colace) OTC	**Cap:** 50mg, 100mg; **Liq:** 10mg/mL; **Syrup:** 20mg/ 5mL	***Adults/Pediatrics:*** **≥12 yrs:** 50-200mg/ day. **(Retention or Flushing Enema)** Add 5-10mL of liquid to enema fluid. Mix Liq/Syr into 6-8 oz of milk or juice. **6-12 yrs:** 40-120mg/day Liq. **3-6 yrs:** 2mL Liq tid. Mix Liq/Syr into 6-8 oz of milk, juice, or formula. **(Retention/ Flushing Enema)** Add 5-10mL of liquid to enema fluid.	**W/P:** Avoid with abdominal pain, nausea, or vomiting. D/C enema if rectal bleeding occurs or fail to have a bowel movement. **P/N:** Safety in pregnancy and nursing not known.	**Bitter taste, throat irritation,** nausea, rash.
Docusate Sodium/ Senna (Peri-Colace) OTC	(Docusate Sodium-Sennosides) **Tab:** 50mg-8.6mg	***Adults/Pediatrics:*** **≥12yrs:** 2-4 tabs daily. **6 to <12yrs:** 1-2 tabs daily. **2 to <6yrs:** Max of 1 tab daily.	**W/P:** Caution with use >1 week. **P/N:** Safety in pregnancy and nursing not known.	—
Glycerin (Fleet Glycerin Laxatives) OTC	**Enema:** (Pedia-Lax) 1g, (Glycerin) 2g, (Liquid Glycerin) 5.6g	***Adults/Pediatrics:*** **≥6 yrs:** 1 glycerin suppository (2g) or 1 liquid glycerin suppository (5.6g) rectally. **2-5 yrs:** (Pedia-Lax) 1 suppository (1g) rectally.	**W/P:** Rectal irritation may occur. Do not use with nausea, vomiting, or abdominal pain. Rectal bleeding or failure to have a bowel movement after use may indicate a serious condition. Do not use longer than 1 week. **P/N:** Safety in pregnancy and nursing is not known.	Rectal discomfort, burning sensation.
Lactulose (Constulose, Enulose, Generlac)	**Sol:** 10g/15mL	***Adults:*** **Constipation:** 15-30mL qd. Max 60mL/day. May mix with fruit juice, water, or milk. **Portal-Systemic Encephalopathy:** 30-45mL tid-qid. Adjust dose every 1 or 2 days to produce 2-3 soft stools daily. **Rectal Use: Reversal of Coma:** Mix 300mL with 700mL of water or saline and retain for 30-60 min. May repeat q4-6h. Oral doses should be started before completely stopping	**W/P:** Caution in DM due to galactose and lactose content. Monitor electrolytes periodically in elderly or debilitated if used >6 months. Potential for explosive reaction with electrocautery procedures during proctoscopy or colonoscopy. **Contra:** Patients who require a low galactose diet. **P/N:** Category B, caution in nursing.	Flatulence, intestinal cramps, diarrhea, N/V.

Table 16.1. PRESCRIBING INFORMATION FOR GASTROINTESTINAL DRUGS *(cont.)*

NAME	FORM/ STRENGTH	DOSAGE	WARNINGS/PRECAUTIONS & CONTRAINDICATIONS	ADVERSE EFFECTS†
LAXATIVES/EVACUANTS *(cont.)*				
Lactulose (Constulose, Enulose, Generlac) *(cont.)*		enema. ***Pediatrics:* Portal-Systemic Encephalopathy: Older Children/Adolescents:** 40-90mL/day divided tid-qid adjusted to produce 2-3 soft stools daily. **Infants:** 2.5-10mL in divided doses to produce 2-3 soft stools daily.		
Lactulose (Kristalose)	**Powder (crystals for suspension):** 10g/pkt, 20g/pkt [1[s], 30[s]]	***Adults:*** 10-20g/day. **Max:** 40g/day. Dissolve pkt contents in 4oz of water.	**W/P:** Caution in DM due to galactose and lactose content. Monitor electrolytes periodically in elderly or debilitated if used for >6 months. Potential for explosive reaction with electrocautery procedures during proctoscopy or colonoscopy. **Contra:** Patients who require a low galactose diet. **P/N:** Category B, caution in nursing.	Flatulence, intestinal cramps, diarrhea, N/V.
Methylnaltrexone Bromide (Relistor)	**Inj:** 12mg/0.6mL	***Adults:*** Inject SQ in upper arm, abdomen, or thigh. **Usual:** One dose every other day prn. **Max:** One dose/24 hrs. **38 to <62kg (84 to <136lbs):** 8mg. **62-114kg (136-251lbs):** 12mg. **Patients Outside These Ranges:** 0.15mg/kg. To calculate inj volume for these patients, multiply wt in lbs by 0.0034 or wt in kg by 0.0075 and round up volume to nearest 0.1mL. **CrCl <30mL/min:** Reduce dose by one-half.	**W/P:** D/C therapy and consult physician if severe or persistent diarrhea occurs during treatment. Use has not been studied in patients with peritoneal catheters. **Contra:** Known or suspected mechanical GI obstruction. **P/N:** Category B, caution in nursing.	Abdominal pain, flatulence, nausea, dizziness, diarrhea.
Polyethylene Glycol 3350 (MiraLax) OTC	**Powder:** 17g/ dose [119g, 238g]	***Adults/Pediatrics:* ≥17 yrs:** Stir and dissolve 17g in 4-8 oz of beverage and drink qd. Use no more than 7 days.	**W/P:** Avoid in kidney disease.	—
Polyethylene Glycol 3350/ Potassium Chloride/Sodium Bicarbonate/ Sodium Chloride (NuLYTELY, Trilyte)	**Sol:** (Polyethylene Glycol-Potassium Chloride-Sodium Bicarbonate-Sodium Chloride) 420g-1.48g-5.72g-11.2g [4000mL]	***Adults:* PO:** 240mL every 10 min until fecal discharge is clear or 4L is consumed. **NG Tube:** 20-30mL/min (1.2-1.8L/hr). Patient should fast at least 3-4 hours before administration. ***Pediatrics:* ≥6 months: PO/NG Tube:** 25mL/kg/hr until fecal discharge is clear. Patient should fast at least 3-4 hours before administration.	**W/P:** Do not add additional ingredients (eg, flavorings). Caution with severe ulcerative colitis. Monitor therapy with impaired gag reflex, unconsciousness/ semiconsciousness, and patients prone to regurgitation and aspiration. Temporarily d/c if develop severe bloating, distention, or abdominal pain. Monitor for hypoglycemia in pediatrics <2 yrs of age. **Contra:** GI obstruction, gastric retention, bowel perforation, toxic colitis, toxic megacolon, ileus. **P/N:** Category C, caution in nursing.	N/V, abdominal fullness/cramps, bloating, anal irritation.
Polyethylene Glycol 3350/ Potassium Chloride/Sodium Bicarbonate/ Sodium Chloride/ Sodium Sulfate (Colyte, Colyte w/ Flavor Packs, Colyte-Flavored)	**Sol:** (Polyethylene Glycol-Potassium Chloride-Sodium Bicarbonate-Sodium Chloride-Sodium Sulfate) 60g-0.745g-1.68g-1.46g-5.68g/L [3754mL, 4000mL]	***Adults:* PO:** 240mL every 10 min until fecal discharge is clear. **NG Tube:** 20-30mL/min (1.2-1.8L/hr). Patient should fast at least 3 hrs before administration, except for clear liquids.	**W/P:** Caution with severe ulcerative colitis. Monitor therapy with impaired gag reflex, semi- or unconsciousness, and risk of regurgitation or aspiration especially with NG tube. **Contra:** Ileus, gastric retention, GI obstruction, bowel perforation, toxic colitis, toxic megacolon. **P/N:** Category C, safety in nursing is unkown.	N/V, abdominal fullness/cramps, bloating, anal irritation.
Polyethylene Glycol 3350/ Potassium Chloride/Sodium Bicarbonate/ Sodium Chloride/ Sodium Sulfate (GoLYTELY)	**Sol:** (Polyethylene Glycol-Potassium Chloride-Sodium Bicarbonate-Sodium Chloride-Sodium Sulfate) 236g-	***Adults:* PO:** 240mL every 10 min until fecal discharge is clear or 4L is consumed. **NG Tube:** 20-30mL/min (1.2-1.8L/hr). Patient should fast at least 3-4 hrs before administration.	**W/P:** Do not add additional ingredients (eg, flavorings). Caution with severe ulcerative colitis. Monitor therapy with impaired gag reflex, unconsciousness/ semiconsciousness, and patients prone to regurgitation or aspiration. Slow administration or temporarily d/c if severe bloating, distention, or abdominal	N/V, abdominal fullness, cramping, bloating, anal irritation.

*Scored. †Bold entries denote special dental considerations.
BB = black box warning; **W/P** = warnings/precautions; **Contra** = contraindications; **P/N** = pregnancy category rating and nursing considerations.

NAME	FORM/ STRENGTH	DOSAGE	WARNINGS/PRECAUTIONS & CONTRAINDICATIONS	ADVERSE EFFECTS†
Polyethylene Glycol 3350/ Potassium Chloride/Sodium Bicarbonate/ Sodium Chloride/ Sodium Sulfate (GoLYTELY) *(cont.)*	2.97g-6.74g-5.86g-22.74g [4000mL]		pain develops. **Contra:** GI obstruction, gastric retention, bowel perforation, toxic colitis, toxic megacolon, ileus. **P/N:** Category C, caution in nursing.	
Senna (Senokot) OTC	**Tab:** (Sennoside A and B) (Senokot) 8.6mg, (SenokotXTRA) 17.2mg; (Docusate Sodium-Sennoside A and B) (Senokot-S) 50mg-8.6mg	***Adults/Pediatrics:* ≥12 yrs:** Take hs. **(Senokot/Senokot-S)** 2 tabs qd. **Max:** 4 tabs bid. **(SenokotXTRA)** 1 tab qd. **Max:** 2 tabs bid. ***Pediatrics:* 6-12 yrs:** Take hs. **(Senokot/Senokot-S)** 1 tab qd. **Max:** 2 tabs bid. **(SenokotXTRA)** 1/2 tab qd. **Max:** 1 tab bid. **2-6 yrs:** Take hs. **(Senokot/Senokot-S)** 1/2 tab qd. **Max:** 1 tab bid.	**W/P:** Do not use with abdominal pain, nausea, or vomiting. Should not be used for longer than 1 week. Rectal bleeding or failure to have a bowel movement after use may indicate serious condition. **P/N:** Safety in pregnancy and nursing not known.	—
Sodium Phosphate (Visicol)	**Tab:** (Sodium Phosphate Monobasic Monohydrate-Sodium Phosphate Dibasic Anhydrous) 1.102g-0.398g*	***Adults:* ≥18 yrs:** Drink only clear liquids 12 hrs before dose. **Evening Before Exam:** 3 tabs with 8 oz clear liquids every 15 min for total of 20 tabs (last dose is 2 tabs). Repeat on day of exam 3-5 hrs before procedure. May retreat after 7 days.	**W/P:** Fatalities reported from electrolyte imbalances and arrhythmias if administered with other sodium phosphate-containing products. May induce QT prolongation, colonic mucosal aphthous ulcerations, and exacerbate IBS. Caution with severe renal insufficiency (creatinine clearance less than 30 mL/minute), CHF, ascites, unstable angina, acute bowel obstruction, bowel perforation, toxic megacolon, gastric retention, ileus, pseudo-obstruction of the bowel, severe chronic constipation, acute colitis, gastric bypass, stapling surgery, or hypomotility syndrome. Correct electrolyte disturbance before use. Caution within 3 months of acute MI or cardiac surgery. Do not use additional enema or laxative. Reports of generalized tonic-clonic seizures and/or loss of consciousness in patients with no prior history of seizures. **Contra:** Patients with biopsy-proven acute phosphate nephropathy. **P/N:** Category C, safety in nursing not known.	N/V, abdominal bloating, dizziness, headache, abdominal pain.
MISCELLANEOUS GASTROINTESTINAL AGENTS				
Adalimumab (Humira)	**Inj:** 20mg/ 0.4mL, 40mg/ 0.8mL	***Adults:* AS/PA/RA:** 40mg SQ every other week. Some patients with RA not taking concomitant MTX may derive additional benefit from increasing the dosing frequency to 40mg every week. **Crohn's Disease: Initial:** 160mg (may be given as 4 injections on Day 1, or 2 injections/day for 2 consecutive days); then 80mg after 2 weeks (Day 15). **Maint:** 40mg every other week beginning at Week 4 (Day 29). **Plaque Psoriasis: Initial:** 80mg. **Maint:** 40mg every other week starting 1 week after initial dose. ***Pediatrics:* JA: 4-17 yrs: 15kg-<30kg:** 20mg every other week. **≥30kg:** 40mg every other week.	**BB:** Reports of TB, invasive fungal infections, and other opportunistic infections. Evaluate for latent TB and treat if necessary prior to initiation of therapy. **W/P:** Caution with serious infections, including sepsis, TB, and opportunistic infections. D/C if serious infection develops. Avoid with active infection. Monitor HBV carriers as reactivation may occur; if reactivation occurs, d/c and start antiviral therapy. Caution with pre-existing or recent-onset CNS demyelinating disorders. May affect host defenses against infections and malignancies. Lymphomas and allergic reactions observed. May result in autoantibody formation; d/c if lupus-like syndrome develops. Rare possibility of anaphylaxis and pancytopenia including aplastic anemia. May cause CHF or worsen pre-existing disease. **P/N:** Category B, not for use in nursing.	URI, injection site pain/reactions, headache, rash, sinusitis, nausea, UTI, flu syndrome, abdominal pain, hyperlipidemia, hypercholesterolemia, back pain, hematuria, HTN, immunogenicity.

Table 16.1. PRESCRIBING INFORMATION FOR GASTROINTESTINAL DRUGS *(cont.)*

NAME	FORM/ STRENGTH	DOSAGE	WARNINGS/PRECAUTIONS & CONTRAINDICATIONS	ADVERSE EFFECTS†
MISCELLANEOUS GASTROINTESTINAL AGENTS *(cont.)*				
Alvimopan (Entereg)	**Cap:** 12mg	***Adults:* ≥18 yrs:** 12mg given 30 min to 5 hrs prior to surgery followed by 12mg bid beginning day after surgery for maximum of 7 days or until discharge. **Max:** 15 doses.	**BB:** Available only for short-term (15 doses) use in hospitalized patients. Only hospitals that have registered and met requirements for the Entereg Access Support and Education (E.A.S.E.) program may use drug. **W/P:** Caution in patients receiving >3 doses of opioid within week prior to surgery and in post-operative ileus. Avoid using in severe hepatic impairment, end-stage renal disease (ESRD), surgery for correction of complete bowel obstruction. MI reported in patients treated with opioids for chronic pain. **Contra:** Therapeutic doses of opioids for >7 consecutive days immediately prior to therapy. **P/N:** Category B, caution in nursing.	Anemia, constipation, dyspepsia, flatulence, hypokalemia, back pain, urinary retention.
Certolizumab pegol (Cimzia)	**Inj:** 200mg	***Adults:* Initial:** 400mg SQ, and at Weeks 2 and 4. **Maint:** 400mg SQ every 4 weeks.	**BB:** Tuberculosis (TB), invasive fungal infections, and other opportunistic infections have occured. Evaluate for latent TB and treat if necessary prior to therapy. Monitor all patients for active TB during treatment, even if initial tuberculin skin test is negative. **W/P:** Serious infections, sepsis, and cases of opportunistic infections, including fatalities reported. Caution with history of recurrent infection, concomitant immunosuppressive therapy, or underlying conditions that may predispose to infections. May increase risk of reactivation of hepatitis B virus; monitor HBV carriers during and several months after therapy. Lymphoma and other malignancies have occurred with TNF-blockers. Anaphylaxis or serious allergic reactions may occur. Caution with pre-existing or recent onset CNS demyelinating disorders. Rare cases of pancytopenia, including aplastic anemia, reported; d/c if significant hematologic abnormalities occur. Caution with heart failure; monitor closely. May cause autoimmune antibodies; d/c if lupus-like syndrome develops. **P/N:** Category B, not for use in nursing.	Upper respiratory tract infection, UTI, arthralgia.
Infliximab (Remicade)	**Inj:** 100mg	***Adults:* RA (Combo with MTX):** 3mg/kg as IV infusion; repeat at 2 and 6 weeks. **Maint:** 3mg/kg every 8 weeks. **Incomplete Response:** May increase to 10mg/kg or give every 4 weeks. **CD/ Fistulizing CD: Induction Regimen:** 5mg/kg IV at 0, 2, and 6 weeks. **Maint:** 5mg/kg every 8 weeks. For patients who respond then lose their response, may increase to 10mg/kg. May d/c if no response by Week 14. **AS:** 5mg/kg as IV infusion; repeat at 2 and 6 weeks. **Maint:** 5mg/kg every 6 weeks. **PA:** 5mg/kg as IV infusion; repeat at 2 and 6 weeks. **Maint:** 5mg/kg every 8 weeks. May be used with or without MTX. **UC:** 5mg/kg at 0, 2, and 6 weeks. **Maint:** 5mg/kg every 8 weeks. **Plaque**	**BB:** Increased risk for developing serious infections may lead to hospitalization or death. Concomitant use of immunosuppresants (eg, methotrexate or corticosteroids) may develop these infections. Reports of TB, invasive fungal infections, and other opportunistic infections. Evaluate for latent TB and treat if necessary prior to initiation of therapy. Hepatosplenic T-cell lymphoma reported. **W/P:** Leukopenia, neutropenia, thrombocytopenia, and pancytopenia reported. Serious infections, including sepsis and pneumonia, reported. Avoid with active infection. D/C if serious infection develops. Hypersensitivity reactions reported. Caution with optic neuritis, chronic and recurrent	Nausea, infections, infusion reactions, headache, sinusitis, **pharyngitis, coughing,** abdominal pain, diarrhea, bronchitis, dyspepsia, fatigue, **laryngeal/pharyngeal edema,** severe brochospasm, seizure.

†Bold entries denote special dental considerations.
BB = black box warning; **W/P** = warnings/precautions; **Contra** = contraindications; **P/N** = pregnancy category rating and nursing considerations.

NAME	FORM/ STRENGTH	DOSAGE	WARNINGS/PRECAUTIONS & CONTRAINDICATIONS	ADVERSE EFFECTS†
Infliximab (Remicade) *(cont.)*		**Psoriasis:** 5mg/kg IV infusion; repeat at 2 and 6 weeks. **Maint:** 5mg/kg every 8 weeks. ***Pediatrics:* ≥6 yrs: CD: Induction Regimen:** 5mg/kg IV at 0, 2, and 6 weeks. **Maint:** 5mg/kg every 8 weeks.	infections, CNS demyelinating disease (eg, MS), and seizure disorder. May result in autoantibody formation; d/c if lupus-like syndrome develops. Monitor closely and d/c if new or worsening symptoms of heart failure appear. Lymphoma reported; caution with malignancies. Severe hepatic reactions, including acute liver failure, jaundice, hepatitis, and cholestasis reported rarely. Caution in elderly. Hepatosplenic T-cell lymphoma (rare) may occur in adolescent and young adult male patients with Crohn's disease or ulcerative colitis. Pediatric Crohn's patients should be brought up to date with all vaccinations prior to therapy with infliximab. **Contra:** Hypersensitivity to murine proteins. Moderate or severe CHF (NYHA Class III/IV) with doses >5mg/kg. **P/N:** Category B, not for use in nursing.	
Lubiprostone (Amitiza)	**Cap:** 8mcg, 24mcg	***Adults:* Chronic Idiopathic Constipation:** 24mcg bid with food. **IBS-C:** 8mcg bid with food.	**W/P:** Potential to cause fetal loss; women who could become pregnant should have a negative pregnancy test prior to initiation of therapy and comply with effective contraceptive measures. May cause nausea. Do not prescribe to patients with severe diarrhea. Dyspnea reported. Confirm absence of mechanical GI obstruction prior to initiating therapy. **Contra:** History of mechanical gastrointestinal obstruction. **P/N:** Category C, not for use in nursing.	N/V, diarrhea, abdominal distention/pain/discomfort, flatulence, loose stools, sinusitis, urinary/upper respiratory tract infections, headache, dizziness, peripheral edema, arthralgia.
Natalizumab (Tysabri)	**Inj:** 300mg/15mL	***Adults:* MS/CD:** 300mg IV infusion over 1 hr every 4 weeks. **CD:** D/C therapy if no therapeutic benefit by 12 weeks, if patient cannot be tapered off corticosteroids within 6 months, or in patients who require additional steroid use that exceeds 3 months within a calendar year to control their CD.	**BB:** Increases risk of progressive multifocal leukoencephalopathy (PML). Because of risk of PML, natalizumab is available only through a special restricted distribution program called the TOUCH™ Prescribing Program. Administer only to patients who are enrolled in and meet all conditions of the TOUCH™ Prescribing Program. Monitor patients for any new signs or symptoms that may be suggestive of PML. Dosing should be withheld immediately at the first sign or symptom suggestive of PML. **W/P:** Possible hypersensitivity reactions, including anaphylaxis. Concurrent use with antineoplastic, immunosuppressive, or immunomodulating agents may further increase the risk of infections. Liver injury reported. Induces increase in circulating lymphocytes, monocytes, eosinophils, basophils, and nucleated RBCs. **Contra:** Progressive multifocal leukoencephalopathy (PML). **P/N:** Category C, caution in nursing.	Headache, fatigue, UTI, depression, lower respiratory tract infection, arthralgia, abdominal discomfort, rash, gastroenteritis, vaginitis, allergic reaction, urinary urgency/frequency, irregular menstruation/dysmenorrhea, dermatitis, abnormal LFTs.
Simethicone (Mylanta Gas Maximum Strength, Mylanta Gas Maximum Strength Chewable Tablets, Mylanta Gas Maximum Strength Softgels) OTC	**Softgels, Maximum Strength:** 125mg; **Tab, Maximum Strength Chewable:** 125mg	***Adults:*** Take pc or hs. Softgels/Tabs, Chew: 1-2 prn. **Max:** 4 per day.	—	—

Table 16.2. DRUG INTERACTIONS FOR GASTROINTESTINAL DRUGS

ANTIDIARRHEALS	
Atropine Sulfate/Diphenoxylate HCl (Lomotil, Lonox) CV	
CNS depressants	May potentiate barbiturates, tranquilizers, and alcohol.
MAOIs	MAOIs may precipitate hypertensive crisis.
Bismuth Subsalicylate (Pepto-Bismol, Pepto-Bismol Maximum Strength) OTC	
Anticoagulants	Caution with anticoagulants.
Antidiabetic agents	Caution with antidiabetic agents.
Antigout agents	Caution with antigout agents.
ASA	May cause ringing in ears with ASA; d/c if this occurs.
Nitazoxanide (Alinia)	
Protein-bound drugs	Highly protein bound; caution with other highly plasma protein-bound drugs with narrow therapeutic indices.
ANTIEMETICS	
Aprepitant, Fosaprepitant (Emend)	
Astemizole	Avoid use with astemizole. Dose-dependent inhibition of CYP3A4 by aprepitant could result in elevated plasma concentrations of astemizole, potentially causing serious or life-threatening reactions.
Cisapride	Avoid use with cisapide. Dose-dependent inhibition of CYP3A4 by aprepitant could result in elevated plasma concentrations of cisapride, potentially causing serious or life-threatening reactions.
Contraceptives, oral	May reduce efficacy of oral contraceptives; use alternative contraception during treatment and for 1 month after last dose.
CYP2C9 substrates	May decrease levels of warfarin, tolbutamide, phenytoin, or other drugs metabolized by CYP2C9.
CYP3A4 inducers	Decreased efficacy with CYP3A4 inducers (eg, rifampin, carbamazepine, phenytoin).
CYP3A4 inhibitors	Caution with strong CYP3A4 inhibitors (eg, ketoconazole, itraconazole, nefazodone, troleandomycin, clarithromycin, ritonavir, nelfinavir) and moderate CYP3A4 inhibitors (eg, diltiazem).
CYP3A4 substrates	May increase levels of drugs metabolized by CYP3A4 including chemotherapy agents (eg, docetaxel, paclitaxel, etoposide, irinotecan, ifosfamide, imatinib, vinblastine, vincristine), dexamethasone, methylprednisolone, and certain benzodiazepines (eg, midazolam, alprazolam, triazolam).
Paroxetine	Concomitant paroxetine may decrease levels of both drugs.
Pimozide	Avoid use with pimozide. Dose-dependent inhibition of CYP3A4 by aprepitant could result in elevated plasma concentrations of pimozide, potentially causing serious or life-threatening reactions.
Terfenadine	Avoid use with terfenadine. Dose-dependent inhibition of CYP3A4 by aprepitant could result in elevated plasma concentrations of terfenadine, potentially causing serious or life-threatening reactions.

Table 16.2. DRUG INTERACTIONS FOR GASTROINTESTINAL DRUGS *(cont.)*

ANTIEMETICS *(cont.)*

Dolasetron Mesylate (Anzemet)	
Anthracycline	Increased risk of prolongation of cardiac conduction intervals with cumulative high-dose anthracycline therapy.
Antiarrhythmics	Increased risk of prolongation of cardiac conduction intervals with antiarrhythmics.
Atenolol, IV	Decreased clearance with IV atenolol.
Cimetidine	Cimetidine increases levels of dolasetron.
Diuretics	Increased risk of prolongation of cardiac conduction intervals with diuretics.
QTc interval, drugs prolonging	Increased risk of prolongation of cardiac conduction intervals with drugs that prolong QTc interval.
Rifampin	Rifampin decreases levels of dolasetron.
Dronabinol (Marinol) CIII	
Amphetamines	Additive HTN, tachycardia, and possible cardiotoxicity with amphetamines.
Anticholinergic agents	Increased tachycardia, and drowsiness with anticholinergic agents.
Antipyrine	Decreases clearance of antipyrine.
Barbiturates	Decreases clearance of barbiturates.
CNS depressants	Potentiates effects of CNS depressants.
Cocaine	Additive HTN, tachycardia, and possible cardiotoxicity with cocaine.
Protein-bound drugs	Highly protein-bound drugs may require dosage changes.
Psychoactive drugs	Additive effects with alcohol, sedatives, hypnotics, or other psychoactive drugs.
Sympathomimetics	Additive HTN, tachycardia, and possible cardiotoxicity with sympathomimetics.
TCAs	Potentiates effects of TCAs.
Droperidol (Inapsine)	
Alcohol	Caution with alcohol.
Analgesics, parenteral	Increased BP with fentanyl citrate or other parenteral analgesics.
Anesthesia, conduction	Caution with conduction anesthesia (eg, spinal, peridural).
CNS depressants	May potentiate and be potentiated by CNS depressants (eg, barbiturates, benzodiazepines, tranquilizers, opioids, general anesthetics); use lower doses.
Diuretics	Caution with diuretics.
Electrolyte disturbances, drugs inducing	Caution with drugs that induce hypokalemia, hypomagnesemia.
Epinephrine	Epinephrine may paradoxically decrease BP.
MAOIs	Caution with MAOIs.
QT interval, drugs prolonging	Avoid drugs that prolong the QT interval (eg, antimalarials, CCBs, antidepressants, Class I and III antiarrhythmics, certain antihistamines, neuroleptics).

ANTIEMETICS *(cont.)*

Granisetron HCl (Kytril)	
CYP450 enzyme inducers or inhibitors	Hepatic CYP450 enzyme inducers or inhibitors may alter clearance.
Meclizine HCl (Antivert)	
Alcohol	Avoid alcoholic beverages.
Metoclopramide HCl (Reglan, Reglan Injection)	
Anticholinergics	Antagonized by anticholinergics.
CNS depressants	Additive sedation with alcohol, hypnotics, narcotics, or tranquilizers.
Extrapyramidal reactions, drugs causing	Caution with use of other drugs causing extrapyramidal reactions; frequency and severity of seizures or extrapyramidal reactions may be increased.
Insulin	Insulin dose or timing of dose may need adjustment to prevent hypoglycemia.
Intestine, drugs absorbed from	The rate of and/or extent of absorption of drugs from the small bowel may be increased (eg, APAP, tetracycline, levodopa, ethanol, cyclosporine).
MAOIs	Caution with MAOIs.
Opioids	Antagonized by opioids.
Stomach, drugs absorbed from	Absorption of drugs from the stomach may be diminished (eg, digoxin)
Nabilone (Cesamet) CII	
Alcohol	Alcohol may increase the positive subjective mood effects.
Amphetamines	Additive HTN, tachycardia, and possible cardiotoxicity with amphetamines.
Anticholinergics	Additive or super-additive tachycardia, drowsiness may occur with atropine, scopolamine, antihistamines, other anticholinergics.
Antihistamines	Additive drowsiness and CNS depression may occur with antihistamines.
Antipyrine	Decreases clearance of antipyrine.
Barbiturates	Decreases clearance of barbiturates; additive CNS depression may occur.
Benzodiazepines	Additive drowsiness and CNS depression may occur with benzodiazepines.
Buspirone	Additive drowsiness and CNS depression may occur with buspirone.
CNS depressants	Additive drowsiness and CNS depression may occur with other CNS depressants, including alcohol.
Cocaine	Additive HTN, tachycardia, and possible cardiotoxicity with cocaine.
Disulfiram	Hypomanic reaction reported with disulfiram.
Fluoxetine	Hypomanic reaction reported with fluoxetine.
Lithium	Additive drowsiness and CNS depression may occur with lithium.
Muscle relaxants	Additive drowsiness and CNS depression may occur with muscle relaxants.
Naltrexone	Effects may be enhanced by opioid-receptor blockade.
Opioids	Cross-tolerance and mutual potentiation with opioids; additive CNS depression may occur.
Sympathomimetics	Additive HTN, tachycardia, and possible cardiotoxicity with sympathomimetics.

Table 16.2. DRUG INTERACTIONS FOR GASTROINTESTINAL DRUGS *(cont.)*

ANTIEMETICS *(cont.)*	
Nabilone (Cesamet) CII *(cont.)*	
TCAs	Additive tachycardia, HTN, drowsiness may occur with TCAs.
Theophylline	May increase metabolism of theophylline.
Ondansetron (Zofran)	
CYP450 inducers or inhibitors	Ondansetron is metabolized by CYP450 enzymes; inducers or inhibitors of these enzymes may change the clearance and half-life of ondansetron.
Prochlorperazine	
Anticoagulants, oral	May decrease oral anticoagulant effects.
Anticonvulsants	Anticonvulsants may need adjustment.
β-Blockers	May potentiate β-adrenergic blockade.
Diuretics, thiazide	Thiazide diuretics potentiate orthostatic hypotension.
Guanethidine	May antagonize antihypertensive effects of guanethidine and related compounds.
Lithium	Risk of encephalopathic syndrome with lithium.
Propranolol	Increased levels of both drugs with propranolol.
Promethazine HCl Injection	
Anesthetics, general	Additive sedative effects with general anesthetics; reduce dose of anesthetic or d/c.
Anticholinergics	Caution with anticholinergics.
Barbiturates	Additive sedative effects with barbiturates; reduce barbiturate dose by 1/2.
CNS depressants	Additive sedative effects with other CNS depressants, including alcohol; reduce dose or eliminate these agents.
Epinephrine	Do not use epinephrine for promethazine injection overdose.
MAOIs	Possible increased extrapyramidal effects.
Opioid analgesics	Additive sedative effects with opioid analgesics; reduce opioid dose by 1/4 to 1/2.
Sedative-hypnotics	Additive sedative effects with sedative-hypnotics; reduce dose of sedative-hypnotic or d/c.
Seizure threshold, drugs altering	Caution with drugs that alter seizure threshold (eg, narcotics, local anesthetics).
TCAs	Additive sedative effects with TCAs; reduce dose of TCA or d/c.
Tranquilizers	Additive sedative effects with tranquilizers; reduce dose of tranquilizer or d/c.
Scopolamine (Transderm Scop)	
Anticholinergics	Caution with anticholinergic drugs (eg, other belladonna alkaloids, antihistamines, TCAs, muscle relaxants).
CNS depressants	Increased CNS effects with sedatives, tranquilizers, and alcohol.
Medications, oral	May decrease absorption of oral medications due to delayed gastric emptying or decreased gastric motility.

ANTIEMETICS *(cont.)*

Trimethobenzamide HCl (Tigan)	
Alcohol	Adverse drug interactions reported with alcohol.
CNS agents	Caution with CNS agents (eg, phenothiazines, barbiturates, belladonna derivatives) in acute febrile illness, encephalitides, gastroenteritis, dehydration, and electrolyte imbalance.

ANTISPASMODICS/IBS AGENTS

Alosetron HCl (Lotronex)	
Cimetidine	Avoid with cimetidine.
CYP inducers and inhibitors	Inducers and inhibitors of hepatic CYP drug-metabolizing enzymes may change the clearance of alosetron.
CYP1A2 inhibitors, moderate	Avoid concomitant administration.
CYP3A4 inhibitors	Caution with CYP3A4 inhibitors (ketoconazole, clarithromycin, telithromycin, protease inhibitors, voriconazole, itraconazole).
Fluvoxamine	Fluvoxamine increases AUC; concomitant administration is contraindicated.
GI motility, drugs decreasing	Increased risk of constipation with medications that decrease GI motility.
Quinolones	Avoid with quinolone antibiotics.
Atropine Sulfate/Hyoscyamine Sulfate/Phenobarbital/Scopolamine Hydrobromide (Donnatal, Donnatal Extentabs)	
Phenobarbital	Phenobarbital may decrease anticoagulant effects; adjust dose.
Chlordiazepoxide HCl/Clidinium Bromide (Librax) CIV	
Anticoagulants, oral	Altered coagulation effects with oral anticoagulants.
CNS depressants	Caution with alcohol and other CNS depressants.
Psychotropics	Avoid with other psychotropics; if combination is indicated, use caution, especially with MAOIs and phenothiazines.
Dicyclomine HCl (Bentyl)	
Achlorhydria, drugs treating	Antagonized by drugs treating achlorhydria and those used to test gastric secretion.
Amantadine	Potentiated by amantadine.
Antacids	Decreased absorption with antacids.
Antiarrhythmics, Class I	Potentiated by Class I antiarrhythmics (eg, quinidine).
Anticholinergic activity, drugs having	Potentiated by other drugs having anticholinergic activity.
Antiglaucoma agents	Antagonizes the effects of antiglaucoma agents.
Antihistamines	Potentiated by antihistamines.
Antipsychotics	Potentiated by antipsychotics (eg, phenothiazines).
Benzodiazepines	Potentiated by benzodiazepines.
Corticosteroid eye drops	Do not give with corticosteroid eye drops.

Table 16.2. DRUG INTERACTIONS FOR GASTROINTESTINAL DRUGS *(cont.)*

ANTISPASMODICS/IBS AGENTS *(cont.)*	
Dicyclomine HCl (Bentyl) *(cont.)*	
Digoxin	May effect the GI absorption of delayed-release digoxin.
MAOIs	Potentiated by MAOIs.
Metoclopramide	Antagonizes the effect of metoclopramide.
Nitrates/nitrites	Potentiated by nitrates/nitrites.
Opioid analgesics	Potentiated by opioid analgesics (eg, meperidine).
Sympathomimetics	Potentiated by sympathomimetics.
TCAs	Potentiated by TCAs.
Hyoscyamine Sulfate (IB-Stat, Levbid, Levsin, Levsinex)	
Amantadine	Additive effects with amantadine.
Antacids	Antacids interfere with absorption; take ac and antacids pc.
Antihistamines	Additive effects with some antihistamines.
Antimuscarinics	Additive effects with other antimuscarinics.
Haloperidol	Additive effects with haloperidol.
MAOIs	Additive effects with MAOIs.
Phenothiazines	Additive effects with phenothiazines.
TCAs	Additive effects with TCAs.
ANTIULCER/GERD AGENTS	
Aluminum Hydroxide OTC	
Prescription drugs	Antacids may interact with certain prescription drugs.
Tetracycline	Avoid with tetracycline.
Amoxicillin/Clarithromycin/Lansoprazole (Prevpac)	
Antiarrhythmics	QTc prolongation has occurred with coadministration of clarithromycin and antiarrhythmics (eg, quinidine, disopyramide).
Anticoagulants, oral	Clarithromycin potentiates oral anticoagulants.
Astemizole	Contraindicated with astemizole.
Carbamazepine	Clarithromycin increases plasma levels of carbamazepine.
Cisapride	Contraindicated with cisapride.
Colchicine	Concomitant clarithromycin and colchicine may lead to increased exposure to colchicine.
CYP450 substrates	Caution with drugs metabolized by CYP450 (eg, cyclosporine, tacrolimus, phenytoin); monitor levels.
Digoxin	Clarithromycin increases plasma levels of digoxin.
Ergot derivatives	Contraindicated; erythromycin or clarithromycin can cause acute ergot toxicity with ergotamine or dihydroergotamine.

ANTIULCER/GERD AGENTS *(cont.)*

Amoxicillin/Clarithromycin/Lansoprazole (Prevpac) *(cont.)*	
Gastric pH, drugs depending on	May interfere with absorption of drugs dependent on gastric pH for bioavailability (eg, atazanavir, ketoconazole, ampicillin esters, iron salts, digoxin).
HMG CoA reductase inhibitors	Clarithromycin increases levels of HMG CoA reductase inhibitors (eg, lovastatin, simvastatin).
Pimozide	Contraindicated with pimozide.
Sucralfate	Take lansoprazole and other proton pump inhibitors 30 minutes before sucralfate.
Terfenadine	Contraindicated with terfenadine.
Theophylline	Theophylline may need dose adjustment.
Triazolam	Clarithromycin may decrease triazolam clearance.
Bismuth Subsalicylate/Metronidazole/Tetracycline HCl (Helidac)	
Alcohol	Avoid alcohol during and at least 1 day after metronidazole.
Antacids	Tetracycline can cause impaired absorption with antacids containing aluminum, calcium, magnesium.
Anticoagulants	Monitor anticoagulants; possible risk of bleeding and/or decreased prothrombin activity.
Antidiabetic agents	Caution with antidiabetic agents; possible enhanced hypoglycemic effect.
ASA	Caution with ASA.
Calcium carbonate	Possible reduced absorption with calcium carbonate.
Contraceptives, oral	May antagonize oral contraceptive effects.
Dairy products	Possible reduced absorption with dairy products.
Disulfiram	Psychotic reactions reported in alcoholics with concomitant disulfiram and metronidazole; space metronidazole and disulfiram dosing by 2 weeks.
Lithium	May increase lithium levels.
Metabolism inducers	Increased elimination with drugs that induce metabolism (eg, phenytoin, phenobarbital).
Metabolism inhibitors	Metronidazole can cause decreased plasma clearance with drugs that decrease metabolism (eg, cimetidine).
Metal cations	Tetracycline can cause impaired absorption with agents containing iron or zinc.
Methoxyflurane	Fatal renal toxicity with methoxyflurane reported.
Penicillin	May interfere with bactericidal action of penicillin; avoid concomitant use.
Phenytoin	May impair phenytoin clearance.
Probenecid	Caution with probenecid.
Sodium bicarbonate	Tetracycline can cause impaired absorption with agents containing sodium bicarbonate.
Sulfinpyrazone	Caution with sulfinpyrazone.

Table 16.2. DRUG INTERACTIONS FOR GASTROINTESTINAL DRUGS *(cont.)*

ANTIULCER/GERD AGENTS *(cont.)*	
Calcium Carbonate (Children's Mylanta) OTC	
Prescription drugs	Antacids may interact with certain prescription drugs.
Calcium Carbonate/Magnesium Hydroxide (Mylanta Gelcaps Antacid, Mylanta Supreme, Mylanta Ultra Tabs) OTC	
Prescription drugs	Antacids may interact with other prescription drugs.
Cimetidine (Tagamet)	
Antacids	Antacids may interfer with absorption of cimetidine; space the dosing.
Anticoagulants	Reduces metabolism of warfarin-type anticoagulants. Monitor PT/INR.
Chlordiazepoxide	Reduces metabolism of chlordiazepoxide.
Diazepam	Reduces metabolism of diazepam.
Gastric pH, drugs affected by	May affect absorption of drugs (eg, ketoconazole) affected by gastric pH; give 2 hrs before cimetidine.
Lidocaine	Adverse effects reported with lidocaine; monitor levels.
Metronidazole	Reduces metabolism of metronidazole.
Nifedipine	Reduces metabolism of nifedipine.
Phenytoin	Reduces metabolism of phenytoin. Adverse effects reported with phenytoin; monitor levels.
Propranolol	Reduces metabolism of propranolol.
TCAs	Reduces metabolism of TCAs.
Theophylline	Reduces metabolism of theophylline. Adverse effects reported with theophylline; monitor levels.
Esomeprazole Magnesium (Nexium, Nexium IV)	
Antibiotics	Increased levels with amoxicillin and clarithromycin coadministration. Clarithromycin is contraindicated with pimozide.
Atazanavir	May reduce levels of atazanavir when used concomitantly.
CYP substrates	Concomitant use with CYP2C19 and CYP3A4 substrates (eg, voriconazole) may result in doubling of plasma exposure.
Diazepam	Potentiates diazepam.
pH-dependent drugs	May alter absorption of pH-dependent drugs (eg, ketoconazole, digoxin, iron salts).
Warfarin	Concomitant use with warfarin may increase INR and PT.
Famotidine OTC (Pepcid AC)	
Acid reducers	Avoid with other acid reducers.
Glycopyrrolate (Robinul Injection)	
Anticholinergics	Increased anticholinergic side effects with other anticholinergics.
Antiparkinson drugs	Increased anticholinergic side effects with antiparkinson drugs.
Phenothiazines	Increased anticholinergic side effects with phenothiazines.
Potassium chloride	Increased severity of GI lesions with potassium chloride in a wax matrix.
TCAs	Increased anticholinergic side effects with TCAs.

ANTIULCER/GERD AGENTS *(cont.)*

Lansoprazole (Prevacid, Prevacid IV, Prevacid Solutab)	
pH-dependent drugs	May alter absorption of pH-dependent drugs (eg, ketoconazole, ampicillin esters, digoxin, and iron salts).
Sucralfate	Give at least 30 minutes prior to sucralfate.
Theophylline	Theophylline may need dose adjustment; may cause a minor increase in theophylline clearance.
Warfarin	Concomitant use with warfarin may increase INR and prothrombin time.
Methscopolamine Bromide (Pamine, Pamine Forte)	
Antacids	Antacids may interfere with absorption.
Anticholinergic effects, drugs with	Additive effects with other drugs with anticholinergic effects.
Antipsychotics	Additive anticholinergic effects with antipsychotics.
TCAs	Additive anticholinergic effects with TCAs.
Misoprostol (Cytotec)	
Antacids, magnesium-containing	Avoid with magnesium-containing antacids to decrease incidence of diarrhea.
Nizatidine (Axid, Axid Oral Solution)	
ASA	May elevate serum salicylate levels with high-dose ASA.
Omeprazole (Prilosec)	
Atazanavir	May reduce plasma levels of atazanavir.
Clarithromycin	Increased levels of clarithromycin and omeprazole.
CYP450 substrates	Monitor drugs metabolized by CYP450 (eg, cyclosporine, disulfiram, benzodiazepines).
Diazepam	May potentiate diazepam.
pH-dependent drugs	May alter absorption of pH-dependent drugs (eg, ketoconazole, ampicillin esters, iron salts).
Phenytoin	May potentiate phenytoin.
Tacrolimus	May increase levels of tacrolimus.
Voriconazole	Voriconazole may increase levels.
Warfarin	May potentiate warfarin.
Omeprazole Magnesium (Prilosec OTC) OTC	
Antifungals	Caution with antifungals.
Atazanavir	Caution with atazanavir.
Diazepam	Caution with diazepam.
Digoxin	Caution with digoxin.
Tacrolimus	Caution with tacrolimus.
Warfarin	Caution with warfarin.

Table 16.2. DRUG INTERACTIONS FOR GASTROINTESTINAL DRUGS *(cont.)*

ANTIULCER/GERD AGENTS *(cont.)*

Omeprazole/Sodium Bicarbonate (Zegerid)	
Atazanavir	May reduce levels of atazanavir.
Clarithromycin	Increased levels of clarithromycin and omeprazole.
CYP450 substrates	Monitor when given with drugs metabolized by CYP450 (eg, cyclosporine, disulfiram, benzodiazepines).
Diazepam	May prolong elimination of diazepam.
pH-dependent drugs	May alter absorption of pH-dependent drugs (eg, ketoconazole, ampicillin esters, and iron salts).
Phenytoin	May prolong elimination of phenytoin.
Tacrolimus	May increase levels of tacrolimus.
Warfarin	May prolong elimination of warfarin. May increase PT and INR if given concomitantly with warfarin.
Pantoprazole Sodium (Protonix, Protonix IV)	
Atazanavir	May substantially decrease atazanavir levels; avoid concomitant use.
pH-dependent drugs	May alter absorption of pH-dependent drugs (eg, ketoconazole, ampicillin esters, and iron salts).
Warfarin	May increase INR and prothrombin time with concomitant warfarin therapy.
Rabeprazole Sodium (Aciphex)	
Clarithromycin	Increased rabeprazole and clarithromycin levels with triple therapy.
Cyclosporine	May inhibit cyclosporine metabolism.
Digoxin	May increase digoxin plasma levels.
Ketoconazole	May decrease ketoconazole levels.
pH-dependent drugs	May alter absorption of pH-dependent drugs (eg, ketoconazole, digoxin).
Warfarin	Concomitant use with warfarin increases the INR and PT time; monitor PT/INR.
Ranitidine HCl (Zantac)	
Anticoagulants	Monitor anticoagulants.
Triazolam	Increases plasma levels of triazolam.
Ranitidine HCl (Zantac 150, Zantac 75, Zantac OTC) OTC	
Acid reducers	Avoid other acid reducers.
Sucralfate (Carafate)	
Aluminum	Additive aluminum absorption with aluminum-containing products.
Antacids	Antacids should not be taken within 1/2 hr before or after sucralfate.
Cimetidine	Reduced absorption of cimetidine; dose concomitant drugs 2 hrs before sucralfate.
Digoxin	Reduced absorption of digoxin; dose concomitant drugs 2 hrs before sucralfate.
Fluoroquinolones	Reduced absorption of fluoroquinolones; dose concomitant drugs 2 hrs before sucralfate.

ANTIULCER/GERD AGENTS *(cont.)*

Sucralfate (Carafate) *(cont.)*	
Ketoconazole	Reduced absorption of ketoconazole; dose concomitant drugs 2 hrs before sucralfate.
Levothyroxine	Reduced absorption of levothyroxine; dose concomitant drugs 2 hrs before sucralfate.
Phenytoin	Reduced absorption of phenytoin; dose concomitant drugs 2 hrs before sucralfate.
Quinidine	Reduced absorption of quinidine; dose concomitant drugs 2 hrs before sucralfate.
Ranitidine	Reduced absorption of ranitidine; dose concomitant drugs 2 hrs before sucralfate.
Tetracycline	Reduced absorption of tetracycline; dose concomitant drugs 2 hrs before sucralfate.
Theophylline	Reduced absorption of theophylline; dose concomitant drugs 2 hrs before sucralfate.
Warfarin	Monitor warfarin. Possible subtherapeutic prothrombin times (rare).

COLORECTAL AGENTS

Balsalazide Disodium (Colazal)	
Antibiotics, oral	Oral antibiotics may interfere with the release of mesalamine in the colon.
Budesonide (Entocort EC)	
CYP3A4 inhibitors	Increased levels with CYP3A4 inhibitors (eg, ketoconazole, itraconazole, saquinavir, erythromycin, grapefruit, grapefruit juice); reduce budesonide dose.
Hydrocortisone (Colocort)	
ASA	Caution with ASA in hypoprothrombinemia.
Vaccinations	Avoid vaccinations.
Hydrocortisone Acetate (Cortifoam)	
Aminoglutethimide	Caution with aminoglutethimide.
Amphotericin B	Risk of hypokalemia with amphotericin B injection.
Anticholinesterase	Withdraw anticholinesterase agents 24 hrs prior to initiation.
Antidiabetic agents	May increase blood glucose levels; may need to adjust antidiabetic agents.
Cholestyramine	Increased clearance with cholestyramine.
Cyclosporine	Cyclosporine may increase activity of both drugs; convulsions reported with concomitant use.
Digitalis glycosides	Risk of hypokalemia with digitalis glycosides.
Estrogens	Decreased clearance or metabolism with estrogens.
Hepatic enzyme inducers	Increased metabolism with hepatic enzyme inducers (eg, barbiturates, phenytoin, carbamazepine, rifampin).
Isoniazid	May decrease isoniazid and salicylate levels.

Table 16.2. DRUG INTERACTIONS FOR GASTROINTESTINAL DRUGS *(cont.)*

COLORECTAL AGENTS *(cont.)*	
Hydrocortisone Acetate (Cortifoam) *(cont.)*	
Ketoconazole	Decreased clearance or metabolism with ketoconazole.
Macrolides	Decreased clearance or metabolism with macrolide antibiotics.
Neuromuscular blockers	Caution with neuromuscular blockers.
Potassium-depleting agents	Risk of hypokalemia with potassium-depleting agents.
Salicylates	May decrease salicylate levels. Caution with ASA in hypoprothrombinemia. Increased risk for GI side effects with ASA and other NSAIDs.
Vaccines, live	Avoid live vaccines with immunosuppressive doses.
Warfarin	Inhibits response to warfarin; monitor PT/INR.
Hydrocortisone Acetate/Lidocaine HCl (AnaMantle HC)	
Antiarrhythmics	Additive adverse effects with Class I antiarrhythmics.
Mesalamine (Lialda)	
6-mercaptopurine	Concurrent 6-mercaptopurine can increase potential for blood disorders.
Azathioprine	Concurrent azathioprine can increase potential for blood disorders.
Nephrotoxic agents	Concurrent use with nephrotoxic agents (eg, NSAIDs) may increase risk of renal reactions.
Olsalazine Sodium (Dipentum)	
6-mercaptopurine	May increase risk of myelosuppression with 6-mercaptopurine.
Heparin products	Increased risk of bleeding when coadministered with LMW heparins or heparinoids.
Salicylates	Increased risk of bleeding when coadministered with salicylates.
Thioguanine	May increase risk of myelosuppression with thioguanine.
Vaccine, varicella	Avoid salicylates for 6 weeks after varicella vaccine; may increase risk of Reye's syndrome.
Warfarin	Increased PT time with warfarin.
Sulfasalazine (Azulfidine, Azulfidine EN)	
Digoxin	Reduces absorption of digoxin.
Folic acid	Reduces absorption of folic acid.
Methotrexate (MTX)	Increased incidence of GI adverse events with combination of sulfasalazine (2g/day) and MTX (7.5mg/week).
DIGESTIVE ENZYMES/BILE ACIDS	
Amylase/Lipase/Protease (Creon)	
Food	Do not add capsule contents to food with pH >5.5.
Ursodiol (Actigall)	
Antacids	Decreased absorption with aluminum-based antacids.
Bile acid sequestrants	Decreased absorption with bile acid sequestrants.
Clofibrate	Clofibrate encourages gallstone formation.

DIGESTIVE ENZYMES/BILE ACIDS *(cont.)*

Ursodiol (Actigall) *(cont.)*	
Contraceptives, oral	Oral contraceptives encourage gallstone formation.
Estrogens	Estrogens encourage gallstone formation.
Ursodiol (Urso 250, Urso Forte)	
Antacids	Decreased absorption with aluminum-based antacids.
Bile acid sequestrants	Decreased absorption with bile acid sequestering agents (eg, cholestyramine, colestipol).
Cholesterol-lowering agents	Clofibrate and perhaps other cholesterol-lowering agents may counteract effectiveness.
Contraceptives, oral	Oral contraceptives may counteract effectiveness.
Estrogens	Estrogens may counteract effectiveness.

LAXATIVES/EVACUANTS

Ascorbic Acid/Polyethylene Glycol 3350/Potassium Chloride/Sodium Ascorbate/Sodium Chloride/Sodium Sulfate (MoviPrep)	
Medications, oral	Oral medications given within 1 hr of administration may be flushed from GI tract and may not be absorbed.
Bisacodyl (Dulcolax, Fleet Bisacodyl) OTC	
Antacids	Do not administer tabs within 1 hr after taking an antacid.
Milk	Do not administer tabs within 1 hr after taking milk or milk products.
Bisacodyl/Polyethylene Glycol 3350/Potassium Chloride/Sodium Bicarbonate/Sodium Chloride (HalfLytely)	
Antacids	Avoid bisacodyl delayed-release tablets within 1 hr of taking an antacid.
Medications, oral	Oral medications taken within 1 hr of start of administration may not be absorbed from GI tract.
Docusate Sodium/Senna OTC (Peri-Colace)	
Mineral oil	Caution with mineral oil.
Lactulose (Constulose, Enulose, Generlac)	
Antacids	Decreased effect with nonabsorbable antacids.
Polyethylene Glycol 3350/Potassium Chloride/Sodium Bicarbonate/Sodium Chloride (NuLYTELY, Trilyte, Colyte, Colyte w/ Flavor Packs, Colyte-Flavored, GoLYTELY)	
Medications, oral	Oral medications taken within 1 hr of start of administration may not be absorbed from GI tract.
Senna OTC (Senokot)	
Mineral oil	Avoid mineral oil with Senokot-S (docusate sodium and senna).
Sodium Phosphate (Visicol)	
Drugs, other	May reduce absorption of other drugs.
Electrolytes, agents affecting	Caution with agents that affect electrolyte levels.
QT interval, agents prolonging	Caution with agents that prolong QT interval.
Sodium phosphate products	Caution with sodium phosphate-containing products.

Table 16.2. DRUG INTERACTIONS FOR GASTROINTESTINAL DRUGS *(cont.)*

MISCELLANEOUS GASTROINTESTINAL AGENTS

Adalimumab (Humira)	
Anakinra	Do not give anakinra concurrently due to increased risk of serious infections.
Methotrexate (MTX)	Reduced clearance with MTX.
Vaccines, live	Do not give live vaccines concurrently.
Certolizumab pegol (Cimzia)	
Anakinra	Avoid combination treatment with anakinra.
Vaccines, live	Do not give live vaccines concurrently.
Infliximab (Remicade)	
Anakinra	Do not give anakinra concurrently due to increased risk of serious infections and neutropenia.
Immunosuppressants	Concurrent use with corticosteroids may lead to development of infections.
Methotrexate (MTX)	Concurrent use with MTX may lead to development of infections.
Vaccines, live	Do not give live vaccines concurrently.
Natalizumab (Tysabri)	
Immunomodulators	Avoid concurrent use with other inhibitors of TNF-α.
Immunosuppressants	Avoid concurrent use with 6-mercaptopurine, azathioprine, and cyclosporine. Taper corticosteroids in Crohn's disease patients before starting therapy.

Chapter 17

Neurological Drugs

Steven Ganzberg, D.M.D., M.S.; Jennifer P. Bassiur, D.D.S.

Patients who are receiving ongoing treatment of neurological conditions may consult a dentist for oral health care. One of the more common neurological conditions dentists see among these patients is seizure disorders; they also may encounter other conditions such as Parkinson's disease, multiple sclerosis, Alzheimer's disease, myasthenia gravis and other myopathies, spasticity resulting from spinal cord injury, and poststroke syndrome. Long-term medication management is common. The dentist also may prescribe neurological drugs for the treatment of orofacial pain of neuropathic origin as well as for primary headache syndromes, such as migraine, cluster, and tension-type headaches. Undertaking treatment of these disorders requires advanced training or experience in diagnosis and management of these disorders. For general information on neurological drugs, see **Tables 17.1 and 17.2**.

Clinicians should review the condition and level of disease control (for example, quality of seizure control) of patients who have neurological conditions. If warranted, it may be prudent to delay elective dental treatment pending medical consultation. Perform a preoperative evaluation of vital signs, including respiratory status. Adverse effects and precautions/contraindications are provided in **Table 17.1**.

ANTICONVULSANT DRUGS

Anticonvulsant drugs typically are used to control epilepsy, a convulsive disorder characterized by intermittent excessive discharges of neurons. This dysregulation of neural function is frequently associated with altered or lost consciousness. Seizure disorders have been characterized as generalized, including tonic-clonic (grand mal) seizures, absence, partial, atonic, and other forms. Specific anticonvulsant agents have been shown to be superior for some types of seizures. None has been proved to be antiepileptogenic.

In orofacial pain management, anticonvulsants are useful in treating trigeminal neuralgia and other posttraumatic trigeminal neuropathies. Carbamazepine, phenytoin, valproic acid and its derivatives, clonazepam, gabapentin, and lamotrigine (as well as baclofen, an antispastic) have been reported to be useful. Other agents are being investigated in this regard. Certain anticonvulsants have been reported to provide some benefit for fibromyalgia and migraine headache as well. These medications have numerous side effects, some life-threatening. The dentist prescribing an anticonvulsant drug is presumed to be fully aware of the drug's interactions, adverse effects, monitoring requirements and contraindications.

See **Tables 17.1** and **17.2** for basic information on anticonvulsant drugs, both commonly and rarely used (owing to pronounced side effects or inferior efficacy compared to that of newer agents).

Special Dental Considerations

Many commonly prescribed anticonvulsants can cause blood dyscrasias, especially carbamazepine, phenytoin, and valproic acid. Stevens-Johnson syndrome can occur with many anticonvulsants, especially lamotrigine. Xerostomia and taste changes are common with many anticonvulsants. Topiramate can cause gingivitis. Consider these agents in the differential diagnosis of oral complaints if signs or symptoms warrant. Valproic acid/divalproex sodium may inhibit platelet aggregation.

Drug Interactions of Dental Interest

Anticonvulsants are frequently sedating. Sedative agents, including opioids, may potentiate this effect. Meperidine, especially when used in multiple doses, can promote seizures in patients with otherwise well-controlled seizure disorders due to accumulation of its metabolite.

Many anticonvulsants induce hepatic microsomal enzymes, causing decreased effectiveness or shorter duration of action of certain concomitantly prescribed drugs. Patients taking anticonvulsants may experience increased metabolism of concomitantly administered corticosteroids, benzodiazepines, and barbiturates, a situation that leads to decreased effectiveness of these agents.

Prolonged use of acetaminophen may increase the risk of anticonvulsant-induced hepatic toxicity.

Propoxyphene, erythromycin, and clarithromycin may result in decreased metabolism of carbamazepine and increased risk of toxicity.

Fluconazole, ketoconazole, and metronidazole may result in decreased metabolism of phenytoin and related hydantoins and increased risk of toxicity. Aspirin may increase plasma concentrations of hydantoins, thereby leading to toxicity. For phenytoin, high doses of lidocaine may have additive cardiac depressant effects.

Laboratory Value Alterations

- With most anticonvulsants (except benzodiazepines, acetazolamide, and gabapentin), leukopenia, thrombocytopenia, anemia, or pancytopenia is possible.
- With hydantoin derivatives, an increase in serum glucose is possible.
- With acetazolamide, an increase in serum glucose is possible.
- With valproic acid/divalproex sodium, bleeding time may be increased.
- With zonisamide and topiramate, a decrease in sodium bicarbonate is possible.

Special Patients

Pediatric patients

Pediatric patients taking hydantoin derivatives are more prone than adults to gingival enlargement, coarsening of facial features (widening of nasal tip, thickening of lips), and facial hair growth.

Pharmacology

Anticonvulsants' primary action is to prevent the spread of abnormal neuronal depolarization from an epileptic focus without completely suppressing that focus. The pharmacological mechanisms of action are varied but generally involve, alone or in combination, stabilization of neuronal sodium channels, increasing γ-aminobutyric acid (GABA) tone, alteration of excitatory amino acid neurotransmission, and alteration of calcium ion influx. In many cases, the exact mechanism of action remains unknown.

ANTIMYASTHENIC AND ALZHEIMER'S-TYPE DEMENTIA DRUGS

Myasthenia gravis is a progressive disease characterized by a decreased number of functional acetylcholine receptors at the neuromuscular junction, resulting in muscular weakness. Drugs to combat this disease impair acetylcholinesterase, the enzyme that degrades acetylcholine, thus increasing the relative concentration of available acetylcholine.

Alzheimer's disease is an age-associated neurodegenerative disorder characterized by intracellular neurofibrillary tangles and extracellular amyloid plaque accumulation in the brain, resulting in cognitive, behavioral, and functional disturbances. The Alzheimer's-type dementia drugs included in this discussion are either reversible centrally acting anticholinesterase drugs or NMDA receptor antagonists.

Current theories of Alzheimer's disease attribute some of the symptoms to a deficiency in central nervous system (CNS) cholinergic transmission or to glutamate excitotoxicity, as well as to additional proposed mechanisms. The use of these drugs for mild to moderate Alzheimer's disease shows variable, but clinically measurable, improvement in some patients.

See **Tables 17.1** and **17.2** for basic information on antimyasthenic and Alzheimer's-type dementia drugs.

Special Dental Considerations

Monitor vital signs, including respiratory status, before beginning dental treatment. Also evaluate the patient for possible postural hypotension by having him or her sit in the dental chair for a minute or two after being in a supine position and then evaluating him or her when standing.

These drugs may cause decreased salivation.

Drug Interactions of Dental Interest

There may be a reduced rate of metabolism of ester local anesthetics.

High doses of local anesthetic may depress muscle function.

CNS depressants should be used with caution.

Pharmacology

Antimyasthenic drugs increase the amount of acetylcholine present at the neuromuscular junction by inhibition of acetylcholinesterase, the enzyme that degrades acetylcholine. The increase in acetylcholine concentration improves muscular function.

The Alzheimer's-type dementia drugs included in this section increase CNS cholinergic function by inhibiting the cholinesterase enzyme or by blocking the pathologic neural toxicity associated with prolonged glutamate release by noncompetitive blocking of the NMDA receptor. These symptomatic treatments work to slow the progression of the cognitive, behavioral, and functional symptoms. In some patients, the cognitive indices improve.

ANTIPARKINSON DRUGS

Parkinson's disease is a CNS disorder characterized by compromised cognition and resting tremor, and is frequently accompanied by involuntary mouth and tongue movements, rigidity of the limbs and trunk, postural instability, and bradykinesia, including loss of facial expressions (mask-like facies). Drooling is common, owing to swallowing incoordination. A relative imbalance between dopamine, acetylcholine, and GABA neurotransmission in the basal ganglia and related areas plays a significant role in the pathophysiology of this disorder. Antiparkinson drugs attempt to alter this neurotransmitter imbalance.

See **Tables 17.1** and **17.2** for basic information on antiparkinson drugs.

Special Dental Considerations

Many of these drugs can cause xerostomia. Consider them in the differential diagnosis of caries, periodontal disease, or oral candidiasis.

If newly diagnosed mouthing movements (involuntary mouth and tongue movements and/or drooling) are seen, which may indicate a serious medication side effect, consultation with the patient's physician may be appropriate.

Selegiline may cause circumoral burning.

Monitor the patient's vital signs during all dental visits. Have the patient sit upright in the dental chair for a minute or two after being in a supine position and then monitor the patient when standing.

Sedation or general anesthesia may be required for dental care.

Drug Interactions of Dental Interest

Patients taking levodopa, entacapone, tolcapone, and high doses of selegiline may exhibit an exaggerated hemodynamic response to vasoconstrictors in local anesthetic solutions. Employ careful aspiration technique with limited vasoconstrictor (0.04 mg epinephrine). Additional vasoconstrictor may be used after monitoring of vital signs.

Dopamine antagonist medications, such as chlorpromazine, metoclopramide, and promethazine, which may be prescribed for nausea, are contraindicated in patients with Parkinson's disease.

Anticholinergics may have an additive oral drying effect and should be used with caution.

In patients taking high doses of selegiline, meperidine, and possibly other opioids, a hyperthermic and possibly hypertensive crisis may occur.

Pharmacology

Parkinson's disease is classically characterized by an imbalance in dopaminergic and cholinergic neurotransmission with contributions involving GABA neurotransmission in the nigrastriatum. Medications that act on dopamine increase its availability either by increasing the concentration of dopamine precursors (levodopa), decreasing the breakdown of precursors (carbidopa), acting as agonists at the dopamine receptor (bromocriptine and amantadine) or decreasing the degradation of dopamine by MAO-B (selegiline). The catechol-O-methyl-transferase (COMT) inhibitor drugs entacapone and tolcapone are used with carbidopa-levodopa (Sinemet) to decrease levodopa degradation, thus increasing levodopa plasma levels. Centrally acting anticholinergic drugs or antihistamines with some degree of anticholinergic activity decrease cholinergic tone by blocking cholinergic receptors and improving the balance between dopaminergic and cholinergic transmission. GABA agonists, such as clonazepam, and other drugs, such as β-blockers, are also useful in some cases.

MUSCLE RELAXANTS AND ANTISPASTIC DRUGS

Muscle relaxants are generally used for acute muscle spasm, including that associated with temporomandibular disorders. The efficacy in chronic muscular disorders is not well established. Patients taking antispastic drugs typically have spinal cord or other CNS lesions. Spasticity can occur in some neurological disorders, such as multiple sclerosis.

Baclofen also may be effective for the treatment of trigeminal neuralgia and other trigeminal neuropathies.

See **Tables 17.1** and **17.2** for basic information on antispastic drugs.

Special Dental Considerations

Baclofen and orphenadrine may cause dry mouth. Carisoprodol has some potential for abuse and abstinence syndrome on discontinuation. Carisoprodol should be used for no more than two weeks except for those dentists with training and/or experience in chronic pain management. Dantrolene can infrequently cause blood dyscrasias. Consider these drugs in the differential diagnosis if oral signs and symptoms warrant it. Tizanidine may cause hypotension.

Drug Interactions of Dental Interest

These drugs may be sedating. Sedative agents, including opioids, may potentiate this effect.

Laboratory Value Alterations

- Dantrolene may infrequently cause blood dyscrasias.

Pharmacology

Muscle relaxants do not produce any direct effect on muscle. Muscle-relaxing effects are due to either generalized sedative effects or effects on CNS motor or reflex activity. Orphenadrine citrate may have mild analgesic effects. Antispastic drugs work directly on the muscle by decreasing calcium release from the sarcoplasmic reticulum (dantrolene) in the CNS by increasing GABA tone (baclofen), or by a CNS α_2-agonist effect (tizanidine).

HEADACHE SUPPRESSANTS

There are numerous conditions that cause headache or facial pain. The majority of patients who list headache as a primary condition on their medical history will be diagnosed with migraine, tension-type, or cluster headache. Numerous drugs are used to treat these conditions. They can be divided into symptomatic medications, abortive medications, and preventive medications. Symptomatic medications include analgesics and antiemetics, both of which have been covered in other chapters and will not be listed here. These drugs generally are taken intermittently for severe head pain, as continued use can aggravate headache conditions.

Abortive medications include those drugs which, when taken at onset of or during a severe headache (such as migraine or cluster headache), will arrest the headache process and, in some cases, the associated symptoms (such as nausea and photophobia). These medications include ergotamines, triptans, isometheptene mucate combinations and, in some cases, phenothiazines. These medications can have adverse cardiovascular consequences, but because they generally are taken on an intermittent basis not associated with a dental visit, they should not be of concern in dental care.

Preventive medications are varied and frequently draw from other drug categories. Various cardiovascular medications—including calcium channel blockers and β-blockers—are used for management of chronic headache. Likewise, most antidepressants and some anticonvulsants have been used for headache prevention.

Neuropathic facial pains, if they respond to medical treatment, are usually treated with anticonvulsant or antidepressant medications. Specific conditions may respond to baclofen, β-blockers, or clonidine.

See **Tables 17.1** and **17.2** for basic information on vascular headache suppressants. A thorough discussion of the pharmacological management of headache and facial pain is beyond the scope of this book. Headache suppressant medications, which have not been covered elsewhere in this text, will be presented.

Special Dental Considerations

Abortive headache medications are used only when needed for moderate-to-severe headache and generally not on the day of a dental appointment. If an ergot preparation or a triptan is used within 12 to 24 hours of a dental procedure, follow vasoconstrictor precautions similar to those for hypertensive patients. For preventive medications—for example, antidepressants, anticonvulsants, or antihypertensives—follow precautions listed for that specific category of drug.

The dentist who undertakes primary treatment of head and face pain is presumed to have established a proper diagnosis and to be fully aware of the interactions, adverse effects, and contraindications of headache medications.

Drug Interactions of Dental Interest

Ergot derivatives may have hypertensive effects, in which case, vasoconstrictors in local anesthetic solutions should be used cautiously.

For preventive medications, see the appropriate drug category.

Laboratory Value Alterations

- For preventive medications, see the appropriate drug category.
- Methysergide may cause blood dyscrasias and fibrotic disorders.

Pharmacology

Numerous drugs are used for the management of headache and facial pain. The pharmacology reflects the condition that is to be treated. For example, migraine headache is thought to involve abnormal serotonergic transmission. Varied medications, such as antidepressants, ergots, and specific antihistamines, alter serotonin neurotransmission and can be effective in the acute or preventive treatment of migraine. Trigeminal neuralgia responds to anticonvulsant medications by decreasing hyperactive neuronal function.

Treatment of headache and facial pain is beyond the scope of this text. For a more complete review of the pharmacological basis of headache and facial pain management, consult appropriate references.

Adverse Effects, Precautions, and Contraindications

Table 17.1 presents adverse effects and precautions/contraindications of neurological drugs.

SUGGESTED READING

Calne DB. Treatment of Parkinson's disease. *N Engl J Med*. 1993;329:1021-1027.

Factor SA. Current status of symptomatic medical therapy in Parkinson's disease. *Neurotherapeutics*. 2008;5(2):164-180.

Fraser AD. New drugs for the treatment of epilepsy. *Clin Biochem*. 1996:29(2):97-110.

Kalia LV, Kalia SK, Salter MW. NMDA receptors in clinical neurology: excitatory times ahead. *Lancet Neurol*. 2008;7:742-755.

McQuay H, Carrol D, et al. Anticonvulsant drugs for the management of pain: a systematic review. *BMJ*. 1995;311(7012):1047-1052.

Millard CB, Broomfield CA. Anticholinesterases: medical applications of neuro-chemical principles. *J Neurochem*. 1995;64(5):1909-1918.

Saper JR, Siberstein S, et al. *Handbook of Headache Management*. Baltimore: Williams & Wilkins; 1993.

Shah RS, Lee H, et al. Current approaches in the treatment of Alzheimer's disease. *Biomed Pharmacotherapy*. 2008;62:199-207.

The United States Pharmacopeial Convention. *Drug Information for the Health Care Professional*. 23rd ed. Rockville, MD: The United States Pharmacopeial Convention, Inc; 2003.

Table 17.1. PRESCRIBING INFORMATION FOR NEUROLOGICAL AGENTS

NAME	FORM/ STRENGTH	DOSAGE	WARNINGS/PRECAUTIONS & CONTRAINDICATIONS	ADVERSE EFFECTS†
ALZHEIMER'S AGENTS				
Donepezil HCl (Aricept, Aricept ODT)	**Tab:** 5mg, 10mg; **Tab, Disintegrating:** 5mg, 10mg	***Adults:*** Take hs. **Mild-to-Moderate Alzheimer's Disease: Usual:** 5-10mg qd. **Initial:** 5mg qd. **Titrate:** May increase to 10mg after 4-6 weeks. **Severe Alzheimer's Disease: Usual:** 10mg qd. **Initial:** 5mg qd. **Titrate:** May increase to 10mg after 4-6 weeks. Swallow tab whole with water or dissolve ODT tab on tongue and follow with water.	**W/P:** May exaggerate succinylcholine-type muscle relaxation during anesthesia. May have vagotonic effects on sinoatrial and atrioventricular node; may cause bradycardia or heart block. May increase gastric acid secretion; monitor for GI bleeding. May cause bladder outflow obstruction or seizures. Caution with asthma or COPD. **Contra:** Hypersensitivity to piperidine derivatives. **P/N:** Category C, not for use in nursing.	N/V, diarrhea, insomnia, muscle cramps, fatigue, anorexia, dizziness, depression, weight decrease, infection, HTN, back pain, abnormal dreams, ecchymosis.
Ergoloid Mesylates	**Tab:** 1mg	***Adults:* Usual:** 1mg tid.	**W/P:** Because symptoms are of unknown etiology, careful diagnosis should be attempted before prescribing. **Contra:** Acute or chronic psychosis. **P/N:** Safety in pregnancy and nursing is not known.	Transient nausea, gastric disturbances.
Galantamine Hydrobromide (Razadyne, Razadyne ER)	**Sol:** (Razadyne) 4mg/mL [100mL]; **Tab:** (Razadyne) 4mg, 8mg, 12mg **Cap, Extended-Release:** (Razadyne ER) 8mg, 16mg, 24mg	***Adults:*** (Sol, Tab) **Initial:** 4mg bid with am and pm meals. **Titrate:** Increase to 8mg bid after 4 weeks if tolerated, then increase to 12mg bid after 4 weeks if tolerated. **Usual:** 16-24mg/day. **Max:** 24mg/day. (Cap, ER) **Initial:** 8mg qd with am meal. **Titrate:** Increase to 16mg qd after 4 weeks, then increase to 24mg qd after 4 weeks if tolerated. **Usual:** 16-24mg/day. **Max:** 24mg/day. If therapy is interrupted, restart at lowest dose and increase to current dose. **Moderate Renal/Hepatic Impairment (Child-Pugh: 7-9):** Caution during dose titration. **Max:** 16mg/day. Avoid use with severe renal (CrCl <9mL/min) and severe hepatic impairment (Child-Pugh: 10-15).	**W/P:** Vagotonic effects; caution with supraventricular conduction disorder. May cause bradycardia and/or heart block. Caution with asthma or obstructive pulmonary disease. Monitor for active or occult GI bleeding and ulcers due to increased gastric acid secretion. Risk of generalized convulsions or bladder outflow obstruction. Ensure adequate fluid intake during treatment. Deaths reported with mild cognitive impairment. **P/N:** Category B, not for use in nursing.	N/V, diarrhea, anorexia, weight loss, fatigue, dizziness, headache, depression, insomnia, abdominal pain, dyspepsia, UTI.
Memantine HCl (Namenda)	**Sol:** 2mg/mL; **Tab:** 5mg, 10mg; **Titration-Pak:** 5mg [28[s]], 10mg [21[s]]	***Adults:* Target Dose:** 20mg/day. **Initial:** 5mg qd. **Titrate:** In 5mg-increments at intervals of at least one week, increase to 5mg bid (10mg/day), then one separate 5mg- and 10mg-dose per day (15mg/day), then to 10mg bid (20mg/day). **Severe Renal Impairment (5-29mL/min): Target Dose:** 5mg bid.	**W/P:** Use not evaluated with seizure disorders. Alkalinized urine (eg, renal tubular acidosis, severe urinary tract infections) may increase levels. Reduce dose with severe renal impairment. Should be administered with caution to patients with severe hepatic impairment. **P/N:** Category B, caution in nursing.	Dizziness, confusion, headache, constipation, coughing, HTN, pain, vomiting, somnolence, hallucinations.
Rivastigmine Tartrate (Exelon)	**Cap:** 1.5mg, 3mg, 4.5mg, 6mg; **Sol:** 2mg/mL [120mL]; **Patch:** 4.6mg/24 hrs, 9.5mg/24 hrs [30[s]]	***Adults:* Alzheimer's Dementia:** (Cap, Sol) **Initial:** 1.5mg bid. **Titrate:** May increase by 1.5mg bid every 2 weeks. **Max:** 12mg/day. If not tolerating, suspend therapy for several doses and restart at same or next lower dose. If interrupted longer than several days, reinitiate with lowest daily dose and titrate as above. **Dementia Associated with Parkinson's Disease:** (Cap, Sol) **Initial:** 1.5mg bid. **Titrate:** May increase by 1.5mg every 4 weeks. **Max:** 12mg/day. Take with food in am and pm. May mix solution with water, cold fruit juice, or soda. (Patch) **Alzheimer's Dementia/ Dementia Associated with Parkinson's Disease: Initial:** Apply 4.6mg/24 hrs patch qd to clean, dry, hairless intact skin. **Maint:** Increase dose after 4 weeks. **Max:** 9.5mg/24 hrs if well tolerated. **Switching from Capsules/ Oral Sol: Total Oral Daily Dose <6mg:** Switch to 4.6mg/24 hrs patch. **Total Oral Daily Dose 6-12mg:** Switch to 9.5mg/24 hrs patch. Apply first patch on day following last oral dose.	**W/P:** Significant GI intolerance (eg, nausea, vomiting, anorexia, and weight loss); always follow dosing guidelines. Vagotonic effect on HR (bradycardia), especially in sick sinus syndrome or supraventricular conduction abnormalities. May cause urinary obstruction and seizures. Monitor for peptic ulcers/GI bleeds. Caution in asthma and COPD. May exacerbate or induce extrapyramidal symptoms. (Patch) May impair mental/physical capabilities. Titrate dose with caution in patients with body weight below 50kg. **Contra:** Hypersensitivity to carbamate derivatives. **P/N:** Category B, not for use in nursing.	N/V, abdominal pain, dyspepsia, constipation, somnolence, anorexia, asthenia, headache, dizziness, fatigue, diarrhea, tremor, depression.

†Bold entries denote special dental considerations.
BB = black box warning; **W/P** = warnings/precautions; **Contra** = contraindications; **P/N** = pregnancy category rating and nursing considerations.

Table 17.1. PRESCRIBING INFORMATION FOR NEUROLOGICAL AGENTS *(cont.)*

NAME	FORM/ STRENGTH	DOSAGE	WARNINGS/PRECAUTIONS & CONTRAINDICATIONS	ADVERSE EFFECTS†
ALZHEIMER'S AGENTS *(cont.)*				
Tacrine HCl (Cognex)	**Cap:** 10mg, 20mg, 30mg, 40mg	***Adults:*** **Initial:** 10mg qid. **Titrate:** Increase to 20mg qid after 4 weeks, then increase at 4-week intervals to 30mg qid then to 40mg qid. **ALT/SGPT: >3 to ≤5x ULN:** Reduce dose by 40mg/day and resume dose titration when levels are normal. **>5x ULN:** Stop therapy and monitor; may rechallenge when ALT/SGPT levels are normal. D/C and do not rechallenge if jaundice and/or signs of hypersensitivity. **Rechallenge:** 10mg qid, may titrate if normal ALT/SGPT after 6 weeks. Monitor weekly for 16 weeks, then monthly for 2 months, and every 3 months thereafter. Take between meals.	**W/P:** Vagotonic effects; caution with conduction abnormalities, bradyarrhythmia, sick sinus syndrome. May increase risk of developing ulcers. Monitor LFTs every other week from weeks 4 to 16 from start of therapy, then every 3 months. Modify LFT monitoring based on LFTs (see dosage). Higher incidence of LFTs elevation in females. May cause seizures, bladder outflow obstruction, neutrophil abnormalities. May worsen cognitive function with abrupt withdrawal. Caution with liver disease, ulcers, asthma. D/C with clinical jaundice or hypersensitivity with ALT/SGPT elevations. **Contra:** Hypersensitivity to acridine derivatives, history of tacrine-associated jaundice (bilirubin >3mg/dL), or signs of hypersensitivity associated with ALT/SGPT elevations. **P/N:** Category C, caution in nursing.	Elevated LFTs, N/V, diarrhea, dyspepsia, myalgia, anorexia, ataxia, dizziness.
ANTICONVULSANTS				
Acetazolamide	**Inj:** 500mg; **Tab:** 125mg*, 250mg*	***Adults:*** **Epilepsy: Monotherapy:** 8-30mg/kg/day in divided doses. **Usual:** 375mg-1g/day. **Max:** 1g/day. **Combination Therapy: Initial:** 250mg qd. **Titrate:** If needed up to 1g/day. **Conversion to Monotherapy:** Should be gradual and in accordance with usual practice in epilepsy therapy.	**W/P:** Rare reports of fatal sulfonamide hypersensitivity reactions (eg, Stevens-Johnson syndrome, toxic epidermal necrolysis, fulminant hepatic necrosis, anaphylaxis, agranulocytosis, aplastic anemia, other blood dyscrasias) have occurred. D/C drug if this occurs. Sensitizations may recur when a sulfonamide is readministered irrespective of the route of administration. Dose increase does not increase diuresis and may result in decreased diuresis and increased drowsiness. Use with caution if patient predisposed to acid/base imbalances (elderly with renal impairment), DM, or impaired alveolar ventilation. Monitor serum electrolytes. Obtain CBC and platelet count before therapy and at regular intervals during therapy. **Contra:** In sodium- or potassium-depleted patients, marked hepatic or kidney impairment, cirrhosis, suprarenal gland failure, hyperchloremic acidosis, (with long-term therapy) chronic noncongestive angle-closure glaucoma. **P/N:** Category C, not for use in nursing.	Paresthesia, hearing dysfunction, tinnitus, loss of appetite, **taste alteration,** GI disturbances, polyuria, drowsiness, confusion, metabolic acidosis, electrolyte imbalance, transient myopia.
Carbamazepine (Carbatrol, Tegretol, Tegretol-XR)	**Cap, Extended-Release:** (Carbatrol) 100mg, 200mg, 300mg; **Sus:** 100mg/5mL [450mL]; **Tab:** (Tegretol) 200mg*; **Tab, Chewable:** 100mg*; **Tab, Extended-Release:** (Tegretol-XR) 100mg, 200mg, 400mg	***Adults/Pediatrics:*** **>12 yrs: Epilepsy: Initial:** (Immediate- or Extended-Release Tabs or Caps) 200mg bid or (Sus) 100mg qid. **Titrate:** (Immediate-Release Tabs/Sus) Increase weekly by 200mg/day given tid-qid. (Extended-Release Tabs) Increase weekly by 200mg/day given bid. Extended-Release Tabs should be swallowed whole and not crushed or chewed. (Extended-Release Caps) Increase weekly by 200mg/day. **Maint:** 800-1200mg/day. **Max: 12-15 yrs:** 1000mg/day; **>15yrs:** 1200mg/day. **Trigeminal Neuralgia: Initial (Day 1):** (Immediate-or Extended-Release Tabs) 100mg bid or (Extended-Release Caps) 200mg	**BB:** Serious and fatal dermatologic reactions, including toxic epidermal necrolysis (TEN) and Stevens-Johnson syndrome (SJS); increased risk with the presence of HLA-B*1502 allele reported. Aplastic anemia and agranulocytosis reported. Obtain complete pretreatment hematological testing as a baseline. D/C if evidence of bone marrow depression develops. **W/P:** Caution with history of adverse hematologic reaction to any drug, increased IOP, the elderly, mixed seizure disorder with atypical absence seizure. Fetal harm with pregnancy. May activate latent psychosis. Caution with cardiac (eg, conduction disturbance including second and 3rd-degree AV block),	Dizziness, drowsiness, unsteadiness, N/V, bone marrow depression, rash, urticaria, photosensitivity reactions, CHF, edema, HTN, hypotension, Stevens-Johnson syndrome, toxic epidermal necrolysis.

*Scored. †Bold entries denote special dental considerations.
BB = black box warning; **W/P** = warnings/precautions; **Contra** = contraindications; **P/N** = pregnancy category rating and nursing considerations.

NAME	FORM/ STRENGTH	DOSAGE	WARNINGS/PRECAUTIONS & CONTRAINDICATIONS	ADVERSE EFFECTS†
Carbamazepine (Carbatrol, Tegretol, Tegretol-XR) *(cont.)*		qd or (Sus) 50mg qid. **Titrate:** May increase to 200mg q12h (Caps/Tabs) or 100mg qid (Sus). **Maint:** 400-800mg/day. **Max:** 1200mg/day. Re-evaluate every 3 months. Extended-Release tabs should be swallowed whole and not crushed or chewed. ***Pediatrics:* Epilepsy: 6-12 yrs: Initial:** (Immediate- or Extended-Release Tabs) 100mg bid or (Sus) 50mg qid. **Titrate:** (Immediate-Release Tabs/Sus) Increase weekly by 100mg/day given tid-qid. (Extended-Release Tabs) Increase weekly by 100mg/day given bid. **Maint:** 400-800mg/day. **Max:** 1000mg/day. **6 months-6 yrs: Initial:** (Immediate-Release Tabs) 10-20mg/kg/day given bid-tid or (Sus) 10-20mg/kg/day given qid. **Titrate:** (Immediate-Release Tabs/Sus) Increase weekly tid-qid. **Max:** 35mg/kg/day. (Extended-Release Caps) May convert immediate-release dose ≥400mg/day to equal daily dose using bid regimen. **Usual/Max:** ≤35mg/kg/day.	hepatic, or renal damage. Perform eye exam and monitor LFTs and renal function at baseline and periodically. Suspension produces higher peak levels than the tablet. Avoid in hepatic porphyria (eg, acute intermittent porphyria, variegate porphyria, porphyria cutanea tarda). Withdraw gradually to minimize the potential of increased seizure frequency. **Contra:** History of bone marrow depression, MAOI use within 14 days, hypersensitivity to TCAs. Coadministration with nefazodone. **P/N:** Category D, not for use in nursing.	
Clonazepam (Klonopin, Klonopin Wafers) CIV	**Tab:** 0.5mg*, 1mg, 2mg; **Tab, Disintegrating (Wafer):** 0.125mg, 0.25mg, 0.5mg, 1mg, 2mg	***Adults:* Seizure Disorders: Initial:** Not to exceed 1.5mg/day given tid. **Titrate:** May increase by 0.5-1mg every 3 days. **Max:** 20mg qd. **Panic Disorder: Initial:** 0.25mg bid. **Titrate:** Increase to 1mg/day after 3 days, then may increase by 0.125-0.25mg bid every 3 days. **Max:** 4mg/day. **Wafer:** Dissolve in mouth with or without water. ***Pediatrics:* <10 yrs or 30kg: Seizure Disorders: Initial:** 0.01-0.03mg/kg/day up to 0.05mg/kg/day given bid-tid. **Titrate:** Increase by no more than 0.25-0.5mg every 3 days. **Maint:** 0.1-0.2mg/kg/day given tid. **Wafer:** Dissolve in mouth with or without water.	**W/P:** May increase incidence of generalized tonic-clonic seizures. Monitor blood counts and LFTs periodically with long-term therapy. Caution with renal dysfunction, chronic respiratory depression. Increased fetal risks during pregnancy. Avoid abrupt withdrawal. Hypersalivation reported. Caution may alter mental alertness. **Contra:** Significant liver disease, acute narrow-angle glaucoma, untreated open-angle glaucoma. **P/N:** Category D, not for use in nursing.	Somnolence, depression, ataxia, CNS depression, upper respiratory tract infection, fatigue, dizziness, sinusitis, colpitis.
Diazepam (Diastat) CIV	**Kit:** 2.5mg, 5mg, 10mg, 15mg, 20mg	***Adults/Pediatrics:* ≥12 yrs:** 0.2mg/kg rectally. Calculate amount and round upwards to next available dose. May give 2nd dose 4-12 hrs later. **Max:** 5 episodes/month or 1 episode every 5 days. **6-11yrs:** 0.3mg/kg. **2-5 yrs:** 0.5mg/kg. Calculate amount and round upwards to next available dose. May give 2nd dose 4-12 hrs later. For rectal administration. **Max:** 5 episodes/month and 1 episode every 5 days.	**W/P:** Produces CNS depression. Avoid abrupt withdrawal. Caution with elderly, hepatic/renal dysfunction, compromised respiratory function, neurologic damage. Not for daily chronic use. Withdrawal symptoms reported with discontinuation. **Contra:** Acute narrow-angle glaucoma, untreated open-angle glaucoma. **P/N:** Category D, not for use in nursing.	Somnolence, dizziness, headache, pain, abdominal pain, nervousness, vasodilation, diarrhea, ataxia, euphoria, incoordination, asthma, rhinitis, rash.
Divalproex Sodium (Depakote, Depakote ER)	**Cap, Delayed-Release (Sprinkle):** (Depakote) 125mg; **Tab, Delayed-Release:** (Depakote) 125mg, 250mg, 500mg; **Tab, Extended-Release:** (Depakote ER) 250mg, 500mg	***Adults:* (Depakote) Complex Partial Seizures: Initial:** 10-15mg/kg/day. **Titrate:** Increase by 5-10mg/kg/week. **Max:** 60mg/kg/day. **Absence Seizures: Initial:** 15mg/kg/day. **Titrate:** Increase weekly by 5-10mg/kg/day. **Max:** 60mg/kg/day. Give in divided doses if >250mg/day. **(Tab, DR) Migraine: Initial: ≥16 yrs:** 250mg bid. **Max:** 1000mg/day. **Mania:** 750mg daily in divided doses. **Titrate:** Increase dose rapidly to clinical effect. **Max:** 60mg/kg/day. **Elderly:** Reduce initial dose and titrate slowly. Decrease dose or d/c if decreased food or fluid intake or if excessive somnolence occurs.	**BB:** Fatal hepatic failure (<2 yrs at considerable risk), teratogenic effects (eg, neural tube defects), and life-threatening pancreatitis reported. **W/P:** Hyperammonemic encephalopathy in UCD patients; d/c if this occurs. Prior to therapy, evaluate for UCD in high-risk patients (eg, history of unexplained encephalopathy, coma, etc). Measure ammonia levels if develop unexplained lethargy, vomiting, or mental status changes. Caution with hepatic disease. Check LFTs prior to therapy, then frequently during first 6 months. Dose-related thrombocytopenia and elevated liver enzymes reported. Thrombocytopenia significantly	Diarrhea, N/V, somnolence, dyspepsia, thrombocytopenia, asthenia, abdominal pain, tremor, headache, anorexia, diplopia, blurred vision, weight gain, ataxia, nystagmus, increased appetite, asthenia, somnolence, infection, dizziness, back pain, alopecia.

Table 17.1. PRESCRIBING INFORMATION FOR NEUROLOGICAL AGENTS *(cont.)*

NAME	FORM/ STRENGTH	DOSAGE	WARNINGS/PRECAUTIONS & CONTRAINDICATIONS	ADVERSE EFFECTS†
ANTICONVULSANTS *(cont.)*				
Divalproex Sodium (Depakote, Depakote ER) *(cont.)*		**(Depakote ER)** For qd dosing. **Migraine: Initial:** 500mg qd for 1 week. **Titrate:** Increase to 1000mg qd. **Max:** 1000mg/day. **Complex Partial Seizures: Monotherapy/ Adjunct Therapy: Initial:** 10-15mg/kg/day. **Titrate:** Increase by 5-10mg/kg/week to optimal response. **Usual:** Less than 60mg/kg/day (accepted therapeutic range 50-100mcg/mL). When converting to monotherapy, reduce concomitant antiepilepsy drug by 25% every 2 weeks starting at initiation or delay 1-2 weeks after start of therapy. **Simple and Complex Absence Seizures: Initial:** 15mg/kg/day. **Titrate:** Increase weekly by 5-10mg/kg/day to optimal response. **Max:** 60mg/kg/day. **Bipolar Disorder: Initial:** 25mg/kg/day given once daily. **Titrate:** Increase dose rapidly to clinical effect. **Max:** 60mg/kg/day. **Conversion from Depakote:** Administer Depakote ER qd using a dose 8-20% higher than the total daily dose of Depakote. If cannot directly convert to Depakote ER, consider increasing to next higher Depakote total daily dose before converting to appropriate total daily Depakote ER dose. **Elderly:** Give lower initial dose and titrate slowly. Decrease dose or d/c if decreased food or fluid intake or if excessive somnolence occurs. Swallow whole; do not crush or chew. ***Pediatrics:*** **≥10 yrs: (Depakote) Complex Partial Seizures: Initial:** 10-15mg/kg/day. **Titrate:** Increase by 5-10mg/kg/week. **Max:** 60mg/kg/day. **Absence Seizures: Initial:** 15mg/kg/day. **Titrate:** Increase weekly by 5-10mg/kg/day. **Max:** 60mg/kg/day. Give in divided doses if >250mg/day. **(Depakote ER)** For qd dosing. **Complex Partial Seizures: Monotherapy/Adjunct Therapy: Initial:** 10-15mg/kg/day. **Titrate:** Increase by 5-10mg/kg/week to optimal response. **Usual:** Less than 60mg/kg/day (accepted therapeutic range 50-100mcg/mL). When converting to monotherapy, reduce concomitant antiepilepsy drug by 25% every 2 weeks starting at initiation or delay 1-2 weeks after start of therapy. **Simple and Complex Absence Seizures: Initial:** 15mg/kg/day. **Titrate:** Increase weekly by 5-10mg/kg/day to optimal response. **Max:** 60mg/kg/day.	increases with plasma trough levels >110mcg/mL in females and >135mcg/mL in males. Monitor platelet and coagulation tests prior to therapy, then periodically. Altered thyroid function tests and urine ketone test. May stimulate replication of HIV and CMV viruses. Avoid abrupt discontinuation. **Contra:** Hepatic disease, significant hepatic dysfunction, known urea cycle disorders (UCD). **P/N:** Category D, not for use in nursing.	
Ethosuximide (Zarontin)	**Cap:** 250mg; **Syrup:** 250mg/5mL	***Adults/Pediatrics:*** **≥6 yrs: Initial:** 500mg qd. **3-6 yrs: Initial:** 250mg qd. **Titrate:** May increase daily dose by 250mg every 4-7 days. **Optimal Pediatric Dose:** 20mg/kg/day. **Max:** 1.5g/day.	**W/P:** Extreme caution in liver and renal dysfunction. Monitor blood counts, liver and renal function periodically. SLE, blood dyscrasias reported. Adjust dose slowly and avoid abrupt withdrawal. May increase grand mal seizures in mixed types of epilepsy when used alone. Caution with mental/physical activities. **P/N:** Safety in pregnancy and nursing not known.	Anorexia, N/V, abdominal pain, blood dyscrasias, drowsiness, headache, urticaria, SLE, myopia.

*Scored. †Bold entries denote special dental considerations.
BB = black box warning; **W/P** = warnings/precautions; **Contra** = contraindications; **P/N** = pregnancy category rating and nursing considerations.

NAME	FORM/ STRENGTH	DOSAGE	WARNINGS/PRECAUTIONS & CONTRAINDICATIONS	ADVERSE EFFECTS†
Felbamate (Felbatol)	**Sus:** 600mg/5mL [240mL, 960mL]; **Tab:** 400mg*, 600mg*	***Adults/Pediatrics:* ≥14 yrs: Initial Monotherapy:** 300mg qid or 400mg tid. **Titrate:** Increase by 600mg every 2 weeks to 2.4g/day. **Max:** 3.6g/day. **Conversion to Monotherapy from Combination Therapy:** 300mg qid or 400mg tid while reducing present AED. **Titrate:** Increase at Week 2 to 2.4g/day, at Week 3 up to 3.6g/day, while continuing to decrease other AEDs. **Adjunctive Therapy: Initial:** 300mg qid or 400mg tid while reducing present AEDs by 20% to control drug concentrations. **Titrate:** Increase by 1.2g/day every week up to a daily dose of 3.6mg/day. **Renal Dysfunction:** May need to reduce dose with concomitant AEDs. ***Pediatrics:* 2-14 yrs: Lennox-Gastaut Syndrome: Adjunct Therapy:** 15mg/kg/day in 3-4 divided doses while reducing present AED by 20% to control drug concentrations. **Titrate:** Increase by 15mg/kg/day increments at weekly intervals to 45mg/kg/day.	**BB:** Associated with aplastic anemia and fatal hepatic failure. Monitor blood, LFTs. Avoid in history of hepatic dysfunction. **W/P:** Avoid abrupt discontinuation. Caution with renal dysfunction. Obtain written, informed consent. Obtain full hematologic evaluations and LFTs before, during, and after discontinuation. D/C if bone marrow depression or liver abnormalities occur. **Contra:** History of blood dyscrasias, hepatic dysfunction. **P/N:** Category C, safety in nursing not known.	Anorexia, N/V, insomnia, headache, anemias, hepatic failure.
Fosphenytoin Sodium (Cerebyx)	**Inj:** 50mg PE/mL (2mL, 10mL)	***Adults:*** Doses, concentration in dosing solutions, and infusion rates are expressed as phenytoin sodium equivalents (PE). **Status Epilepticus: LD:** 15-20 PE/kg IV at 100-150mg PE/min then switch to maintenance dose. **Nonemergent Cases: LD:** 10-20mg PE/kg IV (max 150mg PE/min) or IM. **Maint: Initial:** 4-6mg PE/kg/day. May substitute for oral phenytoin sodium at the same total daily dose.	**W/P:** Avoid abrupt discontinuation. Not for use in absence seizures. Hypotension and severe cardiovascular reactions and fatalities reported; continuously monitor ECG, BP, and respiration during and for at least 20 min after IV infusion and monitor phenytoin levels at least 2 hrs after IV infusion or 4 hrs after IM injection. Caution with severe myocardial insufficiency, porphyria, hepatic/renal dysfunction, hypoalbuminemia, elderly, and diabetes. Acute hepatotoxicity, lymphadenopathy, hemopoietic complications, hyperglycemia reported. D/C if rash or acute hepatotoxicity occurs. Neonatal postpartum bleeding disorder, congenital malformations, and increased seizure frequency reported with use during pregnancy. Avoid use with seizures due to hypoglycemia or other metabolic causes. Caution with phosphate restriction because of phosphate load (0.0037mmol phosphate/mg PE). May lower folate levels. **Contra:** Sinus bradycardia, sino-atrial block, 2nd- and 3rd-degree AV block, Adams-Stokes syndrome. **P/N:** Category D, not for use in nursing.	Nystagmus, dizziness, pruritus, paresthesia, headache, somnolence, ataxia, tinnitus, stupor, nausea, hypotension, vasodilation, tremor, incoordination, **dry mouth.**
Gabapentin (Neurontin)	**Cap:** 100mg, 300mg, 400mg; **Sol:** 250mg/5mL; **Tab:** 600mg*, 800mg*	***Adults:* Epilepsy: Initial:** 300mg tid. **Titrate:** Increase up to 1800mg/day. **Max:** 3600mg/day. **PHN:** 300mg single dose on Day 1, then 300mg bid on Day 2, and 300mg tid on Day 3. Increase further prn for pain. **Max:** 600mg tid. **Renal Impairment: CrCl 30-59mL/min:** 400-1400 mg/day. **CrCl 15-29mL/min:** 200-700 mg/day. **CrCl 15mL/min:** 100-300mg/day. **CrCl <15 mL/min:** Reduce dose in proportion to CrCl. **Hemodialysis: Maint:** Base on CrCl. Give supplemental dose (125-350mg) after 4 hrs of hemodialysis. Refer to prescribing information for dose-adjustment. ***Pediatrics:* Epilepsy: >12 yrs: Initial:** 300mg tid. **Titrate:** Increase up to 1800mg/day. **Max:** 3600mg/day.	**W/P:** Avoid abrupt withdrawal. Possible tumorigenic potential. Sudden and unexplained deaths reported. Neuropsychiatric adverse events in pediatrics (3-12 yrs). **P/N:** Category C, caution in nursing.	Somnolence, dizziness, ataxia, nystagmus, fatigue, tremor, rhinitis, weight gain, N/V, viral infection, fever, dysarthria, diplopia.

Table 17.1. PRESCRIBING INFORMATION FOR NEUROLOGICAL AGENTS *(cont.)*

NAME	FORM/ STRENGTH	DOSAGE	WARNINGS/PRECAUTIONS & CONTRAINDICATIONS	ADVERSE EFFECTS†
ANTICONVULSANTS *(cont.)*				
Gabapentin (Neurontin) *(cont.)*		**3-12 yrs: Initial:** 10-15mg/kg/day given tid. **Titrate:** Increase over 3 days. **Usual: 3-4 yrs:** 40mg/kg/day given tid. **≥5 yrs:** 25-35mg/kg/day given tid. **Max:** 50mg/kg/day. **Renal Impairment: ≥12 yrs: CrCl 30-59mL/min:** 400-1400 mg/day. **CrCl 15-29mL/min:** 200-700 mg/day. **CrCl 15mL/min:** 100-300mg/day. **CrCl <15 mL/min:** Reduce dose in proportion to CrCl. **Hemodialysis: Maint:** Base on CrCl. Give supplemental dose (125-350 mg) after 4 hrs of hemodialysis. Refer to prescribing information for dose-adjustment.		
Lamotrigine (Lamictal, Lamictal CD)	**Tab:** 25mg*, 100mg*, 150mg*, 200mg*; **Tab, Chewable:** (Lamictal CD) 2mg, 5mg, 25mg	***Adults:* Epilepsy: Concomitant AEDs with Valproate (VPA): Weeks 1 and 2:** 25mg every other day. **Weeks 3 and 4:** 25mg qd. **Titrate:** Increase every 1-2 weeks by 25-50mg/day. **Maint:** 100-400mg/day, given qd or bid; 100-200mg/day when added to VPA alone. **Concomitant EIAEDs without VPA: Weeks 1 and 2:** 50mg qd. **Weeks 3 and 4:** 50mg bid. **Titrate:** Increase every 1-2 weeks by 100mg/day. **Maint:** 150-250mg bid. **Conversion to Monotherapy From Single EIAED: ≥16 yrs: Weeks 1 and 2:** 50mg qd. **Weeks 3 and 4:** 50mg bid. **Titrate:** Increase every 1-2 weeks by 100mg/day. **Maint:** 250mg bid. Withdraw EIAED over 4 weeks. **Conversion to Monotherapy From VPA: ≥16 yrs: Step 1:** Follow Concomitant AEDs with VPA dosing regimen to achieve lamotrigine dose of 200mg/day. Maintain previous VPA dose. **Step 2:** Maintain lamotrigine 200mg/day. Decrease VPA to 500mg/day by decrements of ≤500mg/day per week. Maintain VPA 500mg/day for 1 week. **Step 3:** Increase to lamotrigine 300mg/day for 1 week. Decrease VPA simultaneously to 250mg/day for 1 week. **Step 4:** D/C VPA. Increase lamotrigine 100mg/day every week to maint dose of 500mg/day. **Bipolar Disorder: Patients Not Taking Carbamazepine, Other Enzyme-Inducing Drugs (EIDs) or VPA: Weeks 1 and 2:** 25mg qd. **Weeks 3 and 4:** 50mg qd. **Week 5:** 100mg qd. **Weeks 6 and 7:** 200mg qd. **Patients Taking VPA: Weeks 1 and 2:** 25mg every other day. **Weeks 3 and 4:** 25mg qd. **Week 5:** 50mg qd. **Weeks 6 and 7:** 100mg qd. **Patients Taking Carbamazepine (Or Other EIDs) and Not Taking VPA: Weeks 1 and 2:** 50mg qd. **Weeks 3 and 4:** 100mg qd (divided doses). **Week 5:** 200mg qd (divided doses). **Week 6:** 300mg qd (divided doses). **Week 7:** up to 400mg qd (divided doses). **After D/C of Psychotropic Drugs Excluding VPA, Carbamazepine, or Other EIDs:** Maintain current dose. **After D/C of VPA and current lamotrigine dose of 100mg qd: Week 1:** 150mg qd. **Week 2 and onward:** 200mg qd. **After D/C of**	**BB:** Serious, life-threatening rash, including Stevens-Johnson syndrome and toxic epidermal necrolysis, reported. Occurs more often in pediatrics than adults. D/C at first sign of rash. **W/P:** Risk of serious life-threatening rash; d/c if rash occurs. Multiorgan failure, sudden unexplained death, hypersensitivity reactions, and pure red cell aplasia reported. Avoid abrupt withdrawal. Caution with renal, hepatic, or cardiac functional impairment. May cause ophthalmic toxicity. Do not exceed recommended initial dose and dose escalations. Caution in elderly. Chewable tabs may be swallowed whole, chewed (with water/diluted fruit juice), or dispersed in water/diluted fruit juice; do administer partial quantities. **P/N:** Category C, not for use in nursing.	Serious rash, dizziness, ataxia, somnolence, headache, diplopia, blurred vision, N/V, insomnia, back/abdominal pain, fatigue, xerostomia, rhinitis.

*Scored. †Bold entries denote special dental considerations.
BB = black box warning; **W/P** = warnings/precautions; **Contra** = contraindications; **P/N** = pregnancy category rating and nursing considerations.

NAME	FORM/ STRENGTH	DOSAGE	WARNINGS/PRECAUTIONS & CONTRAINDICATIONS	ADVERSE EFFECTS†
Lamotrigine (Lamictal, Lamictal CD) *(cont.)*		**Carbamazepine or Other EIDs and current Lamotrigine Dose of 400mg qd: Week 1:** 400mg qd. **Week 2:** 300mg qd. **Week 3 and Onward:** 200mg qd. **Concomitant or Starting Estrogen-Containing Oral Contraceptives:** not taking carbamazepine, phenytoin, phenobarbital, primidone, or rifampin, lamotrigine should be increased by as much as 2-fold over the recommended target maintenance dose; the dose increase should start at the same time as the initiation and continuation of contraceptives. **Stopping Estrogen-Containing Oral Contraceptives:** may decrease lamictal by as much as 50%. **Hepatic Impairment: Initial/ Titrate/Maint:** Reduce by 50% for moderate (Child-Pugh Grade B) and 75% for severe (Child-Pugh Grade C) impairment. **Significant Renal Impairment: Maint:** Reduce dose. **Elderly:** Start at low end of dosing range. ***Pediatrics:*** Round dose down to nearest whole tab. **2-12 yrs: ≥6.7kg: Lennox-Gastaut/Partial Seizures: Concomitant AEDs w/ VPA: Weeks 1 and 2:** 0.15mg/kg/day given qd-bid. **Weeks 3 and 4:** 0.3mg/kg/day given qd or bid. **Titrate:** Increase q1-2 weeks by 0.3mg/ kg/day. **Maint:** 1-5mg/kg/day given qd or bid; 1-3mg/kg/day when added to VPA alone. **Max:** 200mg/day. **Concomitant AEDs w/o VPA: Weeks 1 and 2:** 0.3mg/ kg/day given qd or bid. **Weeks 3 and 4:** 0.6mg/kg/day given bid. **Titrate:** Increase q1-2 weeks by 0.6mg/kg/day. **Maint:** 4.5-7.5mg/kg/day given bid. **Max:** 300mg/day. **Concomitant EIAEDs w/o VPA: Weeks 1 and 2:** 0.6mg/kg/day given bid. **Weeks 3 and 4:** 1.2mg/kg/day given bid. **Titrate:** Increase q1-2 weeks by 1.2mg/kg/day. **Maint:** 5-15mg/kg/day given bid. **Max:** 400mg/day. **>12 yrs: Concomitant AEDs w/ VPA: Weeks 1 and 2:** 25mg every other day. **Weeks 3 and 4:** 25mg qd. **Titrate:** Increase q1-2 weeks by 25-50mg/ day. **Maint:** 100-400mg/day, given qd or bid; 100-200mg/day when added to VPA alone. **Concomitant AEDs w/o VPA: Weeks 1 and 2:** 25mg qd. **Weeks 3 and 4:** 50mg qd. **Titrate:** Increase q1-2 weeks by 50mg/day. **Maint:** 225 to 375mg/day given bid. **Concomitant EIAEDs w/o VPA: Weeks 1 and 2:** 50mg qd. **Weeks 3 and 4:** 50mg bid. **Titrate:** Increase q1-2 weeks by 100mg/day. **Maint:** 150-250mg bid. **Hepatic Impairment: Initial/Titrate/Maint:** Reduce by 50% for moderate (Child-Pugh Grade B) and 75% for severe (Child-Pugh Grade C) impairment. **Significant Renal Impairment: Maint:** Reduce dose.		
Levetiracetam (Keppra)	**Inj:** 500mg/5mL; **Sol:** 100mg/mL; **Tab:** 250mg*, 500mg*, 750mg*, 1000mg*	***Adults:*** **Inj/PO: Initial:** 500mg bid. **Titrate:** Increase by 1000mg/day every 2 weeks. **Max:** 3000mg/day. **Inj: Replacement Therapy:** Initial total daily dosage and frequency should equal total daily dosage and frequency of oral therapy. Dilute injection in 100mL of compatible diluent and give as 15-min IV infusion. **Individualize Dose: CrCl >80mL/min:** 500mg-1500mg q12h. **CrCl 50-80mL/ min:** 500mg-1000mg q12h. **CrCl 30-50mL/min:** 250mg-750mg q12h. **CrCl <30mL/min:** 250mg-500mg q12h. **ESRD with Dialysis:** 500-1000mg q24h. A supplemental dose of 250mg-500mg	**W/P:** Associated with somnolence, fatigue, coordination difficulties, and behavioral abnormalities (eg, psychotic symptoms, suicide ideation, and other abnormalities). Avoid abrupt withdrawal. Hematologic abnormalities reported. Caution in renal dysfunction. Myoclonic seizures reported. **P/N:** Category C, not for use in nursing.	Somnolence, asthenia, headache, infection, pain, anorexia, dizziness, nervousness, vertigo, ataxia, **pharyngitis**, rhinitis, irritability, hepatic failure.

Table 17.1. PRESCRIBING INFORMATION FOR NEUROLOGICAL AGENTS *(cont.)*

NAME	FORM/ STRENGTH	DOSAGE	WARNINGS/PRECAUTIONS & CONTRAINDICATIONS	ADVERSE EFFECTS†
ANTICONVULSANTS *(cont.)*				
Levetiracetam (Keppra) *(cont.)*		after dialysis is recommended. ***Pediatrics:*** **PO: Partial-Onset Seizures/PGTC: ≥16 yrs or JME: ≥12 yrs: Initial:** 500mg bid. **Titrate:** Increase by 1000mg/day every 2 weeks. **Max:** 3000mg/day. **Partial-Onset Seizures: 4 to <16 yrs or PGTC: 6-16 yrs: Initial:** 10mg/kg bid: **Titrate:** Increase by 20mg/kg/day every 2 weeks. **Max:** 60mg/kg/day. **Inj: Partial-Onset Seizures: Initial:** 500mg bid. **Titrate:** Increase by 1000mg/day every 2 weeks. **Max:** 3000mg/day. **Replacement Therapy:** Initial total daily dosage and frequency should equal total daily dosage and frequency of oral therapy. Dilute injection in 100mL of compatible diluent and give as 15-min IV infusion. **CrCl >80mL/min:** 500mg-1500mg q12h. **CrCl 50-80mL/min:** 500mg-1000mg q12h. **CrCl 30-50mL/min:** 250mg-750mg q12h. **CrCl <30mL/min:** 250mg-500mg q12h. **ESRD with Dialysis:** 500mg-1000mg q24h. A supplemental dose of 250mg-500mg after dialysis is recommended.		
Mephobarbital (Mebaral) CIV	**Tab:** 32mg*, 50mg*, 100mg	***Adults:*** **Epilepsy:** 400-600mg/day. Start with small dose, gradually increase over 4-5 days until optimum dose. **Elderly/Debilitated/Renal or Hepatic Dysfunction:** Reduce dose. **Concomitant Phenobarbital:** Give 50% of each drug. **Concomitant Phenytoin:** Reduce phenytoin dose. **Sedation:** 32-100mg tid-qid. **Optimum Dose:** 50mg tid-qid. ***Pediatrics:*** **Epilepsy: >5 yrs:** 32-64mg tid-qid. **<5 yrs:** 16-32mg tid-qid. Start with small dose, gradually increase over 4-5 days until optimum dose. **Sedation:** 16-32mg tid-qid.	**W/P:** May be habit forming; tolerance and dependence may occur with continued use. Avoid abrupt withdrawal. Caution in acute/chronic pain; paradoxical excitement may occur or symptoms masked. Can cause fetal damage. May cause marked excitement, depression, and confusion in elderly or debilitated. Reduce initial dose with hepatic damage. Careful adjustment in impaired renal, cardiac, or respiratory function, myasthenia gravis, and myxedema. May increase vitamin D requirements. Caution with depression, suicidal tendencies, and history of drug abuse. **Contra:** Manifest or latent porphyria. **P/N:** Category D, caution with nursing.	Somnolence, agitation, confusion, hyperkinesia, ataxia, CNS depression, hypoventilation, apnea, bradycardia, hypotension, syncope, N/V, headache.
Methsuximide (Celontin)	**Cap:** 150mg, 300mg	***Adults/Pediatrics:*** **Initial:** 300mg qd for 7 days. **Titrate:** Increase weekly by 300mg/day for 3 weeks if needed. **Max:** 1.2g/day. Use 150mg caps in small children.	**W/P:** Fatal blood dyscrasias reported; monitor blood counts periodically or if signs of infection. SLE reported. Withdraw slowly if altered behavior appears. May increase frequency of grand mal seizures if given alone in mixed type of seizures. Avoid abrupt withdrawal. Caution with renal/hepatic disease. May impair mental/physical abilities. **P/N:** Safety in pregnancy and nursing not known.	GI effects, blood dyscrasias, dermatologic manifestations, drowsiness, ataxia, dizziness, hyperemia, proteinuria, periorbital edema.
Oxcarbazepine (Trileptal)	**Sus:** 300mg/5mL [250mL]; **Tab:** 150mg*, 300mg*, 600mg*	***Adults:*** **Monotherapy: Initial:** 300mg bid. **Titrate:** Increase by 300mg/day every 3rd day. **Maint:** 1200mg/day. **Adjunct Therapy: Initial:** 300mg bid. **Titrate:** Increase weekly by a maximum of 600mg/day. **Maint:** 600mg bid. **Conversion to Monotherapy: Initial:**	**W/P:** Risk of hyponatremia. Cross sensitivity with carbamazepine. Avoid abrupt withdrawal. Adjust dose in renal impairment. Reports of serious dermatologic reactions (eg, Stevens-Johnson syndrome, toxic epidermal necrolysis). CNS effects reported (eg, psychomotor	Dizziness, somnolence, diplopia, N/V, asthenia, nystagmus, ataxia, abnormal vision, tremor, abnormal gait, headache.

*Scored. †Bold entries denote special dental considerations.
BB = black box warning; **W/P** = warnings/precautions; **Contra** = contraindications; **P/N** = pregnancy category rating and nursing considerations.

NAME	FORM/ STRENGTH	DOSAGE	WARNINGS/PRECAUTIONS & CONTRAINDICATIONS	ADVERSE EFFECTS†
Oxcarbazepine (Trileptal) *(cont.)*		300mg bid while reducing other AEDs. **Titrate:** Increase weekly by 600mg/day. Withdraw other AEDs over 3-6 weeks. **Maint:** 2400mg/day. **Renal Impairment: CrCl <30mL/min: Initial:** 300mg qd. **Titrate:** Increase gradually. ***Pediatrics:* 4-16 yrs: Monotherapy: Initial:** 4-5mg/kg bid. **Titrate:** Increase by 5mg/kg/day every 3rd day. **Maint (mg/day): 20kg: Initial:** 600mg. **Max:** 900mg. **25-30kg: Initial:** 900mg. **Max:** 1200mg. **35-40kg: Initial:** 900mg. **Max:** 1500mg. **45kg: Initial:** 1200mg. **Max:** 1500mg. **50-55kg: Initial:** 1200mg. **Max:** 1800mg. **60-65kg: Initial:** 1200mg. **Max:** 2100mg. **70kg: Initial:** 1500mg. **Max:** 2100mg. **Adjunct Therapy: Initial:** 4-5mg/kg bid. **Max:** 600mg/day. **Titrate:** Increase over 2 weeks. **Maint (mg/day): 20-29kg:** 900mg. **29.1-39kg:** 1200mg. **>39kg:** 1800mg. **Conversion to Monotherapy: Initial:** 4-5mg/kg bid while reducing other AEDs. **Titrate:** Increase weekly by max of 10mg/kg/day to target dose. Withdraw other AEDs over 3-6 weeks. **Renal Impairment: CrCl <30mL/min: Initial:** 300mg qd. **Titrate:** Increase gradually.	slowing, concentration difficulty, speech or language problems, somnolence or fatigue, coordination abnormalities). Reports of multiorgan hypersensitivity reactions in close temporal association to initiation of therapy. Rare cases of anaphylaxis and angioedema involving the larynx, glottis, lips, and eyelids reported. **P/N:** Category C, not for use in nursing.	
Pentobarbital Sodium (Nembutal Sodium)	**Inj:** 50mg/mL	***Adults:* Usual: IM:** 150-200mg as a single IM injection. **IV:** 100mg (commonly used initial dose for 70kg adult); if needed additional small increments may be given up to 200-500mg total dose. Rate of IV injection should not exceed 50mg/min. **Elderly/Debilitated/Renal or Hepatic Impairment:** Reduce dose. ***Pediatrics:* IM:** 2-6mg/kg as a single IM injection. **Max:** 100mg. **IV:** Proportional reduction in dosage. Slow IV injection is essential.	**W/P:** May be habit-forming; avoid abrupt cessation after prolonged use. Avoid rapid administration. Tolerance to hypnotic effect can occur. Prehepatic coma use not recommended. Use with caution in patients with chronic or acute pain, mental depression, suicidal tendencies, history of drug abuse, or hepatic impairment. Monitor blood, liver and renal function. May impair mental/physical abilities. Avoid alcohol. **Contra:** History of manifest or latent porphyria. **P/N:** Category D, caution with nursing.	Agitation, confusion, hyperkinesia, ataxia, CNS depression, somnolence, bradycardia, hypotension, NV, constipation, headache, hypersensitivity reactions, liver damage.
Phenobarbital CIV	**Elixir:** 20mg/5mL; **Tab:** 15mg, 30mg, 32.4mg, 60mg, 64.8mg, 100mg	***Adults:* Sedation:** 30-120mg/day given bid-tid. **Max:** 400mg/24h. **Hypnotic:** 100-200mg. **Seizures:** 60-200mg/day. **Elderly/Debilitated/Renal or Hepatic Dysfunction:** Reduce dosage. ***Pediatrics:* Seizures:** 3-6mg/kg/day.	**W/P:** May be habit forming. Avoid abrupt withdrawal. Caution with acute or chronic pain; may mask symptoms or paradoxical excitement may occur. Cognitive deficits reported in children with febrile seizures. May cause excitement in children and excitement, depression, or confusion in elderly and debilitated. Caution with hepatic dysfunction, borderline hypoadrenal function, depression. **Contra:** Respiratory disease with dyspnea or obstruction, porphyria, severe liver dysfunction. Large doses with nephritic patients. **P/N:** Category D, caution in nursing.	Drowsiness, residual sedation, lethargy, vertigo, somnolence, respiratory depression, hypersensitivity reactions, N/V, headache.
Phenytoin Sodium (Dilantin, Phenytek)	**Cap, Extended-Release (CER):** (Dilantin) 30mg, 100mg; (Phenytek) 200mg, 300mg; **Sus:** 125mg/5mL	***Adults:*** (CER) **Initial:** 100mg tid. **Titrate:** May increase at 7-10 day intervals. **Max:** 200mg tid. May give once daily with extended-release if controlled on 300mg daily. **LD (clinic/hospital):** 1g in 3 divided doses (400mg, 300mg, 300mg) given 2 hrs apart. Start	**W/P:** Avoid abrupt discontinuation. Caution with porphyria, hepatic dysfunction, elderly, diabetes, debilitated. D/C if rash occurs. Lymphadenopathy reported. Serum sickness may occur with lymph node involvement. Gingival hyperplasia reported; maintain proper dental	Nystagmus, ataxia, slurred speech, decreased coordination, confusion, dizziness, insomnia, transient nervousness,

Table 17.1. PRESCRIBING INFORMATION FOR NEUROLOGICAL AGENTS *(cont.)*

NAME	FORM/ STRENGTH	DOSAGE	WARNINGS/PRECAUTIONS & CONTRAINDICATIONS	ADVERSE EFFECTS†
ANTICONVULSANTS *(cont.)*				
Phenytoin Sodium (Dilantin, Phenytek) *(cont.)*	[237mL]; **Tab, Chewable (CTB):** 50mg*	maintenance 24 hrs later. Avoid LD with renal and hepatic disease. (CTB) **Initial:** 100mg tid. **Titrate:** May increase at 7-10 day intervals. **Usual:** 300-400mg/day. **Max:** 600mg/day. May chew or swallow tab whole. Not for once daily dosing. (Sus) **Initial:** 125mg tid. **Titrate:** May increase at 7-10 day intervals. **Max:** 625mg/day. ***Pediatrics:*** (CER, CTB, Sus) **Initial:** 5mg/kg/day given bid-tid. **Titrate:** May increase at 7-10 day intervals. **Maint:** 4-8mg/kg/day. **Max:** 300mg/day. **>6 yrs:** May require the minimum adult dose (300mg/day).	hygiene. Hyperglycemia, birth defects, and osteomalacia reported. Monitor levels. Confusional states reported with increased levels. Increased seizure frequency during pregnancy. Neonatal coagulation defects reported within first 24 hrs of birth. Give vitamin K to mother before delivery and to neonate after birth. Avoid use with seizures due to hypoglycemia or other metabolic causes. **P/N:** Possibly teratogenic, weigh benefits versus risk; not for use in nursing.	motor twitchings, headaches, N/V, constipation, rash, hypersensitivity reactions.
Pregabalin (Lyrica) CV	**Cap:** 25mg, 50mg, 75mg, 100mg, 150mg, 200mg, 225mg, 300mg	***Adults:*** **Neuropathic Pain: Initial:** 50mg tid (150mg/day). **Titrate:** May increase to 300mg/day within 1 week. **Max:** 100mg tid (300mg/day). **Postherpetic Neuralgia: Initial:** 150mg/day divided bid or tid. **Max:** 600mg/day divided bid or tid. **Epilepsy: Initial:** 150mg/day divided bid-tid. **Max:** 600mg/day. **Fibromyalgia: Initial:** 75mg bid (150mg/day). **Titrate:** May increase to 150mg bid (300mg/day) within 1 week based on efficacy and tolerability. May further increase to 225mg bid (450mg/day) if needed. **Max:** 450mg/day. **Renal Impairment: CrCl 30-60 mL/min:** 75-300mg/day divided bid or tid. **CrCl 15-30 mL/min:** 25-150mg/day divided qd or bid. **CrCl <15mL/min:** 25-75mg/day given qd. Give supplemental dose (25-150mg) immediately after every 4-hr hemodialysis treatment. Refer to prescribing information for further details. **D/C:** Taper over minimum of 1 week.	**W/P:** Avoid abrupt withdrawal. Gradually taper over 1 week. Possible tumorigenic potential. May impair physical/mental abilities. May cause weight gain; blurred vision, monitor for ophthalmic changes; peripheral edema, caution in heart failure; elevated creatine kinase, d/c if myopathy or markedly elevated creatine kinase levels occur; decreased platelet count; and mild PR-interval prolongation. Angioedema reported in initial and chronic treatment. **P/N:** Category C, not for use in nursing.	Somnolence, dizziness, **dry mouth,** edema, blurred vision, weight gain, abnormal thinking (difficulty with concentration/attention), headache, nausea, diarrhea.
Primidone (Mysoline)	**Tab:** 50mg*, 250mg*	***Adults/Pediatrics:*** **≥8 yrs: Initial: Day 1-3:** 100-125mg qhs. **Day 4-6:** 100-125mg bid. **Day 7-9:** 100-125mg tid. **Day 10-Maint:** 250mg tid. **Max:** 500mg qid. Effective serum level is 5-12mcg/mL. **Prior Anticonvulsant Therapy: Initial:** 100-125mg qhs. **Titrate:** Increase gradually to maintenance dose as other drug is discontinued over 2 weeks. **<8 yrs: Day 1-3:** 50mg qhs. **Day 4-6:** 50mg bid. **Day 7-9:** 100mg bid. **Day 10-Maint:** 125-250mg tid or 10-25mg/kg/day in divided doses. Effective serum level is 5-12mcg/mL.	**W/P:** Avoid abrupt withdrawal. May take several weeks to assess therapeutic efficacy. Pregnant women should receive prophylactic vitamin K_1 therapy for 1 month prior to and during delivery. Perform CBC and SMA-12 test every 6 months. Phenobarbital is a metabolite of primidone. **Contra:** Porphyria, phenobarbital hypersensitivity. **P/N:** Safety in pregnancy not known, caution in nursing.	Ataxia, vertigo, N/V, anorexia, fatigue, hyperirritability, emotional disturbances, sexual impotency, diplopia, nystagmus, drowsiness, morbilliform skin eruptions.
Tiagabine HCl (Gabitril)	**Tab:** 2mg, 4mg, 12mg, 16mg	***Adults:*** **Initial:** 4mg qd. **Titrate:** May increase weekly by 4-8mg until clinical response. **Max:** 56mg/day given bid-qid. Take with food. ***Pediatrics:*** **≥12 yrs: Initial:** 4mg qd. **Titrate:** May increase to 8mg qd at beginning of Week 2, then increase weekly by 4-8mg until clinical response. **Max:** 32mg/day. Take with food.	**W/P:** Reports of new-onset seizure or status epilepticus in patients without epilepsy. D/C and evaluate for underlying seizure disorder. Avoid abrupt withdrawal. Monitor during initial titration for impaired concentration, speech problem, somnolence, fatigue; may require hospitalization if reaction is severe. May exacerbate EEG abnormalities; adjust dose. Status epilepticus and sudden death reported. Reduce dose or d/c if generalized weakness occurs. Reduce dose with hepatic impairment. Serious skin rash reported. **P/N:** Category C, caution in nursing.	Dizziness, asthenia, somnolence, N/V, nervousness, tremor, abdominal pain, abnormal thinking, depression, confusion, **pharyngitis,** rash.

*Scored. †Bold entries denote special dental considerations.
BB = black box warning; **W/P** = warnings/precautions; **Contra** = contraindications; **P/N** = pregnancy category rating and nursing considerations.

NAME	FORM/ STRENGTH	DOSAGE	WARNINGS/PRECAUTIONS & CONTRAINDICATIONS	ADVERSE EFFECTS†
Topiramate (Topamax, Topamax Sprinkle Capsules)	**Cap, Sprinkle:** 15mg, 25mg; **Tab:** 25mg, 50mg, 100mg, 200mg	***Adults:* Seizures: Monotherapy: Initial:** 25mg qam and qpm for 1 week. **Titrate:** Increase am and pm dose by 25mg every week until 200mg/day, then increase by 50mg every week until 400mg/day. **Adjunct Therapy: ≥17 yrs: Initial:** 25-50mg/day. **Titrate:** Increase by 25-50mg/week. **Usual: Partial:** 100-200mg bid. **Tonic-Clonic:** 200mg bid. **Max:** 1600mg/day. **Migraine Prophylaxis: Titrate: Week 1:** 25mg qpm. **Week 2:** 25mg bid. **Week 3:** 25mg qam and 50mg qpm. **Week 4:** 50mg bid. **Usual:** 50mg bid. **Renal Dysfunction:** 50% of usual dose. Swallow caps whole or sprinkle over food. ***Pediatrics:* Seizures: Monotherapy: ≥10 yrs: Initial:** 25mg qam and qpm for 1 week. **Titrate:** Increase am and pm dose by 25mg every week until 200mg/day, then increase by 50mg every week until 400mg/day. **Adjunct Therapy: 2-16 yrs: Initial:** 1-3mg/kg nightly for 1 week. **Titrate:** Increase by 1-3mg/kg/day every 1-2 weeks. **Usual:** 2.5-4.5mg/kg bid. Swallow caps whole or sprinkle over food.	**W/P:** Hyperchloremic, nonanion gap, metabolic acidosis reported; obtain baseline and periodic serum bicarbonate levels. Withdraw gradually. Psychomotor slowing, difficulty with concentration, speech/language problems, paresthesia, acute myopia with secondary angle closure glaucoma, oligohidrosis, hyperthermia, and dose-related depression or mood problems reported. May cause hyperammonemia and encephalopathy if used concomitantly with valproic acid. Risk of kidney stones; maintain adequate fluid intake. Caution with renal or hepatic dysfunction. **P/N:** Category C, caution in nursing.	Somnolence, fatigue, dizziness, ataxia, speech disorders, psychomotor slowing, abnormal vision, memory difficulty, paresthesia, diplopia, depression, anorexia, anxiety, mood problems, pancreatitis, hepatic failure.
Valproate Sodium (Depacon)	**Inj:** 100mg/mL	***Adults/Pediatrics:* Simple/Complex Absence Seizure: ≥2 yrs: Initial:** 15mg/kg/day. **Titrate:** Increase weekly by 5-10mg/kg/day until optimal response. **Max:** 60mg/kg/day. **Complex Partial Seizure: ≥10 yrs: Initial:** 10-15mg/kg/day. **Titrate:** Increase weekly by 5-10mg/kg/day until optimal response. **Max:** 60mg/kg/day. **Conversion to Monotherapy:** Reduce concomitant antiepileptic drug (AED) dosage by 25% q2 weeks; withdrawal of AED highly variable, monitor closely for seizure frequency. **Elderly:** Reduce initial dose and titrate slowly. If dose >250mg/day, give in divided doses. Administer as 60 min IV infusion, not >20mg/min. Not for use >14 days; switch to oral route as soon as clinically feasible. Decrease dose or d/c if decreased food or fluid intake or if excessive somnolence occurs.	**BB:** Fatal hepatic failure (<2 yrs at considerable risk), teratogenic effects (eg, neural tube defects), and life-threatening pancreatitis reported. **W/P:** Hyperammonemic encephalopathy in UCD patients; d/c if this occurs. Prior to therapy, evaluate for UCD in high risk patients (eg, history of unexplained encephalopathy, coma, etc.). Measure ammonia levels if develop unexplained lethargy, vomiting, or mental status changes. Caution in elderly; monitor for fluid/nutritional intake, dehydration, somnolence. Monitor LFTs before therapy and during first 6 months. D/C if develop hepatic dysfunction, pancreatitis. Increased risk of hepatotoxicity with multiple anticonvulsants, congenital metabolic disorders, severe seizure disorder with mental retardation, organic brain disease, children <2 yrs. Avoid abrupt withdrawal. Monitor platelets and coagulation tests before therapy and periodically thereafter. Elevated liver enzymes and thrombocytopenia may be dose-related. Not for prophylaxis of posttraumatic seizures in acute head trauma. May interfere with urine ketone and thyroid function tests. **Contra:** Hepatic disease, significant hepatic dysfunction, known urea cycle disorders (UCD). **P/N:** Category D, not for use in nursing.	Dizziness, headache, nausea, local reactions.
Valproic Acid (Depakene, Stavzor)	**Cap:** (Depakene) 250mg; **Cap, Delayed-Release:** (Stavzor) 125mg, 250mg, and 500mg. **Syrup:** (Depakene) 250mg/5mL	**(Depakene/Stavzor) *Adults/Pediatrics:* ≥10 yrs: Complex Partial Seizures (monotheraphy/adjunctive): Initial:** 10-15mg/kg/day. **Titrate:** Increase weekly by 5-10mg/kg/day until optimal response. **Max:** 60mg/kg/day. If dose >250mg/day, give in divided doses. **Conversion to Monotherapy:** Reduce concomitant antiepileptic drug (AED) dosage by 25% q2 weeks; withdrawal of AED highly variable, monitor closely for seizure frequency. **Elderly:** Reduce	**BB:** Fatal hepatotoxicity, usually during first 6 months, reported (children <2 yrs are at higher risk); monitor closely and perform LFTs prior to therapy and periodically thereafter. Teratogenic effects (eg, neural tube defects) and life-threatening pancreatitis reported. **W/P:** Monitor LFTs before therapy and during first 6 months; d/c if hepatic dysfunction and hemorrhagic pancreatitis occur. Increased risk of hepatotoxicity with multiple anticonvulsants, congenital	Headache, asthenia, rash, ataxia, N/V, abdominal pain, dyspepsia, diarrhea, anorexia, somnolence, tremor, dizziness, diplopia, asthenia, thrombocytopenia, ecchymosis, nystagmus, alopecia, flu syndrome.

Table 17.1. PRESCRIBING INFORMATION FOR NEUROLOGICAL AGENTS *(cont.)*

NAME	FORM/ STRENGTH	DOSAGE	WARNINGS/PRECAUTIONS & CONTRAINDICATIONS	ADVERSE EFFECTS†
ANTICONVULSANTS *(cont.)*				
Valproic Acid (Depakene, Stavzor) *(cont.)*		initial dose. Swallow caps whole, do not chew. **Simple/Complex Absence Seizure: Initial:** 15mg/kg/day. **Titrate:** Increase weekly by 5-10mg/kg/day until optimal response. **Max:** 60mg/kg/day. **(Stavzor)** ***Adults:*** **Mania: Initial:** 750mg daily in divided doses. **Titrate:** Increase rapidly to produce the desired clinical effect or plasma level (50-125mcg/mL). **Max:** 60mg/kg/day. **Migraine: Initial:** 250mg bid. **Max:** 1000mg/day. **Elderly:** Reduce initial dose. Swallow whole.	metabolic disorders, severe seizure disorders with mental retardation, organic brain disease, and in children <2 yrs. Avoid abrupt withdrawal. Fatal hyperammonemic encephalopathy observed with UCD; d/c if ammonia levels increase. Prior to therapy, evaluate for UCD in high-risk patients (eg, history of unexplained encephalopathy, coma). Dose-related thrombocytopenia may occur; measure platelets and coagulation tests prior to initiation and periodically thereafter. Measure ammonia levels if unexplained lethargy, vomiting, or mental status changes develop. Somnolence in elderly may occur; increase dose slowly and monitor for fluid and nutritional intake. Hyperammonemia, hypothermia, multiorgan hypersensitivity reactions reported. May interfere with urine ketone and thyroid function tests. **Contra:** Hepatic disease, significant hepatic dysfunction, and known urea cycle disorders (UCD). **P/N:** Category D, not for use in nursing.	
Zonisamide (Zonegran)	**Cap:** 25mg, 100mg	***Adults/Pediatrics:*** **≥16 yrs: Initial:** 100mg qd for 2 weeks. **Titrate:** May increase to 200mg/day for at least 2 weeks. May then increase to 300mg/day, then to 400mg/day for at least 2-week intervals. **Max:** 600mg/day (No apparent benefit from doses >400mg/day).	**W/P:** Sulfonamide hypersensitivity reactions (eg, Stevens-Johnson syndrome, toxic epidermal necrolysis, fulminant hepatic necrosis, blood dyscrasias), cognitive/neuropsychiatric effects, kidney stones, sudden death reported. D/C with unexplained rash. Increased risk of oligohidrosis and hyperthermia in pediatrics; monitor for decreased sweating and increased body temperature. Metabolic acidosis reported. Advise females to use contraceptives to prevent pregnancy. Caution with renal/hepatic impairment. Avoid abrupt withdrawal. May cause cognitive/neuropsychiatric adverse events. Caution while driving, operating machinery, or performing hazardous tasks. Taper and d/c if CPK levels elevated or if patient manifests clinical signs and symptoms of pancreatitis. **Contra:** Sulfonamide hypersensitivity. **P/N:** Category C, not for use in nursing.	Headache, abdominal pain, anorexia, nausea, dizziness, ataxia, confusion, difficulty concentrating, memory difficulties, agitation/irritability, depression, insomnia, somnolence, fatigue, tiredness.
ANTIPARKINSON AGENTS				
Amantadine Hydrochloride (Symmetrel)	**Syrup:** 50mg/5mL; **Tab:** 100mg	***Adults:*** **Parkinsonism: Initial:** 100mg bid. **Serious Associated Illness/ Concomitant High Dose Antiparkinson Agent: Initial:** 100mg qd. **Titrate:** May increase to 100mg bid after 1 to several weeks. **Max:** 400mg/day. **Drug-Induced Extrapyramidal Reactions:** 100mg bid. **Titrate:** May increase to 300mg/day in divided doses. **CrCl 30-50mL/min:** 200mg on Day 1, then 100mg qd. **CrCl 15-29mL/min:** 200mg on Day 1, then 100mg every other day. **CrCl <15mL/min/Hemodialysis:** 200mg every 7 days.	**W/P:** Deaths reported from overdose. Suicide attempts, neuroleptic malignant syndrome (NMS) reported. Caution with CHF, peripheral edema, orthostatic hypotension, renal or hepatic dysfunction, recurrent eczematoid rash, uncontrolled psychosis or severe psychoneurosis. Avoid in untreated angle closure glaucoma. Do not d/c abruptly in Parkinson's disease. May increase seizure activity. Increase risk of melanoma with Parkinson's disease; monitor periodically. May impair mental/physical abilities. **P/N:** Category C, not for use in nursing.	Nausea, dizziness, insomnia, depression, anxiety, hallucinations, confusion, anorexia, **dry mouth,** constipation, ataxia, livedo reticularis, peripheral edema, orthostatic hypotension, irritability, headache.

*Scored. †Bold entries denote special dental considerations.
BB = black box warning; **W/P** = warnings/precautions; **Contra** = contraindications; **P/N** = pregnancy category rating and nursing considerations.

NAME	FORM/ STRENGTH	DOSAGE	WARNINGS/PRECAUTIONS & CONTRAINDICATIONS	ADVERSE EFFECTS†
Apomorphine HCl (Apokyn)	**Inj:** 10mg/mL [3mL]	***Adults:*** **Test Dose:** 0.2mL SC to patients in an 'off' state; closely monitor BP. If 0.2mL is tolerated but ineffective, give 0.4mL at the next 'off' period (no sooner than 2 hrs after the first test dose). If 0.4mL is tolerated, initiate with a starting dose of 0.3mL prn. If 0.4mL is not tolerated, administer 0.3mL at the next off period (no sooner than 2 hrs after the prior test dose). If 0.3mL is tolerated, initiate with a starting dose of 0.2mL prn. **Titrate:** Increase by 0.1mL every few days, as necessary; assess efficacy/tolerability. Do not give a second dose for an 'off' period if the first was ineffective. **Max:** 2mL/day. Trimethobenzamide (300mg tid orally) should be started 3 days prior to initial apomorphine dose and for at least during the first two months of therapy. **Renal Impairment: Test Dose/Initial:** 0.1mL SC.	**W/P:** Avoid IV administration; serious adverse events reported (thrombus formation and PE). Nausea, vomiting, syncope, symptomatic hypotension, falls, hallucinations, falling asleep during activities of daily living, coronary events (eg, angina, MI, cardiac arrest, suddden death) reported. May prolong QT interval; potential proarrhythmic effects; caution with drugs that prolong QT/QTc interval. Caution with sulfite sensitivity. May cause or worsen dyskinesias. Withdrawal-emergent hyperpyrexia and confusion reported with rapid dose reduction/withdrawal/changes in therapy. Fibrotic complications (eg, retroperitoneal fibrosis, pulmonary infiltrates, pleural effusion/thickening, cardiac valvulopathy) reported. May cause priapism. Caution with hepatic/ renal impairment. **Contra:** Concomitant use with 5-HT_3 antagonists (eg, ondansetron, granisetron, dolasetron, palonosetron, alosetron). **P/N:** Category C, not for use in nursing.	Yawning, somnolence, dizziness, rhinorrhea, edema, chest pain, increased sweating, flushing, pallor.
Benztropine Mesylate (Cogentin)	**Inj:** 1mg/mL; **Tab:** 0.5mg, 1mg, 2mg	***Adults:*** **Parkinsonism: Initial:** 0.5-1mg PO/IV/IM qhs. **Titrate:** May increase every 5-6 days by 0.5mg. **Usual:** 1-2mg PO/IV/IM qhs. **Max:** 6mg/day. **Extrapyramidal Disorders:** 1-4mg PO/IV/IM qd-bid. **Acute Dystonic Reactions:** 1-2mg IM/IV, then 1-2mg PO bid.	**W/P:** May produce anhidrosis, caution in hot weather. Muscle weakness and dysuria may occur. Caution in pediatrics >3 years of age. Not recommended for tardive dyskinesia. Avoid with angle-closure glaucoma. Caution with CNS disease, mental disorders, tachycardia, prostatic hypertrophy, alcoholics, chronically ill, and those exposed to hot environments. **Contra:** Patients <3 yrs. **P/N:** Safety in pregnancy and nursing not known.	Tachycardia, paralytic ileus, constipation, N/V, **dry mouth,** confusion, blurred vision, urinary retention, heat stroke, hyperthermia, fever.
Bromocriptine Mesylate (Parlodel)	**Cap:** 5mg; **Tab:** 2.5mg*	***Adults:*** Take with food. **Parkinson's Disease: Initial:** 1.25mg bid. **Titrate:** if needed, increase by 2.5mg/day every 2-4 weeks. **Max:** 100mg/day. **Hyperprolactinemia: Initial:** 1.25mg-2.5mg qd. **Titrate:** If needed, increase by 2.5mg every 2-7 days. **Usual:** 2.5-15mg/ day. **Acromegaly: Initial:** 1.25-2.5mg qhs for 3 days. **Titrate:** Increase by 1.25-2.5mg every 3-7 days until optimal response. **Usual:** 20-30mg/ day. **Max:** 100mg/day. Withdraw for 4-8 weeks every year in patients treated with pituitary irradiation. ***Pediatrics:*** Take with food. **11-15 yrs: Prolactin-Secreting Pituitary Adenomas: Initial:** 1.25-2.5mg/day. **Titrate:** Increase as tolerated. **Usual:** 2.5-10mg/day.	**W/P:** Caution with renal or hepatic dysfunction, psychosis, CVD, peptic ulcer, dementia. D/C with macroadenomas associated with rapid regrowth of tumor and increased prolactin levels and if severe headache or HTN develops. Risk of pulmonary infiltrates, pleural effusion, thickening of pleura, and retroperitoneal fibrosis with long-term use. Not for prevention of physiological lactation. Monitor BP for symptomatic hypotension and HTN. **Contra:** Uncontrolled HTN, ergot alkaloid sensitivity, postpartum with CVD unless withdrawal is medically contraindicated, pregnancy if treating hyperprolactinemia, HTN in pregnancy. **P/N:** Category B, not for use in nursing.	Headache, dizziness, GI effects, orthostatic hypotension, fatigue, arrhythmia, insomnia, hallucinations, abnormal involuntary movements, depression, syncope.
Carbidopa/ Entacapone/ Levodopa (Stalevo)	(Carbidopa/ Levodopa/Entacapone) **Tab: Stalevo 50:** 12.5mg/ 50mg/ 200mg; **Stalevo 75:** 18.75mg/ 75mg/ 200mg; **Stalevo 100:** 25mg/ 100mg/ 200mg; **Stalevo 125:** 31.25mg/ 125mg/ 200mg;	***Adults:*** **Currently Taking Carbidopa/ Levodopa and Entacapone:** May switch directly to corresponding strength of carbidopa/levodopa. **Currently Taking Carbidopa/Levodopa but not Entacapone:** First titrate individually with carbidopa/levodopa product and entacapone product then transfer to corresponding dose. **Max: Stalevo 50/ Stalevo 75/Stalevo 100/Stalevo 125/ Stalevo 150:** 8 tabs/day. **Stalevo 200:** 6 tabs/day.	**W/P:** Dyskinesia, mental disturbances, hypotension/syncope, hallucinations, rhabdomyolysis, hyperpyrexia, confusion, and fibrotic complications reported. Caution with biliary obstruction, severe cardiovascular or pulmonary disease, bronchial asthma, renal, hepatic, or endocrine disease, chronic wide-angle glaucoma, history of MI with residual arrhythmias, peptic ulcer. Neuroleptic malignant syndrome reported with dose reductions or withdrawal. Avoid rapid withdrawal or abrupt dose	Dyskinesia, hyperkinesia, hypokinesia, dizziness, N/V, diarrhea, abdominal pain, constipation, urine discoloration, back pain, fatigue.

Table 17.1. PRESCRIBING INFORMATION FOR NEUROLOGICAL AGENTS *(cont.)*

NAME	FORM/ STRENGTH	DOSAGE	WARNINGS/PRECAUTIONS & CONTRAINDICATIONS	ADVERSE EFFECTS†
ANTIPARKINSON AGENTS *(cont.)*				
Carbidopa/ Entacapone/ Levodopa (Stalevo) *(cont.)*	**Stalevo 150:** 37.5mg/ 150mg/ 200mg; **Stalevo 200:** 50mg/ 200mg/ 200mg		reduction. May cause dark color to appear in saliva, urine, or sweat. May cause false-positive ketonuria, false-negative glucosuria (glucose-oxidase method), elevated LFTs, abnormal BUN, positive Coombs test. May depress prolactin secretion and increase growth hormone levels. **Contra:** MAOIs during or within 14 days of use, narrow-angle glaucoma, undiagnosed skin lesions, history of melanoma. **P/N:** Category C, caution in nursing.	
Carbidopa/ Levodopa (Parcopa, Sinemet, Sinemet CR)	**Tab:** (Sinemet) 10mg-100mg*, 25mg-100mg*, 25mg-250mg*; **Tab, Disintegrating:** (Parcopa) 10mg-100mg*, 25mg-100mg*, 25mg-250mg* **Tab, Extended-Release:** (Sinemet CR) 25mg-100mg, 50mg-200mg*	***Adults:* ≥18 yrs: Parcopa, Sinemet: 25mg-100mg Tab: Initial:** 1 tab tid. **Titrate:** Increase by 1 tab qd or every other day until 8 tabs/day. **10mg-100mg Tab: Initial:** 1 tab tid-qid. **Titrate:** Increase 1 tab qd or every other day until 2 tabs qid. 70-100mg/day carbidopa required. **Max:** 200mg/day carbidopa. **Conversion from Levodopa:** D/C levodopa at least 12hrs before starting carbidopa-levodopa. Choose a dose that will provide approximately 25% of the previous levodopa dose. **Initial: Levodopa Dose <1500mg:** 25mg-100mg tid-qid. **Levodopa Dose >1500mg:** 25mg-250mg tid-qid. **Sinemet CR: No Prior Levodopa Use: Initial:** 1 tab 50mg-200mg bid at intervals >6 hrs. **Titrate:** Increase or decrease dose or interval accordingly. Adjust dose every 3 days. **Usual:** 400-1600mg/day levodopa, given in 4-8 hr intervals while awake. **Conversion from Levodopa:** D/C levodopa at least 12hrs before starting carbidopa-levodopa. Choose a dose that will provide approximately 25% of the previous levodopa dose. **Conversion from Immediate-Release Levodopa:** Refer to PI.	**W/P:** Dyskinesias and mental disturbances may occur. Caution with severe cardiovascular or pulmonary disease, bronchial asthma, renal or hepatic disease, endocrine disease, chronic wide-angle glaucoma, peptic ulcer, and MI with residual arrhythmias. NMS reported during dose reduction or withdrawal. Dark color may appear in saliva, urine, or sweat. May cause false-positive ketonuria or false-negative glucosuria (glucose-oxidase method). **Contra:** MAOIs within 14 days, narrow-angle glaucoma, suspicious/undiagnosed skin lesions, history of melanoma. **P/N:** Category C, caution in nursing.	Dyskinesias, nausea, cardiac irregularities, hypotension, **dark saliva,** GI bleeding, psychotic episodes, NMS, confusion, agitation, dizziness, somnolence, dream abnormalities.
Entacapone (Comtan)	**Tab:** 200mg	***Adults:*** 200mg with each levodopa/ carbidopa dose. **Max:** 1600mg/day. Withdraw slowly for discontinuation.	**W/P:** Hypotension/syncope, diarrhea, hallucinations, dyskinesia, rhabdomyolysis, hyperpyrexia, confusion, and fibrotic complications may occur due to increased dopaminergic activity. Caution with hepatic impairment, biliary obstruction. Avoid rapid withdrawal or abrupt dose reduction. May impair mental and/ or motor performance. **P/N:** Category C, caution with nursing.	Sweating, back pain, dyskinesia, hyperkinesia, hypokinesia, nausea, diarrhea, abdominal pain, urine discoloration.
Pramipexole Dihydrochloride (Mirapex)	**Tab:** 0.125mg, 0.25mg*, 0.5mg*, 0.75mg, 1mg*, 1.5mg*	***Adults:* Parkinson's Disease: Initial:** 0.125mg tid. **Titrate:** May increase every 5-7 days (eg, **Week 2:** 0.25mg tid; **Week 3:** 0.5mg tid; **Week 4:** 0.75mg tid; **Week 5:** 1mg tid; **Week 6:** 1.25mg tid; **Week 7:** 1.5mg tid). **Maint:** 0.5-1.5mg tid. **Max:** 1.5mg tid. **CrCl >60mL/min: Initial:** 0.125mg tid. **Max:** 1.5mg tid. **CrCl 35-59mL/min: Initial:** 0.125mg bid. **Max:** 1.5mg bid. **CrCl 15-34mL/min: Initial:** 0.125mg qd. **Max:** 1.5mg qd. **RLS: Initial:** 0.125mg once daily, 2-3 hours before bedtime. **Titrate:** May double dose every 4-7 days up to 0.5mg/day.	**W/P:** Somnolence, symptomatic hypotension, hallucinations, and rhabdomyolysis reported. Caution with renal insufficiency. May potentiate dyskinesia. May cause retinal pathology, fibrotic complications, withdrawal-emergent hyperpyrexia, and confusion. Consider discontinuation if significant daytime sleepiness or sudden onset of sleep occurs during daily activities. Cases of pathological gambling, hypersexuality, and compulsive eating reported. Rebound and augmentation in RLS reported. Falling asleep during activities of daily living. **P/N:** Category C, not for use in nursing.	Nausea, dizziness, somnolence, insomnia, constipation, asthenia, hallucination, vision abnormalities, peripheral edema, arthritis, **dry mouth,** postural hypotension, chest pain, malaise.

*Scored. †Bold entries denote special dental considerations.

BB = black box warning; **W/P** = warnings/precautions; **Contra** = contraindications; **P/N** = pregnancy category rating and nursing considerations.

NAME	FORM/ STRENGTH	DOSAGE	WARNINGS/PRECAUTIONS & CONTRAINDICATIONS	ADVERSE EFFECTS†
Rasagiline Mesylate (Azilect)	**Tab:** 0.5mg, 1mg	***Adults:*** **Monotherapy:** 1mg qd. **Adjunctive Therapy: Initial:** 0.5mg qd. **Titrate:** May increase to 1mg qd. Adjust dose of levodopa with concomitant use. **Concomitant Ciprofloxacin or Other CYP1A2 Inhibitors/Hepatic Impairment:** 0.5mg qd.	**W/P:** May increase incidence of melanoma. Concomitant use with levodopa may potentiate dopaminergic side effects and exacerbate preexisting dyskinesia. Postural hypotension reported. Patients should be warned to restrict dietary tyramines and avoid amine-containing medications for 2 weeks after discontinuation. **Contra:** Pheochromocytoma. Concomitant use with meperidine, tramadol, methadone, propoxyphene, dextromethorphan, St. John's wort, mirtazapine, cyclobenzaprine, sympathomimetic amines (eg, amphetamines, cold products containing pseudoephedrine, phenylephrine, phenylpropanolamine, and ephedrine), other MAOIs, cocaine, general anesthesia, local anesthesia containing vasoconstrictors. **P/N:** Category C, caution in nursing.	Headache, arthralgia, depression, falls, flu syndrome, dyskinesia, accidental injury, N/V, weight loss, constipation, postural hypotension, **dry mouth,** rash, somnolence.
Ropinirole HCl (Requip, Requip XL)	**Tab:** 0.25mg, 0.5mg, 1mg, 2mg, 3mg, 4mg, 5mg; **Tab, Extended-Release:** (XL) 2mg, 4mg, 8mg	***Adults:*** **Parkinson's Disease: Tab: Initial:** 0.25mg tid. **Titrate:** May increase weekly by 0.25mg tid (0.75mg/day) for 4 weeks. After week 4, may increase weekly by 1.5mg/day up to 9mg/day, then by 3mg/day weekly to 24mg/day. **Max:** 24mg/day. **Withdrawal:** Decrease dose to bid for 4 days, then qd for 3 days. **Tab, Extended-Release: Initial:** 2mg qd for 1-2 weeks. **Titrate:** May increase by 2mg/day at ≥1 week intervals, depending on therapeutic response and tolerability. **Max:** 24mg/day. Swallow whole; do not chew, crush, or divide. **Switching from Immediate-Release (IR) to XL:** Initial dose should match total daily dose of IR formulation. See PI for more info. **RLS: Tab: Initial:** 0.25mg qd, 1-3 hours before bedtime. **Titrate:** 0.5mg qd days 3-7, 1mg qd week 2, then increase by 0.5mg weekly. **Max:** 4mg.	**W/P:** (Tab/Tab, Extended-Release) Falling asleep during activities of daily living reported; if significant, d/c or warn patient to refrain from dangerous activities. Syncope, symptomatic hypotension, and hallucinations reported. Caution with severe renal or hepatic dysfunction. May cause or exacerbate preexisting dyskinesia. Neuroleptic malignant syndrome, fibrotic complications, and melanoma reported. Augmentation and rebound in RLS reported. Avoid rapid dose reduction or abrupt withdrawal. Compulsive behaviors reported. (Tab, Extended-Release) May cause elevation of BP and changes in HR. **P/N:** Category C, not for use in nursing.	(Tab) Neuralgia, increased BUN, hallucinations, somnolence, vomiting, headache, sweating, asthenia, edema, fatigue, syncope, orthostatic symptoms. (Tab, Extended-Release) Nausea, somnolence, dizziness, constipation, abdominal pain/ discomfort.
Selegiline HCl (Eldepryl, Zelapar)	**Cap:** (Eldepryl) 5mg; **Tab, Disintigrating:** (Zelapar) 1.25mg	***Adults:*** **Eldepryl:** 5mg bid, at breakfast and lunch. **Max:** 10mg/day. May reduce levodopa/carbidopa by 10-30% after 2-3 days of therapy. May reduce further with continued therapy. **Zelapar:** 1.25mg every morning without liquid for 6 weeks. **Titrate:** After 6 weeks, may increase to 2.5mg if desired benefit not achieved. **Max:** 2.5mg/day.	**W/P:** Greater risk of orthostatic hypotension and dizziness in geriatric patients. Decrease levodopa/carbidopa to prevent exacerbation of levodopa side effects. Perform periodic dermatologic screening. May increase frequency of mild oropharyngeal abnormality. Caution with renal or hepatic impairment. Neuroleptic malignant syndrome reported in association with rapid dose reduction, withdrawal of, or changes in antiparkinsonian therapy. (Eldepryl) Do not exceed 10mg/day due to nonselective MAO inhibition. (Zelepar) Do not exceed 2.5mg/day; risk of nonselective MAO inhibition. **Contra:** Concomitant meperidine, tramadol, methadone, propoxyphene, dextromethorphan, and other MAOIs. **P/N:** Category C, not for use in nursing.	Nausea, dizziness, pain, headache, insomnia, rhinitis, skin disorders, dyskinesia, backache, lightheadedness, fainting, confusion, dyspepsia, stomatitis, constipation, hallucinations, **pharyngitis,** rash, **xerostomia.**
Tolcapone (Tasmar)	**Tab:** 100mg, 200mg	***Adults:*** **Initial:** 100mg tid. **Titrate:** Use 200mg tid only if clinical benefit is justified. May need to decrease levodopa dose.	**BB:** Risk of fatal, acute fulminant liver failure. Withdraw if patients fail to show benefit within 3 weeks of initiation. D/C if hepatotoxicity develops, and do not consider retreatment. Perform LFTs before therapy, then every 2 weeks for first year, every 4 weeks for next 6 months, then every 8 weeks thereafter. Perform	Dyskinesia, N/V, dystonia, excessive dreaming, anorexia, muscle cramps, orthostatic complaints, diarrhea, confusion, hallucination,

Table 17.1. PRESCRIBING INFORMATION FOR NEUROLOGICAL AGENTS *(cont.)*

NAME	FORM/ STRENGTH	DOSAGE	WARNINGS/PRECAUTIONS & CONTRAINDICATIONS	ADVERSE EFFECTS†
ANTIPARKINSON AGENTS *(cont.)*				
Tolcapone (Tasmar) *(cont.)*			LFTs before increase dose to 200mg tid. Avoid with liver disease or if LFTs ≥2x ULN. Caution with severe dyskinesia or dystonia. **W/P:** Hypotension/syncope, rhabdomyolysis, hallucinations, confusion, diarrhea, hematuria reported. Fibrotic complications can occur. Avoid with liver dysfunction. Caution with severe renal dysfunction. Closely monitor when discontinuing therapy. **Contra:** Liver disease, patients withdrawn from therapy due to drug-induced hepatocellular injury. History of nontraumatic rhabdomyolysis, hyperpyrexia, or confusion related to medication. **P/N:** Category C, caution in nursing.	constipation, fatigue, increased sweating, **dry mouth,** urine discoloration, hepatotoxicity.
Trihexyphenidyl HCl	**Sol:** 2mg/5mL; **Tab:** 2mg, 5mg	***Adults:*** **Idiopathic Parkinsonism:** 1mg on Day 1. **Titrate:** Increase by 2mg every 3-5 days. **Usual:** 6-10mg/day. **Max:** 15mg/day. **Drug-Induced Parkinsonism: Initial:** 1mg. If extrapyramidal manifestations not controlled in a few hrs, increase dose until achieve control. **Usual:** 5-15mg/day. **Concomitant Levodopa:** Trihexyphenidyl dose may need reduction. **Usual:** 3-6mg/day. Divide total daily dose into 3 doses. May divide doses >10mg/day into 4 doses; 3 doses with meals and 1 at bedtime.	**W/P:** Monitor IOP. Caution with exposure in hot weather (esp., alcoholics), glaucoma, obstructive disease of GI or GU tract, prostatic hypertrophy, HTN, and cardiac, liver, or kidney disorders. Angle-closure glaucoma reported with long-term treatment. Neuroleptic malignant syndrome (NMS) reported with dose reduction or discontinuation. Avoid in tardive dyskinesia except in Parkinson's Disease. Use low initial dose with history of idiosyncrasy to other drugs or arteriosclerosis. Avoid abrupt withdrawal. **P/N:** Safety in pregnancy not known, caution in nursing.	**Dry mouth,** blurred vision, dizziness, N/V, nervousness, constipation, drowsiness, urinary hesitancy/retention, tachycardia, pupil dilation, increased intraocular tension, headache.
MIGRAINE THERAPY/TENSION HEADACHE				
Acetaminophen/ Aspirin/Caffeine (Excedrin Migraine) OTC	**Tab:** (APAP-ASA-Caffeine) 250mg-250mg-65mg	***Adults:*** Take 2 tabs with water. **Max:** 2 tabs/day.	**W/P:** Children and teenagers should not use for viral illnesses. APAP and ASA may cause liver damage and GI bleeding. **P/N:** Safety in pregnancy and nursing not known.	
Acetaminophen/ Butalbital (Phrenilin, Phrenilin Forte)	(Butalbital-APAP) **Cap:** (Phrenilin Forte) 50mg-650mg; **Tab:** (Phrenilin) 50mg-325mg.	***Adults/Pediatrics:*** **≥12 yrs: Tension Headache: Phrenilin Forte:** 1 cap q4h. **Phrenilin:** 1-2 tabs q4h. **Max:** 6 caps/tabs/day.	**W/P:** May be habit-forming; potential for abuse. Not for long-term use. May impair mental and/or physical abilities. Caution in elderly, debilitated, severe renal or hepatic impairment, acute abdominal conditions. **Contra:** Porphyria. **P/N:** Category C, not for use in nursing.	Drowsiness, lightheadedness, dizziness, sedation, SOB, N/V, abdominal pain, intoxicated feeling.
Acetaminophen/ Butalbital/Caffeine (Esgic-Plus, Fioricet)	(Butalbital-APAP-Caffeine) **Cap/Tab:**(Esgic-Plus) 50mg-500mg-40mg* **Tab:** (Fioricet) 50mg-325mg-40mg	***Adults/Pediatrics:*** **≥12 yrs: Fioricet:** 1-2 tabs q4h prn. **Esgic-Plus:** 1 cap/tab q4h prn. **Max:** 6 caps/tabs/day.	**W/P:** May be habit-forming; potential for abuse. Not for long-term use. May impair mental and/or physical abilities. Caution in elderly, debilitated, severe renal or hepatic impairment, acute abdominal conditions. **Contra:** Porphyria. **P/N:** Category C, not for use in nursing.	Drowsiness, lightheadedness, dizziness, sedation, SOB, N/V, abdominal pain, intoxicated feeling.
Acetaminophen/ Butalbital/Caffeine/ Codeine Phosphate (Fioricet with Codeine) CIII	**Cap:** (Butalbital-APAP-Caffeine-Codeine) 50mg-325mg-40mg-30mg	***Adults:*** 1-2 caps q4h prn. **Max:** 6 caps/day. Not for extended use.	**W/P:** May be habit forming. Not for extended use. Respiratory depression and CSF pressure enhanced with head injury or intracranial lesions. Caution in elderly, debilitated, severe renal or hepatic impairment, hypothyroidism, urethral stricture, Addison's disease, BPH, and history of drug abuse. May mask signs of acute abdominal conditions. **Contra:** Porphyria. **P/N:** Category C, not for use in nursing.	Drowsiness, lightheadedness, dizziness, sedation, SOB, N/V, abdominal pain, intoxicated feeling.

*Scored. †Bold entries denote special dental considerations.
BB = black box warning; **W/P** = warnings/precautions; **Contra** = contraindications; **P/N** = pregnancy category rating and nursing considerations.

NAME	FORM/ STRENGTH	DOSAGE	WARNINGS/PRECAUTIONS & CONTRAINDICATIONS	ADVERSE EFFECTS†
Acetaminophen/ Dichloral-phenazone/ Isometheptene Mucate (Amidrine, Duradrin, Midrin, Migquin, Migrazone) CIV	**Cap:** (APAP-Dichloral-phenazone-Isometheptene) 325mg-100mg-65mg	***Adults:*** **Migraine:** 2 caps, then 1 cap every hr until relieved. **Max:** 5 caps/12hrs. **Tension Headache:** 1-2 caps q4h. **Max:** 8 caps/day.	**W/P:** Caution with HTN, peripheral vascular disease, or recent cardiovascular attacks. **Contra:** Glaucoma, severe renal disease, HTN, organic heart disease, hepatic disease, concomitant MAOI therapy. **P/N:** Safety in pregnancy and nursing are not known.	Transient dizziness, skin rash.
Almotriptan Malate (Axert)	**Tab:** 6.25mg, 12.5mg	***Adults:*** **≥18 yrs: Initial:** 6.25-12.5mg at onset of headache. May repeat after 2 hrs. **Max:** 2 doses/24 hrs. **Hepatic/ Renal Impairment:** 6.25mg at onset of headache. **Max:** 12.5mg/24 hrs. Safety of treating >4 headaches/30 days not known.	**W/P:** Confirm diagnosis. Supervise first dose and monitor cardiac function in those at risk of CAD (eg, HTN, hypercholesterolemia, smoker, obesity, diabetes, CAD family history, post-menopausal women, males >40 yrs). Monitor cardiovascular function with long-term intermittent use. May cause vasospastic reactions or cerebrovascular events. Caution with renal or hepatic dysfunction. Avoid in elderly. **Contra:** Ischemic heart disease, coronary artery vasospasm, other significant CVD, uncontrolled HTN, within 24 hrs of another 5-HT_1 agonist or ergot-type agent, hemiplegic or basilar migraine. **P/N:** Category C, caution in nursing.	Nausea, somnolence, headache, paresthesia, **dry mouth,** coronary artery vasospasm, MI, ventricular tachycardia, fibrillation.
Aspirin/Butalbital/ Caffeine (Fiorinal) CIII	**Cap:** (Butalbital-ASA-Caffeine) 50mg-325mg-40mg	***Adults:*** 1-2 caps q4h prn. **Max:** 6 caps/ day. Not for extended use.	**W/P:** May be habit-forming. Not for extended use. Caution in elderly, debilitated, severe renal or hepatic impairment, hypothyroidism, urethral stricture, head injuries, elevated ICP, acute abdominal conditions, Addison's disease, prostatic hypertrophy, peptic ulcer, coagulation disorders. Avoid with ASA allergy. Risk of ASA hypersensitivity with nasal polyps and asthma. Caution in children with chickenpox or flu. Preoperative ASA may prolong bleeding time. **Contra:** Porphyria, peptic ulcer disease, serious GI lesions, hemorrhagic diathesis. Syndrome of nasal polyps, angioedema, and bronchospastic reactivity to ASA or NSAIDs. **P/N:** Category C, not for use in nursing.	Drowsiness, lightheadedness, dizziness, sedation, N/V, flatulence.
Aspirin/Butalbital/ Caffeine/Codeine Phosphate (Fiorinal with Codeine) CIII	**Cap:** (Butalbital-ASA-Caffeine-Codeine) 50mg-325mg-40mg-30mg	***Adults:*** 1-2 caps q4h prn. **Max:** 6 caps/ day. Not for extended use.	**W/P:** May be habit-forming. Not for extended use. Respiratory depression and CSF pressure may be enhanced with head injury or intracranial lesions. Caution in elderly, debilitated, severe renal or hepatic impairment, hypothyroidism, urethral stricture, head injuries, elevated ICP, acute abdominal conditions, Addison's disease, prostatic hypertrophy, peptic ulcer, coagulation disorders. Caution in children with chickenpox or flu. May obscure acute abdominal conditions. Preoperative ASA may prolong bleeding time. Avoid with ASA allergy. Risk of ASA hypersensitivity with nasal polyps and asthma. **Contra:** Porphyria, peptic ulcer disease, serious GI lesions, hemorrhagic diathesis. Syndrome of nasal polyps, angioedema and bronchospastic reactivity to ASA or NSAIDs. **P/N:** Category C, not for use in nursing.	Drowsiness, lightheadedness, dizziness, sedation, SOB, N/V, abdominal pain, intoxicated feeling.

Table 17.1. PRESCRIBING INFORMATION FOR NEUROLOGICAL AGENTS *(cont.)*

NAME	FORM/ STRENGTH	DOSAGE	WARNINGS/PRECAUTIONS & CONTRAINDICATIONS	ADVERSE EFFECTS†
MIGRAINE THERAPY/TENSION HEADACHE *(cont.)*				
Caffeine/ Ergotamine Tartrate (Cafergot Tablets)	**Tab:** (Ergotamine-Caffeine) 1mg-100mg	***Adults:*** 2 tabs at start of attack. Repeat 1 tab every 1/2 hr prn. **Max:** 6 tabs/attack, 10 tabs/week. May give at bedtime as short-term preventive measure.	**BB:** Serious and/or life-threatening peripheral ischemia has been associated with coadministration of Cafergot with potent CYP3A4 inhibitors (eg, protease inhibitors, macrolide antibiotics). Because CYP3A4 inhibition elevates serum levels of Cafergot, the risk for vasospasm leading to cerebral ischemia and/or ischemia of the extremities is increased. Concomitant use of these medications is contraindicated. **W/P:** Do not exceed recommended dosage; ergotism may develop. Fibrotic complications (eg, retroperitoneal and/or pleuropulmonary fibrosis) reported. **Contra:** Pregnancy, peripheral vascular disease, CHD, HTN, hepatic/renal dysfunction, coadministration with potent CYP3A4 inhibitors (eg, ritonavir, nelfinavir, erythromycin, clarithromycin, troleandomycin, ketoconazole, itraonazole). **P/N:** Category X, not for use in nursing.	Precordial distress, transient tachycardia or bradycardia, N/V, localized edema, itching, numbness/tingling of fingers/toes, muscle pain, leg weakness.
Dihydroergotamine Mesylate (D.H.E. 45, Migranal)	**Inj:** (D.H.E. 45) 1mg/mL; **Nasal Spray:** (Migranal) 0.5mg/spray [3.5mL]	***Adults:*** (Inj) 1mL IV/IM/SQ. May repeat at 1 hr intervals. **Max:** 3mL/24hrs IM/SC or 2mL/24hrs IV and 6mL/week. (Spray) 1 spray per nostril, repeat in 15 min. **Max:** 6 sprays/24 hrs or 8 sprays/week.	**BB:** Serious and life-threatening peripheral ischemia reported with potent CYP3A4 inhibitors (eg, protease inhibitors, macrolides). Elevated levels of dihydroergotamine increases risk of vasospasm leading to cerebral ischemia or ischemia of the extremities. Concomitant use with CYP3A4 inhibitors is contraindicated. **W/P:** Confirm migraine diagnosis. Inform of risks of adverse cardiac, cerebrovascular, and vasospastic events and fatalities. Avoid with cardiac risk factors (eg, HTN, hypercholesterolemia, smoker, obesity, DM, strong family history of CAD, females who are surgically/physiologically postmenopausal, or males >40 yrs) unless cardiovascular evaluation is done. Perform cardiovascular monitoring with long-term use. Significant BP elevations reported. **Contra:** Ergot alkaloids hypersensitivity, ischemic heart disease, coronary artery vasospasm (eg, Prinzmetal's variant angina), uncontrolled HTN, hemiplegic or basilar migraine, peripheral artery disease, sepsis, following vascular surgery, severe renal/hepatic dysfunction, pregnancy, nursing, with potent CYP3A4 inhibitors (eg, ritonavir, nelfinavir, indinavir, erythromycin, clarithromycin, troleandomycin, ketoconazole, itraconazole), concomitant peripheral and central vasoconstrictors, and within 24 hrs after taking 5-HT_1 agonists, methysergide, ergotamine-containing or ergot-type agents. **P/N:** Category X, contraindicated in nursing.	(Inj) Vasospasm, angina, paraesthesia, HTN, dizziness, anxiety, dyspnea, headache, flushing, diarrhea, rash, increased sweating. (Spray) Rhinitis, **altered taste,** application-site reactions, dizziness, N/V, pharyngitis, somnolence.
Eletriptan Hydrobromide (Relpax)	**Tab:** 20mg, 40mg	***Adults:* ≥18 yrs: Initial:** 20 or 40mg at onset of headache. If recurs after initial relief, may repeat after 2 hrs. **Max:** 40mg/dose or 80mg/day. Safety of treating >3 headaches/30 days not known. **Severe Hepatic Impairment:** Avoid use. Avoid within 72 hrs of potent CYP3A4 inhibitors.	**W/P:** Confirm diagnosis. Supervise first dose and monitor cardiac function in those at risk of CAD (eg, HTN, hypercholesterolemia, smoker, obesity, diabetes, CAD family history, postmenopausal women, males >40 yrs). Consider ECG during interval immediately following initial administration in patients with CAD risk factors. Monitor cardiac	Asthenia, chest tightness, dizziness, **dry mouth,** headache, nausea, paresthesia, somnolence, **pain/pressure/heaviness in precordium/throat/jaw.**

†Bold entries denote special dental considerations.
BB = black box warning; **W/P** = warnings/precautions; **Contra** = contraindications; **P/N** = pregnancy category rating and nursing considerations.

NAME	FORM/ STRENGTH	DOSAGE	WARNINGS/PRECAUTIONS & CONTRAINDICATIONS	ADVERSE EFFECTS†
Eletriptan Hydrobromide (Relpax) *(cont.)*			function in intermittent long-term users with CAD risk factors. Serious adverse cardiac events, increased BP, cerebrovascular events, vasospastic reactions reported. Caution in elderly. Possible long-term ophthalmic effects. **Contra:** Ischemic heart disease, coronary artery vasospasm (eg, Prinzmetal's angina), or other significant underlying cardiovascular disease, peripheral vascular disease, cerebrovascular syndromes, uncontrolled HTN, hemiplegic or basilar migraine, use within 24 hrs of other 5-HT_1 agonist or ergot-type agent (eg, dihydroergotamine, methysergide), severe hepatic impairment. **P/N:** Category C, caution in nursing.	
Frovatriptan Succinate (Frova)	**Tab:** 2.5mg	***Adults:*** **≥18 yrs:** 2.5mg with fluids. If headache recurs after initial relief, may repeat after 2 hrs. **Max:** 7.5mg/day. Safety of treating >4 headaches/30 days not known.	**W/P:** Confirm diagnosis. Supervise first dose and monitor cardiac function in those at risk of CAD (eg, HTN, hypercholesterolemia, smoker, obesity, diabetes, CAD family history, postmenopausal women, males >40 yrs). Serious adverse cardiac events, cerebrovascular events, vasospastic reactions reported with 5-HT_1 agonists. May bind to melanin in the eye; possibility of long-term effects. **Contra:** Ischemic heart disease, coronary artery vasospasm (eg, Prinzmetal's angina), significant cardiovascular disease, cerebrovascular syndromes, peripheral vascular disease, uncontrolled HTN, hemiplegic or basilar migraine, use within 24 hrs of treatment with another 5-HT_1 agonist or ergot-type agent. **P/N:** Category C, caution in nursing.	Dizziness, headache, paresthesia, **dry mouth,** dyspepsia, fatigue, hot or cold sensation, chest pain, skeletal pain, flushing.
Ibuprofen (Advil Migraine) OTC	**Cap:** 200mg	***Adults:*** 2 caps with water. **Max:** 2 caps/24hrs.	**W/P:** May cause severe allergic reaction (eg, hives, facial swelling, asthma, shock). **P/N:** Safety in pregnancy and nursing not known.	—
Naproxen Sodium/ Sumatriptan Succinate (Treximet)	**Tab:** (Naproxen-Sumatriptan): 500mg-85mg [9[s]]	***Adults:*** **≥18 yrs: Initial:** 1 tab; may repeat after 2 hrs. **Max:** 2 tabs/24 hrs. Do not split, crush, or chew.	**BB:** Treximet may cause an increased risk of serious cardiovascular thrombotic events, MI, stroke, and serious GI adverse events including bleeding, ulceration, and perforation of the stomach or intestines. **W/P:** Establish clear diagnosis. Caution in patients with uncontrolled HTN; monitor closely during initiation and throughout course of therapy. Caution in patients with fluid retention and heart failure. Serotonin syndrome may occur. Caution in those with prior history of ulcer disease or GI bleed; impaired renal function; heart failure; liver dysfunction; elderly; taking ACE-inhibitors or diuretics; with diseases that may alter absorption, metabolism, excretion of drugs; history of epilepsy or condition that lowers seizure threshold. Not recommended in patients with advanced renal disease. Anaphylactic/anaphylactoid reactions, serious skin reaction such as exfoliative dermatitis, Stevens-Johnson syndrome, and toxic epidermal necrosis may occur. Chest, jaw, or neck pain/discomfort reported. May cause vision disturbances. Caution in those with coagulation disorders, or	Dizziness, somnolence, paresthesia, nausea, dyspepsia, **dry mouth, chest/ neck/throat/jaw pain, tightness, pressure.**

Table 17.1. PRESCRIBING INFORMATION FOR NEUROLOGICAL AGENTS *(cont.)*

NAME	FORM/ STRENGTH	DOSAGE	WARNINGS/PRECAUTIONS & CONTRAINDICATIONS	ADVERSE EFFECTS†
MIGRAINE THERAPY/TENSION HEADACHE *(cont.)*				
Naproxen Sodium/ Sumatriptan Succinate (Treximet) *(cont.)*			receiving anticoagulants, and preexisting asthma. **Contra:** History, symptoms, or signs of ischemic cardiac, cerebrovascular, or peripheral vascular syndromes. Other significant CVD; uncontrolled HTN; hemiplegic or basilar migraine; severe hepatic impairment; MAOIs during or within 2 weeks of use; within 24 hrs of ergotamine-containing agents, ergot-type agents, or other 5-HT_1 agonists; allergy to naproxen/asthma; nasal polyps; urticaria; and hypotension associated with NSAIDs. **P/N:** Category C, not for use in nursing.	
Naratriptan HCl (Amerge)	**Tab:** 1mg, 2.5mg	***Adults:*** **≥18 yrs:** 1mg or 2.5mg taken with fluids; may repeat dose once after 4 hrs. **Max:** 5mg/24 hrs. **Mild-Moderate Renal/Hepatic Impairment. Initial:** Lower dose. **Max:** 2.5mg/24 hrs. Safety of treating >4 headaches/30 days not known.	**W/P:** Confirm diagnosis. Supervise first dose and monitor cardiac function in those at risk of CAD (eg, HTN, hypercholesterolemia, smoker, obesity, diabetes, CAD family history, postmenopausal women, males >40 yrs). Monitor cardiovascular function with long-term intermittent use. May cause vasospastic reactions or cerebrovascular events. Caution with renal or hepatic dysfunction. Avoid in elderly. **Contra:** Uncontrolled HTN, ischemic cardiac, cerebrovascular, or peripheral vascular syndromes, other significant CVD, severe renal or hepatic impairment, and basilar or hemiplegic migraine. Within 24 hrs of another 5-HT_1 agonist, ergotamine-containing or ergot-containing drug (dihydroergotamine or methysergide). **P/N:** Category C, caution in nursing.	Paresthesias, dizziness, drowsiness, malaise/fatigue, **throat and neck symptoms (eg, pain/pressure sensation).**
Rizatriptan Benzoate (Maxalt, Maxalt-MLT)	**Tab:** 5mg, 10mg; **Tab, Disintegrating:** (MLT) 5mg, 10mg	***Adults:*** **≥18 yrs:** 5-10mg, may repeat q2h. **Max:** 30mg/24 hrs. Safety of treating >4 headaches/30 days not known. (MLT) Dissolve on tongue without water. **Concomitant Propranolol:** 5mg, up to 3 doses/24 hrs.	**W/P:** Confirm diagnosis. Supervise first dose and monitor cardiac function in those at risk of CAD (eg, HTN, hypercholesterolemia, smoker, obesity, diabetes, CAD family history, postmenopausal women, males >40 yrs). Serious adverse cardiac events, cerebrovascular events, vasospastic reactions, hypertensive crisis, and fatalities reported with 5-HT1 agonists. Disintegrating tabs contain phenylalanine. Caution with renal dialysis and hepatic dysfunction. **Contra:** Ischemic heart disease, coronary artery vasospasm (eg, Prinzmetal's angina), uncontrolled HTN, significant cardiovascular disease, hemiplegic or basilar migraine, MAOI use within 14 days, other 5-HT1 agonist or ergot-type agent use within 24 hrs. **P/N:** Category C, caution in nursing.	Paresthesia, **dry mouth,** nausea, dizziness, somnolence, asthenia/fatigue.
Sumatriptan (Imitrex)	**Inj:** 6mg/0.5mL; **Nasal Spray:** 5mg, 20mg [0.1mL 6[s]]; **Tab:** 25mg, 50mg, 100mg [9[s]]	***Adults:*** **≥18 yrs: (Inj) Initial:** 6mg SQ; may repeat after 1 hr. **Max:** 12mg/24 hrs. **(Spray)** 5mg, 10mg, or 20mg single dose; may repeat after 2 hrs. **Max:** 40mg/24 hrs. **(Tab) Initial:** 25-100mg; may repeat after 2 hrs. **Max:** 200mg/24 hrs. May give up to 100mg/day of tabs after initial inj dose. **Hepatic Disease: Max:** 50mg/single dose. Safety of treating >4 headaches/30 days not known.	**W/P:** Confirm diagnosis. Supervise first dose and monitor cardiac function in those at risk of CAD (eg, HTN, hypercholesterolemia, smoker, obesity, diabetes, CAD family history, postmenopausal women, males >40 yrs). Monitor cardiac function in intermittent long-term users with CAD risk factors. Serious adverse cardiac events, cerebrovascular events, vasospastic reactions reported. Avoid in elderly. Caution with hepatic or renal	Tingling, burning sensation, flushing, **chest/mouth/ tongue discomfort,** injection-site reaction, numbness, weakness, neck pain/stiffness.

*Scored. †Bold entries denote special dental considerations.
BB = black box warning; **W/P** = warnings/precautions; **Contra** = contraindications; **P/N** = pregnancy category rating and nursing considerations.

NAME	FORM/ STRENGTH	DOSAGE	WARNINGS/PRECAUTIONS & CONTRAINDICATIONS	ADVERSE EFFECTS†
Sumatriptan (Imitrex) *(cont.)*			impairment, history of seizures or brain lesions. Possible long-term ophthalmic effects. Reconsider diagnosis before second dose. **Contra:** History, symptoms, or signs of ischemic cardiac, cerebrovascular, or peripheral vascular syndromes. Other significant CVD, uncontrolled HTN, hemiplegic or basilar migraine, severe hepatic impairment, MAOIs during or within 2 weeks of use, within 24 hrs of ergotamine-containing agents, ergot-type agents, or other 5-HT_1 agonists. **P/N:** Category C, caution in nursing	
Zolmitriptan (Zomig, Zomig Nasal Spray, Zomig-ZMT)	**Nasal Spray:** 5mg [0.1mL, 6[S]]; **Tab:** 2.5mg*; 5mg; **Tab, Disintegrating:** (ZMT) 2.5mg, 5mg	***Adults:*** **≥18 yrs:** (Spray) 5mg single dose; may repeat once after 2 hrs. **Max:** 10mg/24 hrs. Safety of treating >4 headaches/30 days unknown. (Tab) **Initial:** 2.5mg or lower (2.5mg tab may be broken in 1/2), may repeat after 2 hrs. **Max:** 10mg/24 hrs. Safety of treating >3 headaches in 30 days is unknown. (ZMT) Dissolve on tongue without water. **Hepatic Impairment:** Use low dose and monitor blood pressure.	**W/P:** Confirm migraine diagnosis. Supervise first dose and monitor cardiac function in those at risk of CAD (eg, HTN, hypercholesterolemia, smoker, obesity, diabetes, CAD family history, postmenopausal women, males >40 yrs). Serious adverse cardiac events, cerebrovascular events, vasospastic reactions reported with 5-HT_1 agonists. Disintegrating tabs contain phenylalanine. Caution with hepatic dysfunction. Reconsider diagnosis before second dose, if no response seen after first dose. **Contra:** Ischemic heart disease, coronary artery vasospasm (eg, Prinzmetal's angina), uncontrolled HTN, other significant cardiovascular disease, hemiplegic or basilar migraine, MAOI use during or within 14 days, other 5-HT_1 agonist or ergot-type agent (eg, dihydroergotamine, methysergide) use within 24 hrs. **P/N:** Category C, caution in nursing.	Paresthesia, asthenia, warm/cold sensation, **neck/ throat/jaw pain, dry mouth,** nausea, dizziness, somnolence, **unusual taste** (nasal spray).
MUSCLE ANALGESICS/RELAXANTS				
Aspirin/Caffeine/ Orphenadrine Citrate	**Tab:** (ASA-Caffeine-Orphenadrine Citrate) 385mg-30mg-25mg; 770mg-60mg-50mg*	***Adults:*** (385mg-30mg-25mg) 1-2 tabs tid-qid. (770mg-60mg-50mg) 1/2-1 tab tid-qid.	**W/P:** Reye's Syndrome may develop with chickenpox, influenza, or flu symptoms. Extreme caution with peptic ulcers and coagulation abnormalities. Monitor blood, urine, and LFT's periodically with prolonged use. **Contra:** Glaucoma, pyloric or duodenal obstruction, achalasia, prostatic hypertrophy, bladder neck obstruction, myasthenia gravis. **P/N:** Safety in pregnancy and nursing not known.	Tachycardia, palpitation, urinary hesitancy/retention, **dry mouth,** blurred vision, increased intraocular tension, N/V, headache, dizziness, constipation, drowsiness, urticaria, GI hemorrhage.
Aspirin/ Carisoprodol (Soma Compound)	**Tab:** (Carisoprodol-ASA) 200mg-325mg	***Adults:*** **≤65 yrs/Pediatrics ≥16 yrs: Usual:** 1-2 tabs qid. **Max:** 2 tabs qid. Do not take for ≥2-3 weeks.	**W/P:** First-dose idiosyncratic reactions reported (rare). Caution with liver or renal dysfunction, elderly, peptic ulcer, gastritis, addiction-prone patients, and anticoagulant therapy. **Contra:** Acute intermittent porphyria, hypersensitivity to a carbamate, history of a serious GI complication due to aspirin or aspirin induced asthma. **P/N:** Category D, not for use in nursing.	Drowsiness, dizziness, vertigo, ataxia, N/V, gastritis, occult bleeding, constipation, diarrhea.
Aspirin/ Carisoprodol/ Codeine Phosphate (Soma Compound/ Codeine) CIII	**Tab:** (Carisoprodol-Codeine-Aspirin) 200mg-16mg-325mg	***Adults:*** **≤65 yrs/Pediatrics ≥16 yrs: Usual:** 1-2 tabs qid. **Max:** 2 tabs qid. Do not take for ≥2-3 weeks.	**W/P:** First-dose idiosyncratic reactions reported (rare). Contains sodium metabisulfate; may cause allergic-type reactions. Caution with liver or renal dysfunction, elderly, peptic ulcer, gastritis, addiction-prone patients, and anticoagulant therapy. Caution in individuals who are ultra rapid	Drowsiness, dizziness, vertigo, ataxia, N/V, gastritis, occult bleeding, constipation, diarrhea, miosis, allergic-skin rash, postural hypotension.

Table 17.1. PRESCRIBING INFORMATION FOR NEUROLOGICAL AGENTS *(cont.)*

NAME	FORM/ STRENGTH	DOSAGE	WARNINGS/PRECAUTIONS & CONTRAINDICATIONS	ADVERSE EFFECTS†
MUSCLE ANALGESICS/RELAXANTS *(cont.)*				
Aspirin/ Carisoprodol/ Codeine Phosphate (Soma Compound/ Codeine) CIII *(cont.)*			metabolizers of codeine. **Contra:** Acute intermittent porphyria, hypersensitivity to a carbamate, history of a serious GI complication due to aspirin or aspirin-induced asthma. **P/N:** Category D, not for use in nursing.	
Baclofen (Kemstro)	**Tab:** (Generic) 10mg*, 20mg*; **Tab, Disintegrating (ODT):** (Kemstro) 10mg*, 20mg*	***Adults/Pediatrics:*** **≥12 yrs: Initial:** 5mg tid for 3 days. **Titrate:** May increase dose by 5mg tid every 3 days. **Usual:** 40-80mg/day. **Max:** 80mg/day (20mg qid). **Renal Impairment:** Reduce dose.	**W/P:** Caution with psychosis, schizophrenia, confusional states; may exacerbate conditions. Caution with bladder sphincter hypertonia, peptic ulceration, seizures, elderly, cerebrovascular disorder, respiratory failure, hepatic or renal failure. Abnormal AST, alkaline phosphatase, and blood glucose reported. Caution when used to maintain locomotion or to obtain increased function. Decreased alertness with operating machinery. Has not significantly benefited stroke patients. Avoid abrupt discontinuation; reduce dose slowly over 1-2 weeks. **P/N:** Category C, caution in nursing.	Drowsiness, dizziness, weakness, fatigue, confusion, daytime sedation, headache, insomnia, hypotension, nausea, constipation, urinary frequency.
Carisoprodol (Soma)	**Tab:** 250mg, 350mg	***Adults:*** **≤65 yrs/Pediatrics ≥16 yrs:** 250-350mg tid and hs for 2-3 weeks. **Max:** ≤2-3 weeks.	**W/P:** May have sedative properties. Cases of drug abuse, dependence and withdrawal reported. Caution in addiction-prone patients. First-dose idiosyncratic reactions reported (rare). Occasionally within period of 1st-4th dose, allergic reactions have occured. Rare reports of seizures in postmarketing surveillance. Caution with liver or renal dysfunction. Seizures reported. **Contra:** Acute intermittent porphyria and hypersensitivity to a carbamate. **P/N:** Category C, caution in nursing.	Drowsiness, dizziness, headache, N/V, tachycardia, postural hypotension, agitation, irritability, insomnia, seizures.
Chlorzoxazone (Parafon Forte DSC)	**Tab:** 500mg*	***Adults:*** **Usual:** 500mg tid-qid. **Titrate:** May increase to 750mg tid-qid.	**W/P:** Serious (including fatal) hepatocellular toxicity reported. D/C if signs of hepatotoxicity develop. Caution with history of drug allergies. **P/N:** Safety in pregnancy and nursing not known.	Drowsiness, dizziness, malaise, lightheadedness, overstimulation.
Cyclobenzaprine HCl (Amrix, Flexeril)	**Cap, Extended-Release:** (Amrix) 15mg, 30mg; **Tab:** (Flexeril) 5mg, 10mg	***Adults:*** **Amrix: Usual:** 15mg qd. **Titrate:** May increase to 30mg qd if needed. **Max:** Use for longer than 2-3 weeks not recommended. ***Adults/ Pediatrics*** **≥15 yrs: Flexeril: Usual:** 5mg tid. **Titrate:** May increase to 10mg tid. **Max:** Use for longer than 2-3 weeks not recommended. **Mild Hepatic Dysfunction/Elderly: Initial:** 5mg qd, then titrate slowly. **Moderate/Severe Hepatic Dysfunction:** Avoid use.	**W/P:** Caution with history of urinary retention, angle-closure glaucoma, increased IOP, hepatic dysfunction. Caution in elderly due to increased risk of CNS effects. May produce arrhythmias, sinus tachycardia, and conduction time prolongation. May impair mental/ physical abilities. **Contra:** Acute recovery phase of MI, arrhythmias, heart block or conduction disturbances, CHF, hyperthyroidism, MAOI use during or within 14 days. **P/N:** Category B, caution in nursing.	Drowsiness, **dry mouth,** headache, dizziness, somnolence, fatigue.
Dantrolene Sodium (Dantrium IV)	**Inj:** 20mg	***Adults/Pediatrics:*** **Malignant Hyperthermia: Initial:** Minimum 1mg/ kg IV push. Continue until symptoms subside or max cumulative dose 10mg/ kg. ***Adults:*** **Pre-Op Malignant Hyperthermia Prophylaxis:** 2.5mg/kg 1.25 hrs before anesthesia and infuse over 1 hr. May need additional therapy during anesthesia/surgery if symptoms arise. **Post-Op Prophylaxis: Initial:** 1mg/kg or more as clinical situation dictates.	**W/P:** Use with supportive therapies to treat malignant hyperthermia. Take steps to prevent extravasation. Fatal and non-fatal hepatic disorders reported. Do not operate automobile or engage in hazardous activity for 48 hrs after therapy. Caution at meals on day of administration because difficulty in swallowing/choking reported. Monitor vital signs if receive preoperatively. **P/N:** Category C, safety in nursing not known.	Loss of grip strength, weakness in legs, drowsiness, dizziness, pulmonary edema, thrombophlebitis, urticaria, erythema.

*Scored. †Bold entries denote special dental considerations.
BB = black box warning; **W/P** = warnings/precautions; **Contra** = contraindications; **P/N** = pregnancy category rating and nursing considerations.

NAME	FORM/ STRENGTH	DOSAGE	WARNINGS/PRECAUTIONS & CONTRAINDICATIONS	ADVERSE EFFECTS†
Dantrolene Sodium (Dantrium)	**Cap:** 25mg, 50mg, 100mg	***Adults:* Chronic Spasticity: Initial:** 25mg qd for 7 days. **Titrate:** Increase to 25mg tid for 7 days, then 50mg tid for 7 days, then 100mg tid. **Max:** 100mg qid. If no further benefit at next higher dose, decrease to previous lower dose. **Malignant Hyperthermia: Pre-Op:** 4-8mg/kg/day given tid-qid for 1-2 days before surgery, with last dose given 3-4 hrs before surgery. **Post-Op Following Malignant Hyperthermia Crisis:** 4-8mg/kg/day given qid for 1-3 days. ***Pediatrics:* ≥5 yrs: Chronic Spasticity: Initial:** 0.5mg/kg qd for 7 days. **Titrate:** Increase to 0.5mg/kg tid for 7 days, then 1mg/kg tid for 7 days, then 2mg/kg tid. **Max:** 100mg qid. If no further benefit at next higher dose, decrease to previous lower dose.	**BB:** Associated with hepatotoxicity; monitor hepatic function. Discontinue if no benefit after 45 days. **W/P:** Monitor LFTs at baseline, then periodically. Increased risk of hepatocellular disease in females and patients >35 yrs. Caution with pulmonary, cardiac, and liver dysfunction. Photosensitivity reaction may occur; limit sunlight exposure. **Contra:** Active hepatic disease, where spasticity is utilized to sustain upright posture and balance in locomotion, when spasticity is utilized to obtain or maintain increased function. **P/N:** Safety in nursing not known. Not for use in nursing.	Drowsiness, dizziness, weakness, malaise, fatigue, diarrhea, hepatitis, tachycardia, aplastic anemia, thrombocytopenia, depression, seizure.
Metaxalone (Skelaxin)	**Tab:** 800mg*	***Adults/Pediatrics:* >12 yrs:** 800mg tid-qid.	**W/P:** Caution with preexisting liver damage. Monitor hepatic function. False-positive Benedict's test reported. **Contra:** Tendency for drug-induced, hemolytic, and other anemias. Significant renal or hepatic impairment. **P/N:** Not for use in pregnancy or nursing.	N/V, GI upset, drowsiness, dizziness, headache, nervousness, leukopenia, hemolytic anemia, jaundice.
Methocarbamol (Robaxin, Robaxin Injection, Robaxin-750)	**Inj:** 100mg/mL [10mL]; **Tab:** 500mg, 750mg	***Adults:* (PO) Initial: (500mg tab)** 1500mg qid for 2-3 days. **Maint:** 1000mg qid. **Initial: (750mg tab)** 1500mg qid for 2-3 days. **Maint:** 750mg q4h or 1500mg tid. **Max:** 6g/d for 2-3 days; 8g/d if severe. **(Inj) Moderate Symptoms:** 10mL IV/IM. **IV Max Rate:** 3mL undiluted drug/min. **IM Max:** 5mL into each gluteal region. **Severe/Post-Op Condition: Max:** 20-30mL/day up to 3 consecutive days. If feasible, continue with PO. **Tetanus:** 10-20mL up to 30mL. May repeat q6h until NG tube can be inserted. Continue with crushed tabs. **Max:** 24g/day PO. ***Pediatrics:* Tetanus: Initial:** 15mg/kg or 500mg/m^2. Repeat q6h prn. **Max:** 1.8g/m^2 for three consecutive days. Administer by injection into tubing or IV infusion.	**W/P:** May impair mental/physical abilities required for operating machinery or driving a motor vehicle. May cause color interference in certain screening tests for 5-hydroxy-indoleacetic acid (5-HIAA) and vanillylmandelic acid (VMA). Caution in epilepsy with the injection. Injection rate should not exceed 3mL/min. Avoid extravasation with injection. Avoid use of injection particularly during early pregnancy. **Contra:** (Inj) Renal pathology with injection due to propylene glycol content. **P/N:** Category C, caution in nursing.	Lightheadedness, dizziness, drowsiness, nausea, urticaria, pruritus, rash, conjunctivitis, nasal congestion, blurred vision, headache, fever, seizures, syncope, flushing.
Orphenadrine Citrate	**Inj:** 30mg/mL [2mL]; **Tab, Extended-Release:** 100mg	***Adults:*** (Tab) 100mg bid, in the am and pm. (Inj) 60mg IM/IV q12h.	**W/P:** Caution with tachycardia, cardiac decompensation, coronary insufficiency, cardiac arrhythmias. Monitor blood, urine, and LFTs periodically with prolonged use. Injection contains sodium bisulfite. **Contra:** Glaucoma, pyloric or duodenal obstruction, stenosing peptic ulcers, prostatic hypertrophy, bladder neck obstruction, cardiospasm, myasthenia gravis. **P/N:** Category C, safety in nursing not known.	**Dry mouth,** tachycardia, palpitation, urinary hesitancy/retention, blurred vision, pupil dilation, increased ocular tension, weakness, dizziness, constipation.
Tizanidine HCl (Zanaflex)	**Cap:** 2mg, 4mg, 6mg; **Tab:** 2mg*, 4mg*	***Adults:* Initial:** 4mg single dose q6-8h. **Titrate:** Increase by 2-4mg. **Usual:** 8mg single dose q6-8h. **Max:** 3 doses/24h or 36mg/day.	**W/P:** May prolong QT interval. May cause liver damage; monitor baseline LFTs and at 1, 3, and 6 months. Retinal degeneration and corneal opacities reported. Caution with renal impairment or elderly. May cause hypotension, caution with antihypertensives; avoid ciprofloxacin and fluvoxamine. Use with extreme cautions in patients with hepatic impairment. May cause sedation and hallucinations. Avoid concomitant use	**Dry mouth,** somnolence, asthenia, dizziness, UTI, urinary frequency, flu-like syndrome, rhinitis.

Table 17.1. PRESCRIBING INFORMATION FOR NEUROLOGICAL AGENTS *(cont.)*

NAME	FORM/ STRENGTH	DOSAGE	WARNINGS/PRECAUTIONS & CONTRAINDICATIONS	ADVERSE EFFECTS†
MUSCLE ANALGESICS/RELAXANTS *(cont.)*				
Tizanidine HCl (Zanaflex) *(cont.)*			with oral contraceptives. When discontinuing, taper dose to avoid withdrawal and rebound HTN, tachycardia, and hypertonia. **Contra:** Concomitant use with fluvoxamine, ciprofloxacin, or potent inhibitors of CYP1A2. **P/N:** Category C, caution in nursing	
MISCELLANEOUS NEUROLOGICAL AGENTS				
Atropine Sulfate	**Inj:** 0.05mg/mL, 0.1mg/mL, 0.4mg/mL, 0.5mg/mL, 1mg/mL	***Adults:*** **Usual:** 0.5mg IM/IV/SC. **Range:** 0.4-0.6mg. If used as an antisialagogue, inject IM prior to anesthesia induction. **Bradyarrhythmias:** 0.4-1mg every 1-2 hrs prn. **Max:** 2mg/dose. May be used as antidote for cardiovascular collapse resulting from injudicious administration of choline ester. When cardiac arrest has occurred, external cardiac massage or other method of resuscitation is required to distribute the drug after IV injection. **Anticholinesterase Poisoning From Insecticide Poisoning:** 2-3mg IV. Repeat until signs of atropine intoxication appear. **Mushroom Poisoning:** Administer sufficient doses to control parasympathomimetic signs before coma and cardiovascular collapse supervene. ***Pediatrics:*** **Range:** 0.1mg (newborn) to 0.6mg (>12 yrs). Inject SC 30 min before surgery. **Bradyarrhythmias: Range:** 0.01-0.03mg/kg IV.	**W/P:** Avoid overdose in IV administration. Increased susceptibility to toxic effects in children. Caution in patients >40 yrs. Conventional doses may precipitate glaucoma in susceptible patients, convert partial organic pyloric stenosis into complete obstruction, lead to complete urinary retention in patients with prostatic hypertrophy or cause inspissation of bronchial secretions and formation of dangerous viscid plugs in patients with chronic lung disease. **Contra:** Glaucoma, pyloric stenosis, or prostatic hypertrophy except in doses used for preanesthetic medication. **P/N:** Category C, safety in nursing not known.	**Dryness of the mouth,** blurred vision, photophobia, tachycardia, anhidrosis.
Riluzole (Rilutek)	**Tab:** 50mg	***Adults:*** 50mg q12h. Take 1 hr before or 2 hrs after meals.	**W/P:** Caution in elderly, and hepatic or renal dysfunction. Perform baseline LFT's before therapy, every month during first 3 months, every 3 months for next 9 months, then periodically thereafter. Neutropenia reported; obtain WBC count with febrile illness. **P/N:** Category C, not for use in nursing.	Asthenia, N/V, dizziness, decreased lung function, diarrhea, abdominal pain, pneumonia, vertigo, paresthesia, anorexia, somnolence

†Bold entries denote special dental considerations.
BB = black box warning; **W/P** = warnings/precautions; **Contra** = contraindications; **P/N** = pregnancy category rating and nursing considerations.

Table 17.2. DRUG INTERACTIONS FOR NEUROLOGICAL AGENTS

ALZHEIMER'S AGENTS	
Donepezil HCl (Aricept, Aricept ODT)	
Anticholinergics	May interfere with anticholinergic medications.
Cholinergic agonists	Synergistic effect with cholinergic agonists (eg, bethanechol).
CYP inducers	CYP2D6 and CYP3A4 inducers (eg, phenytoin, carbamazepine, dexamethasone, rifampin, phenobarbital) may increase elimination rate.
CYP inhibitors	Ketoconazole and quinidine, inhibitors of CYP450, 3A4, and 2D6, inhibit donepezil metabolism.
Neuromuscular blockers	Synergistic effect with neuromuscular blocking agents (eg, succinylcholine).
Galantamine Hydrobromide (Razadyne, Razadyne ER)	
Anticholinergics	May interfere with anticholinergic medications.
Cholinergic agonists	Synergistic effect with cholinergic agonists (eg, bethanechol).
Cholinesterase inhibitors	Synergistic effect with other cholinesterase inhibitors.
Cimetidine	Increased levels with cimetidine.
Drugs that slow heart rate	Caution with drugs that slow heart rate due to vagotonic effects.
Ketoconazole	Increased levels with ketoconazole.
Neuromuscular blockers	Synergistic effect with neuromuscular blocking agents (eg, succinylcholine).
NSAIDs	Monitor for GI bleeding with NSAIDs.
Paroxetine	Increased levels with paroxetine.
Succinylcholine	Synergistic effect with succinylcholine.
Memantine HCl (Namenda)	
NMDA antagonists	Caution with other NMDA antagonists (eg, amantadine, ketamine, dextromethorphan).
Renally-excreted drugs	Other renally-excreted drugs (eg, HCTZ, triamterene, metformin, cimetidine, ranitidine, quinidine, nicotine) may alter levels of both agents.
Urinary alkalinizers	Caution with urinary alkalinizers (eg, carbonic anhydrase inhibitors, sodium bicarbonate).
Rivastigmine Tartrate (Exelon)	
Anticholinergics	May interfere with anticholinergic medications.
Cholinergic agonists	Synergistic effect with cholinergic agonists (eg, bethanechol).
Neuromuscular blockers	Synergistic effect with neuromuscular blocking agents (eg, succinylcholine).
Succinylcholine	May be synergistic with succinylcholine. May exaggerate succinylcholine-type muscle relaxation during anesthesia.
Tacrine HCl (Cognex)	
Anticholinergics	May interfere with anticholinergic medications.
Cholinergic agonists	Synergistic effect with cholinergic agonists (eg, bethanechol).
Cholinesterase inhibitors	Synergistic effect with cholinesterase inhibitors.
Cimetidine	Increased levels with cimetidine.
CYP450 substrates	May interact with drugs metabolized by CYP450.

Table 17.2. DRUG INTERACTIONS FOR NEUROLOGICAL AGENTS *(cont.)*

ALZHEIMER'S AGENTS *(cont.)*	
Tacrine HCl (Cognex) *(cont.)*	
Fluvoxamine	Fluvoxamine increases levels.
Neuromuscular blockers	Synergistic effect with neuromuscular blocking agents (eg, succinylcholine).
NSAIDs	Monitor for GI bleeding with NSAIDs.
Theophylline	May potentiate theophylline.
ANTICONVULSANTS	
Acetazolamide	
Amphetamines	Acetazolamide decreases the urinary excretion of amphetamines and may enhance their effects.
Aspirin	Caution with high-dose ASA as anorexia, tachypnea, lethargy, coma, and death have been reported.
Carbonic anhydrase inhibitors	May increase effects of other carbonic anhydrase inhibitors.
Cyclosporine	May increase levels of cyclosporine.
Folic acid antagonists	May increase effects of folic acid antagonists.
Hypoglycemic agents	Caution with hypoglycemic agents; acetazolamide may increase or decrease blood glucose levels.
Lithium	Acetazolamide increases the urinary excretion of lithium and may decrease its levels.
Methenamine	May prevent urinary antiseptic effect of methenamine.
Phenytoin	May increase phenytoin levels; may increase occurrence of osteomalacia.
Primidone	May decrease gastrointestinal absorption of primidone.
Quinidine	Acetazolamide decreases the urinary excretion of quinidine and may enhance its effects.
Sodium bicarbonate	Increased risk of renal calculus formation with sodium bicarbonate.
Carbamazepine (Carbatrol, Tegretol, Tegretol-XR)	
Acetaminophen	Decreases levels of APAP.
Anticonvulsants	Decreases levels of other anticonvulsants (eg, ethosuximide, felbamate, oxcarbazepine, etc.).
Antipsychotics	Decreases levels of clozapine, haloperidol, olanzapine, quetiapine, risperidone, and ziprasidone.
Benzodiazepines	Decreases levels of alprazolam, clonazepam, diazepam, lorazepam, midazolam, and triazolam.
Bupropion	Carbatrol: Decreases levels of bupropion.
Buspirone	Carbatrol: Decreases levels of buspirone.
Calcium channel blockers, dihydropyridine	Decreases levels of dihydropyridine calcium channel blockers (eg, felodipine).
Citalopram	Decreases levels of citalopram.

ANTICONVULSANTS *(cont.)*

Carbamazepine (Carbatrol, Tegretol, Tegretol-XR) *(cont.)*	
Clomipramine	Increases plasma levels of clomipramine.
Contraceptives, oral	Decreases the levels and effectiveness of oral contraceptives.
Cyclosporine	Decreases levels of cyclosporine.
CYP1A2 substrates	Carbamazepine potentiates metabolism of drugs by CYP1A2.
CYP3A4 inducers	Metabolism is induced by CYP3A4 inducers (eg, rifampin, phenytoin, trazodone, etc.).
CYP3A4 inhibitors	Metabolism is inhibited by CYP3A4 inhibitors (eg, azole antifungals, cimetidine, macrolides, etc.).
CYP3A4 substrates	Carbamazepine potentiates metabolism of drugs by CYP3A4.
Delaviridine	Decreases levels of delaviridine.
Dicumarol	Decreases levels of dicumarol.
Diluents	Tegretol, Tegretol-XR: Do not give suspension with diluents.
Doxycycline	Decreases levels of doxycycline.
Epoxide hydrolase inhibitors	Increased levels of carbamezepine with drugs that inhibit epoxide hydrolase (eg, clarithromycin).
Glucocorticoids	Decreases levels of glucocorticoids.
Itraconazole	Decreases levels of itraconazole.
Levothyroxine	Decreases levels of levothyroxine.
Lithium	Increased risk of neurotoxic side effects with lithium.
MAOIs	MAOI use should be discontinued for a minimum of 14 days before use of carbamazepine.
Medicinal liquids	Tegretol, Tegretol-XR: Do not give suspension with other medicinal liquids.
Methadone	Decreases levels of methadone.
Mirtazapine	Decreases levels of mirtazapine.
Phenytoin	Increases/decreases levels of phenytoin.
Protease inhibitors	Increased levels of carbamazepine and decreased levels of protease inhibitors.
Theophylline	Decreases levels of theophylline.
Tramadol	Decreases levels of tramadol.
Tricyclic antidepressants (TCAs)	Contraindicated if sensitive to TCAs.
Warfarin	Decreases levels of warfarin.
Clonazepam (Klonopin, Klonopin Wafers) CIV	
Alcohol	Alcohol potentiates CNS-depressant effects.
Anticonvulsants	Other anticonvulsant drugs potentiate CNS-depressant effects.
Antipsychotic, butyrophenone	Butyrophenone antipsychotics potentiate CNS-depressant effects.
Anxiolytics	Anxiolytics potentiate CNS-depressant effects.

Table 17.2. DRUG INTERACTIONS FOR NEUROLOGICAL AGENTS *(cont.)*

ANTICONVULSANTS *(cont.)*	
Clonazepam (Klonopin, Klonopin Wafers) CIV *(cont.)*	
Barbiturates	Barbiturates potentiate CNS-depressant effects.
CYP3A inhibitors	Caution with CYP3A inhibitors (eg, oral antifungals).
CYP450 inducers	Decreased serum levels with CYP450 inducers (eg, phenytoin, carbamazepine, phenobarbital).
Hypnotics, nonbarbiturate	Nonbarbiturate hypnotics potentiate CNS-depressant effects.
MAOIs	MAOIs potentiate CNS-depressant effects.
Narcotics	Narcotics potentiate CNS-depressant effects.
Phenothiazines	Phenothiazines potentiate CNS-depressant effects.
Thioxanthene	Thioxanthene potentiates CNS-depressant effects.
Tricyclic antidepressants (TCAs)	TCAs potentiate CNS-depressant effects.
Diazepam (Diastat) CIV	
Antidepressants	Potentiated by other antidepressants.
Barbiturates	Potentiated by barbiturates.
CYP450 inducers	CYP450 2C19 (eg, rifampin) and CYP450 3A4 (eg, carbamazepine, phenytoin, dexamethasone, phenobarbital) inducers could increase elimination.
CYP450 inhibitors	Potential inhibitors of CYP450 2C19 (eg, cimetidine, quinidine, tranylcypromine) and CYP450 3A4 (eg, ketoconazole, troleandomycin, clotrimazole) may decrease elimination.
CYP450 substrates	May interfere with metabolism of substrates for CYP450 2C19 (eg, omeprazole, propranolol, imipramine) and CYP450 3A4 (eg, cyclosporine, paclitaxel, terfenadine, theophylline, warfarin).
Monoamine oxidase inhibitors	Potentiated by MAOIs.
Narcotics	Potentiated by narcotics.
Phenothiazines	Potentiated by phenothiazines.
Valproate	Potentiated by valproate.
Divalproex Sodium (Depakote, Depakote ER)	
Amitriptyline	Potentiates amitriptyline.
Aspirin	Efficacy potentiated by ASA.
Carbamazepine	Potentiates carbamazepine. Efficacy reduced by carbamazepine.
Clonazepam	Clonazepam may induce absence status in patients with history of absence type seizures.
CNS depressants	CNS depression with alcohol and other CNS depressants.
Diazepam	Potentiates diazepam.
Ethosuximide	Potentiates ethosuximide.
Felbamate	Efficacy potentiated by felbamate.
Lamotrigine	Potentiates lamotrigine.
Lorazepam	Potentiates lorazepam.

ANTICONVULSANTS *(cont.)*

Divalproex Sodium (Depakote, Depakote ER) *(cont.)*	
Nortriptyline	Potentiates nortriptyline.
Phenobarbital	Potentiates phenobarbital. Efficacy reduced by phenobarbital.
Phenytoin	Potentiates phenytoin. Efficacy reduced by phenytoin.
Primidone	Potentiates primidone. Efficacy reduced by primidone.
Rifampin	Efficacy reduced by rifampin.
Tolbutamide	Potentiates tolbutamide.
Warfarin	Monitor PT/INR with warfarin.
Zidovudine	Potentiates zidovudine.
Ethosuximide (Zarontin)	
Phenytoin	May increase phenytoin levels.
Valproic acid	Valproic acid may alter levels.
Felbamate (Felbatol)	
Carbamazepine	Increases plasma levels of active carbamazepine metabolite. Decreases carbamazepine levels. Decreased felbamate levels with carbamazepine.
Contraceptives, oral	Caution with oral contraceptives.
Phenobarbital	Increases plasma levels of phenobarbital. Decreased felbamate levels with phenobarbital.
Phenytoin	Increases plasma levels of phenytoin. Decreased felbamate levels with phenytoin.
Valproate	Increases plasma levels of valproate.
Fosphenytoin Sodium (Cerebyx)	
Alcohol	Increased levels with acute alcohol intake. Decreased levels with chronic alcohol abuse.
Amiodarone	Increased levels with amiodarone.
Anticoagulants	Decreases efficacy of anticoagulants.
Carbamazepine	Decreased levels with carbamazepine.
Chloramphenicol	Increased levels with chloramphenicaol.
Chlordiazepoxide	Increased levels with chlordiazepoxide.
Cimetidine	Increased levels with cimetidine.
Contraceptives, oral	Decreases efficacy of oral contraceptives.
Corticosteroids	Decreases efficacy of corticosteroids.
Coumarin	Decreases efficacy of coumarin.
Diazepam	Increased levels with diazepam.
Dicumarol	Increased levels with dicumarol.
Digitoxin	Decreases efficacy of digitoxin.
Disulfiram	Increased levels with disulfiram.

Table 17.2. DRUG INTERACTIONS FOR NEUROLOGICAL AGENTS *(cont.)*

ANTICONVULSANTS *(cont.)*

Fosphenytoin Sodium (Cerebyx) *(cont.)*	
Doxycyline	Decreases efficacy of doxycycline.
Estrogens	Increased levels with estrogens. Decreases efficacy of estrogens.
Ethosuximide	Increased levels with ethosuximide.
Fluoxetine	Increased levels with fluoxetine.
Furosemide	Decreases efficacy of furosemide.
H_2-Antagonists	Increased levels with H_2-antagonists.
Halothane	Increased levels with halothane.
Isoniazid	Increased levels with isoniazid.
Methylphenidate	Increased levels with methylphenidate.
Phenobarbital	Variable effects (increased or decreased levels) with phenobarbital.
Phenothiazines	Increased levels with phenothiazines.
Phenylbutazone	Increased levels with phenylbutazone.
Protein-bound drugs	Caution with drugs highly bound to serum albumin.
Quinidine	Decreases efficacy of quinidine.
Reserpine	Decreased levels with reserpine.
Rifampin	Decreases efficacy of rifampin.
Salicylates	Increased levels with salicylates.
Sodium valproate	Variable effects (increased or decreased levels) with sodium valproate.
Succinimides	Increased levels with succinimides.
Sulfonamides	Increased levels with sulfonamides.
Theophylline	Decreases efficacy of theophylline.
Tolbutamide	Increased levels with tolbutamide.
Trazadone	Increased levels with trazadone.
Tricyclic antidepressants (TCAs)	TCAs may precipitate seizures.
Valproic acid	Variable effects (increased or decreased levels) with valproic acid.
Vitamin D	Decreases efficacy of vitamin D.
Gabapentin (Neurontin)	
Antacids	Take 2 hrs after antacids.
Morphine	Increased levels with controlled-release morphine.
Lamotrigine (Lamictal, Lamictal CD)	
Carbamazepine	Decreased levels by 40% with carbamazepine.
Contraceptives, oral	Decreased levels about 50% with estrogen-containing oral contraceptives.
Folate inhibitors	Inhibits dihydrofolate reductase; may potentiate folate inhibitors.
Phenobarbital	Decreased levels by 40% with phenobarbital.
Phenytoin	Decreased levels by 40% with phenytoin.

ANTICONVULSANTS *(cont.)*

Lamotrigine (Lamictal, Lamictal CD) *(cont.)*	
Primidone	Decreased levels by 40% with primidone.
Rifampin	Decreased levels about 50% with rifampin.
Valproic acid	Risk of life-threatening rash with valproic acid. Lamotrigine decreases valproic acid levels; valproic acid increases lamotrigine levels slightly more than 2-fold.
Mephobarbital (Mebaral) CIV	
Alcohol	Additive CNS depression with alcohol.
Anticoagulants, oral	Decreases effects of oral anticoagulants.
CNS depressants	May produce additive CNS depression with other CNS depressants (eg, other sedative-hypnotics, antihistamines, tranquilizers).
Contraceptives, oral	Decreases effects of oral contraceptives.
Corticosteroids	Increases corticosteroid metabolism.
Doxycycline	Decreases half-life of doxycycline.
Griseofulvin	Interferes with griseofulvin absorption.
MAOIs	MAOIs may prolong effects.
Phenytoin	May alter phenytoin metabolism.
Sodium valproate	Sodium valproate decreases metabolism.
Valproic acid	Valproic acid decreases metabolism.
Methsuximide (Celontin)	
Anticonvulsants	May interact with other anticonvulsants; monitor serum levels periodically.
Phenobarbital	May increase phenobarbital levels.
Phenytoin	May increase phenytoin levels.
Oxcarbazepine (Trileptal)	
Alcohol	Additive sedative effect with alcohol.
Carbamazepine	Carbamazepine may decrease levels.
Contraceptives, oral	Decreased plasma levels of oral contraceptives.
Felodipine	Decreased plasma levels of felodipine.
Phenobarbital	Phenobarbital may decrease levels. Increased plasma levels of phenobarbital.
Phenytoin	Phenytoin may decrease levels. Increased plasma levels of phenytoin.
Valproic acid	Valproic acid may decrease levels.
Verapamil	Verapamil may decrease levels.
Pentobarbital Sodium (Nembutal Sodium) CII	
Alcohol	Additive CNS depression with alcohol.
Anticoagulants, oral	May decrease levels of oral anticoagulants. May require dosage adjustments for anticoagulants.
Antihistamines	May produce additive CNS depression with antihistamines.

Table 17.2. DRUG INTERACTIONS FOR NEUROLOGICAL AGENTS *(cont.)*

ANTICONVULSANTS *(cont.)*

Pentobarbital Sodium (Nembutal Sodium) CII *(cont.)*	
CNS depressants	May produce additive CNS depression with other CNS depressants.
Contraceptives, oral	May decrease effects of estradiol, estrone, progesterone, and other steroidal hormones; alternative contraceptive method should be suggested.
Corticosteroids	May decrease levels of corticosteroids. May require dosage adjustments for corticosteroids.
Doxycycline	May decrease levels of doxycycline.
Griseofulvin	May decrease levels of griseofulvin.
MAOIs	Prolonged effect with MAOIs.
Phenytoin	Variable effects on phenytoin; monitor blood levels and adjust dose appropriately.
Sedative-hypnotics	May produce additive CNS depression with sedative-hypnotics.
Sodium valproate	Increased levels with sodium valproate; monitor blood levels and adjust dose appropriately.
Tranquilizers	May produce additive CNS depression with tranquilizers.
Valproic acid	Increased levels with sodium valproate; monitor blood levels and adjust dose appropriately.
Phenobarbital CIV	
Alcohol	Additive CNS depression with alcohol.
Anticoagulants, oral	Decreases effects of oral anticoagulants.
Antihistamines	May be potentiated by antihistamines.
CNS depressants	May be potentiated by other CNS depressants.
Contraceptives, oral	Decreases effects of oral contraceptives.
Corticosteroids	Increases corticosteroid metabolism.
Doxycycline	Decreases half-life of doxycycline.
Griseofulvin	Decreases absorption of griseofulvin.
MAOIs	May be potentiated by MAOIs.
Phenytoin	May alter phenytoin metabolism.
Sedative-hypnotics	May be potentiated by sedative-hypnotics.
Sodium valproate	Increased levels with sodium valproate.
Tranquilizers	May be potentiated by tranquilizers.
Valproic acid	Increased levels with valproic acid.
Phenytoin Sodium (Dilantin, Phenytek)	
Alcohol	Increased levels with acute alcohol intake. Decreased levels with chronic alcohol abuse.
Amiodarone	Increased levels with amiodarone.
Antacids	Calcium antacids decrease absorption; space dosing.

ANTICONVULSANTS *(cont.)*

Phenytoin Sodium (Dilantin, Phenytek) *(cont.)*	
Barbiturates	Increased risk of phenytoin hypersensitivity with barbiturates.
Carbamazepine	Decreased levels with carbamazepine.
Chloramphenicol	Increased levels with chloramphenicol.
Chlordiazepoxide	Increased levels with chlordiazepoxide.
Contraceptives, oral	Decreases effects of oral contraceptives.
Corticosteroids	Decreases effects of corticosteroids.
Coumarin anticoagulants	Decreases effects of coumarin anticoagulants.
Diazepam	Increased levels with diazepam.
Dicumarol	Increased levels with dicumarol.
Digitoxin	Decreases effects of digitoxin.
Disulfiram	Increased levels with disulfiram.
Doxycycline	Decreases effects of doxycycline.
Estrogens	Increased levels with estrogens. Decreases effects of estrogens.
Furosemide	Decreases effects of furosemide.
H_2 Antagonists	Increased levels with H_2 antagonists.
Halothane	Increased levels with halothane.
Isoniazid	Increased levels with isoniazid.
Methylphenidate	Increased levels with methylphenidate.
Moban	Moban contains calcium ions that interfere with absorption.
Oxazolidinediones	Increased risk of phenytoin hypersensitivity with oxazolidinediones.
Phenobarbital	May increase or decrease levels of phenobarbital or phenytoin.
Phenothiazines	Increased levels with phenothiazines.
Phenylbutazone	Increased levels with phenylbutazone.
Quinidine	Decreases effects of quinidine.
Reserpine	Decreased levels with reserpine.
Rifampin	Decreases effects of rifampin.
Salicylates	Increased levels with salicylates.
Sodium valproate	May increase or decrease levels of sodium valproate or phenytoin.
Succinamides	Increased levels with succinamides. Increased risk of phenytoin hypersensitivity with succinamides.
Sucralfate	Decreased levels with sucralfate.
Sulfonamides	Increased levels with sulfonamides.
Theophylline	Decreases effects of theophylline.
Tolbutamide	Increased levels with tolbutamide.
Trazodone	Increased levels with trazodone.

Table 17.2. DRUG INTERACTIONS FOR NEUROLOGICAL AGENTS *(cont.)*

ANTICONVULSANTS *(cont.)*

Phenytoin Sodium (Dilantin, Phenytek) *(cont.)*	
Tricyclic antidepressants (TCAs)	TCAs may precipitate seizures.
Valproic acid	May increase or decrease levels of valproic acid or phenytoin.
Vitamin D	Decreases effects of vitamin D.
Pregabalin (Lyrica) CV	
Alcohol	Additive CNS depression with alcohol.
CNS depressants	Additive CNS side effects with CNS depressants (eg, opiates, benzodiazepines).
Tiagabine HCl (Gabitril)	
Alcohol	Additive CNS depression with alcohol.
Carbamazepine	Diminished effects with carbamazepine.
CNS depressants	Additive CNS depression with CNS depressants.
Phenytoin	Diminished effects with phenytoin.
Triazolam	Additive CNS depression with triazolam.
Valproate levels	May reduce valproate levels.
Topiramate (Topamax, Topamax Sprinkle Capsules)	
Alcohol	Additive CNS depression with alcohol.
Carbamazepine	Carbamazepine decreases levels.
Carbonic anhydrase inhibitors	Increased risk of kidney stones with carbonic anhydrase inhibitors.
CNS depressants	May potentiate CNS depression with other CNS depressants.
Digoxin	May decrease AUC of digoxin.
Metformin	May increase metformin levels; monitor diabetics regularly.
Phenytoin	Phenytoin decreases levels. Increases phenytoin levels.
Valproic acid	Valproic acid decreases levels. Decreases valproic acid levels.
Valproate Sodium (Depacon)	
Alcohol	Additive CNS depression with alcohol.
Amitriptyline	Potentiates amitriptyline.
Aspirin	Potentiated by ASA.
Carbamazepine	Potentiates carbamazepine. Antagonized by carbamazepine.
Clonazepam	Clonazepam may induce absence status in patients with absence seizures.
CNS depressants	Additive CNS depression with other CNS depressants.
Diazepam	Potentiates diazepam.
Ethosuximide	Potentiates ethosuximide.
Felbamate	Potentiated by felbamate.
Lamotrigine	Potentiates lamotrigine.
Nortriptyline	Potentiates nortriptyline.
Phenobarbital	Potentiates phenobarbital. Antagonized by phenobarbital.

ANTICONVULSANTS *(cont.)*

Valproate Sodium (Depacon) *(cont.)*	
Phenytoin	Potentiates phenytoin. Antagonized by phenytoin.
Primidone	Potentiates primidone.
Rifampin	Antagonized by rifampin.
Tolbutamide	Potentiates tolbutamide.
Warfarin	Potentiates warfarin.
Zidovudine	Potentiates zidovudine.
Valproic Acid (Depakene, Stavzor)	
Alcohol	Additive CNS depression with alcohol.
Carbamazepine	May potentiate carbamazepine. Antagonized by carbamazepine.
Carbapenems	Carbapenem antibiotics may reduce serum levels.
Clonazepam	Clonazepam may induce absence status in patients with absence seizures.
CNS depressants	Additive CNS depression with other CNS depressants.
Diazepam	May potentiate diazepam.
Ethosuximide	May potentiate ethosuximide.
Felbamate	Potentiated by felbamate.
Lamotrigine	May potentiate lamotrigine.
Phenobarbital	Phenobarbital may increase clearance. Antagonized by phenobarbital.
Phenytoin	Phenytoin may increase clearance. Antagonized by phenytoin.
Primidone	Primidone may increase clearance.
Rifampin	Antagonized by rifampin.
Tolbutamide	May potentiate tolbutamide. Antagonized by tolbutamide.
Topiramate	Concomitant topiramate may induce hyperammonemia.
Tricyclic antidepressants (TCAs)	May potentiate amitriptyline/nortriptyline.
Warfarin	May potentiate warfarin. Antagonized by warfarin.
Zidovudine	May potentiate zidovudine.
Zonisamide (Zonegran)	
Enzyme inducers	Liver enzyme inducers increase metabolism and clearance and decrease half-life.
Heat disorders, drugs predisposing	Caution with drugs that predispose patients to heat-related disorders (eg, carbonic anhydrase inhibitors, anticholinergic drugs).

ANTIPARKINSON AGENTS

Amantadine HCl (Symmetrel)	
Anticholinergics	Anticholinergic agents may potentiate the anticholinergic-like side effects.
CNS stimulants	Caution with CNS stimulants.

Table 17.2. DRUG INTERACTIONS FOR NEUROLOGICAL AGENTS *(cont.)*

ANTIPARKINSON AGENTS *(cont.)*

Amantadine HCl (Symmetrel) *(cont.)*	
Flu vaccine, live-attenuated (LAIV)	LAIV should not be administered within 2 weeks before or 48 hours after taking amantadine, unless medically indicated
Quinidine	Increased plasma levels with quinidine.
Quinine	Increased plasma levels with quinine.
Thioridazine	Increased tremor in elderly Parkinson's disease patients with thioridazine.
Triamterene/HCTZ	May increase plasma levels of amantadine (rare).
Apomorphine HCl (Apokyn)	
5-HT_3 antagonists	Contraindicated; may cause profound hypotension and loss of consciousness. Do not administer with 5-HT_3 antagonists (ondansetron, granisetron, dolasetron, palonosetron, and alosetron).
Antihypertensives	Antihypertensives may increase risk of hypotension, MI, serious pneumonia, falls, bone and joint injuries.
Dopamine antagonists	Dopamine antagonists (eg, phenothiazines, butyrophenones, thioxanthenes, metoclopramide) may diminish effectiveness.
QTc interval, drugs prolonging	Caution with drugs prolonging the QTc interval.
Vasodilators	Vasodilators (especially nitrates) may increase risk of hypotension, MI, serious pneumonia, falls, bone and joint injuries.
Benztropine Mesylate (Cogentin)	
Atropine-like agents	Caution with other atropine-like agents.
Phenothiazines	Paralytic ileus, hyperthermia, and heat stroke reported with phenothiazines.
Tricyclic antidepressants (TCAs)	Paralytic ileus, hyperthermia, and heat stroke reported with TCAs.
Bromocriptine Mesylate (Parlodel)	
Alcohol	Alcohol may potentiate side effects.
Antihypertensives	Caution with antihypertensives.
Dopamine antagonists	Decreased effects with dopamine antagonists (eg, butyrophenones, haloperidol, phenothiazines, pimozide, metoclopramide).
Ergot alkaloids	Not for use with other ergot alkaloids.
Levodopa	Levodopa may cause hallucinations.
Carbidopa/Entacapone/Levodopa (Stalevo)	
Antibiotics	Some antibiotics (eg, erythromycin, rifampicin, ampicillin, chloramphenicol) may interfere with biliary excretion.
Antihypertensives	Risk of postural hypotension with antihypertensives.
Cholestyramine	Cholestyramine may interfere with biliary excretion.
COMT substrates	Increased HR, arrhythmias, and BP changes with drugs metabolized by COMT (eg, isoproterenol, epinephrine, norepinephrine, dopamine, dobutamine, alpha-methyldopa, apomorphine, isoetherine, bitolterol).
Dopamine D_2 antagonists	Reduced effect with dopamine D_2 antagonists (eg, phenothiazines, butyrophenones, risperidone).

ANTIPARKINSON AGENTS *(cont.)*

Carbidopa/Entacapone/Levodopa (Stalevo) *(cont.)*	
Iron salts	Reduced bioavailability with iron salts.
Isoniazid	Reduced effect with isoniazid.
MAOIs	MAOIs are contraindicated during or within 14 days of administration.
Metoclopramide	Reduced effect with metoclopramide.
Papaverine	Reduced effect with papaverine.
Phenytoin	Reduced effect with phenytoin.
Probenecid	Probenecid may interfere with biliary excretion.
Protein bound drugs, highly	Caution with highly protein-bound drugs (eg, warfarin, salicylic acid, phenylbutazone, diazepam).
Selegiline	Risk of postural hypotension with selegiline.
Tricyclic antidepressants (TCAs)	HTN and dyskinesia may occur with TCAs.
Carbidopa/Levodopa (Parcopa, Sinemet, Sinemet CR)	
Antihypertensives	Risk of postural hypotension with antihypertensives.
Dopamine D_2 antagonists	Reduced effects with dopamine D_2 antagonists (eg, phenothiazines, butyrophenones, risperidone).
High-protein diets	Reduced bioavailability with high-protein diets.
Iron salts	Reduced bioavailability with iron salts.
Isoniazid	Reduced effects with isoniazid.
MAOIs	MAOIs are contraindicated during or within 14 days of administration.
Metoclopramide	Antagonized by metoclopramide.
Papaverine	Antagonized by papaverine.
Phenytoin	Antagonized by phenytoin.
Selegiline	Risk of postural hypotension with selegiline.
Tricyclic antidepressants (TCAs)	HTN and dyskinesia may occur with TCAs.
Entacapone (Comtan)	
Antibiotics	Some antibiotics (eg, erythromycin, rifamipicin, ampicillin, chloramphenicol) may interfere with biliary excretion.
Cholestyramine	Cholestyramine may interfere with biliary excretion.
CNS depressants	Additive sedative effects with CNS depressants.
COMT substrates	Caution with drugs metabolized by COMT (eg, isoproterenol, epinephrine, norepinephrine, dopamine, dobutamine, alpha-methyldopa, apomorphine, isoetherine, bitolterol); increased HR, arrhythmias, and BP changes may occur.
MAOIs, non-selective	Avoid non-selective MAOIs (eg, phenelzine, tranylcypromine).
Probenecid	Probenecid may interfere with biliary excretion.
Pramipexole Dihydrochloride (Mirapex)	
Cimetidine	Cimetidine may decrease clearance.

Table 17.2. DRUG INTERACTIONS FOR NEUROLOGICAL AGENTS *(cont.)*

ANTIPARKINSON AGENTS *(cont.)*

Pramipexole Dihydrochloride (Mirapex) *(cont.)*	
Diltiazem	Diltiazem may decrease clearance.
Dopamine antagonists	Dopamine antagonists (eg, phenothiazines, butyrophenones, thioxanthenes, metoclopramide) may decrease effects.
Quinidine	Quinidine may decrease clearance.
Quinine	Quinine may decrease clearance.
Ranitidine	Ranitidine may decrease clearance.
Triamterene	Triamterene may decrease clearance.
Verapamil	Verapamil may decrease clearance.
Rasagiline Mesylate (Azilect)	
Anesthesia, general	Concomitant use with general anesthesia is contraindicated.
Anesthesia, local	Concomitant use with local anesthesia containing vasoconstrictors is contraindicated.
Antidepressants	Concomitant use with tricyclic and tetracyclic antidepressants is not recommended due to severe CNS toxicity.
Cocaine	Concomitant use with cocaine is contraindicated.
Cyclobenzaprine	Concomitant use with cyclobenzaprine is contraindicated.
CYP1A2 inhibitors	Increased plasma concentrations up to 2-fold with concomitant ciprofloxacin and other CYP1A2 inhibitors.
Dextromethorphan	Concomitant use with dextromethorphan is contraindicated.
MAOIs	Concomitant use with MAOIs is contraindicated.
Meperidine	Concomitant use with meperidine is contraindicated.
Methadone	Concomitant use with methadone is contraindicated.
Mirtazapine	Concomitant use with mirtazapine is contraindicated.
Propoxyphene	Concomitant use with propoxyphene is contraindicated.
SNRIs	Concomitant use with SNRIs is not recommended due to severe CNS toxicity.
SSRIs	Concomitant use with SSRIs is not recommended due to severe CNS toxicity.
St John's wort	Concomitant use with St John's wort is contraindicated.
Sympathomimetic amines	Concomitant use with sympathomimetic amines is contraindicated. Severe hypertensive reactions reported with concomitant use of sympathomimetics.
Tramadol	Concomitant use with tramadol is contraindicated.
Ropinirole HCl (Requip, Requip XL)	
Alcohol	Caution with alcohol.
Ciprofloxacin	Potentiated by ciprofloxacin.
CYP1A2 inhibitor	Adjust dose if CYP1A2 inhibitor is stopped or started during treatment.
Dopamine antagonists	Decreased effects with dopamine antagonists (eg, phenothiazines, butyrophenones, thioxanthenes, metoclopramide). Caution with dopamine antagonists.

ANTIPARKINSON AGENTS *(cont.)*

Ropinirole HCl (Requip, Requip XL) *(cont.)*	
Estrogen	Adjust dose if estrogen is stopped or started during treatment.
Sedatives	Drowsiness increased with sedatives.
Selegiline HCl (Eldepryl)	
Fluoxetine	Allow 5 weeks for fluoxetine due to a longer half-life.
Meperidine	Contraindicated with meperidine; stupor, muscular rigidity, severe agitation, and elevated temperature reported.
Opioids	Contraindicated for use with other opioids beyond meperidine.
SSRIs	Avoid SSRIs; severe toxicity reported. Allow 2 weeks between discontinuation of selegiline and initiation of SSRIs.
Sympathomimetics	Caution with sympathomimetics.
Tricyclic antidepressants (TCAs)	Avoid TCAs; severe toxicity reported. Allow 2 weeks between discontinuation of selegiline and initiation of TCAs.
Tyramine-containing food	Caution with tyramine-containing food.
Selegiline HCl (Zelapar)	
CYP3A4 inducers	Caution with CYP3A4 inducers (eg, phenytoin, carbamazepine, nafcillin, phenobarbital, and rifampin).
Dextromethorphan	Contraindicated; episodes of psychosis or bizarre behavior reported with dextromethorphan.
Fluoxetine	Allow 5 weeks for fluoxetine due to a longer half-life.
MAOIs	MAOIs are contraindicated during or within 14 days of administration.
Meperidine	Contraindicated; serious, sometimes fatal, reactions have been precipitated with meperidine.
Methadone	Contraindicated; serious, sometimes fatal, reactions have been precipitated with methadone.
Propoxyphene	Contraindicated; serious, sometimes fatal, reactions have been precipitated with propoxyphene.
SSRIs	Severe toxicity reported with SSRIs; avoid concurrent use and allow 2 weeks between discontinuation of selegiline and initiation of SSRIs.
Sympathomimetics	Caution with sympathomimetics.
Tramadol	Contraindicated; serious, sometimes fatal, reactions have been precipitated with tramadol.
Tricyclic antidepressants (TCAs)	Severe toxicity reported with TCAs; avoid concurrent use and allow 2 weeks between discontinuation of selegiline and initiation of TCAs.
Tolcapone (Tasmar)	
Apomorphine	Apomorphine may need a dose reduction.
Desipramine	Caution with desipramine.
Dobutamine	Dobutamine may need a dose reduction.
Isoproterenol	Isoproterenol may need a dose reduction.

Table 17.2. DRUG INTERACTIONS FOR NEUROLOGICAL AGENTS *(cont.)*

ANTIPARKINSON AGENTS *(cont.)*

Tolcapone (Tasmar) *(cont.)*	
Levodopa	May increase risk of orthostatic hypotension and dyskinesia with levodopa.
MAOIs, non-selective	Avoid non-selective MAOIs (eg, phenelzine, tranylcypromine).
Tolbutamide	Caution with tolbutamide.
Warfarin	Caution with warfarin.
Trihexyphenidyl HCl	
Alcohol	Additive effects with alcohol.
Barbiturates	Additive effects with barbiturates.
Cannabinoids	Additive effects with cannabinoids.
CNS depressants	Additive effects with other CNS depressants.
Levodopa	May need to reduce concomitant levodopa dose.
MAOIs	MAOIs intensify anticholinergic effects.
Neuroleptics	Increased risk of tardive dyskinesia with neuroleptics.
Opiates	Additive effects with opiates.
Tricyclic antidepressants (TCAs)	TCAs may intensify anticholinergic effects.

MIGRAINE THERAPY/TENSION HEADACHE

Acetaminophen/Aspirin/Caffeine (Excedrin Migraine) OTC	
Alcohol	Caution with alcohol.
Caffeine	Limit caffeine-containing medications, foods, or beverages.
Acetaminophen/Butalbital (Phrenilin, Phrenilin Forte)	
Alcohol	May enhance CNS depression effects of alcohol.
Anesthetics, general	May enhance CNS depression effects of general anesthetics.
MAOIs	Enhanced CNS effects with MAOIs.
Opioid analgesics	May enhance CNS depression effects of opioid analgesics.
Tranquilizers	May enhance CNS depression effects of tranquilizers (eg, chlordiazepoxide, sedative hypnotics, CNS depressants).
Acetaminophen/Butalbital/Caffeine (Esgic-Plus, Fioricet)	
Alcohol	May enhance CNS depression effects of alcohol.
Anesthetics, general	May enhance CNS depression effects of general anesthetics.
MAOIs	Enhanced CNS effects with MAOIs.
Opioid analgesics	May enhance CNS depression effects of opioid analgesics.
Tranquilizers	May enhance CNS depression effects of tranquilizers (eg, chlordiazepoxide, sedative hypnotics, CNS depressants).
Acetaminophen/Butalbital/Caffeine/Codeine Phosphate (Fioricet with Codeine) CIII	
Alcohol	May enhance CNS depression effects of alcohol.
Anesthetics, general	May enhance CNS depression effects of general anesthetics.

MIGRAINE THERAPY/TENSION HEADACHE *(cont.)*

Acetaminophen/Butalbital/Caffeine/Codeine Phosphate (Fioricet with Codeine) CIII *(cont.)*	
MAOIs	Enhanced CNS effects with MAOIs.
Opioid analgesics	May enhance CNS depression effects of opioid analgesics.
Tranquilizers	May enhance CNS depression effects of tranquilizers.
Almotriptan Malate (Axert)	
5-HT_1 agonists	Avoid other 5-HT_1 agonist drugs within 24-hr period.
CYP3A4 inhibitors	Increased levels possible with CYP3A4 inhibitors (eg, ketoconazole).
Ergot-containing drugs	Prolonged vasospastic reactions reported with ergot-containing drugs; avoid within 24 hours of each other.
MAOIs	Clearance may be decreased by MAOIs.
SSRIs	SSRIs may cause weakness, hyperreflexia, and incoordination.
Aspirin/Butalbital/Caffeine (Fiorinal) CIII	
6-Mercaptopurine (6-MP)	May cause bone marrow toxicity and blood dyscrasias with 6-MP.
Alcohol	Additive CNS depression with alcohol.
Anesthetics, general	Additive CNS depression with general anesthetics.
Anticoagulants	May enhance effects of anticoagulants.
Antidiabetic agents, oral	May cause hypoglycemia with oral antidiabetic agents.
ASA	Withdrawal of corticosteroids may cause salicylism with chronic ASA use.
CNS depressants	Additive CNS depression with other CNS depressants.
Insulin	May cause hypoglycemia with insulin.
MAOIs	CNS effects enhanced by MAOIs.
Methotrexate	May cause bone marrow toxicity and blood dyscrasias with methotrexate.
NSAIDs	Increased risk of peptic ulceration and bleeding with NSAIDs.
Opioid analgesics	Additive CNS depression with other opioid analgesics.
Sedative-hypnotics	Additive CNS depression with sedative-hypnotics.
Tranquilizers	Additive CNS depression with tranquilizers (eg, chloral hydrate).
Uricosuric agents	Decreased effects of uricosuric agents (eg, probenecid, sulfinpyrazone).
Aspirin/Butalbital/Caffeine/Codeine Phosphate (Fiorinal with Codeine) CIII	
6-Mercaptopurine (6-MP)	May cause bone marrow toxicity and blood dyscrasias with 6-MP.
Alcohol	Additive CNS depression with alcohol.
Anesthetics, general	Additive CNS depression with general anesthetics.
Anticoagulants	May enhance effects of anticoagulants.
Antidiabetic	May cause hypoglycemia with oral antidiabetic agents.
ASA	Withdrawal of corticosteroids may cause salicylism with chronic ASA use.
CNS depressants	Additive CNS depression with other CNS depressants.
Insulin	May cause hypoglycemia with insulin.

Table 17.2. DRUG INTERACTIONS FOR NEUROLOGICAL AGENTS *(cont.)*

MIGRAINE THERAPY/TENSION HEADACHE *(cont.)*

Aspirin/Butalbital/Caffeine/Codeine Phosphate (Fiorinal with Codeine) CIII *(cont.)*	
MAOIs	CNS effects enhanced by MAOIs.
Methotrexate	May cause bone marrow toxicity and blood dyscrasias with methotrexate.
NSAIDs	Increased risk of peptic ulceration and bleeding with NSAIDs.
Opioid analgesics	Additive CNS depression with other opioid analgesics.
Sedative-hypnotics	Additive CNS depression with sedative-hypnotics.
Tranquilizers	Additive CNS depression with tranquilizers (eg, chloral hydrate).
Uricosuric agents	Decreased effects of uricosuric agents (eg, probenecid, sulfinpyrazone).
Caffeine/Ergotamine Tartrate (Cafergot Tablets)	
CYP3A4 inhibitors, less potent	Coadministration with less potent CYP3A4 inhibitors (eg, saquinavir, nefazodone, fluconazole, fluoxetine, grapefruit juice, fluvoxamine, zileuton, metronidazole, clotrimazole) may lead to potential risk for serious toxicity, including vasospasm.
CYP3A4 inhibitors, more potent	Use with potent CYP3A4 inhibitors (eg, protease inhibitors, macrolide anitbiotics) is contraindicated. CYP3A4 inhibition elevates serum levels of Cafergot, risk for vasospasm leading to cerebral ischemia, and/or serious and life-threatening ischemia of the extremities is increased.
Nicotine	Nicotine may provoke vasoconstriction, predisposing to greater ischemic response.
Propranolol	Propranolol may potentiate vasoconstrictive action.
Sympathomimetics	Use with sympathomimetics (pressor agents) may cause extreme BP elevation.
Vasoconstrictors	Avoid coadministration with other vasoconstrictors.
Dihydroergotamine Mesylate (D.H.E. 45, Migranal)	
CYP3A4 inhibitors	Contraindicated with CYP3A4 inhibitors (eg, macrolides, protease inhibitors). Caution with less potent CYP3A4 inhibitors (eg, saquinavir, nefazodone, fluconazole, grapefruit juice, fluoxetine, fluvoxamine, zileuton, clotrimazole).
Macrolides	Increased plasma levels and peripheral vasoconstriction with macrolides.
Nicotine	Nicotine may potentiate the vasoconstrictive action.
Propranolol	Propranolol may potentiate the vasoconstrictive action.
Sumatriptan	Additive coronary vasospastic effect with sumatriptan; avoid within 24 hrs of each other.
Vasoconstrictors	Potentiated BP elevation with peripheral and central vasoconstrictors.
Eletriptan Hydrobromide (Relpax)	
5-HT_1 agonists	Avoid other 5-HT_1 agonist drugs within 24-hr period due to additive effects.
CYP3A4 inhibitors	Avoid within 72 hrs of potent CYP3A4 inhibitors (eg, ketoconazole, itraconazole, nefazodone, troleandomycin, clarithromycin, ritonavir, nelfinavir).
Ergot-containing drugs	Prolonged vasospastic reactions reported with ergot-containing drugs; avoid within 24 hours of each other.
Erythromycin	Erythromycin may increase levels.

MIGRAINE THERAPY/TENSION HEADACHE *(cont.)*

Eletriptan Hydrobromide (Relpax) *(cont.)*	
Fluconazole	Fluconazole may increase levels.
Propranolol	Propranolol may increase levels.
Verapamil	Verapamil may increase levels.
Frovatriptan Succinate (Frova)	
5-HT-$_{1B/1D}$ agonists	Avoid within 24 hours of other 5-HT-$_{1B/1D}$ agonists.
Ergot-containing drugs	Prolonged vasospastic reactions reported with ergot-containing drugs; avoid use within 24 hours.
SSRIs	Weakness, hyperreflexia, and incoordination reported with SSRIs (rare).
Ibuprofen (Advil Migraine) **OTC**	
Alcohol	Risk of stomach bleeding with alcohol.
Naproxen Sodium/Sumatriptan Succinate (Treximet)	
5-HT$_1$ agonists	Other 5-HT$_1$ agonists are contraindicated.
ACE inhibitors	Use with ACE inhibitors may potentiate renal disease states.
ASA	Avoid use with ASA.
β-Blockers	May reduce the antihypertensive effect of propranolol and other β-blockers.
Ergot-containing drugs	Contraindicated for use within 24 hrs of ergotamine-containing agents and ergot-type drugs.
Lithium	May cause lithium toxicity when administered concurrently with lithium.
MAOIs	MAOIs are contraindicated during or within 14 days of administration.
Methotrexate (MTX)	Caution when administered concomitantly with MTX due to elevated and prolonged serum MTX levels.
Probenecid	Probenecid may extend naproxen plasma half-life.
SNRIs	Combined use with SNRIs may cause serotonin syndrome.
SSRIs	Combined use with SSRIs may cause serotonin syndrome.
Triptans	Combined use with triptans may cause serotonin syndrome.
Warfarin	Increases GI bleed with warfarin.
Naratriptan HCl (Amerge)	
5-HT$_1$ agonists	Avoid other 5-HT$_1$ agonist drugs within 24-hr period due to additive effects.
Ergot-containing drugs	Prolonged vasospastic reactions reported with ergot-containing drugs; avoid use within 24 hours.
SSRIs	SSRIs may cause weakness, hyperreflexia, and incoordination.
Rizatriptan Benzoate (Maxalt, Maxalt-MLT)	
5-HT$_1$ agonists	Avoid other 5-HT$_1$ agonist drugs within 24-hr period due to additive effects.
Ergot-containing drugs	Prolonged vasospastic reactions reported with ergot-containing drugs; avoid use within 24 hours.
MAOIs	MAOIs are contraindicated during or within 14 days of administration.

Table 17.2. DRUG INTERACTIONS FOR NEUROLOGICAL AGENTS *(cont.)*

MIGRAINE THERAPY/TENSION HEADACHE *(cont.)*

Rizatriptan Benzoate (Maxalt, Maxalt-MLT) *(cont.)*	
Propranolol	Increased plasma levels with propranolol.
SSRIs	SSRIs may cause weakness, hyperreflexia, and incoordination (rare).
Sumatriptan (Imitrex)	
5-HT_1 agonists	Avoid other 5-HT_1 agonist drugs within 24-hr period due to additive effects.
Ergot-containing drugs	Prolonged vasospastic reactions reported with ergot-containing drugs; avoid use within 24 hours.
MAOIs	MAOIs are contraindicated during or within 14 days of administration.
SSRIs	Weakness, hyperreflexia, and incoordination reported with SSRIs (rare).
Zolmitriptan (Zomig, Zomig Nasal Spray, Zomig-ZMT)	
5-$HT_{1B/1D}$ agonists	Avoid within 24 hours of other 5-$HT_{1B/1D}$ agonists.
Cimetidine	Half-life and AUC doubled with cimetidine.
Ergot-containing drugs	Prolonged vasospastic reactions reported with ergot-containing drugs; avoid use within 24 hours.
MAOIs	MAOIs are contraindicated during or within 14 days of administration.
SNRIs	Serotonin syndrome reported with combined use of an SNRI.
SSRIs	Serotonin syndrome reported with combined use of an SSRI.

MUSCLE ANALGESICS/RELAXANTS

Aspirin/Caffeine/Orphenadrine Citrate	
Propoxyphene	Confusion, tremor, anxiety reported with propoxyphene.
Aspirin/Carisoprodol (Soma Compound)	
Alcohol	Increases GI bleeding risk with alcohol. Additive effects with alcohol.
Antacids	Antacids decrease plasma levels.
Anticoagulants	Increases bleeding risk with anticoagulants.
Antidiabetics, oral	Enhances hypoglycemia with oral antidiabetics.
CNS depressants	Additive effects with other CNS depressants.
Corticosteroids	Corticosteroids decrease plasma levels.
Methotrexate	Enhances methotrexate toxicity.
Probenecid	Antagonizes uricosuric effects of probenecid.
Psychotropic drugs	Additive effects with psychotropic drugs.
Sulfinpyrazone	Antagonizes uricosuric effects of sulfinpyrazone.
Urine acidifiers	Potentiated by urine acidifiers (eg, ammonium chloride).
Aspirin/Carisoprodol/Codeine Phosphate (Soma Compound/Codeine) CIII	
Alcohol	Increases GI bleeding risk with alcohol. Additive effects with alcohol.
Antacids	Antacids decrease plasma levels.
Anticoagulants	Increases bleeding risk with anticoagulants.

MUSCLE ANALGESICS/RELAXANTS *(cont.)*

Aspirin/Carisoprodol/Codeine Phosphate (Soma Compound/Codeine) CIII *(cont.)*	
Antidiabetics, oral	Enhances hypoglycemia with oral antidiabetics.
CNS depressants	Additive effects with other CNS depressants.
Corticosteroids	Corticosteroids decrease plasma levels.
Methotrexate	Enhances methotrexate toxicity.
Probenecid	Antagonizes uricosuric effects of probenecid.
Psychotropic drugs	Additive effects with psychotropic drugs.
Sulfinpyrazone	Antagonizes uricosuric effects of sulfinpyrazone.
Urine acidifiers	Potentiated by urine acidifiers (eg, ammonium chloride).
Baclofen (Kemstro)	
Alcohol	Additive CNS depression with alcohol.
Antidiabetic agents	May increase blood glucose and require dosage adjustment of antidiabetic agents.
Antihypertensives	May potentiate antihypertensives.
CNS depressants	Additive CNS effects with other CNS depressants.
Levodopa/carbidopa	Mental confusion, hallucinations, and agitation with levodopa plus carbidopa therapy.
Magnesium sulfate	Synergistic effects with magnesium sulfate.
MAOIs	May increase CNS depressant effects with MAO inhibitors.
Neuromuscular blockers	Synergistic effects with other neuromuscular blockers.
Tricyclic antidepressants (TCAs)	Potentiated by TCAs.
Carisoprodol (Soma)	
Alcohol	Additive CNS depression with alcohol.
CNS depressants	Additive CNS effects with other CNS depressants.
CYP2C19 inducers	Coadministration with CYP2C19 inducers (eg, St. John's wort, rifampin) may decrease levels.
CYP2C19 inhibitors	Coadministration with CYP2C19 inhibitors (eg, omeprazole, fluvoxamine) may increase levels.
Meprobamate	Concomitant use with meprobamate not recommended.
Psychotropics	Additive effects with psychotropic drugs.
Chlorzoxazone (Parafon Forte DSC)	
Alcohol	Additive CNS depression with alcohol.
CNS depressants	Additive CNS effects with other CNS depressants.
Cyclobenzaprine HCl (Amrix, Flexeril)	
Alcohol	Additive CNS depression with alcohol.
Anticholingerics	Caution with anticholinergic medication.
Barbiturates	Enhances effects of barbiturates.

Table 17.2. DRUG INTERACTIONS FOR NEUROLOGICAL AGENTS *(cont.)*

MUSCLE ANALGESICS/RELAXANTS *(cont.)*	
Cyclobenzaprine HCl (Amrix, Flexeril) *(cont.)*	
CNS depressants	Additive CNS effects with other CNS depressants.
Guanethidine	May block antihypertensive action of guanethidine and similar compounds.
MAOIs	Contraindicated with MAOIs.
Tramadol	May enhance seizure risk with tramadol.
Dantrolene Sodium (Dantrium)	
CCBs	Avoid with CCBs; risk of cardiovascular collapse.
CNS depressants	Additive CNS effects with other CNS depressants.
Estrogens	Caution with estrogens; risk of hepatotoxicity.
Vecuronium	May potentiate vecuronium-induced neuromuscular block.
Dantrolene Sodium (Dantrium IV)	
CCBs	Avoid with CCBs; possible risk of cardiovascular collapse.
Clofibrate	Plasma protein-binding reduced by clofibrate.
Hepatic enzyme inducers	Possible increased metabolism by drugs known to induce hepatic microsomal enzymes.
Tolbutamide	Plasma protein-binding increased by tolbutamide.
Tranquilizers	Caution with tranquilizers.
Vecuronium	May potentiate vecuronium-induced neuromuscular block.
Warfarin	Plasma protein-binding reduced by warfarin.
Metaxalone (Skelaxin)	
Alcohol	Additive CNS depression with alcohol.
Barbiturates	Additive CNS effects with barbiturates.
CNS depressants	Additive CNS effects with other CNS depressants.
Methocarbamol (Robaxin, Robaxin Injection, Robaxin-750)	
Alcohol	Additive CNS depression with alcohol.
Anticholinergics	Caution in patients with myasthenia gravis receiving anticholinergics.
CNS depressants	Additive adverse effects with other CNS depressants.
Pyridostigmine	May inhibit effect of pyridostigmine.
Orphenadrine Citrate	
Propoxyphene	Confusion, anxiety, and tremors reported with propoxyphene.
Tizanidine HCl (Zanaflex)	
Alcohol	Additive CNS depression with alcohol.
Alpha-adrenergic agonists	Avoid alpha-adrenergic agonists.
Ciprofloxacin	Concomitant use with ciprofloxacin is contraindicated.
Contraceptives, oral	Potentiated by oral contraceptives.
CYP1A2 inhibitors	Contraindicated; avoid with CYP1A2 inhibitors.
Fluvoxamine	Concomitant use with fluvoxamine is contraindicated.

Chapter 18

Psychoactive Drugs

Steven Ganzberg, D.M.D., M.S.; Robert L. Merrill, D.D.S., M.S.

Approximately one of every three people will suffer from a mental illness at some point in his or her life. Many of these people will be placed on a regimen of psychoactive drugs, which may influence dental management. Psychiatric medications partially include antidepressant, antianxiety, antipsychotic, and mood stabilizing drugs for bipolar disorders, drugs for attention deficit/hyperactivity disorders as well as sedatives and "sleeping pills." Drugs that have psychological activity include not only drugs listed above, but other classes of drugs such as antiepileptic drugs that may be also used to stabilize depression and bipolar disorder.

When members of the dental team are treating a patient taking psychoactive medications, common sense dictates that they should take care in their personal interactions with the patient. Efforts to minimize anxiety, although routine in dental practice, should be given high priority.

General psychiatric drug information is provided in **Tables 18.1** and **18.2**, including adverse effects, precautions/contraindications, and interactions with other drugs.

Use of Psychoactive Drugs in Dental Practice

The prescription of psychoactive agents by dentists is indicated for a number of conditions, including acute anxiety associated with dental or oral surgery, management of bruxism, and management of various orofacial pain conditions. These agents also have a place in dentistry for sedation (see **Chapter 2**) and general anesthesia (see **Appendix L**).

Anxiety Associated with Dental or Oral Surgery

The benzodiazepines are generally regarded as the drugs of choice for oral preoperative anxiolysis, termed minimal sedation, in dental practice. These drugs have a high margin of safety, especially when used as a single dose 30 minutes to 1 hour before a dental visit. Diazepam historically has been used in this regard, but with the advent of newer agents with different phamacokinetic properties, other agents may be preferred. Diazepam is an inexpensive drug, with a rapid onset of action, and a long half-life with active metabolites. At a dose of 5 mg to 10 mg given 1 hour before a dental appointment, most adult patients will have some element of anxiolysis/minimal sedation. Another drug, triazolam, has a more rapid onset of action and the shortest half-life of any oral benzodiazepine: 1.5 to 5 hours without active metabolites. This agent may provide less postoperative sedation, which may be desirable. The typical adult oral preoperative minimal sedation dosage for triazolam would be 0.25 mg to 0.5 mg given 1 hour before the dental appointment. The IV drug midazolam has a similar pharmacokinetic profile to that of triazolam. This medication is FDA-approved for oral sedation in children.

Recently, attention has focused on the use of multiple dosing of triazolam or other sedatives on the same treatment day in an effort to achieve a desired level of *moderate* sedation, similar to what is achieved with titration of IV sedatives. Since orally administered drugs have unpredictable rates of absorption, this route of administration may result in unpredictable levels of sedation and, possibly, deeper levels of sedation than the dentist is trained to manage. Refer to the ADA Guidelines for the Use of Sedation and General Anesthesia for Dentists and the Guidelines for Teaching Pain Control and Sedation to Dentists and Dental Students for current training requirements, preoperative preparation, dosing guidelines, monitoring, postoperative care, and emergency management recommendations. In addition, many state dental boards already have in place or will develop policies and rules regarding the use of oral sedatives in dental practice, which should be followed before proceeding with oral sedation. Specific policies or rules may also be established for pediatric sedation, usually for patients ≤12 years, that are different from the rules for oral sedation of adults.

When used for minimal sedation, benzodiazepines result in minimal respiratory or cardiac depression when used alone. In elderly, medically compromised, or smaller adult patients, the lower dose range should be prescribed initially. Some patients may experience significant sedation even at low doses. If an oral sedative is prescribed, the patient must have a responsible adult escort present at all times until the effects of the sedative have worn off sufficiently. Patients who have taken an oral sedative before a dental appointment must not drive to or from the dental office. Caution patients about lingering sedative effects during the day and to avoid other central nervous system (CNS) depressants such as alcohol and opioids.

Management of Nocturnal Bruxism

If an acute anxiety-producing circumstance leads to severe bruxism, a short course of a benzodiazepine at bedtime, and possibly during the day, can be efficacious. Typically, diazepam 5 mg to 10 mg at bedtime has been used owing to its muscle-relaxing properties and anxiolytic effect. Other benzodiazepines are also effective. In general, this type of benzodiazepine use should be limited to no more than 2 weeks to avoid issues of dependence, rebound insomnia, and alteration of sleep architecture. Benzodiazepines are relatively contraindicated in a depressed patient unless approved by the patient's psychiatrist in advance. Caution patients about lingering sedative effects during the day and to avoid other CNS depressants such as alcohol and opioids.

The tricyclic antidepressants have come into increasing use for the long-term management of nocturnal bruxism unresponsive to intraoral orthotic therapy. Although not fully understood, bruxism appears to occur during transitional stages of sleep or during rapid-eye-movement (REM) sleep. The tricyclic antidepressants decrease the number of awakenings, shorten time spent in transitional stages of sleep, increase stage N3 sleep, decrease time spent in REM sleep, and increase total sleep time. These effects may be beneficial for some patients with bruxism or pain. Common agents used include amitriptyline, nortriptyline, or doxepin. These drugs are usually started at 10 mg at bedtime and gradually titrated upward every few days. It is uncommon for most patients to require more than 50 mg at bedtime, which is substantially below the effective dose for use as an antidepressant.

These drugs are not benign. They have significant anticholinergic and antihistaminic side effects. They can cause cardiac dysrhythmias and may lower the seizure threshold.

In patients >40 years, pretreatment electrocardiogram evaluation may be appropriate. In addition, all antidepressants can induce a manic episode in bipolar patients, so the drugs should be used with caution in this patient population. The dentist prescribing antidepressants for pain or bruxism is presumed to have established a proper diagnosis and to be fully aware of the drug's interactions, adverse effects, and contraindications. When used as antidepressants, these drugs should be prescribed only by clinicians who have had special training in the diagnosis and management of depression.

Management of Orofacial Pain

Psychotropic drugs have a long history of use for chronic pain conditions. A full listing of indications and prescribing information is not appropriate for this text. For the properly trained dentist, the use of psychoactive drugs is appropriate for the management of orofacial conditions such as primary headaches and neuropathic and musculoskeletal pain.

Antidepressants are commonly used for a variety of chronic pain conditions (including myofascial pain syndrome and migraine headache). Phenothiazines can be a useful adjunct for some types of neuropathic pains, and lithium is indicated for cluster headaches. The dentist using these drugs as therapeutic agents is presumed to be proficient in prescribing and managing these medications.

ANTIANXIETY AGENTS

Anxiety is a state of uneasiness of mind that resembles fear, but usually has no identifiable source. Anxiety has both physiological and psychological components. The anxious patient may be tachycardic, nauseated, diaphoretic, or light-headed. Although a patient may be diagnosed with a generalized anxiety disorder, at times clearly defined categories of anxiety apply. These categories include phobia, agoraphobia, panic attacks, obsessive-compulsive disorder, post-traumatic stress disorder, and performance anxiety. Benzodiazepines, agonists on γ-aminobutyric acid-A ($GABA_A$) specific receptors, are commonly prescribed for these disorders. GABA is an inhibitory neurotransmitter; potentiation of the ion-channel linked $GABA_A$ receptor modulates pain, providing another useful characteristic for the benzodiazepines. The development of dependence with these agents may limit their long-term use. Oral overdose of benzodiazepines is rarely fatal unless combined with other CNS depressants such as opioids, barbiturates, or alcohol. Buspirone, a selective serotonin agonist, has a lower dependence-producing profile and may be effective for some generalized anxiety disorders. Antidepressants are frequently prescribed as primary therapy for anxiety or for those patients with coexisting anxiety and depression.

β-Blockers more recently have been prescribed as an adjunct to benzodiazepine treatment and for control of performance anxiety. The antihistamine hydroxyzine is sometimes used for selected cases of anxiety disorders and combined with other agents for pediatric oral sedation.

See **Tables 18.1** and **18.2** for general information on antianxiety agents. Other agents listed as sleep adjuncts, although not FDA-approved for treatment of anxiety, may be prescribed for these disorders. More information on sleep adjuncts appears later in this chapter.

Special Dental Considerations

Antianxiety agents may cause xerostomia and should be considered in the differential diagnosis of caries, periodontal disease, or candidiasis. They also may cause orthostatic hypotension, hence after supine positioning, ask the patient to sit upright in the dental chair for a minute or two and then monitor the patient when he or she is standing.

If these drugs are used for oral preoperative anxiolysis for dental procedures, a competent adult should drive the patient to and from the dental office. Assistance to and from the dental chair may be needed, especially for elderly patients.

Drug Interactions of Dental Interest

Antianxiety agents may have an additive sedative effect with concomitantly administered CNS depressants.

Absorption of diazepam and chlordiazepoxide is delayed with antacids. The metabolism of chlordiazepoxide, diazepam, and triazolam is decreased if they are administered with cimetidine and erythromycin. The clearance of diazepam is decreased if it is administered with some selective serotonin reuptake inhibitor (SSRI) antidepressants.

Special Patients

In elderly, medically compromised, or smaller adult patients, the lower dose range should be prescribed initially. Some of these patients may experience significant sedation even at low doses.

Pharmacology

These agents are mainly benzodiazepines, which act at the $GABA_A$ receptor, an ion-gated chloride channel that has specific benzodiazepine and barbiturate receptor sites. Binding of benzodiazepines to the receptor complex opens the chloride channel to allow influx of chloride. Chloride causes hyperpolarization of the neuron, inhibiting the formation of action potentials. GABA, therefore, is the main inhibitory neurotransmitter of the CNS. Activity of the GABA system provides antianxiety, sedative, anticonvulsant, amnestic, and muscle-relaxing actions. Long-term use of benzodiazepines can lead to a withdrawal syndrome if abruptly discontinued. The sedative and antianxiety effects of these drugs are used to advantage in promoting short-term sleep improvement. These drugs are hepatically metabolized to active or inactive metabolites for excretion in the bile or urine.

Buspirone, a serotonin ($5HT1_A$) receptor partial agonist with weak dopamine receptor activity, has shown some utility in the management of generalized anxiety. Its onset of action is delayed, thus making this drug a poor choice for management of acute anxiety. Antidepressant pharmacology is discussed in the section below.

The antihistamines hydroxyzine and diphenhydramine are seldom-used older agents that have sedative and anticholinergic effects independent of GABA action.

ANTIDEPRESSANTS

Depression is a common mental illness that will affect at least 5% of the population at some time in life. A great number of these patients will be placed on antidepressants. Antidepressants are classified as heterocyclic (tricyclic, tetracyclic), monoamine oxidase inhibitors (MAOIs), selective serotonin reuptake inhibitors (SSRIs), serotonin/norepinephrine reuptake inhibitors (SNRIs), and other miscellaneous agents. These drugs work by affecting neurotransmitter balance between serotonin, norepinephrine and, in some cases, dopamine in the CNS. Some of the SSRI antidepressants are also used for obsessive-compulsive disorder and are listed separately in the tables. The SNRIs and tricyclic agents are commonly prescribed for chronic pain management as well.

Implications in dental and oral surgery revolve around the use of vasoconstrictors in local anesthetics, medication side effects and issues of patient management.

See **Tables 18.1** and **18.2** for basic information on antidepressants and for epinephrine/levonordefrin interaction information.

Special Dental Considerations

Most of these drugs have mild to moderate anticholinergic side effects and may cause decreased salivary flow. Consider this in the differential diagnosis of caries, periodontal disease, or oral candidiasis.

The SSRIs (such as fluoxetine and sertraline) can initiate bruxism. Consider this in the differential diagnosis of bruxism-related signs and symptoms.

These drugs, in rare cases, cause blood dyscrasias and should be considered in the differential diagnosis of oral signs and symptoms.

Many of these drugs can cause orthostatic hypotension. Ask the patient to sit upright in the dental chair for a minute or two after being in a supine position and then monitor the patient when standing.

Amoxapine, and less commonly other antidepressants, can cause tardive dyskinesia or extrapyramidal symptoms, which are manifested as involuntary oral or facial movements. Management of bruxism, occlusal adjustments, and bite registrations may be difficult to obtain. If newly diagnosed mouthing movements (involuntary mouth and tongue movements and/or drooling) are seen, which may indicate a serious medication side effect, consultation with the patient's physician may be appropriate.

Venlafaxine can, rarely, cause trismus.

Drug Interactions of Dental Interest

There has been much misunderstanding about the use of local anesthetics with vasoconstrictors for patients taking antidepressants. Local anesthetics with epinephrine or other vasoconstrictors are not absolutely contraindicated for any patient taking any antidepressant—including tricyclic or MAOI agents, all of which increase the concentration of norepinephrine in the synaptic cleft. The potential concern is that these drug combinations might lead to a hypertensive/tachycardic crisis. Because a major route of metabolism of exogenously administered catecholamines (such as epinephrine) involves catechol-O-methyl transferase (COMT), use of epinephrine or levonordefrin in patients taking MAOIs is not likely to be of concern. Antidepressants that block norepinephrine reuptake (eg, tricyclics, tetracyclics, venlafaxine, nefazodone, desvenlafaxine, sibutramine, duloxetine) could cause unwanted cardiovascular effects when vasoconstrictor-containing local anesthetics are administered. It is prudent, therefore, to monitor vital signs for dental patients taking antidepressants that affect norepinephrine reuptake blockade or monoamine oxidase A (MAO-A) activity.

For patients taking these agents, it is reasonable to administer small doses of vasoconstrictor in local anesthetic solutions (eg, no more than 40 µg of epinephrine, two cartridges with 1:100,000 epinephrine, or preferably less if the patient's preoperative vital signs reveal hypertension or tachycardia) within a short period with careful aspiration technique. Additional anesthetic with a vasoconstrictor may be administered if vital signs are acceptable. No vasoconstrictor contraindication exists for the SSRI antidepressants. *Gingival retraction cord with epinephrine is contraindicated for all patients taking antidepressants other than an SSRI* and should be used with caution, if at all, in other patients.

Use anticholinergics and antihistamines with caution due to additive xerostomia and CNS sedative effects.

CNS depressants (eg, alcohol, opioids, and benzodiazepines) may potentiate sedative side effects.

Meperidine and dextromethorphan are specifically contraindicated in patients taking MAOIs. Hypermetabolic crisis may occur. Caution with other opioids may be warranted.

Tricyclic antidepressants (which might be used for bruxism and pain such as atypical odontalgia or postherpetic neuralgia) are contraindicated with MAOIs and should be used cautiously with SSRIs unless their use is cleared by the patient's prescribing physician.

The anticoagulant effect of coumarin agents is increased when most antidepressants, including tricyclic agents, are administered concomitantly.

Antidepressants may lower the seizure threshold.

The therapeutic effect of tricyclic antidepressants may be decreased by concurrent administration of barbiturates, anticonvulsants, or other hepatic enzyme–inducing drugs.

With cimetidine, fluoxetine, methylphenidate, and some estrogens (ie, oral contraceptives), there is increased plasma concentration of tricyclic antidepressants.

Laboratory Value Alterations

- Blood glucose levels may increase or decrease.
- ECG changes are possible with tricyclic antidepressants, especially with pre-existing conduction abnormalities.

Special Patients

Side effects, such as xerostomia and orthostatic hypotension, are more pronounced in elderly patients.

Pharmacology

Antidepressants affect mood by altering the balance between serotonin, norepinephrine, and dopamine in critical brain centers. Antidepressants, in general, increase the availability of neurotransmitters in the synaptic cleft, changing postsynaptic receptor activity. These changes take some time to develop, thus accounting for the delay in action of two to four weeks or longer for these drugs' mood-altering effects to become apparent. Due to the side-effect profile of many of the tricyclic and MAOI agents, the SSRIs are frequently chosen as first-line therapy for depression. In pain management, both norepinephrine and serotonin reuptake blockade appear to be important for an analgesic effect, so the tricyclics, venlafaxine, desvenlafaxine, and duloxetine remain the preferred initial agents. Analgesia occurs well before the antidepressant effect and at lower doses that are not effective for management of depression in many patients with chronic pain.

The heterocyclic (tricyclic and tetracyclic) and SSRI antidepressants block the reuptake of the neurotransmitters into the presynaptic neuron, a partial mechanism by which neurotransmitter activity is modulated. The SSRIs, as their name implies, are selective for serotonin reuptake blockade. Because of the receptor selectivity of these agents, they generally possess the fewest side effects of any antidepressant type. SNRIs inhibit the reuptake of serotonin and norepinephrine with few effects at other receptors. The heterocyclic (tricyclic, tetracyclic) antidepressants affect norepinephrine and serotonin, as well as a number of other important neurotransmitters, but to varying degrees. Amoxapine possesses strong dopamine reuptake blocking effects. The MAOIs block the action of MAO-A, an enzyme found in the presynaptic neuron, which degrades serotonin and norepinephrine after reuptake. Bupropion is a weak reuptake blocker of dopamine and, to a lesser extent, norepinephrine and serotonin. Mirtazapine is an α_2 antagonist affecting norepinephrine and, indirectly, serotonin.

ANTIMANIC/BIPOLAR DISORDER DRUGS

Mania is a state of excessive excitement or enthusiasm and is frequently associated with hyperactivity or aggressive behavior. Approximately 90% of people who experience mania alternate these experiences with episodes of depression; this condition is termed "bipolar disorder" (manic-depression). Lithium carbonate has historically been the most prescribed agent, but now various antiepileptic and antipsychotic agents are also being used as first-line treatments.

As noted above, antidepressants may cause a manic episode in bipolar patients and should be used with caution and in consultation with the physician who is following the patient's psychiatric condition.

See **Tables 18.1** and **18.2** for general information on antimanic/bipolar disorder drugs.

Special Dental Considerations: Lithium and Other Agents

Lithium can cause decreased salivary flow. Consider in the differential diagnosis of caries, periodontal disease, or oral candidiasis.

Lithium can cause blood dyscrasias and should be considered in the differential diagnosis of oral signs and symptoms.

Lithium can cause orthostatic hypotension. Monitor vital signs and, after supine positioning, ask the patient to sit upright in the dental chair for a minute or two and then monitor the patient when standing.

Antipsychotic agents are discussed in the sections below. Anti-epileptic agents are discussed in **Chapter 17** (Neurological Drugs).

Drug Interactions of Dental Interest: Lithium and Other Agents

Vasoconstrictors in local anesthetics should be used with caution owing to lithium's hypotensive effects. Opioids, alcohol, and other hypotension-producing agents have additive hypotensive effects. NSAIDs, except aspirin and sulindac, increase lithium's plasma concentration because of decreased renal clearance and should be prescribed, if at all, in consultations with the patient's psychiatrist. Metronidazole increases plasma lithium concentration because of decreased renal clearance. Tricyclic antidepressants (which may be used for bruxism) may lead to manic episodes.

Antipsychotic agents are discussed in the sections below. Anti-epileptic agents are discussed in **Chapter 17** (Neurological Drugs).

Laboratory Value Alterations: Lithium

- Blood glucose may be increased.

Pharmacology

Lithium remains a primary treatment for prevention of mania and treatment of bipolar disorder. Although the mechanism of action is incompletely understood, the mood-stabilizing effects may be due to enhancement of the Na^+/K^+ ATPase pump, catecholamine neurotransmission, interference with inositol turnover in the brain, or decreased activity of cyclic AMP. Lithium, a monovalent cation, is almost completely dependent on renal excretion for elimination. Coadministered drugs that affect renal function, such as NSAIDs, can increase the plasma concentration of this agent, which has a narrow therapeutic plasma concentration range.

Other agents useful for the treatment of mania include various antiepileptic and antipsychotic agents. Antipsychotic pharmacology is discussed below. The pharmacology of the antiepileptic agents is discussed in **Chapter 17** (Neurological Drugs).

ANTIPSYCHOTIC AGENTS

The term "psychotic" refers to behavior in which a person cannot distinguish between the real and the unreal. Although the term "psychotic state" denotes mental illness, it does not identify the etiology, such as schizophrenia, major depression, brain tumor, or adverse drug reaction. Hallucinations, delusions, and thought disorders are characteristic of a psychotic state. Antipsychotic drugs are prescribed to help patients organize chaotic and disorganized thinking. In the past, the terms "major tranquilizers" (denoting prominent sedative side effects) and "neuroleptics" (denoting parkinsonian-like side effects) were used, but the term "antipsychotic" is now preferred.

See **Tables 18.1** and **18.2** for general information on antipsychotic agents.

Special Dental Considerations

Many of these drugs can cause decreased salivary flow; the dentist should consider this in the differential diagnosis of caries, periodontal disease, or oral candidiasis.

These drugs can cause blood dycrasias (although this is less likely with risperidone and molindone). Consider this in the differential diagnosis of oral signs and symptoms.

Many of these drugs can cause orthostatic hypotension. After supine positioning, have the patient to sit upright in the dental chair for a minute or two and then monitor once standing.

Extrapyramidal effects can cause involuntary oral or facial movements (although this is less likely with risperidone and clozapine). Management of bruxism, occlusal adjustments, and bite registrations may be difficult. If newly diagnosed oral movements (eg, involuntary mouth and tongue movements and/or drooling) are seen, this may indicate a serious medication side effect and the need for consultation with the patient's physician.

Some of the antipsychotic drugs are routinely used for their antiemetic capability. This is particularly true with migraine patients or patients undergoing chemotherapy. Dentists who treat headache disorders as part of the TMD/facial pain complex should be aware of the potential for some of these drugs to cause acute dystonic reactions when used acutely for the management of nausea and/or vomiting.

Drug Interactions of Dental Interest

With epinephrine

Many antipsychotic agents can cause α-adrenergic receptor blockade. Use of epinephrine-containing local anesthetic solutions may cause, although rarely, hypotension and tachycardia. It is prudent, therefore, to monitor vital signs for dental patients taking these medications. It is reasonable to administer no more than 40 μg of epinephrine in local anesthetic solutions (approximately one cartridge of local anesthetic with 1:50,000 epinephrine, two cartridges with 1:100,000 epinephrine, or four cartridges with 1:200,000 epinephrine) within a short period with careful aspiration technique. Additional anesthetic with vasoconstrictor may be administered if vital signs are acceptable.

CNS depressants such as alcohol, opioids, and barbiturates have additive sedative effects.

Anticholinergic drugs have additive anticholinergic effects.

Tricyclic antidepressants (which may be used for bruxism) have additive anticholinergic effects; combined use of these drugs can lead to alteration of plasma concentration of either drug. Also, they are associated with a possible increased risk of neuroleptic malignant syndrome.

Laboratory Value Alterations

- ECG changes (Q, T wave changes, QT interval, ST depression, AV conduction changes) are possible.

Special Patients

If antipsychotic drugs are being used in elderly patients for an antiemetic effect, USE lower doses.

Pharmacology

All antipsychotic drugs appear to produce a reduction of dopamine synaptic activity in limbic forebrain centers as a common pathway of antipsychotic activity. It appears that action at the dopamine-2 receptor is particularly important. Some of the newer agents, such as clozapine, have significant influences at serotonergic receptors as well, which suggests that other neurotransmitters also play a role in affected midbrain dopamine neurotransmission. Many of the side effects of these drugs relate to interaction at other receptor sites. α-Adrenergic receptor blockade (causing orthostatic hypotension, reflex tachycardia, and epinephrine interactions), antihistaminic effects (causing sedation), metabolic effects (causing weight gain), and anticholinergic effects (causing dry mouth, constipation, tachycardia, and difficulty in focusing the eyes) are common with many of these drugs.

Because these drugs produce effects on nigrostriatal pathways—an important area in Parkinson's disease—side effects such as tardive dyskinesia and neuroleptic malignant syndrome can occur with these agents. Other extrapyramidal reactions, such as akathisia (restlessness usually associated with some component of motor hyperactivity) or acute dystonic reactions such as oculogyric crisis (uncontrolled eye, face, or neck movements), can occur. Bruxism or other excessive oral movement disorders can be a drug-induced side effect.

These drugs typically undergo extensive hepatic metabolism by oxidation and glucuronidation to inactive metabolites, which are then excreted in the urine.

DRUGS USED FOR ADD/ADHD

Children with attention deficit disorder (ADD) have difficulty concentrating on tasks and are easily distracted. Those who also exhibit hyperactive symptoms (ADHD) have difficulty keeping still for even a few minutes or may display impulsive behaviors. These diagnoses should not be cavalierly applied to any child who is difficult to manage or is distracted easily; rather, a thorough medical and psychological evaluation, including an evaluation of the child's psychosocial functioning, is needed to render the diagnosis of ADD and/or ADHD. Interestingly, stimulant medications, with or without psychotherapy, are frequently used for treatment. α_2-Agonists, such as clonidine, are commonly used at bedtime to counteract the common adverse effect of insomnia. There is increasing recognition of this disorder in adults.

These drugs are also used for disorders of excessive somnolence, such as narcolepsy. Another drug for this indication is modafinil.

See **Tables 18.1** and **18.2** for general information on drugs used for ADD/ADHD and narcolepsy.

Special Dental Considerations

Determine if the patient is taking any drug for ADD or narcolepsy. Monitor vital signs because of possible sympathomimetic effects.

Many of these drugs can cause decreased salivary flow and should be considered in the differential diagnosis of caries, periodontal disease, or oral candidiasis.

Amphetamines may cause gingival enlargement, which dentists should monitor.

These drugs can, rarely, cause blood dyscrasias; consider this in the differential diagnosis of oral signs and symptoms.

Drug Interactions of Dental Interest

Vasoconstrictors in local anesthetics have possible additive sympathomimetic effects. Depending on vital signs, it is reasonable to administer no more than 40 μg of epinephrine in local anesthetic solutions (approximately one cartridge of local anesthetic with 1:50,000 epinephrine, two cartridges with 1:100,000 epinephrine, or four cartridges with 1:200,000 epinephrine) within a short period with careful aspiration technique. If vital signs warrant, less vasoconstrictor should be used. Additional anesthetic with vasoconstrictor may be administered if vital signs are acceptable after a short period.

Use tricyclic antidepressants (which may be used for bruxism) with caution, because their metabolism is decreased by methylphenidate. Increased sympathomimetic effects are possible when tricyclic antidepressants are prescribed to patients taking dextroamphetamine because of norepinephrine reuptake blockade by tricyclics.

Anticholinergics have additive oral drying effects.

Pharmacology
Methylphenidate and pemoline appear to act by blocking dopamine reuptake. These drugs increase children's ability to pay attention and decrease their motor restlessness. Dextroamphetamine/amphetamine are sympathomimetic amines that block the reuptake of dopamine and norepinephrine, inhibit MAO, and release catecholamines. Atomoxepine selectively blocks the reuptake of norepinephrine. Because of the stimulant effects, use of these drugs may result in weight loss, insomnia, and tachycardia. These effects are particularly prominent with dextroamphetamine. These drugs are also used to treat narcolepsy.

OBESITY AGENTS

Obesity is defined as a Body Mass Index (BMI), a measure of weight in respect to height, >30. Obesity can lead to a number of medical complications including diabetes mellitus, hypertension, coronary artery disease, stroke, obstructive sleep apnea as well as many other conditions. While exercise and calorie reduction remain the mainstay of treatment, some patients require surgery and/or medication to help achieve weight reduction goals. Most medications are in the stimulant/amphetamine classification although sibutramine, an SNRI, has recently been approved by the FDA for treating obesity. Other antidepressant medications, particularly the SSRIs, may also be used in conjunction with stimulant medications.

Special Dental Considerations
Monitor vital signs because of possible sympathomimetic effects. Many of these drugs can cause decreased salivary flow and should be considered in the differential diagnosis of caries, periodontal disease, or oral candidiasis. Rarely, these drugs can cause blood dyscrasias; consider this in the differential diagnosis of oral signs and symptoms.

Drug Interactions of Dental Interest
Vasoconstrictors in local anesthetics have possible additive sympathomimetic effects. Depending on vital signs, it is reasonable to administer no more than 40 µg of epinephrine in local anesthetic solutions (approximately one cartridge of local anesthetic with 1:50,000 epinephrine, two cartridges with 1:100,000 epinephrine, or four cartridges with 1:200,000 epinephrine) within a short period with careful aspiration technique. If vital signs warrant, less vasoconstrictor should be used. Additional anesthetic with vasoconstrictor may be administered if vital signs are acceptable after a short period.

Use tricyclic antidepressants (which may be used for bruxism) with caution, as increased sympathomimetic effects are possible. Anticholinergics have additive oral drying effects.

Pharmacology
Most drugs that help manage obesity are appetite suppressants of the amphetamine family. They block the reuptake of norepinephrine and dopamine and may also release these catecholamines from presynaptic nerves. Because of this, use of epinephrine in local anesthetic solutions may produce exaggerated cardiovascular effects.

SLEEP ADJUNCTS

Surveys undertaken by the National Sleep Foundation in 1989 and 1991 found that approximately 36% of the respondents reported having current sleep problems in the previous year and 10% to 20% reported that the problem was severe. Insomnia is the most prevalent of the sleep problems, with estimates of 69% in a primary care population. This higher incidence was consistent with increased psychiatric and medical illness. The incidence of sleep apnea is estimated to be 3% to 5% of the population. The significance of these statistics relates to the fact that these patients have an increased likelihood of taking medications that could have an impact on their dental health and dental care. Drugs commonly prescribed for insomnia include benzodiazepines and antidepressants such as the tricyclic antidepressants, trazodone, and mirtazapine (discussed in sections above). They are used because they decrease sleep-onset latency and can increase slow wave sleep (delta sleep), or restorative sleep. However, the medications can decrease rapid eye-movement sleep and some may be habituating.

Sleep disorders include difficulty in initiating or maintaining sleep, excessive somnolence, disorders of sleep-wake schedule, and parasomnias (including nocturnal bruxism). Disorders of initiating and maintaining sleep are by far the most common complaints and will be addressed in this section.

Since sleep disorders are common in the general population and over-the-counter (OTC) medications that affect sleep are readily available, self-medication for sleep is very common. The most common OTC sleep aids are alcohol, herbal remedies such as St. John's wort, melatonin, and antihistamines.

The most commonly prescribed medications to enhance sleep are the antihistamines, benzodiazepines, hypnotics, and antidepressants. The antihistamines are H_1 receptor antagonists. The benzodiazepines, $GABA_A$ agonists, are the drugs most commonly prescribed for insomnia. Unfortunately, prolonged use can interfere with normal sleep architecture and be detrimental in the long term. The FDA indication for these drugs is for short-term use only, although they are frequently prescribed for many months or years. Dependence and rebound insomnia are frequently observed. Nevertheless, for short-term use, these agents are generally effective. The nonbenzodiazepine $GABA_A$ agonists—zolpidem, zaleplon, and eszopiclone—are hypnotics that produce less disruption of sleep architecture and may have some effect in treating bruxism.

The more sedating tricyclic antidepressants, trazadone and mirtazapine, also have been used for some patients who require long-term treatment. Clonidine is also used for some forms of insomnia. The older barbiturate drugs, such as secobarbital and pentobarbital, are rarely used today for insomnia.

See **Tables 18.1** and **18.2** for general information on sleep adjuncts.

Special Dental Considerations

These drugs can cause xerostomia. Consider this in the differential diagnosis of caries, periodontal disease, or candidiasis.

These drugs may cause orthostatic hypotension. Monitor vital signs and ask the patient to sit upright in the dental chair for 1 to 2 minutes after being in a supine position, then monitor the patient once standing.

If these drugs are used for preoperative anxiolysis for dental procedures, ensure that a competent adult drives the patient to and from the dental office. Assistance to and from the dental chair may be needed, especially for elderly patients.

Drug Interactions of Dental Interest

CNS depressants will have an additive effect with concomitantly administered CNS depressants.

Diazepam and chlordiazepoxide have delayed absorption with antacids.

The metabolism of chlordiazepoxide, diazepam, and triazolam is decreased if they are administered with cimetidine and erythromycin.

The clearance of diazepam is decreased if it is administered with SSRI antidepressants.

Special Patients

In elderly, medically compromised, or smaller adult patients, the lower dose range should be prescribed initially. Some of these patients may experience significant sedation even at low doses.

Pharmacology

See the description for antianxiety agents discussed earlier in this chapter.

Adverse Effects, Precautions, and Contraindications

Table 18.1 provides adverse effects, precautions, and contraindications of psychoactive drugs.

SUGGESTED READING

American Psychiatric Association. *Diagnostic and Statistical Manual of Mental Disorders (DSM-IV).* 4th ed. Washington, D.C. American Psychiatric Association; 1994.

Brown RS, Bottomley WK. The utilization and mechanism of action of tricyclic antidepressants in the treatment of chronic facial pain: a review of the literature. *Anesth Prog.* 1990;37:223-229.

Eschalier A, Mestre C, Dubray C, et al. Why are antidepressants effective as pain relief? *CNS Drugs.* 1994;2:261-267.

Hasan AA, Ciancio S. Relationship between amphetamine ingestion and gingival enlargement. *Pediatr Dent.* 2004 Sep-Oct;26(5):396-400.

Mortimer AM. Newer and older antipsychotics: a comparative review of appropriate use. *CNS Drugs.* 1994;2:381-386.

Okeson JP, ed. *Orofacial Pain: Guidelines for Assessment, Diagnosis and Management.* Lombard, Ill.: Quintessence; 1996.

Tucker GJ. Psychiatric disorders in medical practice. In: Wyngaarden JB, Smith LH Jr., Bennett JC, eds. *Cecil Textbook of Medicine.* 19th ed. Philadelphia: Saunders; 1992.

The United States Pharmacopeial Convention. *Drug Information for the Health Care Professional.* 23rd ed. Rockville, MD: The United States Pharmacopeial Convention, Inc.; 2003.

Table 18.1. PRESCRIBING INFORMATION FOR PSYCHOACTIVE DRUGS

NAME	FORM/ STRENGTH	DOSAGE	WARNINGS/PRECAUTIONS & CONTRAINDICATIONS	ADVERSE EFFECTS†
ANTIANXIETY/HYPNOTIC AGENTS				
BENZODIAZEPINES				
Alprazolam (Niravam, Xanax, Xanax XR) CIV	**Tab:** (Xanax) 0.25mg*, 0.5mg*, 1mg*, 2mg*; **Tab, Extended-Release:** (Xanax XR) 0.5mg, 1mg, 2mg, 3mg; **Tab, Orally Disintegrating:** (Niravam) 0.25mg*, 0.5mg*, 1mg*, 2mg*	***Adults:*** (Tab/Tab, OD) **Anxiety: Initial:** 0.25-0.5mg tid. **Titrate:** May increase every 3-4 days. **Max:** 4mg/day. **Panic Disorder: Initial:** 0.5mg tid. **Titrate:** Increase by no more than 1mg/day every 3-4 days; slower titration if ≥4mg/day. **Usual:** 1-10mg/day. Decrease dose slowly (no more than 0.5mg every 3 days). **Elderly/Advanced Liver Disease/Debilitated: Initial:** 0.25mg bid-tid. **Titrate:** Increase gradually as tolerated. (Tab, ER) **Panic Disorder: Initial:** 0.5-1mg qd, preferably in the am. **Titrate:** Increase by no more than 1mg/day every 3-4 days. **Maint:** 1-10mg/day. **Usual:** 3-6mg/day. Decrease dose slowly (no more than 0.5mg every 3 days). **Elderly/Advanced Liver Disease/Debilitated: Initial:** 0.5mg qd.	**W/P:** Risk of dependence. Withdrawal symptoms, including seizure, reported with dose reduction or abrupt discontinuation; avoid abrupt withdrawal. Risk of CNS depression and impaired performance. May cause fetal harm. Caution with impaired renal, hepatic, or pulmonary function, severe depression, obesity, elderly and debilitated. Hypomania/mania reported with depression. Weak uricosuric effect. **Contra:** Acute narrow-angle glaucoma, untreated open-angle glaucoma, concomitant ketoconazole or itraconazole. **P/N:** Category D, not for use in nursing.	Drowsiness, fatigue/tiredness, impaired coordination, irritability, memory impairment, cognitive disorder, dysarthria, decreased libido, confusional state, light-headedness, **dry mouth,** hypotension, diarrhea, N/V, tachycardia/palpitations, blurred vision, nasal congestion, sedation, somnolence, depression, constipation, mental impairment, ataxia, increased/decreased appetite, (Tab, OD) **increased salivation.**
Chlordiazepoxide HCl (Librium) CIV	**Cap:** 5mg, 10mg, 25mg	***Adults:*** **Mild-Moderate Anxiety:** 5-10mg tid-qid. **Severe Anxiety:** 20-25mg tid-qid. **Alcohol Withdrawal:** 50-100mg; repeat until agitation controlled. **Max:** 300mg/day. **Pre-op Anxiety:** 5-10mg PO tid-qid on days prior to surgery. **Elderly/Debilitated:** 5mg bid-qid. ***Pediatrics:*** **≥6 yrs:** 5mg bid-qid. May increase to 10mg bid-tid.	**W/P:** Avoid in pregnancy. Paradoxical reactions reported in psychiatric patients and in hyperactive aggressive pediatrics. Caution with porphyria, renal or hepatic dysfunction. Reduce dose in elderly, debilitated. Avoid abrupt withdrawal after extended therapy. May impair mental/physical abilities. **P/N:** Not for use in pregnancy, safety in nursing not known.	Drowsiness, ataxia, confusion, skin eruptions, edema, nausea, constipation, extrapyramidal symptoms, libido changes, EEG changes.
Clorazepate Dipotassium (Tranxene T-Tab) CIV	**Tab:** 3.75mg*, 7.5mg*, 15mg*	***Adults:*** **Anxiety: Usual:** 30mg/day in divided doses or as a single dose qhs, starting at 15mg qhs. Adjust dosage based on individual patient responses. **Max:** 60mg/day. **Elderly/Debilitated: Initial:** 7.5-15mg/day. **Alcohol Withdrawal: Day 1:** 30mg initially, then 30-60mg in divided doses. **Day 2:** 45-90mg in divided doses. **Day 3:** 22.5-45mg in divided doses. **Day 4:** 15-30mg in divided doses. After, gradually reduce dose to 7.5-15mg/day; discontinue when stable. **Max:** 90mg/day. ***Adults/Pediatrics:*** **>12yrs: Antiepileptic Adjunct: Initial:** 7.5mg tid. **Titrate:** Increase by no more than 7.5mg/week. **Max:** 90mg/day. **9-12 yrs: Initial:** 7.5mg bid. **Titrate:** Increase by no more than 7.5mg/week. **Max:** 60mg/day.	**W/P:** Avoid with depressive neuroses or psychotic reactions. Withdrawal symptoms with abrupt withdrawal; taper gradually. Caution with known drug dependency, renal/hepatic impairment. Suicidal tendencies reported; give lowest effective dose. Monitor LFTs and blood counts periodically with long-term therapy. Use lowest effective dose in elderly. **Contra:** Acute narrow-angle glaucoma. **P/N:** Safety in pregnancy not known, not for use in nursing.	Drowsiness, dizziness, GI complaints, nervousness, blurred vision, **dry mouth,** headache, mental confusion.
Diazepam (Valium) CIV	**Inj:** 5mg/mL; **Tab:** (Valium) 2mg*, 5mg*, 10mg*	(Inj) ***Adults:*** **Anxiety (moderate):** 2-5mg IM/IV, may repeat in 3-4 hrs. **Anxiety (severe):** 5-10mg IM/IV, may repeat in 3-4 hrs. **Alcohol Withdrawal (acute):** 10mg IM/IV, then 5-10mg in 3-4 hrs if needed. **Endoscopic Procedures: Usual:** ≤10mg IV (up to 20mg) or 5-10mg IM 30 min prior to procedure. **Muscle Spasm:** 5-10mg IM/IV, then 5-10mg in 3-4 hrs if needed. **Status Epilepticus/Severe Seizures: Initial:** 5-10mg IV. **Maint:** May repeat at 10-15 min intervals. **Max:** 30mg. **Pre-op:** 10mg IM. **Cardioversion:** 5-15mg	**W/P:** Monitor blood counts and LFTs in long-term use. Neutropenia and jaundice reported. Increase in grand mal seizures reported. Avoid abrupt withdrawal. Caution with kidney or hepatic dysfunction. (Diazepam Injection): Inject slowly and avoid small veins with IV. Do not mix or dilute with other products in syringe or infusion flask. Extreme caution in elderly, severely ill and those with limited pulmonary reserve. Avoid if in shock, coma, or acute alcohol intoxication with depressed vital signs. May impair mental/physical abilities. Increase	Drowsiness, fatigue, ataxia, paradoxical reactions, minor EEG changes, (Injection) venous thrombosis, and phlebitis (injection site).

*Scored. †Bold entries denote special dental considerations.
BB = black box warning; **W/P** = warnings/precautions; **Contra** = contraindications; **P/N** = pregnancy category rating and nursing considerations.

Table 18.1. PRESCRIBING INFORMATION FOR PSYCHOACTIVE DRUGS *(cont.)*

NAME	FORM/ STRENGTH	DOSAGE	WARNINGS/PRECAUTIONS & CONTRAINDICATIONS	ADVERSE EFFECTS†
ANTIANXIETY/HYPNOTIC AGENTS *(cont.)*				
BENZODIAZEPINES *(cont.)*				
Diazepam (Valium) CIV *(cont.)*		IV, 5-10 min prior to procedure. **Elderly/Debilitated: Usual:** 2-5mg. ***Pediatrics:* Tetanus: 30 days-5 yrs:** 1-2mg IM/IV (slowly), may repeat every 3-4 hrs prn. **≥5 yrs:** 5-10mg IM/IV, may repeat every 3-4 hrs. **Status Epilepticus/Severe Seizures: 30 days-5 yrs:** 0.2-0.5mg IV (slowly) every 2-5 min up to 5mg. ≥5 yrs: 1mg IV (slowly) every 2-5 min up to 10mg, may repeat in 2-4 hrs. (Tab) ***Adults:* Anxiety:** 2-10mg bid-qid. **Alcohol Withdrawal:** 10mg tid-qid for 24 hours. **Maint:** 5mg tid-qid prn. **Skeletal Muscle Spasm:** 2-10mg tid-qid: **Seizure Disorders:** 2-10mg bid-qid. **Elderly/Debilitated:** 2-2.5mg qd-bid initially; may increase gradually as needed and tolerated. ***Pediatrics:* ≥6 months: Initial:** 1-2.5mg tid-qid. **Titrate:** May increase gradually as needed and tolerated.	in grand mal seizures reported. Not for obstetrical use. Withdrawal symptoms may occur. Hypotension and muscular weakness reported. Not for maintenance of seizures once controlled. **Contra:** Acute narrow-angle glaucoma, untreated open-angle glaucoma; additional contraindications with oral diazepam therapy: patients <6 months. **P/N:** Not for use during pregnancy, safety in nursing unknown.	
Estazolam CIV	**Tab:** 1mg*, 2mg*	***Adults:* Initial:** 1mg qhs. May increase to 2mg qhs. **Small/Debilitated/Elderly: Initial:** 0.5mg qhs.	**W/P:** Avoid abrupt withdrawal after prolonged use. Caution with depression, elderly/debilitated, renal/hepatic impairment. May cause respiratory depression. May impair mental/physical abilities. **Contra:** Pregnancy. **P/N:** Category X, not for use in nursing.	Somnolence, hypokinesia, dizziness, abnormal coordination, headache, malaise, nervousness, cold symptoms, asthenia.
Flurazepam HCl (Dalmane) CIV	**Cap:** 15mg, 30mg	***Adults/Pediatrics:* ≥15 yrs: Usual:** 15-30mg hs. **Elderly/Debilitated: Initial:** 15mg hs.	**W/P:** Caution in elderly, debilitated, severely depressed, those with suicidal tendencies, hepatic/renal impairment, respiratory disease. Ataxia and falls reported in elderly and debilitated. Withdrawal symptoms after discontinuation; avoid abrupt discontinuation. Rare cases of angioedema involving the tongue, glottis, or larynx reported. Complex behaviors such as sleep driving, and other complex behaviors (eg, preparing and eating food, making phone calls, and having sex) reported. **Contra:** Pregnancy. **P/N:** Not for use in pregnancy or nursing.	Confusion, dizziness, drowsiness, lightheadedness, ataxia.
Lorazepam (Ativan) CIV	**Inj:** 2mg/mL, 4mg/mL **Tab:** 0.5mg, 1mg*, 2mg*	(Inj) ***Adults:* ≥18 yrs: Status Epilepticus:** 4mg IV (given slowly at 2mg/min); may repeat one dose after 10-15 min if seizures recur or fail to cease. **Preanesthetic Sedation: Usual:** 0.05mg/kg IM; 2mg or 0.044mg/kg IV (whichever is smaller). **Max:** 4mg IM/IV. (Tab) ***Adults/ Pediatrics:* >12 yrs: Initial:** 2-3mg/day given bid-tid. **Usual:** 2-6mg/day in divided doses. **Insomnia:** 2-4mg qhs. **Elderly/Debilitated:** 1-2mg/day in divided doses.	**W/P:** (Inj) Monitor all parameters to maintain vital function. Risk of respiratory depression or airway obstruction in heavily sedated patients. May cause fetal damage during pregnancy. Increased risk of CNS and respiratory depression in elderly. Avoid with hepatic/renal failure. Caution with mild-to-moderate hepatic/renal disease. Avoid outpatient endoscopic procedures. Possible propylene glycol toxicity in renal impairment. Extreme caution when administering injections to elderly, very ill, or to patients with limited pulmonary reserve; hypoventilation and/or hypoxic cardiac arrest may occur. Gasping syndrome, characterized by CNS depression, metabolic acidosis, gasping respirations, and high levels of benzyl alcohol, may occur.	(Inj) Respiratory depression/failure, hypotension, somnolence, headache, hypoventilation; (Tab) Sedation, dizziness, weakness, unsteadiness, transient amnesia, memory impairment, visual disturbance, depression, respiratory depression, constipation, vertigo, change in appetite, headache.

*Scored. †Bold entries denote special dental considerations.
BB = black box warning; **W/P** = warnings/precautions; **Contra** = contraindications; **P/N** = pregnancy category rating and nursing considerations.

NAME	FORM/ STRENGTH	DOSAGE	WARNINGS/PRECAUTIONS & CONTRAINDICATIONS	ADVERSE EFFECTS†
Lorazepam (Ativan) CIV *(cont.)*			(Tab): Avoid with primary depression or psychosis. Withdrawal symptoms with abrupt discontinuation. Careful supervision if addiction-prone. Caution in patients with compromised respiratory function. Caution with elderly, and renal or hepatic dysfunction. Monitor for GI disease with prolonged therapy. Periodic blood counts and LFTs with long-term therapy. **Contra:** Acute narrow-angle glaucoma; additional contraindications with lorazepam injection: sleep apnea syndrome, severe respiratory insufficiency. Not for intraarterial injection. **P/N:** Category D, not for use in nursing.	
Midazolam HCl CIV	**Inj:** 1mg/mL, 5mg/mL; **Syr:** 2mg/mL [118mL]	***Adults:*** (IV) **Sedation/Anxiolysis/Amnesia Induction: <60 yrs: Initial:** 1-2.5mg IV over 2 min. **Max:** 5mg. **Titrate:** In small increments at 2 min intervals if needed. **Concomitant Narcotics/Other CNS Depressants:** Reduce by 30%. **≥60 yrs/Debilitated/Chronically Ill: Initial:** 1-1.5mg IV over 2 min. **Max:** 3.5mg. **Titrate:** In small increments at 2 min intervals if needed. Concomitant Narcotics/Other CNS Depressants: Reduce by 50%. **Maint:** 25% of sedation dose by slow titration. (IM) **Preoperative Sedation/Anxiolysis/Amnesia: <60 yrs:** 0.07-0.08mg/kg IM up to 1 hr before surgery. **≥60 yrs/Debilitated:** 1-3mg IM. **Anesthesia Induction: Unpremedicated: <55 yrs: Initially:** 0.3-0.35mg/kg IV over 20-30 seconds. May give additional doses of 25% of initial dose to complete induction. **≥55 yrs: Initial:** 0.3mg/kg IV. **Debilitated: Initial:** 0.15-0.25mg/kg IV. **Premedicated: <55 yrs: Initial:** 0.25mg/kg IV over 20-30 seconds. **≥55 yrs: Initial:** 0.2mg/kg IV. **Debilitated:** 0.15mg/kg IV. **Maintenance Sedation:** LD: 0.01-0.05mg/kg IV. May repeat dose at 10-15 min intervals until adequate sedation. **Maint:** 0.02-0.1mg/kg/hr. Titrate to desired level of sedation using 25-50% adjustments. Infusion rate should be decreased 10-25% every few hrs to find minimum effective infusion rate. ***Pediatrics:*** (IV) **Sedation/Anxiolysis/Amnesia Induction: <6 months:** Limited information; titrate with small increments and monitor. **6 months-5 yrs: Initial:** 0.05-0.1mg/kg IV over 2-3 min, up to 0.6mg/kg if needed. **Max:** 6mg. 6-12 yrs: **Initial:** 0.025-0.05mg/kg IV over 2-3 min, up to 0.4mg/kg if needed. **Max:** 10mg. **12-16 yrs:** 1-2.5mg IV over 2 min. **Titrate:** In small increments at 2 min intervals if needed. **Max:** 10mg. (IM) 0.1-0.15mg/kg IM, up to 0.5mg/kg if needed. **Max:** 10mg. **Sedation:** LD: 0.05-0.2mg/kg IV infusion over 2-3 min. **Maint:** 0.06-0.12mg/kg/hr IV infusion. May adjust dose by 25%. **Sedation in Critical Care: Neonatal Dose: <32 weeks: Initial:** 0.03mg/kg/hr IV infusion. **>32**	**BB:** Associated with respiratory depression and respiratory arrest especially when used for sedation in noncritical care settings. Do not administer by rapid injection to neonates. Continuous monitoring required. **W/P:** Agitation, involuntary movements, hyperactivity, and combativeness reported. Caution with CHF, cardiac or respiratory compromised patients, chronic renal failure, chronic hepatic disease, pulmonary disease, uncompensated acute illnesses (eg, severe fluid or electrolyte disturbances), elderly or debilitated. Avoid use with shock or coma, or in acute alcohol intoxication with depression of vital signs. Monitor for respiratory adverse events and paradoxical reactions. (Inj) Contains benzyl alcohol. Administer IM or IV only. **Contra:** Acute narrow-angle glaucoma, (Inj) untreated open-angle glaucoma, intrathecal or epidural use. **P/N:** Category D, caution in nursing.	(Inj) Decreased tidal volume and/or respiratory rate, BP/HR variations, apnea, hypotension, pain and local reactions at injection site, hiccoughs, N/V; (Syr) Emesis, nausea, agitation, hypoxia, **laryngospasm,** agitation.

Table 18.1. PRESCRIBING INFORMATION FOR PSYCHOACTIVE DRUGS *(cont.)*

NAME	FORM/ STRENGTH	DOSAGE	WARNINGS/PRECAUTIONS & CONTRAINDICATIONS	ADVERSE EFFECTS†
ANTIANXIETY/HYPNOTIC AGENTS *(cont.)*				
BENZODIAZEPINES *(cont.)*				
Midazolam HCl CIV *(cont.)*		**weeks: Initial:** 0.06mg/kg/hr IV infusion. Adjust to lowest effective dose. (Syr) ***Pediatrics:*** Single dose of 0.25-1mg/kg. **6 months-5 yrs or less cooperative patients:** 1mg/kg. **Max:** 20mg. **6-15 yrs or cooperative patients:** 0.25mg/kg. **Max:** 20mg. **Cardiac/ Respiratory Compromised, Higher-Risk Surgical Patients, Concomitant Narcotics/Other CNS Depressants:** 0.25mg/kg. **Max:** 20mg.		
Oxazepam CIV	**Cap:** 10mg, 15mg, 30mg; **Tab:** 15mg	***Adults:*** **Anxiety: Mild-Moderate:** 10-15mg tid-qid. **Severe:** 15-30mg tid-qid. **Elderly: Initial:** 10mg tid. **Titrate:** Increase to 15mg tid-qid. **Alcohol Withdrawal:** 15-30mg tid-qid.	**W/P:** May impair mental/physical abilities. Withdrawal symptoms with abrupt discontinuation. Caution in sensitivity to hypotension, elderly. Caution with tablets in tartrazine or ASA allergy. Risk of congenital malformations; avoid in pregnancy. **Contra:** Psychoses. **P/N:** Not for use in pregnancy or nursing.	Drowsiness, dizziness, vertigo, headache, paradoxical excitement, transient amnesia, memory impairment.
Temazepam (Restoril) CIV	**Cap:** 7.5mg, 15mg, 22.5mg, 30mg	***Adults:*** **Usual:** 15mg qhs. **Range:** 7.5-30mg qhs. **Transient Insomnia:** 7.5mg qhs. **Elderly/Debilitated: Initial:** 7.5mg qhs.	**W/P:** Caution in elderly, debilitated, severely depressed, those with suicidal tendencies, hepatic/renal impairment, pulmonary insufficiency. Avoid abrupt discontinuation. If no improvement after 7-10 days, may indicate primary psychiatric and/or medical condition. **Contra:** Pregnancy. **P/N:** Category X, caution in nursing.	Headache, dizziness, drowsiness, fatigue, nervousness, nausea, lethargy, hangover.
Triazolam (Halcion) CIV	**Tab:** 0.125mg, 0.25mg*	***Adults:*** 0.25mg qhs. **Max:** 0.5mg. **Elderly/Debilitated: Initial:** 0.125mg. **Max:** 0.25mg.	**W/P:** Worsening or failure of response after 7-10 days may indicate other medical conditions. Increased daytime anxiety, abnormal thinking, and behavioral changes have occurred. May impair mental/physical abilities. Anterograde amnesia reported with therapeutic doses. Caution with baseline depression, suicidal tendencies, history of drug dependence, elderly/debilitated, renal/hepatic impairment, chronic pulmonary insufficiency, and sleep apnea. Withdrawal symptoms after discontinuation; avoid abrupt withdrawal. **Contra:** Pregnancy. With ketoconazole, itraconazole, nefazodone, medications that impair CYP3A. **P/N:** Category X, not for use in nursing.	Drowsiness, dizziness, lightheadedness, headache, N/V, coordination disorders, ataxia.
NONBENZODIAZEPINES				
Amitriptyline HCl/ Chlordiazepoxide (Limbitrol, Limbitrol DS) CIV	(Chlordiazepoxide-Amitriptyline) **Tab:** (Limbitrol) 5mg-12.5mg, (Limbitrol DS) 10mg-25mg	***Adults:*** **Initial:** 3-4 tabs/day in divided doses. **Max:** (Limbitrol DS) 6 tabs/ day. **Elderly:** Start at low end of dosing range.	**BB:** Antidepressants increased the risk of suicidal thinking and behavior (suicidality) in short-term studies in children, adolescents, and young adults with major depressive disorder (MDD) and other psychiatric disorders. Limbitrol is not approved for use in pediatric patients. **W/P:** Caution with urinary retention, angle-closure glaucoma, cardiovascular disorder, history of seizures, hyperthyroidism, renal or hepatic dysfunction. May produce arrhythmia, sinus tachycardia, and conduction time	Drowsiness, **dry mouth,** constipation, blurred vision, dizziness, bloating, anorexia, fatigue, weakness, restlessness, lethargy.

*Scored. †Bold entries denote special dental considerations.
BB = black box warning; **W/P** = warnings/precautions; **Contra** = contraindications; **P/N** = pregnancy category rating and nursing considerations.

NAME	FORM/ STRENGTH	DOSAGE	WARNINGS/PRECAUTIONS & CONTRAINDICATIONS	ADVERSE EFFECTS†
Amitriptyline HCl/ Chlordiazepoxide (Limbitrol, Limbitrol DS) CIV *(cont.)*			prolongation. May impair mental alertness. Caution in elderly. Avoid abrupt withdrawal. Monitor blood and LFTs periodically with long-term therapy. **Contra:** MAOI use during or within 14 days, acute recovery period following MI. **P/N:** Not for use in pregnancy or nursing.	
Amitriptyline HCl/ Perphenazine	**Tab:** (Amitriptyline-Perphenazine) 10mg-2mg, 10mg-4mg, 25mg-2mg, 25mg-4mg, 50mg-4mg	***Adults:*** **Initial:** 25mg-2mg tab or 25mg-4mg tab tid-qid or 50mg-4mg bid. **Maint:** 25mg-2mg tab or 25mg-4mg tab bid-qid or 50mg-4mg bid. **Max:** 4 tabs/day of 50mg-4mg or 8 tabs/day any other strength. **Severe Illness with Schizophrenia: Initial:** 2 tabs of 25mg-4mg tid and hs prn. **Elderly/Adolescents: Initial:** 10mg-4mg tab tid-qid.	**BB:** Antidepressants increased the risk of suicidal thinking and behavior (suicidality) in short-term studies in children and adolescents with major depressive disorder (MDD) and other psychiatric disorders. **W/P:** Tardive dyskinesia may develop. NMS reported. May alter blood glucose levels. D/C before elective surgery. Caution with urinary retention, angle-closure glaucoma, increased IOP, hyperthyroidism, convulsive disorders, hepatic dysfunction and cardiovascular disorders. May increase prolactin levels. May obscure diagnosis of brain tumor or intestinal obstruction due to antiemetic effects. D/C if significant increase in body temperature develops. May impair mental/physical abilities. **Contra:** CNS depression from drugs, bone marrow depression, MAOI use within 14 days, acute recovery phase following MI. **P/N:** Not for use in pregnancy or nursing.	Sedation, hypotension, HTN, neurological impairment, **dry mouth**.
Buspirone HCl (BuSpar)	**Tab:** 5mg*, 10mg*, 15mg*, 30mg*	***Adults:*** **Usual:** 7.5mg bid. **Titrate:** May increase by 5mg/day every 2-3 days. **Usual:** 20-30mg/day. **Max:** 60mg/day. Use low dose with potent CYP450 3A4 inhibitors (eg, 2.5mg qd with nefazodone). Take consistently with or without food; bioavailability increased with food.	**W/P:** Avoid with hepatic or renal impairment. **P/N:** Category B, not for use in nursing.	Dizziness, nausea, headache, nervousness, lightheadedness, excitement, dystonia, fatigue, parkinsonism, akathisia, restless leg syndrome, restlessness.
Chloral Hydrate CIV	**Syrup:** 500mg/5mL	***Adults:*** Dilute in half glass of water, fruit juice, or ginger ale. **Hypnotic: Usual:** 500mg-1g 15-30 min before bedtime. **Sedative: Usual:** 250mg tid pc. **Alcohol Withdrawal: Usual:** 500mg-1g q6h prn. **Max:** 2g/day. ***Pediatrics:*** **Hypnotic:** 50mg/kg. **Max:** 1g/dose. **Sedative:** 8mg/kg tid. **Max:** 500mg tid. Prior to EEG: 20-25mg/kg.	**W/P:** May be habit forming. Caution with depression, suicidal tendencies, history of drug abuse. Avoid with esophagitis, gastritis, or gastric or duodenal ulcers, large doses with severe cardiac disease. May impair mental/physical abilities. Risk of gastritis, skin eruptions, parenchymatous renal damage with prolonged use. Withdraw gradually with chronic use. **Contra:** Marked hepatic or renal impairment. **P/N:** Category C, caution in nursing.	N/V, diarrhea, ataxia, dizziness.
Diphenhydramine HCl	**Cap:** 50mg	***Adults/Pediatrics:*** **≥12 yrs: Sleep Aid:** 50mg HS.	**W/P:** Caution with narrow-angle glaucoma, stenosing peptic ulcer, pyloroduodenal obstruction, symptomatic prostatic hypertrophy, or bladder-neck obstruction. May cause excitation in pediatrics. Increased risk of dizziness, sedation, and hypotension in elderly. Caution with lower respiratory diseases, bronchial asthma, increased IOP, hyperthyroidism, cardiovascular disease, or HTN. **Contra:** Neonates, premature infants, nursing. **P/N:** Category B, contraindicated in nursing.	Sedation, drowsiness, dizziness, disturbed coordination, epigastric distress, thickening of bronchial secretions.

Table 18.1. PRESCRIBING INFORMATION FOR PSYCHOACTIVE DRUGS *(cont.)*

NAME	FORM/ STRENGTH	DOSAGE	WARNINGS/PRECAUTIONS & CONTRAINDICATIONS	ADVERSE EFFECTS†
ANTIANXIETY/HYPNOTIC AGENTS *(cont.)*				
NONBENZODIAZEPINES *(cont.)*				
Doxylamine Succinate (Unisom) OTC	**Tab:** 25mg	***Adults/Pediatrics:* ≥12 yrs:** 1 tab 30 min prior to going to bed. **Max:** 1 tab qhs.	**W/P:** Caution in emphysema, chronic bronchitis, glaucoma, and difficulty in urination due to BPH. Caution with alcohol. Reevaluate therapy if sleeplessness persists >2 weeks. **Contra:** Pregnancy, nursing, asthma, glaucoma, prostate enlargement. **P/N:** Not for use in pregnancy or nursing.	Anticholinergic effects.
Eszopiclone (Lunesta) CIV	**Tab:** 1mg, 2mg, 3mg	***Adults:*** **Initial:** 2mg qhs. **Max:** 3mg qhs. **Elderly: Difficulty Falling Asleep: Initial:** 1mg qhs. **Max:** 2mg qhs. **Difficulty Staying Asleep: Initial/Max:** 2mg qhs. Avoid high-fat meal.	**W/P:** Abnormal thinking and behavioral changes reported. Amnesia and other neuropsychiatric symptoms may occur. Worsening of depression including suicidal thinking reported in primarily depressed patients. Avoid rapid dose decrease or abrupt discontinuation. Should only be taken immediately prior to bed or after going to bed and experiencing difficulty falling asleep. Avoid hazardous occupations. Caution in elderly, debilitated, or conditions affecting metabolism or hemodynamic responses. Reduce dose with severe hepatic impairment or concurrent use of potent CYP3A4 inhibitors. Caution with signs and symptoms of depression or suicidal tendencies. **P/N:** Category C, caution in nursing.	Headache, **unpleasant taste,** somnolence, **dry mouth,** dizziness, infection, rash, chest pain, peripheral edema, migraine.
Hydroxyzine HCl	**Inj:** 25mg/mL, 50mg/mL; **Syrup:** 10mg/ 5mL; **Tab:** 10mg, 25mg, 50mg, 100mg	***Adults:*** (PO) **Anxiety:** 50-100mg qid. **Pruritus:** 25mg tid-qid. **Sedation:** 50-100mg. IM: **Nausea/Vomiting:** 25-100mg. **Pre-/Postoperative and Pre-/Postpartum Adjunct:** 25-100mg. **Psychiatric/Emotional Emergencies:** 50-100mg q4-6h prn. ***Pediatrics:*** (PO) **Anxiety/Pruritus: <6 yrs:** 50mg/day in divided doses. **≥6 yrs:** 50-100mg in divided doses. **Sedation:** 0.6mg/kg. IM: **Nausea/Vomiting:** 0.5mg/lb. **Pre-/ Post-op Adjunct:** 0.5mg/lb.	**W/P:** Caution in elderly. May impair mental/physical abilities. Effectiveness as an antianxiety agent for long-term use (>4 months) has not been established. **Contra:** Early pregnancy. Injection is intended only for IM administration and should not, under any circumstances, be injected SQ, intra-arterially, or IV. **P/N:** Not for use in pregnancy or nursing.	**Dry mouth,** drowsiness, involuntary motor activity.
Meprobamate CIV	**Tab:** 200mg, 400mg	***Adults:*** **Usual:** 1200-1600mg/day given tid-qid. **Max:** 2400mg/day. **Elderly: >65 yrs:** Start at low end of dosing range. ***Pediatrics:*** **6-12 yrs:** 200-600mg/day given bid-tid.	**W/P:** Physical and psychological dependence reported. Avoid abrupt withdrawal after prolonged or excessive use. Increased risk of congenital malformations with use during first trimester of pregnancy. Caution with liver or renal dysfunction, and in elderly. May precipitate seizures in epileptic patients. Prescribe small quantities in suicidal patients. **Contra:** Porphyria, allergic or idiosyncratic reactions to carisoprodol, mebutamate, tybamate, carbromal. **P/N:** Safety in pregnancy and nursing not known.	Drowsiness, ataxia, slurred speech, vertigo, weakness, N/V, diarrhea, tachycardia, transient ECG changes, rash, leukopenia, petechiae.
Pentobarbital Sodium (Nembutal Sodium Solution) CII	**Inj:** 50mg/mL	***Adults:*** **Usual:** 150-200mg as a single IM injection. (IV) 100mg (commonly used initial dose for 70kg adult); if needed additional small increments may be given up to 200-500mg total dose. Rate of IV injection should not exceed 50mg/min. **Elderly/Debilitated/ Renal or Hepatic Impairment:** Reduce dose. ***Pediatrics:*** (IM) 2-6mg/kg as a	**W/P:** May be habit forming; avoid abrupt cessation after prolonged use. Avoid rapid administration. Tolerance to hypnotic effect can occur. Prehepatic coma use not recommended. Use with caution in patients with chronic or acute pain, mental depression, suicidal tendencies, history of drug abuse or hepatic impairment. Monitor blood, liver	Agitation, confusion, hyperkinesia, ataxia, CNS depression, somnolence, bradycardia, hypotension, N/V, constipation, headache, hypersensitivity reactions, liver damage.

†Bold entries denote special dental considerations.
BB = black box warning; **W/P** = warnings/precautions; **Contra** = contraindications; **P/N** = pregnancy category rating and nursing considerations.

NAME	FORM/ STRENGTH	DOSAGE	WARNINGS/PRECAUTIONS & CONTRAINDICATIONS	ADVERSE EFFECTS†
Pentobarbital Sodium (Nembutal Sodium Solution) CII *(cont.)*		single IM injection. **Max:** 100mg. (IV) Proportional reduction in dosage. Slow IV injection is essential.	and renal function. May impair mental/ physical abilities. Avoid alcohol. **Contra:** History of manifest or latent porphyria. **P/N:** Category D, caution with nursing.	
Ramelteon (Rozerem)	**Tab:** 8mg	***Adults:*** 8mg within 30 min of bedtime. Do not take with or after high-fat meal.	**W/P:** Severe anaphylactic and anaphylactoid reactions reported. Sleep disturbances may manifest as a physical and/or psychiatric disorder, symptomatic treatment of insomnia should be initiated after evaluation. Abnormal thinking, behavioral changes, hallucinations, complex behaviors, (eg, sleep driving), worsening depression, suicidal ideation reported. D/C therapy if complex sleep behavior occurs. May impair physical/mental abilities. May affect reproductive hormones. Avoid with severe hepatic impairment, severe sleep apnea, and severe COPD. Caution in moderate hepatic impairment. **Contra:** Avoid with fluvoxamine. **P/N:** Category C, caution in nursing.	Headache, somnolence, fatigue, dizziness, nausea, exacerbated insomnia, upper respiratory tract infection.
Secobarbital Sodium CII	**Cap:** 100mg	***Adults:*** **Hypnotic:** 100mg hs; **Preoperatively:** 200-300mg, 1-2 hrs before surgery; **Elderly/Debilitated/Renal or Hepatic Dysfunction:** Reduce dose. ***Pediatrics:*** **Preoperatively:** 2-6mg/kg. **Max:** 100mg.	**W/P:** May be habit-forming; avoid abrupt cessation after prolonged use. Tolerance, psychological and physical dependence may occur with continued use. Use with caution, if at all, in patients who are mentally depressed, have suicidal tendencies, or have a history of drug abuse. In patients with hepatic damage, use with caution and initially reduce dose. Caution when administering to patients with acute or chronic pain. May impair mental and/or physical abilities. Avoid alcohol. **Contra:** History of manifest or latent porphyria, marked impairment of liver function, or respiratory disease in which dyspnea or obstruction is evident. **P/N:** Category D, caution in nursing.	Agitation, confusion, hyperkinesia, ataxia, CNS depression, somnolence, bradycardia, hypotension, N/V, constipation, headache, hypersensitivity reactions, liver damage.
Zaleplon (Sonata) CIV	**Cap:** 5mg, 10mg	***Adults:*** **Insomnia:** 10mg qhs. **Low-Weight Patients:** Start with 5mg hs. **Max:** 20mg/day. **Elderly/Debilitated/ Concomitant Cimetidine:** 5mg qhs. **Max:** 10mg/day. **Mild-to-Moderate Hepatic Dysfunction:** 5mg qhs. Take immediately prior to bedtime.	**W/P:** Monitor elderly/debilitated closely. Abnormal thinking and behavioral changes reported. Avoid abrupt withdrawal. Abuse potential exists. Caution in respiratory disorders, depression, conditions affecting metabolism or hemodynamic responses, and mild-to-moderate hepatic insufficiency. Not for use in severe hepatic impairment. May cause impaired coordination even the following day. Reevaluate if no improvement of insomnia after 7-10 days of therapy. Contains tartrazine. **P/N:** Category C, not for use in nursing.	Headache, asthenia, nausea, dizziness, amnesia, somnolence, eye pain, dysmenorrhea, abdominal pain.
Zolpidem Tartrate (Ambien, Ambien CR) CIV	**Tab:** (Ambien) 5mg, 10mg; **Tab, Extended-Release:** (Ambien CR) 6.25mg, 12.5mg	***Adults:*** (Tab) **Usual:** 10mg qhs. **Elderly/Debilitated/Hepatic Insufficiency: Initial:** 5mg. Decrease dose with other CNS depressants. **Max:** 10mg qd. Re-evaluate if insomnia persists after 7-10 days. (Tab, ER) **Usual:** 12.5mg qhs. **Elderly/Debilitated/Hepatic Insufficiency:** 6.25mg qhs. Swallow whole; do not divide, crush, or chew.	**W/P:** Abnormal thinking, behavior changes and complex behaviors (eg, sleep driving) reported. Worsening of depression or suicidal thinking may occur; use lowest feasible amount to avoid intentional overdose. Withdrawal symptoms may occur with rapid dose reduction or discontinuation. Monitor elderly and debilitated patients for impaired motor performance. Severe anaphylactic/anaphylactoid reactions reported. Potential impairment of activities requiring complete mental alertness (eg, operating machinery) after	Drowsiness, dizziness, headache, nausea, diarrhea, drugged feeling, dyspepsia, myalgia, lethargy, memory loss, anxiety, abnormal thoughts and behavior, **tongue or throat swelling.**

Table 18.1. PRESCRIBING INFORMATION FOR PSYCHOACTIVE DRUGS *(cont.)*

NAME	FORM/ STRENGTH	DOSAGE	WARNINGS/PRECAUTIONS & CONTRAINDICATIONS	ADVERSE EFFECTS†
ANTIANXIETY/HYPNOTIC AGENTS *(cont.)*				
NONBENZODIAZEPINES *(cont.)*				
Zolpidem Tartrate (Ambien, Ambien CR) CIV *(cont.)*			ingestion and following day. Avoid with alcohol. Caution with hepatic impairment, mild-to-moderate COPD or sleep apnea, impaired drug metabolism or hemodynamic responses. Avoid if you cannot get a full night's sleep. **P/N:** Category C, not for use in nursing.	
ANTIDEPRESSANT/OCD AGENTS				
MONOAMINE OXIDASE INHIBITORS				
Phenelzine Sulfate (Nardil)	**Tab:** 15mg	***Adults:*** **Initial:** 15mg tid. **Titrate:** Increase to 60-90mg/day at a fairly rapid pace until maximum benefit. **Maint:** Reduce slowly over several weeks to 15mg qd or 15mg qod.	**BB:** Antidepressants increased the risk of suicidal thinking and behavior (suicidality) in short-term studies in children, adolescents, and young adults with major depressive disorder (MDD) and other psychiatric disorders. Phenelzine is not approved for use in pediatric patients. **W/P:** Hypertensive crisis, postural hypotension reported; monitor BP frequently. Caution with epilepsy, asthma, DM, or psychosis. D/C if palpitations or headache occur. Excessive stimulation in schizophrenics. D/C 10 days prior to elective surgery. Avoid abrupt withdrawal. **Contra:** Pheochromocytoma, CHF, history of liver disease, abnormal LFTs, severe renal impairment or renal disease, meperidine, MAOIs, dextromethorphan, CNS depressants, alcohol, certain narcotics, sympathomimetic drugs (eg, amphetamines, cocaine, methylphenidate, dopamine, epinephrine, norepinephrine), or related compounds (eg, methyldopa, L-dopa, L-tryptophan, L-tyrosine, phenylalanine), high tyramine-containing food (eg, cheese, pickled herring, beer, wine, yeast extract, salami, yogurt), excessive caffeine and chocolate, dextromethorphan, CNS depressants, buspirone, serotoninergic agents (eg, dexfenfluramine, fluoxetine, fluvoxamine, paroxetine, sertraline, venlafaxine), bupropion, guanethidine. **P/N:** Safety in pregnancy and nursing not known.	Dizziness, headache, drowsiness, sleep disturbances, constipation, **dry mouth,** GI disturbances, elevated serum transaminases, weight gain, edema, sexual disturbances.
Selegiline (Emsam)	**Patch:** 6mg/24 hrs, 9mg/24 hrs, 12mg/24 hrs [30[s]]	***Adults:*** **MDD:** Apply to dry, intact skin on the upper torso, upper thigh, or outer surface of upper arm once every 24 hrs. **Initial/Target Dose:** 6mg/24hrs. **Titrate:** May increase in increments of 3mg/24hrs at intervals no less than 2 weeks. **Max:** 12mg/24hrs. **Elderly:** 6mg/24hrs. Increase dose cautiously and monitor closely.	**BB:** Antidepressants increased the risk of suicidal thinking and behavior (suicidality) in short-term studies in children, adolescents, and young adults with major depressive disorder and other psychiatric disorders. Selegiline transdermal system is not approved for use in pediatric patients. **W/P:** Hypertensive crisis may occur with ingestion of foods with a high concentration of tyramine. Postural hypotension may occur; consider dosage adjustment with orthostatic symptoms. Activation of mania/hypomania may occur; caution with history of mania. Caution with disorders or conditions that can produce altered metabolism or hemodynamic responses. Avoid elective surgery requiring general anesthesia. **Contra:** Pheochromocytoma. Concomitant SSRIs	Headache, diarrhea, dyspepsia, insomnia, **dry mouth, pharyngitis,** sinusitis, application-site reaction, rash.

*Scored. †Bold entries denote special dental considerations.
BB = black box warning; **W/P** = warnings/precautions; **Contra** = contraindications; **P/N** = pregnancy category rating and nursing considerations.

NAME	FORM/ STRENGTH	DOSAGE	WARNINGS/PRECAUTIONS & CONTRAINDICATIONS	ADVERSE EFFECTS†
Selegiline (Emsam) *(cont.)*			(eg, fluoxetine, sertraline, paroxetine), dual serotonin and norepinephrine reuptake inhibitors (eg, venlafaxine, duloxetine), TCAs (eg, imipramine, amitriptyline), bupropion, buspirone, meperidine, analgesic agents (eg, tramadol, methadone, and propoxyphene), dextromethorphan, St. John's wort, mirtazapine, cyclobenzaprine, carbamazepine, oxcarbazepine, sympathetic amines (including amphetamines), cold products and weight-reducing preparations that contain vasoconstrictors (eg, pseudoephedrine, phenylephrine, phenylpropanolamine, ephedrine), oral selegiline, other MAOIs (eg, isocarboxazid, phenelzine, tranylcypromine), general anesthesia agents, cocaine, or local anesthesia containing sympathomimetic vasoconstrictors. Dietary modifications required with 9mg/24hrs and 12mg/24hrs systems. **P/N:** Category C, caution in nursing.	
Tranylcypromine Sulfate (Parnate)	**Tab:** 10mg	***Adults:*** **MDD: Usual:** 30mg/day in divided doses. **Titrate:** After 2 weeks, may increase by 10mg/day every 1-3 weeks depending on signs of improvement. **Max:** 60mg/day.	**BB:** Antidepressants increased the risk of suicidal thinking and behavior (suicidality) in short-term studies in children, adolescents, and young adults with major depressive disorder and other psychiatric disorders. Tranylcypromine is not approved for use in pediatric patients. **W/P:** Use in patients who are resistant to other therapies. Hypotension reported. Drug dependency possible in doses excessive of the therapeutic range. May suppress anginal pain in myocardial ischemia. Caution with hyperthyroidism, renal dysfunction, diabetes, elderly. May aggravate depression symptoms. May lower seizure threshold. Inhibits MAO 10 days after discontinuation. D/C at least 10 days before elective surgery. D/C if palpitations or frequent headaches occur. **Contra:** Cardiovascular or cerebrovascular disorder, HTN, history of headache, pheochromocytoma. Concomitant MAOIs, dibenzazepine derivatives, sympathomimetics (including amphetamines), some CNS depressants (including narcotics and alcohol), antihypertensives, diuretics, antihistamines, sedatives, anesthetics, bupropion, buspirone, meperidine, SSRIs, dexfenfluramine, dextromethorphan, foods with high tyramine content (cheese) and excessive quantities of caffeine. Elective surgery requiring general anesthesia. History of liver disease or abnormal LFTs. Caution with antiparkinsonism drugs. **P/N:** Safety in pregnancy and nursing not known.	Restlessness, insomnia, weakness, drowsiness, nausea, diarrhea, tachycardia, anorexia, edema, tinnitis, muscle spasm, overstimulation, dizziness, **dry mouth,** blood dyscrasias.
SELECTIVE SEROTONIN REUPTAKE INHIBITORS				
Citalopram Hydrobromide (Celexa)	**Sol:** 10mg/5mL [240mL]; **Tab:** 10mg, 20mg*, 40mg*	***Adults:*** **Initial:** 20mg qd, in the am or pm. **Titrate:** Increase by 20mg at intervals of no less than 1 week. **Max:** 40mg/day (nonresponders may require 60mg/day). **Elderly/Hepatic Impairment:** 20mg/day; titrate to 40mg/day in nonresponders.	**BB:** Antidepressants increased the risk of suicidal thinking and behavior (suicidality) in short-term studies in children, adolescents, and young adults with major depressive disorder (MDD) and other psychiatric disorders. Citalopram is not approved for use in pediatric patients. **W/P:** Activation of mania/hypomania, SIADH, hyponatremia reported.	N/V, dyspepsia, diarrhea, **dry mouth,** somnolence, insomnia, increased sweating, ejaculation disorder, rhinitis, anxiety, anorexia, skeletal pain, agitation.

Table 18.1. PRESCRIBING INFORMATION FOR PSYCHOACTIVE DRUGS *(cont.)*

NAME	FORM/ STRENGTH	DOSAGE	WARNINGS/PRECAUTIONS & CONTRAINDICATIONS	ADVERSE EFFECTS†
ANTIDEPRESSANT/OCD AGENTS *(cont.)*				
SELECTIVE SEROTONIN REUPTAKE INHIBITORS *(cont.)*				
Citalopram Hydrobromide (Celexa) *(cont.)*			Close supervision with high-risk suicide patients. Caution with history of mania or seizures, hepatic impairment, severe renal impairment, conditions that alter metabolism or hemodynamic responses. May impair judgment, thinking, or motor skills. **Contra:** Concomitant MAOI or pimozide therapy. **P/N:** Category C, not for use in nursing.	
Escitalopram Oxalate (Lexapro)	**Sol:** 5mg/5mL [240mL]; **Tab:** 5mg, 10mg*, 20mg*	***Adults:* Initial:** 10mg qd, in am or pm. **Titrate:** May increase to 20mg after a minimum of 1 week. **Elderly/Hepatic Impairment:** 10mg qd. Reevaluate periodically.	**BB:** Antidepressants increased the risk of suicidal thinking and behavior (suicidality) in short-term studies in children, adolescents, and young adults with major depressive disorder (MDD) and other psychiatric disorders. Escitalopram is not approved for use in pediatric patients. **W/P:** Avoid abrupt withdrawal. Activation of mania/ hypomania, hyponatremia reported. SIADH reported with citalopram. Caution with history of mania or seizures, hepatic impairment, severe renal impairment, conditions that alter metabolism or hemodynamic responses, suicidal tendencies. May impair mental/physical abilities. Consider tapering dose during third trimester of pregnancy. **Contra:** Concomitant MAOI or pimozide therapy. **P/N:** Category C, not for use in nursing.	Nausea, insomnia, ejaculation disorder, increased sweating, somnolence, fatigue, diarrhea.
Fluoxetine HCl (Prozac, Prozac Weekly)	**Cap, Extended-Release:** (Prozac Weekly) 90mg; **Cap:** (Prozac) 10mg, 20mg, 40mg; **Sol:** (Prozac) 20mg/5mL [120mL]	(Cap, ER) ***Adults:*** One 90mg cap every week starting 7 days after last daily dose of fluoxetine 20mg. (Cap/ Sol) ***Adults:* MDD: Daily Dosing: Initial:** 20mg qam; increase dose if no improvement after several weeks. Doses >20mg/day, give qam or bid (am and noon). **Max:** 80mg/day. **OCD: Initial:** 20mg qam; may increase dose if no significant improvement after several weeks. **Maint:** 20-60mg/day given qd-bid, am and noon. **Max:** 80mg/day. **Bulimia Nervosa:** 60mg qam. **Max:** 60mg/ day. **Panic Disorder: Initial:** 10mg/day. May increase to 20mg/day after 1 week. May increase further after several weeks if no clinical improvement. **Max:** 60mg/ day. **Hepatic Impairment/Elderly:** Use lower or less frequent dosage. ***Pediatrics:* MDD: ≥8 yrs: Higher-Weight Peds: Initial:** 10 or 20mg/day. After 1 week at 10mg/day, may increase to 20mg/day. **Lower-Weight Peds: Initial:** 10mg/day. **Titrate:** May increase to 20mg/day after several weeks if clinical improvement is not observed. **OCD: ≥7 yrs: Adolescents and Higher-Weight Peds: Initial:** 10mg/day. **Titrate:** Increase to 20mg/day after 2 weeks. Consider additional dose increases after several more weeks if clinical improvement is not observed. **Usual:** 20-60mg/ day. **Lower-Weight Peds: Initial:** 10mg/ day. **Titrate:** Consider additional dose increases after several weeks if clinical improvement is not observed. **Usual:** 20-30mg/day. **Max:** 60mg/day.	**BB:** Antidepressants increased the risk of suicidal thinking and behavior (suicidality) in short-term studies in children, adolescents, and young adults with major depressive disorder (MDD) and other psychiatric disorders. Fluoxetine is approved for use in pediatric patients with MDD and obsessive-compulsive disorder (OCD). **W/P:** Rash with systemic involvement and urticaria reported. Anxiety, nervousness, insomnia or activation of mania/hypomania reported. Weight loss and altered appetite; monitor weight changes. Caution with diseases or conditions that could affect metabolism or hemodynamic responses, diabetes, or history of seizures. May impair judgment, thinking or motor skills. Altered platelet function and hyponatremia reported. Monitor for clinical worsening and/or suicidality, especially at initiation of therapy or dose changes. Avoid abrupt withdrawal. Monitor for discontinuation symptoms. Caution in third trimester of pregnancy due to risk of neonatal complications. **Contra:** During or within 14 days of MAOI therapy. Thioridazine during or within 5 weeks of discontinuation. Concomitant use of pimozide. **P/N:** Category C, not for use in nursing.	Nausea, diarrhea, insomnia, anxiety, nervousness, dizziness, somnolence, tremor, decreased libido, sweating, anorexia, asthenia, **dry mouth,** dyspepsia, headache.

*Scored. †Bold entries denote special dental considerations.
BB = black box warning; **W/P** = warnings/precautions; **Contra** = contraindications; **P/N** = pregnancy category rating and nursing considerations.

NAME	FORM/ STRENGTH	DOSAGE	WARNINGS/PRECAUTIONS & CONTRAINDICATIONS	ADVERSE EFFECTS†
Fluvoxamine Maleate (Luvox, Luvox CR)	**Cap, Extended-Release:** (Luvox CR) 100mg, 150mg; **Tab:** (Luvox) 25mg, 50mg*, 100mg*	***Adults:*** (Tab) **Initial:** 50mg qhs. **Titrate:** Increase by 50mg every 4-7 days. **Maint:** 100-300mg/day. Give bid if total dose >100mg daily. **Max:** 300mg/day. **Elderly/Hepatic Impairment:** Modify initial dose and titration. (Cap, ER) **Initial:** 100mg qhs. **Titrate:** May increase by 50mg every week. **Maint:** 100-300mg/day. **Max:** 300mg/day. **Elderly/Hepatic Impairment:** Titrate slowly following initial dose. ***Pediatrics:*** (Tab) **8-17 yrs: Initial:** 25mg qhs. **Titrate:** Increase by 25mg every 4-7 days. **Maint:** 50-200mg/day. **Max: 8-11 yrs:** 200mg/day. **Adolescents:** 300mg/day. Give bid if total dose >50mg daily.	**BB:** Antidepressants increased the risk of suicidal thinking and behavior (suicidality) in short-term studies in children, adolescents, and young adults with major depressive disorder (MDD) and other psychiatric disorders. Fluvoxamine is not approved for use in pediatric patients. **W/P:** May experience worsening of depression and/or emergence of suicidal behavior. Close supervision with high-risk suicide patients. Activation of mania/hypomania, seizures, and hyponatremia reported. Serious discontinuation symptoms reported. Caution with history of MI or unstable heart disease, liver dysfunction, or conditions altering metabolism or hemodynamic responses. Interference with cognitive or motor performance. Serotonin syndrome reported with concomitant use of triptans and MAOIs. Reduce dose gradually and do not d/c abruptly. May increase risk of bleeding events with ASA, NSAIDs, and other anticoagulants. Neuroleptic malignant syndrome (NMS) or NMS-like events may occur with concomitant antipsychotics. Smoking increases metabolism. **Contra:** Coadministration of alosetron, tizanidine, thioridazine, or pimozide. Concurrent use of MAOIs or MAOI usage within 14 days of discontinuing treatment with Luvox CR. **P/N:** Category C, not for use in nursing.	Headache, asthenia, N/V, diarrhea, anorexia, dyspepsia, insomnia, somnolence, nervousness, agitation, dizziness, anxiety, **dry mouth,** sweating, tremor, abnormal ejaculation.
Paroxetine HCl (Paxil, Paxil CR)	**Sus:** (Paxil) 10mg/5mL [250mL]; **Tab:** (Paxil) 10mg*, 20mg*, 30mg, 40mg; **Tab, Controlled-Release:** (Paxil CR) 12.5mg, 25mg, 37.5mg	***Adults:*** (Tab, CR) Give qd, usually in the am. Swallow whole. **MDD: Initial:** 25mg/day. **Titrate:** May increase weekly by 12.5mg/day. **Max:** 62.5mg/day. **Panic Disorder: Initial:** 12.5mg/day. May increase weekly by 12.5mg/day. **Max:** 75mg/day. **SAD: Initial:** 12.5mg/day. May increase weekly by 12.5mg/day. **Max:** 37.5mg/day. **PMDD: Initial:** 12.5mg/day continuous or limited to luteal phase of cycle. May increase weekly by 12.5mg/day. **Elderly/Debilitated/Severe Renal/Hepatic Impairment: Initial:** 12.5mg/day. **Max:** 50mg/day. (Sus/Tab) Give qd, usually in the am. **MDD: Initial:** 20mg/day. **Max:** 50mg/day. **OCD: Initial:** 20mg qd. **Usual:** 40mg qd. **Max:** 60mg/day. **Panic Disorder: Initial:** 10mg qd. **Usual:** 40mg/day. **Max:** 60mg/day. **GAD: Initial:** 20mg/day. **Usual:** 20-50mg/day. **SAD: Initial/Usual:** 20mg/day. **Max:** 60mg/day. **PTSD: Initial:** 20mg/day. **Usual:** 20-50mg/day. To titrate, may increase weekly by 10mg/day. **Elderly/Debilitated/Severe Renal/Hepatic Impairment: Initial:** 10mg qd. **Max:** 40mg/day.	**BB:** Antidepressants increased the risk of suicidal thinking and behavior (suicidality) in short-term studies in children, adolescents, and young adults with major depressive disorder (MDD) and other psychiatric disorders. Paroxetine is not approved for use in pediatric patients. **W/P:** Caution with history of mania or seizures, conditions that affect metabolism or hemodynamic responses, narrow-angle glaucoma. D/C if seizures occur. Hyponatremia, mydriasis reported. Avoid abrupt withdrawal. Reevaluate periodically. Monitor for clinical worsening and/or suicidality, especially at initiation of therapy or dose changes. **Contra:** Concomitant MAOIs, thioridazine, or pimozide. **P/N:** Category C, caution in nursing.	Somnolence, insomnia, nausea, asthenia, abnormal ejaculation, **dry mouth,** constipation, dizziness, diarrhea, decreased libido, sweating.
Paroxetine Mesylate (Pexeva)	**Tab:** 10mg, 20mg, 30mg, 40mg	***Adults:*** **MDD: Initial:** 20mg/day. **Max:** 50mg/day. **OCD: Initial:** 20mg/day. **Titrate:** Increase by 10mg/day. **Usual:** 40mg/day. **Max:** 60mg/day. **Panic Disorder: Initial:** 10mg/day. **Titrate:** 10mg/day increments at intervals of at least 1 week. **Max:** 60mg/day. **GAD: Initial:** 20mg/day. **Titrate:** Increase by 10mg/day. **Max:** 50mg/day.	**BB:** Antidepressants increased the risk of suicidal thinking and behavior (suicidality) in short-term studies in children, adolescents, and young adults with major depressive disorder (MDD) and other psychiatric disorders. Pexeva is not approved for use in pediatric patients. **W/P:** Caution with history of mania, seizures, history of suicidal	Asthenia, sweating, nausea, decreased appetite, somnolence, dizziness, insomnia, tremor, nervousness, abnormal ejaculation, **dry mouth,** constipation,

Table 18.1. PRESCRIBING INFORMATION FOR PSYCHOACTIVE DRUGS *(cont.)*

NAME	FORM/ STRENGTH	DOSAGE	WARNINGS/PRECAUTIONS & CONTRAINDICATIONS	ADVERSE EFFECTS†
ANTIDEPRESSANT/OCD AGENTS *(cont.)*				
SELECTIVE SEROTONIN REUPTAKE INHIBITORS *(cont.)*				
Paroxetine Mesylate (Pexeva) *(cont.)*		**Elderly/Debilitated/Severe Renal or Hepatic Impairment: Initial:** 10mg qd. **Max:** 40mg/day.	thoughts or attempts (adolescents have an increased risk of suicidal thoughts and/or attempts), conditions that affect metabolism or hemodynamic responses, narrow-angle glaucoma. Risk of serotonin syndrome with concomitant use of triptans, tramadol, and other serotonergic agents. D/C if seizures occur. Altered platelet function, hyponatremia, mydriasis reported. Avoid abrupt withdrawal. Reevaluate periodically. Monitor for clinical worsening and/or suicidality, especially at initiation of therapy or dose changes. **Contra:** Concomitant MAOIs, thioridazine, and pimozide. **P/N:** Category D, caution in nursing.	decreased libido, impotence, headache, tinnitus.
Sertraline HCl (Zoloft)	**Sol:** 20mg/mL [60mL]; **Tab:** 25mg*, 50mg*, 100mg*	***Adults:*** **MDD/OCD:** 50mg qd. **Titrate:** Adjust dose at 1 week intervals. **Max:** 200mg/day. **Panic Disorder/PTSD/ SAD: Initial:** 25mg qd. **Titrate:** Increase to 50mg qd after 1 week. Adjust dose at 1-week intervals. **Max:** 200mg/day. **PMDD: Initial:** 50mg qd continuous or limited to luteal phase of cycle. **Titrate:** Increase 50mg/cycle if needed up to 150mg/day for continuous or 100mg/day for luteal phase dosing. If 100mg/day is established for luteal phase dosing, a 50mg/day titration step for 3 days should take place at the beginning of each luteal phase dosing period. **Hepatic Impairment:** Use lower or less frequent doses. Dilute sol with 4oz water, ginger ale, lemon/lime soda, lemonade or orange juice. Take immediately after mixing. ***Pediatrics:*** **OCD: Initial: 6-12 yrs:** 25mg qd. **13-17 yrs:** 50mg qd. **Titrate:** Adjust dose at 1-week intervals. **Max:** 200mg/day. **Hepatic Impairment:** Use lower or less frequent doses. Dilute sol with 4oz water, ginger ale, lemon/lime soda, lemonade or orange juice. Take immediately after mixing.	**BB:** Antidepressants increased the risk of suicidal thinking and behavior (suicidality) in short-term studies in children, adolescents, and young adults with major depressive disorder (MDD) and other psychiatric disorders. Sertraline HCl is not approved for use in pediatric patients except for patients with obsessive-compulsive disorder (OCD).**W/P:** Activation of mania/hypomania reported. Monitor weight loss. Caution with conditions that could affect metabolism or hemodynamic responses, seizure disorder. Adjust dose with liver dysfunction. Altered platelet function and hyponatremia reported. Weak uricosuric effects reported. Caution with latex sensitivity; solution dropper dispenser contains rubber. Monitor for clinical worsening and/or suicidality, especially at initiation of therapy or dose changes. Avoid abrupt withdrawal. Monitor for discontinuation symptoms. **Contra:** Concomitant use with MAOIs or pimozide. Concomitant disulfiram with solution. **P/N:** Category C, caution in nursing.	Ejaculation failure, **dry mouth,** increased sweating, somnolence, tremor, anorexia, dizziness, headache, N/V, diarrhea, dyspepsia,agitation, insomnia, nervousness, abnormal vision.
SELECTIVE SEROTONIN REUPTAKE INHIBITOR/ ATYPICAL ANTIPSYCHOTIC COMBINATION				
Fluoxetine HCl/ Olanzapine (Symbyax)	**Cap:** (Olanzapine-Fluoxetine): 3mg-25mg, 6mg-25mg, 6mg-50mg, 12mg-25mg, 12mg-50mg	***Adults:*** **≥18 yrs: Treatment Resistant Depression/Depressive Episodes Associated with Bipolar I Disorder: Initial:** 6-25mg qd in evening. **Titrate:** Adjust dose based on efficacy and tolerability. **Max:** 18mg/75mg. **Hypotension Risk/Hepatic Impairment/ Slow Metabolizers: Initial:** 3-25mg to 6-25mg qd in evening. **Titrate:** Increase cautiously. Reevaluate periodically.	**BB:** Antidepressants increased the risk of suicidal thinking and behavior (suicidality) in short-term studies in children, adolescents, and young adults with major depressive disorder (MDD) and other psychiatric disorders. Symbyax is not approved for use in pediatric patients. Elderly patients with dementia-related psychosis treated with atypical antipsychotic drugs are at an increased risk of death; most appeared to be cardiovascular (eg, heart failure, sudden death) or infectious (eg, pneumonia) in nature. Symbyax is not approved for the treatment of patients with dementia-related psychosis.	Asthenia, somnolence, weight gain, edema, increased appetite, peripheral edema, **pharyngitis,** abnormal thinking, tremor, diarrhea, **dry mouth,** amblyopia, twitching, arthralgia, abnormal ejaculation.

*Scored. †Bold entries denote special dental considerations.
BB = black box warning; **W/P** = warnings/precautions; **Contra** = contraindications; **P/N** = pregnancy category rating and nursing considerations.

NAME	FORM/ STRENGTH	DOSAGE	WARNINGS/PRECAUTIONS & CONTRAINDICATIONS	ADVERSE EFFECTS†
Fluoxetine HCl/ Olanzapine (Symbyax) *(cont.)*			**W/P:** Monitor for clinical worsening and/or suicidality. Monitor for hyperglycemia, worsening of glucose control with DM, FBG levels with diabetes risk. Not for use with dementia-related psychosis. Risk of orthostatic hypotension, NMS, tardive dyskinesia, hyperprolactinemia, hyponatremia, seizures. Caution with cardio- or cerebrovascular disease, hypotension risk (eg, dehydration, hypovolemia), history of seizures or conditions that lower seizure threshold, elderly (especially with dementia), hepatic impairment, risk of aspiration pneumonia, conditions that affect metabolism or hemodynamic responses, prostatic hypertrophy, narrow-angle glaucoma, history of paralytic ileus, suicidal tendencies. D/C if unexplained allergic reaction occurs. Elevated transaminases, bleeding episodes reported. Monitor for symptoms of mania/ hypomania. May cause disruption of body temperature regulation. Serotonin syndrome reported; caution with MAOIs, other serotonergic drugs. Caution when prescribing olanzapine and fluoxetine products concomitantly. May impair judgment, thinking, or motor skills. **Contra:** During or within 14 days of MAOI use; during or within 5 weeks of discontinuation of thioridazine use; concomitant pimozide use. **P/N:** Category C, not for use in nursing.	
SEROTONIN/NOREPINEPHRINE REUPTAKE INHIBITORS				
Desvenlafaxine (Pristiq)	**Tab, Extended-Release:** 50mg, 100mg	***Adults:*** **≥18 yrs:** 50mg qd. **Renal Impairment (CrCl<30mL/min) or ESRD:** 50mg every other day. Supplemental doses should not be given to patients after dialysis. **Hepatic Impairment: Max:** 100mg/day. **Upon discontinuation:** Gradually reduce dose (giving 50mg less frequently) rather than abrupt cessation. Do not divide, crush, chew, or place in water.	**BB:** Antidepressants increased the risk of suicidal thinking and behavior (suicidality) in short-term studies in children, adolescents, and young adults with major depressive disorder (MDD) and other psychiatric disorders. Desvenlafaxine is not approved for use in pediatric patients. **W/P:** Worsening of depression and/or emergence of suicidal behavior may occur. Serotonin syndrome reported; caution with concomitant serotonergic drugs. May cause sustained increases in BP; monitor BP regularly. May increase risk of bleeding events. Monitor with increased IOP or if at risk of acute narrow-angle glaucoma. Activation of mania/hypomania reported. Caution with cardiovascular or cerebrovascular disease, recent MI, renal impairment, and seizure disorder. Cholesterol and triglyceride elevation may occur; consider monitoring. Discontinuation symptoms may occur; taper dose and monitor symptoms. Hyponatremia, interstitial lung disease, and eosinophilic pneumonia may occur. **Contra:** Concomitant MAOI or within 14 days of stopping. **P/N:** Category C, not for use in nursing.	Headache, N/V, **dry mouth,** diarrhea, dizziness, insomnia, somnolence, hyperhidrosis, fatigue, constipation, palpitations, anxiety, decreased appetite, specific male sexual disorders.

Table 18.1. PRESCRIBING INFORMATION FOR PSYCHOACTIVE DRUGS *(cont.)*

NAME	FORM/ STRENGTH	DOSAGE	WARNINGS/PRECAUTIONS & CONTRAINDICATIONS	ADVERSE EFFECTS†
ANTIDEPRESSANT/OCD AGENTS *(cont.)*				
SEROTONIN/NOREPINEPHRINE REUPTAKE INHIBITORS *(cont.)*				
Duloxetine HCl (Cymbalta)	**Cap, Delayed-Release:** 20mg, 30mg, 60mg	***Adults:*** **MDD: Initial:** 40mg/day (given as 20mg bid) to 60mg/day (given qd or as 30mg bid) or 30mg qd for 1 week before increasing to 60mg qd. **Max:** 120mg. Reevaluate periodically. **Diabetic Peripheral Neuropathic Pain:** 60mg/day given qd. May lower starting dose if tolerability a concern. **Renal Impairment:** Consider lower starting dose with gradual increase. **GAD: Initial:** 60mg qd or 30mg qd for 1 week to adjust before increasing to 60mg qd. **Titrate:** May increase by increments of 30mg qd if needed. **Max:** 120 mg qd. **FM: Initial:** 30mg qd for 1 week to adjust before increasing to 60mg qd. **Max:** 60mg qd. Do not chew or crush.	**BB:** Antidepressants increased the risk of suicidal thinking and behavior (suicidality) in short-term studies in children, adolescents, and young adults with major depressive disorder (MDD) and other psychiatric disorders. Not approved for use in pediatric patients. **W/P:** Monitor for clinical worsening and/or suicidality. May cause hepatotoxicity. Avoid with chronic liver disease. May increase BP; obtain baseline and monitor periodically. Orthostatic hypotension and syncope reported. Avoid abrupt cessation and with severe renal impairment/ESRD or hepatic insufficiency. Caution with conditions that may slow gastric emptying, history of mania or seizures. May increase risk of mydriasis; caution in patients with controlled narrow-angle glaucoma. Serotonin syndrome may occur; caution with concomitant use of serotonergic drugs. Hyponatremia reported. May affect urethral resistance. May increase risk of abnormal bleeding; caution with aspirin, NSAIDs, warfarin. May increase risk of serum transaminase elevations. **Contra:** Concomitant use of MAOIs, uncontrolled narrow-angle glaucoma. **P/N:** Category C, not for use in nursing.	N/V, **dry mouth,** constipation, diarrhea, decreased appetite, fatigue, dizziness, somnolence, increased sweating, blurred vision, insomnia, agitation, erectile dysfunction.
Venlafaxine HCl (Effexor, Effexor XR)	**Cap, Extended-Release:** (Effexor XR) 37.5mg, 75mg, 150mg; **Tab:** (Effexor) 25mg*, 37.5mg*, 50mg*, 75mg*, 100mg*	(Tab) ***Adults:*** **≥18 yrs: Initial:** 75mg/day given bid-tid with food. **Titrate:** Increase by 75mg/day at no less than 4-day intervals. **Max:** 375mg/day. **Hepatic Impairment (moderate):** Reduce dose by 50%. **Renal Impairment (mild to moderate):** Reduce dose by 25%. **Hemodialysis:** Reduce dose by 50%. Withhold dose until after hemodialysis treatment completed. If drug used 6 weeks or longer, taper gradually (over 2 weeks or more) when discontinuing treatment. (Cap, ER) ***Adults:*** **MDD/GAD/SAD: Initial:** 75mg qd, or 37.5mg qd; increase to 75mg qd after 4-7 days. **Titrate:** May increase by 75mg/day at no less than 4-day intervals. **Max:** 225mg/day. **PD: Initial:** 37.5mg qd for 7 days. **Titrate:** May increase 75mg/day, as needed, at no less than 7-day intervals. **Max:** 225mg/day. **Moderate Hepatic Impairment:** Reduce initial dose by 50%. **Renal Impairment:** Reduce total daily dose by 25-50%. **Hemodialysis:** Reduce total daily dose by 50%. Withhold dose until after hemodialysis treatment completed. If drug used 6 weeks or longer, taper gradually (over 2 weeks or more) when discontinuing treatment. Periodically reassess need for maintenance therapy. Take with food in the am or pm, the same time each day. May sprinkle on spoonful of applesauce. Do not divide, crush, chew, or place in water.	**BB:** Antidepressants increased the risk of suicidal thinking and behavior (suicidality) in short-term studies in children, adolescents, and young adults with major depressive disorder (MDD) and other psychiatric disorders. Venlafaxine is not approved for use in pediatric patients. **W/P:** May cause sustained increases in BP; monitor BP regularly. Treatment-emergent nervousness, insomnia and anorexia reported. Caution with seizures, conditions affecting hemodynamic responses or metabolism, volume-depletion, the elderly. Risk of mydriasis; monitor those with raised IOP or risk of acute narrow angle glaucoma. Abnormal bleeding (eg, ecchymosis) and activation of mania/hypomania reported. Risk of hyponatremia, SIADH. Caution with recent MI, hyperthyroidism, heart failure, renal or hepatic impairment. Serotonin syndrome may occur; caution with concomitant use of serotonergic drugs. Patients who present with progressive dyspnea, cough or chest discomfort should consider the possibility of interstitial lung disease and eosinophilic pneumonia. D/C if impaired balance occurs. Cases of clinically significant hyponatremia in elderly. **Contra:** Concomitant MAOI therapy. **P/N:** Category C, not for use in nursing.	Asthenia, sweating, N/V, constipation, anorexia, insomnia, somnolence, **dry mouth,** dizziness, nervousness, anxiety, tremor, blurred vision, abnormal ejaculation/orgasm, impotence in men.

*Scored. †Bold entries denote special dental considerations.
BB = black box warning; **W/P** = warnings/precautions; **Contra** = contraindications; **P/N** = pregnancy category rating and nursing considerations.

NAME	FORM/ STRENGTH	DOSAGE	WARNINGS/PRECAUTIONS & CONTRAINDICATIONS	ADVERSE EFFECTS†
TETRACYCLIC ANTIDEPRESSANTS				
Amoxapine	**Tab:** 25mg*, 50mg*, 100mg*, 150mg*	***Adults:*** **Initial:** 50mg bid-tid. **Titrate:** May increase to 100mg bid-tid by end of first week. **Usual:** 200-300mg/day. **Max: Outpatients:** 400mg/day; **Inpatients:** 600mg/day. **Elderly: Initial:** 25mg bid-tid. **Titrate:** May increase to 50mg bid-tid by end of first week. **Max:** 300mg/day. Doses ≤300mg/day may be given as single dose at bedtime.	**BB:** Antidepressants increased the risk of suicidal thinking and behavior (suicidality) in short-term studies in children, adolescents, and young adults with major depressive disorder (MDD) and other psychiatric disorders. **W/P:** D/C if NMS, TD, rash, and/or drug fever occur. Caution with history of urinary retention, angle-closure glaucoma, increased IOP, suicidal tendencies. May induce sinus tachycardia, changes in conduction time, arrhythmias. MI, stroke reported. Extreme caution with history of seizure disorders. Activation of mania, increased psychosis reported. May impair mental/physical abilities. **Contra:** During or within 14 days of MAOIs; recent MI. **P/N:** Category C, caution in nursing.	Drowsiness, **dry mouth,** constipation, blurred vision, tardive dykinesia, extrapyramidal symptoms.
Mirtazapine (Remeron, Remeron SolTab)	**Tab:** 15mg*, 30mg*, 45mg; **Tab, Disintegrating:** 15mg, 30mg, 45mg	***Adults:*** **Initial:** 15mg qhs. **Titrate:** May increase every 1-2 weeks. **Max:** 45mg/day. Disintegrating tabs disintegrate rapidly on tongue and can be swallowed with saliva; no water needed. Do not cut tabs in half.	**BB:** Antidepressants increased the risk of suicidal thinking and behavior (suicidality) in short-term studies in children, adolescents, and young adults with major depressive disorder (MDD) and other psychiatric disorders. Mirtazapine is not approved for use in pediatric patients. **W/P:** Risk of agranulocytosis. D/C if sore throat, fever, or stomatitis, along with low WBC count, develops. May increase appetite, cholesterol, and triglycerides. Caution in history of seizures, mania/hypomania, hepatic or renal impairment, altered metabolic or hemodynamic conditions, elderly. Somnolence, dizziness reported. Close supervision with high-risk suicide patients. May impair judgment, thinking, or motor skills. **P/N:** Category C, caution in nursing.	Somnolence, appetite increase, weight gain, dizziness, **dry mouth,** constipation, asthenia, flu syndrome, abnormal dreams.
TRICYCLIC ANTIDEPRESSANTS				
Amitriptyline HCl	**Inj:** 10mg/mL; **Tab:** 10mg, 25mg, 50mg, 75mg, 100mg, 150mg	***Adults:*** **PO: Initial: (Outpatient)** 75mg/day in divided doses or 50-100mg qhs. **(Inpatient)** 100mg/day. **Titrate: (Outpatient)** Increase by 25-50mg qhs. **(Inpatient)** Increase to 200mg/day. **Maint:** 50-100mg qhs. **Max: (Outpatient)** 150mg/day. **(Inpatient)** 300mg/day. **IM: Initial:** 20-30mg qid. **Elderly:** 10mg tid and 20mg qhs.	**BB:** Antidepressants increased the risk of suicidal thinking and behavior (suicidality) in short-term studies in children, adolescents, and young adults with major depressive disorder (MDD) and other psychiatric disorders. **W/P:** Caution with history of seizures, urinary retention, angle-closure glaucoma, increased IOP, hyperthyroidism, cardiovascular disorders, liver dysfunction. Increases symptoms with schizophrenia and manic-depression. D/C several weeks before elective surgery. May alter blood glucose levels. **Contra:** MAOI use or within 14 days; acute recovery period following MI; concurrent cisapride. **P/N:** Category C, not for use in nursing.	MI, stroke, seizure, paralytic ileus, urinary retention, constipation, blurred vision, **dry mouth,** hyperpyrexia, rash, bone marrow depression, testicular swelling, gynecomastia (male), breast enlargement (female), alopecia, edema.
Clomipramine HCl (Anafranil)	**Cap:** 25mg, 50mg, 75mg	***Adults:*** **Initial:** 25mg/day with meals. **Titrate:** Increase within 2 weeks to 100mg/day. Increase further over several weeks. **Max:** 250mg/day. **Maint:** May give total daily dose at bedtime. ***Pediatrics:*** **>10 yrs: Initial:** 25mg/day with meals. **Titrate:** Increase within 2 weeks to 3mg/kg or 100mg/day, whichever is smaller. Increase further over several weeks. **Max:** 3mg/kg/day or 200mg/day. **Maint:** May give total daily dose at bedtime.	**BB:** Antidepressants increased the risk of suicidal thinking and behavior (suicidality) in short-term studies in children, adolescents, and young adults with major depressive disorder (MDD) and other psychiatric disorders. Clomipramine is not approved for use in pediatric patients except for patients with OCD. **W/P:** Pooled analyses of short-term placebo-controlled trials of antidepressant drugs showed that these drugs increase the risk of suicidal	**Dry mouth,** constipation, nausea, dyspepsia, anorexia, weight gain, increased sweating, increased appetite, myoclonus, nervousness, libido change, dizziness, tremor, somnolence, impotence, visual changes.

Table 18.1. PRESCRIBING INFORMATION FOR PSYCHOACTIVE DRUGS *(cont.)*

NAME	FORM/ STRENGTH	DOSAGE	WARNINGS/PRECAUTIONS & CONTRAINDICATIONS	ADVERSE EFFECTS†
ANTIDEPRESSANT/OCD AGENTS *(cont.)*				
TRICYCLIC ANTIDEPRESSANTS *(cont.)*				
Clomipramine HCl (Anafranil) *(cont.)*			thinking and behavior (suicidality) in children, adolescents, and young adults (ages 18-24) with major depressive disorder (MDD) and other psychiatric disorders. Increased risks with electro-convulsive therapy. D/C prior to elective surgery. Avoid abrupt withdrawal. Caution with seizure disorder, conditions predisposing to seizures (eg, brain damage, alcoholism), urinary retention, narrow-angle glaucoma, adrenal medulla tumors, increased IOP, hyperthyroidism, cardiovascular disorders, liver dysfunction, significant renal dysfunction. Monitor hepatic enzymes with liver dysfunction. Weight changes, sexual dysfunction, blood dyscrasias, elevated liver enzymes reported. Hypomania/mania reported with affective disorder. Psychosis reported with schizophrenia. All patients being treated with antidepressants for any indication should be monitored appropriately and observed closely for clinical worsening, suicidality, and unusual changes in behavior, especially during the initial few months of therapy or at times of dose changes. **Contra:** MAOI use within 14 days, acute recovery period following MI. **P/N:** Category C, not for use in nursing.	
Desipramine HCl (Norpramin)	**Tab:** 10mg, 25mg, 50mg, 75mg, 100mg, 150mg	***Adults:*** **Usual:** 100-200mg/day given qd or in divided doses. **Max:** 300mg/day. **Elderly/Adolescents: Usual:** 25-100mg/day given qd or in divided doses. **Max:** 150mg/day.	**BB:** Antidepressants increased the risk of suicidal thinking and behavior (suicidality) in short-term studies in children, adolescents, and young adults with major depressive disorder (MDD) and other psychiatric disorders. Desipramine is not approved for use in pediatric patients. **W/P:** Hypomania with manic-depressive disease. D/C prior to elective surgery. Do not withdraw abruptly. Extreme caution with urinary retention, glaucoma, seizure disorders, cardiovascular disease, thyroid disease, alcohol abuse. May exacerbate psychosis; caution with schizophrenia. May impair mental or physical abilities. May alter blood glucose levels. **Contra:** MAOI use within 14 days, acute recovery period following MI. **P/N:** Safety in pregnancy and nursing not known.	Arrhythmias, hypotension, HTN, tachycardia, confusion, hallucination, dizziness, anxiety, numbness, tingling, ataxia, tremors, **dry mouth,** urinary retention, urticaria, photosensitivity, SIADH, altered libido.
Doxepin HCl (Sinequan)	**Cap:** 10mg, 25mg, 50mg, 75mg, 100mg, 150mg; **Sol, Concentrate:** 10mg/mL [120mL]	***Adults:*** **Very Mild Illness: Usual:** 25-50mg/day. **Mild-to-Moderate Severity: Initial:** 75mg/day. **Usual:** 75-150mg/day. **Severely Ill:** May increase up to 300mg/day. Dilute solution with 120mL of water, milk or juice. Give once daily or in divided doses. Divide dose if >150mg. **Elderly:** Use lower doses and monitor closely.	**BB:** Antidepressants increased the risk of suicidal thinking and behavior (suicidality) in short-term studies in children, adolescents, and young adults with major depressive disorder (MDD) and other psychiatric disorders. Doxepin is not approved for use in pediatric patients. **W/P:** Monitor for suicidal tendencies and increased symptoms of psychosis. Avoid abrupt discontinuation. **Contra:** Glaucoma, urinary retention. **P/N:** Safety in pregnancy and nursing not known.	Drowsiness, **dry mouth,** blurred vision, constipation, urinary retention, hypotension, tachycardia, rash, edema, photosensitization, pruritus, eosinophilia, nausea, dizziness.

†Bold entries denote special dental considerations.
BB = black box warning; **W/P** = warnings/precautions; **Contra** = contraindications; **P/N** = pregnancy category rating and nursing considerations.

NAME	FORM/ STRENGTH	DOSAGE	WARNINGS/PRECAUTIONS & CONTRAINDICATIONS	ADVERSE EFFECTS†
Imipramine HCl (Tofranil) **Imipramine Pamoate** (Tofranil-PM)	**Cap:** (Tofranil-PM) 75mg, 100mg, 125mg, 150mg; **Tab:** (Tofranil) 10mg, 25mg, 50mg	(Tab) ***Adults:*** **Depression: Initial: Inpatient:** 100mg/day in divided doses. **Titrate:** Increase to 200mg/day; up to 250-300mg/day after 2 weeks if needed. **Outpatient:** 75mg/day. **Titrate:** Increase to 150mg/day. **Maint:** 50-150mg/day. **Max:** 200mg/day. **Elderly/ Adolescents: Initial:** 30-40mg/day. **Max:** 100mg/day. ***Pediatrics:*** **Depression: Adolescents: Initial:** 30-40mg/day. **Max:** 100mg/day. **Enuresis: ≥6 yrs: Initial:** 25mg/day 1 hour before bedtime. **Titrate: 6-12 yrs:** If inadequate response in 1 week, increase to 50mg before bedtime. **≥12 yrs:** Increase to 75mg before bedtime after 1 week if needed. **Max:** 2.5mg/kg/day. (Cap) ***Adults:*** **Inpatient: Initial:** 100-150mg/day. **Titrate:** May increase to 200mg/day. After 2 weeks may increase up to 250-300mg/day if needed. **Outpatient: Initial:** 75mg/day. **Titrate:** May increase to 150mg/day. **Max:** 200mg/day. **Inpatient/Outpatient: Maint:** Following remission, maintain at lowest possible dose. **Usual:** 75-150mg/day. **Elderly/ Adolescents:** Initiate with Tofranil 25-50mg/day. Switch to Tofranil-PM with doses ≥75mg. **Max:** 100mg/day.	**BB:** Antidepressants increased the risk of suicidal thinking and behavior (suicidality) in short-term studies in children, adolescents, and young adults with major depressive disorder (MDD) and other psychiatric disorders. Imipramine HCl is not approved for use in pediatric patients except for patients with nocturnal enuresis. Imipramine pamoate is not approved for use in pediatric patients. **W/P:** Caution with elderly, serious depression, cardiovascular disease, hyperthyroidism, urinary retention, narrow-angle glaucoma, increased IOP, seizure disorders, renal and hepatic impairment. May activate psychosis in schizophrenia; reduce dose. Limit electroshock therapy. May alter blood glucose levels. Photosensitivity reported. D/C prior to elective surgery, or with hypomanic or manic episodes. D/C with pathological neutrophil depression. **Contra:** Within 14 days of MAOI therapy, or during acute recovery period following MI. **P/N:** Safety in pregnancy not known; not for use in nursing.	Orthostatic hypotension, HTN, confusion, hallucinations, numbness, tremors, **dry mouth,** urticaria, N/V, diarrhea, gynecomastia (male), breast enlargement (female), galactorrhea.
Nortriptyline HCl (Pamelor)	**Cap:** 10mg, 25mg, 50mg, 75mg; **Sol:** 10mg/5mL	***Adults:*** 25mg tid-qid. **Max:** 150mg/day. Total daily dose may be given once a day. Monitor serum levels if dose >100mg/day. **Elderly/Adolescents:** 30-50mg/day in single or divided doses.	**BB:** Antidepressants increased the risk of suicidal thinking and behavior (suicidality) in short-term studies in children, adolescents, and young adults with major depressive disorder (MDD) and other psychiatric disorders. Nortriptyline is not approved for use in pediatric patients. **W/P:** MI, arrhythmia, strokes have occurred. Caution with cardiovascular disease, glaucoma, history of urinary retention, hyperthyroidism. May lower seizure threshold, exacerbate psychosis or activate schizophrenia, cause symptoms of mania in bipolar disease, or alter glucose levels. D/C several days prior to elective surgery. **Contra:** MAOI use within 14 days, acute recovery period following MI. **P/N:** Safety during pregnancy and nursing not known.	Arrhythmias, hypotension, HTN, tachycardia, MI, heart block, stroke, confusion, hallucination, insomnia, tremors, ataxia, anxiety, **dry mouth,** blurred vision, skin rash, extrapyramidal symptoms, photosensitivity, SIADH, anorexia.
Protriptyline HCl (Vivactil)	**Tab:** 5mg, 10mg	***Adults:*** **Usual:** 15-40mg/day taken tid-qid. **Titrate:** May increase to 60mg/day. **Max:** 60mg/day. **Elderly: Initial:** 5mg tid. **Titrate:** Increase gradually if needed. Monitor cardiovascular system with doses >20mg/day. ***Pediatrics:*** **Adolescents: Initial:** 5mg tid. **Titrate:** Increase gradually if needed.	**BB:** Antidepressants increased the risk of suicidal thinking and behavior (suicidality) in short-term studies in children, adolescents, and young adults with major depressive disorder (MDD) and other psychiatric disorders. Protriptyline is not approved for use in pediatric patients. **W/P:** Caution with history of seizures, urinary retention, increased IOP, cardiovascular disorders, hyperthyroidism, elderly. May aggravate psychotic symptoms in schizophrenia, manic symptoms in manic-depressive psychosis, and anxiety/agitation in overactive/agitated patients. D/C several days before elective surgery. Both elevation and lowering of blood sugar levels reported. **Contra:** Within 14 days of MAOI therapy, cisapride, acute recovery period following MI. **P/N:** Safety in pregnancy and nursing not known.	Tachycardia, hypotension, confusion, anxiety, insomnia, nightmares, seizures, EPS, dizziness, headache, anticholinergic effects, rash, photosensitivity, blood dyscrasias, GI effects, impotence, decreased libido, flushing.

Table 18.1. PRESCRIBING INFORMATION FOR PSYCHOACTIVE DRUGS *(cont.)*

NAME	FORM/ STRENGTH	DOSAGE	WARNINGS/PRECAUTIONS & CONTRAINDICATIONS	ADVERSE EFFECTS†
ANTIDEPRESSANT/OCD AGENTS *(cont.)*				
TRICYCLIC ANTIDEPRESSANTS *(cont.)*				
Trimipramine Maleate (Surmontil)	**Cap:** 25mg, 50mg, 100mg	***Adults:*** **Outpatient: Initial:** 75mg/day in divided doses. **Titrate:** Increase to 150mg/day. **Maint:** 50-150mg/day. **Max:** 200mg/day. **Inpatient: Initial:** 100mg/day in divided doses. **Titrate:** Increase gradually to 200mg/day. If no improvement after 2-3 weeks, may increase up to 250-300mg/day. **Elderly: Initial:** 50mg/day. **Titrate:** Increase gradually to 100mg/day. Take hs for at least 3 months. ***Pediatrics:*** **Adolescents: Initial:** 50mg/day. **Titrate:** Increase gradually to 100mg/day. Take hs for at least 3 months.	**BB:** Antidepressants increased the risk of suicidal thinking and behavior (suicidality) in short-term studies in children, adolescents, and young adults with major depressive disorder (MDD) and other psychiatric disorders. Trimipramine is not approved for use in pediatric patients. **W/P:** Caution with cardiovascular disease, increased IOP, urinary retention, narrow-angle glaucoma, hyperthyroidism, seizure disorder, liver dysfunction. May impair ability to operate machinery. May alter glucose levels. May activate psychosis in schizophrenia. Manic or hypomanic episodes may occur. May increase hazards with electroshock therapy. **Contra:** Acute recovery period post-MI, within 14 days of MAOI therapy. **P/N:** Category C, safety in nursing not known.	Hypotension, HTN, arrhythmia, confusion, insomnia, incoordination, GI complaints, allergic reactions, gynecomastia, blood dyscrasias, **dry mouth,** blurred vision, urinary retention.
MISCELLANEOUS ANTIDEPRESSANTS				
Bupropion HCl (Wellbutrin, Wellbutrin SR, Wellbutrin XL)	**Tab:** (Wellbutrin) 75mg, 100mg; **Tab, Extended-Release:** (Wellbutrin SR) 100mg, 150mg, 200mg; (Wellbutrin XL) 150mg, 300mg	***Adults:*** **≥18 yrs:** (Wellbutrin) **Initial:** 100mg bid, may increase to 100mg tid after 3 days. **Usual:** 100mg tid. **Max:** 450mg/day, given in divided doses of not more than 150mg each. **Severe Hepatic Cirrhosis: Max:** 75mg qd. (Wellbutrin SR) **Initial:** 150mg qd, may increase to 150mg bid after 3 days. **Usual:** 150mg bid. **Max:** 200mg bid. Separate doses by at least 8 hrs. **Severe Hepatic Cirrhosis:** 100mg/day or 150mg every other day. **Mild-Moderate Hepatic Cirrhosis/Renal Impairment:** Reduce frequency and/or dose. (Wellbutrin XL) Give in AM. Swallow whole. **MDD: Initial:** 150mg qd. May increase to 300mg qd on Day 4. **Usual:** 300mg qd. **Max:** 450mg qd. **SAD:** Start in autumn; stop in early spring. **Initial:** 150mg qd. May increase to 300mg after 1 week. **Usual/Max:** 300mg qd. Taper dose for 2 weeks prior to discontinuation. **Mild-Moderate Hepatic Cirrhosis/Renal Impairment:** Reduce frequency and/or dose. **Severe Hepatic Cirrhosis: Max:** 150mg every other day.	**BB:** Antidepressants increased the risk of suicidal thinking and behavior (suicidality) in short-term studies in children, adolescents, and young adults with major depressive disorder (MDD) and other psychiatric disorders. Bupropion is not approved for use in pediatric patients. **W/P:** Dose-related risk of seizures. D/C and do not restart if seizure occurs. Extreme caution with history of seizure, cranial trauma, severe hepatic cirrhosis. Agitation, insomnia, psychosis, confusion and other neuro-psychiatric signs reported. Caution with bipolar disorder, recent MI, unstable heart disease, renal impairment. Altered appetite/weight, allergic reactions, HTN reported. Monitor for clinical worsening and/or suicidality, especially at initiation of therapy or dose changes. **Contra:** Seizure disorder, bulimia or anorexia nervosa, within 14 days of MAOIs, other forms of bupropion, abrupt discontinuation of alcohol or sedatives. **P/N:** Category C, not for use in nursing.	Headache, **dry mouth,** nausea, insomnia, dizziness, **pharyngitis,** abdominal pain, agitation, diarrhea, palpitations, myalgia, anxiety, tinnitus, constipation, sweating, rash.
Bupropion Hydrobromide (Aplenzin)	**Tab, Extended-Release:** 174mg, 348mg, 522mg	***Adults:*** **≥18 yrs:** Give in morning. Swallow whole. **Initial:** 174mg qd. **Titrate:** May increase to 348mg qd on Day 4 if tolerated. **Max:** 522mg/day given as single dose if no clinical improvement after several weeks. **Switching from Wellbutrin, Wellbutrin SR, or Wellbutrin XL:** Give equivalent dose. 522mg bupropion HBr = 450mg bupropion HCl, 348mg bupropion HBr = 300mg bupropion HCl, 174mg bupropion HBr = 150mg bupropion HCl. **Mild-Moderate Hepatic Cirrhosis/Renal Impairment:** Reduce frequency and/or dose. **Severe Hepatic Cirrhosis: Max:** 174mg every other day.	**BB:** Antidepressants increased the risk of suicidal thinking and behavior (suicidality) in short-term studies in children, adolescents, and young adults with major depressive disorder (MDD) and other psychiatric disorders. Bupropion is not approved for use in pediatric patients. **W/P:** May worsen depression and/or emergence of suicidal ideation and behavior; monitor closely. May precipitate manic episodes in bipolar disorder. Dose-related risk of seizures; d/c and do not restart if seizure occurs. Extreme caution with history of seizure, cranial trauma, severe hepatic cirrhosis, concomitant medications that lower	**Dry mouth,** nausea, insomnia, dizziness, **pharyngitis,** abdominal pain, agitation, anxiety, tremor, palpitation, sweating, tinnitus, myalgia, anorexia, urinary frequency, rash.

*Scored. †Bold entries denote special dental considerations.
BB = black box warning; **W/P** = warnings/precautions; **Contra** = contraindications; **P/N** = pregnancy category rating and nursing considerations.

NAME	FORM/ STRENGTH	DOSAGE	WARNINGS/PRECAUTIONS & CONTRAINDICATIONS	ADVERSE EFFECTS†
Bupropion Hydrobromide (Aplenzin) *(cont.)*			seizure threshold. Agitation, insomnia, psychosis, confusion, and other neuropsychiatric signs reported. Caution with hepatic impairment (including mild-to-moderate hepatic cirrhosis). Anorexia/weight loss may occur. HTN reported; caution with recent history of MI or unstable heart disease. Anaphylactoid/anaphylactic reactions reported; d/c if any occur. **Contra:** Seizure disorder, bulimia or anorexia nervosa, within 14 days of MAOIs, other forms of bupropion, abrupt discontinuation of alcohol or sedatives (including benzodiazepines). **P/N:** Category C, not for use in nursing.	
Nefazodone HCl	**Tab:** 50mg, 100mg*, 150mg*, 200mg, 250mg	***Adults:*** **Initial:** 100mg bid. **Usual:** 300-600mg/day. **Titrate:** May increase by 100-200mg/day at intervals of no less than 1 week. **Elderly/Debilitated: Initial:** 50mg bid.	**BB:** Antidepressants increased the risk of suicidal thinking and behavior (suicidality) in short-term studies in children, adolescents, and young adults with major depressive disorder (MDD) and other psychiatric disorders. Nefazodone is not approved for use in pediatric patients. Life-threatening hepatic failure reported. Avoid with active liver disease or elevated serum transaminases. D/C and do not retreat if symptoms of hepatic disease develop or if ALT/AST ≥3x ULN. **W/P:** May cause postural hypotension. Caution with cardiovascular or cerebrovascular disease that could be exacerbated by hypotension and conditions with predisposition to hypotension (eg, dehydration, hypotension). May activate mania/hypomania. Priapism reported. Caution with history of MI, unstable heart disease, seizures, liver cirrhosis. Avoid with active liver disease. **Contra:** Coadministration of terfenadine, astemizole, cisapride, pimozide, carbamazepine, triazolam. Liver injury from previous treatment. **P/N:** Category C, caution in nursing.	Hepatic failure, somnolence, **dry mouth,** nausea, dizziness, insomnia, agitation, constipation, asthenia, lightheadedness, blurred vision, confusion, abnormal vision.
Trazodone HCl	**Tab:** 50mg*, 100mg*, 150mg*, 300mg*	***Adults:*** **Initial:** 150mg/day in divided doses pc. **Titrate:** May increase by 50mg/day every 3-4 days. **Max: Outpatient:** 400mg/day; **Inpatient:** 600mg/day.	**BB:** Antidepressants increased the risk of suicidal thinking and behavior (suicidality) in short-term studies in children and adolescents with major depressive disorder (MDD) and other psychiatric disorders. Trazodone is not approved for use in pediatric patients. **W/P:** Avoid during initial recovery phase of MI. Caution in cardiac disease. D/C prior to elective surgery. **P/N:** Category C, caution in nursing.	**Dry mouth,** edema, constipation, blurred vision, fatigue, nervousness, drowsiness, dizziness, headache, insomnia, N/V, musculoskeletal pain, hypotension, confusion, priapism.
ANTIMANIC/BIPOLAR DISORDER DRUGS				
Carbamazepine (Equetro)	**Cap, Extended-Release:** 100mg, 200mg, 300mg	***Adults:*** **Initial:** 400mg/day, given in divided doses, bid. **Titrate:** 200mg qd. **Max:** 1600mg/day. Do not crush or chew.	**BB:** Serious and fatal dermatologic reactions, including toxic epidermal necrolysis (TEN) and Stevens-Johnson syndrome (SJS); increased risk with presence of HLA-B*1502 allele reported. Aplastic anemia and agranulocytosis reported. Obtain complete pretreatment hematological testing as baseline. D/C if evidence of bone marrow depression develops. **W/P:** Severe dermatologic reactions associated with HLA-B* 1502 allele; requires appropriate testing for gene variation prior to therapy. D/C at	Dizziness, somnolence, N/V, ataxia, headache, infection, pain, rash, diarrhea, dyspepsia, asthenia, amnesia, toxic epidermal necrolysis, Stevens-Johnson syndrome.

Table 18.1. PRESCRIBING INFORMATION FOR PSYCHOACTIVE DRUGS *(cont.)*

NAME	FORM/ STRENGTH	DOSAGE	WARNINGS/PRECAUTIONS & CONTRAINDICATIONS	ADVERSE EFFECTS†
ANTIMANIC/BIPOLAR DISORDER DRUGS *(cont.)*				
Carbamazepine (Equetro) *(cont.)*			first sign of rash, unless clearly not drug-related. Increased risk of suicidal thoughts or behavior; monitor emergence or worsening of depression, suicidal thoughts or behavior, and/or any unusual changes in mood or behavior. Mild anticholinergic activity may occur; observe closely with increased IOP. Caution in patients with a history of cardiac, hepatic, or renal damage, or with interrupted courses of therapy. Previous adverse hematologic reaction to other drugs may increase risk of bone marrow depression. May cause activate latent psychosis. May cause confusion/ agitation in elderly. Perform eye exam and monitor LFTs and renal function at baseline and periodically. May impair physical/ mental ability. **Contra:** Avoid in patients with a history of previous bone marrow depression, hypersensitivity to any tricyclic compounds. Use of MAOIs is not recommended; d/c MAOIs for a minimum of 14 days prior to use. **P/N:** Category D, not for use in nursing.	
Divalproex Sodium (Depakote, Depakote ER)	**Tab, Delayed-Release:** (Depakote) 125mg, 250mg, 500mg; **Tab, Extended-Release:** (Depakote ER) 250mg, 500mg	***Adults:*** (Tab, DR) **Mania:** 750mg daily in divided doses. **Titrate:** Increase dose rapidly to clinical effect. **Max:** 60mg/ kg/day. **Elderly:** Reduce initial dose and titrate slowly. Decrease dose or d/c if decreased food or fluid intake or if excessive somnolence occurs. (Tab, ER) **Bipolar Disorder: Initial:** 25mg/kg/day given once daily. **Titrate:** Increase dose rapidly to clinical effect. **Max:** 60mg/kg/ day. **Conversion from Depakote:** Administer Depakote ER qd using a dose 8-20% higher than the total daily dose of Depakote. If cannot directly convert to Depakote ER, consider increasing to next higher Depakote total daily dose before converting to appropriate total daily Depakote ER dose. **Elderly:** Give lower initial dose and titrate slowly. Decrease dose or d/c if decreased food or fluid intake or if excessive somnolence occurs. Swallow whole; do not crush or chew.	**BB:** Fatal hepatic failure (<2 yrs at considerable risk), teratogenic effects (eg, neural tube defects), and life-threatening pancreatitis reported. **W/P:** Hyperammonemic encephalopathy in UCD patients; d/c if this occurs. Prior to therapy, evaluate for UCD in high risk patients (eg, history of unexplained encephalopathy, coma, etc). Measure ammonia levels if develop unexplained lethargy, vomiting, or mental status changes. Caution with hepatic disease. Check LFTs prior to therapy, then frequently during first 6 months. Dose-related thrombocytopenia and elevated liver enzymes reported. Thrombocytopenia significantly increases with plasma trough levels >110mcg/mL in females and >135mcg/mL in males. Monitor platelet and coagulation tests prior to therapy, then periodically. Altered thyroid function tests and urine ketone test. May stimulate replication of HIV and CMV viruses. Avoid abrupt discontinuation. **Contra:** Hepatic disease, significant hepatic dysfunction, known urea cycle disorders (UCD). **P/N:** Category D, not for use in nursing.	Diarrhea, N/V, somnolence, dyspepsia, thrombocytopenia, asthenia, abdominal pain, tremor, headache, anorexia, diplopia, blurred vision, weight gain, ataxia, nystagmus, increased appetite, asthenia, somnolence, infection, dizziness, back pain, alopecia.
Lithium Carbonate (Lithobid), **Lithium Citrate**	**Cap:** (Lithium Carbonate) 150mg, 300mg, 600mg; **Sol:** (Lithium Citrate) 8mEq/5mL; **Tab:** (Lithium Carbonate)	***Adults/Pediatrics:* ≥12 yrs:** (Cap/Sol/ Tab) **Acute Mania:** (Cap/Tab) 600mg tid or (Sol) 10mL tid to achieve effective serum levels of 1-1.5mEq/L; monitor levels twice weekly until stabilized. **Long-Term Control:** (Cap/Tab) 300mg tid-qid or (Sol) 5mL tid-qid to maintain serum levels of 0.6-1.2 mEq/L; monitor	**BB:** Lithium toxicity is related to serum lithium levels and can occur at doses close to therapeutic levels. **W/P:** May cause fetal harm; if possible withdraw for at least the 1st trimester of pregnancy. Caution in the elderly. Maintain normal diet, adequate salt/fluid intake. Assess kidney function prior to and	Fine hand tremor, polyuria, mild thirst, nausea, incoordination, diarrhea, vomiting, drowsiness, muscular weakness.

*Scored. †Bold entries denote special dental considerations.
BB = black box warning; **W/P** = warnings/precautions; **Contra** = contraindications; **P/N** = pregnancy category rating and nursing considerations.

NAME	FORM/ STRENGTH	DOSAGE	WARNINGS/PRECAUTIONS & CONTRAINDICATIONS	ADVERSE EFFECTS†
Lithium Carbonate (Lithobid), **Lithium Citrate** *(cont.)*	300mg; **Tab, Extended-Release:** 450mg*; (Lithobid) 300mg	levels every 2 months. **Elderly:** Reduce dose. (Tab, ER) **Acute Mania: Initial:** 900mg bid or 600mg tid to achieve effective serum levels of 1-1.5mEq/L; monitor levels twice weekly until stabilized. **Long-Term Control:** 900-1200mg/day, given bid-tid to maintain serum levels of 0.6-1.2mEq/L; monitor levels every 2 months. **Elderly:** Reduce dose. **Conversion from Immediate-Release to 450mg Extended-Release Tabs:** Give same total daily dose when possible. If the previous dosage of immediate-release lithium is not a multiple of 450 mg, initiate extended-release at the multiple of 450 mg nearest to, but below, the original daily dose.	during therapy. May impair mental/physical abilities. Reduce dose or d/c with sweating, diarrhea, infection with elevated temperatures. Caution with thyroid disorders; monitor thyroid function. Chronic therapy associated with diminution of renal concentrating ability (eg, diabetes insipidus), glomerular and interstitial fibrosis, and nephron atrophy. **Contra:** Renal or cardiovascular disease, severe debilitation or dehydration, sodium depletion, and diuretic use. **P/N:** Category D, not for use in nursing.	
Valproic Acid (Stavzor)	**Cap, Delayed-Release:** (Stavzor) 125mg, 250mg, 500mg	***Adults:*** **Mania: Initial:** 750mg daily in divided doses. **Titrate:** Increase rapidly to produce the desired clinical effect or plasma level (50-125mcg/mL). **Max:** 60mg/kg/day. **Migraine: Initial:** 250mg bid. **Max:** 1000mg/day. **Elderly:** Reduce initial dose. Swallow whole.	**BB:** Fatal hepatoxicity, usually during first 6 months, reported (children <2 yrs are at higher risk); monitor closely and perform LFTs prior to therapy and periodically thereafter. Teratogenic effects (eg, neural tube defects) and life-threatening pancreatitis reported. **W/P:** Monitor LFTs before therapy and during first 6 months; d/c if hepatic dysfunction and hemorrhagic pancreatitis occur. Increased risk of hepatotoxicity with multiple anticonvulsants, congenital metabolic disorders, severe seizure disorders with mental retardation, organic brain disease, and in children <2 yrs. Avoid abrupt withdrawal. Fatal hyperammonemic encephalopathy observed with UCD; d/c if ammonia levels increase. Prior to therapy, evaluate for UCD in high-risk patients (eg, history of unexplained encephalopathy, coma). Dose-related thrombocytopenia may occur; measure platelets and coagulation tests prior to initiation and periodically thereafter. Measure ammonia levels if unexplained lethargy, vomiting or mental status changes develop. Somnolence in elderly may occur; increase dose slowly and monitor for fluid and nutritional intake. Hyperammonemia, hypothermia, multiorgan hypersensitivity reactions reported. May interfere with urine ketone and thyroid function tests. **Contra:** Hepatic disease, significant hepatic dysfunction, and known urea cycle disorders (UCD). **P/N:** Category D, not for use in nursing.	Headache, asthenia, rash, ataxia, N/V, abdominal pain, dyspepsia, diarrhea, anorexia, somnolence, tremor, dizziness, diplopia, asthenia, thrombocytopenia, ecchymosis, nystagmus, alopecia, flu syndrome.
ANTIPSYCHOTIC AGENTS				
FIRST-GENERATION ANTIPSYCHOTICS				
Chlorpromazine	**Cap, Extended-Release:** 30mg, 75mg, 150mg; **Inj:** 25mg/mL; **Sup:** 25mg, 100mg; **Syrup:** 10mg/5mL [120mL]; **Tab:** 10mg, 25mg, 50mg, 100mg, 200mg	***Adults:*** **Severe Behavioral Problems: Inpatient: Acute Schizophrenic/Manic State:** 25mg IM, then 25-50mg IM in 1 hr if needed. **Titrate:** Increase over several days up to 400mg q4-6h until controlled then switch to PO. **Usual:** 500mg/day PO. **Max:** 1000mg/day PO. **Less Acutely Disturbed:** 25mg PO tid. **Titrate:** Increase gradually to 400mg/day. **Outpatient:** 10mg PO tid-qid or 25mg PO bid-tid. **More Severe:** 25mg PO tid. **Titrate:** After 1-2 days, increase	**W/P:** Tardive dyskinesia, NMS may occur. Caution with chronic respiratory disorders, acute respiratory infections (especially in children), glaucoma, cardiovascular, hepatic, or renal disease, history of hepatic encephalopathy due to cirrhosis. Suppresses cough reflex; aspiration of vomitus possible. Caution if exposed to extreme heat or organophosphates. Avoid in children/adolescents with signs of Reye's syndrome. Lowers seizure threshold. Reduce dose	Drowsiness, jaundice, agranulocytosis, hypotensive effects, EKG changes, dystonias, motor restlessness, pseudo-parkinsonism, tardive dyskinesia, anticholinergic effects, NMS, ocular changes.

Table 18.1. PRESCRIBING INFORMATION FOR PSYCHOACTIVE DRUGS *(cont.)*

NAME	FORM/ STRENGTH	DOSAGE	WARNINGS/PRECAUTIONS & CONTRAINDICATIONS	ADVERSE EFFECTS†
ANTIPSYCHOTIC AGENTS *(cont.)*				
FIRST-GENERATION ANTIPSYCHOTICS *(cont.)*				
Chlorpromazine *(cont.)*		by 20-50mg twice weekly until calm. **Prompt Control of Severe Symptoms:** 25mg IM, may repeat in 1 hr then 25-50mg PO tid. **Nausea/Vomiting: Usual:** 10-25mg PO q4-6h prn; 25mg IM then, if no hypotension, 25-50mg q3-4h prn until vomiting stops then switch to PO; 100mg rectally q6-8h prn. **Nausea/ Vomiting in Surgery:** 12.5mg IM, may repeat in 1/2 hr; 2mg IV per fractional injection at 2-min intervals. **Max:** 25mg. **Presurgical Apprehension:** 25-50mg PO 2-3 hrs pre-op; 12.5-25mg IM 1-2 hrs pre-op. **Intractable Hiccups:** 25-50mg PO tid-qid; if symptoms persist after 2-3 days, give 25-50mg IM; if symptoms still persist, give 25-50mg slow IV. **Porphyria:** 25-50mg PO tid-qid; 25mg IM tid-qid until PO therapy. **Tetanus:** 25-50mg IM tid-qid; 25-50mg IV. **Elderly:** Use lower doses, increase dose more gradually, monitor closely. ***Pediatrics:* 6 months-12 yrs: Severe Behavioral Problems: Outpatient:** 0.25mg/lb PO q4-6h prn; 0.5mg/lb sup rectally q6-8h prn; 0.25mg/lb IM q6-8h prn. **Inpatient:** Start low and increase gradually to 50-100mg/day; ≥200mg/ day in older children. **Max:** 500mg/day. **<5 yrs (<50lbs): Max:** ≤40mg/day IM; **5-12 yrs (50-100lbs): Max:** ≤75mg/ day IM. **Nausea/Vomiting:** 0.25mg/lb PO q4-6h; 0.5mg/lb sup rectally q6-8 prn. 0.25mg/lb IM q6-8h prn. **Max: 6 months-5 yrs (or 50 lbs):** <40mg/day. **5-12 yrs (or 50-100lbs):** <75mg/day except in severe cases. **During Surgery:** 0.125mg/lb IM repeat in 1/2 hr if needed; 1mg IV per fractional injection at 2-min intervals and not exceeding recommended IM dosage. **Presurgical Apprehension:** 0.25mg/lb PO 2-3 hrs (or IM 1-2 hrs) before operation. **Tetanus:** 0.25mg/lb IM/IV q6-8h. **<50lbs: Max:** ≤40mg/day; **50-100lbs: Max:** ≤75mg/day.	gradually to prevent side effects. May mask signs of overdose to other drugs and obscure diagnosis of other conditions (eg, intestinal obstruction, brain tumor, Reye's syndrome). May produce false-positive PKU test. May elevate prolactin levels. Injection contains sulfites. **Contra:** Comatose states, or with large amounts of CNS depressants. Hypersensitivity to phenothiazines. **P/N:** Safety in pregnancy not known. Not for use in nursing.	
Fluphenazine HCl	**Inj:** 2.5mg/ mL; **Elixir:** 2.5mg/5mL; **Sol, Concentrate:** 5mg/mL; **Tab:** 1mg, 2.5mg, 5mg, 10mg	***Adults:*** (PO) **Initial:** 2.5-10mg/day in divided doses q6-8h. **Titrate:** May increase up to 40mg/day. **Maint:** 1-5mg qd. **Elderly: Initial:** 1-2.5mg/day. (Inj) **Initial:** 1.25mg IM q6-8h. **Max:** 10mg/day.	**W/P:** May develop tardive dyskinesia, NMS. Caution with history of cholestatic jaundice, dermatoses or allergic reactions to phenothiazine derivatives. Elevated prolactin levels reported. Avoid abrupt withdrawal. Caution if exposed to extreme heat or phosphorous insecticides, seizure disorder, cardiovascular disease, pheochromocytoma. May develop liver damage, pigmentary retinopathy, lenticular and corneal dyskinesias with prolonged therapy. Monitor for hypotension in patients on large doses undergoing surgery. May impair mental/physical abilities. **Contra:** Comatose state, severe depression, concomitant large dose hypnotics, blood dyscrasia, hepatic impairment, subcortical brain damage, cross-sensitivity to phenothiazine derivatives. **P/N:** Safety in pregnancy or nursing not known.	Extrapyramidal symptoms, tardive dyskinesia, HTN, hypotension, allergic reactions, nausea, loss of appetite, **dry mouth,** headache, constipation, perspiration, **salivation,** polyuria, hepatic dysfunction.

*Scored. †Bold entries denote special dental considerations.
BB = black box warning; **W/P** = warnings/precautions; **Contra** = contraindications; **P/N** = pregnancy category rating and nursing considerations.

NAME	FORM/ STRENGTH	DOSAGE	WARNINGS/PRECAUTIONS & CONTRAINDICATIONS	ADVERSE EFFECTS†
Haloperidol (Haldol, Haldol Decanoate)	**Inj:** 5mg/mL; **Inj:** (Decanoate) 50mg/mL, 100mg/mL; **Sol:** 2mg/mL; **Tab:** 0.5mg*, 1mg*, 2mg*, 5mg*, 10mg*, 20mg*	***Adults:*** (Immediate-Release) **PO: Moderate Symptoms/Elderly/Debilitated:** 0.5-2mg bid-tid. **Severe Symptoms/ Resistant Patients:** 3-5mg bid-tid. **Max:** 100mg/day. **IM: Acute Agitation:** 2-5mg every 4-8 hrs or hourly as needed for moderately severe or very severe symptoms. **Max:** 100mg/day. (Decanoate) For IM inj only. Give every 4 weeks or monthly. **Initial:** 10-20 times daily oral dose up to 100mg. Give remainder of dose 3-7 days later if initial dose >100mg. **Usual:** 10-15 times daily oral dose. **Max:** 450mg/ month. **Elderly/Debilitated: Initial:** 10-15 times daily oral dose. ***Pediatrics:*** **3-12 yrs: (15-40kg): PO: Psychosis: Initial:** 0.05-0.15mg/kg/day given bid-tid. **Nonpsychotic Disorder/Tourette's:** 0.05-0.075mg/kg/day given bid-tid. **Max:** 6mg/day.	**W/P:** Risk of tardive dyskinesia, especially in elderly. NMS, hyperpyrexia, heat stroke, bronchopneumonia reported. Decreased cholesterol, cutaneous, and/ or ocular changes may occur. Neurotoxicity may occur with thyrotoxicosis. Caution with CV disease, seizures, EEG abnormalities, QT-prolonging conditions, elderly. Do not administer IV. Cases of sudden death and Torsades de Pointes reported. **Contra:** Comatose states, severe toxic CNS depression, Parkinson's disease. **P/N:** Category C, not for use in nursing.	Extrapyramidal symptoms, tardive dyskinesia, tardive dystonia, ECG changes, QT prolongation, ventricular arrhythmias, tachycardia, hypotension, HTN, N/V, constipation, diarrhea, **dry mouth,** blurred vision, urinary retention.
Loxapine Succinate (Loxitane)	**Cap:** 5mg, 10mg, 25mg, 50mg	***Adults:*** **Initial:** 10mg bid, up to 50mg/ day for severely disturbed. **Titrate:** Increase rapidly over 7-10 days. **Maint:** 60-100mg/day. **Max:** 250mg/day.	**W/P:** Extrapyramidal symptoms, tardive dyskinesia, NMS can occur. May lower seizure threshold. May mask symptoms of overdose of other drugs. May obscure diagnosis of intestinal obstruction, brain tumor. Ocular toxicity reported. Caution in cardiovascular disease, glaucoma, urinary retention. Elevates prolactin levels. Caution with activities requiring alertness. **Contra:** Comatose states, severe drug-induced depressed states (eg, alcohol, barbiturates, narcotics). **P/N:** Safety in pregnancy not known. Not for use in nursing.	Drowsiness, weakness, NMS, tachycardia, hypotension, HTN, syncope, edema, **dry mouth,** constipation, blurred vision.
Molindone HCl (Moban)	**Tab:** 5mg, 10mg, 25mg*, 50mg*	***Adults/Pediatric:*** **≥12 yrs: Initial:** 50-75mg/day. **Titrate:** Increase to 100mg/ day in 3-4 days; adjust to patient response. **Maint: Mild:** 5-15mg tid-qid. **Moderate:** 10-25mg tid-qid. **Severe:** 225mg/day.	**W/P:** Tardive dyskinesia, NMS may occur. Caution with activities requiring alertness. Convulsions, increased activity reported. May obscure signs of intestinal obstruction or brain tumor. May elevate prolactin levels. **Contra:** Severe CNS depression (alcohol, barbiturates, narcotics), comatose states. **P/N:** Safety in pregnancy and nursing not known.	Drowsiness, depression, hyperactivity, euphoria, extrapyramidal reactions, akathisia, Parkinson's syndrome, blurred vision, nausea, **dry mouth**.
Perphenazine	**Tab:** 2mg, 4mg, 8mg, 16mg	***Adults:*** **Moderately Disturbed Nonhospitalized With Schizophrenia: Initial:** 4-8mg tid. **Maint:** Reduce to minimum effective dose. **Hospitalized Psychotic Patients With Schizophrenia:** 8-16mg bid-qid. **Max:** 64mg/day. **Severe Nausea/Vomiting:** 8-16mg/ day in divided doses. **Max:** 24mg/day. **Elderly:** Lower dosages recommended. ***Pediatrics:*** **≥12 yrs:** Use lowest limits of adult dose.	**W/P:** Tardive dyskinesia may develop. NMS, photosensitivity reported. May lower convulsive threshold; caution with alcohol withdrawal. Caution with psychic depression, renal impairment, respiratory impairment. May impair mental/ physical abilities. May mask signs of overdosage to other drugs. May obscure diagnosis of intestinal obstruction, brain tumor. Severe hypotension may occur in surgery. May elevate prolactin levels. Monitor hepatic/renal functions, blood counts. Increased risk of liver damage, jaundice, corneal and lenticular deposits, and irreversible dyskinesias with long-term use. **Contra:** Comatose or greatly obtunded patients, large doses of CNS depressants (eg, barbiturates, alcohol, narcotics, analgesics, or antihistamines), blood dyscrasias, bone marrow depression, liver damage, subcortical brain damage with or without hypothalamic involvement. **P/N:** Safety in pregnancy and nursing not known.	Extrapyramidal reactions, tardive dyskinesia, cerebral edema, seizures, drowsiness, **dry mouth, salivation**, N/V, diarrhea, anorexia, constipation, urticaria, erythema, eczema, postural hypotension, tachycardia.

Table 18.1. PRESCRIBING INFORMATION FOR PSYCHOACTIVE DRUGS *(cont.)*

NAME	FORM/ STRENGTH	DOSAGE	WARNINGS/PRECAUTIONS & CONTRAINDICATIONS	ADVERSE EFFECTS†
ANTIPSYCHOTIC AGENTS *(cont.)*				
FIRST-GENERATION ANTIPSYCHOTICS *(cont.)*				
Pimozide (Orap)	**Tab:** 1mg*, 2mg*	***Adults:*** **Initial:** 1-2mg/day in divided doses. May increase every other day. **Maint:** <0.2mg/kg/day or 10mg/day, whichever is less. **Max:** 0.2mg/kg/day or 10mg/day. ***Pediatrics:*** **>12 yrs: Initial:** 0.05mg/kg qhs. **Titrate:** May increase every 3 days. **Max:** 0.2mg/kg/day or 10mg/day.	**W/P:** May cause tardive dyskinesia, NMS, hyperpyrexia. Caution with history of seizures, EEG abnormalities, severe hepatic/renal impairment. Perform ECG before therapy, periodically thereafter, with dose adjustment. Produces anticholinergic effects. Sudden death reported. May impair mental/physical abilities. **Contra:** Severe CNS depression, comatose states, congenital long QT syndrome, history of cardiac arrhythmias, hypokalemia, hypomagnesemia, simple tics or tics not associated with Tourette's syndrome. CYP3A4 inhibitors (eg, nefazadone, macrolide antibiotics, azole antifungals, protease inhibitors), sertraline, and drugs that cause motor and phonic tics (eg, pemoline, methylphenidate, amphetamines) or prolong the QT interval. **P/N:** Category C, not for use in nursing.	Akinesia, QT prolongation, tardive dyskinesia, sedation, loss of libido, constipation, **dry mouth,** visual disturbances, headache, asthenia, **increased salivation**.
Thioridazine HCl	**Tab:** 10mg, 15mg, 25mg, 50mg, 100mg, 150mg, 200mg	***Adults:*** **Initial:** 50-100mg tid. **Titrate:** Increase gradually. **Usual:** 200-800mg/day given bid-qid. **Max:** 800mg/day. ***Pediatrics:*** **Initial:** 0.6mg/kg/day given in divided doses. **Titrate:** Increase gradually. **Max:** 3mg/kg/day.	**BB:** Prolongation of QTc interval reported in a dose related manner. Associated with torsade de pointes and sudden death; reserve for patients who fail to respond to or cannot tolerate other antipsychotics. **W/P:** Perform baseline ECG and measure baseline potassium level; monitor periodically thereafter. May develop tardive dyskinesia. NMS, seizures, leukopenia, agranulocytosis reported. Caution with activities requiring alertness. May elevate prolactin levels. **Contra:** Severe CNS depression, comatose states, severe hypo- or hypertensive heart disease. Drugs that prolong QTc interval, congenital long QT syndrome, cardiac arrhythmias, drugs that inhibit CYP450 2D6 (eg, fluoxetine, paroxetine), patients with reduced activity of CYP450 2D6. **P/N:** Safety in pregnancy and nursing not known.	Tardive dyskinesia, ECG changes, drowsiness, **dry mouth,** blurred vision, peripheral edema, galactorrhea, NV, gynecomastia, impotence, constipation, diarrhea.
Thiothixene (Navane)	**Cap:** 1mg, 2mg, 5mg, 10mg, 20mg	***Adults/Pediatrics:*** **≥12 yrs: Mild Condition: Initial:** 2mg tid. **Titrate:** May increase to 15mg/day. **Severe Condition: Initial:** 5mg bid. **Usual:** 20-30mg/day. **Max:** 60mg/day.	**W/P:** May develop tardive dyskinesia, NMS. May mask symptoms of overdose of toxic drugs. May obscure conditions such as intestinal obstruction and brain tumor. May lower seizure threshold. Monitor for pigmentary retinopathy and lenticular pigmentation. Caution with cardiovascular disease, extreme heat exposure, activities requiring alertness. May elevate prolactin levels. **Contra:** Circulatory collapse, comatose states, CNS depression, blood dyscrasias. **P/N:** Safety in pregnancy and nursing not known.	Tachycardia, hypotension, lightheadedness, syncope, drowsiness, agitation, insomnia, hyperreflexia, cerebral edema, pseudoparkinsonism, LFT elevation, blood dyscrasias, rash, photosensitivity, **dry mouth,** blurred vision.

*Scored. †Bold entries denote special dental considerations.
BB = black box warning; **W/P** = warnings/precautions; **Contra** = contraindications; **P/N** = pregnancy category rating and nursing considerations.

NAME	FORM/ STRENGTH	DOSAGE	WARNINGS/PRECAUTIONS & CONTRAINDICATIONS	ADVERSE EFFECTS†
Trifluoperazine HCl	**Tab:** 1mg, 2mg, 5mg, 10mg	***Adults:* Psychotic Disorders: Initial:** 2-5mg PO bid. **Usual:** 15-20mg/day. **Max:** 40mg/day or more if needed. **Non-Psychotic Anxiety:** 1-2mg bid. **Max:** 6mg/day or >12 weeks. **Elderly:** Lower dose and increase more gradually. ***Pediatrics:* Psychotic Disorders: 6-12 yrs: Initial:** 1mg PO qd-bid. **Titrate:** Increase gradually until symptoms controlled. **Usual:** 15mg/day.	**W/P:** May develop tardive dyskinesia, neuroleptic malignant syndrome. May elevate prolactin levels; caution with prolactin-dependent tumors. May mask drug toxicity and drug overdose due to antiemetic effects. May obscure diagnosis and treatment of intestinal obstruction, brain tumor, and Reye's syndrome. Risk of hypotension; avoid large doses and IV use with cardiovascular disease. Caution with glaucoma, angina, and elderly. May cause retinopathy; d/c if retinal changes occur. Evaluate therapy periodically with prolonged use. May interfere with thermoregulatory mechanism; caution in extreme heat. Jaundice, hepatic damage reported. May cause false-positive PKU test. **Contra:** Comatose or greatly depressed states due to CNS depressants, bone marrow depression, blood dyscrasias, hepatic damage. **P/N:** Safety in pregnancy not known. Not for use in nursing.	EPS, motor restlessness, dystonias, pseudoparkinsonism, tardive dyskinesia, convulsions, **dry mouth,** headache, nausea, blood dycrasias.
SECOND-GENERATION ANTIPSYCHOTICS				
Aripiprazole (Abilify, Abilify Discmelt)	**Tab, Orally Disintegrating:** (Discmelt) 10mg, 15mg; **Tab:** 2mg, 5mg, 10mg, 15mg, 20mg, 30mg; **Sol:** 1mg/mL [150mL]; **Inj:** 7.5mg/mL	***Adults:*** (PO) **Schizophrenia: Initial/ Target:** 10-15mg qd. **Titrate:** Should not increase before 2 weeks. **Max:** 30mg/day. **Bipolar Disorder (Monotherapy or Adjunct): Initial/Target:** 15mg/day. **Max:** 30mg/day. **MDD: Initial:** 2-5mg/day. **Titrate:** May adjust dose at increments of ≤5mg/day at intervals ≥1 week. **Range:** 2-15mg/day. **Max:** 15mg/day. Periodically reassess need for maintenance therapy. Oral sol can be given on mg-per-mg basis up to 25mg. Patients receiving 30mg tabs should receive 25mg of oral sol. (Inj) **Agitation:** 9.75mg IM. **Range:** 5.25-15mg IM. **Max:** 30mg/day; initiate PO therapy as soon as possible. **Concomitant Strong CYP3A4 Inhibitors (eg, ketoconazole, clarithromycin):** Reduce usual aripiprazole dose by 50%. **Concomitant CYP2D6 Inhibitors (eg, quinidine, fluoxetine, paroxetine):** Reduce usual aripiprazole dose by 50%. **Concomitant CYP3A4 Inducers (eg, carbamazepine):** Double aripiprazole dose. ***Pediatrics:*** (PO) **Schizophrenia (13-17 yrs)/Bipolar Disorder (Monotherapy or Adjunct) (10-17 yrs): Initial:** 2mg/day. **Titrate:** 5mg after 2 days. May adjust dose in 5mg/day increments. **Usual:** 10mg/day. **Max:** 30mg/day. Periodically reassess need for maintenance therapy. Oral sol can be given on mg-per-mg basis up to 25mg. Patients receiving 30mg tabs should receive 25mg of oral sol. **Concomitant Strong CYP3A4 Inhibitors (eg, ketoconazole, clarithromycin):** Reduce usual aripiprazole dose by 50%. **Concomitant CYP2D6 Inhibitors (eg, quinidine, fluoxetine, paroxetine):** Reduce usual aripiprazole dose by 50%. **Concomitant CYP3A4 Inducers (eg, carbamazepine):** Double aripiprazole dose.	**BB:** Elderly patients with dementia-related psychosis treated with atypical antipsychotic drugs are at an increased risk of death; most appeared to be cardiovascular (eg, heart failure, sudden death) or infectious (eg, pneumonia) in nature. Aripiprazole is not approved for the treatment of patients with dementia-related psychosis. Children, adolescents, and young adults taking antidepressants for major depressive disorder and other psychiatric disorders are at increased risk of suicidal thinking and behavior. **W/P:** May develop tardive dyskinesia, NMS. Monitor for hyperglycemia, worsening of glucose control with DM, FBG levels with diabetes risk. Increased incidence of cerebrovascular adverse events (stroke) in elderly dementia patients. Orthostatic hypotension reported; caution with cardiovascular disease, conditions predisposed to hypotension (eg, dehydration, hypovolemia). May lower seizure threshold. Potential for cognitive and motor impairment. May disrupt body's temperature regulation. Possible esophageal dysmotility and aspiration; caution in patients at risk for aspiration pneumonia. Observe vigilance in treating psychosis associated with Alzheimer's disease. **P/N:** Category C, not for use in nursing.	Headache, asthenia, rash, blurred vision, rhinitis, **cough,** tremor, anxiety, insomnia, N/V, lightheadedness, somnolence, constipation, akathisia, extrapyramidal disorder, somnolence, **oropharyngeal spasm,** grand mal seizure, jaundice, **nasopharyngitis,** dizziness.

Table 18.1. PRESCRIBING INFORMATION FOR PSYCHOACTIVE DRUGS *(cont.)*

NAME	FORM/ STRENGTH	DOSAGE	WARNINGS/PRECAUTIONS & CONTRAINDICATIONS	ADVERSE EFFECTS†
ANTIPSYCHOTIC AGENTS *(cont.)*				
SECOND-GENERATION ANTIPSYCHOTICS *(cont.)*				
Clozapine (Clozaril, Fazaclo)	**Tab:** 12.5mg, 25mg, 100mg; (Clozaril) 25mg*, 100mg*; **Tab, Disintegrating:** (Fazaclo) 12.5mg, 25mg*, 50mg, 100mg*	***Adults:*** **Initial:** 12.5mg qd-bid. **Titrate:** Increase by 25-50mg/day, up to 300-450mg/day by end of 2nd week, then increase weekly or bi-weekly by up to 100mg. **Usual:** 100-900mg/day given tid. **Max:** 900mg/day. To d/c, gradually reduce dose over 1-2 weeks. Monitor for psychotic symptoms if abrupt discontinuation warranted (eg, leukopenia).	**BB:** Risk of agranulocytosis, seizures, myocarditis, and other cardiovascular and respiratory effects. Obtain baseline WBC and ANC before initiation of therapy, regularly during therapy, and for 4 weeks after discontinuation. Elderly patients with dementia-related psychosis treated with atypical antipsychotic drugs are at an increased risk of death; most deaths appeared to be cardiovascular (eg, heart failure, sudden death) or infectious (eg, pneumonia) in nature. Clozapine is not approved for the treatment of patients with dementia-related psychosis. **W/P:** Reserve treatment for severely ill patients unresponsive to other schizophrenia therapies. Monitor for hyperglycemia, worsening of glucose control with DM, FBG levels with diabetes risk. Significant risk of orthostatic hypotension, and tachycardia. May impair alertness with initial doses. May cause high fever, hyperglycemia, or pulmonary embolism. Cardiomyopathy reported; d/c unless benefit outweighs risk. Caution with prostatic enlargement, narrow angle glaucoma, and renal, hepatic, or cardiac/pulmonary disease. NMS and tardive dyskinesia reported. Acquire WBC and ANC at baseline, then weekly for first 6 months of therapy, then every 2 weeks for 6 months, and then every 4 weeks thereafter if WBCs and ANC are acceptable. Avoid initiation of treatment if WBCs <3500/mm^3, ANC <2000/mm^3, history of myeloproliferative disorder, previous clozapine-induced agranulocytosis or granulocytopenia. D/C treatment if WBCs <3000/mm^3, ANC <1500/mm^3, eosinophils >4000/mm^3, or if myocarditis develops. D/C over 1-2 weeks. Varying degrees of intestinal peristalsis impairment (eg, constipation, intestinal obstruction, paralytic ileus), ECG changes reported. **Contra:** Myeloproliferative disorders, uncontrolled epilepsy, paralytic ileus, history of clozapine-induced agranulocytosis or severe granulocytopenia, severe CNS depression, coma, with agents with potential to cause agranulocytosis or suppress bone marrow function. **P/N:** Category B, not for use in nursing.	Drowsiness, vertigo, headache, tremor, **salivation,** sweating, **dry mouth,** visual disturbances, tachycardia, hypotension, syncope, constipation, nausea, blood dyscrasias, fever.
Olanzapine (Zyprexa, Zyprexa IntraMuscular, Zyprexa Zydis)	**Inj:** 10mg; **Tab:** 2.5mg, 5mg, 7.5mg, 10mg, 15mg, 20mg; **Tab, Disintegrating:** (Zydis) 5mg, 10mg, 15mg, 20mg	***Adults:*** (PO) **Schizophrenia: Initial/ Usual:** 5-10mg qd. **Titrate:** Adjust by 5mg daily at weekly intervals. **Max:** 20mg/day. **Bipolar Disorder: Initial:** 10-15mg qd. **Titrate:** May increase/ decrease dose by 5mg daily. **Max:** 20mg/day. **With Lithium or Valproate: Initial/Usual:** 10mg qd. **Max:** 20mg/ day. **Debilitated/Hypotension Risk/Slow Metabolizers/Sensitivity to Olanzapine Effects: Initial:** 5mg qd. **Titrate:**	**BB:** Elderly patients with dementia-related psychosis treated with atypical antipsychotic drugs are at an increased risk of death; most appeared to be cardiovascular (eg, heart failure, sudden death) or infectious (eg, pneumonia) in nature. Olanzapine is not approved for the treatment of patients with dementia-related psychosis. **W/P:** Monitor for hyperglycemia, worsening of glucose control with DM, FBG levels	Postural hypotension, constipation, **dry mouth,** weight gain, somnolence, dizziness, personality disorder, akathisia, asthenia, dyspepsia, tremor, increased appetite, ecchymosis, rhinitis, joint pain.

*Scored. †Bold entries denote special dental considerations.
BB = black box warning; **W/P** = warnings/precautions; **Contra** = contraindications; **P/N** = pregnancy category rating and nursing considerations.

NAME	FORM/ STRENGTH	DOSAGE	WARNINGS/PRECAUTIONS & CONTRAINDICATIONS	ADVERSE EFFECTS†
Olanzapine (Zyprexa, Zyprexa IntraMuscular, Zyprexa Zydis) *(cont.)*		Increase cautiously. (IM) **Agitation: Initial:** 10mg IM. **Usual:** 2.5-10mg IM. **Max:** 3 doses of 10mg q 2-4h. **Elderly:** 5mg IM. **Debilitated/Hypotension Risk/Sensitivity to Olanzapine Effects:** 2.5mg IM. May initiate PO therapy when clinically appropriate.	with diabetes risk. Risk of NMS, tardive dyskinesia, orthostatic hypotension, seizures. Caution in hepatic impairment, prostatic hypertrophy, narrow-angle glaucoma, history of paralytic ileus, elderly patients with dementia, cardio- or cerebrovascular disease, hypotension risk (eg, hypovolemia, dehydration), risk for aspiration pneumonia, suicidal tendencies. May cause alterations in lipid levels and weight gain; monitor regularly. May cause cognitive and motor impairment. Elevated transaminases, hyperprolactinemia reported. May cause disruption of body temperature regulation. Reevaluate periodically. **P/N:** Category C, not for use in nursing.	
Paliperidone (Invega)	**Tab, Extended-Release:** 1.5mg, 3mg, 6mg, 9mg	***Adults:*** 6mg qd in am. **Range:** 3-12mg/day. **Titrate:** May increase by 3mg/day at intervals of >5 days. **Max:** 12mg/day. Swallow whole; do not chew, divide, or crush. **CrCl ≥50 to <80mL/min: Initial:** 3mg qd. Max of 6mg/day. **CrCl ≥10 to <50mL/min: Initial:** 1.5mg qd. **Max:** 3mg/day. Evaluate periodically for long-term use.	**BB:** Elderly patients with dementia-related psychosis treated with atypical antipsychotic drugs are at an increased risk of death; most appeared to be cardiovascular (eg, heart failure, sudden death) or infectious (eg, pneumonia) in nature. Paliperidone is not approved for the treatment of patients with dementia-related psychosis. **W/P:** May increase QTc interval; avoid with congenital long QT syndrome and with a history of cardiac arrhythmias. Neuroleptic malignant syndrome (NMS) and tardive dyskinesia (TD) may occur. Monitor for hyperglycemia; perform fasting blood glucose testing if symptoms develop or with risk factors for DM. Avoid with preexisting severe GI narrowing. Cerebrovascular events (eg, stroke, TIA) reported in elderly with dementia-related psychosis. Not approved for the treatment of dementia-related psychosis. May induce priapism. May induce orthostatic hypotension and syncope; monitor closely in those vulnerable to hypotension. Caution with history of seizures or other conditions that may lower seizure threshold. May elevate prolactin levels. May cause esophageal dysmotility and aspiration; caution in those at risk for aspiration pneumonia. May disrupt body's ability to reduce core body temperature; caution in those who may experience conditions that may contribute to an elevation in core body temperature. Caution with known suicidal tendencies, cardiovascular disease, elderly, and renal impairment. May impair mental/physical abilities. Reevaluate periodically. **P/N:** Category C, caution in nursing.	Tachycardia, nausea, akathisia, dizziness, extrapyramidal disorder, headache, somnolence, anxiety, parkinsonism, dyskinesia, hyperkinesia.
Quetiapine Fumarate (Seroquel, Seroquel XR)	**Tab:** (Seroquel) 25mg, 50mg, 100mg, 200mg, 300mg, 400mg; **Tab, Extended-Release:** (Seroquel XR) 50mg, 150mg, 200mg, 300mg, 400mg	***Adults:*** (Tab) **Schizophrenia: Initial:** 25mg bid. **Titrate:** Increase by 25-50mg bid-tid on the 2nd and 3rd day to 300-400mg/day given bid-tid by the 4th day. Adjust doses by 25-50mg bid at intervals of at least 2 days. **Maint:** Lowest effective dose. **Max:** 800mg/day. **Bipolar Disorder: Depressive Episodes:** Give once daily hs. **Day 1:** 50mg/day. **Day 2:** 100mg/day. **Day 3:** 200mg/day. **Day 4:** 300mg/day. **Bipolar Mania: Monotherapy/Adjunctive:**	**BB:** Elderly patients with dementia-related psychosis treated with atypical antipsychotic drugs are at an increased risk of death; most deaths appeared to be cardiovascular (eg, heart failure, sudden death) or infectious (eg, pneumonia) in nature. Quetiapine is not approved for the treatment of patients with dementia-related psychosis. Antidepressants increased the risk of suicidal thinking and behavior (suicidality) in short-term studies in children, adolescents, and young	**Dry mouth,** constipation, dyspepsia, somnolence, dizziness, orthostatic hypotension, weight gain, increased appetite, fatigue, dysarthria, nasal congestion, insomnia, headache.

Table 18.1. PRESCRIBING INFORMATION FOR PSYCHOACTIVE DRUGS *(cont.)*

NAME	FORM/ STRENGTH	DOSAGE	WARNINGS/PRECAUTIONS & CONTRAINDICATIONS	ADVERSE EFFECTS†
ANTIPSYCHOTIC AGENTS *(cont.)*				
SECOND-GENERATION ANTIPSYCHOTICS *(cont.)*				
Quetiapine Fumarate (Seroquel, Seroquel XR) *(cont.)*		Give bid. **Initial:** 100mg/day on Day 1. **Titrate:** Increase to 400mg/day on Day 4 in increments of up to 100mg/day in bid divided doses. Adjust doses up to 800mg/day by Day 6 in increments ≤200mg/day. **Max:** 800mg/day. **Maintenance for Bipolar I Disorder:** Give bid. 400-800mg/day. **Hepatic Impairment: Initial:** 25mg/day. **Titrate:** Increase by 25-50mg/day to effective dose. **Elderly/Debilitated/Predisposition to Hypotension:** Consider slower rate of dose titration and lower target dose. (Tab, ER) **Schizophrenia:** Give once daily, preferably in evening. **Initial:** 300mg/day. **Titrate:** Within range of 400-800mg/day depending on response and tolerance. Dose increases may be made at intervals as short as 1 day and in increments up to 300mg/day. **Maint:** 400-800mg/day for 16 weeks. **Bipolar Disorder: Depressive Episodes:** Give once daily in evening. **Day 1:** 50mg/day. **Day 2:** 100mg/day. **Day 3:** 200mg/day. **Day 4:** 300mg/day. **Bipolar Mania: Monotherapy/Adjunct:** Give once daily in evening. **Day 1:** 300mg. **Day 2:** 600mg. **Titrate:** May adjust dose between 400-800mg beginning on Day 3 depending on response and tolerance. **Maintenance of Bipolar I Disorder:** 400-800mg/day given bid. Take without food or with light meal. Reevaluate periodically. **Elderly/Hepatic Impairment: Initial:** 50mg/day; may increase in increments of 50mg/day depending on response and tolerance. **Switching from Seroquel:** May switch to Seroquel XR at equivalent total daily dose given once daily. Swallow tab whole; do not split, crush, or chew.	adults with major depressive disorder (MDD) and other psychiatric disorders. Seroquel XR is not approved for use in pediatric patients. **W/P:** Hyperglycemia reported; monitor DM patients regularly for worsening of glucose control and all patients for symptoms of hyperglycemia. NMS reported. May develop tardive dyskinesia. May induce orthostatic hypotension. Caution with cardiovascular or cerebrovascular disease, conditions that predispose to hypotension (eg, dehydration, hypovolemia, treatment with antihypertensives), history of seizures. Leukopenia, neutropenia, and agranulocytosis reported. Monitor for cataracts at initiation, then every 6 months. Possible hypothyroidism. Hepatic enzyme, cholesterol, and triglyceride elevations reported. May impair judgment, thinking, and motor skills. Priapism reported. May disrupt body's ability to reduce core temperature. Caution in patients at risk for aspiration, elderly, debilitated. Depression may worsen in patients or suicidal thoughts and behaviors may also arise. May increase prolactin levels. Acute withdrawal symptoms (eg, N/V, insomnia) may occur after abrupt cessation. **P/N:** Category C, caution in nursing.	
Risperidone (Risperdal Consta)	**Inj:** 12.5mg, 25mg, 37.5mg, 50mg	***Adults:*** 25mg IM every 2 weeks. **Max:** 50mg every 2 weeks. Give first injection with oral dosage form or other oral antipsychotic. Continue for 3 weeks, then d/c oral. **Titrate:** Increase at intervals of no more than every 4 weeks. **Hepatic or Renal Impairment/Certain Drug Interactions/Poor Tolerability to Psychotropic Meds: Premedication: Initial:** 0.5mg PO bid during the first week of risperidone. **Titrate:** May increase to 1mg bid or 2mg qd during the second week. Give first injection with oral dosage form. Continue for 3 weeks. **Treatment: Initial:** 12.5mg. **Elderly:** Start 25mg every 2 weeks. Give first injection with oral dosage form or other oral antipsychotic. Continue for 3 weeks.	**BB:** Elderly patients with dementia-related psychosis treated with atypical antipsychotic drugs are at an increased risk of death; most appeared to be cardiovascular (eg, heart failure, sudden death) or infectious (eg, pneumonia) in nature. Risperidone is not approved for the treatment of patients with dementia-related psychosis. **W/P:** Cerebrovascular events (eg, stroke, TIA) reported in elderly with dementia-related psychosis. Not approved for the treatment of dementia-related psychosis. Neuroleptic malignant syndrome and/or tardive dyskinesia may occur. Monitor for hyperglycemia; perform fasting blood glucose testing if symptoms develop or with risk factors for DM. May elevate prolactin levels, induce orthostatic hypotension, have an antiemetic effect. May impair physical/mental ability. Caution in elderly, renal/hepatic impairment, history of seizures, cardio- or cerebrovascular	Headache, dizziness, constipation dyspepsia, akathisia, parkinsonism, weight increased, **dry mouth,** fatigue, pain in extremity.

†Bold entries denote special dental considerations.
BB = black box warning; **W/P** = warnings/precautions; **Contra** = contraindications; **P/N** = pregnancy category rating and nursing considerations.

NAME	FORM/ STRENGTH	DOSAGE	WARNINGS/PRECAUTIONS & CONTRAINDICATIONS	ADVERSE EFFECTS†
Risperidone (Risperdal Consta) *(cont.)*			disease, suicidal tendencies, esophageal dysmotility, risk of aspiration pneumonia, conditions predisposing to hypotension (eg, hypovolemia, dehydration) or affecting metabolism or hemodynamic responses. Severe priapism and TTP reported. May disrupt body temperature regulation; caution in patients exposed to temperature extremes. Must inject into the gluteal muscle; avoid injection into blood vessel. Monitor for suicidal attempts in high risk patients. Reevaluate periodically. Patients who receive antipsychotics are reported to have an increased sensitivity to antipsychotic medications. Osteodystrophy, renal tubular tumors, and adrenomedullary pheochromocytomas reported in animal studies. **P/N:** Category C, not for use in nursing.	
Risperidone (Risperdal, Risperdal M-Tab)	**Sol:** 1mg/mL [30mL]; **Tab:** 0.25mg, 0.5mg, 1mg, 2mg, 3mg, 4mg; **Tab, Disintegrating:** (M-Tab) 0.5mg, 1mg, 2mg, 3mg, 4mg	***Adults:*** **Schizophrenia: Initial:** 2mg/day given once or twice daily. **Titrate:** Adjust dose at intervals not <24 hrs, in increments of 1-2mg/day, as tolerated, to recommended dose of 4-8mg/day. **Range:** 4-16mg/day. **Max:** 16mg/day. **Bipolar Disorder: Initial:** 2-3mg qd. **Titrate:** Adjust dose at intervals not <24 hrs and in increments/decrements of 1mg/day. **Range:** 1-6mg/day. **Max:** 6mg/day. **Elderly/Debilitated/ Hypotension/Severe Renal or Hepatic Impairment: Initial:** 0.5mg bid. **Titrate:** Adjust dose in increments not >0.5mg bid. Increases to doses >1.5mg bid should occur at intervals of ≥1 week. Periodically reassess to determine maintenance treatment. ***Pediatrics:*** **Schizophrenia: 13-17 yrs: Initial:** 0.5mg qd in morning or evening. **Titrate:** Adjust dose, if needed, in increments of 0.5 or 1mg/day and at intervals not <24 hrs, as tolerated, to recommended dose of 3mg/day. **Max:** 6mg/day. **Bipolar Disorder: 10-17 yrs: Initial:** 0.5mg qd in morning or evening. **Titrate:** Adjust dose, if needed, in increments of 0.5 or 1mg/day and at intervals not <24 hrs, as tolerated, to recommended dose of 2.5mg/day. **Max:** 6mg/day. **Irritability with Autistic Disorder: 5-16 yrs: Initial: <20kg:** 0.25mg/day; **≥20kg:** 0.5mg/day. **Titrate:** After at least 4 days, may increase dose by 0.5mg/day (<20kg) or 1mg/day (≥20kg). **Maint:** Minimum of 14 days. **Inadequate Response: Increase at ≥2-wk intervals: <20kg:** Increase by 0.25mg/day; **≥20kg:** Increase by 0.5mg/day. Caution in patients <15kg. **Max: <20kg:** 1mg/day; **≥20kg:** 2.5mg/day; **>45kg:** 3mg/day.	**BB:** Elderly patients with dementia-related psychosis treated with atypical antipsychotic drugs are at an increased risk of death; most appeared to be cardiovascular (eg, heart failure, sudden death) or infectious (eg, pneumonia) in nature. Risperidone is not approved for the treatment of patients with dementia-related psychosis. **W/P:** Neuroleptic malignant syndrome and/or tardive dyskinesia may occur. Monitor for hyperglycemia; perform fasting blood glucose testing if symptoms develop or with risk factors for DM. Cerebrovascular events (eg, stroke, TIA) reported in elderly with dementia-related psychosis. Not approved for the treatment of dementia-related psychosis. May induce orthostatic hypotension, elevate prolactin levels, have an antiemetic effect. Caution in elderly, renal/hepatic impairment, history of seizures, cardio- or cerebrovascular disease, suicidal tendencies, risk of aspiration pneumonia, conditions predisposing to hypotension (eg, hypovolemia, dehydration) or affecting metabolism or hemodynamic responses. May impair judgement, thinking, or motor skills; caution when operating hazardous machinery. May disrupt body temperature regulation; caution in patients exposed to temperature extremes. Reevaluate periodically. Patients with Parkinson's disease or dementia with Lewy bodies who receive antipsychotics are reported to have an increased sensitivity to antipsychotic medications. **Contra:** Anaphylactic reactions and angioedema. **P/N:** Category C, not for use in nursing.	Somnolence, increased appetite, fatigue, N/V, **cough,** urinary incontinence, constipation, fever, parkinsonism, abdominal pain, anxiety, dizziness, tremor, dyspepsia.
Ziprasidone HCl (Geodon, Geodon for Injection)	**Cap:** (HCl) 20mg, 40mg, 60mg, 80mg; **Inj:** (Mesylate) 20mg/mL	***Adults:*** **Schizophrenia:** (Cap) **Initial:** 20mg bid with food. **Titrate:** May increase up to 80mg bid; adjust dose at intervals of not less than 2 days. **Maint:** 20-80mg bid for up to 52 weeks. (Inj) 10-20mg IM up to max 40mg/day. May give 10mg q2h or 20mg q4h up to 40mg/day for 3 days. **Bipolar Mania:** (Cap) **Initial:** 40mg bid with	**BB:** Elderly patients with dementia-related psychosis treated with atypical antipsychotic drugs are at an increased risk of death; most appeared to be cardiovascular (eg, heart failure, sudden death) or infectious (eg, pneumonia) in nature. Ziprasidone is not approved for the treatment of patients with dementia-related psychosis. **W/P:** D/C if persistent	Asthenia, N/V, constipation, dyspepsia, diarrhea, **dry mouth,** rash, somnolence, akathisia, dizziness, EPS, dystonia, hypertonia, respiratory disorder, upper respiratory

Table 18.1. PRESCRIBING INFORMATION FOR PSYCHOACTIVE DRUGS *(cont.)*

NAME	FORM/ STRENGTH	DOSAGE	WARNINGS/PRECAUTIONS & CONTRAINDICATIONS	ADVERSE EFFECTS†
ANTIPSYCHOTIC AGENTS *(cont.)*				
SECOND-GENERATION ANTIPSYCHOTICS *(cont.)*				
Ziprasidone HCl (Geodon, Geodon for Injection) *(cont.)*		food. **Titrate:** Increase to 60-80mg bid on second day of treatment. **Maint:** 40-80mg bid.	QTc measurements >500 msec, NMS, tardive dyskinesia occurs. Monitor for hyperglycemia in patients with DM or at risk for DM. Avoid with congenital long QT syndrome, history of arrhythmia. Caution in history of seizures. Esophageal dysmotility and aspiration reported. May elevate prolactin levels. Orthostatic hypotension reported; caution with cardiovascular or cerebrovascular disease, conditions predisposed to hypotension (eg, dehydration, hypovolemia). Caution with IM use in renal dysfunction. **Contra:** Concomitant dofetilide, sotalol, quinidine, Class Ia/III antiarrhythmics, mesoridazine, thioridazine, chlorpromazine, droperidol, pimozide, sparfloxacin, gatifloxacin, moxifloxacin, halofantrine, mefloquine, pentamidine, arsenic trioxide, levomethadyl acetate, dolasetron, probucol, tacrolimus, and drugs that prolong QT interval. History of QT prolongation, recent acute MI, uncompensated heart failure. **P/N:** Category C, not for use in nursing.	infection, headache, injection-site pain, **swollen tongue,** facial droop, tardive dyskinesia, enuresis, urinary incontinence.
ATTENTION DEFICIT HYPERACTIVITY DISORDER/NARCOLEPSY AGENTS				
Amphetamine Salt Combo (Adderall, Adderall XR) CII	**Cap, Extended-Release:** (Adderall XR) 5mg, 10mg, 15mg, 20mg, 25mg, 30mg; **Tab:** (Adderall) 5mg*, 7.5mg*, 10mg*, 12.5mg*, 15mg*, 20mg*, 30mg*	(Tab) ***Adults/Pediatrics:*** **≥12 yrs: Narcolepsy: Initial:** 10mg/day. **Titrate:** May increase by 10mg/day every week. **Usual:** 5-60mg/day. Give first dose upon awakening, and additional doses q4-6h. ***Pediatrics:*** **ADHD: 3-5 yrs: Initial:** 2.5mg qd. **Titrate:** May increase by 2.5mg weekly. **≥6 yrs:** 5mg qd-bid. May increase by 5mg weekly. **Max (usual):** 40mg/day. **Narcolepsy: 6-12 yrs: Initial:** 5mg/day. May increase by 5mg weekly. (Tab, ER) ***Adults:*** **Initial:** 20mg qam. ***Pediatrics:*** **13 to 17 yrs: Initial:** 10mg/day. **Titrate:** May increase to 20mg/day after one week. **≥6 yrs: Initial:** 10mg qam. **Titrate:** May increase weekly by 5-10mg/day. **Max:** 30mg/day. **Currently Using Adderall:** Switch to Adderall XR at the same total daily dose, taken once daily. Titrate at weekly intervals as needed. Swallow cap whole or open cap and sprinkle contents on applesauce; do not chew beads.	**BB:** High potential for abuse; avoid prolonged use. Misuse of amphetamines may cause sudden death and serious CV adverse events. **W/P:** May exacerbate symptoms of behavior disturbance and thought disorder in psychotic patients. Caution when using stimulants to treat patients with comorbid bipolar disorder because of concern for possible induction of mixed/manic episode in such patients. Stimulants at usual doses can cause treatment emergent psychotic or manic symptoms (eg, hallucinations, delusional thinking, mania) in children and adolescents without prior history of psychotic illness. Aggressive behavior or hostility reported in clinical trials and postmarketing experience of some medications indicated for the treatment of ADHD. Monitor growth in children. May lower convulsive threshold; d/c in presence of seizures. Visual disturbances reported with stimulant treatment. May exacerbate Tourette's syndrome and phonic or motor tics. Caution with HTN and monitor BP. Interrupt occasionally to determine if patient requires continued therapy. Sudden death reported in children with structural cardiac abnormalities; avoid use in children or adults with structural cardiac abnormalities. May decrease appetite. **Contra:** Advanced arteriosclerosis, symptomatic cardiovascular disease, moderate to severe HTN, hyperthyroidism, glaucoma, agitated states, history of drug abuse, during or within 14 days of MAOI use. **P/N:** Category C, not for use in nursing.	Abdominal pain, asthenia, fever, infection, viral infection, loss of appetite, diarrhea, N/V, emotional lability, insomnia, nervousness, weight loss, **dry mouth,** headache, urticaria, anaphylaxis, HTN, tachycardia, palpitations, CNS overstimulation, anorexia, impotence, rash, angioedema, anaphylaxis, Stevens-Johnson syndrome.

*Scored. †Bold entries denote special dental considerations.

BB = black box warning; **W/P** = warnings/precautions; **Contra** = contraindications; **P/N** = pregnancy category rating and nursing considerations.

NAME	FORM/ STRENGTH	DOSAGE	WARNINGS/PRECAUTIONS & CONTRAINDICATIONS	ADVERSE EFFECTS†
Armodafinil (Nuvigil) CIV	**Tab:** 50mg, 150mg, 250mg	***Adults:*** **OSAHS/Narcolepsy:** 150mg or 250mg qd in AM. **SWSD:** 150mg qd 1 hr prior to work shift. **Hepatic Dysfunction:** Reduce dose. **Elderly:** Consider dose reduction.	**W/P:** May cause serious rash, including Stevens-Johnson syndrome, anaphylactoid reactions, angioedema, and multiorgan hypersensitivity. May impair mental/physical abilities. Psychiatric adverse experiences reported; consider discontinuing treatment if psychiatric symptoms develop and use caution with history of psychosis, depression, or mania. Caution with history of MI or unstable angina. Avoid with history of left ventricular hypertrophy, ischemic ECG changes, chest pain, arrhythmia, or other manifestations of mitral valve prolapse with CNS stimulants. Monitor hypertensive patients. **P/N:** Category C, caution in nursing.	Headache, nausea, dizziness, insomnia, diarrhea, **dry mouth,** anxiety, depression, rash.
Atomoxetine HCl (Strattera)	**Cap:** 10mg, 18mg, 25mg, 40mg, 60mg, 80mg, 100mg	***Adults:*** **Initial:** 40mg/day given qam or evenly divided doses in the am and late afternoon/early evening. **Titrate:** Increase after minimum of 3 days to target dose of about 80mg/day. After 2-4 weeks, may increase to max of 100mg/day. **Max:** 100mg/day. **Hepatic Insufficiency: Moderate (Child-Pugh Class B):** Reduce initial and target doses to 50% of normal dose. **Severe (Child-Pugh Class C):** Reduce initial and target doses to 25% of normal dose. **Concomitant CYP450 2D6 inhibitor (eg, paroxetine, fluoxetine, quinidine): Initial:** 40mg/day. **Titrate:** Only increase to 80mg/day if symptoms fail to improve after 4 weeks. ***Pediatrics:*** **≥6 yrs: ≤70kg: Initial:** 0.5mg/kg/day given qam or evenly divided doses in the am and late afternoon or early evening. **Titrate:** Increase after minimum of 3 days to target dose of about 1.2mg/kg/day. **Max:** 1.4mg/kg/day or 100mg, whichever is less. **>70kg: Initial:** 40mg/day given qam or evenly divided doses in the am and late afternoon/early evening. **Titrate:** Increase after minimum of 3 days to target dose of about 80mg/day. After 2-4 weeks, may increase to max of 100mg/day. **Max:** 100mg/day. **Hepatic Insufficiency: Moderate (Child-Pugh Class B):** Reduce initial and target doses to 50% of the normal dose. **Severe (Child-Pugh Class C):** Reduce initial and target doses to 25% of normal dose. **Concomitant CYP450 2D6 inhibitor (eg, paroxetine, fluoxetine, quinidine): ≥6 yrs: ≤70kg: Initial:** 0.5mg/kg/day. **Titrate:** Only increase to 1.2mg/kg/day if symptoms fail to improve after 4 weeks. **>70kg: Initial:** 40mg/day. **Titrate:** Only increase to 80mg/day if symptoms fail to improve after 4 weeks.	**BB:** Increased risk of suicidal ideation in short-term studies in children or adolescents with ADHD. Closely monitor for suicidality, clinical worsening, or unusual changes in behavior. Close observation/communication with prescriber by families and caregivers is advised. **W/P:** Monitor for clinical worsening and/or suicidality. Allergic reactions, orthostatic hypotension and syncope reported. Monitor growth. May increase BP and HR; caution with HTN, tachycardia, cardiovascular or cerebrovascular disease. May increase urinary retention and urinary hesitation. Rare cases of priapism reported. May cause severe liver injury in rare cases; monitor liver enzymes and d/c with jaundice or liver injury. Reports of MI, stroke and sudden death in adults. Avoid with known structural cardiac abnormalities or other serious cardiac problems. Physical exam and evaluation of patient history is necessary. Stimulants at usual doses can cause treatment-emergent psychotic or manic symptoms (eg, hallucinations, delusional thinking, mania) in children and adolescents without prior history of psychotic illness. Monitor for appearance or worsening of aggressive behavior or hostility. **Contra:** During or within 14 days of MAOI use; narrow angle glaucoma. **P/N:** Category C, caution in nursing.	(Adults) **Dry mouth,** headache, insomnia, N/V, decreased appetite, constipation, dysmenorrhea, erectile disturbance, urinary retention. (Pediatrics) Upper abdominal pain, headache, decreased appetite, irritability, dizziness, somnolence.
Dexmethylphenidate HCl (Focalin, Focalin XR) CII	**Cap, Extended-Release:** (Focalin XR) 5mg, 10mg, 15mg, 20mg; **Tab:** (Focalin) 2.5mg, 5mg, 10mg.	(Tab) ***Adults/Pediatrics:*** **≥6 yrs:** Take bid at least 4 hrs apart. **Methylphenidate Naive: Initial:** 2.5mg bid. **Titrate:** Increase weekly by 2.5-5mg/week. **Max:** 20mg/day. **Currently on Methylphenidate: Initial:** Take 1/2 of methylphenidate dose. **Max:** 20mg/day. Reduce or d/c if paradoxical aggravation of symptoms. D/C if no improvement after appropriate	**BB:** Caution with previous history of drug dependence or alcoholism. Marked tolerance and psychological dependence with varying degrees of abnormal behavior may occur with chronic abusive use. Careful supervision is necessary during withdrawal from abusive use to avoid severe depression. **W/P:** Avoid with known serious structural cardiac abnormalities, cardiomyopathy, serious	(Tab) Abdominal pain, fever, anorexia, nausea, nervousness, insomnia. (Pediatrics) Loss of appetite, weight loss, tachycardia. (Cap, ER) Dyspepsia, headache, anxiety. (Adults)

Table 18.1. PRESCRIBING INFORMATION FOR PSYCHOACTIVE DRUGS *(cont.)*

NAME	FORM/ STRENGTH	DOSAGE	WARNINGS/PRECAUTIONS & CONTRAINDICATIONS	ADVERSE EFFECTS†
ATTENTION DEFICIT HYPERACTIVITY DISORDER/NARCOLEPSY AGENTS *(cont.)*				
Dexmethylphenidate HCl (Focalin, Focalin XR) CII *(cont.)*		dosage adjustments over 1 month. (Cap, ER) ***Adults:* Individualize Dose: Methylphenidate Naive: Initial:** 10mg/day. **Titrate:** May adjust weekly by 10mg-20mg qd. **Max:** 20mg/day. **Currently on Methylphenidate: Initial:** Take 1/2 of methylphenidate dose. **Max:** 20mg/day. **Currently on Dexmethylphenidate Immediate-Release:** Switch to same daily dose of XR. **Max:** 20mg/day. Reduce or d/c if paradoxical aggravation of symptoms. Swallow capsule whole or sprinkle contents on applesauce. Contents should not be crushed, chewed, or divided. D/C if no improvement after appropriate dosage adjustments over 1 month. ***Pediatrics:* ≥6 yrs: Individualize Dose: Methylphenidate Naive: Initial:** 5mg/day. **Titrate:** May adjust weekly by 5mg. **Max:** 20mg/day. **Currently on Methylphenidate: Initial:** Take 1/2 of methylphenidate dose. **Max:** 20mg/day. Currently on **Dexmethylphenidate Immediate-Release:** Switch to same daily dose of XR. **Max:** 20mg/day. Reduce or d/c if paradoxical aggravation of symptoms. Swallow capsule whole or sprinkle contents on applesauce; contents should not be crushed, chewed, or divided. D/C if no improvement after appropriate dosage adjustments over 1 month.	heart rhythm abnormalities, CAD, or other serious cardiac problems. May cause modest increase in BP; caution with HTN, heart failure, recent MI, or ventricular arrhythmia. May exacerbate symptoms of behavior disturbance and thought disorder with preexisting psychotic disorder. Caution when using stimulants to treat patients with comorbid bipolar disorder because of concern for possible induction of mixed/manic episodes in such patients. Stimulants at usual doses may cause treatment-emergent psychotic or manic symptoms (eg, hallucinations, delusional thinking, mania) in children and adolescents without prior history of psychotic illness or mania. Aggressive behavior or hostility reported in clinical trials and the postmarketing experience of some medications indicated for the treatment of ADHD. Suppression of growth reported with long-term use; monitor growth. May lower convulsive threshold; d/c in the presence of seizures. Visual disturbances reported. Monitor CBC, differential, and platelets with prolonged therapy. **Contra:** Marked anxiety, tension, and agitation; glaucoma; motor tics or family history or diagnosis of Tourette's syndrome; during or within 14 days of MAOI use. **P/N:** Category C, caution in nursing.	**Dry mouth, pharyngolaryngeal pain,** feeling jittery, dizziness. (Pediatrics) Decreased appetite, nausea.
Dextroamphetamine Sulfate (Dexedrine, Dexedrine Spansules, DextroStat) CII	**Cap, Extended-Release:** (Spansules) 5mg, 10mg, 15mg; **Tab:** (Dexedrine) 5mg* (DextroStat) 5mg*, 10mg*	***Adults/Pediatrics:* ≥12 yrs: Narcolepsy: Initial:** 10mg/day. **Titrate:** May increase by 10mg/day every week. **Usual:** 5-60mg/day. For tabs, give first dose upon awakening and additional every 4-6 hrs. May give caps once daily. ***Pediatrics:* Narcolepsy: 6-12 yrs: Initial:** 5mg qd. **Titrate:** Increase weekly by 5mg/day. **ADHD: Initial: 3-5 yrs:** 2.5mg qd. **Titrate:** Increase weekly by 2.5mg/day. **≥6 yrs:** 5mg qd-bid. **Titrate:** Increase weekly by 5mg/day. **Max:** 40mg/day. For tabs, give first dose upon awakening and additional every 4-6 hrs. May give caps once daily.	**BB:** High potential for abuse; avoid prolonged use. Misuse of amphetamines may cause sudden death and serious CV adverse events. **W/P:** May exacerbate symptoms of behavior disturbance and thought disorder in psychotic patients. Caution when using stimulants to treat patients with comorbid bipolar disorder because of concern for possible induction of mixed/manic episode in such patients. Stimulants at usual doses can cause treatment emergent psychotic or manic symptoms (eg, hallucinations, delusional thinking, mania) in children and adolescents without prior history of psychotic illness. Aggressive behavior or hostility reported in clinical trials and the postmarketing experience of some medications indicated for the treatment of ADHD. Caution with HTN. Tablets contain tartrazine; may cause allergy reactions. Exacerbation of motor and phonic tics and Tourette's syndrome. Monitor growth in children. Avoid with serious structural cardiac abnormalities, cardiomyopathy, serious heart rhythm abnormalities, CAD, or other serious cardiac problems. Avoid use in the presence of seizure. Visual disturbances	Palpitations, tachycardia, BP elevation, CNS overstimulation, restlessness, insomnia, **dry mouth,** GI disturbances, anorexia, urticaria, impotence.

*Scored. †Bold entries denote special dental considerations.
BB = black box warning; **W/P** = warnings/precautions; **Contra** = contraindications; **P/N** = pregnancy category rating and nursing considerations.

NAME	FORM/ STRENGTH	DOSAGE	WARNINGS/PRECAUTIONS & CONTRAINDICATIONS	ADVERSE EFFECTS†
Dextroamphetamine Sulfate (Dexedrine, Dexedrine Spansules, DextroStat) CII *(cont.)*			reported with stimulant treatment. **Contra:** Advanced arteriosclerosis, symptomatic cardiovascular disease, moderate-to-severe HTN, hyperthyroidism, glaucoma, agitated states, history of drug abuse, during or within 14 days of MAOI use. **P/N:** Category C, not for use in nursing.	
Lisdexamfetamine Dimesylate (Vyvanse) CII	**Cap:** 20mg, 30mg, 40mg, 50mg, 60mg, 70mg	***Pediatrics:* 6-12 yrs:** Individualize dose. **Usual:** 30mg qam. **Titrate:** If needed, may increase in increments of 10mg or 20mg at weekly intervals. **Max:** 70mg/day. Swallow caps or dissolve contents in glass of water; do not store once dissolved. Reevaluate periodically.	**BB:** High potential for abuse; avoid prolonged use. Misuse of amphetamines may cause sudden death and serious CV adverse events. **W/P:** Avoid use with structural cardiac abnormalities, cardiomyopathy, serious heart rhythm abnormalities, or other serious cardiac problems; sudden death reported. Assess presence of cardiac disease through cardiac evaluation. Caution with HTN, heart failure, recent MI, or ventricular arrhythmia; monitor BP and HR. May exacerbate symptoms of behavior disturbance and thought disorder in psychotic patients. Caution with comorbid bipolar disorder; concern for possible induction of mixed/manic episode. Treatment emergent psychotic or manic symptoms (eg, hallucinations, delusional thinking, or mania, without prior history of psychotic illness) may occur; d/c treatment if needed. Aggressive behavior or hostility reported; monitor condition as it worsens. Monitor growth in children. Stimulants may lower the convulsive threshold; d/c in the presence of seizures. Difficulties with accommodation and blurring of vision reported. May exacerbate motor or phonic tics and Tourette's syndrome. **Contra:** Advanced arteriosclerosis, symptomatic CVD, moderate to severe HTN, hyperthyroidism, glaucoma, agitated states, history of drug abuse, during or within 14 days of MAOI use. **P/N:** Category C, not for use in nursing.	Ventricular hypertrophy, tic, N/V, psychomotor hyperactivity, insomnia, rash, upper abdominal pain, decreased appetite, dizziness, **dry mouth,** irritability, weight loss, headache, affect lability.
Methamphetamine HCl (Desoxyn) CII	**Tab:** 5mg	***Adults/Pediatrics:* ≥12 yrs: Obesity:** 5mg, 1/2 hr before each meal. Do not exceed a few weeks of treatment. ***Pediatrics:* ADHD: ≥6 yrs: Initial:** 5mg qd-bid. **Titrate:** Increase by 5mg/week until optimum response. **Usual:** 20-25mg/day given as a single dose or two divided doses.	**BB:** High potential for abuse; reserve only for use in weight reduction programs. Avoid prolonged use. Misuse of amphetamines may cause sudden death and serious CV adverse events. **W/P:** Tolerance to anorectic effect develops within a few weeks, do not exceed recommended dose to increase effect. Monitor growth in children. Caution with HTN. Do not use to combat fatigue or replace rest. Exacerbation of motor and phonic tics and Tourette's syndrome. May exacerbate behavior disturbance and thought disorder in psychotic pediatrics. Emergence of new psychotic symptoms may warrant discontinuation of therapy. Monitor for the appearance or worsening of aggressive behavior in children. Therapy may lower the convulsive threshold and cause blurred vision and difficulty with accommodation. Interrupt occasionally to determine if patient requires continued therapy. Misuse may cause sudden death and serious cardiovascular adverse events. Caution in patients with underlying.	BP elevation, tachycardia, palpitation, dizziness, insomnia, tremor, diarrhea, constipation, **dry mouth,** urticaria, impotence, changes in libido.

Table 18.1. PRESCRIBING INFORMATION FOR PSYCHOACTIVE DRUGS *(cont.)*

NAME	FORM/ STRENGTH	DOSAGE	WARNINGS/PRECAUTIONS & CONTRAINDICATIONS	ADVERSE EFFECTS†
ATTENTION DEFICIT HYPERACTIVITY DISORDER/NARCOLEPSY AGENTS *(cont.)*				
Methamphetamine HCl (Desoxyn) CII *(cont.)*			cardiovascular conditions and comorbid bipolar disorder. **Contra:** Advanced arteriosclerosis, symptomatic cardiovascular disease, moderate-to-severe HTN, hyperthyroidism, glaucoma, agitated states, history of drug abuse, during or within 14 days of MAOI use. **P/N:** Category C, not for use in nursing	
Methylphenidate (Daytrana) CII **Methylphenidate HCl** (Metadate CD, Metadate ER, Methylin, Methylin ER, Ritalin, Ritalin LA, Ritalin SR) CII	**Cap, Extended-Release:** (Metadate CD): 10mg, 20mg, 30mg, 40mg, 50mg, 60mg; (Ritalin LA): 10mg, 20mg, 30mg, 40mg; **Patch:** (Daytrana) 10mg/9 hrs, 15mg/9 hrs, 20mg/9 hrs, 30mg/9 hrs [10[s], 30[s]]; **Sol:** (Methylin) 5mg/5mL [500mL], 10mg/5mL [500mL]; **Tab:** (Ritalin): 5mg, 10mg*, 20mg* (Methylin): 5mg, 10mg, 20mg; **Tab, Chewable:** (Methylin): 2.5mg, 5mg, 10mg; **Tab, Extended-Release:** (Concerta): 18mg, 27mg, 36mg, 54mg; (Ritalin SR) 20mg (Mathylin ER) 10mg, 20mg	(Daytrana) ***Adults/Pediatrics:*** **≥6 yrs:** Individualize dose. Apply to hip area 2 hrs before effect is needed and remove 9 hrs after application. **Recommended Titration Schedule: Week 1:** 10mg/9 hrs. **Week 2:** 15mg/9 hrs. **Week 3:** 20mg/9 hrs. **Week 4:** 30mg/9 hrs. (Concerta) ***Adults/Pediatrics:*** **≥6 yrs: Methylphenidate-Naive or Receiving Other Stimulant: Initial:** 18mg qam with food. **Titrate:** Adjust dose at weekly intervals. **Max: 6-12 yrs:** 54mg/day; **13-17 yrs:** 72mg/day not to exceed 2mg/kg/day. **Previous Methylphenidate Use: Initial:** 18mg qam if previous dose 10-15mg/day; 36mg qam if previous dose 20-30mg/day; 54mg qam if previous dose 30-45mg/day. Initial conversion should not exceed 54mg/day. **Titrate:** Adjust dose at weekly intervals. **Max:** 72mg/day. Reduce dose or discontinue if paradoxical aggravation of symptoms occurs. Discontinue if no improvement after appropriate dosage adjustments over 1 month. Swallow whole with liquids. Do not crush, chew, or divide. (Metadate CD) ***Pediatrics:*** **≥6 yrs: Usual:** 20mg qam before breakfast. **Titrate:** Increase weekly by 20mg depending on tolerability/efficacy. **Max:** 60mg/day. Reduce dose or discontinue if paradoxical aggravation of symptoms occur. D/C if no improvement after appropriate dose adjustments over 1 month. Swallow whole with liquids or open and sprinkle on 1 tbsp applesauce followed by water. Do not crush, chew, or divide. (Metadate ER, Methylin, Methylin ER, Ritalin, Ritalin LA, Ritalin SR) ***Adults:*** (Methylin, Ritalin) 10-60mg/day given bid-tid 30-45 min ac. Take last dose before 6 pm if insomnia occurs. (Metadate ER, Methylin ER, Ritalin SR) May use in place of immediate release (IR) when the 8-hr dose corresponds to the titrated 8-hr IR dose. Swallow whole; do not chew or crush. (Ritalin LA) **Initial:** 20mg qam. **Titrate:** Adjust weekly by 10mg. **Max:** 60mg qam. ***Pediatrics:*** **≥6 yrs:** (Methylin, Ritalin) **Initial:** 5mg bid before breakfast and lunch. **Titrate:** Increase gradually by 5-10mg weekly. **Max:** 60mg/day.	**BB:** Caution with previous history of drug dependence or alcoholism. Marked tolerance and psychological dependence with varying degrees of abnormal behavior may occur with chronic abusive use. Careful supervision is necessary during withdrawal from abusive use to avoid severe depression. **W/P:** Monitor growth in children. Not for severe depression or fatigue. May exacerbate symptoms of behavior disturbance and thought disorder in psychotic children. Care should be taken in using stimulants to treat patients with comorbid bipolar disorder because of concern for possible induction of mixed/manic episode in such patients. Stimulants at usual doses can cause treatment emergent psychotic or manic symptoms (hallucinations, delusional thinking, mania) in children and adolescents without prior history of psychotic illness. Aggressive behavior or hostility reported in clinical trials and the postmarketing experience of some medications indicated for the treatment of ADHD. May lower seizure threshold, especially with prior history of seizures or with prior EEG abnormalities; d/c if seizures occur. Caution with HTN and other underlying conditions that may be compromised such as heart failure, recent MI, or hyperthyroidism. Visual disturbances may occur (rare). Monitor CBC, differential, and platelets with prolonged use. Caution with emotionally unstable patients or prior history of drug dependence or alcoholism; chronic use may lead to tolerance and psychological dependence. Monitor during withdrawal. Periodically d/c to assess condition. Avoid with known structural cardiac abnormalities or other serious cardiac problems. **Contra:** Marked anxiety, tension, and agitation; glaucoma; motor tics or family history or diagnosis of Tourette's syndrome; during or within 14 days of MAOI use. Additional contraindications during treatment with Metadate CD, Metadate ER, and Methylin ER: severe HTN, angina pectoris, cardiac arrhythmias, heart failure, recent MI, hyperthyroidism, or thyrotoxicosis. **P/N:** Category C, caution in nursing.	(Daytrana) N/V, **nasopharyngitis,** weight decrease, anorexia, decreased appetite, affect lability, insomnia, tics, nasal congestion. (Concerta) Loss of appetite, headache, **dry mouth,** nausea, insomnia, tics, anxiety, dizziness, weight reduction, irritability, upper abdominal pain, hyperhidrosis, tachycardia, palpitations. (Metadate CD) Headache, abdominal pain, anorexia, insomnia. (Metadate ER, Methylin, Methylin ER, Ritalin, Ritalin LA, Ritalin SR) Nervousness, insomnia, hypersensitivity reactions, anorexia, nausea, dizziness, palpitations, headache, dyskinesia, drowsiness, BP and pulse changes, tachycardia, angina, arrhythmia, abdominal pain.

*Scored. †Bold entries denote special dental considerations.
BB = black box warning; **W/P** = warnings/precautions; **Contra** = contraindications; **P/N** = pregnancy category rating and nursing considerations.

NAME	FORM/ STRENGTH	DOSAGE	WARNINGS/PRECAUTIONS & CONTRAINDICATIONS	ADVERSE EFFECTS†
Methylphenidate (Daytrana) CII **Methylphenidate HCl** (Metadate CD, Metadate ER, Methylin, Methylin ER, Ritalin, Ritalin LA, Ritalin SR) CII *(cont.)*		(Metadate ER, Methylin ER, Ritalin SR) May use in place of IR when the 8-hr dose corresponds to the titrated 8-hr IR dose. Swallow whole; do not chew or crush. (Ritalin LA) **Initial:** 20mg qam. **Titrate:** Adjust weekly by 10mg. **Max:** 60mg qam. **Previous Methylphenidate Use:** May use as qd in place of IR dosed bid or daily dose of methylphenidate SR. Swallow whole or sprinkle over spoonful of applesauce. Do not crush, chew, or divide. Reduce dose or d/c if paradoxical aggravation of symptoms occurs. D/C if no improvement after appropriate dose adjustment over 1 month.		
Modafinil (Provigil) CIV	**Tab:** 100mg, 200mg*	***Adults:*** 200mg qd. **Narcolepsy/OSAHS:** Take in AM. **SWSD:** Take 1 hr prior to start of work shift. **Hepatic Dysfunction:** 100mg qd. **Elderly:** Consider dose reduction.	**W/P:** Avoid in history of left ventricular hypertrophy, ischemic ECG changes, chest pain, arrhythmia or other manifestations of mitral valve prolapse with CNS stimulants. Caution if recent MI, unstable angina, history of psychosis. Monitor hypertensive patients. Rare cases of severe or life-threatening rash, including Stevens-Johnson syndrome (SJS), toxic epidermal necrolysis (TEN), and drug rash with eosinophilia and systemic symptoms (DRESS) have been reported with the use of modafinil. Angioedema and anaphylactoid reactions reported. **P/N:** Category C, caution in nursing.	Headache, infection, nausea, nervousness, anxiety, insomnia, rhinitis, diarrhea, back pain, dizziness, dyspepsia, hostility.
OBESITY AGENTS/APPETITE MODIFIERS				
Benzphetamine HCl (Didrex) CIII	**Tab:** 50mg*	***Adults/Pediatrics:*** **≥12 yrs: Initial:** 25-50mg qd. **Usual:** 25-50mg qd-tid.	**W/P:** Caution with mild HTN. D/C if tolerance develops. Psychological disturbances reported with restrictive dietary regimen. **Contra:** Advanced arteriosclerosis, symptomatic cardiovascular disease, moderate to severe HTN, agitated states, hyperthyroidism, glaucoma, history of drug abuse, concomitant CNS stimulants, MAOI use within 14 days, pregnancy. **P/N:** Category X, not for use in nursing.	Palpitations, tachycardia, BP elevation, restlessness, dizziness, insomnia, headache, tremor, sweating, **dry mouth,** nausea, diarrhea, **unpleasant tastes,** urticaria, altered libido.
Diethylpropion HCl (Tenuate, Tenuate Dospan) CIV	**Tab:** (Tenuate) 25mg; **Tab, Extended Release:** (Tenuate Dospan)75mg	***Adults/Pediatrics:*** **≥16 yrs: Tab:** 25mg tid 1 hour before meals, and mid-evening if needed for night hunger. **Tab, ER:** 75mg at qd in mid-morning, swallowed whole.	**W/P:** Possible risk of pulmonary HTN and valvular heart disease. Caution with HTN, symptomatic cardiovascular disease. Avoid with heart murmur, valvular heart disease, severe HTN. May increase convulsions with epilepsy. Prolonged use may induce dependence with withdrawal symptoms. D/C if tolerance develops or insignificant weight loss after 4 weeks of therapy. **Contra:** Advanced arteriosclerosis, hyperthyroidism, glaucoma, pulmonary HTN, severe HTN, within 14 days of MAOI use, agitated states, history of drug abuse, other concomitant anorectics. **P/N:** Category B, caution in nursing.	Palpitations, tachycardia, arrhythmias, blurred vision, dizziness, anxiety, insomnia, depression, urticaria, gynecomastia, N/V, GI disturbances, bone marrow depression, impotence.

Table 18.1. PRESCRIBING INFORMATION FOR PSYCHOACTIVE DRUGS *(cont.)*

NAME	FORM/ STRENGTH	DOSAGE	WARNINGS/PRECAUTIONS & CONTRAINDICATIONS	ADVERSE EFFECTS†
OBESITY AGENTS/APPETITE MODIFIERS *(cont.)*				
Phendimetrazine Tartrate (Bontril PDM, Bontril Slow-Release) CIII	**Cap, Extended-Release:** (Slow-Release) 105mg; **Tab:** (PDM) 35mg*	***Adults/Pediatrics:*** **≥12 yrs: (Slow-Release)** 105mg qam, 30-60 min before breakfast. **(PDM)** 35mg bid-tid, 1 hr before meals; may reduce to 17.5mg/dose. **Max:** 70mg tid.	**W/P:** Tolerance to anorectic effect develops within a few weeks, d/c if this occurs. Fatigue and depression with abrupt withdrawal after prolonged high dose therapy. Caution with mild HTN. **Contra:** Advanced arteriosclerosis, symptomatic cardiovascular disease, moderate and severe HTN, hyperthyroidism, glaucoma, agitated states, history of drug abuse, concomitant CNS stimulants including MAOIs. **P/N:** Not for use in pregnancy, safety in nursing not known.	Palpitation, tachycardia, BP elevation, overstimulation, restlessness, dizziness, **dry mouth,** diarrhea, constipation, nausea, libido changes, dysuria, insomnia.
Phentermine HCl (Adipex-P) CIV	**Cap:** 37.5mg; **Tab:** 37.5mg*	***Adults/Pediatrics:*** **>16 yrs: Usual:** 37.5mg before breakfast or 1-2 hrs after breakfast. **Alternate Schedule:** (Tab) 18.75mg qd-bid. Avoid late evening dosing.	**W/P:** Only for short-term therapy. Primary pulmonary HTN and valvular heart disease reported. Abuse potential. Caution with mild HTN. Tolerance may develop. **Contra:** Advanced arteriosclerosis, cardiovascular disease, moderate-to-severe HTN, hyperthyroidism, glaucoma, agitated states, history of drug abuse, within 14 days of MAOI use. **P/N:** Category C, not for use in nursing.	Primary pulmonary hypertension, regurgitant valvular heart disease, palpitation, tachycardia, BP elevation, CNS overstimulation, **dry mouth,** impotence, urticaria.
Sibutramine HCl Monohydrate (Meridia) CIV	**Cap:** 5mg, 10mg, 15mg	***Adults/Pediatrics:*** **≥16 yrs: Initial:** 10mg qd. **Titrate:** May increase after 4 weeks to 15mg qd. **Max:** 15mg/day. Use 5mg/day in patients unable to tolerate 10mg/day. May continue for up to 2 yrs.	**W/P:** May increase BP and/or pulse. Avoid with uncontrolled or poorly controlled HTN, CAD, CHF, arrhythmias, stroke, severe hepatic or renal dysfunction. Monitor BP and pulse before therapy and regularly thereafter. Caution with narrow-angle glaucoma, mild-to-moderate renal impairment, seizures, and if predisposed to bleeding. Exclude organic causes of obesity. Gallstones precipitated with weight loss. **Contra:** Concomitant MAOIs or centrally acting appetite suppressants, eating disorders (eg, anorexia/bulimia nervosa). **P/N:** Category C, not for use in nursing.	Anorexia, constipation, increased appetite, nausea, dyspepsia, **dry mouth,** insomnia, dizziness, nervousness, HTN, tachycardia, dysmenorrhea, headache.

*Scored. †Bold entries denote special dental considerations.
BB = black box warning; **W/P** = warnings/precautions; **Contra** = contraindications; **P/N** = pregnancy category rating and nursing considerations.

Table 18.2. DRUG INTERACTIONS FOR PSYCHOACTIVE DRUGS

ANTIANXIETY/HYPNOTIC AGENTS

Benzodiazepines

Alprazolam (Niravam, Xanax, Xanax XR) CIV	
Alcohol	May have additive CNS depressant effects.
Amiodarone	Caution with amiodarone.
Anticonvulsants	May have additive CNS depressant effects.
Antihistamines	May have additive CNS depressant effects.
Antisialogogues	Concomitant drugs that cause dry mouth might slow disintegration or dissolution, resulting in slowed or decreased absorption (Niravam).
Azole antifungals	Avoid concomitant use with azole antifungals.
Carbamazepine	Carbamazepine may induce metabolism and decrease levels.
Cimetidine	Cimetidine may increase levels.
CNS depressants	May have additive CNS depressant effects.
Contraceptives, oral	Oral contraceptives may increase levels.
Cyclosporine	Caution with cyclosporine.
CYP3A inducers	CYP3A inducers may decrease levels.
CYP3A inhibitors	Avoid coadministration with potent CYP3A inhibitors (eg, azole antifungals); caution with moderate and weak CYP3A inhibitors.
Desipramine	May increase levels of desipramine.
Diltiazem	Caution with diltiazem.
Ergotamine	Caution with ergotamine.
Fluoxetine	Fluoxetine may increase levels and potentiate CNS depressant effects.
Fluvoxamine	Fluvoxamine may increase levels and potentiate CNS depressant effects.
GI alkalinizing agents	Concomitant drugs that raise stomach pH might slow disintegration or dissolution, resulting in slowed or decreased absorption.
Grapefruit juice	Caution with grapefruit juice.
Imipramine	May increase levels of imipramine.
Isoniazid	Caution with isoniazid.
Itraconazole	Concomitant use with itraconazole is contraindicated.
Ketoconazole	Concomitant use with ketoconazole is contraindicated.
Macrolides	Caution with macrolide antibiotics (eg, erythromycin, clarithromycin).
Nefazodone	Nefazodone may increase levels.
Nicardipine	Caution with nicardipine.
Nifedipine	Caution with nifedipine.
Paroxetine	Caution with paroxetine.
Propoxyphene	Propoxyphene may increase levels.

Table 18.2. DRUG INTERACTIONS FOR PSYCHOACTIVE DRUGS *(cont.)*

ANTIANXIETY/HYPNOTIC AGENTS *(cont.)*

Benzodiazepines

Alprazolam (Niravam, Xanax, Xanax XR) CIV *(cont.)*	
Psychotropics	May have additive CNS depressant effects.
Sertraline	Caution with sertraline.
Chlordiazepoxide HCl (Librium) CIV	
Alcohol	May have additive CNS depressant effects.
Anticoagulants, oral	May have variable effects on anticoagulation.
CNS depressants	May have additive CNS depressant effects.
Psychotropics	Avoid concomitant use with other psychotropic agents.
Clorazepate Dipotassium (Tranxene T-Tab) CIV	
Alcohol	May have additive CNS depressant effects.
Antidepressants	Antidepressants may potentiate effects.
Barbiturates	Barbiturates may potentiate effects.
CNS depressants	May have additive CNS depressant effects.
Hypnotics	Concomitant use with hypnotic drugs may result in increased sedation.
MAOIs	MAOIs may potentiate effects.
Opioids	Opioids may potentiate effects.
Phenothiazines	Phenothiazines may potentiate effects.
Psychotropics	Caution with psychotropic agents.
Diazepam (Valium) CIV	
Alcohol	May have additive CNS depressant effects and increase risk of apnea; the injection may cause hypotension or muscle weakness when given concomitantly with alcohol.
Anesthetics	Anesthetics may potentiate or may be potentiated by diazepam.
Antacids	Antacids may slow the rate of absorption.
Anticonvulsants	Abrupt discontinuation of diazepam may result in a temporary increase in the frequency of seizures; anticonvulsants may potentiate or may be potentiated by diazepam.
Antidepressants	Antidepressants may potentiate or may be potentiated by diazepam.
Antihistamines	Antihistamines may potentiate or may be potentiated by diazepam.
Antipsychotics	Antipsychotics may potentiate or may be potentiated by diazepam.
Anxiolytics	Anxiolytics may potentiate or may be potentiated by diazepam.
Barbiturates	May have additive CNS depressant effects and increase risk of apnea. The injection may cause hypotension or muscle weakness when given concomitantly with barbiturates.
Cimetidine	May delay clearance.
CNS depressants	May have additive CNS depressant effects and increase risk of apnea.

ANTIANXIETY/HYPNOTIC AGENTS *(cont.)*

Benzodiazepines

Diazepam (Valium) CIV *(cont.)*	
CYP2C19 inhibitors	CYP2C19 inhibitors may increase levels leading to increased and prolonged sedation.
CYP3A inhibitors	CYP3A inhibitors may increase levels leading to increased and prolonged sedation.
Hypnotics	Hypnotics may potentiate or may be potentiated by diazepam.
MAOIs	MAOIs may potentiate or may be potentiated by diazepam.
Opioids	Opioids may potentiate effects; reduce the dose of concomitant narcotic analgesics by at least 1/3 and administer it slowly. The injection may cause hypotension or muscle weakness when given concomitantly with narcotics.
Phenothiazines	Phenothiazines may potentiate or may be potentiated by diazepam.
Phenytoin	May decrease the metabolic elimination of phenytoin.
Psychotropics	Caution with psychotropic agents.
Sedatives	Sedatives may potentiate or may be potentiated by diazepam.
Estazolam CIV	
Alcohol	Alcohol may potentiate effects.
Anticonvulsants	Anticonvulsants may potentiate effects.
Antidepressants	Antidepressants may potentiate effects.
Antihistamines	Antihistamines may potentiate effects.
Barbiturates	Barbiturates may potentiate effects.
CNS depressants	May have additive CNS depressant effects.
CYP1A2 inducers	CYP1A2 inducers (eg, smoking) may increase clearance.
MAOIs	MAOIs may potentiate effects.
Opioids	Opioids may potentiate effects.
Phenothiazines	Phenothiazines may potentiate effects.
Psychotropics	Caution with psychotropic agents.
Flurazepam HCl (Dalmane) CIV	
Alcohol	May have additive CNS depressant effects.
CNS depressants	May have additive CNS depressant effects.
Hypnotics	May have additive CNS depressant effects.
Lorazepam (Ativan, Ativan Injection) CIV	
Alcohol	May have additive CNS depressant effects.
Anesthetics	May interfere with patient cooperation in determining levels of anesthesia when given as a preanesthetic; may have additive CNS depressant effects.
Anticonvulsants	May have additive CNS depressant effects.

Table 18.2. DRUG INTERACTIONS FOR PSYCHOACTIVE DRUGS *(cont.)*

ANTIANXIETY/HYPNOTIC AGENTS *(cont.)*

Benzodiazepines

Lorazepam (Ativan, Ativan Injection) CIV *(cont.)*	
Antidepressants	May have additive CNS depressant effects.
Antihistamines	May have additive CNS depressant effects.
Antipsychotics	May have additive CNS depressant effects.
Anxiolytics	May have additive CNS depressant effects.
Barbiturates	May have additive CNS depressant effects.
Clozapine	Concomitant use with clozapine may cause marked sedation, excessive salivation, ataxia, delirium, and respiratory arrest.
CNS depressants	May have additive CNS depressant effects leading to potentially fatal respiratory depression.
Contraceptives, oral	Oral contraceptives may increase clearance; may need to increase dose of lorazepam.
Haloperidol	Concomitant use with haloperidol may cause apnea, coma, bradycardia, arrhythmia, cardiac arrest, and death.
Hypnotics	May have additive CNS depressant effects.
Loxapine	Concomitant use with loxapine may cause significant respiratory depression, stupor, and/or hypotension.
Methylxanthines	Methylxanthines (theophylline, aminophylline) may reduce the sedative effects of lorazepam.
MAOIs	May have additive CNS depressant effects.
Opioids	May have additive CNS depressant effects.
Phenothiazines	May have additive CNS depressant effects.
Probenecid	Probenecid may increase levels; decrease dose of lorazepam by 50%.
Scopolamine	Concomitant use with scopolamine may increase incidence of sedation, hallucinations, and irrational behavior.
Sedatives	May have additive CNS depressant effects.
Valproate	Valproate may increase levels; decrease dose of lorazepam by 50%.
Midazolam HCl CIV	
Alcohol	Increased sedative and respiratory effects with alcohol.
Anesthetics	Caution with anesthetics; may decrease concentration of halothane and thiopental required for anesthesia.
Barbiturates	Increased sedative and respiratory effects with barbiturates.
CNS depressants	Increased sedative effects with morphine, meperidine, fentanyl, secobarbital, droperidol, or other CNS depressants.
CYP3A4 inducers	Decreased levels with CYP3A4 inducers (eg, rifampin, carbamazepine, phenytoin).

ANTIANXIETY/HYPNOTIC AGENTS *(cont.)*

Benzodiazepines

Midazolam HCl CIV *(cont.)*	
CYP3A4 inhibitors	Increased levels and prolonged sedation with CYP3A4 inhibitors (eg, azole antimycotics, protease inhibitors, CCBs, macrolide antibiotics, cimetidine).
Droperidol	Increased sedative and respiratory effects with droperidol.
Fentanyl	May cause severe hypotension with concomitant use of fentanyl in neonates.
Ketamine	Increased sedative and respiratory effects with ketamine.
Nitrous oxide	Increased sedative and respiratory effects with nitrous oxide.
Opioids	Increased sedative and respiratory effects with opioids.
Propofol	Increased sedative and respiratory effects with propofol.
Oxazepam CIV	
CNS depressants	Additive effects with alcohol and other CNS depressants.
Temazepam (Restoril) CIV	
CNS depressants	Additive CNS depressant effects with alcohol and CNS depressants.
Diphenhydramine	May be synergistic with diphenhydramine.
Triazolam (Halcion) CIV	
Cimetidine	Caution with cimetidine.
Contraceptives, oral	Potentiated by oral contraceptives.
Cyclosporine	Caution with cyclosporine.
CYP3A inhibitors	Avoid the concomitant use with inhibitors of the CYP3A.
Diltiazem	Caution with diltiazem.
Ergotamine	Caution with ergotamine.
Fluvoxamine	Caution with fluvoxamine.
Grapefruit juice	Potentiated by grapefruit juice.
Isoniazid	Potentiated by isoniazid.
Itraconazole	Use is contraindicated.
Ketoconazole	Use is contraindicated.
Macrolides	Caution with macrolides.
Nefazodone	Use is contraindicated.
Nicardipine	Caution with nicardipine.
Nifedipine	Caution with nifedipine.
Paroxetine	Caution with paroxetine.
Ranitidine	Potentiated by ranitidine.
Sertraline	Caution with sertraline.
Verapamil	Caution with verapamil.

Table 18.2. DRUG INTERACTIONS FOR PSYCHOACTIVE DRUGS *(cont.)*

ANTIANXIETY/HYPNOTIC AGENTS *(cont.)*

Nonbenzodiazepines

Amitriptyline HCl/Chlordiazepoxide (Limbitrol, Limbitrol DS) CIV	
Alcohol	May have additive CNS depressant effects.
Antiarrhythmics, Class IC	Class IC antiarrhythmics (eg, propafenone, flecainide) may increase TCA levels resulting in toxicity.
Anticholinergic agents	May cause severe constipation with anticholinergic agents.
Antidepressants	Antidepressants may increase TCA levels resuling in toxicity.
Cimetidine	Cimetidine may increase TCA levels.
CNS depressants	May have additive CNS depressant effects.
CYP2D6 inhibitors	CYP2D6 inhibitors (eg, quinidine, cimetidine) may increase TCA levels resulting in toxicity; dose adjustment may be warranted.
CYP2D6 substrates	CYP2D6 substrates may increase TCA levels resulting in toxicity.
Fluoxetine	Avoid initiating TCAs for at least 5 weeks after stopping fluoxetine.
Guanethidine	May decrease the hypotensive effect of guanethidine.
MAOIs	Use with or 2 weeks after an MAOI is contraindicated.
Phenothiazines	Phenothiazines may increase TCA levels resulting in toxicity.
Psychotropics	May have additive CNS depressant effects.
SSRIs	Caution with SSRIs and also when switching between TCAs and SSRIs.
Amitriptyline HCl/Perphenazine	
Alcohol	Avoid with alcohol due to increased hypotension and additive CNS depressant effects.
Analgesics	May potentiate CNS depressant effects of analgesics.
Antiarrhythmics, Class IC	Class IC antiarrhythmics (eg, propafenone, flecainide) may increase TCA levels resulting in toxicity.
Anticholinergic agents	Caution with anticholinergic agents (eg, atropine, organic phosphate insecticides); may cause hyperpyrexia or paralytic ileus.
Antidepressants	Antidepressants may increase TCA levels resulting in toxicity.
Antihistamines	May potentiate CNS depressant effects of antihistamines.
Barbiturates	May have additive CNS depressant effects.
Cimetidine	Cimetidine may increase TCA levels.
CNS depressants	May have additive CNS depressant effects.
CYP2D6 inhibitors	CYP2D6 inhibitors (eg, quinidine, cimetidine) may increase TCA levels resulting in toxicity; dose adjustment may be warranted.
CYP2D6 substrates	CYP2D6 substrates may increase TCA levels resulting in toxicity.
Ethchlorvynol	Caution with ethchlorvynol; may cause transient delirium.
Fluoxetine	Avoid initiating TCAs for at least 5 weeks after discontinuing fluoxetine.
Guanethidine	May decrease the hypotensive effect of guanethidine.

ANTIANXIETY/HYPNOTIC AGENTS *(cont.)*

Nonbenzodiazepines

Amitriptyline HCl/Perphenazine *(cont.)*	
MAOIs	Use with or 2 weeks after an MAOI is contraindicated.
Neuroleptics	May cause hyperpyrexia with neuroleptic drugs.
Opiates	May potentiate CNS depressant effects of opiates.
Phenothiazines	Phenothiazines may increase TCA levels resulting in toxicity.
SSRIs	Caution with SSRIs and also when switching between TCAs and SSRIs.
Sympathomimetics	Caution with sympathomimetic drugs, including epinephrine combined with local anesthetics.
Buspirone HCl (BuSpar)	
Cimetidine	Cimetidine may increase levels.
CYP3A4/5 inducers	Potent CYP3A4/5 inducers (eg, dexamethasone, phenytoin, phenobarbital, carbamazepine) may decrease levels.
CYP3A4/5 inhibitors	Potent CYP3A4/5 inhibitors (eg, ketoconazole, ritonavir) may increase levels.
Diazepam	Concomitant administration may lead to an increase in diazepam-associated adverse events (dizziness, headache, nausea).
Digoxin	Digoxin and other weakly protein-bound drugs may be displaced by buspirone.
Diltiazem	Diltiazem may increase levels; concomitant administration may lead to an increase in diltiazem-associated adverse events.
Erythromycin	Erythromycin may increase levels; concomitant administration may lead to an increase in buspirone-associated adverse events.
Grapefruit juice	Grapefruit juice may increase levels.
Haloperidol	May increase levels of haloperidol.
Itraconazole	Itraconazole may increase levels; concomitant administration may lead to an increase in buspirone-associated adverse events.
MAOIs	Avoid concomitant use with MAOIs.
Nefazodone	Concomitant use may lead to an increase in the levels of both buspirone and nefazodone.
Psychotropics	Caution with other CNS-active drugs.
Rifampin	Rifampin may decrease levels.
Trazodone	May elevate ALT with trazodone.
Verapamil	Verapamil may increase levels; concomitant administration may lead to an increase in verapamil-associated adverse events.
Chloral Hydrate CIV	
Anticoagulants, coumarin	May reduce the efficacy of coumarin anticoagulants.
CNS depressants	May have additive effects with other CNS depressants (eg, paraldehyde, barbiturates, alcohol).

Table 18.2. DRUG INTERACTIONS FOR PSYCHOACTIVE DRUGS *(cont.)*

ANTIANXIETY/HYPNOTIC AGENTS *(cont.)*

Nonbenzodiazepines

Chloral Hydrate CIV *(cont.)*	
Furosemide	Concomitant use with IV furosemide may result in diaphoresis, flushing, and variable BP; use an alternate hypnotic.
Warfarin	May temporarily potentiate warfarin-induced hypoprothombinemia.
Diphenhydramine Hydrochloride	
Alcohol	May have additive CNS depressant effects.
Antihistamines	May cause additive CNS depresion with antihistamines.
CNS depressants	May cause additive CNS depression with other CNS depressants, including alcohol.
MAOIs	MAOIs prolong and intensify anticholinergic effects.
Sedative-hypnotics	May cause additive CNS depression with sedative-hypnotics.
Tranquilizers	May cause additive CNS depression with tranquilizers.
Doxylamine Succinate (Unisom) OTC	
Alcohol	Avoid concomitant use with alcohol.
Eszopiclone (Lunesta) CIV	
Alcohol	May have additive CNS depressant effects.
CYP3A4 inducers	CYP3A4 inducers (eg, rifampicin) may decrease levels.
CYP3A4 inhibitors	CYP3A4 inhibitors (eg, ketoconazole, itraconazole, clarithromycin, nefazodone, troleandomycin, ritonavir, nelfinavir) may increase levels.
Fat	The effects of sleep onset may be reduced if it is taken with or immediately after a high-fat/heavy meal.
Olanzapine	Coadministration with olanzapine produced a decrease in DSST score.
Hydroxyzine Hydrochloride	
Alcohol	May have additive CNS depressant effects.
Antihistamines	May cause additive CNS depression with antihistamines.
CNS depressants	May cause additive CNS depression with other CNS depressants.
Sedative-hypnotics	May cause additive CNS depression with sedative-hypnotics.
Tranquilizers	May cause additive CNS depression with tranquilizers.
Meprobamate CIV	
Alcohol	May have additive CNS depressant effects.
CNS depressants	May have additive CNS depressant effects.
Psychotropics	May have additive CNS depressant effects.
Pentobarbital Sodium (Nembutal Sodium Solution) CII	
Anticoagulants, oral	May decrease levels of oral anticoagulants.
CNS depressants	May produce additive CNS depression with other CNS depressants (eg, other sedatives/hypnotics, antihistamines, tranquilizers, alcohol).

ANTIANXIETY/HYPNOTIC AGENTS *(cont.)*

Nonbenzodiazepines

Pentobarbital Sodium (Nembutal Sodium Solution) CII *(cont.)*	
Corticosteroids	May decrease levels of corticosteroids.
Doxycycline	May decrease levels of doxycycline.
Estradiol	May decrease effects of estradiol; alternative contraceptive method should be suggested.
Griseofulvin	May decrease levels of griseofulvin.
MAOIs	Prolonged effect with MAOIs.
Phenytoin	Variable effects on phenytoin metabolism; monitor levels of both drugs more frequently during concomitant administration.
Sodium valproate	Sodium valproate may decrease barbiturate metabolism; monitor pentobarbital blood levels and make dosage adjustments as indicated.
Valproic acid	Valproic acid may decrease barbiturate metabolism; monitor pentobarbital blood levels and make dosage adjustments as indicated.
Ramelteon (Rozerem)	
CNS depressants	Additive effect with alcohol and CNS depressants.
CYP450 inducers	Decreased efficacy with strong CYP inducers (eg, rifampin).
CYP450 inhibitors	Caution with less strong CYP1A2 inhibitors, strong CYP3A4 inhibitors (eg, ketoconazole), strong CYP2C9 inhibitors (eg, fluconazole).
Fluvoxamine	Fluvoxamine increases AUC for ramelteon; use is contraindicated.
Secobarbital Sodium (Seconal Sodium) CII	
Anticoagulants, oral	May increase metabolism and decrease response to oral anticoagulants.
Anticonvulsants	Variable effect on phenytoin and increased levels with sodium valproate and valproic acid; monitor blood levels and adjust dose appropriately.
Antihistamines	May cause additive depressant effects with antihistamines.
CNS depressants	May cause additive depressant effects with other CNS depressants, including alcohol.
Corticosteroids	May enhance metabolism of exogenous corticosteroids.
Doxycycline	May shorten half-life of doxycycline for up to 2 weeks after being discontinued.
Estradiol	May decrease effect of estradiol; alternative contraceptive methods should be suggested.
Griseofulvin	Avoid concomitant administration; decreases griseofulvin absorption.
MAOIs	Prolonged effects with MAOIs.
Sedative-hypnotics	May cause additive depressant effects with sedative-hypnotics.
Tranquilizers	May cause additive depressant effects with tranquilizers.
Zaleplon (Sonata) CIV	
Anticonvulsants	Potentiates CNS depression with anticonvulsants.
Antihistamines	Potentiates CNS depression with antihistamines.
Cimetidine	Potentiated by cimetidine.

Table 18.2. DRUG INTERACTIONS FOR PSYCHOACTIVE DRUGS *(cont.)*

ANTIANXIETY/HYPNOTIC AGENTS *(cont.)*

Nonbenzodiazepines

Zaleplon (Sonata) CIV *(cont.)*	
CNS depressants	Potentiates CNS depression with alcohol and other CNS depressants.
CYP3A4 inducers	CYP3A4 inducers (eg, rifampin, phenytoin, carbamazepine, phenobarbital) decrease levels.
Promethazine	Coadministration may decrease plasma levels of zaleplon.
Psychotropics	Potentiates CNS depression with psychotropics (eg, thioridazine, imipramine).
Zolpidem Tartrate (Ambien, Ambien CR) CIV	
Chlorpromazine	Impaired alertness and psychomotor performance with chlorpromazine.
CNS depressants	Additive psychomotor impairment with alcohol and other CNS depressants.
Flumazenil	Flumazenil may reverse effect.
Imipramine	Decreased alertness with imipramine.
Rifampin	Rifampin may decrease effects.

ANTIDEPRESSANTS/OCD AGENTS

MAOIs

Phenelzine Sulfate (Nardil)	
Alkaloids	Caution with rauwolfia alkaloids.
Anesthetics	Use contraindicated with general and spinal anethesia, cocaine, and local anesthetics containing sympathomimetic amines.
Antidepressants	Allow 14 days between starting another antidepressant.
Antihypertensives	Exaggerated hypotensive effects with antihypertensives.
Barbiturates	Reduce dose of barbiturates.
Bupropion	Use is contraindicated; allow 14 days between discontinuing phenelzine and starting bupropion.
Buspirone	Use is contraindicated; allow 14 days between discontinuing phenelzine and starting buspirone.
CNS depressants	Use is contraindicated with CNS depressants, including alcohol and certain opioids.
Dextromethorphan	Use is contraindicated.
Fluoxetine	Allow 5 weeks after discontinuing fluoxetine before starting therapy. Allow 14 days between discontinuation of phenelzine and starting fluoxetine.
Food	Ingesting excessive amounts of caffeine and chocolate is contraindicated; may cause hypertensive crisis.
Guanethidine	Use is contrainidicated.
MAOIs	MAOI use during or within 14 days of administration is contraindicated; allow 14 days between discontinuing phenelzine and starting buspirone.
Meperidine	Use is contraindicated.
Serotonergic drugs	Use is contraindicated.
SSRIs	Allow 14 days between discontinuing phenelzine and starting an SSRI and vice versa.

ANTIDEPRESSANTS/OCD AGENTS *(cont.)*

MAOIs

Phenelzine Sulfate (Nardil) *(cont.)*	
Sympathomimetics	Use is contraindicated with sympathomimetics or related compounds.
Tyramine-containing foods	Use is contraindicated (eg, cheese, beer, wine, and high-protein food).
Selegiline (Emsam)	
Alcohol	Avoid alcohol.
Analgesic agents	Use is contraindicated (eg, tramadol, methadone, propoxyphene).
Anesthetics	Use of general anesthetic agents, cocaine, or local anesthesia containing sympathomimetic vasoconstrictors is contraindicated.
Bupropion	Use is contraindicated.
Buspirone	Use is contraindicated.
Carbamazepine	Use is contraindicated.
Cyclobenzaprine	Use is contraindicated.
Dextromethorphan	Use is contraindicated.
MAOIs	Use of other MAOIs is contraindicated.
Meperidine	Use is contraindicated.
Mirtazapine	Use is contraindicated.
Oxcarbazepine	Use is contraindicated.
Selegiline, oral	Use is contraindicated.
SNRIs	Use is contraindicated.
SSRIs	Use is contraindicated.
St. John's wort	Use is contraindicated.
Sympathetic amines	Use is contraindicated.
TCAs	Use is contraindicated.
Vasocontrictors, products containing	Cold products and weight-reducing preparations that contain vasoconstrictors are contraindicated.
Tranylcypromine Sulfate (Parnate)	
Anesthetics	Use is contraindicated.
Antihistamines	Use is contraindicated.
Antihypertensives	Use is contraindicated.
Bupropion	Use is contraindicated.
Buspirone	Use is contraindicated.
Caffeine	Excessive quantities of caffeine are contraindicated.
CNS depressants	Some CNS depressants are contraindicated, including alcohol and opioids.
Dexfenfluramine	Use is contraindicated.
Dextromethorphan	Use is contraindicated.

Table 18.2. DRUG INTERACTIONS FOR PSYCHOACTIVE DRUGS *(cont.)*

ANTIDEPRESSANTS/OCD AGENTS *(cont.)*

MAOIs

Tranylcypromine Sulfate (Parnate) *(cont.)*	
Dibenzazepine derivatives	Use is contraindicated.
Disulfiram	Caution with disulfiram.
Diuretics	Use is contraindicated.
MAOIs	Use is contraindicated.
Meperidine	Use is contraindicated.
Metrizamide	Avoid metrizamide; d/c 48 hrs before myelography and may resume 24 hrs post-procedure.
Phenothiazines	Additive hypotensive effects with phenothiazines.
Sedatives	Use is contraindicated.
SSRIs	Use is contraindicated.
Sympathomimetics	Use is contraindicated.
Tryptophan	Tryptophan may precipitate disorientation, memory impairment, and other neurological and behavioral signs.
Tyramine-containing foods	Use is contraindicated (eg, cheese).

SELECTIVE SEROTONIN REUPTAKE INHIBITORS

Citalopram Hydrobromide (Celexa)	
Alcohol	Avoid alcohol.
ASA	Increased risk of bleeding with ASA.
Carbamazepine	Caution with carbamazepine.
Cimetidine	Caution with cimetidine.
CNS drugs	Caution with other CNS drugs.
CYP2C19 inhibitors	Clearance may be decreased with potent CYP2C19 (eg, omeprazole) inhibitors.
CYP3A4 inhibitors	Clearance may be decreased with potent CYP3A4 (eg, ketoconazole, itraconazole, fluconazole, erythromycin) inhibitors.
Lithium	Caution with lithium.
MAOIs	MAOI use during or within 14 days of administration is contraindicated.
Metoprolol	May increase metoprolol levels which leads to decreased cardioselectivity.
NSAIDs	Caution with NSAIDs.
Pimozide	Use is contraindicated.
SSRIs	Rare reports of weakness, hyperreflexia, incoordination with SSRIs.
Sumatriptan	Rare reports of weakness, hyperreflexia, incoordination with sumatriptan.
TCAs	Caution with TCAs.
Warfarin	Increased risk of bleeding with warfarin.

ANTIDEPRESSANTS/OCD AGENTS *(cont.)*

SELECTIVE SEROTONIN REUPTAKE INHIBITORS

Escitalopram Oxalate (Lexapro)	
Alcohol	Avoid alcohol.
ASA	Increased risk of bleeding with ASA.
Carbamazepine	Caution with carbamazepine.
Citalopram	Avoid citalopram.
CNS drugs	Caution with CNS drugs.
CYP2D6 substrates	Caution with drugs metabolized by CYP2D6 (eg, desipramine).
Linezolid	Serotonin syndrome reported with linezolid.
Lithium	Caution with lithium.
MAOIs	MAOI use during or within 14 days of administration is contraindicated; upon discontinuation, wait at least 5 days before starting MAOI therapy.
Metoprolol	May increase metoprolol levels which leads to decreased cardioselectivity.
NSAIDs	Increased risk of bleeding with NSAIDs.
Pimozide	Concomitant use is contraindicated.
SSRIs	Rare reports of weakness, hyperreflexia, incoordination with SSRIs.
Sumatriptan	Rare reports of weakness, hyperreflexia, incoordination with sumatriptan.
Warfarin	Increased risk of bleeding with warfarin.
Fluoxetine HCl (Prozac, Prozac Weekly)	
Alcohol	Avoid alcohol.
Antidepressants	May potentiate antidepressants.
Antidiabetic drugs	Antidiabetic drugs may need adjustment.
Antipsychotics	May potentiate antipsychotics.
Benzodiazepines	May increase benzodiazepine levels.
Carbamazepine	May increase carbamazepine levels.
CNS drugs	Caution with CNS drugs.
CYP2D6 substrates	May potentiate CYP2D6 substrates.
Hemostasis, drugs affecting	Caution with drugs that interfere with hemostasis (eg, non-selective NSAIDs, ASA, warfarin) due to increased risk of bleeding.
Lithium	Lithium levels may increase/decrease; monitor lithium levels.
MAOIs	MAOI use during or within 14 days of administration is contraindicated; upon discontinuation, wait at least 5 days before starting MAOI therapy.
Phenytoin	May increase phenytoin levels.
Pimozide	Concomitant use is contraindicated.
Plasma-bound drugs	May shift concentrations with plasma-bound drugs (eg, coumadin, digitoxin).

Table 18.2. DRUG INTERACTIONS FOR PSYCHOACTIVE DRUGS *(cont.)*

ANTIDEPRESSANTS/OCD AGENTS *(cont.)*

Selective Serotonin Reuptake Inhibitors

Fluoxetine HCl (Prozac, Prozac Weekly) *(cont.)*	
Thioridazine	Thiordazine use during or within 5 weeks of discontinuation.
Triptans	Serotonin syndrome reported with use of an SSRI and a triptan; monitor closely.
Warfarin	May alter warfarin effects.
Fluvoxamine Maleate (Luvox, Luvox CR)	
Alcohol	Avoid alcohol.
Alosetron	Use is contraindicated.
ASA	Caution with ASA.
Astemizole	Avoid astemizole.
Benzodiazepines	Reduces clearance of benzodiazepines metabolized by hepatic oxidation (eg, alprazolam, midazolam, triazolam).
β-Blockers	Increases serum levels of β-blockers.
Carbamazepine	Increases serum levels of carbamazepine.
Clozapine	Increases serum levels of clozapine.
Diltiazem	Bradycardia with diltiazem.
Linezolid	Caution with linezolid.
Lithium	Lithium may increase serotonergic effects.
MAOIs	MAOI use during or within 14 days of administration is contraindicated; potential for serious, fatal interactions with MAOIs
Methadone	Increases serum levels of methadone.
Metoprolol	May potentiate metoprolol.
Mexiletine	Reduces clearance of mexiletine.
NSAIDs	Caution with NSAIDs.
Pimozide	Use is contraindicated.
Propranolol	Increases serum levels of propranolol.
Ramelteon	Avoid ramelteon.
St. John's wort	Caution with St. John's wort.
Sumatriptan	Caution with sumatriptan.
Tacrine	Increases serum levels of tacrine.
TCAs	Caution with TCAs.
Terfenadine	Avoid terfenadine.
Theophylline	Increases serum levels of theophylline.
Thioridazine	Use is contraindicated.
Tizanidine	Use is contraindicated.

ANTIDEPRESSANTS/OCD AGENTS *(cont.)*

Selective Serotonin Reuptake Inhibitors

Fluvoxamine Maleate (Luvox, Luvox CR) *(cont.)*	
Tramadol	Caution with tramadol.
Tryptophan	Caution with tryptophan.
Warfarin	Increases serum levels of warfarin.
Paroxetine HCl (Paxil, Paxil CR), **Paroxetine Mesylate** (Pexeva)	
Alcohol	Avoid alcohol.
Anticoagulants, oral	Increased risk of bleeding with oral anticoagulants.
ASA	Increased risk of bleeding with ASA.
Atomoxetine	Paroxetine may increase levels of atomoxetine; initiate atomoxetine at reduced dose and adjust dose as necessary.
Cimetidine	Increased levels of cimetidine.
CYP2D6 inhibitors	Caution with drugs that inhibit CYP2D6 (eg, quinidine).
CYP2D6 substrates	Caution with drugs metabolized by CYP2D6 (eg, antidepressants, phenothiazines, Class Ic antiarrhythmics).
Digoxin	Caution with digoxin.
Diuretics	Caution with diuretics.
Lithium	Caution with lithium.
MAOIs	MAOI use during or within 14 days of administration is contraindicated; this includes linezolid.
NSAIDs	Increased risk of bleeding with NSAIDs.
Phenobarbital	Caution with phenobarbital.
Phenytoin	Caution with phenytoin.
Pimozide	Use is contraindicated.
Plasma-bound drugs	May shift concentrations with plasma-bound drugs.
Procyclidine	Reduce procyclidine dose if anticholinergic effects occur.
Protease inhibitors	Fosamprenavir/ritonavir may decrease levels.
Risperidone	May increase levels of risperidone.
Serotonergic drugs	Caution with other serotonergic drugs (eg, tryptophan, triptans, SSRIs, linezolid, lithium, tramadol, or St. John's wort); increased risk of serotonin syndrome.
SSRIs	Rare reports of weakness, hyperreflexia, incoordination with SSRIs.
Sumatriptan	Rare reports of weakness, hyperreflexia, incoordination with sumatriptan.
TCAs	May inhibit metabolism of TCAs; caution with TCAs.
Theophylline	Monitor theophylline.
Thioridazine	Use is contraindicated.

Table 18.2. DRUG INTERACTIONS FOR PSYCHOACTIVE DRUGS *(cont.)*

ANTIDEPRESSANTS/OCD AGENTS *(cont.)*

SELECTIVE SEROTONIN REUPTAKE INHIBITORS

Paroxetine HCl (Paxil, Paxil CR), **Paroxetine Mesylate (Pexeva)** *(cont.)*	
Trytophan	Avoid tryptophan.
Warfarin	Caution with warfarin.
Sertraline HCl (Zoloft)	
Alcohol	Avoid alcohol.
Cimetidine	Increased levels with cimetidine.
Cisapride	May induce metabolism of cisapride.
CNS drugs	Caution with CNS drugs (eg, diazepam).
CYP2D6 substrates	May potentiate drugs metabolized by CYP2D6 (eg, TCAs, Class Ic antiarrhythmics).
Disulfiram	Contraindicated with disulfiram due to alcohol content (oral concentrate solution).
Hemostasis, drugs affecting	Caution with drugs that interfere with hemostasis (eg, non-selective NSAIDs, ASA, warfarin) due to increased risk of bleeding.
Lithium	Monitor lithium.
MAOIs	Concomitant use is contraindicated.
OTC products	Caution with OTC products.
Pimozide	Concomitant use is contraindicated.
Protein-bound drugs	May shift concentrations with plasma protein-bound drugs (eg, warfarin, digitoxin).
SSRIs	Rare reports of weakness, hyperreflexia, incoordination with an SSRI.
Sumatriptan	Rare reports of weakness, hyperreflexia, incoordination with a sumatriptan.
TCAs	Caution with TCAs; may need dose adjustment.
Tolbutamide	Decreases clearance of tolbutamide.
Warfarin	Monitor PT with warfarin.

SELECTIVE SEROTONIN REUPTAKE INHIBITOR/ATYPICAL ANTIPSYCHOTIC COMBINATION

Fluoxetine HCl/Olanzapine (Symbyax)	
Refer to the interactions of each individual drug.	

SEROTONIN/NOREPINEPHRINE REUPTAKE INHIBITORS

Desvenlafaxine (Pristiq)	
Alcohol	Avoid alcohol.
Anticoagulants	May increase risk of bleeding.
Aspirin	May increase risk of bleeding.
CNS-active drugs	Caution with CNS-active drugs (eg, triptans, SSRIs, lithium).
CYP inhibitors	Caution with potent inhibitors of CYP3A4 and CYP2D6.

ANTIDEPRESSANTS/OCD AGENTS *(cont.)*

SEROTONIN/NOREPINEPHRINE REUPTAKE INHIBITORS

Desvenlafaxine (Pristiq) *(cont.)*	
Desvenlafaxine	Avoid products containing desvenlafaxine.
MAOIs	MAOI use during or within 14 days of administration is contraindicated.
NSAIDs	May increase risk of bleeding.
Serotonergic drugs	Caution with serotonergic drugs (eg, tramadol, tryptophans, SNRIs).
Venlafaxine	Avoid products containing venlafaxine.
Warfarin	May increase risk of bleeding.
Duloxetine HCl (Cymbalta)	
Alcohol	Avoid substantial alcohol use.
CNS-active drugs	Caution with CNS-active drugs.
CYP1A2 inhibitors	Avoid CYP1A2 inhibitors (eg, fluvoxamine, some quinolone antibiotics).
CYP2D6 inhibitors	Increased levels with potent CYP2D6 inhibitors (eg, paroxetine, fluoxetine, quinidine).
CYP2D6 substrates	Caution with drugs metabolized by CYP2D6 having a narrow therapeutic index (eg, TCAs, phenothiazines, Class Ic antiarrhythmics).
Gastric acidity, drugs affecting	Potential for interaction with drugs that affect gastric acidity.
MAOIs	MAOI use during or within 14 days of administration is contraindicated; upon discontinuation, wait at least 5 days before starting MAOI therapy.
Protein-bound drugs	May increase free concentration levels of highly protein-bound drugs.
Serotonergic drugs	Caution with serotonergic drugs (including triptans, tramadol, SNRIs).
Thioridazine	Avoid thioridazine.
Venlafaxine HCl (Effexor, Effexor XR)	
Alcohol	Avoid alcohol.
Cimetidine	Caution with cimetidine in elderly, hepatic dysfunction, or pre-existing HTN.
CNS-active drugs	Caution with CNS-active drugs (eg, triptans, SSRIs, lithium).
CYP inhibitors	Caution with potent inhibitors of CYP3A4 and CYP2D6.
Desipramine	Increases desipramine plasma levels.
Diuretics	Caution with diuretics.
Epinephrine	Administer no more than 40μg epinephrine in local anesthetic solutions (two cartridges of 2% liodocaine with 1:100,000 epinephrine or its equivalent) within short period with careful aspiration technique; additional anesthetic with vasoconstrictor may be given if vital signs are acceptable.
Haloperidol	Decreases clearance of haloperidol.
Indinavir	Decreases indinavir plasma levels.
MAOIs	MAOI use during or within 14 days of administration is contraindicated. Upon discontinuation, wait at least 7 days before starting MAOI therapy.
Risperidone	Increases risperidone plasma levels.
Serotonergic drugs	Caution with serotonergic drugs.

Table 18.2. DRUG INTERACTIONS FOR PSYCHOACTIVE DRUGS *(cont.)*

ANTIDEPRESSANTS/OCD AGENTS *(cont.)*

Tetracyclic Antidepressants

Amoxapine	
CNS depressants	Additive effects with alcohol, barbiturates, and other CNS depressants.
CYP2D6 inhibitors	Increased levels with CYP2D6 inhibitors (eg, quinidine, cimetidine).
CYP2D6, poor metabolizers of	Increased levels in poor metabolizers of CYP2D6.
CYP2D6 substrates	Increased levels with CYP2D6 substrates (eg, other antidepressants, phenothiazines, propafenone, flecainide).
MAOIs	MAOIs are contraindicated (during or within 14 days of therapy).
SSRIs	Caution with SSRIs.
Mirtazapine (Remeron, Remeron SolTab)	
Alcohol	Alcohol increases cognitive and motor skill impairment.
Diazepam	Diazepam increases cognitive and motor skill impairment.
Epinephrine	Administer no more than 40μg epinephrine in local anesthetic solutions (two cartridges of 2% liodocaine with 1:100,000 epinephrine or its equivalent) within short period with careful aspiration technique; additional anesthetic with vasoconstrictor may be given if vital signs are acceptable.
MAOIs	Avoid MAOIs within 14 days of use.

Tricyclic Antidepressants

Amitriptyline HCl	
Anticholinergics	Paralytic ileus and hyperpyrexia with anticholinergics
Cimetidine	Increased plasma levels with cimetidine.
Cisapride	Concomitant use is contraindicated.
CNS depressants	Potentiates other CNS depressants (eg, alcohol, barbiturates).
CYP2D6 inhibitors	Increased levels with CYP2D6 inhibitors (eg, quinidine, cimetidine, SSRIs) and enzyme substrates (eg, phenothiazines, propafenone, flecainide).
Disulfiram	Delirium reported with disulfiram.
Epinephrine	Administer no more than 40μg epinephrine in local anesthetic solutions (two cartridges of 2% liodocaine with 1:100,000 epinephrine or its equivalent) within short period with careful aspiration technique; additional anesthetic with vasoconstrictor may be given if vital signs are acceptable.
Ethchlorvynol	Delirium reported with ethchlorvynol.
Fluoxetine	Avoid within 5 weeks of fluoxetine use.
Guanethidine	May block antihypertensive effects of guanethidine.
MAOIs	MAOI use during or within 14 days of administration is contraindicated.
Neuroleptics	Monitor with neuroleptics.
Sympathomimetics	Monitor with sympathomimetics.
Thyroid drugs	Caution with thyroid drugs.

ANTIDEPRESSANTS/OCD AGENTS *(cont.)*

Tricyclic Antidepressants

Clomipramine HCl (Anafranil)	
Anticholinergics	Caution with anticholinergics.
Clonidine	May block effects of clonidine.
CNS depressants	Additive effects with CNS depressants (eg, barbiturates, alcohol).
CNS drugs	Caution with CNS drugs.
CYP2D6 inhibitors	Increased levels with CYP2D6 inhibitors (eg, quinidine, cimetidine, SSRIs).
CYP2D6 substrates	Increased levels with CYP2D6 substrates (eg, phenothiazines, propafenone, flecainide).
Enzyme inducers	Decreased levels with enzyme inducers (eg, barbiturates, phenytoin).
Fluoxetine	At least 5 weeks must elapse before starting TCA therapy after fluoxetine discontinuation.
Guanethidine	May block effects of guanethidine.
Haloperidol	Increased levels with haloperidol.
MAOIs	MAOI use during or within 14 days of administration is contraindicated.
Methylphenidate	Increased levels with methylphenidate.
Neuroleptics	NMS reported with neuroleptics.
Phenobarbital	Increases phenobarbital plasma levels.
Protein-bound drugs	Increased levels of highly protein-bound drugs (eg, warfarin, digoxin).
Sympathomimetics	Caution with sympathomimetics.
Thyroid drugs	Caution with thyroid drugs.
Desipramine HCl (Norpramin)	
Alcohol	Exaggerates response to alcohol.
Anticholinergics	Monitor with other anticholinergics.
Benzodiazepines	Additive sedative effects with benzodiazepines (eg, diazepam, chlordiazepoxide).
CNS depressants	Additive sedative effects with other CNS depressants (eg, sedative-hypnotics, psychotropics).
CYP2D6 inhibitors	Increased levels with CYP2D6 inhibitors (eg, quinidine, cimetidine, SSRIs).
CYP2D6 substrates	Potentiated by substrates of CYP2D6 (eg, other antidepressants, phenothiazines, propafenone, flecainide).
Guanethidine	May block effects of guanethidine.
MAOIs	MAOI use during or within 14 days of administration is contraindicated.
Sympathomimetics	Monitor with other sympathomimetic drugs.
Thyroid drugs	Caution with thyroid medications.
Doxepin HCl (Sinequan)	
Alcohol	Increased danger of overdose with alcohol.
Anticholinergics	Increased side effects with anticholinergics.

Table 18.2. DRUG INTERACTIONS FOR PSYCHOACTIVE DRUGS *(cont.)*

ANTIDEPRESSANTS/OCD AGENTS *(cont.)*

Tricyclic Antidepressants

Doxepin HCl (Sinequan) *(cont.)*	
CYP2D6 inhibitors	Potentiated by CYP2D6 inhibitors (eg, cimetidine, quinidine, SSRIs).
CYP2D6 substrates	Potentiated by CYP2D6 substrates (eg, other antidepressants, phenothiazines, propafenone, flecainide); use caution with coadministration.
MAOIs	Avoid within 2 weeks of MAOI therapy.
TCAs	Caution when switching from TCAs to SSRIs (≥5 weeks may be needed before initiating TCA treatment after withdrawal from fluoxetine).
Tolazamide	Hypoglycemia reported with fluoxetine.
Imipramine HCl (Tofranil), **Imipramine Pamoate** (Tofranil-PM)	
Alcohol	Additive effects with alcohol.
Anticholinergics	Additive effects with anticholinergics. Paralytic ileus with anticholinergics.
Blood pressure lowering drugs	Caution with drugs that lower BP.
Clonidine	May block effects of clonidine
CNS depressants	Additive effects with CNS depressants.
CYP2D6 inhibitors	Increased levels with CYP2D6 inhibitors (eg, quinidine, cimetidine, SSRIs).
CYP2D6 substrates	Increased levels with CYP2D6 substrates (eg, phenothiazines, other antidepressants, propafenone, flecainide).
Enzyme inducers	Decreased levels with enzyme inducers (eg, barbiturates, phenytoin).
Guanethidine	May block effects of guanethidine.
MAOIs	MAOI use during or within 14 days of administration is contraindicated.
Methylphenidate	Increased levels with methylphenidate.
SSRIs	Wait 5 weeks after discontinuing SSRIs before initiating TCAs.
Sympathomimetic amines	Avoid preparations that contain sympathomimetic amines (eg, epinephrine, norepinephrine); may potentiate catecholamine effect.
Thyroid drugs	Caution with thyroid drugs.
Nortriptyline HCl (Pamelor)	
Alcohol	Alcohol may potentiate effects.
Anticholinergics	Monitor with anticholinergics.
Antidepressants	May potentiate effects.
Chlorpropamide	Hypoglycemia reported with chlorpropamide.
Cimetidine	Increased plasma levels with cimetidine.
CYP2D6 inhibitors	May potentiate effects.
Flecainide	May potentiate effects.
Guanethidine	May block guanethidine effects.
MAOIs	MAOI use during or within 14 days of administration is contraindicated.
Phenothiazines	May potentiate effects.
Propafenone	May potentiate effects.

ANTIDEPRESSANTS/OCD AGENTS *(cont.)*

Tricyclic Antidepressants

Nortriptyline HCl (Pamelor) *(cont.)*	
Quinidine	Decreased clearance with quinidine.
Reserpine	Stimulating effect with reserpine.
SSRIs	May potentiate effects.
Sympathomimetics	Monitor with sympathomimetics.
Thyroid agents	Arrhythmia risk with thyroid agents.
Protriptyline HCl (Vivactil)	
Anticholinergics	Risk of hyperpyrexia with anticholinergics.
Cimetidine	Reduced hepatic metabolism with cimetidine.
Cisapride	Use is contraindicated.
CNS depressants	Enhanced response to alcohol, barbiturates, other CNS depressants.
CYP2D6 inhibitors	Use with CYP2D6 enzyme inhibitors (eg, quinidine, cimetidine, other antidepressants, phenothiazines, propafenone, flecainide, SSRIs) requires lower doses for either TCA or other drug.
Guanethidine	May block antihypertensive effect of guanethidine, or similarly acting compounds.
MAOIs	MAOI use during or within 14 days of administration is contraindicated.
Neuroleptics	Risk of hyperpyrexia with neuroleptics.
Tramadol	Enhanced seizure risk with tramadol.
Trimipramine Maleate (Surmontil)	
Alcohol	Alcohol may exaggerate effects.
Anticholinergics	May potentiate anticholinergic effects.
Catecholamines	May potentiate catecholamine effects.
Cimetidine	Cimetidine inhibits elimination.
CYP2D6 inhibitors	Potentiated by CYP2D6 inhibitors (eg, quinidine) and substrates (eg, other antidepressants, phenothiazines, propafenone, fleccainide).
MAOIs	MAOI use during or within 14 days of administration is contraindicated.
SSRIs	Caution with SSRIs; wait 5 weeks after fluoxetine withdrawal before initiating therapy.

Miscellaneous Antidepressants

Bupropion HCl (Aplenzin, Wellbutrin, Wellbutrin SR, Wellbutrin XL)	
Alcohol	Minimize or avoid alcohol; increased seizure risk with excessive use or abrupt discontinuation of alcohol.
Amantadine	Caution with amantadine; use low initial dose and gradually titrate bupropion.
Anorectics	Increased seizure risk.
Bupropion-containing drugs	Avoid other bupropion-containing drugs.
Carbamazepine	May induce metabolism of bupropion; caution with carbamazepine.

Table 18.2. DRUG INTERACTIONS FOR PSYCHOACTIVE DRUGS *(cont.)*

ANTIDEPRESSANTS/OCD AGENTS *(cont.)*

Miscellaneous Antidepressants

Bupropion HCl (Aplenzin, Wellbutrin, Wellbutrin SR, Wellbutrin XL) *(cont.)*	
Cimetidine	May induce metabolism of bupropion.
Cocaine	Increased seizure risk.
CYP2B6 substrates/inhibitors	Caution with CYP2B6 substrates or inhibitors (eg, orphenadrine, cyclophosphamide, thiotepa).
CYP2D6 substrates	Caution with drugs metabolized by CYP2D6 (eg, SSRIs, TCAs, antipsychotics, β-blockers, Class IC antiarrhythmics); use low initial dose and gradually titrate bupropion.
Hypoglycemics, oral	Increased seizure risk.
Insulin	Increased seizure risk.
Levodopa	Caution with levodopa; use low initial dose and gradually titrate bupropion.
MAOIs	MAOI use during or within 14 days of administration is contraindicated.
Nicotine, transdermal	Monitor hypertension with transdermal nicotine.
Opioids	Increased seizure risk.
Phenobarbital	May induce metabolism of bupropion.
Phenytoin	May induce metabolism of bupropion.
Sedatives	Increased seizure risk with excessive use or abrupt discontinuation of sedatives (eg, benzodiazepines).
Seizure threshold, drugs lowering	Extreme caution with drugs that lower seizure threshold (eg, antidepressants, antipsychotics, theophylline, systemic steroids).
Stimulants	Increased seizure risk with stimulants.
Nefazodone HCl	
Alcohol	Avoid alcohol.
Alprazolam	Reduce alprazolam dose by 50%.
Anesthetics, general	Discontinue prior to general anesthesia.
Astemizole	Avoid astemizole.
Buspirone	May increase buspirone levels; decrease buspirone dose to 2.5mg qd.
Carbamazepine	Effects antagonized by carbamazepine.
Cisapride	Avoid cisapride.
CNS-active drugs	Caution with CNS-active drugs.
Cyclosporine	Increases plasma levels of cyclosporine.
CYP3A4 substrates	Caution with drugs metabolized by CYP3A4.
Digoxin	Monitor digoxin.
Epinephrine	Administer no more than 40μg epinephrine in local anesthetic solutions (two cartridges of 2% liodocaine with 1:100,000 epinephrine or its equivalent) within short period with careful aspiration technique; additional anesthetic with vasoconstrictor may be given if vital signs are acceptable.

ANTIDEPRESSANTS/OCD AGENTS *(cont.)*

MISCELLANEOUS ANTIDEPRESSANTS

Nefazodone HCl *(cont.)*	
Fluoxetine	Institute a wash-out period and lower doses if used after fluoxetine therapy.
Haloperidol	Haloperidol may need dose adjustment.
MAOIs	Avoid MAOIs within 14 days of use.
Pimozide	Avoid pimozide.
Protein-bound drugs	Caution with highly protein-bound drugs.
Statins	Rhabdomyolysis (rare) reported with simvastatin and lovastatin.
Tacrolimus	Increases plasma levels of tacrolimus.
Terfenadine	Avoid terfenadine.
Triazolam	Reduce triazolam dose by 75% and avoid in elderly.
Trazodone HCl	
Antihypertensives	Caution with antihypertensives.
Carbamazepine	Carbamazepine decreases levels.
CNS depressants	May enhance response to alcohol, barbiturates, and other CNS depressants.
CYP3A4 inhibitors	Potent CYP3A4 inhibitors (eg, ritonavir, ketoconazole, indinavir, itraconazole, nefazodone) may increase levels.
Digoxin	Increases digoxin serum levels.
MAOIs	Caution with MAOIs.
Phenytoin	Increases phenytoin serum levels.
Warfarin	May affect PT in patients on warfarin.

ANTIMANIC/BIPOLAR DISORDER DRUGS

Carbamazepine (Equetro)	
Anti-malarial drugs	Anti-malarial drugs may antagonize the activity of carbamazepine.
Centrally-acting drugs	Caution with other centrally-acting drugs and/or alcohol.
Clomipramine	May increase plasma levels of clomipramine.
CYP substrates	May induce CYP1A2 and CYP3A4; may interact with any agent metabolized by these enzymes.
CYP3A4 inducers	CYP3A4 inducers may decrease plasma levels.
CYP3A4 inhibitors	CYP3A4 inhibitors may increase plasma levels.
Delavirdine	Co-administration with delavirdine may lead to loss of virologic response and possible resistance to non-nucleoside reverse transcriptase inhibitors.
Lithium	May increase risk of neurotoxic side effects of lithium.
MAOIs	MAOI use during or within 14 days of administration is contraindicated.
Phenytoin	May increase plasma levels of phenytoin.
Primidone	May increase plasma levels of primidone.
Trazodone	Decreases levels of trazodone with concomitant administration.

Table 18.2. DRUG INTERACTIONS FOR PSYCHOACTIVE DRUGS *(cont.)*

ANTIDEPRESSANTS/OCD AGENTS *(cont.)*

Antimanic/Bipolar Disorder Drugs

Divalproex Sodium (Depakote, Depakote ER)	
Amitriptyline	Potentiates amitriptyline.
ASA	Efficacy potentiated by ASA.
Carbamazepine	Potentiates carbamazepine. Efficacy reduced by carbamazepine.
Clonazepam	Clonazepam may induce absence status in patients with history of absence type seizures.
CNS depressants	CNS depression with alcohol and other CNS depressants.
Diazepam	Potentiates diazepam.
Ethosuximide	Potentiates ethosuximide.
Felbamate	Efficacy potentiated by felbamate.
Lamotrigine	Potentiates lamotrigine.
Lorazepam	Potentiates lorazepam.
Nortriptyline	Potentiates nortriptyline.
Phenobarbital	Potentiates phenobarbital. Efficacy reduced by phenobarbital.
Phenytoin	Potentiates phenytoin. Efficacy reduced by phenytoin.
Primidone	Potentiates primidone. Efficacy reduced by primidone.
Rifampin	Efficacy reduced by rifampin.
Tolbutamide	Potentiates tolbutamide.
Warfarin	Monitor PT/INR with warfarin.
Zidovudine	Potentiates zidovudine.
Lithium Carbonate (Lithobid), **Lithium Citrate**	
ACE inhibitors	Avoid ACE inhibitors; risk of lithium toxicity due to reduced renal clearance.
Acetazolamide	Decreased levels of acetazolamide.
Alkalinizing agents	Decreased levels of alkalinizing agents.
Angiotensin II receptor antagonists (ARBs)	Increased plasma levels of ARBs.
Antipsychotics	Risk of encephalopathic syndrome (eg, weakness, lethargy, fever, tremulousness, confusion, EPS) with haloperidol and other antipsychotics; discontinue therapy if such signs occur.
Carbamazepine	Increased risk of neurotoxic effects with carbamazepine.
CCBs	Increased risk of neurotoxicity with CCBs.
COX-2 inhibitors	Increased plasma levels of COX-2 inhibitors.
Diuretics	Avoid diuretics; risk of lithium toxicity due to reduced renal clearance.
Fluoxetine	Fluoxetine may increase and/or decrease lithium levels.
Indomethacin	Increased plasma levels of indomethacin.
Iodide preparations	May produce hypothyroidism with iodide preparations.

ANTIDEPRESSANTS/OCD AGENTS *(cont.)*

ANTIMANIC/BIPOLAR DISORDER DRUGS

Lithium Carbonate (Lithobid), **Lithium Citrate** *(cont.)*	
Metronidazole	Increased risk of toxicity with metronidazole.
Neuromuscular blockers	May prolong effects of neuromuscular blockers.
NSAIDs	Increased plasma levels of NSAIDs.
Piroxicam	Increased plasma levels of piroxicam.
Urea	Decreased levels of urea.
Xanthine preparations	Decreased levels of xanthine preparations.
Valproic Acid (Stavzor)	
Alcohol	Additive CNS depression with alcohol.
Carbamazepine	Carbamazepine may increase clearance. Antagonized by carbamazepine. May potentiate carbamazepine.
Carbapenems	Carbapenem antibiotics may reduce serum levels.
Clonazepam	Clonazepam may induce absence status in patients with absence seizures.
CNS depressants	Additive CNS depression with other CNS depressants.
Diazepam	May potentiate diazepam.
Ethosuximide	May potentiate ethosuximide.
Felbamate	Potentiated by felbamate.
Lamotrigine	May potentiate lamotrigine.
Phenobarbital	Phenobarbital may increase clearance. Antagonized by phenobarbital.
Phenytoin	Phenytoin may increase clearance. Antagonized by phenytoin.
Primidone	Primidone may increase clearance.
Rifampin	Antagonized by rifampin.
TCAs	May potentiate amitriptyline/nortriptyline.
Tolbutamide	May potentiate tolbutamide. Antagonized by tolbutamide.
Topiramate	Concomitant topiramate may induce hyperammonemia.
Warfarin	May potentiate warfarin. Antagonized by warfarin.
Zidovudine	May potentiate zidovudine.

ANTIPSYCHOTIC AGENTS

ATYPICAL ANTIPSYCHOTICS

Aripiprazole (Abilify, Abilify Discmelt)	
Alcohol	Avoid alcohol.
Anticholinergics	Caution with anticholinergic agents, other centrally-acting drugs.
Antihypertensives	May potentiate effect of antihypertensives.
CYP3A4 inducers	CYP3A4 inducers (eg, carbamazepine) may lower blood levels.
CYP3A4 inhibitors	CYP3A4 inhibitors (eg, ketoconazole, itraconazole) or 2D6 inhibitors (eg, quinidine, fluoxetine, paroxetine) can increase blood levels.

Table 18.2. DRUG INTERACTIONS FOR PSYCHOACTIVE DRUGS *(cont.)*

ANTIPSYCHOTIC AGENTS *(cont.)*

Atypical Antipsychotics

Clozapine (Clozaril, Fazaclo)	
Alcohol	Use caution.
Anesthesia	Use caution.
Antihypertensives	Potentiates hypotensive effects of antihypertensives.
Atropine-type drugs	Potentiates anticholinergic effects of atropine-type drugs.
Benzodiazepines	Use caution.
Bone marrow suppressants	Avoid bone marrow suppressants.
Carbamazepine	Avoid carbamazepine.
CNS-active drugs	Use caution.
CYP inhibitors/inducers	Use caution with inhibitors/inducers of CYP1A2, 2D6, and 3A4.
CYP2D6 substrates	Decrease dose with drugs metabolized by CYP2D6.
CYP450 inducers	CYP450 inducers (eg, phenytoin, nicotine, rifampin) decrease plasma levels.
CYP450 inhibitors	CYP450 inhibitors (eg, cimetidine, caffeine, erythromycin, citalopram) increase plasma levels.
Epinephrine	Avoid epinephrine.
Fluvoxamine	Use caution.
Paroxetine	Use caution.
Psychotropics	Use caution with other psychotropics.
Sertraline	Use caution.
Olanzapine (Zyprexa, Zyprexa IntraMuscular, Zyprexa Zydis)	
Activated charcoal	Decreased levels with activated charcoal.
Alcohol	Caution with alcohol.
Antihypertensives	May potentiate antihypertensives.
Carbamazepine	Increased clearance with carbamazepine.
CNS drug	Caution with other CNS drugs.
CYP1A2 inducers	Inducers of CYP1A2 may increase clearance.
CYP1A2 inhibitors	Inhibitors of CYP1A2 may decrease clearance.
Dopamine agonists	May antagonize dopamine agonists.
Fluvoxamine	Increased levels with fluvoxamine; lower olanzapine dose.
Glucuronyl transferase	Inducers of glucuronyl transferase (eg, omeprazole, rifampin) may increase clearance.
Levodopa	May antagonize levodopa.
Paliperidone (Invega)	
Alcohol	Caution with alcohol.
CNS drugs	Caution with other CNS drugs.

ANTIPSYCHOTIC AGENTS *(cont.)*

Atypical Antipsychotics

Paliperidone (Invega) *(cont.)*	
Dopamine agonists	May antagonize the other dopamine agonists.
Levodopa	May antagonize the effect of levodopa.
QTc interval, drugs prolonging	Avoid in combination with other drugs known to prolong QTc interval including Class 1A (eg, quinidine, procainamide) or Class III (eg, amiodarone, sotalol) antiarrhythmics, antipsychotic medications (eg, chlopromazine, thioridazine), antibiotics (eg, gatifloxacin, moxifloxacin), or any other class of drugs known to prolong the QTc interval.
Quetiapine Fumarate (Seroquel, Seroquel XR)	
Alcohol	May increase cognitive and motor effects of alcohol.
Antihypertensives	May enhance effects of antihypertensives.
CNS drugs	Caution with other CNS drugs.
CYP3A inhibitors	Caution with CYP3A inhibitors (eg, itraconazole, ketoconazole, fluconazole, erythromycin).
Divalproex	Divalproex may increase mean maximum plasma levels without affecting absorption or mean oral clearance.
Hepatic enzyme inducers	Phenytoin or other hepatic enzyme inducers (eg, carbamazepine, barbiturates, glucocorticoids) may reduce levels.
Levodopa	May antagonize effects of levodopa and dopamine agonists.
Lorazepam	May reduce oral clearance of lorazepam.
Thioridazine	Thioridazine may increase clearance.
Risperidone (Risperdal, Risperdal M-Tab, Risperdal Consta)	
Alcohol	Caution with alcohol.
Antihypertensives	May potentiate antihypertensives.
Clozapine	Clozapine may increase levels.
CNS drugs	Caution with other CNS drugs.
CYP3A4 inducers	CYP3A4 inducers (eg, carbamazepine, phenytoin, rifampin, phenobarbital) may decrease levels.
Fluoxetine	Fluoxetine may increase levels.
Furosemide	Increased mortality with furosemide in elderly patients.
Levodopa	May antagonize levodopa and dopamine agonists.
Paroxetine	Paroxetine may increase levels.
Valproate	May increase valproate levels.
Ziprasidone HCl (Geodon, Geodon for Injection)	
Antihypertensives	May enhance effects of antihypertensives.
Arsenic trioxide	Use is contraindicated.
Carbamazepine	Carbamazepine may decrease levels.

Table 18.2. DRUG INTERACTIONS FOR PSYCHOACTIVE DRUGS *(cont.)*

ANTIPSYCHOTIC AGENTS *(cont.)*

Atypical Antipsychotics

Ziprasidone HCl (Geodon, Geodon for Injection) *(cont.)*	
Centrally acting drugs	Caution with centrally acting drugs.
Chlorpromazine	Use is contraindicated.
Class IA/III antiarrhythmics	Use is contraindicated.
CYP3A4 inhibitors	CYP3A4 inhibitors may increase levels.
Dofetilide	Use is contraindicated.
Dolasetron	Use is contraindicated.
Droperidol	Use is contraindicated.
Gatifloxacin	Use is contraindicated.
Halfantrine	Use is contraindicated.
Levodopa	May antagonize effects of levodopa and dopamine agonists.
Levomethadyl acetate	Use is contraindicated.
Mefloquine	Use is contraindicated.
Mesoridazine	Use is contraindicated.
Moxifloxacin	Use is contraindicated.
Pentamidine	Use is contraindicated.
Pimozide	Use is contraindicated.
Probucol	Use is contraindicated.
QTc interval, drugs prolonging	Use is contraindicated.
Quinidine	Use is contraindicated.
Sotalol	Use is contraindicated.
Sparfloxacin	Use is contraindicated.
Tacrolimus	Use is contraindicated.
Thioridazine	Use is contraindicated.

Typical Antipsychotics

Chlorpromazine	
α-Adrenergic blockade	Can cause α-adrenergic blockade.
Anesthetics	Potentiates the depressant effects of anesthetics; reduce dose of anesthetics by 1/4 to 1/2.
Anticoagulants, oral	May decrease effects of oral anticoagulants.
Anticonvulsants	Anticonvulsants may need adjustment; phenytoin toxicity reported.
Atropine	Caution with atropine or related drugs.
Barbiturates	Potentiates the depressant effects of barbiturates; reduce dose of barbiturates by 1/4 to 1/2.

ANTIPSYCHOTIC AGENTS *(cont.)*

Typical Antipsychotics

Chlorpromazine *(cont.)*	
CNS depressants	Potentiates effects of other CNS depressants; reduce doses of these drugs by 1/4 to 1/2. Contraindicated with large amounts of CNS depressants.
Guanethidine	May decrease effects of oral guanethidine.
Lithium	Encephalopathic syndrome reported with lithium.
Metrizamide	Do not use with metrizamide (Amipaque®); d/c at least 48 hrs before myelography and resume at least 24 hrs after.
Opioids	Potentiates depressant effects of opioids; reduce dose of opioids by 1/4 to 1/2.
Propranolol	Propranolol increases plasma levels of both agents.
Thiazide diuretics	Thiazide diuretics may potentiate orthostatic hypotension.
Fluphenazine HCl	
Alcohol	May potentiate alcohol effects.
Anesthetics	Reduce dose of anesthetics.
Anticholinergics	May potentiate anticholinergic effects.
CNS depressants	Reduce dose of CNS depressants prior to surgery.
Haloperidol (Haldol, Haldol Decanoate)	
Alcohol	Avoid concomitant alcohol use.
Anticholinergics	Caution with anticholinergics
Anticoagulants	Caution with anticoagulants.
Anticonvulsants	Caution with anticonvulsants.
Antiparkinson agents	Caution with antiparkinson agents.
Epinephrine	Antagonizes epinephrine.
Lithium	Monitor for neurological toxicity with lithium.
Rifampin	Caution with rifampin.
Loxapine Succinate (Loxitane)	
CNS-active drugs	Caution with CNS-active drugs, including alcohol.
Epinephrine	Antagonizes epinephrine.
Lorazepam	Significant respiratory depression and hypotension reported with lorazepam (rare).
Molindone HCl (Moban)	
Calcium sulfate	Tabs contain calcium sulfate; may interfere with phenytoin sodium and tetracycline absorption.
Perphenazine	
Anticholinergic effects	Additive anticholinergic effects with atropine/atropine-like drugs, and exposure to phosphorous insecticide.
CNS depressants	Additive effects with CNS depressants; use reduced amount of added drug. Contraindicated with large amounts of CNS depressants.

Table 18.2. DRUG INTERACTIONS FOR PSYCHOACTIVE DRUGS *(cont.)*

ANTIPSYCHOTIC AGENTS *(cont.)*

Typical Antipsychotics

Perphenazine *(cont.)*	
CYP2D6 inhibitors	Cytochrome P450 2D6 inhibitors (TCAs, SSRIs) may increase levels; lower doses may be required.
Phenothiazines	Additive effects with phenothiazines; use reduced amount of added drug.
Pimozide (Orap)	
CNS depressants	May potentiate CNS depressants (eg, analgesics, sedatives, anxiolytics, alcohol).
CYP1A2 inhibitors	May interact with CYP1A2 inhibitors.
CYP3A4 inhibitors	Avoid CYP3A4 inhibitors (eg, azole antifungal drugs, macrolides, protease inhibitors, zileuton, fluvoxamine).
Fluoxetine	Bradycardia reported with fluoxetine.
Grapefruit juice	Avoid grapefruit juice.
QT prolongation, drugs that potentiate	Avoid other drugs that may potentiate QT prolongation (eg, phenothiazines, TCAs, antiarrhythmics, sparfloxacin, gatifloxacin, moxifloxacin, halofantrine, mefloquine, pentamidine, arsenic trioxide, levomethadyl acetate, dolasetron mesylate, probucol, tacrolimus, ziprasidone).
Sertraline	Avoid sertraline.
Thioridazine HCl	
Alcohol	May potentiate alcohol.
Atropine	May potentiate atropine.
CNS depressants	May potentiate CNS depressants.
CYP2D6 inhibitors	Use is contraindicated.
CYP2D6, reduced activity	Use is contraindicated in patients with reduced CYP2D6 activity.
Fluvoxamine	Increases thioridazine plasma levels; avoid concomitant use.
Phosphorous insecticides	May potentiate insecticides.
Pindolol	Increases thioridazine plasma levels; avoid concomitant use.
Propranolol	Increases thioridazine plasma levels; avoid concomitant use.
QTc interval, drugs prolonging	Use is contraindicated.
Thiothixene (Navane)	
Alcohol	Possible additive effects including hypotension with alcohol.
CNS depressants	Possible additive effects including hypotension with CNS depressants.
Pressor agents	Paradoxical effects with pressor agents.
Trifluoperazine HCl	
α-Adrenergic blockade	May potentiate α-adrenergic blockade.
Anticoagulants, oral	May decrease effects of oral anticoagulants.
Anticonvulsants	May lower seizure threshold; adjust anticonvulsants.

ANTIPSYCHOTIC AGENTS *(cont.)*

Typical Antipsychotics

Trifluoperazine HCl *(cont.)*	
CNS depressants	Additive CNS depression with other CNS depressants (eg, sedatives, narcotics, anesthetics, tranquilizers, alcohol).
Guanethidine	May decrease effects of guanethidine.
Lithium	Risk of encephalopathic syndrome with lithium.
Metrizamide	Avoid with metrizamide (Amipaque®); d/c 48 hrs before myelography, resume 24 hrs post-procedure.
Phenytoin	May cause phenytoin toxicity.
Propranolol	Propranolol may increase levels of both drugs.
Thiazide diuretics	Thiazide diuretics may potentiate orthostatic hypotension.

ATTENTION DEFICIT HYPERACTIVITY DISORDER/NARCOLEPSY AGENTS

Amphetamine Salt Combo (Adderall, Adderall XR) CII	
Adrenergic blockers	Antagonizes adrenergic blockers.
Antihistamines	May counteract the sedative effects of antihistamines.
Antihypertensives	May antagonize the hypotensive effects of antihypertensives.
Chlorpromazine	Chlorpromazine may inhibit the central stimulant effects of amphetamines.
Ethosuximide	May delay the absorption of ethosuximide.
GI acidifying agents	GI acidifying agents (eg, guanethidine, reserpine, glutamic acid, ascorbic acid, etc.) may decrease absorption and decrease efficacy.
GI alkalinizing agents	GI alkalinizing agents (eg, antacids, sodium bicarbonate, etc.) may increase absorption and potentiate effects.
Haloperidol	Haloperidol may inhibit the central stimulant effects of amphetamines.
Lithium carbonate	Lithium carbonate may inhibit the stimulant effects of amphetamines.
MAOIs	MAOIs slow metabolism potentiating effects and possibly leading to adverse effects (eg, toxic neurological effects, hypertensive crisis).
Meperidine	May potentiate the analgesic effects of meperidine.
Norepinepherine	May enhance the adrenergic effects of norepinepherine.
Phenobarbital	May delay the absorption of phenobarbital; concomitant use may have a synergistic anticonvulsant effect.
Phenytoin	May delay the absorption of phenytoin; concomitant use may have a synergistic anticonvulsant effect.
Propoxyphene	May potentiate amphetamine CNS stimulation and can cause fatal convulsions in cases of propoxyphene overdose.
TCAs	Concomitant use may lead to the effects of both amphetamines and TCAs being enhanced.

Table 18.2. DRUG INTERACTIONS FOR PSYCHOACTIVE DRUGS *(cont.)*

ATTENTION DEFICIT HYPERACTIVITY DISORDER/NARCOLEPSY AGENTS *(cont.)*	
Amphetamine Salt Combo (Adderall, Adderall XR) CII *(cont.)*	
Urinary acidifying agents	Urinary acidifying agents (eg, ammonium chloride, sodium phosphate, methenamine therapy, etc.) may increase excretion and decrease efficacy.
Urinary alkalinizing agents	Urinary alkalinizing agents (eg, acetazolamide, some thiazides) may decrease excretion and potentiate effects.
Veratrum alkaloids	May antagonize the hypotensive effects of veratrum alkaloids.
Armodafinil (Nuvigil) CIV	
Cyclosporine	May decrease levels of cyclosporine.
CYP2C19 substrates	May induce CYP2C19 activity and reduce the efficacy of CYP2C19 substrates (eg, phenytoin, diazepam, and propranolol, omeprazole, and clomipramine); dose adjustment may be required.
CYP3A4/5 inducers, potent	Potent CYP3A4/5 inducers (eg, carbamazepine, phenobarbital, rifampin) may decrease levels.
CYP3A4/5 inhibitors, potent	Potent CYP3A4/5 inhibitors (eg, ketoconazole, erythromycin) may increase levels.
CYP3A4/5 substrates	May induce CYP3A4/5 activity and reduce the efficacy of CYP3A4/5 substrates (eg, cyclosporine, ethinyl estradiol, midazolam, and triazolam); dose adjustment may be required.
Dextroamphetamine	Dextroamphetamine may delay absorption.
MAOIs	Caution with MAOIs.
Methylphenidate	Methylphenidate may delay absorption.
Steroidal contraceptives	May reduce the efficacy of steroidal contraceptives during and for 1 month after the discontinuation of therapy.
Warfarin	Monitor PT/INR with warfarin.
Atomoxetine HCl (Strattera)	
β-$_2$ agonists, systemic	Caution with systemic β-$_2$ agonists (eg, albuterol) due to the potentiation of cardiovascular effects resulting in increased heart rate and blood pressure.
CYP2D6 inhibitors	Concomitant use with CYP2D6 inhibitors (eg, paroxetine, fluoxetine, quinidine) may increase levels in extensive metabolizers; atomoxetine may need dose adjustment.
MAOIs	Use with or 2 weeks after an MAOI is contraindicated.
Pressor agents	Caution with pressor agents (eg, dopamine, dobutamine) due to possible effects on blood pressure.
Dexmethylphenidate HCl (Focalin, Focalin XR) CII	
Acid suppressants	Acid suppressants may alter the release of dexmethylphenidate (Focalin XR).
Antacids	Antacids may alter the release of dexmethylphenidate (Focalin XR).
Anticoagulants, coumarin	May inhibit the metabolism of coumarin anticoagulants; dose adjustment may be required.
Anticonvulsants	May inhibit the metabolism of anticonvulsants (eg, phenobarbital, phenytoin, primidone); dose adjustment may be required.

ATTENTION DEFICIT HYPERACTIVITY DISORDER/NARCOLEPSY AGENTS *(cont.)*

Dexmethylphenidate HCl (Focalin, Focalin XR) CII *(cont.)*	
Antihypertensives	May decrease the efficacy of antihypertensives.
Clonidine	Concomitant use with clonidine may lead to serious adverse events.
MAOIs	Avoid use with or 2 weeks after an MAOI.
Pressor agents	Caution with pressor agents (eg, dopamine, dobutamine) due to possible effects on blood pressure.
TCAs	May inhibit the metabolism of TCAs (eg, imipramine, clomipramine, desipramine); dose adjustment may be required.
Dextroamphetamine Sulfate (Dexedrine, Dexedrine Spansules, DextroStat) CII	
Adrenergic blockers	Antagonizes adrenergic blockers.
Antihistamines	May counteract the sedative effects of antihistamines.
Antihypertensives	May antagonize the hypotensive effects of antihypertensives.
Chlorpromazine	Chlorpromazine may inhibit the central stimulant effects of amphetamines.
Ethosuximide	May delay the absorption of ethosuximide.
GI acidifying agents	GI acidifying agents (eg, guanethidine, reserpine, glutamic acid, ascorbic acid, fruit juices, etc.) may decrease absorption and decrease efficacy.
GI alkalinizing agents	GI alkalinizing agents (eg, antacids, sodium bicarbonate, etc.) may increase absorption and potentiate effects.
Haloperidol	Haloperidol may inhibit the central stimulant effects of amphetamines.
Lithium carbonate	Lithium carbonate may inhibit the stimulant effects of amphetamines.
MAOIs	MAOIs slow the metabolism of dextroamphetamine, potentiating its effects and possibly leading to adverse effects (eg, toxic neurological effects, hypertensive crisis).
Meperidine	May potentiate the analgesic effects of meperidine.
Norepinepherine	May enhance the adrenergic effects of norepinepherine.
Phenobarbital	May delay the absorption of phenobarbital; concomitant use may have a synergistic anticonvulsant effect.
Phenytoin	May delay the absorption of phenytoin; concomitant use may have a synergistic anticonvulsant effect.
Propoxyphene	May potentiate amphetamine CNS stimulation and can cause fatal convulsions in cases of propoxyphene overdose.
TCAs	Concomitant use may lead to the effects of both amphetamines and TCAs being enhanced.
Urinary acidifying agents	Urinary acidifying agents (eg, ammonium chloride, sodium phosphate, methenamine therapy, etc.) may increase excretion and decrease efficacy.
Urinary alkalinizing agents	Urinary alkalinizing agents (eg, acetazolamide, some thiazides) may decrease excretion and potentiate effects.
Veratrum alkaloids	May antagonize the hypotensive effects of veratrum alkaloids.

Table 18.2. DRUG INTERACTIONS FOR PSYCHOACTIVE DRUGS *(cont.)*

ATTENTION DEFICIT HYPERACTIVITY DISORDER/NARCOLEPSY AGENTS *(cont.)*	
Lisdexamfetamine Dimesylate (Vyvanse) CII	
Adrenergic blockers	Antagonizes adrenergic blockers.
Antihistamines	May counteract the sedative effects of antihistamines.
Antihypertensives	May antagonize the hypotensive effects of antihypertensives.
Chlorpromazine	Chlorpromazine may inhibit the central stimulant effects of amphetamines.
Ethosuximide	May delay the absorption of ethosuximide.
GI acidifying agents	GI acidifying agents (eg, guanethidine, reserpine, glutamic acid, ascorbic acid, fruit juices, etc.) may decrease absorption and decrease efficacy.
GI alkalinizing agents	GI alkalinizing agents (eg, antacids, sodium bicarbonate, etc.) may increase absorption and potentiate effects.
Haloperidol	Haloperidol may inhibit the central stimulant effects of amphetamines.
Lithium carbonate	Lithium carbonate may inhibit the stimulant effects of amphetamines.
MAOIs	MAOIs slow the metabolism of lisdexamfetamine, potentiating its effects and possibly leading to adverse effects (eg, toxic neurological effects, hypertensive crisis).
Meperidine	May potentiate the analgesic effects of meperidine.
Norepinepherine	May enhance the adrenergic effects of norepinepherine.
Phenobarbital	May delay the absorption of phenobarbital; concomitant use may have a synergistic anticonvulsant effect.
Phenytoin	May delay the absorption of phenytoin; concomitant use may have a synergistic anticonvulsant effect.
Propoxyphene	May potentiate amphetamine CNS stimulation and can cause fatal convulsions in cases of propoxyphene overdose.
TCAs	Concomitant use may lead to the effects of both amphetamines and TCAs being enhanced.
Urinary acidifying agents	Urinary acidifying agents (eg, ammonium chloride, sodium phosphate, methenamine therapy, etc.) may increase excretion and decrease efficacy.
Urinary alkalinizing agents	Urinary alkalinizing agents (eg, acetazolamide, some thiazides) may decrease excretion and potentiate effects.
Veratrum alkaloids	May antagonize the hypotensive effects of veratrum alkaloids.
Methamphetamine HCl (Desoxyn) CII	
Guanethidine	May decrease the hypotensive effect of guanethidine.
Insulin	May alter insulin requirements in patients with diabetes mellitus.
MAOIs	Use with or 2 weeks after an MAOI is contraindicated.
Phenothiazines	Phenothiazines may antagonize the CNS stimulant action of amphetamines.
TCAs	Caution with TCAs; monitor closely and adjust dosages carefully.

ATTENTION DEFICIT HYPERACTIVITY DISORDER/NARCOLEPSY AGENTS *(cont.)*

Methylphenidate (Daytrana), **Methylphenidate HCl** (Concerta, Metadate CD, Metadate ER, Methylin, Methylin ER, Ritalin, Ritalin LA, Ritalin SR) CII	
Anesthetics, halogenated	May lead to a sudden increase in blood pressure during surgery; avoid methylphenidate on the day of surgery.
Antacids	Antacids may alter the release of methylphenidate (Ritalin LA).
Anticoagulants, coumarin	May inhibit the metabolism of coumarin anticoagulants; dose adjustment may be required.
Anticonvulsants	May inhibit the metabolism of anticonvulsants (eg, phenobarbital, phenytoin, primidone); dose adjustment may be required.
Antihypertensives	May decrease the efficacy of antihypertensives.
Clonidine	Concomitant use with clonidine may lead to serious adverse events.
Guanethidine	May decrease the hypotensive effect of guanethidine.
MAOIs	Use with or 2 weeks after an MAOI is contraindicated.
Pressor agents	Caution with pressor agents (eg, dopamine, dobutamine) due to possible effects on blood pressure.
TCAs	May inhibit the metabolism of TCAs (eg, imipramine, clomipramine, desipramine); dose adjustment may be required.
Urinary acidifying agents	Urinary acidifying agents (eg, ammonium chloride, sodium phosphate, methenamine therapy, etc.) may increase excretion and decrease efficacy.
Urinary alkalinizing agents	Urinary alkalinizing agents (eg, acetazolamide, some thiazides) may decrease excretion and potentiate effects.
Modafinil (Provigil) CIV	
Clomipramine	May increase levels of clomipramine.
Cyclosporine	May decrease levels of cyclosporine.
CYP1A2 substrates	May induce CYP1A2 activity and reduce the efficacy of CYP1A2 substrates.
CYP2B6 substrates	May induce CYP2B6 activity and reduce the efficacy of CYP2B6 substrates.
CYP2C9 substrates	May inhibit CYP2C9 activity and potentiate the effects of CYP2C9 substrates (eg, phenytoin, S-warfarin).
CYP2C19 substrates	May induce CYP2C19 activity and reduce the efficacy of CYP2C19 substrates (eg, phenytoin, diazepam, and propranolol, omeprazole, and clomipramine); dose adjustment may be required.
CYP3A4 inducers, potent	Potent CYP3A4 inducers (eg, carbamazepine, phenobarbital, rifampin) may decrease levels.
CYP3A4 inhibitors, potent	Potent CYP3A4 inhibitors (eg, ketoconazole, erythromycin) may increase levels.
CYP3A4 substrates	May induce CYP3A4 activity and reduce the efficacy of CYP3A4 substrates.
Dextroamphetamine	Dextroamphetamine may delay absorption.
MAOIs	Caution with MAOIs.
Methylphenidate	Methylphenidate may delay absorption.

Table 18.2. DRUG INTERACTIONS FOR PSYCHOACTIVE DRUGS *(cont.)*

ATTENTION DEFICIT HYPERACTIVITY DISORDER/NARCOLEPSY AGENTS *(cont.)*

Modafinil (Provigil) CIV *(cont.)*	
Steroidal contraceptives	May reduce the efficacy of steroidal contraceptives during and for 1 month after the discontinuation of therapy.
Triazolam	May decrease levels of triazolam.
TCAs	May inhibit the metabolism of TCAs in CYP2D6-deficient patients (eg, poor metabolizers of debrisoquine) due to inhibition of 2C19.
Warfarin	Monitor PT/INR with warfarin.

OBESITY AGENTS/APPETITE MODIFIERS

Benzphetamine HCl (Didrex) CIII	
Antihypertensives	Decreases effects of antihypertensives.
CNS stimulants	Avoid with other CNS stimulants.
Insulin	May alter insulin requirements.
MAOIs	MAOI use during or within 14 days of administration is contraindicated. Hypertensive crisis risk if used within 14 days of MAOIs.
TCAs	Potentiates TCAs.
Urinary acidifying agents	Potentiated by urinary acidifying agents.
Urinary alkalinizing agents	Potentiated by urinary alkalinizing agents.
Diethylpropion HCl CIV	
Alcohol	Adverse reactions with alcohol.
Anesthetics, general	Potential for arrhythmias with general anesthetics.
Anorectics	Avoid with other anorectic agents (prescription, OTC, herbal products) or if used within prior year.
Antidiabetic drugs	Antidiabetic drug requirements may be altered.
Antihypertensives	May interfere with antihypertensives (eg, guanethidine, methyldopa).
Dexfenfluramine	Valvular heart disease reported with dexfenfluramine.
Fenfluramine	Valvular heart disease reported with fenfluramine.
MAOIs	MAOI use during or within 14 days of administration is contraindicated.
Phenothiazines	Phenothiazines may antagonize anorectic effects.
Phendimetrazine Tartrate (Bontril PDM, Bontril Slow-Release) CIII	
CNS stimulants	Concomitant CNS stimulants are contraindicated; including MAOIs.
Guanethidine	May decrease hypotensive effects of guanethidine.
Insulin	May alter insulin requirements.
Phentermine HCl (Adipex-P) CIV	
Dexfenfluramine	Valvular heart disease reported with dexfenfluramine.
Fenfluramine	Valvular heart disease reported with fenfluramine.
Guanethidine	May decrease effects of guanethidine.

ATTENTION DEFICIT HYPERACTIVITY DISORDER/NARCOLEPSY AGENTS *(cont.)*

Phentermine HCl (Adipex-P) CIV *(cont.)*	
Insulin	May alter insulin requirements.
MAOIs	MAOI use during or within 14 days of administration is contraindicated.
Sibutramine HCl Monohydrate (Meridia) CIV	
Alcohol	Avoid excess alcohol.
Blood pressure increasing drugs	Caution with ephedrine, pseudoephedrine, and other agents that increase BP and heart rate.
CNS-active drugs	Avoid CNS-active drugs.
Erythromycin	Possible decreased metabolism with erythromycin.
Hemostasis, drugs affecting	Caution with drugs affecting hemostasis or platelet function.
Ketoconazole	Possible decreased metabolism with ketoconazole.
MAOIs	MAOI use during or within 14 days of administration of sibutramine is contraindicated and vice versa.
Serotonergic drugs	Avoid other serotonergic drugs (eg, SSRIs, migraine therapy agents, certain opioids).

Chapter 19

Hematologic Drugs

Angelo J. Mariotti, D.D.S., Ph.D.

Hematologic disturbances involve a wide variety of diseases that affect erythrocyte production (anemia or erythrocytosis), leukocytes (leukopenia or leukocytosis), platelets (thrombocytopenia or thrombocytosis), homeostasis (hemorrhage), and normal growth of the lymphoreticular system.

Because various drugs, including hormones, growth factors, vitamins, and minerals, can directly or indirectly influence the blood as well as blood-forming organs, the treatment of hematologic disorders should always be directed to the specific cause of the disorder. Accordingly, proper testing is an important factor in diagnosing the hematologic disturbance. In addition to hematologic disturbances, a variety of locally applied hemostatic agents can also be used to stop troublesome bleeding following surgical treatment.

ANTIANEMIC AGENTS

Special Dental Considerations

Clinical signs of iron toxicity sometimes include bluish-colored lips, fingernails, or palms of hands.

Drug Interactions of Dental Interest

Use of iron supplements reduces the absorption of tetracyclines.

Laboratory Value Alterations

The normal daily recommended intake of elemental iron for adolescent and adult males is 10 mg; for nonpregnant adolescent and adult females, the amount ranges from 10 mg to 15 mg. Common methods to ascertain iron levels in the human body usually measure iron indirectly via hemoglobin levels or hematocrits. For adult males, the normal range of hemoglobin is 14 mg/dL to 18 mg/dL and the normal hematocrit is 42% to 52%. For adult females, the normal range of hemoglobin is 12 mg/dL to 16 mg/dL and the normal hematocrit range is 37% to 47%. Laboratory values falling below these ranges may indicate anemia.

See **Tables 19.1** and **19.2** for general information on antianemic agents.

Pharmacology

Iron supplements provide adequate amounts of iron necessary for erythropoeisis and increased oxygen transport capacity in the blood. Epoetin alfa induces erythropoeisis by stimulating erythroid progenitor cells to divide and differentiate into mature red blood cells.

ANTICOAGULANT AGENTS

Special Dental Considerations

Early signs of overdose include bleeding from noninflamed gingivae on brushing or unexplained bruising on skin or in the mouth. In addition, the patient may exhibit purplish areas on the skin, unprovoked nosebleeds, prolonged and intense bleeding from minor cuts or wounds, or all of these. There is some controversy about whether patients receiving therapeutic levels of continuous anticoagulant therapy need to be removed from drug therapy before undergoing dental treatment (such as root planing or extractions). Although sound reasons exist to continue anticoagulation therapy during dental treatment, there also is a risk of hemorrhage in patients who are at therapeutic levels of anticoagulation. Generally, a patient who is taking anticoagulants and has an international normalized ratio (INR) of <3.0 is considered safe to undergo scaling and root planing. Nonetheless, as the risk of localized bleeding after dental procedures (such as scaling, root planing, and surgical procedures) can increase in a patient who is taking anticoagulants, consult with the patient's physician to determine whether temporary reduction or withdrawal of the drug is advisable.

Drug Interactions of Dental Interest

All drug interactions affecting anticoagulants have not been identified; therefore, monitoring INR is recommended when any drug is added to or withdrawn from a patient's regimen.

Special Patients

Women of childbearing age should use additional nonhormonal birth control to prevent pregnancy when using anticoagulant agents. Anticoagulant use is not recommended during pregnancy or labor and delivery.

See **Tables 19.1** and **19.2** for general information on anticoagulant agents.

Pharmacology

These agents inhibit vitamin K γ-carboxylation of procoagulation factors II, VII, IX, and X in the liver. Heparin potentiates the effects of antithrombin III and neutralizes thrombin.

ANTIDOTES

Special Dental Considerations

In most cases, patients who receive folinic acid are suffering from toxicity (symptoms such as gastrointestinal bleeding and thrombocytopenia) owing to methotrexate, pyrimethamine, or trimethoprim therapy for a neoplasm.

See **Tables 19.1** and **19.2** for general information on the antidote leucovorin.

Pharmacology

The principal use of leucovorin is to circumvent the actions of dihydrofolate reductase inhibitors.

ANTIFIBRINOLYTIC AGENT

Special Dental Considerations

Aminocaproic acid has been used for postsurgical hemorrhage after oral procedures. See **Chapter 4** for further discussion of this and other agents that modify blood coagulation.

Drug Interactions of Dental Interest

Aminocaproic acid and drugs containing estrogen may increase thrombus formation.

Special Patients

In women using oral contraceptives, concurrent use of aminocaproic acid increases the chance of thrombus formation.

See **Tables 19.1** and **19.2** for general information on the antifibrinolytic agent aminocaproic acid.

Pharmacology

This agent inhibits the activation of plasminogen.

ANTITHROMBOTIC AGENTS

Special Dental Considerations

As increased risk of localized bleeding can occur after dental procedures (such as scaling, root planing, and surgical procedures), consider consulting the patient's physician to determine whether temporary reduction or withdrawal of the drug is advisable. It is recommended that these drugs be discontinued 10 to 14 days before any dental surgery. Ticlopidine also may induce neutropenia, leading to microbial infections, delayed healing, and gingival bleeding. Delay dental work if severe neutropenia occurs.

Drug Interactions of Dental Interest

There are additive effects of dipyridamole with aspirin on platelet aggregation. Therefore, there is a risk of increased bleeding when these agents are used with aspirin or nonsteroidal anti-inflammatory drugs (NSAIDs).

Laboratory Value Alterations

- Monitor blood pressure and bleeding times. Normal bleeding times range between 3 and 10 minutes, depending on the method used to determine bleeding times. Normal neutrophil levels are 3,000/cm^3 to 7,000/cm^3.

See **Tables 19.1** and **19.2** for general information on antithrombotic agents.

Pharmacology

These agents either decrease or increase platelet aggregation.

NUTRITIONAL SUPPLEMENTS

Special Dental Considerations

Anemic patients may exhibit pallor in the mouth. Cyanocobalamin and folic acid are dietary supplements used to treat anemia.

Drug Interactions of Dental Interest

Antibiotics can interfere with the assay of serum vitamin B_{12} concentrations or serum folic acid concentrations. Sulfonamides will inhibit the absorption of folate.

See **Tables 19.1** and **19.2** for general information on nutritional supplements.

Pharmacology

These supplements provide adequate amounts of vitamin K or folic acid to prevent anemia.

THROMBOLYTIC AGENTS

Special Dental Considerations

These agents are used intensively for short periods in a hospital setting; therefore, drug interactions are not normally observed in a dental office.

Drug Interactions of Dental Interest

Certain antibiotics (eg, cefamandole, cefoperazone, cefotetan), aspirin, and NSAIDs may increase the risk of bleeding when used in conjunction with thrombolytic agents.

See **Tables 19.1** and **19.2** for general information on thrombolytic agents.

Pharmacology

These agents activate the endogenous fibrinolytic system by converting plasminogen to plasmin.

Adverse Effects, Precautions, and Contraindications

Dental care professionals should be aware of the possible adverse effects of hematologic drugs, as well as precautions and contraindications for their use (**Table 19.1**).

TOPICAL HEMOSTATIC AGENTS

Special Dental Considerations

Bleeding can be an expected sequela of many oral, soft-tissue surgical procedures. Although hemostasis following surgery can often be controlled by direct pressure, electrocoagulation, or suture ligation, other agents are available when the aforementioned procedures are ineffective. These agents can play an important role in helping the dental surgeon to effectively manage post-operative bleeding.

Drug Interactions of Dental Interest

Some of the agents used for topical hemostasis include acrylates, silver nitrate, microfibrillar collagen, epinephrine, thrombin, and more. Any potential drug interaction will be dependent on the agent used to promote hemostasis. For more information regarding possible interactions, see **Table 19.2** for general information on topical hemostatic agents.

Pharmacology

The mechanism of action of these agents can include physical or mechanical barriers against hemorrhage leading to tamponade; caustic agents producing tissue destruction that results in protein coagulation and precipitation; biologic physical hemostatic agents that mimic biological molecules and proteins; and physiologic agents that initiate vasoconstriction or mimic the later stages of the coagulation cascade.

Adverse Effects, Precautions, and Contraindications

Since different topical hemostatic agents have a variety of actions, dental care professionals should be aware of the possible adverse effects, precautions, and contraindications for the particular topical hemostatic drug that they use (see **Table 19.1**).

SUGGESTED READING

Angiolillo DJ, Bhatt DL, Gurbel PA, Jennings LK. Advances in antiplatelet therapy: agents in clinical development. *Am J Cardiol.* 2009;103(suppl 3):40A-51A.

Johnson BS. Antianemic and hematopoietic stimulating drugs. In: *Pharmacology and Therapeutics for Dentistry.* 6th ed. Yagiela JA, Dowd FJ, Mariotti, A, Johnson, BS, Neidle EA (eds). Elsevier Mosby, St. Louis, MO, 2009, pp. 483-502.

Johnson BS. Procoagulant, anticoagulant and thrombolytic drugs. In: *Pharmacology and Therapeutics for Dentistry.* 6th ed. Yagiela JA, Dowd FJ, Mariotti, A, Johnson, BS, Neidle EA (eds). Elsevier Mosby, St. Louis, MO, 2009, pp. 503-527.

Mariotti A. Laboratory testing of patients for systemic conditions in periodontal practice. *Periodontol 2000.* 2004;34:84-108.

O'Donnell M, Kearon C. Perioperative management of oral coagulation. *Clin Geriatr Med.* 2006;22:199-213.

Seyednejad H, Imani M, Jaieson T, Seifalian AM. Topical haemostatic agents. *Br J Surg.* 2008;95:1197-1225.

Stern R, Karlis V, Kinney L, et al. Using the international normalized ratio to standardize prothrombin time. *JADA.* 1997;128:1121-1122.

Wahl MJ. Myths of dental surgery in patients receiving anticoagulant therapy. *JADA.* 2000;131:77-81.

Table 19.1. PRESCRIBING INFORMATION FOR HEMATOLOGIC DRUGS

NAME	FORM/ STRENGTH	DOSAGE	WARNINGS/PRECAUTIONS & CONTRAINDICATIONS	ADVERSE EFFECTS†
COAGULATION MODIFIERS				
Abciximab (ReoPro)	**Inj:** 2mg/mL	***Adults:*** **PCI:** 0.25mg/kg IV bolus given 10-60 min before start PCI, followed by 0.125mcg/kg/min IV infusion. **Max:** 10mcg/min for 12 hrs. **Unstable Angina:** 0.25mg/kg IV bolus followed by 10mcg/min infusion for 18-24 hrs, concluding 1 hr after PCI.	**W/P:** Increased risk of bleeding. Monitor all potential bleeding sites (eg, catheter insertion sites, arterial and venous puncture sites, cutdown sites). Minimize vascular and other trauma. D/C if serious, uncontrollable bleeding, thrombocytopenia, or emergency surgery occurs. Anaphylaxis may occur. Antibody (HACA) formation may occur; risk of hypersensitivity, thrombocytopenia, decreased benefit with readministration. Monitor platelets, PT, APTT, ACT before infusion. **Contra:** Active internal bleeding, recent (within 6 weeks) significant GI or GU bleeding, CVA within 2 yrs, CVA with significant residual neurological deficit, bleeding diathesis, oral anticoagulants within 7 days (unless PT ≤1.2x control), thrombocytopenia, recent (within 6 weeks) major surgery or trauma, intracranial neoplasm, arteriovenous malformation, aneurysm, severe uncontrolled HTN, history of vasculitis, IV dextran use before PCI or during an intervention. Hypersensitivity to murine proteins. **P/N:** Category C, caution in nursing.	Bleeding, thrombocytopenia, hypotension, bradycardia, N/V, back/chest pain, headache.
Alteplase (Activase)	**Inj:** 50mg, 100mg	***Adults:*** **AMI: Accelerated Infusion: >67kg:** 15mg IV bolus, then 50mg over next 30 min, and then 35mg over next 60 min. **≤67kg:** 15mg IV bolus, then 0.75mg/kg (max 50mg) over next 30 min, then 0.5mg/kg (max 35mg) over next 60 min. **Max:** 100mg total dose. **3-Hr Infusion: ≥65kg:** 60mg in 1st hr (give 6-10mg as IV bolus), then 20mg over 2nd hr, then 20mg over 3rd hr. **<65kg:** 1.25mg/kg over 3 hrs as described above. **Stroke:** 0.9mg/kg IV over 1 hr (max 90mg total dose). Administer 10% of total dose as IV bolus over 1 min. **PE:** 100mg IV over 2 hrs. Start heparin at end or immediately after infusion when PTT or PT ≤2x normal.	**W/P:** Weigh benefits/risks with recent major surgery, cerebrovascular disease, recent GI or GU bleeding, recent trauma, HTN, left heart thrombus, acute pericarditis, subacute bacterial endocarditis, hemostatic defects, severe hepatic dysfunction, pregnancy, diabetic hemorrhagic retinopathy or other hemorrhagic ophthalmic conditions, septic thrombophlebitis or occluded AV cannula at a seriously infected site, elderly, any other bleeding condition that is difficult to manage. For stroke, also weigh benefits/risks with severe neurological deficit or major early infarct signs on CT. Cholesterol embolism and internal/superficial bleeding reported. Arrhythmias may occur with reperfusion. Avoid IM injection, noncompressible arterial puncture, and internal jugular or subclavian venous puncture. Caution with readministration. **Contra:** (AMI, PE) Active internal bleeding, history of cerebrovascular accident (CVA), recent intracranial/intraspinal surgery or trauma, intracranial neoplasm, arteriovenous (AV) malformation, aneurysm, bleeding diathesis, severe uncontrolled HTN. (Stroke) Active internal bleeding, AV malformation, intracranial neoplasm or hemorrhage, aneurysm, bleeding diathesis, uncontrolled HTN, subarachnoid hemorrhage, seizure at stroke onset. Recent intracranial or intraspinal surgery, serious head trauma, previous stroke. **P/N:** Category C, caution in nursing.	Bleeding.

†Bold entries denote special dental considerations.
BB = black box warning; **W/P** = warnings/precautions; **Contra** = contraindications; **P/N** = pregnancy category rating and nursing considerations.

Table 19.1. PRESCRIBING INFORMATION FOR HEMATOLOGIC DRUGS *(cont.)*

NAME	FORM/ STRENGTH	DOSAGE	WARNINGS/PRECAUTIONS & CONTRAINDICATIONS	ADVERSE EFFECTS†
COAGULATION MODIFIERS *(cont.)*				
Alteplase (Cathflo Activase)	**Inj:** 2mg	***Adults/Pediatrics:* ≥2 yrs: ≥30kg:** 2mg in 2mL. **<30kg:** 110% of catheter internal lumen volume, not to exceed 2mg in 2mL. If function not restored after 120 min, may instill 2nd dose. **Max:** 2mg/dose. Reconstitute to final concentration of 1mg/mL.	**W/P:** Before therapy, consider catheter dysfunction due to causes other than thrombus formation. Avoid excessive pressure when instilling alteplase into catheter. D/C and withdraw drug from catheter if serious bleeding in critical location occurs. Caution if active internal bleeding, infection in the catheter, any bleeding condition that is difficult to manage, thrombocytopenia, hemostatic defects, or if high risk for emobolic complications. Caution if any of the following occurred within 48 hrs: surgery, OB delivery, percutaneous biopsy of viscera or deep tissues, or puncture of non-compressible vessels. **P/N:** Category C, caution in nursing.	Sepsis, GI bleeding, venous thrombosis.
Aminocaproic Acid (Amicar)	**Syrup:** 1.25g/5mL; **Tab:** 500mg*, 1000mg*	***Adults:*** 5g during 1st hr, then 5mL (syr) or 1g (tabs) per hr. Continue therapy for 8 hrs or until bleeding is controlled.	**W/P:** Avoid in hematuria of upper urinary tract origin due to risk of intrarenal obstruction from glomerular capillary thrombosis or clots in renal pelvis and ureters. Skeletal muscle weakness with necrosis of muscle fibers reported after prolonged therapy. Consider cardiac muscle damage with skeletal myopathy. Thrombophlebitis may occur. Do not administer without a definite diagnosis of hyperfibrinolysis. **Contra:** Active intravascular clotting process, disseminated intravascular coagulation without concomitant heparin. **P/N:** Category C, caution in nursing.	Edema, headache, anaphylactoid reactions, pain, bradycardia, hypotension, abdominal pain, diarrhea, N/V, agranulocytosis, increased CPK, confusion, dyspnea, pruritus, tinnitus.
Anagrelide HCl (Agrylin)	**Cap:** 0.5mg	***Adults:* Initial:** 0.5mg qid or 1mg bid for at least 1 week. **Moderate Hepatic Impairment: Initial:** 0.5mg qd for at least 1 week. **Titrate:** Increase by no more than 0.5mg/day per week. **Max:** 10mg/day or 2.5mg/dose. Adjust lowest effective dose to reduce and maintain platelets <600,000/mcL. Monitor platelets every 2 days during first week, then weekly thereafter until reach maintenance dose. ***Pediatrics:* Initial:** 0.5mg qd. **Titrate:** Increase by no more than 0.5mg/day per week. **Max:** 10mg/day or 2.5mg/dose. Adjust to lowest effective dose to reduce and maintain platelets <600,000/mcL. Monitor platelets every 2 days during first week, then weekly thereafter until reach maintenance dose.	**W/P:** Caution with heart disease, renal or hepatic dysfunction. Perform pre-treatment cardiovascular exam and monitor during treatment; may cause cardiovascular effects (eg, vasodilation, tachycardia, palpitations, CHF). Monitor closely for renal toxicity if creatinine ≥2mg/dL or hepatic toxicity if bilirubin, SGOT, or LFTs >1.5x ULN. Monitor blood counts, renal and hepatic function while platelets are lowered. Increase in platelets after therapy interruption. Reduce dose in moderate hepatic impairment. **Contra:** Severe hepatic impairment. **P/N:** Category C, not for use in nursing.	Headache, palpitations, asthenia, edema, GI effects, dizziness, pain, dyspnea, fever, chest pain, rash, tachycardia, malaise, **pharyngitis,** cough, paresthesia.
Argatroban	**Inj:** 100mg/mL	***Adults:* Thrombosis:** D/C heparin and obtain baseline aPTT. **Initial:** 2mcg/kg/min IV. Check aPTT after 2 hrs. **Titrate:** Increase dose until aPTT is 1.5-3x initial baseline. **Max:** 10mcg/kg/min. **Moderate Hepatic Impairment: Initial:** 0.5mcg/kg/min. **PCI: Initial:** 350mcg/kg bolus with 25mcg/kg/min IV. Check activated clotting time (ACT) 5-10 min after bolus. Proceed with PCI if ACT >300 sec. If ACT <300 sec, give additional 150mcg/kg bolus and increase infusion to 30mcg/kg/min. Check ACT 5-10 min later. If ACT >450 sec, decrease to 15mcg/kg/min and check ACT 5-10 min later. Continue infusion	**W/P:** D/C all parenteral anticoagulants before administering. Extreme caution in conditions associated with an increased danger of hemorrhage (eg, severe HTN, immediately following lumbar puncture, bleeding disorder, GI lesions, spinal anesthesia, major surgery, etc). Caution in hepatic impairment. Avoid high doses in PCI patients with significant hepatic disease or AST/ALT ≥3x ULN. Monitor aPTT. For PCI, obtain ACT before dose, 5-10 min after bolus and infusion rate change, at the end of PCI, and every 20-30 min during prolonged procedures. **Contra:** Overt major bleeding. **P/N:** Category B, not for use in nursing.	GI bleed, GU bleed, Hct/Hgb decrease, hypotension, fever, diarrhea, sepsis, cardiac arrest, N/V, ventricular tachycardia, allergic reactions, chest pain (in PCI).

*Scored. †Bold entries denote special dental considerations.
BB = black box warning; **W/P** = warnings/precautions; **Contra** = contraindications; **P/N** = pregnancy category rating and nursing considerations.

NAME	FORM/ STRENGTH	DOSAGE	WARNINGS/PRECAUTIONS & CONTRAINDICATIONS	ADVERSE EFFECTS†
Argatroban *(cont.)*		dose at therapeutic ACT (300-450 sec) during procedure. May give additional 150mcg/kg bolus and increase infusion to 40mcg/kg/min if dissection, impending abrupt closure, thrombus formation, or inability to achieve/ maintain ACT >300 sec. After PCI, may use lower infusion rate if anticoagulation is needed.		
Aspirin (Halfprin) OTC	**Tab, Delayed-Release:** 81mg, 162mg	***Adults:*** 162mg as soon as MI suspected; continue qd for 30 days. May need to continue as prophylaxis for recurrent MI. Crush, chew, or suck the 1st dose.	**W/P:** Caution with marked HTN or renal dysfunction; monitor renal function with long-term therapy. **P/N:** Safety in pregnancy and nursing not known.	Stomach pain, heartburn, N/V, GI bleeding, small increases in BP.
Aspirin/ Dipyridamole (Aggrenox)	**Cap:** (Dipyridamole Extended-Release/ASA) 200mg-25mg	***Adults:*** 1 cap bid (am and pm).	**W/P:** Increased risk of bleeding with chronic, heavy alcohol use. Caution with inherited or acquired bleeding disorders, severe CAD, and hypotension. Monitor for signs of GI ulcers and bleeding. Avoid with history of peptic ulcer disease, severe renal failure (CrCl <10mL/ min). Risk of hepatic dysfunction. Not interchangeable with individual components of ASA and Persantine tabs. Avoid in 3rd trimester of pregnancy. **Contra:** NSAID allergy, children or teenagers with viral infections, syndrome of asthma, rhinitis, nasal polyps. **P/N:** Category D, caution in nursing.	Headache, dyspepsia, abdominal pain, N/V, diarrhea, fatigue, arthralgia, pain, hemorrhage.
Bivalirudin (Angiomax)	**Inj:** 250mg	***Adults:*** **Initial:** 0.75mg/kg IV bolus, then 1.75mg/kg/hr for duration of PCI procedure. Additional bolus of 0.3mg/ kg can be given if needed based on ACT. Continuation of infusion for up to 4 hrs post-procedure is optional. After 4 hrs, if needed, an additional 0.2mg/kg/hr IV for up to 20 hrs may be initiated. **Renal Impairment: CrCl <30mL/min:** 1mg/kg/hr infusion. **Hemodialysis:** 0.25mg/kg/hr infusion. Reduction in bolus dose not necessary; monitor anticoagulation.	**W/P:** Not for IM administration. Hemorrhage can occur at any site. D/C with unexplained symptom, fall in BP or Hct. There is no known antidote to treatment, but can be hemodialyzable. Caution when used during brachytherapy procedures. **Contra:** Active major bleeding. **P/N:** Category B, caution in nursing.	Bleeding, back pain, pain, N/V, headache, hypotension, HTN, bradycardia, dyspepsia, urinary retention, insomnia, anxiety, abdominal pain, fever, nervousness.
Cilostazol (Pletal)	**Tab:** 50mg, 100mg	***Adults:*** 100mg bid, 1/2 hr before or 2 hrs after breakfast and dinner. **Concomitant CYP3A4 and CYP2C19 Inhibitors:** Consider 50mg bid.	**BB:** Contraindicated with CHF of any severity due to possible decrease in survival. **W/P:** Risks not known in patients with severe underlying heart disease, moderate or severe hepatic impairment, or with long-term use. Rare cases of thrombocytopenia or leukopenia reported. **Contra:** CHF of any severity. Hemostatic disorders or active pathologic bleeding (eg, peptic ulcer, intracranial bleeding). **P/N:** Category C, not for use in nursing.	Headache, palpitation, tachycardia, abnormal stool, diarrhea, peripheral edema, dizziness, infection, rhinitis, blood pressure increase, aplastic anemia.
Clopidogrel Bisulfate (Plavix)	**Tab:** 75mg, 300mg	***Adults:*** **MI/Stroke/PAD:** 75mg qd. **Acute Coronary Syndrome:** Take with 75-325mg ASA qd. **LD:** 300mg. **Maint:** 75mg qd. **STEMI:** 75mg, with 75-325mg ASA, qd with or without LD.	**W/P:** Caution with risk of increased bleeding, ulcers or lesions with a propensity to bleed, severe hepatic or renal impairment. D/C 5 days before surgery if antiplatelet effect is not desired. Monitor blood cell count and other appropriate tests if symptoms of bleeding or undesirable hematological effects arise. Thrombotic thrombocytopenic purpura (TTP) reported (rare). **Contra:** Active pathological bleeding (eg, peptic ulcer, intracranial hemorrhage). **P/N:** Category B, not for use in nursing.	Chest pain, influenza-like symptoms, pain, edema, HTN, headache, dizziness, abdominal pain, dyspepsia, diarrhea, arthralgia, purpura, upper respiratory tract infection, back pain, dyspnea.

Table 19.1. PRESCRIBING INFORMATION FOR HEMATOLOGIC DRUGS *(cont.)*

NAME	FORM/ STRENGTH	DOSAGE	WARNINGS/PRECAUTIONS & CONTRAINDICATIONS	ADVERSE EFFECTS†
COAGULATION MODIFIERS *(cont.)*				
Dalteparin Sodium (Fragmin)	**Inj:** (Syringe) 2500 IU/0.2mL, 5000 IU/0.2mL, 7500 IU/0.3mL, 10,000 IU/0.4mL, 10,000 IU/1mL, 12,500 IU/0.5mL, 15,000 IU/0.6mL, 18,000 IU/0.72mL; (MDV) 10,000 IU/mL [9.5mL], 25,000 IU/mL [3.8mL]	***Adults:*** Administer SQ. **Unstable Angina/Non-Q-Wave MI:** 120 IU/kg up to 10,000 IU q12h with ASA (75-165mg/day) for 5-8 days. **Hip Surgery: Pre-Op Start: Initial (if start 2 hrs pre-op):** 2500 IU within 2 hrs pre-op, then 2500 IU 4-8 hrs post-op. **Initial (if start 10-14 hrs pre-op):** 5000 IU 10-14 hrs pre-op, then 5000 IU 4-8 hrs post-op. **Maint (for either initial dose):** 5000 IU SQ qd for 5-10 days post-op (up to 14 days). **Post-Op Start:** 2500 IU 4-8 hrs post-op. **Maint:** 5000 IU qd. **Abdominal Surgery:** 2500 IU 1-2 hrs pre-op. **Maint:** 2500 IU qd for 5-10 days post-op. **Abdominal Surgery with High Risk:** 5000 IU evening before surgery. **Maint:** 5000 IU qd for 5-10 days post-op. **Abdominal Surgery with Malignancy: Initial:** 2500 IU 1-2 hrs pre-op, then 2500 IU 12 hrs later. **Maint:** 5000 IU qd for 5-10 days post-op. **Severely Restricted Mobility During Acute Illness:** 5000 IU qd for 12-14 days. **Symptomatic VTE in Cancer Patients:** 200 IU/kg qd for first 30 days, then 150 IU/kg qd for months 2-6. **Max:** 18,000 IU/day. **Platelet Count 50,000-100,000/mm^3:** Reduce dose by 2500 IU until platelet count ≥100,000/mm^3. **Platelet Count <50,000/mm^3:** D/C therapy until platelet count >50,000/mm^3. **Renal Impairment (CrCl <30mL/min):** Monitor anti-Xa levels to determine appropriate dose.	**BB:** Risk of paralysis by spinal/epidural hematoma with neuraxial anesthesia or spinal puncture. Increased risk with in-dwelling epidural catheters for analgesia, drugs affecting hemostasis (eg, NSAIDs, platelet inhibitors, anticoagulants), and traumatic or repeated epidural or spinal puncture. Frequently monitor for signs and symptoms of neurological impairment. **W/P:** Not for IM injection. Cannot use interchangeably unit for unit with heparin or other low molecular weight heparins. Extreme caution with HIT, conditions with increased risk of hemorrhage (eg, bacterial endocarditis, hemorrhagic stroke, etc.). Hemorrhage, thrombocytopenia, HIT may occur. May increase risk of thrombocytopenia with cancer or acute venous thromboembolism. Caution with bleeding diathesis, platelet defects, severe hepatic/kidney dysfunction, hypertensive or diabetic retinopathy, recent GI bleeding or in elderly with low body weight (<45kg) and predisposed to decreased renal function. D/C if thromboembolic event occurs. Perform periodic CBC, platelets, stool occult blood test. May increase LFTs. Multiple dose vial contains benzyl alcohol. Do not mix with other injections or infusions unless compatibility data available. **Contra:** Heparin or pork allergy, regional anesthesia with unstable angina, non-Q-wave MI, or patients with cancer, active major bleeding, thrombocytopenia with a positive in vitro test for antiplatelet antibody. **P/N:** Category B, caution in nursing.	Hemorrhage, injection-site pain, allergic reactions, thrombocytopenia.
Dipyridamole (Persantine)	**Tab:** 25mg, 50mg, 75mg	***Adults:*** 75-100mg qid.	**W/P:** Caution with hypotension or severe CAD (eg, unstable angina or recent MI); may aggravate chest pain. Elevated hepatic enzymes and hepatic failure reported. **P/N:** Category B, caution in nursing.	Dizziness, abdominal distress.
Enoxaparin Sodium (Lovenox)	**Inj:** (MDV) 300mg/3mL; (Syringe) 30mg/0.3mL, 40mg/0.4mL, 60mg/0.6mL, 80mg/0.8mL, 100mg/mL, 120mg/0.8mL, 150mg/mL	***Adults:*** **Hip/Knee Surgery:** 30mg SQ q12h, starting 12-24 hrs post-op, for 7-10 days (up to 12 days) or 40mg SQ qd for hip surgery for 3 weeks. **Abdominal Surgery:** 40mg SQ qd, starting 2 hrs pre-op, for 7-10 days (up to 14 days). **DVT with or without PE treatment:** (inpatient/outpatient) 1mg/kg SQ q12h, or (inpatient) 1.5mg/kg qd with warfarin (start within 72 hrs) for 7 days (up to 17 days). **Acute Illness:** 40mg SQ qd for 6-11 days (up to 14 days). **Unstable Angina/Non-Q-Wave MI:** 1mg/kg SQ q12h with 100-325mg/day of ASA for 2-8 days (up to 12.5 days). **Acute STEMI (<75 yrs):** 30mg single IV bolus plus a 1mg/kg SQ dose followed by 1mg/kg SQ q12h with ASA. **Max:** 100mg for 1st 2 doses only. **Acute STEMI (>75 yrs):** 0.75mg/kg SQ q12h (no initial bolus) with ASA. **Max:** 75mg for 1st 2 doses only. When given with thrombolytic, give enoxaparin dose between 15 min before and 30 min	**BB:** Risk of paralysis by spinal/epidural hematoma with neuraxial anesthesia or spinal puncture. Increased risk with in-dwelling epidural catheters for analgesia, drugs affecting hemostasis (eg, NSAIDs, platelet inhibitors, anticoagulants), and traumatic or repeated epidural or spinal puncture. **W/P:** Not for IM injection. Cannot use interchangeably unit for unit with heparin or other low molecular weight heparins. Extreme caution with HIT, conditions with an increased risk of hemorrhage (eg, bacterial endocarditis, hemorrhagic stroke). Major hemorrhages (eg, retroperitoneal, intracranial), thrombocytopenia reported. D/C if platelets <100,000/mm^3. Perform periodic CBC, platelets, and stool occult blood test. Caution with bleeding diathesis, uncontrolled arterial HTN, recent GI ulceration, diabetic retinopathy, hemorrhage. Delayed elimination with elderly or in renal dysfunction. Monitor elderly with low body weight (<45 kg) and	Hemorrhage, thrombocytopenia, local reactions (ecchymosis, erythema), anemia, elevation of aminotransferases.

†Bold entries denote special dental considerations.
BB = black box warning; **W/P** = warnings/precautions; **Contra** = contraindications; **P/N** = pregnancy category rating and nursing considerations.

NAME	FORM/ STRENGTH	DOSAGE	WARNINGS/PRECAUTIONS & CONTRAINDICATIONS	ADVERSE EFFECTS†
Enoxaparin Sodium (Lovenox) *(cont.)*		after start of fibrinolytic therapy. With PCI, if last enoxaparin SQ dose was given >8 hrs before balloon inflation, an IV bolus of 0.3mg/kg of enoxaparin should be given. **CrCl <30mL/min: Surgery/Acute Illness:** 30mg SQ qd. **DVT with or without PE treatment (inpatient/outpatient)/Unstable Angina/ Non-Q-Wave MI:** 1mg/kg SQ qd. **Acute STEMI: <75 yrs:** 30mg single IV bolus plus a 1mg/kg SQ dose followed by 1mg/kg SQ qd. **>75 yrs:** 1mg/kg SQ qd (no initial bolus).	predisposition to decreased renal function. Higher risk of thromboembolism in pregnant women with prosthetic heart valves. Not for thromboprophylaxis in prosthetic heart valve patients. Achieve homeostasis at puncture site before sheath removal after PCI. Caution in hepatic impairment. **Contra:** Heparin or pork allergy, active major bleeding, thrombocytopenia with a positive in vitro test for anti-platelet antibody. Hypersensitivity to benzyl alcohol (multi-dose formulation). **P/N:** Category B, caution in nursing.	
Eptifibatide (Integrilin)	**Sol:** 0.75mg/mL, 2mg/mL	***Adults:* ACS:** 180mcg/kg IV bolus, then 2mcg/kg/min IV infusion until discharge, initiation of CABG, or up to 72 hrs. If undergoing PCI, continue until discharge or 18-24 hrs post-PCI. **CrCl <50mL/min:** 180mcg/kg IV bolus, then 1mcg/kg/min IV infusion. **PCI:** 180mcg/kg IV bolus immediately before PCI, then 2mcg/kg/min IV infusion. Give 2nd bolus of 180mcg/kg 10 min after 1st bolus. Continue until discharge or 18-24 hrs post-PCI. **CrCl <50mL/min:** 180mcg/kg IV bolus immediately before PCI, then 1mcg/kg/min IV infusion. Give 2nd bolus of 180mcg/kg 10 min after 1st bolus. See PI for concomitant ASA and heparin doses.	**W/P:** Bleeding reported. Caution with renal dysfunction, platelets <100,000mm^3, femoral access site in PCI. Minimize vascular and other trauma. D/C if thrombocytopenia occurs. Monitor Hct, Hgb, platelets, SrCr, and PT/aPTT before therapy (and activated clotting time before PCI). D/C before CABG surgery. **Contra:** Active abnormal bleeding, history of bleeding diathesis, or stroke within past 30 days. Severe HTN uncontrolled with antihypertensives, major surgery within preceding 6 weeks, history of hemorrhagic stroke, concomitant parenteral glycoprotein IIb/IIIa inhibitor, renal dialysis dependency. **P/N:** Category B, caution in nursing.	Bleeding, thrombocytopenia, hypotension.
Fondaparinux Sodium (Arixtra)	**Inj:** (Syringe) 2.5mg/0.5mL, 5mg/0.4mL, 7.5mg/0.6mL, 10mg/0.8mL	***Adults:* DVT Prophylaxis:** 2.5mg SQ qd, starting 6-8 hrs post-op for 5-9 days (up to 11 days). **Hip Fracture Surgery:** Extended prophylaxis up to 24 additional days is recommended. **DVT/PE Treatment: <50kg:** 5mg SQ qd. **50-100kg:** 7.5mg SQ qd. **>100kg:** 10mg SQ qd. Add concomitant warfarin ASAP (usually within 72 hrs) and continue for 5-9 days (up to 26 days) until INR=2-3.	**BB:** Risk of paralysis by spinal/epidural hematoma with neuraxial anesthesia or spinal puncture. Increased risk with indwelling epidural catheters for analgesia, drugs affecting hemostasis (eg, NSAIDs, platelet inhibitors, anticoagulants), and traumatic or repeated epidural or spinal puncture. **W/P:** Not for IM injection. Cannot use interchangeably unit for unit with heparin or other low molecular weight heparins. Risk of hemorrhage increases with renal impairment. Caution with moderate renal dysfunction, elderly, history of HIT, bleeding diathesis, uncontrolled arterial HTN, recent GI ulceration, diabetic retinopathy, hemorrhage. Monitor renal function periodically. Extreme caution in conditions with an increased risk of hemorrhage (eg, bleeding disorders, hemorrhagic stroke, etc.). Perform routine CBC, SCr, stool occult blood tests. D/C if platelets <100,000/mm^3. Thrombocytopenia reported. Major bleeding with abdominal surgery reported. **Contra:** Severe renal impairment (CrCl <30mL/min), body weight <50kg undergoing hip fracture, hip/knee replacement or abdominal surgery, bacterial endocarditis, active major bleeding, thrombocytopenia with a positive in vitro test for anti-platelet antibody. **P/N:** Category B, caution in nursing.	Bleeding complications, thrombocytopenia, local reactions (eg, rash, pruritus), anemia, fever, N/V, edema, constipation, insomnia, hypokalemia, UTI, dizziness, pupura, hypotension.
Heparin Sodium	**Inj:** 1000 U/mL, 2500 U/mL, 5000 U/mL, 7500 U/mL, 10,000 U/mL	***Adults:* Based on 68kg: Initial:** 5000 U IV, then 10,000-20,000 U SQ. **Maint:** 8000-10,000 U q8h or 15,000-20,000 U q12h. **Intermittent IV Injection: Initial:** 10,000 U. **Maint:** 5000-10,000 U q4-6h. **Continuous IV Infusion: Initial:** 5000U. **Maint:** 20,000-40,000 U/24 hrs. Adjust to coagulation test results. See PI	**W/P:** Not for IM use. Hemorrhage can occur at any site; caution with increased danger of hemorrhage (severe HTN, bacterial endocarditis, surgery). Monitor blood coagulation tests frequently. Thrombocytopenia reported; d/c if platelets <100,000mm^3 or if recurrent thrombosis develops. Contains benzyl	Hemorrhage, local irritation, erythema, mild pain, hematoma, chills, fever, urticaria.

Table 19.1. PRESCRIBING INFORMATION FOR HEMATOLOGIC DRUGS *(cont.)*

NAME	FORM/ STRENGTH	DOSAGE	WARNINGS/PRECAUTIONS & CONTRAINDICATIONS	ADVERSE EFFECTS†
COAGULATION MODIFIERS *(cont.)*				
Heparin Sodium *(cont.)*		for details in specific disease states. ***Pediatrics:*** **Initial:** 50 U/kg IV drip. **Maint:** 100 U/kg IV drip q4h or 20,000 U/m²/24 hrs continuously.	alcohol. White-clot syndrome reported. Monitor platelets, Hct, and occult blood in the stool. Increased heparin resistance with fever, thrombosis, thrombophlebitis, infections with thrombosing tendencies, MI, cancer, and post-op. Higher bleeding incidence in women >60 yrs. **Contra:** Severe thrombocytopenia, if cannot perform appropriate blood-coagulation tests (with full-dose heparin), uncontrollable active bleeding state (except in DIC). **P/N:** Category C, safe in nursing.	
Lepirudin (Refludan)	**Inj:** 50mg	***Adults*:** **LD:** 0.4mg/kg (max 44mg) IV over 15-20 seconds. **Initial:** 0.15mg/kg/hr (max 16.5mg/hr) continuous infusion for 2-10 days. Adjust dose based on aPTT. If aPTT is above target range, stop infusion for 2 hrs and restart at 50% of previous rate. Check aPTT 4 hrs later. If aPTT is below target range, increase rate in steps of 20% and check aPTT 4 hrs later. Do not exceed 0.21mg/kg/hr. **Renal Impairment: LD:** 0.2mg/kg. **Initial: CrCl 45-60 mL/min:** 0.075mg/kg/hr. **CrCl 30-44mL/min:** 0.045mg/kg/hr. **CrCl 15-29 mL/min:** 0.0225mg/kg/hr. **CrCl <15mL/min/Hemodialysis:** Avoid or stop infusion. **Concomitant Thrombolytic Therapy: LD:** 0.2mg/kg. **Initial:** 0.1mg/kg/hr.	**W/P:** Risk of bleeding. Weigh risks/benefits with recent puncture of large vessels or organ biopsy, anomaly of vessels or organs, recent CVA, stroke, intracerebral surgery or other neuraxial procedures, severe uncontrolled HTN, bacterial endocarditis, advanced renal impairment, hemorrhagic diathesis, recent major surgery or bleeding. Avoid with baseline aPTT ≥2.5. Monitor aPTT 4 hrs after initiate infusion and at least once daily. Liver injury may enhance anticoagulant effects. Antihirudin antibodies reported; may increase anticoagulant effects. **P/N:** Category B, not for use in nursing.	Hemorrhagic events (eg, bleeding, anemia, hematoma, hematuria, epistaxis, hemothorax), fever, liver dysfunction, pneumonia, sepsis, allergic skin reactions, multiorgan failure.
Pentoxifylline (Trental)	**Tab, Extended-Release:** 400mg	***Adults:*** 400mg tid with meals for at least 8 weeks. Reduce to 400mg bid if digestive and GI side effects occur; discontinue if side effects persist.	**W/P:** Monitor Hgb and Hct with risk factors complicated by hemorrhage (eg, recent surgery, peptic ulceration, cerebral/retinal bleeding). Occasional reports of angina, hypotension, and arrhythmia in patients with concurrent coronary artery and cerebrovascular diseases. **Contra:** Recent cerebral and/or retinal hemorrhage, intolerance to methylxanthines (eg, caffeine, theophylline, theobromine). **P/N:** Category C, not for use in nursing.	Bloating, dyspepsia, N/V, dizziness, headache.
Phytonadione (Mephyton)	**Tab:** 5mg*	***Adults:*** **Anticoagulant-Induced Prothrombin Deficiency: Initial:** 2.5-10mg up to 25mg (rarely 50mg). May repeat if PT is still elevated 12-48 hrs after initial dose. **Hypoprothrombinemia Due to Other Causes:** 2.5-25mg or more (rarely up to 50mg). Give bile salts when endogenous bile supply to GIT is deficient.	**W/P:** Does not produce an immediate coagulant effect. Maintain lowest possible dose to prevent original thromboembolic events. Avoid repeated large doses with hepatic disease. Failure to respond may indicate a congenital coagulation defect or a condition unresponsive to vitamin K. Avoid large doses in liver disease. Monitor PT regularly. **P/N:** Category C, caution in nursing.	Severe hypersensitivity reactions (anaphylactoid reactions, death), flushing, **peculiar taste sensations,** dizziness, rapid and weak pulse, profuse sweating, hypotension, dyspnea, cyanosis.
Phytonadione	**Inj:** 1mg/0.5 mL, 10mg/mL	***Adults:*** Administer SQ when possible. **Anticoagulant-Induced PT Deficiency: Initial:** 2.5-10mg up to 25mg (rarely 50mg). May repeat if PT is still elevated 6-8 hrs after initial dose. **Hypoprothrombinemia Due to Other Causes:** 2.5-25mg or more (rarely up to 50mg); route depends on severity of condition and response. ***Pediatrics:*** **Prophylaxis of Hemorrhagic Disease in Newborn:** 0.5-1mg IM within 1 hr of birth.	**BB:** Severe, fatal reactions reported during or immediately after IV or IM use. Only use IV or IM route when SC route is not feasible. **W/P:** Contains benzyl alcohol; toxicity in newborns may occur. Takes 1-2 hrs to observe improvement in PT. Maintain lowest possible dose to prevent original thromboembolic events. Avoid repeated large doses with hepatic disease. Failure to respond may indicate a congenital coagulation defect or a	Anaphylactoid reactions, flushing, **peculiar taste sensations,** dizziness, rapid and weak pulse, profuse sweating, hypotension, dyspnea, cyanosis, injection site tenderness or swelling,

*Scored. †Bold entries denote special dental considerations.
BB = black box warning; **W/P** = warnings/precautions; **Contra** = contraindications; **P/N** = pregnancy category rating and nursing considerations.

NAME	FORM/ STRENGTH	DOSAGE	WARNINGS/PRECAUTIONS & CONTRAINDICATIONS	ADVERSE EFFECTS†
Phytonadione *(cont.)*		**Treatment of Hemorrhagic Disease in Newborn:** 1mg SQ/IM (may need higher dose if mother has received oral anticoagulants).	condition unresponsive to vitamin K. Monitor PT regularly. **P/N:** Category C, caution in nursing.	hyperbilirubinemia (in newborns).
Reteplase (Retavase)	**Inj:** 10.4 U	***Adults:*** 10 U IV over 2 min. Repeat in 30 min.	**W/P:** Weigh benefits/risks with recent major surgery, previous puncture of noncompressible vessels, cerebrovascular disease, recent GI or GU bleeding, recent trauma, HTN, left heart thrombus, acute pericarditis, subacute bacterial endocarditis, hemostatic defects, severe hepatic or renal dysfunction, pregnancy, diabetic hemorrhagic retinopathy or other hemorrhagic ophthalmic conditions, septic thrombophlebitis or occluded AV cannula at a seriously infected site, elderly, any other bleeding condition that is difficult to manage. Cholesterol embolism and internal/superficial bleeding reported. Arrhythmias may occur with reperfusion. Avoid IM injection, noncompressible arterial puncture, and internal jugular or subclavian venous puncture. Cholesterol embolism and internal/superficial bleeding reported. **Contra:** Active internal bleeding, history of CVA, recent intracranial or intraspinal surgery or trauma, intracranial neoplasm, arteriovenous malformation, aneurysm, bleeding diathesis, severe uncontrolled HTN. **P/N:** Category C, caution in nursing.	Bleeding, allergic reactions, dyspnea, hypotension.
Tenecteplase (TNKase)	**Inj:** 50mg	***Adults:*** Administer as single IV bolus over 5 seconds. **<60kg:** 30mg. **60 to <70kg:** 35mg. **70 to <80kg:** 40mg. **80 to <90kg:** 45mg. **≥90kg:** 50mg. **Max:** 50mg/dose.	**W/P:** Weigh benefits/risks with recent major surgery, cerebrovascular disease, recent GI or GU bleeding, recent trauma, HTN, left heart thrombus, acute pericarditis, subacute bacterial endocarditis, hemostatic defects, severe hepatic dysfunction, pregnancy, diabetic hemorrhagic retinopathy or other hemorrhagic ophthalmic conditions, septic thrombophlebitis or occluded AV cannula at a seriously infected site, elderly, any other bleeding condition that is difficult to manage. Cholesterol embolism and internal/superficial bleeding reported. Arrhythmias may occur with reperfusion. Avoid IM injection, noncompressible arterial puncture, and internal jugular or subclavian venous puncture. Caution with readministration. **Contra:** Active internal bleeding, history of CVA, intracranial or intraspinal surgery or trauma within 2 months, intracranial neoplasm, arteriovenous malformation, aneurysm, bleeding diathesis, severe uncontrolled HTN . **P/N:** Category C, caution in nursing.	Bleeding.
Ticlopidine HCl (Ticlid)	**Tab:** 250mg	***Adults:*** Take with food. **Stroke:** 250mg bid. **Coronary Artery Stenting:** 250mg bid with ASA up to 30 days after stent implant.	**BB:** Can cause life-threatening hematological adverse reactions, including neutropenia/agranulocytosis, thrombotic thrombocytopenic purpura (TTP), and aplastic anemia. Monitor for evidence of neutropenia or TTP during first 3 months; d/c if any seen. **W/P:** Monitor for hematologic toxicity before treatment, then every 2 weeks for 1st 3 months, and 2 weeks after discontinuation. Monitor more frequently if signs of hematological adverse reactions; d/c if neutrophils <1200/mm^3, aplastic anemia	Diarrhea, rash, nausea, GI pain, dyspepsia, neutropenia.

Table 19.1. PRESCRIBING INFORMATION FOR HEMATOLOGIC DRUGS *(cont.)*

NAME	FORM/ STRENGTH	DOSAGE	WARNINGS/PRECAUTIONS & CONTRAINDICATIONS	ADVERSE EFFECTS†
COAGULATION MODIFIERS *(cont.)*				
Ticlopidine HCl (Ticlid) *(cont.)*			or TTP occurs. D/C 10-14 days before surgery. Caution in trauma, surgery, bleeding disorders. May need dose adjustment with renal or hepatic impairment. May elevate LFTs, TG, and cholesterol. **Contra:** Hematopoietic disorders (eg, neutropenia, thrombocytopenia), history of TTP or aplastic anemia, hemostatic disorders, active pathological bleeding, severe liver impairment. **P/N:** Category B, not for use in nursing.	
Tinzaparin Sodium (Innohep)	**Inj:** 20,000 anti-Xa IU/mL	***Adults:*** 175 anti-Xa IU/kg SQ qd for at least 6 days and until anticoagulated with warfarin (INR is at least 2 for 2 days). Begin warfarin within 1-3 days of therapy.	**BB:** Risk of paralysis by spinal/epidural hematoma with neuraxial anesthesia or spinal puncture. Increased risk with indwelling epidural catheters for analgesia, drugs affecting hemostasis (eg, NSAIDs, platelet inhibitors, anticoagulants), and traumatic or repeated epidural or spinal puncture. **W/P:** Not for IM injection. Cannot use interchangeably unit for unit with heparin or other low molecular weight heparins. Extreme caution in conditions with an increased risk of hemorrhage (eg, bacterial endocarditis, hemorrhagic stroke). Bleeding can occur at any site during therapy. D/C if severe hemorrhage occurs. Perform periodic CBC, platelets, and stool occult blood test. Asymptomatic increase in AST and ALT. Priapism reported (rare). Thrombocytopenia can occur; d/c if platelets <100,000/mm^3. Multiple dose vial contains benzyl alcohol. Contains sodium metabisulfite. Caution with bleeding diathesis, uncontrolled arterial HTN, recent GI ulceration, diabetic retinopathy, hemorrhage. Reduced elimination with elderly or in renal dysfunction; use with caution. **Contra:** Heparin, sulfite, benzoyl alcohol, or pork allergy. Active major bleeding, with or history of heparin-induced thrombocytopenia (HIT). **P/N:** Category B, caution use in nursing.	Hemorrhage, thrombocytopenia, elevated LFTs, local reactions (ecchymosis, hematoma), hypersensitivity reactions.
Tirofiban HCl (Aggrastat)	**Inj:** 0.05mg/mL, 0.25mg/mL	***Adults:*** **Initial:** 0.4mcg/kg/min IV for 30 min. **Maint:** 0.1mcg/kg/min IV. Continue through angiography and for 12-24 hrs after angioplasty or atherectomy. **CrCl <30mL/min:** Administer at half of usual rate of infusion.	**W/P:** Bleeding reported. Monitor platelets, Hgb, Hct before treatment, within 6 hrs after loading infusion, and daily during therapy. Monitor platelets earlier if previous GP IIb/IIIa inhibitor use. Determine aPTT before and during therapy with heparin. Caution with platelets <150,000/mm^3, hemorrhagic retinopathy, chronic hemodialysis patients, femoral access site in percutaneous coronary intervention. Minimize vascular and other trauma. D/C if thrombocytopenia confirmed or if bleeding cannot be controlled by pressure. **Contra:** Active internal bleeding, acute pericarditis, severe HTN, concomitant parenteral GP IIb/IIIa inhibitor, hemorrhagic stroke, aortic dissection, thrombocytopenia with prior exposure. Bleeding diathesis, stroke, major surgical procedure, or severe physical trauma within past 30 days. History of intracranial hemorrhage or neoplasm, arteriovenous malformation, aneurysm. **P/N:** Category B, not for use in nursing.	Bleeding, nausea, fever, headache, edema, anaphylaxis.

†Bold entries denote special dental considerations.
BB = black box warning; **W/P** = warnings/precautions; **Contra** = contraindications; **P/N** = pregnancy category rating and nursing considerations.

NAME	FORM/ STRENGTH	DOSAGE	WARNINGS/PRECAUTIONS & CONTRAINDICATIONS	ADVERSE EFFECTS†
Urokinase (Abbokinase)	**Inj:** 250,000 IU	***Adults:*** **LD:** 4400 IU/kg IV at 90mL/hr over 10 min. **Maint:** 4400 IU/kg/hr IV at 15mL/hr for 12 hrs. Flush line after each cycle. For IV use only.	**W/P:** Prior to use obtain Hct, platelet count, and aPTT. Increased risk of bleeding; fatalities due to hemorrhage, including intracranial and retroperitoneal, reported. Avoid IM injections, nonessential patient handling, frequent venipunctures. Use upper extremity vessels when performing arterial punctures. Increased risk of bleeding with recent (within 10 days) major surgery, obstetrical delivery, organ biopsy, previous puncture of noncompressible vessels, serious GI bleeding, high likelihood of left heart thrombus, subacute bacterial endocarditis, hemostatic defects including those secondary to severe hepatic or renal disease, pregnancy, cerebrovascular disease, diabetic hemorrhagic retinopathy, and any other condition in which bleeding may be a significant hazard or difficult to manage. May carry risk of transmitting infectious agents. **Contra:** Active internal bleeding, intracranial neoplasm, arteriovenous malformation, aneurysm, bleeding diathesis, severe uncontrolled arterial HTN. Recent (within 2 months) CVA, intracranial or intraspinal surgery, trauma including resuscitation. **P/N:** Category B, caution in nursing.	Bleeding, fatal hemorrhage, anaphylaxis, allergic-type or infusion reactions.
Warfarin Sodium (Coumadin, Jantoven)	**Inj:** (Coumadin) 5mg; **Tab:** (Coumadin, Jantoven) 1mg*, 2mg*, 2.5mg*, 3mg*, 4mg*, 5mg*, 6mg*, 7.5mg*, 10mg*	***Adults:*** **≥18 yrs:** Adjust dose based on PT/INR. Give IV as alternate to PO. **Initial:** 2-5mg qd. **Usual:** 2-10mg qd. **Venous Thromboembolism (including pulmonary embolism):** INR 2-3. **Atrial Fibrillation:** INR 2-3. **Post-MI:** Initiate 2-4 weeks post-infarct and maintain INR 2.5-3.5. **Mechanical/Bioprosthetic Heart Valve:** INR 2-3 for 12 weeks after valve insertion, then INR 2.5-3.5 long term.	**BB:** May cause major or fatal bleeding; monitor INR regularly. **W/P:** Monitor PT/INR; many endogenous and exogenous factors may affect PT/INR. Weigh benefits/risks with severe-moderate hepatic or renal insufficiency, infectious disease, intestinal flora disturbance, lactation, surgery, trauma, severe-moderate HTN, protein C deficiency, polycythemia vera, vasculitis, severe DM, indwelling catheters. D/C if tissue necrosis, systemic cholesterol microembolization (purple toe syndrome) occurs. Caution with HIT, DVT, elderly. Warfarin resistance, allergic reactions reported. **Contra:** Hemorrhagic tendencies, blood dyscrasias, CNS surgery, ophthalmic or traumatic surgery, inadequate lab facility, threatened abortion, eclampsia, preeclampsia, major regional lumbar block anesthesia, malignant HTN, pregnancy, and unsupervised senile, alcoholic, or psychotic patients. Bleeding of GI, GU, or respiratory tract, aneurysms, pericarditis and pericardial effusion, bacterial endocarditis, cerebrovascular hemorrhage, spinal puncture, procedures with potential for uncontrollable bleeding. **P/N:** Category X, weigh benefits/risks with nursing.	Tissue or organ hemorrhage/ necrosis, paresthesia, vasculitis, fever, rash, abdominal pain, hepatic disorders, fatigue, headache, alopecia.
ERYTHROPOIESIS AGENTS				
Darbepoetin Alfa (Aranesp)	**Inj: Syringe:** 0.025mg/ 0.42mL, 0.04mg/ 0.4mL, 0.06mg/ 0.3mL, 0.1mg/ 0.5mL, 0.15mg/ 0.3mL, 0.2mg/ 0.4mL, 0.3mg/ 0.6mL, 0.5mg/mL;	***Adults:*** **CRF: Initial:** 0.45mcg/kg IV/ SQ weekly. **Titrate:** Adjust to target Hgb <12g/dL. If Hgb increases >1g/dL in a 2-week period or is approaching 12g/dL, decrease dose by 25%. If Hgb continues to increase, hold dose until Hgb begins to decrease, and reinitiate at 25% below previous dose. Do not increase more than once monthly. **Conversion from Epoetin Alfa:** Base	**BB:** Increased mortality, serious cardiovascular/thromboembolic events, and increased risk of tumor progession or recurrence. (Renal Failure) Patients experienced greater risks for death and serious cardiovascular events when administered erythropoiesis-stimulating agents (ESAs) to target higher vs lower Hgb levels (13.5 vs 11.3 g/dL; 14 vs 10 g/dL) in 2 clinical studies. Individualize	Thrombic events, infection, myalgia, HTN, hypotension, headache, diarrhea, fatigue, edema, N/V, fever, dyspnea.

Table 19.1. PRESCRIBING INFORMATION FOR HEMATOLOGIC DRUGS *(cont.)*

NAME	FORM/ STRENGTH	DOSAGE	WARNINGS/PRECAUTIONS & CONTRAINDICATIONS	ADVERSE EFFECTS†
ERYTHROPOIESIS AGENTS *(cont.)*				
Darbepoetin Alfa (Aranesp) *(cont.)*	**SDV:** 0.025mg/mL, 0.04mg/mL, 0.06mg/mL, 0.1mg/mL, 0.15mg/0.75mL, 0.2mg/mL, 0.3mg/mL	dose on weekly epoetin dose. Give once weekly if receiving epoetin 2-3x/week. Give every 2 weeks if receiving epoetin once weekly. (See PI for details). **Malignancy: Initial:** 2.25mcg/kg SQ weekly or 500mcg once every 3 weeks. **Titrate:** Increase to 4.5mcg/kg if Hgb increases <1g/dL after 6 weeks of therapy. If Hgb increases by >1g/dL in a 2-week period or if Hgb >12g/dL, decrease dose by 40%. If Hgb >12g/dL, hold dose until Hgb approaches a level where transfusions may be required. Reinitiate at 40% below previous dose. ***Pediatrics:*** **≥1 year: CRF: Conversion from Epoetin Alfa:** Base dose on weekly epoetin dose. Give once weekly if receiving epoetin 2-3x/week. Give every 2 weeks if receiving epoetin once weekly. (See Full Prescribing Information for details).	dosing to achieve and maintain Hgb levels within range of 10-12g/dL. (Cancer) ESAs shortened overall survival and/or increased risk of tumor progression or recurrence in clinical studies in patients with breast, non-small cell lung, head and neck, lymphoid, and cervical cancers. To decrease these risks, as well as risk of serious cardio- and thrombovascular events, use lowest dose needed to avoid RBC transfusions. Use ESAs only for treatment of anemia due to concomitant myelosuppressive chemotherapy. ESAs are not indicated for patients receiving myelosuppressive therapy when anticipated outcome is cure. D/C following completion of chemotherapy course. **W/P:** Pure red cell aplasia and severe anemia (with or without other cytopenias) may occur. Due to increased Hgb, increased risk of cardiovascular events, including death, may occur. This includes MI, stroke, CHF, and hemodialysis vascular access thrombosis. Control BP before therapy. Seizures reported. Increased risk of thrombotic events. Evaluate etiology if lack/loss of response occurs. Permanently d/c if serious allergic reaction occurs. Monitor renal function, fluid, and electrolytes. Albumin solution carries risk of transmission of viral diseases. May need interval of 2-6 weeks between dose adjustment and response. Monitor Hgb weekly until stabilized and maintenance dose is established, and for at least 4 weeks after dosage change. Monitor iron status before and during therapy. Increases RBCs and decreases plasma volume. ESAs shortened time to tumor progression in patients with advanced head and neck cancer receiving radiation therapy. **Contra:** Uncontrolled HTN. **P/N:** Category C, caution in nursing.	
Epoetin Alfa (Epogen)	**Inj:** 2000 U/mL, 3000 U/mL, 4000 U/mL, 10,000 U/mL, 20,000 U/mL, 40,000 U/mL	***Adults:*** **CRF: Initial:** 50-100 U/kg IV/SQ 3x/week. IV is preferred route in dialysis patients. **Maint:** Individually titrate. Reduce dose by 25% when Hgb approaches 12g/dL or increases >1g/dL in any 2 week period. Increase dose by 25% if Hgb is <10g/dL and has not increased by 1g/dL after 4 weeks of therapy. **Zidovudine-Treated HIV Patients:** If serum erythropoietin ≤500 mU/mL and zidovudine ≤4200mg/week give 100 U/kg IV/SQ 3x/week for 8 weeks. **Titrate:** Increase by 50-100 U/kg 3x/week after 8 weeks if necessary. **Max:** 300 U/kg 3x/week **Maint:** If Hgb >12g/dL, d/c until Hgb <11g/dL, then reduce dose by 25% when resume therapy. **Chemotherapy-Induced Anemia: Initial:** 150 U/kg SQ 3x/week. **Titrate:** Reduce by 25% when Hgb approaches 12g/dL or Hgb increases >1g/dL in any 2-week period. If Hgb >12g/dL, withhold and then restart at 25% below	**BB:** Increased mortality, serious cardiovascular/thromboembolic events, and increased risk of tumor progession or recurrence. (Renal Failure) Patients experienced greater risks for death and serious cardiovascular events when administered erythropoiesis-stimulating agents (ESAs) to target higher vs lower Hgb levels (13.5 vs 11.3g/dL; 14 vs 10g/dL) in 2 clinical studies. Individualize dosing to achieve and maintain Hgb levels within range of 10-12g/dL. (Cancer) ESAs shortened overall survival and/or increased risk of tumor progression or recurrence in clinical studies in patients with breast, non-small cell lung, head and neck, lymphoid, and cervical cancers. To decrease these risks, as well as risk of serious cardio- and thrombovascular events, use lowest dose needed to avoid RBC transfusions. Use ESAs only for treatment of anemia due to concomitant myelosuppressive	HTN, headache, fatigue, arthralgias, N/V, diarrhea, edema, rash, pyrexia, clotted vascular access, respiratory congestion, dyspnea, asthenia, dizziness, seizures, thrombotic events.

†Bold entries denote special dental considerations.
BB = black box warning; **W/P** = warnings/precautions; **Contra** = contraindications; **P/N** = pregnancy category rating and nursing considerations.

NAME	FORM/ STRENGTH	DOSAGE	WARNINGS/PRECAUTIONS & CONTRAINDICATIONS	ADVERSE EFFECTS†
Epoetin Alfa (Epogen) *(cont.)*		previous dose. May increase to 300 U/kg 3x/week if no response after 8 weeks of therapy. **Max:** 300 U/kg 3x/week. **Weekly Dosing:** 40,000 U SQ weekly. **Titrate:** If Hgb not increased by ≥1g/dL after 4 weeks, increase to 60,000 U weekly. If Hgb >12g/dL, withhold and then restart at 25% below previous dose. Reduce dose by 25% if very rapid Hgb response (eg, increase >1g/dL in any 2-week period). **Max:** 60,000 U weekly. **Surgery:** 300 U/kg/day SQ for 10 days before, on day of, and 4 days after surgery; or 600 U/kg SQ once weekly on 21, 14, and 7 days before surgery, and a 4th dose on day of surgery. ***Pediatrics:*** **CRF: Initial:** 50 U/kg 3x/week IV/SQ. **Maint:** Individually titrate. Reduce dose by 25% when Hgb approaches 12g/dL or increases >1g/dL in any 2 week period. Increase dose by 25% if Hgb is <10g/dL and has not increased by 1g/dL after 4 weeks of therapy. **Chemotherapy Induced Anemia: Initial:** 600 U/kg IV weekly. **Titrate:** If Hgb not increased by ≥1g/dL after 4 weeks, increase to 900 U/kg IV weekly. If Hgb >12g/dL, withhold and then restart at 25% below previous dose. Reduce dose by 25% if very rapid Hgb response (eg, increase >1g/dL in any 2-week period. **Max:** 60,000 U weekly.	chemotherapy. ESAs are not indicated for patients receiving myelosuppressive therapy when anticipated outcome is cure. D/C following completion of chemotherapy course. (Perisurgery) Epoetin alfa increased the rate of DVT in patients not receiving prophylactic anticoagulation. Consider DVT prophylaxis. **W/P:** Pure red cell aplasia and severe anemia (with or without other cytopenias) may occur. Caution with porphyria, HTN, or a history of seizures. Evaluate iron stores prior to and during therapy. Most patients need iron supplementation. Monitor Hct, BP, iron levels, serum chemistry, and CBC. Menses may resume. Multidose formulation contains benzyl alcohol. Increased mortality, cardiovascular, and thromboembolic events in patients with CRF reported. ESAs shortened the time to tumor progression in patients with advanced head and neck cancer receiving radiation therapy. Dose should be carefully adjusted in patients with CRF or CHF. **Contra:** Uncontrolled HTN. Hypersensitivity to mammalian cell-derived products and albumin (human). **P/N:** Category C, caution in nursing.	
Epoetin Alfa (Procrit)	**Inj:** 2000 U/mL, 3000 U/mL, 4000 U/mL, 10,000 U/mL, 20,000 U/mL, 40,000 U/mL	***Adults:*** **CRF: Initial:** 50-100 U/kg IV/SQ 3x/week. IV is preferred route in dialysis patients. **Maint:** Individually titrate. Reduce if Hgb approaches 12g/dL or if Hgb increases >1g/dL in any 2-week period. Increase when Hgb does not increase by 2g/dL after 8 weeks of therapy and Hgb is below target range (10-12g/dL). **Zidovudine-Treated HIV Patients:** If serum erythropoietin levels ≤500 mU/mL and zidovudine ≤4200mg/week, give 100 U/kg IV/SQ 3x/week for 8 weeks. **Titrate:** Increase by 50-100 U/kg 3x/week after 8 weeks if necessary. **Max:** 300 U/kg 3x/week. **Maint:** If Hgb >13g/dL, d/c until Hgb <12g/dL, then reduce dose by 25% when therapy resumes. **Chemotherapy-Induced Anemia: Initial:** 150 U/kg SQ 3x/week. **Titrate:** Reduce by 25% when Hgb approaches 12g/dL or Hgb increases >1g/dL in any 2-week period. If Hgb >13g/dL, withhold until Hgb <12g/dL then restart at 25% below previous dose. May increase to 300 U/kg 3x/week if no response after 8 weeks of therapy. **Max:** 300 U/kg 3x/week. **Weekly Dosing:** 40,000 U SQ weekly. **Titrate:** If Hgb not increased by ≥1g/dL after 4 weeks, increase to 60,000 U weekly. If Hgb >13g/dL, withhold until Hgb <12g/dL then restart with 25% dose reduction. Reduce dose by 25% if very rapid Hgb response (eg, increase >1g/dL in any 2-week period). **Max:** 60,000 U weekly. **Surgery:** 300 U/kg/day SQ for 10 days before surgery, on surgery day, and 4 days post-op or 600 U/kg SQ once weekly on 21, 14, and 7 days before	**BB:** Increased mortality, serious cardiovascular/thromboembolic events, and increased risk of tumor progession or recurrence. (Renal Failure) Patients experienced greater risks for death and serious cardiovascular events when administered erythropoiesis-stimulating agents (ESAs) to target higher vs lower Hgb levels (13.5 vs 11.3g/dL; 14 vs 10g/dL) in 2 clinical studies. Individualize dosing to achieve and maintain Hgb levels within range of 10-12g/dL. (Cancer) ESAs shortened overall survival and/or increased risk of tumor progression or recurrence in clinical studies in patients with breast, non-small cell lung, head and neck, lymphoid, and cervical cancers. To decrease these risks, as well as risk of serious cardio- and thrombovascular events, use lowest dose needed to avoid RBC transfusions. Use ESAs only for treatment of anemia due to concomitant myelosuppressive chemotherapy. ESAs are not indicated for patients receiving myelosuppressive therapy when anticipated outcome is cure. D/C following completion of chemotherapy course. (Perisurgery) Epoetin alfa increased the rate of DVT in patients not receiving prophylactic anticoagulation. Consider DVT prophylaxis. **W/P:** Pure red cell aplasia and severe anemia (with or without other cytopenias) may occur. Caution with porphyria, HTN, or history of seizures. Monitor patients with pre-existing CV disease closely. Evaluate iron stores before and during therapy; most patients need iron supplementation. Monitor Hgb, BP,	HTN, headache, fatigue, arthralgias, N/V, diarrhea, edema, rash, pyrexia, constipation, respiratory congestion, dyspnea, asthenia, skin reaction.

Table 19.1. PRESCRIBING INFORMATION FOR HEMATOLOGIC DRUGS *(cont.)*

NAME	FORM/ STRENGTH	DOSAGE	WARNINGS/PRECAUTIONS & CONTRAINDICATIONS	ADVERSE EFFECTS†
ERYTHROPOIESIS AGENTS *(cont.)*				
Epoetin Alfa (Procrit) *(cont.)*		surgery and a 4th dose on surgery day, with adequate iron supplement. ***Pediatrics:*** **CRF: Initial:** 50 U/kg 3x/week IV/SQ. **Titrate:** Reduce if Hgb approaches 12g/dL or if Hgb increases by >1g/dL in any 2-week period. Increase if Hgb does not increase by 2g/dL after 8 weeks of therapy and Hgb is below target range (10-12g/dL). **Maint:** Individually titrate. **Chemotherapy Induced Anemia: Initial:** 600 U/kg IV weekly. **Titrate:** If Hgb not increased by ≥1g/dL after 4 weeks, increase to 900 U/kg IV weekly. If Hgb >13g/dL, withhold until Hgb <12g/dL then restart with 25% dose reduction. Reduce dose by 25% if very rapid Hgb response (eg, increase >1g/dL in any 2-week period). **Max:** 60,000 U weekly.	iron levels, serum chemistry, and CBC. Multidose formulation contains benzyl alcohol, which has been associated with an increased incidence of neurological and other complications in premature infants; these compilcations are sometimes fatal. **Contra:** Uncontrolled HTN. Hypersensitivity to mammalian cell-derived products and albumin (human). **P/N:** Category C, caution in nursing.	
Folic Acid	**Inj:** 5mg/mL; **Tab:** (OTC) 0.4mg, 0.8mg, (Rx) 1mg	***Adults:*** **Usual:** Up to 1mg/day. **Maint:** 0.4mg qd. **Pregnancy/Nursing: Maint:** 0.8mg qd. **Max:** 1mg/day. Increase maintenance dose with alcoholism, hemolytic anemia, anticonvulsant therapy, chronic infection. ***Pediatrics:*** **Usual:** Up to 1mg/day. **Maint: Infants:** 0.1mg qd. **<4 yrs:** 0.3mg qd. **≥4 yrs:** 0.4mg qd.	**W/P:** Not for monotherapy in pernicious anemia and other megaloblastic anemias with B_{12} deficiency. May obscure pernicious anemia in dosage >0.1 mg/day. Decreased B_{12} serum levels with prolonged therapy. **P/N:** Category A, requirement increases during nursing.	Allergic sensitization.
HEMATINICS				
Iron Dextran (INFeD)	**Inj:** 50mg/mL	***Adults/Pediatrics:*** ≥**4 months: >15kg: Iron Deficiency Anemia:** Dose (mL)=0.0442 (desired Hgb-observed Hgb) x LBW + (0.26 x LBW); LBW=lean body wt (kg). See PI for details. **Blood Loss:** Replace equivalent amount of iron in blood loss. ***Pediatrics:*** **≥4 months: 5-15kg:** Dose (mL)=0.0442 (desired Hgb-observed Hgb) x wt + (0.26 x wt). See PI for details. **Blood Loss:** Replace equivalent amount of iron in blood loss.	**BB:** Anaphylactic-type reactions and death possible. Only use when indication clearly established and lab investigations confirm iron deficient state not amenable to oral therapy. **W/P:** Large IV doses associated with increased incidence of adverse effects. Caution with serious hepatic impairment, significant allergies, asthma. Avoid during acute phase of infectious kidney disease. May exacerbate cardiovascular complications in pre-existing cardiovascular disease and joint pain or swelling in rheumatoid arthritis. Hypersensitivity reactions reported after uneventful test doses. Unwarranted therapy can cause exogenous hemosiderosis. Have epinephrine (1:1000) available. Risk of carcinogenesis with IM use. Give 0.5mL test dose before IM/IV administration. **Contra:** Anemia not associated with iron deficiency. **P/N:** Category C, caution in nursing.	Anaphylactic reactions, chest pain/tightness, urticaria, pruritus, abdominal pain, nausea, arthralgia, convulsions, respiratory arrest, hematuria, febrile episodes.
Iron Sucrose (Venofer)	**Inj:** 20mg/mL	***Adults:*** **HDD-CKD:** 100mg IV inj over 2-5 min or 100mg infusion over at least 15 min per consecutive HD session for a total cumulative dose of 1000mg. **NDD-CKD:** 1000mg over a 14-day period as a 200mg slow IV inj undiluted over 2-5 min on 5 different occasions within the 14-day period. **PDD-CKD:** 1000mg slow IV infusion in 3 divided doses within a 28-day period (2 infusions of 300mg over 1.5 hrs 14 days apart, then 400mg infusion over 2.5 hrs 14 days later).	**W/P:** Fatal hypersensitivity reactions characterized by anaphylactic shock, collapse, hypotension, and dyspnea reported. Caution with administration; hypotension may occur. Monitor hematologic and hematinic parameters periodically. **Contra:** Iron overload, anemia not caused by iron deficiency. **P/N:** Category B, caution in nursing.	Headache, fever, pain, asthenia, malaise, hypotension, chest pain, HTN, hypervolemia, nausea, vomiting, elevated LFTs, dizziness, cramps, musculoskeletal pain, dyspnea, **cough,** pruritus, application site reaction.

†Bold entries denote special dental considerations.
BB = black box warning; **W/P** = warnings/precautions; **Contra** = contraindications; **P/N** = pregnancy category rating and nursing considerations.

NAME	FORM/ STRENGTH	DOSAGE	WARNINGS/PRECAUTIONS & CONTRAINDICATIONS	ADVERSE EFFECTS†
Sodium Ferric Gluconate Complex (Ferrlecit)	**Inj:** 62.5mg elemental iron/5mL	***Adults:*** 10mL (125mg) as IV infusion (diluted) over 1 hr or as slow IV injection (undiluted) at a rate of up to 12.5mg/min. **Minimum Cumulative Dose:** 1g elemental iron over 8 sequential dialysis sessions. ***Pediatrics:*** **≥6 yrs:** 0.12mL/kg (1.5mg/kg) as IV infusion over 1 hr at 8 sequential dialysis sessions. **Max:** 125mg/dose.	**W/P:** Hypersensitivity reactions and hypotension reported. Iron overload is more common in patients with hemoglobinopathies and other refractory anemia. Should not be administered to patients with iron overload. Contains benzyl alcohol; avoid in neonates. **Contra:** Anemia not associated with iron deficiency. Evidence of iron overload. **P/N:** Category B, caution in nursing.	Injection site reactions, chest pain, pain, asthenia, headache, abdominal pain, cramps, dizziness, dyspnea, hypotension, HTN, N/V, diarrhea, leg cramps, pruritus, abnormal erythrocytes.
HEMATOPOIETIC AGENTS				
Oprelvekin (Neumega)	**Inj:** 5mg	***Adults:*** 50mcg/kg qd SQ. **Severe renal impairment CrCl <30mL/min:** 25mcg/kg qd SQ. Initiate 6-24 hrs after chemotherapy completion. Monitor platelets to assess optimal duration of therapy. Continue therapy until post-nadir platelets ≥50,000 cells/mcL. D/C at least 2 days before next chemotherapy cycle. **Max:** 21 days of therapy.	**BB:** Allergic or hypersensitivity reactions, including anaphylaxis, reported; permanently d/c if an allergic or hypersensitivity reaction develops. **W/P:** Fluid retention reported; caution in CHF and patients receiving aggressive hydration. Capillary leak syndrome, pleural/pericardial effusion, renal failure, visual disturbances, papilledema, stroke, and rash reported. Monitor fluid and electrolyte balance with chronic diuretic therapy. Permanently d/c if significant allergic reactions occur. Moderate decreases in Hgb, Hct, and RBCs reported. Caution with history of atrial arrhythmias. May develop antibodies to therapy. Obtain CBC before therapy, then regularly. Monitor platelets during expected nadir time and until adequate recovery. **P/N:** Category C, not for use in nursing.	Edema, dyspnea, tachycardia, conjunctival injection, palpitations, atrial arrhythmias, pleural effusions, syncope, pneumonia, neutropenic fever, headache, N/V, fever, mucositis, diarrhea.
Romiplostim (Nplate)	**Inj:** 250mcg, 500mcg	***Adults:*** **Initial:** 1mcg/kg SQ based on actual body wt. **Titrate:** Adjust dose by increments of 1mcg/kg until platelet count reaches ≥50 x 10^9/L. **Max:** 10mcg/kg/week. If platelet count <50 x 10^9/L, increase dose by 1mcg/kg. If platelet count >200 x 10^9/L x 2 consecutive weeks, reduce dose by 1mcg/kg. If platelet count >400 x 10^9/L, do not dose; continue assessing platelet count weekly. If platelet count falls to <200 x 10^9/L, resume therapy at a dose reduced by 1mcg/kg. D/C if platelet count does not increase to ≥50 x 10^9/L after 4 weeks of therapy; obtain CBCs and platelet counts weekly for 2 weeks.	**W/P:** May increase risk for development or progression of reticulin fiber deposition within the bone marrow. Examine peripheral blood smear closely to establish baseline level of cellular morphological abnormalities; d/c treatment if new or worsening morphological abnormalities or cytopenia develop. Discontinuation may worsen thrombocytopenia and increase risk of bleeding. Excessive doses may result in thrombotic/thromboembolic complications. D/C if platelet count does not increase to a level sufficient to avoid bleeding after 4 weeks. May increase risk for hematologic malignancies. Monitor CBCs, including platelet counts, and peripheral blood smears prior to initiation, throughout, and following discontinuation of therapy. Caution in renal/hepatic impairment. Available only through restricted distribution program. **P/N:** Category C, not for use in nursing.	Bone marrow reticulin deposition, worsening thrombocytopenia, headache, arthralgia, dizziness, insomnia, myalgia, pain in extremity, abdominal pain, shoulder pain, dyspepsia, paresthesia.
Sargramostim (Leukine)	**Inj:** 250mcg/vial, 500mcg/mL	***Adults:*** **≥55 yrs: Neutrophil Recovery Post-Chemo in AML: Hypoplastic Bone Marrow with <5% Blasts:** 250mcg/m^2/day IV over 4 hrs starting on day 11 or 4 days after completion of induction chemo. If 2nd cycle of induction chemo needed, give 4 days after completion of chemo. Continue until ANC >1500 cells/mm^3 for 3 consecutive days or max of 42 days. D/C immediately if leukemic regrowth occurs; reduce dose by 50% or temporarily d/c if severe adverse reaction occurs. **Mobilization**	**W/P:** Contains benzyl alcohol; avoid use in neonates. Caution with pre-existing fluid retention, pulmonary infiltrate, CHF, hypoxia, cardiac disease, renal/hepatic dysfunction, or myeloid malignancies. Monitor CBC twice weekly and renal/hepatic function every other week with pre-existing dysfunction. **Contra:** Excessive leukemic myeloid blasts in bone marrow or peripheral blood (≥10%), concomitant chemotherapy or radiotherapy. **P/N:** Category C, caution in nursing.	Fever, N/V, diarrhea, alopecia, rash, headache, stomatitis, anorexia, mucous membrane disorder, asthenia, malaise, abdominal pain, edema, HTN.

Table 19.1. PRESCRIBING INFORMATION FOR HEMATOLOGIC DRUGS *(cont.)*

NAME	FORM/ STRENGTH	DOSAGE	WARNINGS/PRECAUTIONS & CONTRAINDICATIONS	ADVERSE EFFECTS†
HEMATOPOIETIC AGENTS *(cont.)*				
Sargramostim (Leukine) *(cont.)*		**of Peripheral Blood Progenitor Cells (PBPC):** 250mcg/m^2/day IV over 24 hrs or SC once daily. Continue through PBPC collection period. Reduce dose by 50% if WBC >50,000 cells/mm^3. **Post Peripheral Blood Progenitor Cell Transplant:** 250mcg/m^2/day IV over 24 hrs or SC once daily. Begin immediately after infusion of progenitor cells and continue until ANC >1500 cells/mm^3 for 3 consecutive days. **Myeloid Reconstitution After BMT:** 250mcg/m^2/day IV over 2 hrs 2-4 hrs post bone marrow infusion and not less than 24 hrs after last dose of chemo- or radiotherapy. Do not give until ANC <500 cells/mm^3. Continue until ANC >1500 cells/mm^3 for 3 consecutive days. May reduce dose by 50% or temporarily d/c if severe adverse reaction occurs. D/C immediately if blast cells appear or disease progression occurs. **BMT Failure/Engraftment Delay:** 250mcg/m^2/day IV over 2 hrs for 14 days. May repeat after 7 days if needed. Give 3rd course after another 7 days of 500mcg/m^2/day IV for 14 days if needed. May reduce dose by 50% or temporarily d/c if severe adverse reaction occurs. D/C immediately if blast cells appear or disease progression occurs. Reduce dose by 50% or interrupt treatment if ANC >20,000 cells/mm^3.		
IRON SUPPLEMENTS				
Dessicated Stomach Substance/Ferrous Fumarate/Vitamin B_{12}/Vitamin C (Anemagen, Chromagen)	**Cap:** Dessicated Stomach Substance 100mg-Ferrous Fumarate 200mg-Vitamin B_{12} 0.01mg-Vitamin C 250mg	***Adults:*** 1 cap qd.	**Contra:** Hemochromatosis, hemosiderosis. **P/N:** Safety in pregnancy and nursing not known.	N/V, rash, diarrhea, precordial pain, flushing.
Docusate Sodium/ Ferrous Fumarate (Ferro-Sequels) OTC	**Tab, Extended-Release:** (Ferrous Fumarate-Docusate Sodium) 50mg-40mg	***Adults:*** 1 tab qd.	**W/P:** Fatal poisoning reported in children <6 yrs with accidental overdose of iron-containing products. **P/N:** Safety in pregnancy and nursing not known.	—
Ferrous Fumarate (Hemocyte) OTC	**Tab:** 324mg (106mg elemental iron)	***Adults:*** 1 tab up to bid, between meals.	**W/P:** May aggravate existing GI disorders. Ineffective with steatorrhea, partial gastrectomy. **Contra:** Hemochromatosis, hemosiderosis, hemolytic anemia.	Anorexia, nausea, diarrhea, constipation.
Ferrous Fumarate/ Folic Acid (Hemocyte F)	**Tab:** (Ferrous Fumarate-Folic Acid) 324mg-1mg	***Adults:*** 1 tab qd. **Elderly:** Start at low end of dosing range.	**W/P:** Toxic when overdoses are ingested by children. Not for the treatment of pernicious anemia and other megaloblastic anemias where vitamin B_{12} is deficient. Folic acid >0.1mg-0.4mg/day may obscure pernicious anemia. Caution with peptic ulcer, regional enteritis, ulcerative colitis. **Contra:** Hemochromatosis, hemosiderosis, hemolytic anemia, pernicious anemia.	GI disturbances, abdominal cramps, diarrhea, constipation, heartburn, N/V, black stools, allergic sensitization.

†Bold entries denote special dental considerations.
BB = black box warning; **W/P** = warnings/precautions; **Contra** = contraindications; **P/N** = pregnancy category rating and nursing considerations.

NAME	FORM/ STRENGTH	DOSAGE	WARNINGS/PRECAUTIONS & CONTRAINDICATIONS	ADVERSE EFFECTS†
Ferrous Fumarate/Folic Acid/ Minerals/Multiple Vitamin (Hematinic Plus)	**Tab:** Ferrous Fumarate 324mg-Calcium 10mg-Copper 0.8mg-Folic Acid 1mg-Niacinamide 30mg-Zinc 18.2mg-Magnesium 6.9mg-Manganese 1.3mg-Vit C 200mg-Vit B_1 10mg-Vit B_2 6mg-Vit B_6 5mg-Vit B_{12} 15mcg	***Adults:*** 1 tab qd between meals.	**W/P:** May mask pernicious anemia. May aggravate existing GI diseases. Ineffective in patients with steatorrhea and partial gastrectomy. **Contra:** Hemochromatosis, hemosiderosis, hemolytic anemia, pernicious anemia.	Anorexia, nausea, diarrhea, constipation.
Ferrous Fumarate/Folic Acid/ Minerals/Multiple Vitamin (Hemocyte Plus)	**Tab:** Copper 0.8mg-Ferrous Fumarate 324mg-Folic acid 1mg-Magnesium 6.9mg-Manganese 1.3mg-Niacinamide 30mg-Pantothenic acid 10mg-Vit B_1 10mg-Vit B_2 6mg-Vit B_6 5mg-Vit B_{12} 15mc-Vit C 200mg-Zinc 18.2mg	***Adults:*** 1 tab qd between meals.	**W/P:** Folic acid doses above 0.1-0.4mg/day may mask pernicious anemia. Accidental iron overdose may lead to fatal poisoning in children <6 yrs. **Contra:** Hemochromatosis, hemosiderosis, hemolytic anemia, pernicious anemia.	Allergic sensitization, anorexia, nausea, diarrhea, constipation.
Ferrous Fumarate/ Folic Acid/Vitamin B_{12}/Vitamin C (Chromagen FA)	**Cap:** Ferrous Fumarate 200mg-Folic Acid 1mg-Vitamin B_{12} 0.01mg-Vitamin C 250mg	***Adults:*** 1 cap qd.	**W/P:** Accidental overdose of iron-containing products is a leading cause of fatal poisoning in children <6 yrs. Avoid folic acid unless the diagnosis of pernicious anemia has been excluded. **Contra:** Hemochromatosis, hemosiderosis. Folic acid is contraindicated in pernicious anemia. **P/N:** Safety in pregnancy and nursing is not known.	N/V, rash, diarrhea, precordial pain, flushing.
Ferrous Fumarate/ Folic Acid/Vitamin B_{12}/Vitamin C (Chromagen Forte)	**Cap:** Ferrous Fumarate 460mg-Folic Acid 1mg-Vitamin B_{12} 0.01mg-Vitamin C 60mg	***Adults:*** 1-2 caps qd.	**W/P:** Accidental overdose of iron-containing products is a leading cause of fatal poisoning in children <6 yrs. Avoid folic acid unless the diagnosis of pernicious anemia has been excluded. **Contra:** Hemochromatosis, hemosiderosis, pernicious anemia. **P/N:** Safety in pregnancy and nursing not known.	N/V, rash, diarrhea, precordial pain, flushing.
Ferrous Sulfate/ Iron Carbonyl (Feosol) OTC	**Tab:** Feosol Caplet (Iron Carbonyl) 50mg (45mg elemental iron), Feosol Tablet (Ferrous Sulfate) 200mg (65mg elemental iron)	***Adult/Pediatrics:*** **≥12 yrs:** 1 tab qd with food.	**W/P:** Keep product out of reach of children. Accidental overdose of iron-containing products is a leading cause of fatal poisoning in children <6 yrs. **P/N:** Safety in pregnancy and nursing not known.	Nausea, GI disturbance, constipation, diarrhea.
Folic Acid/Iron/ Minerals/Multiple Vitamin (Niferex-PN Forte)	**Tab:** Calcium 250mg-Copper 2mg-Folic Acid 1mg-Iodine 0.2mg-Iron 60mg-Magnesium 10mg-Niacinamide 20mg-Vitamin A 5000IU-	***Adults:*** 1 tab qd.	**W/P:** Fatal poisoning reported in children <6 yrs with accidental overdose of iron-containing products. Folic acid >0.1mg/day may obscure pernicious anemia. High doses of vitamin A may be associated with birth defects. **Contra:** Hemochromatosis, hemosiderosis. **P/N:** Safety in pregnancy and nursing not known.	Constipation, diarrhea, N/V, dark stools, abdominal pain.

Table 19.1. PRESCRIBING INFORMATION FOR HEMATOLOGIC DRUGS *(cont.)*

NAME	FORM/ STRENGTH	DOSAGE	WARNINGS/PRECAUTIONS & CONTRAINDICATIONS	ADVERSE EFFECTS†
IRON SUPPLEMENTS *(cont.)*				
Folic Acid/Iron/ Minerals/Multiple Vitamin (Niferex-PN Forte) *(cont.)*	Vitamin B_1 3mg-Vitamin B_2 3.4mg-Vitamin B_6 4mg-Vitamin B_{12} 0.012mg-Vitamin C 80mg-Vitamin D 400IU-Vitamin E 30IU-Zinc 25mg			
Folic Acid/Iron/ Multiple Vitamin (Niferex-PN)	**Tab:** Calcium 125mg-Folic Acid 1mg-Iron 60mg-Niacinamide 10mg-Vitamin A 4000IU-Vitamin B_1 2.43mg-Vitamin B_2 3mg-Vitamin B_6 1.64mg-Vitamin B_{12} 0.003mg-Vitamin C 50mg-Vitamin D 400IU-Zinc 18mg	***Adults:*** 1 tab qd.	**W/P:** Fatal poisoning reported in children <6 yrs with accidental overdose of iron-containing products. Folic acid >0.1mg/day may obscure pernicious anemia. High doses of vitamin A may be associated with birth defects. **Contra:** Hemochromatosis, hemosiderosis. **P/N:** Safety in pregnancy and nursing not known.	Constipation, diarrhea, N/V, dark stools, abdominal pain.
Folic Acid/Iron/ Vitamin B_{12}/ Vitamin C (Fe-Tinic 150 Forte, Niferex-150 Forte)	**Cap:** Folic Acid 1mg-Iron 150mg-Vitamin B_{12} 25mcg-Vitamin C 60mg	***Adults:*** 1 cap qd.	**W/P:** Fatal poisoning reported in children <6 yrs with accidental overdose of iron-containing products. Determination of type, cause of anemia is recommended before starting therapy. Folic acid >0.1mg/day may obscure pernicious anemia. **Contra:** Hemochromatosis, hemosiderosis. **P/N:** Safety in pregnancy and nursing not known.	Constipation, diarrhea, N/V, dark stools, abdominal pain.
Iron (Niferex) OTC	**Cap:** 60mg; **Sol:** 100mg/5mL	***Adults:*** 1-2 tabs bid or 5-10mL qd. ***Pediatrics:*** **>6 yrs:** 1-2 tabs qd or 5mL qd. **<6 yrs: (Sol):** Individualize dose.	**W/P:** Fatal poisoning reported in children <6 yrs with accidental overdose of iron-containing products. **P/N:** Safety in pregnancy and nursing not known.	—
Iron/Vitamin C (Fe-Tinic 150, Niferex-150) OTC	**Cap:** Iron 150mg-Vitamin C 50mg	***Adults:*** 1-2 caps qd.	**W/P:** Fatal poisoning reported in children <6 yrs with accidental overdose of iron-containing products. **P/N:** Safety in pregnancy and nursing not known.	—
NEUTROPENIA AGENTS				
Filgrastim (Neupogen)	**Inj:** 300mcg/0.5mL, 300mcg/mL, 480mcg/0.8mL, 480mcg/1.6mL [10^s]	***Adults:*** **Myelosuppressive Chemotherapy: Initial:** 5mcg/kg qd SQ bolus, short IV infusion, or continuous SQ/IV infusion. Monitor CBCs and platelets before therapy, twice weekly during therapy. **Titrate:** Increase 5mcg/kg for each chemotherapy cycle according to duration and severity of ANC nadir. Avoid 24 hrs before through 24 hrs after cytotoxic chemotherapy. Perform CBC twice weekly during therapy. Continue therapy after chemotherapy until the post nadir ANC =10,000/mm^3. **BMT:** Following BMT, 10mcg/kg/day by IV infusion of 4 or 24 hrs, or by continuous 24-hr SQ infusion. First dose at least 24 hrs after chemotherapy and at least 24 hrs after bone marrow infusion. **Dose Adjustment:** If ANC	**W/P:** Allergic-type reactions may occur. Rare cases of splenic rupture reported, some fatal. Evaluate for enlarged spleen or splenic rupture if complaints of left upper abdominal and/or shoulder tip pain. Acute respiratory distress syndrome reported with sepsis; d/c until resolved. Sickle cell crisis reported with sickle cell disease; keep patient well hydrated. Potential for immunogenicity. The patient may be at greater risk of thromobocytopenia, anemia, and nonhematologic consequences due to the potential of receiving higher doses of chemotherapy. Regular monitoring of Hct and platelet count recommended. Alveolar hemorrhage manifesting as pulmonary infiltrates and hemoptysis requiring hospitalization reported.	Bone pain, N/V, rash, alopecia, diarrhea, neutropenic fever, mucositis, fatigue, anorexia, dyspnea.

†Bold entries denote special dental considerations.
BB = black box warning; **W/P** = warnings/precautions; **Contra** = contraindications; **P/N** = pregnancy category rating and nursing considerations.

NAME	FORM/ STRENGTH	DOSAGE	WARNINGS/PRECAUTIONS & CONTRAINDICATIONS	ADVERSE EFFECTS†
Filgrastim (Neupogen) *(cont.)*		>1000/mm³ for 3 days, 5mcg/kg/day; increase to 10mcg/kg/day if ANC <1000/mm³. If ANC >1000/mm³ for 3 more days, stop therapy. If ANC drops to <1000/mm³, resume 5mcg/kg/day. **PBPC:** 10mcg/kg/day bolus or continuous SQ 4 days before and for 6-7 days with leukapheresis on days 5, 6, and 7. Monitor neutrophils after 4 days and adjust if WBC >100,000/mm³. **Chronic Neutropenia: Congenital Neutropenia: Initial:** 6mcg/kg SQ bid. **Idiopathic or Cyclic Neutropenia: Initial:** 5mcg/kg SQ qd. Adjust dose based on clinical course and ANC.	**Contra:** Hypersensitivity to *E. coli*-derived proteins. **P/N:** Category C, caution in nursing.	
Pegfilgrastim (Neulasta)	**Inj:** 6mg/0.6mL	***Adults:*** 6mg SQ once per chemotherapy cycle. Do not administer in the period between 14 days before and 24 hrs after chemotherapy.	**W/P:** Rare cases of splenic rupture reported, some fatal. Evaluate for enlarged spleen or splenic rupture if complaints of upper abdominal and/or shoulder tip pain. Acute respiratory distress syndrome (ARDS), allergic reactions (eg, anaphylaxis, rash) reported with filgrastim. Caution with sickle cell disease; monitor for sickle cell crises. Obtain CBC, platelets before chemotherapy. Monitor Hct, platelets regularly. Do not use in infants, children, and smaller adolescents <45kg. **Contra:** Hypersensitivity to *E. coli*-derived proteins. **P/N:** Category C, caution in nursing.	Bone pain, myalgia, arthralgia, peripheral edema, N/V, fatigue, alopecia, diarrhea, constipation, fever, anorexia, headache.
NUTRITION AGENTS				
Calcium Carbonate/Fluoride (Monocal) OTC	**Tab:** Calcium 250mg-Fluoride 3mg	***Adults:*** 1 tab qd.	**P/N:** Safety in pregnancy and nursing not known.	—
Copper/L-Glutathione/ Lutein/ Manganese/Niacinamide/Riboflavin/ Selenium/Vitamin A/Vitamin C/ Vitamin E/Zinc (Ocuvite Extra) OTC	**Tab:** Copper 2mg-L-Glutathione 5mg-Lutein 2mg-Manganese 5mg-Niacinamide 40mg-Riboflavin 3mg-Selenium 55mcg-Vitamin A 1000IU-Vitamin C 300mg-Vitamin E 100IU-Zinc 40mg	***Adults:*** 1 tab qd-bid.	**P/N:** Safety in pregnancy or nursing not known.	—
Copper/Lutein/ Selenium/Vitamin A/Vitamin C/ Vitamin E/Zinc (Ocuvite) OTC	**Tab:** Copper 2mg-Lutein 2mg-Selenium 55mcg-Vitamin A 1000IU-Vitamin C 200mg-Vitamin E 60IU-Zinc 40mg	***Adults:*** 1 tab qd-bid.	**P/N:** Safety in pregnancy or nursing not known.	—
Copper/Lutein/ Vitamin C/Vitamin E/Zinc (Ocuvite Lutein) OTC	**Cap:** Copper 2mg-Lutein 6mg-Vitamin C 60mg-Vitamin E 30IU-Zinc 15mg	***Adults:*** 1 cap qd-bid.	**P/N:** Safety in pregnancy or nursing not known.	—
Copper/Vitamin A/ Vitamin C/Vitamin E/Zinc (Ocuvite PreserVision) OTC	**Tab:** Copper 0.4mg-Vitamin A 7160IU-Vitamin C 113mg-Vitamin E 100IU-Zinc 17.4mg	***Adults:*** 2 tabs bid.	**P/N:** Safety in pregnancy or nursing not known.	—

Table 19.1. PRESCRIBING INFORMATION FOR HEMATOLOGIC DRUGS *(cont.)*

NAME	FORM/ STRENGTH	DOSAGE	WARNINGS/PRECAUTIONS & CONTRAINDICATIONS	ADVERSE EFFECTS†
NUTRITION AGENTS *(cont.)*				
Ferrous Sulfate/ Folic Acid/Multiple Vitamin (Iberet-Folic-500)	**Tab, Extended-Release:** Ferrous Sulfate 105mg-Folic Acid 0.8mg-Vitamin B_1 6mg-Vitamin B_2 6mg-Vitamin B_3 30mg-Vitamin B_5 10mg-Vitamin B_6 5mg-Vitamin B_{12} 25mcg-Vitamin C 500mg	***Adults:*** 1 tab qd on empty stomach.	**W/P:** May mask pernicious anemia. **Contra:** Pernicious anemia. **P/N:** Category A, caution in nursing.	Allergic sensitization.
Ferrous Sulfate/Folic Acid/Vitamin C (Fero-Folic 500)	**Tab, Extended-Release:** Ferrous Sulfate 525mg-Folic Acid 0.8mg-Vitamin C 500mg	***Adults:*** 1 tab qd.	**W/P:** May mask pernicious anemia. **Contra:** Pernicious anemia. **P/N:** Category A, safety in nursing not known.	Gastric intolerance, allergic sensitization.
Ferrous Sulfate/ Vitamin C (Fero-Grad-500) OTC	**Tab, Extended-Release:** Ferrous Sulfate 105mg-Vitamin C 500mg	***Adults/Pediatrics:*** **≥4 yrs:** 1 tab qd.	—	—
Folic Acid/ Omega-3 Acids/ Vitamin B_{12}/ Vitamin B_6 (Animi-3)	**Cap:** Folic Acid 1mg-Vitamin B_6 12.5mg-Vitamin B_{12} 500mcg-Omega-3 Acids 500mg-Phytosterols 200mg	***Adults:*** 1-4 caps qd.	**W/P:** Folic acid doses >0.1mg/day may obscure pernicious anemia (hematological remission can occur while neurological manifestations remain progressive).	Allergic sensitization.
Folic Acid/ Polysaccharide Iron Complex (Irofol)	(Folic Acid-Polysaccharide Iron Complex) **Liquid:** 1mg-100mg/5mL; **Tab:** 1mg-150mg	***Adults/Pediatrics:*** **>12 yrs:** 1-2 tabs or 5-10mL qd.	**W/P:** Not for the treatment of pernicious anemia and other megaloblastic anemias. Folic acid >0.1mg/day may obscure pernicious anemia. **P/N:** Safety in pregnancy and nursing not known.	Gastric intolerance, allergic sensitization.
Folic Acid/Vitamin B_{12}/Vitamin B_6 (Folgard RX 2.2)	**Tab:** Folic Acid 2.2mg-Vitamin B_6 25mg-Vitamin B_{12} 0.5mg*	***Adults:*** 1 tab qd.	**W/P:** Folic acid >0.1mg/day may obscure pernicious anemia. **P/N:** Safety in pregnancy and nursing is not known.	Allergic sensitization.
Folic Acid/Vitamin B_{12}/Vitamin B_6 (Foltx)	**Tab:** Folic Acid 2.5mg-Vitamin B_6 25mg-Vitamin B_{12} 2mg	***Adults:*** 1-2 tabs qd.	**W/P:** Folic acid >0.1mg/day may obscure pernicious anemia (may be alleviated by B_{12} component).	Allergic sensitization, paresthesia, somnolence, mild diarrhea, polycythemia vera, peripheral vascular thrombosis, itching, transitory exanthema, feeling of body swelling.
Isoleucyl prolyl proline/Protein/ Sodium/Valyl prolyl proline (Ameal BP) OTC	**Cap:** 2.5mg; **Tab, Chewable:** 2.5mg	***Adults:*** **Cap:** 2 caps qd. **Tab:** Chew 3 tabs qd.	**W/P:** Keep out of reach of children. **Contra:** Allergy to lactropeptides. **P/N:** Safety not known in pregnancy and in nursing.	—

*Scored. †Bold entries denote special dental considerations.

BB = black box warning; **W/P** = warnings/precautions; **Contra** = contraindications; **P/N** = pregnancy category rating and nursing considerations.

NAME	FORM/ STRENGTH	DOSAGE	WARNINGS/PRECAUTIONS & CONTRAINDICATIONS	ADVERSE EFFECTS†
L-methylfolate/ Vitamin B_{12}/ Vitamin B_6 (Metanx)	**Tab:** L-methylfolate 2.8mg-Vitamin B_6 25mg-Vitamin B_{12} 2mg	***Adults:*** 1-2 tabs qd.	**W/P:** Folic acid >0.1mg/day may obscure pernicious anemia (may be alleviated by B_{12} component).	Paresthesia, somnolence, nausea, headache, diarrhea, polycythemia vera, itching, transitory exanthema, feeling of body swelling.
Magnesium Oxide (Mag-Ox) OTC	**Tab:** 400mg	***Adults:*** **Supplement:** 1-2 tabs qd. **Antacid:** 1 tab bid. **Max:** 2 tabs/day or 2 weeks of therapy.	**W/P:** Not for use in amounts over the Recommended Daily Intake (RDI). May have a laxative effect. **P/N:** Safety in pregnancy and nursing not known.	—
Minerals/Multiple Vitamin (Strovite Forte)	**Tab:** Biotin 0.15mg-Calcium Pantothenate 25mg-Chromium 0.05mg-Copper 3mg-Folic Acid 1mg-Iron 10mg-Magnesium 50mg-Molybdenum 0.02mg-Niacin 100mg-Selenium 0.05mg-Vitamin A 4000 IU-Vitamin B_1 20mg-Vitamin B_2 20mg-Vitamin B_6 25mg-Vitamin B_{12} 0.05mg-Vitamin C 500mg-Vitamin D 400 IU-Vitamin E 60 IU-Zinc 15mg*	***Adults:*** 1 tab qd.	**W/P:** Accidental overdose of iron-containing products is a leading cause of fatal poisoning in children <6 yrs. Not for the treatment of pernicious anemia and other megaloblastic anemias where vitamin B_{12} is deficient.	GI intolerance, allergic and idiosyncratic reactions.
Minerals/Multiple Vitamin (Vicon Forte, Vitacon Forte)	**Cap:** Ascorbic Acid 150mg-Calcium Pantothenate 10mg-Folic Acid 1mg-Magnesium 70mg-Manganese 4mg-Niacinamide 25mg-Pyridoxine 2mg-Riboflavin 5mg-Thiamine 10mg-Vitamin A 8000 IU-Vitamin B_{12} 10mcg-Vitamin E 50 IU-Zinc 80mg	***Adults:*** 1 cap qd.	**W/P:** Folic acid may obscure signs of pernicious anemia. **P/N:** Safety in pregnancy and nursing not known.	—
Minerals/Multiple Vitamin (Vitaplex Plus)	**Tab:** Biotin 0.15mg-Chromium 0.1mg-Copper 3mg-Folic Acid 0.8mg-Iron 27mg-Magnesium 50mg-Manganese 5mg-Niacin	***Adults:*** 1 tab qd.	**W/P:** Not for treatment of pernicious anemia or other megoblastic anemias, or severe specific deficiencies.	Allergic and idiosyncratic reactions, GI intolerance.

Table 19.1. PRESCRIBING INFORMATION FOR HEMATOLOGIC DRUGS *(cont.)*

NAME	FORM/ STRENGTH	DOSAGE	WARNINGS/PRECAUTIONS & CONTRAINDICATIONS	ADVERSE EFFECTS†
NUTRITION AGENTS *(cont.)*				
Minerals/Multiple Vitamin (Vitaplex Plus) *(cont.)*	100mg-Pantothenic Acid 25mg-Vitamin A 5000 IU-Vitamin B_1 20mg-Vitamin B_2 20mg-Vitamin B_6 25mg-Vitamin B_{12} 50mcg-Vitamin C 500mg-Vitamin E 30 IU-Zinc 22.5mg			
Multiple Vitamin (Cefol)	**Tab:** Calcium Pantothenate 20mg-Folic Acid 0.5mg-Niacinamide 100mg-Vitamin B_1 15mg-Vitamin B_2 10mg-Vitamin B_6 5mg-Vitamin B_{12} 6mcg-Vitamin C 750mg-Vitamin E 30 IU	***Adults:*** 1 tab qd.	**W/P:** Folic acid alone is improper treatment of pernicious anemia and other megaloblastic anemias with Vitamin B_{12}-deficiency. Folic acid >0.1mg/day may obscure pernicious anemia. **P/N:** Safety in pregnancy and nursing not known.	Allergic sensitization.
Multiple Vitamin (Nephrocaps)	**Cap:** Biotin 0.15mg-Calcium Pantothenate 5mg-Folate 1mg-Niacin 20mg-Vitamin B_1 1.5mg-Vitamin B_2 1.7mg-Vitamin B_6 10mg-Vitamin B_{12} 0.006mg-Vitamin C 100mg	***Adults:*** 1 cap qd. Take after treatment if on dialysis.	**W/P:** Folic acid may mask symptoms of pernicious anemia. **P/N:** Safety in pregnancy and nursing not known.	—
Multiple Vitamin (Nephro-Vite Rx)	**Tab:** Biotin 0.3mg-Calcium Pantothenic Acid 10mg-Folic Acid 1mg-Niacinamide 20mg-Vitamin B_1 1.5mg-Vitamin B_2 1.7mg-Vitamin B_6 10mg-Vitamin B_{12} 0.006mg-Vitamin C 60mg	***Adults:*** 1 tab qd.	**W/P:** Folic acid may partially correct the hematological damage due to vitamin B_{12} deficiency of pernicious anemia, while neurological damage progresses. **P/N:** Safety in pregnancy and nursing not known.	—
Multiple Vitamin (Vitaplex)	**Tab:** Folic Acid 0.5mg-Niacin 100mg-Pantothenic Acid 18mg-Vitamin B_1 15mg-Vitamin B_2 15mg-Vitamin B_6 4mg-Vitamin B_{12} 5mcg-Vitamin C 500mg	***Adults:*** 1 tab qd.	**W/P:** Not for treatment of pernicious anemia or other megoblastic anemias, or severe specific deficiencies.	Allergic and idiosyncratic reactions.

†Bold entries denote special dental considerations.
BB = black box warning; **W/P** = warnings/precautions; **Contra** = contraindications; **P/N** = pregnancy category rating and nursing considerations.

NAME	FORM/ STRENGTH	DOSAGE	WARNINGS/PRECAUTIONS & CONTRAINDICATIONS	ADVERSE EFFECTS†
Multiple Vitamin/ Sodium Fluoride (Poly-Vi-Flor)	**Sol:** Niacin 8mg-Thiamin 0.5mg-Riboflavin 0.6mg-Vitamin A 1500 IU-Vitamin B_6 0.4mg-Vitamin B_{12} 2mcg-Vitamin C 35mg-Vitamin D 400 IU-Vitamin E 5 IU. 0.25mg drops contains 0.25mg Fluoride [50mL], 0.5mg drops contain 0.5mg Fluoride [50mL]; **Tab, Chewable:** Folate 0.3mg-Niacin 13.5mg-Riboflavin 1.2mg-Thiamin 1.05mg-Vitamin A 2500 IU-Vitamin B_6 1.05mg-Vitamin B_{12} 4.5mcg-Vitamin C 60mg-Vitamin D 400 IU-Vitamin E 15 IU. 0.25mg tabs contain 0.25mg Fluoride; 0.5mg tabs contain 0.5mg Fluoride; 1mg tabs contain 1mg Fluoride	***Pediatrics:*** (Sol) **6 months-3 yrs and <0.3 ppm Fluoride or 3-6 yrs and 0.3-0.6 ppm Fluoride:** 1mL (0.25mg) qd. **3-6 yrs and <0.3 ppm Fluoride or >6 yrs and 0.3-0.6 ppm Fluoride:** 1mL (0.5mg) qd. (Tab) **4-6 yrs and 0.3-0.6 ppm Fluoride:** 0.25mg qd. **4-6 yrs and <0.3 ppm Fluoride or ≥6 yrs and 0.3-0.6 ppm Fluoride:** 0.5mg qd. **6-16 yrs and <0.3 ppm Fluoride:** 1mg qd.	**W/P:** Must chew tab; not for pediatrics <4yrs. Risk of dental fluorosis from ingestion of large amounts of fluoride. Children up to 16 yrs, in areas where water contains less than optimal fluoride levels, should receive daily fluoride supplementation. **P/N:** Safety in pregnancy and nursing not known.	Allergic rash.
Sodium Fluoride (Luride)	**Drops:** 0.5mg/mL [50mL]; **Tab, Chewable:** 0.25mg, 0.5mg, 1mg	***Pediatrics:*** (Drops) **<0.3ppm: 6 months-3 yrs:** 0.5mL qd. **3-6 yrs:** 1mL qd. **6-16 yrs:** 2mL qd. **0.3-0.6ppm: 3-6 yrs:** 0.5mL qd. **6-16 yrs:** 1mL qd. (Tab) **<0.3ppm: 6 months-<3 yrs:** 0.25mg qd. **3-6 yrs:** 0.5mg qd. **6-16 yrs:** 1mg qd. **0.3-0.6ppm: 3-6 yrs:** 0.25mg qd. **6-16 yrs:** 0.5mg qd. Dissolve tab in mouth or chew tab before swallowing. Take at bedtime after brushing teeth.	**W/P:** Dental fluorosis may result from daily ingestion of excessive fluoride in pediatrics <6 yrs especially if water fluoride is >0.6ppm. **Contra:** (Drops) Areas where drinking water fluoride is >0.6ppm, pediatrics <6 months. (Tab) **1mg:** Water fluoride is >0.3ppm, pediatrics <6 yrs. **0.5mg:** Water fluoride is >0.6ppm, pediatrics <6 yrs. **0.25mg:** Water fluoride is >0.6ppm. **P/N:** Safety in pregnancy not known. Caution in nursing.	Allergic rash.
TOPICAL HEMOSTATIC AGENTS				
Thrombin (Bovine Origin) (Thrombin-JMI)	**Powder:** 5,000 IU, 20,000 IU; **Kit: Powder:** 20,000 IU [Spray; Syringe Spray]	***Adults:*** Spray topically on surface of bleeding tissue. Reconstitute with sterile isotonic saline at a recommended concentration of 1,000-2,000 IU/mL. **Profuse bleeding:** Use 1,000 IU/mL. **General use (eg, plastic surgery, dental extractions, skin grafting):** 100 IU/mL. Intermediate strengths may be prepared by diluting in appropriate isotonic saline volume if needed. **Oozing surfaces:** Use dry form. May be used with FlowSeal[NT].	**W/P:** The use of topical bovine thrombin preparations has occasionally been associated with abnormalities in hemostasis ranging from asymptomatic alterations in laboratory determinations, such as prothrombin time (PT) and partial thromboplastin time (PTT), to severe bleeding or thrombosis which rarely have been fatal. Consultation with an expert is recommended if patient exhibits abnormal coagulation laboratory values, abnormal bleeding, or abnormal thrombosis. Should not be injected or allowed to enter large blood vessels. Extensive intravascular clotting and even death may result. **Contra:** Sensitivity to material of bovine origin. **P/N:** Category C, safety in nursing is not known.	Inhibitory antibodies which interfere with hemostasis may develop.

Table 19.1. PRESCRIBING INFORMATION FOR HEMATOLOGIC DRUGS *(cont.)*

NAME	FORM/ STRENGTH	DOSAGE	WARNINGS/PRECAUTIONS & CONTRAINDICATIONS	ADVERSE EFFECTS†
MISCELLANEOUS HEMATOLOGY AGENTS				
Albumin (Albuminar, Albuminar-25, Albuminar-5)	**Inj:** 5%, 25%	***Adults:* Shock: Initial:** (5%) 500mL given as rapidly as tolerated. May repeat 30 min later if needed. Guide therapy by clinical response, BP, assessment of relative anemia. (25%) Dose dependent on BP, degree of pulmonary congestion, Hct. May repeat 15-30 min later if needed. **Severe Burns:** (5%) Large volumes of crystalloid with lesser amount of albumin 5%. May increase ratio of albumin to crystalloid after 24 hrs to maintain plasma albumin level 2.5g/100mL or total serum protein level 5.2g/100mL. **Burns:** (25%) Large volumes of crystalloid during 1st 24 hrs. More albumin than crystalloid after 24 hrs is required. **Hypoproteinemia:** (5%) Use to replace protein lost. (25%) 200-300mL to reduce edema and normalize serum protein.	**W/P:** Avoid if turbid or sediment in bottle. Do not begin administration >4 hrs after container has been entered. Made from human plasma; risk of viral disease transmission. Supplement with RBCs or whole blood when administer large quantities. Slower administration with HTN. Observe for bleeding points due to quick response of BP. Caution with low cardiac reserve or with no albumin deficiency. **Contra:** Severe anemia, cardiac failure, history of human albumin allergy. **P/N:** Category C, safety in nursing not known.	Anaphylaxis, N/V, **increased salivation,** chills, febrile reactions, urticaria, pruritus, edema, erythema, hypotension, bronchospasm, rash.
Antihemophilic Factor (Kogenate FS)	**Inj:** 250 IU, 500 IU, 1000 IU, 2000 IU	***Adults/Pediatrics:* Control/Prevention Of Bleeding Episodes: Minor Bleeding/FVIII 20-40 IU/dL:** 10-20 IU/kg IV; repeat as necessary. **Moderate Bleeding/FVIII 30-60 IU/dL:** 15-30 IU/kg; repeat q12-24h. **Major Bleeding/FVIII 80-100 IU/dL: Initial:** 40-50 IU/kg; repeat 20-25 IU/kg q8-12h. **Peri-operative Management: Minor Surgery/FVIII 30-60 IU/dL:** 15-30 IU/kg; repeat q12-24h until bleeding is resolved. **Major Surgery/FVIII 100 IU/dL: Pre-operative:** 50 IU/kg. Repeat as necessary after 6-12 hrs initially, and for 10-14 days until healing is complete. ***Pediatrics:* Routine Prophylaxis:** 25 IU/kg qod.	**W/P:** Anaphylaxis and severe hypersensitivity reactions (eg, rash, urticaria, chest discomfort) reported; d/c therapy if symptoms occur. Development of circulating neutralizing antibodies to FVIII may occur; monitor plasma FVIII activity levels and development of FVIII inhibitors. **Contra:** Known hypersensitivity to mouse or hamster proteins. **P/N:** Category C, caution in nursing.	Bronchospastic reactions, hypotension, anaphylaxis, rash, pruritus, infusion site reactions, urticaria, inflammation, central line infection.
Cyanocobalamin (Nascobal)	**Spray:** 500mcg/0.1mL (per actuation) [2.3mL]	***Adults:*** 500mcg (1 spray) intranasally once weekly. Patients should be in hematologic remission before treatment.	**W/P:** Severe and swift optic atrophy reported with Leber's disease. Hypokalemia and sudden death may occur in severe megaloblastic anemia treated intensely. Folic acid is not a substitute for vitamin B_{12}-deficient anemia. Perform intradermal test dose if sensitivity suspected. Vitamin B_{12} deficiency may suppress signs of polycythemia vera. Hypokalemia and thrombocytosis may occur upon conversion of severe megaloblastic to normal erythropoiesis. Avoid use with nasal congestion, allergic rhinitis, upper respiratory infection. Monitor vitamin B_{12} levels and peripheral blood counts prior to and periodically during therapy. **Contra:** Sensitivity to cobalt. **P/N:** Category C, consume recommended amount by the Food and Nutrition Board during nursing.	Nausea, headache, rhinitis.
Drotrecogin alfa (Xigris)	**Inj:** 5mg, 20mg	***Adults:*** 24mcg/kg/hr IV for 96 hrs.	**W/P:** Increased risk of bleed with platelets <30,000 x 106/L (even if platelets increased by transfusions), PT/INR >3, GI bleed within 6 weeks, ischemic stroke within 3 months, intracranial arteriovenous malformation or aneurysm, known bleeding diathesis, chronic severe hepatic disease, or condition where bleeding is a significant hazard or difficult to manage due to location. If	Bleeding.

†Bold entries denote special dental considerations.
BB = black box warning; **W/P** = warnings/precautions; **Contra** = contraindications; **P/N** = pregnancy category rating and nursing considerations.

NAME	FORM/ STRENGTH	DOSAGE	WARNINGS/PRECAUTIONS & CONTRAINDICATIONS	ADVERSE EFFECTS†
Drotrecogin alfa (Xigris) *(cont.)*			bleeding occurs, stop infusion. D/C 2 hrs before invasive surgical procedures or procedures with risk of bleeding. Avoid noncompressible puncture sites. **Contra:** Active internal bleeding, hemorrhagic stroke within 3 months, intracranial or intraspinal surgery or severe head trauma within 2 months, trauma with an increased risk of life-threatening bleeding, epidural catheter, intracranial neoplasm or mass lesion, evidence of cerebral herniation. **P/N:** Category C, not for use in nursing.	
Hydroxyurea (Droxia)	**Cap:** 200mg, 300mg, 400mg	***Adults:*** **Initial:** 15mg/kg/day as single dose. **Titrate:** If blood counts are in acceptable range, increase by 5mg/kg/day every 12 weeks until maximum tolerated dose or 35mg/kg/day. If blood counts are toxic, d/c until hematologic recovery. May resume treatment after dose reduction by 2.5mg/kg/day from dose associated with hematologic toxicity. May increase every 12 weeks by 2.5mg/kg/day until reaching a stable dose that does not result in toxicity for 24 weeks. **CrCl <60mL/min or ESRD:** 7.5mg/kg/day; administer in ESRD following hemodialysis.	**BB:** Mutagenic, carcinogenic, clastogenic, and causes cellular transformation to tumorigenic phenotypes. May develop secondary leukemia with long-term therapy for myeloproliferative disorders. Administer only under supervision of a physician experienced in the use of antineoplastic agents. **W/P:** Avoid in marked bone marrow depression. Caution with renal dysfunction. Severe, life-threatening myelosuppression reported. Monitor hematologic, liver, kidney function before therapy and repeatedly thereafter. Interrupt therapy if neutrophils <2000/mm^3 or platelets <80,000/mm^3, Hgb <4.5g/dL or reticulocytes <80,000/mm^2 with Hgb <9g/dL. Monitor blood counts every 2 weeks. Cutaneous vasculitic toxicities, including vasculitic ulcerations and gangrene, reported; d/c if cutaneous vasculitic ulcerations develop. Causes macrocytosis, which masks the incidental development of folic acid deficiency. **P/N:** Category D, not for use in nursing.	Neutropenia, low reticulocyte and platelet levels, hair loss, fever, GI disturbances, weight gain, bleeding, melanonychia, dermatological reactions, cutaneous vasculitic toxicities.
Lenalidomide (Revlimid)	**Cap:** 5mg, 10mg, 15mg, 25mg	***Adults:*** **≥18 yrs: Myelodysplastic Syndromes:** 10mg daily with water. **Multiple Myeloma:** 25mg daily with water. Administer as single dose on Days 1-21 of repeated 28-day cycles. Do not break, chew, or open capsules. Adjust dose based on platelet and/or neutrophil counts.	**BB:** Potential for human birth defects, hematological toxicity (neutropenia and thrombocytopenia), deep venous thrombosis (DVT) and pulmonary embolism (PE). Lenalidomide is an analogue of thalidomide. Thalidomide is a known human teratogen that causes severe life-threatening human birth defects. If taken during pregnancy, may cause birth defects or death to an unborn baby. Avoid pregnancy due to potential toxicity and to avoid fetal exposure. Only available under a special restricted distribution program called RevassistSM. Associated with significant neutropenia and thrombocytopenia in patients with del 5q MDS. CBC should be monitored weekly for the first 8 weeks of therapy and at least monthly thereafter. May require dose interruption and/or reduction and the use of blood product support and/or growth factors. Increased risk of DVT and PE in patients with multiple myeloma. Observe for signs and symptoms of thromboembolism. **W/P:** Risk of adverse reactions may be greater in patients with impaired renal function. **Contra:** Pregnancy. **P/N:** Category X, not for use in nursing.	Thrombocytopenia, neutropenia, pruritus, rash, diarrhea, constipation, nausea, nasopharyngitis, fatigue, arthralgia, **cough,** pyrexia, peripheral edema, insomnia, asthenia.

Table 19.1. PRESCRIBING INFORMATION FOR HEMATOLOGIC DRUGS *(cont.)*

NAME	FORM/ STRENGTH	DOSAGE	WARNINGS/PRECAUTIONS & CONTRAINDICATIONS	ADVERSE EFFECTS†
MISCELLANEOUS HEMATOLOGY AGENTS *(cont.)*				
Leucovorin Calcium	**Inj:** 10mg/mL, 50mg, 100mg, 200mg, 350mg, 500mg; **Tab:** 5mg, 10mg, 15mg, 25mg	***Adults:*** **Colorectal Cancer:** 200mg/m^2 slow IV push over 3 min followed by 5-FU 370mg/m^2 IV qd for 5 days, or 20mg/m^2 IV qd followed by 5-FU 425mg/m^2 IV qd for 5 days. May repeat at 4-week intervals for 2 courses then at 4- to 5-week intervals. May increase 5-FU dose by 10% if no toxicity. Reduce 5-FU dose by 20% with moderate GI/hematologic toxicity and by 30% with severe toxicity. **Leucovorin Rescue:** 15mg q6h for 10 doses starting 24 hrs after start of MTX until serum MTX is $<5x10^{-8}$M. Give IV/IM with GI toxicity. See PI for leucovorin adjustments and extended therapy. **Impaired MTX Elimination/Overdose:** 10mg/m^2 IV/IM/PO q6h until serum MTX is $<10^{-8}$M. Increase to 100mg/m^2 q3h if 24-hr serum creatinine is 50% over baseline, or if 24-hr serum MTX is $>5x10^{-6}$M, or the 48-hr level is $>9x10^{-7}$M. Give IV/IM with GI toxicity. Start ASAP after overdose and within 24 hrs of MTX with delayed excretion. **Megaloblastic Anemia:** Up to 1mg/day. **Elderly:** Caution with dose selection.	**W/P:** Do not administer >160mg/min. Do not give intrathecally. Monitor serum MTX. Higher than recommended PO doses must be given IV. Increased risk of severe toxicity in elderly/debilitated colorectal cancer patients taking 5-FU with leucovorin. Monitor renal function in elderly. **Contra:** Improper therapy for pernicious anemia and other megaloblastic anemias secondary to lack of vitamin B_{12}. **P/N:** Category C, caution use in nursing.	Allergic sensitization.
Lymphocyte Immune Globulin, Anti-Thymocyte Globulin (Equine) (Atgam)	**Inj:** 50mg/mL [5mL]	***Adults/Pediatrics:*** **Renal Transplant: Delaying Rejection Onset:** 15mg/kg/day for 14 days, then every other day for 14 days for total of 21 doses in 28 days. Give 1st dose 24 hrs before or after transplant. **Rejection Treatment:** 10-15mg/kg/day for 14 days. May give additional alternate day therapy up to total of 21 doses. May delay 1st dose until diagnosis of 1st rejection episode. **Aplastic Anemia:** 10-20mg/kg/day for 8-14 days. May give additional alternate day therapy up to total of 21 doses.	**BB:** Administer by physician experienced in immunosuppressive therapy in a facility equipped and staffed with adequate lab and supportive medical resources. **W/P:** Potency of agent may vary from lot to lot. D/C if anaphylaxis (eg, respiratory distress, hypotension) occurs, or if severe and unremitting thrombocytopenia or leukopenia occur in renal transplant patients. Risk of infectious transmission due to equine and human blood components. Monitor for leukopenia, thrombocytopenia, or infection (eg, CMV). Decide whether or not to continue therapy based on clinical circumstances (eg, infection). **Contra:** History of severe systemic reaction to this product or other equine gamma globulin agents. **P/N:** Category C, caution in nursing.	Fever, chills, leukopenia, thrombocytopenia, rash, pruritus, urticaria, wheal, flare, arthralgia, headache, phlebitis, chest/back pain, diarrhea, N/V, dyspnea, hypotension, night sweats, stomatitis.

†Bold entries denote special dental considerations.
BB = black box warning; **W/P** = warnings/precautions; **Contra** = contraindications; **P/N** = pregnancy category rating and nursing considerations.

Table 19.2. DRUG INTERACTIONS FOR HEMATOLOGIC DRUGS

COAGULATION MODIFIERS	
Abciximab (ReoPro)	
Anticoagulants	May increase risk of bleeding with anticoagulants, including heparin.
Antiplatelet agents	May increase risk of bleeding.
Dipyridamole	Caution with dipyridamole; may affect hemostasis.
HACA titers	Possible allergic reactions with monoclonal antibody agents.
NSAIDs	Caution with NSAIDs; may affect hemostasis.
Thrombolytics	May increase risk of bleeding.
Ticlopidine	Caution with ticlopidine; may affect hemostasis.
Alteplase (Activase)	
Heparin	May increase risk of bleeding prior to, during, or after alteplase therapy.
Platelet function, drugs altering	May increase risk of bleeding with drugs that alter platelet function (eg, ASA, dipyridamole, abciximab) prior to, during, or after alteplase therapy.
Vitamin K antagonists	May increase risk of bleeding prior to, during, or after alteplase therapy.
Aminocaproic Acid (Amicar)	
Anti-inhibitor coagulant concentrates	Avoid concomitant use; may increase risk of thrombosis.
Factor IX complex concentrates	Avoid concomitant use; may increase risk of thrombosis.
Anagrelide HCl (Agrylin)	
ASA	Slight enhancement of the inhibition of platelet aggregation by ASA observed with coadministration.
cAMP PDE III inhibitors	May exacerbate effects of products that inhibit cAMP PDE III (eg, inotropes: milrinione, enoximone, amrinone, olprinone, cilostazol).
CYP1A2 inhibitors	May inhibit metabolism and decrease clearance of anagrelide with CYP1A2 inhibitors (eg, fluvoxamine).
CYP1A2 substrates	May inhibit metabolism and decrease clearance of CYP1A2 substrates (eg, theophylline).
Sucralfate	May interfere with anagrelide absorption.
Argatroban	
Anticoagulants	May increase risk of bleeding; d/c all anticoagulants prior to argatroban administration.
Antiplatelet agents	May increase risk of bleeding.
Heparin	Avoid coadministration; allow sufficient time after cessation of heparin therapy for its effect on aPTT to decrease prior to initiating argatroban therapy.
Thrombolytics	May increase risk of bleeding.
Warfarin	May prolong PT/INR with concomitant warfarin.
Aspirin/Dipyridamole (Aggrenox)	
ACE inhibitors	Hyponatremic and hypotensive effects of ACE inhibitors may be diminished by concomitant administration of ASA.
Acetazolamide	May increase plasma levels and toxicity of acetazolamide with coadministration.

Table 19.2. DRUG INTERACTIONS FOR HEMATOLOGIC DRUGS *(cont.)*

COAGULATION MODIFIERS *(cont.)*

Aspirin/Dipyridamole (Aggrenox) *(cont.)*	
Adenosine	May increase plasma levels and cardiovascular effects of adenosine; might require adenosine dosage adjustment.
Anticoagulants	May increase risk of bleeding with anticoagulants (eg, heparin, warfarin).
Anticonvulsants	Salicylic acid may displace protein-bound phenytoin and valproic acid, leading to a decrease in the total concentration of phenytoin and an increase in serum valproic acid levels.
β-Blockers	May diminish hypotensive effects of β-blockers with concomitant aspirin.
Cholinesterase inhibitors	May counteract the anticholinesterase effect of cholinesterase inhibitors with dipyridamole; may potentially aggravate myasthenia gravis.
Diuretics	May diminish the effectiveness of diuretics in patients with underlying renal or cardiovascular disease.
Hypoglycemics, oral	May increase effectiveness of oral hypoglycemics with moderate doses of aspirin; may increase risk of hypoglycemia.
Methotrexate (MTX)	Salicylate may inhibit renal clearance of MTX, leading to bone marrow toxicity, especially in the elderly or renal impaired.
NSAIDs	May increase risk of bleeding or decrease renal function with the concurrent use of ASA and other NSAIDs.
Uricosuric agents	May antagonize the uricosuric action of probenecid and sulfinpyrazone.
Bivalirudin (Angiomax)	
Glycoprotein IIb/IIIa inhibitors	May increase risk of major bleeding events with coadministration.
Heparin	May increase risk of major bleeding events with coadministration.
Thrombolytics	May increase risk of major bleeding events with coadministration.
Warfarin	May increase risk of major bleeding events with coadministration.
Cilostazol (Pletal)	
CYP2C19 inhibitors	Caution with CYP2C19 inhibitors (eg, omeprazole); may increase systemic exposure to cilostazole and its major metabolites.
CYP3A4 inhibitors	Caution with CYP3A4 inhibitors (eg, ketoconazole, erythromycin, diltiazem); may increase systemic exposure to cilostazole and its major metabolites.
Clopidogrel Bisulfate (Plavix)	
ASA	May potentiate the effect of ASA on collagen-induced platelet aggregation.
CYP450 substrates	May inhibit CYP450 (2C9); may interfere with the metabolism of phenytoin, tamoxifen, tolbutamide, warfarin, torsemide, fluvastatin, and many NSAIDs.
GI lesions, drugs that induce	Caution with drugs that may induce GI lesions.
NSAIDs	May increase risk of occult GI blood loss with NSAIDs; caution with coadministration.
Warfarin	May increase risk of bleeding with warfarin; caution with coadministration.
Dalteparin Sodium (Fragmin)	
Anticoagulants	May increase risk of bleeding with anticoagulants.

COAGULATION MODIFIERS *(cont.)*

Dalteparin Sodium (Fragmin) *(cont.)*	
Platelet inhibitors	May increase risk of bleeding with platelet inhibitors.
Thrombolytics	May increase risk of bleeding with thrombolytics.
Dipyridamole (Persantine)	
Adenosine	May increase plasma levels and cardiovascular effects of adenosine; may require adenosine dosage adjustment.
Cholinesterase inhibitors	May counteract the anticholinesterase effect of cholinesterase inhibitors with dipyridamole; may potentially aggravate myasthenia gravis.
Enoxaparin Sodium (Lovenox)	
Anticoagulants	May increase risk of hemorrhage with anticoagulants; consider d/c of anticoagulant prior to initiation of enoxaparin therapy.
Antiplatelet agents	May increase risk of hemorrhage with antiplatelet agents (eg, ASA); consider d/c of antiplatelet agent prior to initiation of enoxaparin therapy.
Dipyridamole	May increase risk of hemorrhage with dipyridamole; consider d/c of dipyridamole prior to initiation of enoxaparin therapy.
NSAIDs	May increase risk of hemorrhage with NSAIDs (eg, ketorolac); consider d/c of NSAID prior to initiation of enoxaparin therapy.
Salicylates	May increase risk of hemorrhage with salicylates; consider d/c of salicylate prior to initiation of enoxaparin therapy.
Sulfinpyrazone	May increase risk of hemorrhage with sulfinpyrazone; consider d/c of sulfinpyrazone prior to initiation of enoxaparin therapy.
Eptifibatide (Integrilin)	
Anticoagulants, oral	May affect hemostasis; caution with coadministration.
ASA	Cerebral, pulmonary, GI hemorrhage reported with ASA.
Dipyridamole	May affect hemostasis with dipyridamole; caution with coadministration.
Glycoprotein IIb/IIIa inhibitors	Potentially additive pharmacological effects with concomitant treatment with other inhibitors of platelet receptor GP IIb/IIIa; avoid concomitant use.
Heparin	Cerebral, pulmonary, GI hemorrhage reported with heparin.
NSAIDs	May affect hemostasis; caution with coadministration.
Thrombolytics	May affect hemostasis; caution with coadministration.
Fondaparinux Sodium (Arixtra)	
Hemorrhage, drugs enhancing risk of	D/C agents that may enhance risk of hemorrhage (eg, platelet inhibitors); monitor closely if coadministered.
Heparin Sodium	
Anticoagulants, oral	At least 5 hours should elapse after last IV dose; measure PT when heparin is given with dicumarol or warfarin.
Antihistamines	May partially counteract the anticoagulant action of heparin.
Digitalis	May partially counteract the anticoagulant action of heparin.
Nicotine	May partially counteract the anticoagulant action of heparin.

Table 19.2. DRUG INTERACTIONS FOR HEMATOLOGIC DRUGS *(cont.)*

COAGULATION MODIFIERS *(cont.)*

Heparin Sodium *(cont.)*	
Nitroglycerin, IV	May partially counteract the anticoagulant action of heparin.
Platelet inhibitors	May increase risk of bleeding with platelet inhibitors (eg, acetylsalicylic acid, dextran, phenylbutazone, ibuprofen, indomethacin, dipyridamole, hydroxychloroquine).
Tetracyclines	May partially counteract the anticoagulant action of heparin.
Lepirudin (Refludan)	
Coumarins	May increase risk of bleeding with coumarin derivatives.
Platelet function, drugs that affect	May increase risk of bleeding with drugs that affect platelet function.
Thrombolytics	May increase risk of bleeding and enhance effect of lepirudin on aPTT prolongation.
Pentoxifylline (Trental)	
Antihypertensives	May require dose reduction of antihypertensive agent with pentoxifylline.
Theophylline	May increase plasma levels and toxicity of theophylline; monitor for signs of toxicity and adjust dosage as necessary.
Warfarin	May increase risk of bleeding with warfarin; monitor PT/INR frequently.
Phytonadione (Mephyton)	
Prothrombin-depressing anticoagulants	Temporary resistance to prothrombin-depressing anticoagulants, especially with large doses.
Reteplase (Retavase)	
Anticoagulants, oral	May increase risks of reteplase therapy.
Heparin	May increase risk of bleeding if administered prior to or after reteplase therapy.
Platelet function, drugs altering	May increase risk of bleeding with drugs that alter platelet function (eg, ASA, dipyridamole, abciximab) if administered prior to or after reteplase therapy.
Vitamin K antagonists	May increase risk of bleeding if administered prior to or after reteplase therapy.
Tenecteplase (TNKase)	
Anticoagulants	May increase risk of bleeding with anticoagulants (eg, heparin, vitamin K antagonists, warfarin) prior to, during, or after tenecteplase therapy.
Platelet function, drugs altering	May increase risk of bleeding with drugs that alter platelet function (eg, ASA, dipyridamole, GP IIb/IIIa inhibitors) prior to, during, or after tenecteplase therapy.
Ticlopidine HCl (Ticlid)	
Antacids	May decrease plasma levels of ticlopidine with antacids.
Anticoagulants	D/C anticoagulants prior to ticlopidine administration.
ASA, NSAIDs	Potentiates the effect of ASA on platelet aggregation. Long-term concomitant use of ASA and ticlopidine not recommended.
Cimetidine	May decrease clearance of ticlopidine with chronic administration of cimetidine.
CYP450 substrates	Adjust dose of drugs metabolized by CYP450 with low therapeutic ratios or in patients with hepatic impairment.
Digoxin	May decrease plasma levels of digoxin with coadministration.

COAGULATION MODIFIERS *(cont.)*

Ticlopidine HCl (Ticlid) *(cont.)*	
Fibrinolytics	D/C fibrinolytics prior to ticlopidine administration.
NSAIDs	Potentiates the effect of NSAIDs on platelet aggregation. Long-term concomitant use of ASA and ticlopidine not recommended.
Phenytoin	Caution with phenytoin; increased plasma levels of phenytoin associated with somnolence and lethargy reported with coadministration.
Propranolol	Caution with concomitant propranolol.
Theophylline	May decrease clearance and increase half-life of theophylline with coadministration.
Tinzaparin Sodium (Innohep)	
Anticoagulants, oral	May increase risk of bleeding.
Platelet inhibitors	May increase risk of bleeding with platelet inhibitors (eg, salicylates, dipyridamole, sulfinpyrazone, dextran, NSAIDs, ticlopidine, clopidogrel).
Thrombolytics	May increase risk of bleeding.
Tirofiban HCl (Aggrastat)	
ASA	May increase risk of bleeding.
GP IIb/IIIa inhibitors, parenteral	Avoid coadministration with other parenteral GP IIb/IIIa inhibitors.
Hemostasis, drugs affecting	Caution with other drugs that affect hemostasis (eg, warfarin).
Heparin	May increase risk of bleeding.
Levothyroxine	May increase clearance of tirofiban.
Omeprazole	May increase clearance of tirofiban.
Urokinase (Abbokinase)	
Anticoagulants	May increase risk of serious bleeding with anticoagulants.
Platelet function, agents altering	May increase risk of serious bleeding with agents that alter platelet function (eg, ASA, other NSAIDs, dipyridamole, GP IIb/IIIa inhibitors).
Thrombolytics	May increase risk of bleeding complications with other thrombolytic agents.
Warfarin Sodium (Coumadin, Jantoven)	
Antibiotics	May interact with antibiotics.
Anticonvulsants	May potentiate anticonvulsants (eg, phenytoin, phenobarbital).
Antihyperlipidemic agents	May potentiate antihyperlipidemic agents.
ASA, NSAIDs	Increased risk of GI bleeding. Caution with coadministration; may require dose adjustment of warfarin.
Hepatic enzyme inducers	May interact with hepatic enzyme inducers.
Hepatic enzyme inhibitors	May interact with hepatic enzyme inhibitors.
Hypoglycemic agents	May potentiate hypoglycemic agents (eg, chlorpropamide, tolbutamide).
NSAIDs	Increased risk of GI bleeding. Caution with coadministration; may require dose adjustment of warfarin.
Protein-bound drugs	Interacts with protein-bound drugs.

Table 19.2. DRUG INTERACTIONS FOR HEMATOLOGIC DRUGS *(cont.)*

ERYTHROPOIESIS AGENT

Folic Acid	
Alcohol	May increase loss of folate, resulting in folate deficiency.
Antibiotics	May cause false low serum and red cell folate levels with antibiotics (eg, tetracyclines) due to suppression of *Lactobacillus casei*.
Anticonvulsants	Increased incidence of seizures reported in patients receiving concomitant anticonvulsant and folic acid. Anticonvulsants (eg, diphenylhydantoin, primidone, barbiturates) may increase loss of folate, resulting in folate deficiency.
Methotrexate (MTX)	May increase loss of folate, resulting in folate deficiency with MTX (folic acid antagonist).
Nitrofurantoin	May increase loss of folate, resulting in folate deficiency.
Phenytoin	May antagonize anticonvulsant action of phenytoin.
Pyrimethamine	May increase loss of folate, resulting in folate deficiency.

HEMATINICS

Iron Dextran (INFeD)	
Iron, oral	D/C oral iron prior to administration of iron dextran.
Iron Sucrose (Venofer)	
Iron, oral	May reduce absorption of oral iron preparations.

HEMATOPOIETIC AGENT

Sargramostim (Leukine)	
Chemotherapy	Avoid coadministration 24 hrs prior, during, or 24 hrs following chemotherapy.
Myeloproliferative effects, drugs potentiating	Caution with drugs that may potentiate myeloproliferative effects (eg, lithium, corticosteroids).
Radiation therapy	Avoid coadministration 24 hrs prior, during, or 24 hrs following radiation therapy.

IRON SUPPLEMENT

Ferrous Sulfate/Iron Carbonyl (Feosol) OTC	
Tetracycline	May decrease absorption of tetracycline; space dose by 2 hrs.

NEUTROPENIA AGENTS

Filgrastim (Neupogen)	
Neutrophils, drugs potentiating the release of	Caution with drugs that potentiate the release of neutrophils (eg, lithium).
Pegfilgrastim (Neulasta)	
Neutrophils, drugs potentiating the release of	Caution with drugs that potentiate the release of neutrophils (eg, lithium).

NUTRITION AGENTS

Ferrous Sulfate/Folic Acid/Multiple Vitamin (Iberet-Folic-500)	
Antacids, carbonate-containing	May inhibit iron absorption.
Food	Milk and eggs may inhibit iron absorption.
Levodopa	Pyridoxine may reverse antiparkinson effects of levodopa.
Magnesium trisilicate	May inhibit iron absorption.
Tetracyclines	May interfere with the absorption of tetracyclines.
Ferrous Sulfate/Folic Acid/Vitamin C (Fero-Folic 500)	
Antacids, carbonate-containing	May inhibit iron absorption.
Food	Milk and eggs may inhibit iron absorption.
Magnesium trisilicate	May inhibit iron absorption.
Tetracyclines	May interfere with the absorption of tetracyclines.
Folic Acid/Polysaccharide Iron Complex (Irofol)	
Antacids, carbonate-containing	May inhibit iron absorption.
Food	Milk and eggs may inhibit iron absorption.
Magnesium trisilicate	May inhibit iron absorption.
Folic Acid/Vitamin B_{12}/Vitamin B_6 (Foltx)	
Levodopa	Pyridoxine may antagonize effects of levodopa; avoid concomitant use. (May use concurrently with preparations containing both levodopa and carbidopa.)
Phenytoin	May decrease efficacy of phenytoin.
L-methylfolate/Vitamin B_{12}/Vitamin B_6 (Metanx)	
Alcohol	Excessive alcohol intake may decrease plasma levels of folate.
Antibiotics	May alter intestinal microflora; reduces absorption of methylcobalamin.
Anticonvulsants	High-dose folic acid may decrease plasma levels and efficacy of 1st generation anticonvulsants (eg, carbamazepine, fosphenytoin, phenytoin, phenobarbital, primidone, valproic acid, valproate); caution with coadministration. 1st generation anticonvulsants and 2nd generation lamotrigine may decrease plasma levels of folate.
Cholestyramine	May decrease enterohepatic reabsorption of methylcobalamin.
Colchicine	May decrease enterohepatic reabsorption of methylcobalamin.
Colestipol	May decrease enterohepatic reabsorption of methylcobalamin.
Levodopa	May antagonize action of levodopa; avoid concomitant use. (May use concurrently with preparations containing both levodopa and carbidopa.)
Metformin	May decrease absorption of methylcobalamin.
Methotrexate	May decrease plasma levels of folate.
Methylprednisone	May decrease plasma levels of folate.
NSAIDs	High-dose NSAIDs may decrease plasma levels of folate.

Table 19.2. DRUG INTERACTIONS FOR HEMATOLOGIC DRUGS *(cont.)*

NUTRITION AGENTS *(cont.)*

L-methylfolate/Vitamin B_{12}/Vitamin B_6 (Metanx) *(cont.)*	
Pancreatic enzymes	Pancrelipase or pancreatin may decrease plasma levels of folate.
Para-aminosalicylic acid	May decrease absorption of methylcobalamin.
Potassium chloride	May decrease absorption of methylcobalamin.
Pyrimethamine	High-dose folic acid may decrease plasma levels of pyrimethamine; caution with coadministration.
Triamterene	May decrease plasma levels of folate.
Trimethoprim	May decrease plasma levels of folate.
Magnesium Oxide (Mag-Ox) OTC	
Prescription drugs	May interact with certain prescription drugs.
Minerals/Multiple Vitamin (Strovite Forte)	
Levodopa	Pyridoxine may decrease efficacy of levodopa; avoid concomitant use.
Minerals/Multiple Vitamin (Vitaplex Plus)	
Levodopa	May decrease efficacy of levodopa.
Multiple Vitamin (Vitaplex)	
Levodopa	May decrease efficacy of levodopa.
Sodium Fluoride (Luride)	
Dairy products	Avoid dairy products within 1 hr of administration.

MISCELLANEOUS HEMATOLOGY AGENTS

Cyanocobalamin (vitamin B_{12}) (Nascobal)	
Alcohol	May produce malabsorption of vitamin B_{12} with heavy alcohol intake for longer than 2 wks.
Antibiotics	May invalidate folic acid and vitamin B_{12} diagnostic blood assays.
Colchicine	May produce malabsorption of vitamin B_{12}.
Methotrexate	May invalidate folic acid and vitamin B_{12} diagnostic blood assays.
Para-aminosalicylic acid	May produce malabsorption of vitamin B_{12}.
Pyrimethamine	May invalidate folic acid and vitamin B_{12} diagnostic blood assays.
Drotrecogin alfa (Xigris)	
Anticoagulants, oral	May increase risk of bleeding with recent administration (within 7 days) of oral anticoagulants.
Glycoprotein IIb/IIIa inhibitors	May increase risk of bleeding with recent administration (within 7 days) of glycoprotein IIb/IIIa inhibitors.
Hemostasis, drugs affecting	May increase risk of bleeding with drugs that affect hemostasis.
Heparin	May increase risk of bleeding with concurrent therapeutic dosing of heparin.
Platelet inhibitors	May increase risk of bleeding with recent administration (within 7 days) of ASA >650mg/day or other platelet inhibitors.
Thrombolytics	May increase risk of bleeding with recent administration (within 3 days) of thrombolytic therapy.

MISCELLANEOUS HEMATOLOGY AGENTS *(cont.)*

Hydroxyurea (Droxia)	
Antiretroviral agents	Peripheral neuropathy, hepatotoxicity, and hepatic failure resulting in death reported in HIV-infected patients treated with hydroxyurea and other antiretroviral agents. Fatal hepatic events reported with concomitant hydroxyurea, didanosine, and stavudine; avoid this combination.
Didanosine	Fatal and nonfatal pancreatitis reported in HIV-infected patients treated with hydroxyurea and didanosine, with or without stavudine.
Interferon therapy	Vasculitic toxicities reported with concurrent interferon therapy.
Lenalidomide (Revlimid)	
Digoxin	May increase digoxin C_{max} with coadministration; periodically monitor digoxin levels.
Leucovorin Calcium	
5-FU	May enhance 5-FU toxicity.
Methotrexate (MTX)	May reduce MTX efficacy.
Phenobarbital	Folic acid in large amounts may antagonize phenobarbital and increase seizure frequency in children.
Phenytoin	Folic acid in large amounts may antagonize phenytoin and increase seizure frequency in children.
Primidone	Folic acid in large amounts may antagonize primidone and increase seizure frequency in children.
Lymphocyte Immune Globulin, Anti-Thymocyte Globulin (Equine) (Atgam)	
Acidic infusion solutions	Avoid use with highly acidic infusion solutions; possible physical instability over time.
Immunosuppressants	Previously masked reactions to lymphocyte immune globulin, anti-thymocyte globulin may appear with corticosteroid or other immunosuppressant dose reduction.

Chapter 20

Endocrine/Hormonal and Bone Metabolism Drugs

Angelo J. Mariotti, D.D.S., Ph.D.

Hormones are chemical substances secreted from various organs into the blood stream and have specific regulatory effects on target tissues. The general functions of hormones can be divided into reproduction; growth and development; homeostasis of the internal environment; and energy production, use, and storage.

Although the effects of hormones are diverse and complex, hormones can be divided into two broad categories according to their chemical structure: polypeptides and steroids. The polypeptides or amino acid derivates represent a majority of hormones. This category comprises hormones that are secreted from a variety of organs (such as brain, pancreas, thyroid, and adrenal glands) and include large polypeptides (such as luteinizing hormone), medium-sized peptides (such as insulin), small peptides (such as thyrotropin-releasing hormone), dipeptides (such as thyroxine), and single amino acid by-products (such as histamine).

The remaining hormones are derivatives of cholesterol and are called steroid hormones. Similarly to the polypeptide hormones, steroid hormones are secreted from a variety of organs (such as adrenal glands, testes, and ovaries). But unlike the polypeptide hormones, they are more uniform in their chemical structure, because each steroid hormone must contain a cyclopentanoperhydrophenanthrene ring system (eg, estradiol).

Hormones, regardless of their chemical structure, have common characteristics. First, hormones are found in low concentrations in the blood circulation. Most polypeptide hormone concentrations in the blood range from 1 to 100 femtomolar, while thyroid and steroid hormone concentrations range between picomolar and micromolar concentrations. Second, hormones must be directed to their sites of action; this is most commonly accomplished by special protein molecules (receptors) that recognize specific hormones. Polypeptide hormone receptors are proteins that are fixed on the cell membrane; thyroid and steroid hormone receptors are proteins located inside the cell.

Although most drugs are considered to be substances foreign to the body, naturally occurring hormones, analogs of hormones, and hormone antagonists can be used as drugs and can exert important effects on the body. For example, endocrine drugs can be used to treat osteoporosis. Although the theories regarding the pathogenesis of osteoporosis are diverse, it is known that estrogen deficiency in women is an important factor in bone loss. A variety of endocrine drugs have been used to help treat osteoporosis. Drugs such as androgens, estrogens, oral contraceptives, serum estrogen receptor modulators, and calcitonin have been used.

In addition to these endocrine drugs, other important medications for treating osteoporosis are bone metabolism agents such as bisphosphonates.

ANDROGENS

Special Dental Considerations

Androgens can exacerbate a patient's inflammatory status, causing erythema and an increased tendency toward gingival bleeding. A controlled oral hygiene program that combines professional cleanings and plaque control will minimize androgen-induced sequelae.

Drug Interactions of Dental Interest

Androgens are responsible for the growth and development of male sex organs and for the maintenance of secondary sexual characteristics in males. Androgens can be used for replacement therapy in androgen-deficient men or for treatment of certain neoplasms.

Androgens may enhance the actions of oral anticoagulants, oral hypoglycemic agents, and glucocorticoids.

See **Tables 20.1** and **20.2** for general information on androgens.

Pharmacology

Androgens bind to intracellular androgen receptors that regulate RNA and DNA in target tissues.

ESTROGENS

Special Dental Considerations

High doses of estrogens can exacerbate a patient's inflammatory status, causing erythema and an increased tendency toward gingival bleeding. In some instances, estrogens have been reported to induce gingival enlargements. A controlled oral hygiene program that combines professional cleanings and plaque control will minimize estrogen-induced sequelae.

Drug Interactions of Dental Interest

Estrogens are responsible for the growth and development of female sex organs and for the maintenance of secondary sexual characteristics in women. Estrogens can be used to treat a variety of estrogen-deficiency states, as well as for certain neoplasms. Estrogen may change the requirements for oral anticoagulants, oral hypoglycemics, insulin, or barbiturates.

See **Tables 20.1** and **20.2** for general information on estrogens.

Pharmacology

Estrogens bind to intracellular estrogen receptors that regulate RNA and DNA in target tissues.

SERUM ESTROGEN RECEPTOR MODULATORS

Special Dental Considerations

The effects of serum estrogen receptor modulators (SERMs) on the oral cavity are largely unknown. SERMs can have variable effects depending on the type of estrogen receptor found in the oral cavity. Patients taking raloxifene will have lowered bone mineral density and, as a result, also may be more susceptible to periodontitis. See "Bone Metabolism Agents" in **Tables 20.1** and **20.2** for general information on raloxifene.

Drug Interactions of Dental Interest

Use caution when prescribing diazepam, ibuprofen, or naproxen with raloxifene, as these drugs can affect the binding of raloxifene to plasma proteins.

Pharmacology

Depending on the subtype of estrogen receptor found in a tissue, SERMs (such as raloxifene and tamoxifen) may act as either estrogen receptor agonists or estrogen receptor antagonists.

ORAL CONTRACEPTIVES

Special Dental Considerations

Most studies recording changes in gingival tissues associated with oral contraceptives were completed when contraceptive concentrations were at much higher levels than are available today. These investigations reported an exacerbation of the gingival inflammatory response sometimes leading to a gingival enlargement. Recent studies evaluating the effects of current oral contraceptives on gingival inflammation in young women found these hormonal agents to have no effect on gingival tissues. From these data, it appears that current compositions of oral contraceptives are not harmful to the periodontium in the vast number of women taking these drugs. Like any other patient, a woman using oral contraceptives will benefit from an oral hygiene program that includes regular oral examinations, professional cleanings, and plaque control.

Drug Interactions of Dental Interest

Oral contraceptives are used primarily to prevent ovulation. The effectiveness of oral contraceptives may be decreased by penicillin, chloramphenicol, oral neomycin, sulfonamides, barbiturates, glucocorticoids, griseofulvin, and tetracyclines.

See **Tables 20.1** and **20.2** for general information on oral contraceptives.

Pharmacology

Oral contraceptives prevent conception by suppressing ovulation, preventing implantation, or slowing migration of sperm to the ovum.

PROGESTINS

Special Dental Considerations

High doses of progestins can exacerbate a patient's inflammatory status, causing erythema and an increased tendency toward gingival bleeding. In some instances, progestins have been reported to induce gingival enlargement. A controlled oral hygiene program that includes regular oral examinations, professional cleanings, and plaque control will minimize the possible side effects of progestins.

Drug Interactions of Dental Interest

Progestins are responsible for maintenance of the female reproductive system in pregnant and nonpregnant women. Progestins are used for the treatment of certain female hormone imbalances as well as for the treatment of some neoplasms. Drug interactions with progestins are limited and involve drugs not normally prescribed by dentists.

See **Tables 20.1** and **20.2** for general information on progestins.

Pharmacology

Progestins bind to intracellular progesterone receptors that regulate RNA and DNA in target tissues.

INSULIN

Special Dental Considerations

Patients with diabetes mellitus are at risk of developing periodontal disease. Perform a thorough evaluation of the mouth, followed by a controlled oral hygiene program—including regular oral examinations, professional cleanings, and plaque control. Because diabetics have an increased risk of developing leukopenia and thrombocytopenia, there is a possibility of increased frequency of infections, altered wound healing, and gingival bleeding. Delay dental treatment if leukopenia or cytopenia occurs.

People who have either type 1 or type 2 diabetes mellitus can experience untoward effects in the dental office. These can occur when a patient's insulin dose is not correctly titrated and blood glucose levels are either too low or too high. In patients whose diabetes is well-controlled by insulin (or other hypoglycemic agents), these concerns are minimized by proper medication in conjunction with proper diet. Signs of hypo- and hyperglycemia are listed in **Table 20.3.**

Drug Interactions of Dental Interest

Insulin can be used for the treatment of patients with either type 1 or type 2 diabetes mellitus.

Corticosteroids may enhance blood glucose levels, and large doses of salicylates and nonsteroidal anti-inflammatory drugs may increase the hypoglycemic effect of insulin.

Laboratory Value Alterations

- Values for leukocytes in leukopenia: <4,000 cells/mm^3 opposed to the normal values of 5,000/mm^3 to 10,000 cells/mm^3.
- Values for platelets in thrombocytopenia: <20,000 platelets/mm^3 as opposed to the normal values of 150,000/mm^3 to 350,000 platelets/mm^3.

See **Tables 20.1** and **20.2** for general information on insulin.

Pharmacology

Insulin binds to fixed receptors on the cell membrane to control the storage and metabolism of carbohydrates, proteins, and lipids.

ORAL HYPOGLYCEMIC AGENTS

Special Dental Considerations

Patients with diabetes mellitus are at risk of developing periodontal disease. In patients whose diabetes is well-controlled by hypoglycemic agents, concerns are minimized with proper medication, diet, and oral hygiene. These patients should receive a thorough evaluation of the mouth followed by a controlled oral hygiene program that includes regular oral examinations, professional cleanings, and plaque control. Owing to an increased risk of leukopenia and thrombocytopenia in diabetic patients, there is a possibility of increased frequency of infections, altered wound healing, and gingival bleeding. Delay dental treatment if leukopenia or cytopenia occurs.

Drug Interactions of Dental Interest

Oral hypoglycemic agents can be used only for the treatment of type 2 diabetes mellitus.

Glucocorticoids may decrease the effectiveness of oral hypoglycemic agents. Nonsteroidal anti-inflammatory drugs and salicylates may increase the risk of hypoglycemia. See **Table 20.3** for a listing of signs of hypoglycemia.

Laboratory Value Alterations

- Values for leukocytes in leukopenia: <4,000 cells/mm^3 as opposed to the normal values of 5,000/mm^3 to 10,000 cells/mm^3.
- Values for platelets in thrombocytopenia: <20,000 platelets/mm^3 as opposed to the normal values of 150,000/mm^3 to 350,000 platelets/mm^3.

See **Tables 20.1** and **20.2** for general information on oral hypoglycemic agents.

Pharmacology

Oral hypoglycemics lower blood glucose levels by stimulating the functioning of β cells of the pancreatic islets to secrete insulin.

CALCITONIN

Special Dental Considerations

Calcitonin is administered primarily intranasally to treat Paget's disease, osteoporosis, or hypercalcemia. As a result of the nasal administration, a variety of oral-facial sequelae (such as skin rash, urticaria, flushing, redness, and swelling) can occur. Except for allergic reactions, these signs and symptoms should not require medical attention unless they continue or are bothersome.

See **Tables 20.1** and **20.2** for general information on calcitonin.

Drug Interactions of Dental Interest

When calcitonin is delivered via a nasal route, it can cause nasal symptoms that include the development of crusts, dryness, epistaxis, inflammation, rhinitis, and itching.

Pharmacology

Calcitonin is a polypeptide hormone that is secreted from the C cells of the thyroid gland. Calcitonin binds to the cell surface receptor and inhibits osteoclastic bone resorption while promoting the renal excretion of calcium, phosphate, sodium, magnesium, and potassium. Calcitonin ultimately acts to lower calcium in the bloodstream.

THYROID HORMONES

Special Dental Considerations

Patients with well-controlled hypothyroidism can receive any dental treatment. Delay dental treatment in patients whose thyroid symptoms are not appropriately controlled pharmacologically.

Drug Interactions of Dental Interest

Thyroid hormones, a mixture of liothyroxin and levothyroxine, are necessary for the homeostasis of the human body. Liothyroxin and/or levothyroxine are used for replacement therapy in patients with diminished thyroid function. Glucocorticoids and sympathomimetic agents may interfere with the actions of the drugs.

See **Tables 20.1** and **20.2** for general information on thyroid hormones.

Pharmacology

Thyroid hormones bind to nuclear thyroid hormone receptors that regulate catabolic and anabolic effects necessary for homeostasis.

ANTITHYROID AGENTS

Special Dental Considerations

Delay dental treatment in patients with hyperthyroidism whose symptoms are not appropriately controlled pharmacologically or surgically. Antithyroid hormones are a group of drugs used to decrease the production of thyroid hormones. Because these agents have the potential to depress cells in the bone marrow, the incidence of microbial infections can increase, resulting in delayed healing and gingival bleeding. A patient who is using antithyroid drugs may exhibit leukopenia, thrombocytopenia or both, and any dental work should be deferred until blood counts return to normal.

Drug Interactions of Dental Interest

Methimazole and propylthiouracil are used in the treatment of patients with hyperthyroidism before surgery or radiotherapy. These drugs can cause mouth sores, sialadenopathy, loss of taste, gingival bleeding, and delayed wound healing.

See **Tables 20.1** and **20.2** for general information on antithyroid hormones.

Pharmacology

Antithyroid hormones inhibit the synthesis of thyroid hormones by interfering with the oxidation of iodide to iodine, thereby blocking the synthesis of thyroxine.

BISPHOSPHONATES

Special Dental Considerations

Drugs that are used to treat osteoporosis may be very important to the dentist, since initial studies have suggested that there might be an association between periodontitis and osteoporosis. Additional studies are needed to demonstrate if a causative relationship exists between osteoporosis and tooth loss. Initial short-term studies in patients with periodontitis who are using bisphosphonates have suggested that these agents may play an important role in the maintenance of alveolar bone. Concomitant use of salicylates or salicylate-containing compounds with bisphosphonates is not recommended since an increased incidence of upper gastrointestinal adverse events can occur.

One of the more important considerations with bisphosphonates for the dentist is the reports of osteonecrosis of the jaw associated with the use of these drugs. The majority of cases of bisphosphonate-associated osteonecrosis (BON) have been associated with the intravenous administration of these agents; however, BON has been reported (at a significantly lower prevalence) with the enteral administration of bisphosphonates. Currently, data are limited regarding the incidence and prevalence of this condition and in identifying the risk factors that may influence BON in patients taking these drugs orally. See **Appendix N** for ADA recommendations on the dental management of patients on oral bisphosphonate therapy.

Pharmacology

Bisphosphonates work to inhibit osteoclast activity and help to preserve bone mass.

Adverse Effects, Precautions, and Contraindications

Table 20.1 presents contraindications, precautions, and adverse effects of endocrine/hormonal and bone metabolism drugs.

SUGGESTED READING

Edwards BJ, Hellstein JW, Jacobsen PL, Kaltman S, Mariotti A, Migliorati CA. American Dental Association Council on Scientific Affairs Expert Panel on Bisphosphonate-Associated Osteonecrosis of the Jaw. Updated recommendations for managing the care of patients receiving oral bisphosphonate therapy: an advisory statement from the American Dental Association Council on Scientific Affairs. *JADA.* 2008;139:1674-1677.

Galasko GT. Insulin, oral hypoglycemics, and glucagon. In: *Pharmacology and Therapeutics for Dentistry.* 6th ed. Yagiela JA, Dowd FJ, Mariotti A, Johnson BS, Neidle EA (eds). Elsevier Mosby; St. Louis, MO, 2009:573-582.

Galasko GT. Pituitary, thyroid and parathyroid pharmacology. In: *Pharmacology and Therapeutics for Dentistry.* 6th ed. Yagiela JA, Dowd FJ, Mariotti A, Johnson BS, Neidle EA (eds). Elsevier Mosby; St. Louis, MO, 2009:555-564.

Mariotti A. Sex steroid hormones and cell dynamics in the periodontium. *Crit Rev Oral Biol Med.* 1994;5:27-53.

Mariotti AJ. Steroid hormones of reproduction and sexual development. In: *Pharmacology and Therapeutics for Dentistry.* 6th ed. Yagiela JA, Dowd FJ, Mariotti A, Johnson BS, Neidle EA (eds). Elsevier Mosby; St. Louis, MO, 2009:583-594.

Preshaw PM, Knutsen M, Mariotti A. Experimental gingivitis in women using oral contraceptives. *J Dent Res.* 2001;80:2011-2015.

Table 20.1. PRESCRIBING INFORMATION FOR ENDOCRINE/HORMONAL AND BONE METABOLISM DRUGS

NAME	FORM/ STRENGTH	DOSAGE	WARNINGS/PRECAUTIONS & CONTRAINDICATIONS	ADVERSE EFFECTS†
ANDROGENS				
Fluoxymesterone CIII	**Tab:** 2mg*, 5mg*, 10mg*	***Adults/Pediatrics:* Male Hypogonadism:** 5-20mg/day qd or in divided doses tid-qid. ***Adults:* Breast Cancer:** 10-40mg/day in divided doses tid-qid. Continue therapy for at least 1 month for satisfactory subjective response, and for 2-3 months for objective response. ***Pediatrics:* Delayed Puberty: Initial:** Use low dose, titrate carefully; use for 4-6 months. Caution in children.	**W/P:** D/C if hypercalcemia occurs in breast cancer or immobilized patients; monitor calcium levels. Risk of hepatic adenomas, hepatocellular carcinoma, and peliosis hepatitis with prolonged high doses. D/C if jaundice, cholestatic hepatitis occurs. Caution in the elderly; increased risk of prostatic hypertrophy and prostatic carcinoma. Risk of edema; caution with preexisting cardiac, renal, or hepatic disease. Risk of compromised stature in children; monitor bone growth every 6 months. Should not be used for enhancement of athletic performance. Monitor for virilization in females. Patients with BPH may develop acute urethral obstruction. If priapism occurs, d/c and if restarted use lower dose. Contains tartrazine; may cause allergic type reactions especially in those with ASA hypersensitivity. Monitor LFTs, Hct, Hgb periodically. **Contra:** Males with breast or prostate cancer, pregnancy, serious cardiac, hepatic or renal disease. **P/N:** Category X, not for use in nursing.	Amenorrhea, virilization, menstrual irregularities, gynecomastia, excessive frequency/ duration of penile erections, male pattern baldness, increased/decreased libido, oligospermia, hirsutism, acne, fluid and electrolyte disturbances, nausea, hypercholesterolemia, clotting factor suppression, polycythemia, altered LFTs, oligospermia, priapism, anxiety, depression.
Methyltestosterone (Testred) CIII	**Cap:** 10mg	***Adults:*** Dose based on age, sex, and diagnosis. Adjust dose according to clinical response and adverse events. **Male Replacement Therapy:** 10-50mg/ day. **Breast Carcinoma:** 50-200mg/day. ***Pediatrics:*** Dose based on age, sex and diagnosis. Adjust dose according to clinical response and adverse events. **Delayed Puberty:** Use lower range of 10-50mg/day for 4-6 months. Caution in children.	**W/P:** D/C if hypercalcemia occurs in breast cancer; monitor calcium levels. Monitor for virilization in females. Risk of compromised stature in children; monitor bone growth every 6 months. Risk of hepatic damage with long-term use. D/C if jaundice, cholestatic hepatitis occurs. Risk of edema; caution with preexisting cardiac, renal or hepatic disease. Caution in the elderly; increased risk of prostatic hypertrophy and prostatic carcinoma. Should not be used for enhancement of athletic performance. Monitor LFTs, Hct, and Hgb periodically. **Contra:** Pregnancy. Males with breast or prostate carcinoma. **P/N:** Category X, not for use in nursing.	Amenorrhea, virilization, menstrual irregularities, gynecomastia, excessive frequency/ duration of penile erections, male pattern baldness, increased/decreased libido, oligospermia, hirsutism, acne, fluid and electrolyte disturbances, nausea, hypercholesterolemia, clotting factor suppression, polycythemia, altered LFTs, priapism, anxiety, depression.
Oxandrolone (Oxandrin) CIII	**Tab:** 2.5mg*, 10mg	***Adults:* Usual:** 2.5-20mg/day given bid-qid for 2-4 weeks. May repeat course intermittently as indicated. **Elderly:** 5mg bid. ***Pediatrics:*** ≤0.1mg/kg/day. May repeat intermittently as indicated.	**W/P:** D/C if peliosis hepatis, liver cell tumors, cholestatic hepatitis, jaundice, LFT abnormalities, hypercalcemia or signs of virilization (females) occur. Edema, with or without CHF, may occur with preexisting cardiac, renal, or hepatic disease. Monitor bone growth in children every 6 months. Increased risk of prostatic hypertrophy/carcinoma in the elderly. May decrease levels of thyroxine-binding globulin, suppress clotting factors II, V, VII, and X and increase PT. Caution with CAD and history of MI. Lower dose recommended in elderly. **Contra:** Carcinoma of the prostate or breast, carcinoma of the breast in females with hypercalcemia, pregnancy, nephrosis, hypercalcemia. **P/N:** Category X, not for use in nursing.	Cholestatic jaundice, gynecomastia, edema, CNS effects, acne, phallic enlargement, increased frequency/ persistence of erections, inhibition of testicular function, chronic priapism, epididymitis, impotence, testicular atrophy, oligospermia, bladder irritability, menstrual irregularities, virilization.

*Scored. †Bold entries denote special dental considerations.
BB = black box warning; **W/P** = warnings/precautions; **Contra** = contraindications; **P/N** = pregnancy category rating and nursing considerations.

Table 20.1. PRESCRIBING INFORMATION FOR ENDOCRINE/HORMONAL AND BONE METABOLISM DRUGS *(cont.)*

NAME	FORM/ STRENGTH	DOSAGE	WARNINGS/PRECAUTIONS & CONTRAINDICATIONS	ADVERSE EFFECTS†
ANDROGENS *(cont.)*				
Testosterone (Androderm) CIII	**Patch:** 2.5mg/24 hrs [60[s]], 5mg/24 hrs [30[s]]	***Adults/Pediatrics:* ≥15 yrs: Initial:** 5mg/day. **Maint:** 2.5mg-7.5mg/day. Apply patch nightly to intact skin of back, abdomen, upper arm, or thigh. Rotate sites; avoid same site for 7 days. Do not apply to scrotum or oily, damaged, irritated areas. May apply 2 patches at same time.	**W/P:** Prolonged use is associated with serious hepatic effects. Increased risk for prostatic hyperplasia/carcinoma in elderly. Risk of edema with preexisting cardiac, renal, or hepatic disease; d/c if edema occurs. Risk of virilization of female sex partner. Monitor LFTs, Hgb, Hct, PSA, cholesterol, lipids. **Contra:** Breast or prostate cancer in men. Women. **P/N:** Category X, not for use in nursing.	Gynecomastia, pruritus/erythema/ vesicles/blister at application site, prostate abnormalities, headache, depression.
Testosterone (Androgel, Testim) CIII	**Gel:** (Androgel) 1% [2.5g, 5g pkts; 75g pump]; (Testim) 1% [5g (50mg)/ tube, 30[s]]	***Adults:* (Androgel)** Apply 5g qd to clean, dry, intact skin of shoulders and upper arms and/or abdomen. Allow to dry prior to dressing. **Titrate:** May increase to 7.5g qd, then 10g qd if response not achieved. Do not apply to scrotum/genitals. **Pump:** Four actuations (5g), six actuations (7.5g), eight actuations (10g). **(Testim) ≥18yrs:** Apply 5g qd, preferably in the am, to clean, dry, intact skin of shoulders and/ or upper arms. Allow to dry prior to dressing. **Titrate:** May increase to 10g qd if response not achieved or serum concentration is below normal range. Do not apply to genitals or abdomen. To maintain serum testosterone levels, do not wash site of application for at least 2 hrs.	**W/P:** Caution in elderly; increased risk of prostatic hypertrophy/carcinoma. Risk of edema with preexisting cardiac, renal, or hepatic disease; d/c if edema occurs, diuretic therapy may be required. Risk of gynecomastia. May potentiate sleep apnea especially with obesity or chronic lung diseases. Transfer of testosterone can occur with skin-to-skin contact. Risk of virilization of female partner. Advise patients to report persistent penis erections, changes in skin color, ankle swelling, unexplained N/V, or breathing disturbances. Monitor serum testosterone, LFTs, Hgb, Hct, PSA, cholesterol, lipids. Prolonged use associated with serious hepatic effects (peliosis hepatitis, hepatic neoplasms, cholestatic hepatitis, jaundice). **Contra:** Breast or prostate carcinoma in men. Not for use by women. Pregnant and nursing women should avoid skin contact with application sites on men. Hypersensitivity to soy products. **P/N:** Category X, not for use in nursing.	Application-site reactions, benign prostatic hyperplasia, decreased DBP, increased BP, gynecomastia, headache, Hct/ Hgb increases, hot flushes, insomnia, increased lacrimation, mood swings, smell disorder.
Testosterone (Striant) CIII	**Tab, Buccal:** 30mg [6 blister packs, 10 buccal systems/blister]	***Adults:*** 30mg q12h to gum region, just above the incisor tooth on either side of mouth. Rotate sites with each application. Hold system in place for 30 seconds.	**W/P:** Caution in elderly; increased risk of prostatic hyperplasia/carcinoma. Risk of edema with preexisting cardiac, renal, or hepatic disease; d/c if edema occurs. May potentiate sleep apnea, especially with obesity or chronic lung diseases. Monitor Hgb, Hct, LFTs, PSA, cholesterol, lipids, serum testosterone. **Contra:** Women. Breast or prostate carcinoma in men. Hypersensitivity to soy products. **P/N:** Category X, not for use in nursing.	**Gum/mouth irritation, bitter taste, gum pain/ tenderness,** headache, gynecomastia.
Testosterone Cypionate (Depo-Testosterone) CIII	**Inj:** 100mg/mL, 200mg/mL	***Adults/Pediatrics:* ≥12 yrs: Male Hypogonadism:** 50-400mg IM every 2-4 weeks. Dose based on age, sex, and diagnosis. Adjust dose according to response and adverse reactions.	**W/P:** May accelerate bone maturation without linear growth; monitor bone growth every 6 months. Risk of hepatic damage with long-term use. D/C if hypercalcemia occurs in immobilized patients. D/C with acute urethral obstruction, priapism, excessive sexual stimulation, or oligospermia; restart at lower doses. Risk of edema; caution with preexisting cardiac, renal, or hepatic disease. Caution in the elderly; increased risk of prostatic hypertrophy and prostatic carcinoma. Caution with BPH. Should not be used for enhancement of athletic performance. Do not administer IV. Monitor Hct, Hgb, cholesterol periodically. **Contra:** Severe renal, hepatic, and cardiac disease. Males with carcinoma of the breast or prostate gland. Pregnancy. **P/N:** Category X, not for use in nursing.	Gynecomastia, excessive frequency/ duration of penile erections, male pattern baldness, increased/decreased libido, oligospermia, hirsutism, acne, fluid and electrolyte disturbances, nausea, hypercholesterolemia, clotting factor suppression, polycythemia, altered LFTs, priapism, anxiety, depression.

†Bold entries denote special dental considerations.
BB = black box warning; **W/P** = warnings/precautions; **Contra** = contraindications; **P/N** = pregnancy category rating and nursing considerations.

NAME	FORM/ STRENGTH	DOSAGE	WARNINGS/PRECAUTIONS & CONTRAINDICATIONS	ADVERSE EFFECTS†
Testosterone Enanthate (Delatestryl) CIII	**Inj:** 200mg/mL	***Adults/Pediatrics:*** Dose based on age, sex, and diagnosis. Adjust dose according to response and adverse reactions. **Male Hypogonadism:** 50-400mg IM every 2-4 weeks. **Delayed Puberty:** 50-200mg every 2-4 weeks for a limited duration (eg, 4-6 months). ***Adults:*** **Breast Cancer:** 200-400mg every 2-4 weeks.	**W/P:** D/C if hypercalcemia occurs in breast cancer or immobilized patients; monitor calcium levels. Risk of hepatic adenomas, hepatocellular carcinoma, and peliosis hepatitis with prolonged high doses. D/C if jaundice, cholestatic hepatitis, or abnormal LFTs occur. Avoid use in elderly with age-related hypogonadism. D/C if edema occurs in patients with preexisting cardiac, renal, or hepatic disease; restart at lower dose. Risk of compromised stature in children; monitor bone growth every 6 months. Monitor for virilization in females. Caution with a history of MI or CAD due to altered serum cholesterol levels. Monitor cholesterol, LFTs, Hct, Hgb periodically. **Contra:** Breast or prostate carcinoma in men. Pregnancy. **P/N:** Category X, not for use in nursing.	Amenorrhea, virilization, menstrual irregularities, gynecomastia, excessive frequency/ duration of penile erections, male pattern baldness, increased/decreased libido, oligospermia, hirsutism, acne, fluid and electrolyte disturbances, nausea, hypercholesterolemia, clotting factor suppression, polycythemia, altered LFTs, oligospermia, anxiety, depression.
BONE METABOLISM AGENTS				
Alendronate Sodium (Fosamax)	**Sol:** 70mg [75mL]; **Tab:** 5mg, 10mg, 35mg, 40mg, 70mg	***Adults:*** **Osteoporosis: Treatment:** 70mg once weekly or 10mg qd. **Prevention:** 35mg once weekly or 5mg qd. **Glucocorticoid-Induced:** 5mg qd; 10mg qd for postmenopausal women not on estrogen. **Paget's Disease:** 40mg qd for 6 months. Take at least 30 min before the first food, beverage (other than water), or medication (take tabs with 6-8 oz plain water or 2 oz with oral sol). Do not lie down for at least 30 min and until after first food of day.	**W/P:** Caution with active upper GI problems. May cause local irritation of the upper GI mucosa. Correct hypocalcemia or other mineral metabolism disturbances before initiating therapy. Supplement calcium and vitamin D if needed. Not recommended with renal insufficiency (CrCl <35mL/min). D/C if symptoms of esophageal disease develop. When combined with glucocorticoids, perform BMD test at initiation and 6-12 months later. Reports of severe, incapacitating bone, joint, and/or muscle pain. **Contra:** Esophagus abnormalities which delay esophageal emptying such as stricture or achalasia; inability to stand or sit upright for at least 30 min; hypocalcemia. **P/N:** Category C, caution in nursing.	Abdominal pain, nausea, dyspepsia, constipation, diarrhea, flatulence, acid regurgitation, musculoskeletal pain, gastric ulcers, joint swelling, asthenia, dizziness/ vertigo, and rarely peripheral edema.
Alendronate Sodium/ Cholecalciferol (Fosamax Plus D)	**Tab:** (Alendronate Sodium-Cholecalciferol) 70mg-2800 IU, 70mg-5600 IU	***Adults:*** 1 tab (70mg/5600 IU or 70mg/2800 IU) once weekly. Take at least 30 min before first food, beverage (other than water), or medication. Do not lie down for at least 30 min and until after first food of day.	**W/P:** Caution with active upper GI problems. May cause local irritation of the upper GI mucosa. Correct hypocalcemia or other mineral metabolism disturbances before initiating therapy. Do not use to treat vitamin D deficiency. May worsen hypercalcemia and/or hypercalciuria. Supplement calcium if needed. Not recommended with renal insufficiency (CrCl <35mL/min). D/C if symptoms of esophageal disease develop. Reports of severe, incapacitating bone, joint, and/or muscle pain. **Contra:** Esophagus abnormalities which delay esophageal emptying such as stricture or achalasia; inability to stand or sit upright for at least 30 min; hypocalcemia. **P/N:** Category C, caution in nursing.	Abdominal pain, nausea, dyspepsia, constipation, diarrhea, flatulence, acid regurgitation, musculoskeletal pain, gastric ulcers, joint swelling, asthenia, dizziness/ vertigo, and rarely peripheral edema.
Calcitonin-Salmon (Miacalcin)	**Inj:** 200 IU/mL; **Nasal Spray:** 200 IU/inh [2mL 2[s]]	***Adults:*** **Paget's Disease:** (Inj) **Usual:** 100 IU IM/SQ qd. **Hypercalcemia:** (Inj) **Initial:** 4 IU/kg IM/SQ q12h. **Titrate:** May increase to 8 IU/kg q12h after 1-2 days, then to 8 IU/kg q6h after 2 days if unsatisfactory response. **Postmenopausal Osteoporosis:** (Inj) 100 IU IM/SQ every other day. If >2mL, use IM injection. (Spray) 1 spray (200 IU) intranasally qd. Alternate nostrils daily. Take with supplemental calcium and vitamin D.	**W/P:** Possibility of systemic allergic reactions. Monitor urine sediment periodically with chronic use. If nasal mucosa ulceration occurs, d/c until healed. D/C if severe ulceration of the nasal mucosa occurs. Perform periodic nasal exams. Monitor drug effects. **P/N:** Category C, not for use in nursing.	(Inj) N/V, injection-site inflammation, flushing of face or hands, nocturia, ear lobe pruritus, poor appetite, abdominal pain. (Spray) Nasal symptoms, back pain, headache, arthralgia, epistaxis.

Table 20.1. PRESCRIBING INFORMATION FOR ENDOCRINE/HORMONAL AND BONE METABOLISM DRUGS *(cont.)*

NAME	FORM/ STRENGTH	DOSAGE	WARNINGS/PRECAUTIONS & CONTRAINDICATIONS	ADVERSE EFFECTS†
BONE METABOLISM AGENTS *(cont.)*				
Calcitonin-Salmon (rDNA origin) (Fortical)	**Nasal Spray:** 200 IU/inh	***Adults:*** 200 IU qd intranasally. Alternate nostrils daily.	**W/P:** Possibility of systemic allergic reactions. Consider skin testing if sensitivity suspected. If nasal mucosa ulceration occurs, d/c until healed. D/C if severe ulceration of nasal mucosa occurs. Perform periodic nasal exams. Incidence of rhinitis, irritation, erythema, and excoriation higher in geriatric patients. **Contra:** Clinical allergy to calcitonin-salmon. **P/N:** Category C, not for use in nursing.	Rhinitis, nasal symptoms, back pain, arthralgia, epistaxis, headache
Calcium Carbonate/Risedronate Sodium (Actonel with Calcium)	**Tab:** (Risedronate Sodium) 35mg; **Tab:** (Calcium Carbonate) 1250mg	***Adults:*** **Risedronate:** 35mg once weekly (Day 1 of 7-day treatment cycle). Take at least 30 min before first food or drink of day other than water. Swallow tab in upright position with 6-8 oz of plain water. Do not lie down for 30 min after dose. Calcium: 1250mg qd with food on each of remaining 6 days (Days 2-7 of the 7-day treatment cycle).	**W/P:** (Risedronate) May cause upper GI disorders (eg, dysphagia, esophagitis, esophageal or gastric ulcer). Treat hypocalcemia and other disturbances of bone and mineral metabolism before therapy. May cause osteonecrosis, primarily in jaw. Avoid with severe renal impairment (CrCl <30mL/min). (Calcium) Should not be used to treat hypocalcemia. Daily intake above 2000mg has been associated with increased risk of adverse effects, including hypercalcemia and kidney stones. Patients with achlorhydria may have decreased absorption of calcium. Severe and occasionally incapacitating bone, joint, and/or muscle pain in patient taking bisphosphonates reported. **Contra:** (Risedronate) Hypocalcemia; inability to stand or sit upright for at least 30 min. (Calcium) Hypercalcemia from any cause (eg, hyperparathyroidism, hypercalcemia of malignancy, sarcoidosis). **P/N:** Category C, not for use in nursing.	(Risedronate) infection, pain, flu syndrome, abdominal pain, headache, asthenia, HTN, constipation, dyspepsia, arthralgia, nausea, diarrhea, dizziness, myalgia. (Calcium) constipation, flatulence, nausea, abdominal pain, bloating.
Estradiol (Menostar)	**Patch:** 14mcg/ day [4[s]]	***Adults:*** Apply 1 patch weekly to lower abdomen (avoid breasts, waistline, and areas where sitting would dislodge the patch). Rotate application sites.	**BB:** Estrogens increase the risk of endometrial cancer. Estrogens, with or without progestins, should not be used for the prevention of cardiovascular disease. Increased risks of MI, stroke, invasive breast cancer, PE, and DVT in postmenopausal women (50-79 yrs of age) reported. Increased risk of developing probable dementia in postmenopausal women ≥65 yrs of age reported. **W/P:** May increase risk of cardiovascular events (eg, MI, stroke), venous thrombosis, and PE; d/c immediately if any of these events occur or are suspected. May increase risk of breast/endometrial cancer, and gallbladder disease. May lead to severe hypercalcemia with breast cancer and bone metastases; monitor and d/c if hypercalcemia occurs. Retinal vascular thrombosis reported; monitor and d/c if papilledema or retinal vascular lesions occur. Consider addition of a progestin if no hysterectomy. May elevate BP; monitor at regular intervals. May cause elevations of plasma triglycerides with preexisting hypertriglyceridemia. Caution with history of cholestatic jaundice associated with past estrogen use or with pregnancy; d/c with recurrence.	Pain, leukorrhea, arthralgia, application-site reaction, bronchitis, cervical polyps, constipation, dyspepsia, myalgia, dizziness, breast pain.

*Scored. †Bold entries denote special dental considerations.

BB = black box warning; **W/P** = warnings/precautions; **Contra** = contraindications; **P/N** = pregnancy category rating and nursing considerations.

NAME	FORM/ STRENGTH	DOSAGE	WARNINGS/PRECAUTIONS & CONTRAINDICATIONS	ADVERSE EFFECTS†
Estradiol (Menostar) *(cont.)*			May lead to increased TBG levels; monitor thyroid function. May cause fluid retention; caution with cardiac/renal dysfunction. Caution with severe hypocalcemia. May increase risk of ovarian cancer. May exacerbate endometriosis, asthma, DM, epilepsy, migraine, porphyria, SLE, and hepatic hemangiomas; use with caution. **Contra:** Pregnancy, undiagnosed abnormal genital bleeding, breast cancer, estrogen-dependent neoplasia, DVT/PE, active or recent (eg, within past year) arterial thromboembolic disease (eg, stroke, MI), liver dysfunction or disease. **P/N:** Contraindicated in pregnancy, caution in nursing.	
Etidronate Disodium (Didronel)	**Tab:** 200mg, 400mg*	***Adults:*** Give as single dose (preferred) or in divided doses. **Paget's disease: Initial:** 5-10mg/kg/day up to 6 months or 11-20mg/kg/day up to 3 months. May retreat after drug-free period of 90 days only if evidence of active disease process. **Heterotopic Ossification: Hip Replacement:** 20mg/kg/day 1 month before and 3 months after surgery. **Spinal Cord:** 20mg/kg/day for 2 weeks, followed by 10mg/kg/day for 10 weeks.	**W/P:** Therapy response in Paget's disease may be of slow onset and continue for months after stopping. Maintain adequate dietary intake of calcium and vitamin D. Diarrhea reported with enterocolitis. Monitor with renal impairment. Reduce dose with decreased GFR. Max dose (20mg/day) or long-term therapy (>6 months) may increase fracture risk. Rachitic syndrome reported in children at doses of 10mg/kg/day for prolonged periods (approaching or exceeding 1 year). **Contra:** Overt osteomalacia. **P/N:** Category C, caution with nursing.	Diarrhea, nausea, increased bone pain in Paget's, alopecia, arthropathy, **esophagitis,** hypersensitivity reactions, osteomalacia, amnesia, confusion.
Ibandronate Sodium (Boniva)	**Inj:** 3mg/3mL; **Tab:** 2.5mg, 150mg	***Adults:*** (Inj) 3mg IV over 15-30 sec every 3 months. (PO) 2.5mg qd or 150mg once monthly. Swallow whole with 6-8 oz water. Do not lie down for 60 min after dose. Take at least 60 min before first food, drink (other than water), medication, or supplementation.	**W/P:** (Inj, PO) Not recommended in severe renal impairment (CrCl <30mL/min). Reports of osteonecrosis, primarily in the jaw, and severe, incapacitating bone, joint, and/or muscle pain. Patients must receive supplemental calcium and vitamin D. (PO) May cause upper GI disorders (eg, dysphagia, esophagitis, esophageal or gastric ulcer). **Contra:** (Inj, PO) Hypocalcemia. (PO) Inability to stand or sit upright for at least 60 min. **P/N:** Category C, caution in nursing.	(Inj) Influenza, **nasopharyngitis,** cystitis, gastroenteritis, UTI, abdominal pain, dyspepsia, nausea, constipation, arthralgia, back pain, HTN. (PO) Back pain, extremity pain, infection, dyspepsia, diarrhea, hypercholesterolemia, myalgia, headache, dizziness, upper respiratory infection, bronchitis, pneumonia, UTI.
Pamidronate Disodium (Aredia)	**Inj:** 30mg, 90mg	***Adults:*** **Moderate Hypercalcemia:** 60-90mg IV single dose over 2-24 hrs. **Severe Hypercalcemia:** 90mg IV single dose over 2-24 hrs. **Retreatment:** May repeat after 7 days. **Paget's Disease:** 30mg IV over 4 hrs for 3 consecutive days. **Osteolytic Bone Lesions of Multiple Myeloma:** 90mg IV over 4 hrs once a month. **Osteolytic Bone Metastases of Breast Cancer:** 90mg IV over 2 hrs every 3-4 weeks. **Max:** 90mg/single dose for all indications. **Renal Dysfunction With Bone Metastases:** Withhold dose if SrCr increases by 0.5mg/dL (normal baseline) or by 1mg/dL (abnormal baseline). Resume when SrCr returns to within 10% of baseline.	**W/P:** Associated with renal toxicity; monitor SrCr prior to each treatment. Monitor serum calcium, electrolytes, phosphate, magnesium, CBC with differential, Hct/Hgb closely. Monitor for 2 weeks posttreatment if preexisting anemia, leukopenia, thrombocytopenia. Increased risk of renal adverse reactions with renal impairment; monitor renal function. Avoid treatment of bone metastases in severe renal impairment. Reports of osteonecrosis of jaw in cancer patients treated with bisphosphonates; avoid invasive dental procedures. **P/N:** Category D, caution in nursing.	Malaise, fever, convulsions, hypomagnesemia, hypocalcemia, hypokalemia, fluid overload, hypophosphatemia, nausea, diarrhea, constipation, anorexia, abnormal hepatic function, bone pain, dyspnea.

Table 20.1. PRESCRIBING INFORMATION FOR ENDOCRINE/HORMONAL AND BONE METABOLISM DRUGS *(cont.)*

NAME	FORM/ STRENGTH	DOSAGE	WARNINGS/PRECAUTIONS & CONTRAINDICATIONS	ADVERSE EFFECTS†
BONE METABOLISM AGENTS *(cont.)*				
Raloxifene HCl (Evista)	**Tab:** 60mg	***Adults:*** 60mg qd.	**BB:** Increased risk of DVT and PE reported. Avoid use in women with active or past history of venous thromboembolism. Increased risk of death due to stroke in postmenopausal women with documented coronary heart disease or at increased risk for major coronary events. **W/P:** May increase risk of DVT, PE, and retinal vein thrombosis; d/c 72 hrs prior to and during prolonged immobilization. May increase risk of death due to stroke in postmenopausal women with documented coronary heart disease or in women at increased risk for coronary events. Should not be used for primary or secondary prevention of CV disease. May increase levels of triglycerides with preexisting hypertriglyceridemia. Not for use in premenopausal women or with systemic estrogens. Caution with hepatic impairment or with moderate or severe renal impairment. Venous thromboembolism reported. **Contra:** Nursing, pregnancy, venous thromboembolic events (eg, DVT, PE, retinal vein thrombosis). **P/N:** Category X, contraindicated in nursing.	Hot flashes, leg cramps, abdominal pain, vaginal bleeding, arthralgia, rhinitis, headache.
Risedronate Sodium (Actonel)	**Tab:** 5mg, 30mg, 35mg, 75mg, 150mg	***Adults:*** **Paget's Disease:** 30mg qd for 2 months. May retreat after 2 months. **Postmenopausal Osteoporosis Prevention/Treatment:** 5mg qd or 35mg once weekly or 75mg on 2 consecutive days each month or 150mg once a month. **Glucocorticoid-Induced Osteoporosis:** 5mg qd. **Increase Bone Mass in Men with Osteoporosis:** 35mg once weekly. Take at least 30 min before first food or drink of day other than water. Swallow tab in upright position with 6-8 oz plain water. Do not lie down for 30 min after dose.	**W/P:** May cause upper GI disorders (eg, dysphagia, esophagitis, esophageal or gastric ulcer). Treat hypocalcemia and other disturbances of bone and mineral metabolism before therapy. Give supplemental calcium and vitamin D if dietary intake is inadequate. Avoid with severe renal impairment (CrCl <30mL/min). Osteonecrosis, primarily in the jaw, has been reported. Postmarketing reports of severe and occasionally incapacitating bone, joint, and/or muscle pain, has been reported. **Contra:** Hypocalcemia; inability to stand or sit upright for at least 30 min. **P/N:** Category C, not for use in nursing.	Asthenia, diarrhea, abdominal pain, nausea, constipation, peripheral edema, arthralgia, leg cramps, headache, dizziness, sinusitis, rash, tinnitus.
Teriparatide (Forteo)	**Inj:** 250mcg/mL [3mL pen]	***Adults:*** 20mcg qd SQ into thigh or abdominal wall. Administer initially under circumstances where patient can sit or lie down if symptoms of orthostatic hypotension occur. Discard pen after 28 days. Use for >2 yrs is not recommended.	**BB:** Increased incidence of osteosarcoma seen in rats. Only prescribe when benefits outweigh risks. Not for those at increased baseline risk for osteosarcoma, including Paget's disease or unexplained alkaline phosphatase elevations, open epiphyses, or prior radiation therapy involving the skeleton. **W/P:** Avoid in Paget's disease of the bone, pediatrics, prior external beam or implant radiation therapy, or with bone metastases, or history of skeletal malignancies, metabolic bone diseases other than osteoporosis, or preexisting hypercalcemia (eg, primary hyperparathyroidism). Potential exacerbation of active or recent urolithiasis. Transient episodes of symptomatic orthostatic hypotension observed infrequently. Increases serum uric acid levels. Transient calcium increases. **P/N:** Category C; not for use in nursing.	Pain, arthralgia, asthenia, nausea, rhinitis, dizziness, headache, HTN, increased cough, **pharyngitis**, constipation, diarrhea, dyspepsia.

†Bold entries denote special dental considerations.
BB = black box warning; **W/P** = warnings/precautions; **Contra** = contraindications; **P/N** = pregnancy category rating and nursing considerations.

NAME	FORM/ STRENGTH	DOSAGE	WARNINGS/PRECAUTIONS & CONTRAINDICATIONS	ADVERSE EFFECTS†
Tiludronate Disodium (Skelid)	**Tab:** 200mg	***Adults:*** 400mg qd for 3 months. After therapy, wait 3 months to assess response. Take with 6-8oz of water. Take 2 hrs after food.	**W/P:** May cause GI disorders (eg, dysphagia, esophagitis, esophageal or gastric ulcers). Maintain adequate vitamin D and calcium intake. Avoid in severe renal failure. May cause osteonecrosis, primarily in jaw, and musculoskeletal pain. **P/N:** Category C, caution in nursing.	Pain, headache, dizziness, paresthesia, diarrhea, N/V, dyspepsia, rhinitis, upper respiratory infection.
Zoledronic Acid (Reclast)	**Sol:** 5mg/100mL [100mL]	***Adults:*** **Osteoporosis:** 5mg IV once a year. **Paget's disease:** 5mg IV as single dose. Infuse for >15 mins at constant rate. Hydrate prior to administration.	**W/P:** Increases risk of hypocalcemia; monitor calcium and mineral levels regularly. May need calcium and vitamin D supplements. Not recommended for use in patients with severe renal impairment (CrCl <35mL/min); monitor SrCr before each dose. May cause osteonecrosis of the jaw; routine oral or dental exam needed prior to treatment. Avoid during pregnancy. Musculoskeletal pain may occur; D/C if severe symptoms develop. **Contra:** Hypocalcemia **P/N:** Category D, not for use in nursing.	Influenza, hypocalcemia, headache, lethargy, HTN, A-fib, arthralgia, myalgia, pyrexia, rigors, peripheral edema, paresthesia, dyspnea, angioedema.
CONTRACEPTIVES, MISCELLANEOUS				
Diaphragm (Ortho Diaphragm Kits)	**ALL-FLEX Arcing Spring Diaphragm or ORTHO Coil Spring Diaphragm:** 55mm, 60mm, 65mm, 70mm, 75mm, 80mm, 85mm, 90mm, 95mm	***Adults:*** Use with contraceptive cream/jelly; apply into cup of diaphragm and around the rim. May insert up to 6 hrs before intercourse. Insert additional contraceptive cream/jelly if more than 6 hrs has elapsed; do not remove diaphragm to do this. Keep diaphragm in place for 6 hrs after intercourse and remove as soon as possible thereafter. Cleanse diaphragm with mild, nonperfumed soap and warm water before initial use, and after each use. Rinse and dry carefully.	**W/P:** Avoid continuous use for >24 hrs. Risk of TSS. Increased risk of vaginal tract infection with retention of diaphragm for any period of time. Increased risk of UTI if not properly fitted. Refit diaphragm if lose/gain >10 lbs, same diaphragm for >1 yr, or if have baby or abortion. D/C with spermicide sensitivity. **Contra:** History of toxic shock syndrome (TSS), hypersensitivity to dry natural rubber. **P/N:** Safety in pregnancy and nursing not known.	
Ethinyl Estradiol/ Etonogestrel (NuvaRing)	**Vaginal ring:** (Ethinyl estradiol-Etonogestrel) 0.015mg-0.120mg/day	***Adults:*** Insert ring vaginally on or before the 5th day of cycle. Remove ring after 3 consecutive weeks. Insert new ring 1 week later on same day of the week and same time of day.	**W/P:** Cigarette smoking increases risk of serious cardiovascular side effects. This risk increases with age (especially >35 yrs) and heavy smoking. Increases risk of MI, thromboembolism, stroke, gallbladder disease, and hypertension. Retinal thrombosis and benign hepatic adenomas reported. May decrease glucose tolerance. May increase BP, PT, sex hormone-binding globulins, thyroid hormone, or LDL levels. May cause other lipid changes, fluid retention, breakthrough bleeding and spotting, or exacerbate migraines. May develop visual changes with contact lens. D/C if jaundice, significant depression, severe headaches or migraines develop. Toxic shock syndrome with tampon use reported. Increased risk of morbidity and mortality in certain inherited thrombophilias, obesity, and diabetes. Older women who take hormonal contraceptive should take the lowest possible dose formulation that is effective. **Contra:** Thrombophlebitis, active or history of thromboembolic disorders, history of DVT, cerebrovascular or coronary artery disease, valvular heart disease with complications, severe HTN, diabetes with vascular complications,	Vaginitis, headache, upper respiratory tract infection, leukorrhea, sinusitis, weight gain, nausea.

Table 20.1. PRESCRIBING INFORMATION FOR ENDOCRINE/HORMONAL AND BONE METABOLISM DRUGS *(cont.)*

NAME	FORM/ STRENGTH	DOSAGE	WARNINGS/PRECAUTIONS & CONTRAINDICATIONS	ADVERSE EFFECTS†
CONTRACEPTIVES, MISCELLANEOUS *(cont.)*				
Ethinyl Estradiol/ Etonogestrel (NuvaRing) *(cont.)*			headaches with focal neurological symptoms, major surgery with prolonged immobilization, breast carcinoma, endometrial carcinoma or other estrogen-dependent neoplasia, undiagnosed abnormal genital bleeding, cholestatic jaundice of pregnancy or jaundice with prior hormonal contraceptive use, hepatic tumors, active liver disease, pregnancy, heavy smoking and >35 yrs. **P/N:** Category X, not for use in nursing.	
Ethinyl Estradiol/ Norelgestromin (Ortho Evra)	**Patch:** (Ethinyl Estradiol-Norelgestromin): 0.75mg-6mg [1s, 3[s]]	***Adults:*** Start first Sunday after menses begin or first day of menses. Apply patch every week on same day for 3 weeks. Week 4 is patch-free. Apply to clean, dry intact skin on buttock, abdomen, upper arm, or upper torso.	**W/P:** Cigarette smoking increases risk of serious cardiovascular side effects. This risk increases with age (especially >35 yrs) and heavy smoking. Increased risk of MI, vascular disease, thromboembolism, stroke, and gallbladder disease. Retinal thrombosis, hepatic neoplasia reported. May cause glucose intolerance. May increase BP, elevate LDL levels, or cause other lipid changes, fluid retention, breakthrough bleeding, and spotting. May cause or exacerbate migraine. May develop visual changes with contact lens. Increased risk of MI with HTN, hyperlipidemia, and diabetes. D/C if jaundice or depression develops. Perform annual physical exam. Use before menarche is not indicated. May affect certain endocrine, LFTs, and blood components. May be less effective in women with body weight ≥198 lbs. **Contra:** Thrombophlebitis, DVT, thromboembolic disorders, pregnancy, cerebrovascular or coronary artery disease, valvular heart disease with complications, undiagnosed abnormal genital bleeding, cholestatic jaundice of pregnancy or jaundice with prior pill use, hepatic adenomas or carcinomas, breast cancer, or other estrogen-dependent neoplasia, severe HTN, diabetes with vascular involvement, headaches with focal neurological symptoms, major surgery with prolonged immobilization, acute/chronic hepatocellular disease with abnormal liver function. **P/N:** Category X, not for use in nursing.	Breast symptoms, headache, application-site reaction, nausea, upper respiratory infection, menstrual cramps, abdominal pain.
Levonorgestrel (Jadelle, Norplant II)	**Implant:** 75mg	***Adults:*** Implant 150mg (2 implants) in midportion of upper arm during first 7 days of onset of menses. Place in a V shape 30 in apart. Replace by end of 5th year.	**W/P:** Complications related to insertion and removal of capsules reported. Bleeding irregularities have occurred. Retinal thrombosis leading to partial or complete loss of vision, hepatic neoplasia, carcinoma of breast and reproductive organs reported. Risk of thromboembolic and thrombotic diseases, MI, ectopic pregnancy, ovarian cysts, breast cancer, gall bladder and autoimmune diseases, cerebrovascular	Menorrhagia, amenorrhea, oligomenorrhea, irregular bleeding, pain/itching or infection at implant site, headache, nervousness, GI effects, dizziness, rash, acne, weight gain, cervicitis.

†Bold entries denote special dental considerations.
BB = black box warning; **W/P** = warnings/precautions; **Contra** = contraindications; **P/N** = pregnancy category rating and nursing considerations.

NAME	FORM/ STRENGTH	DOSAGE	WARNINGS/PRECAUTIONS & CONTRAINDICATIONS	ADVERSE EFFECTS†
Levonorgestrel (Jadelle, Norplant II) *(cont.)*			diseases. Cigarette smoking increases risk of serious cardiovascular side effects; risk increases with age (especially >35 yrs) and the extent of smoking. Idiopathic intracranial HTN and increases in BP reported. Caution with fluid retention. Vision changes reported; caution with contact lenses. Weight gain, thrombosis, and thrombophlebitis reported. May worsen depression, increase LDL levels. If jaundice develops, remove implants. Altered glucose tolerance; monitor diabetics. Rare reports of congenital anomalies with use during early pregnancy. **Contra:** Active thrombophlebitis or thromboembolic disorders, undiagnosed abnormal genital bleeding, pregnancy, acute liver disease or liver tumors, carcinoma of the breast, and idiopathic intracranial HTN. **P/N:** Use in pregnancy not known, caution in nursing.	
Levonorgestrel (Mirena)	**Intrauterine Insert:** 52mg	***Adults:*** Insert intravaginally for contraception. Initial insertion is recommended within 7 days of the onset of menses. Replacement may be done at any time in the cycle. May insert 6 weeks postpartum or until involution of uterus is complete, and immediately after first trimester abortion. Reexamine within 3 months after insertion. Replace every 5 yrs.	**W/P:** Risk of ectopic pregnancy, glucose intolerance. Pregnancy with IUD in place, increased risk of septic abortion, congenital anomalies, premature labor, miscarriage. Increased risk of PID, sepsis, ovarian cysts. Can alter bleeding patterns. Partial penetration or embedment in myometrium may decrease effectiveness. May perforate the uterus or cervix during insertion. Displacement may occur. **Contra:** Pregnancy, congenital or acquired uterine anomaly, acute or history of PID, postpartum endometriosis, infected abortion in the past 3 months, uterine or cervical neoplasia, abnormal Pap smear, genital bleeding of unknown etiology, untreated acute cervicitis or vaginitis, acute liver disease, liver tumor, women or partner with multiple sexual partners, conditions associated with increased susceptibility to microorganisms, genital actinomycosis, previously inserted IUD that is not removed, breast carcinoma, and predisposition to ectopic pregnancy. **P/N:** Category X, not for use in nursing.	Abdominal pain, leukorrhea, headache, vaginitis, back pain, breast pain, acne, depression, HTN, upper respiratory infection, nausea, dysmenorrhea, weight increase, skin disorder, decreased libido, abnormal pap smear.
Levonorgestrel (Plan B)	**Tab:** 0.75mg	***Adults:*** One tab as soon as possible, within 72 hrs after unprotected intercourse, then one tab 12 hrs after first dose. May use during menstrual cycle.	**W/P:** Not for routine use as a contraceptive. Risk of glucose intolerance; monitor women with DM. Not effective in terminating an existing pregnancy. Risk of ectopic pregnancy. Irregular menstrual bleeding may occur. Vomiting within 1 hr after doses may decrease effectiveness. **Contra:** Pregnancy and undiagnosed abnormal genital bleeding. **P/N:** Pregnancy category unknown, caution in nursing.	N/V, abdominal pain, fatigue, headache, menstrual changes, dizziness, breast tenderness, diarrhea.
Medroxyprogesterone Acetate (Depo-Provera Contraceptive, depo-subQ provera 104)	**Inj:** (Depo-Provera Contraceptive) 150mg/mL; (depo-subQ provera 104) 104mg/0.65mL	***Adults:*** 150mg IM every 3 months (13 weeks) in gluteal or deltoid muscle. Give first injection during first 5 days of menses; within first 5 days postpartum if not nursing; or 6 weeks postpartum if nursing.	**BB:** May cause significant loss of bone mineral density (BMD); greater with increasing duration of use and may not be completely reversible. Should be used as long-term birth control (>2 yrs) only if other birth control methods	Menstrual irregularities, weight changes, abdominal pain, dizziness, headache, asthenia, nervousness,

Table 20.1. PRESCRIBING INFORMATION FOR ENDOCRINE/HORMONAL AND BONE METABOLISM DRUGS *(cont.)*

NAME	FORM/ STRENGTH	DOSAGE	WARNINGS/PRECAUTIONS & CONTRAINDICATIONS	ADVERSE EFFECTS†
CONTRACEPTIVES, MISCELLANEOUS *(cont.)*				
Medroxyprogesterone Acetate (Depo-Provera Contraceptive, depo-subQ provera 104) *(cont.)*			are inadequate. Unknown if use during adolescence or early adulthood will reduce peak bone mass and increase risk of osteoporotic fractures in later life. **W/P:** Loss of BMD, may cause bleeding irregularities, cancer risk, thromboembolic disorders, ocular disorders, unexpected pregnancies, ectopic pregnancy, anaphylaxis and anaphylactoid reaction, fluid retention, return of fertility, decrease in glucose metabolism. Caution with CNS or convulsive disorders. D/C if jaundice develops. **Contra:** Pregnancy, undiagnosed vaginal bleeding, breast malignancy, thrombophlebitis, thromboembolic disorders, cerebral vascular disease, liver dysfunction. **P/N:** (Depo-Provera Contraceptive) Category X, safety in nursing not known; (depo-subQ provera 104) not for use in pregnancy, safety in nursing not known.	decreased libido, depression, nausea, insomnia, leukorrhea, acne, vaginitis, pelvic pain.
Mifepristone (Mifeprex)	**Tab:** 200mg	***Adults:* Day 1:** 600mg single dose. **Day 3:** Unless abortion is confirmed, give 400mcg PO of misoprostol. **Day 14:** Assess if complete termination of pregnancy has occurred. Perform surgical termination if Mifeprex and misoprostol fail.	**BB:** Serious and sometimes fatal infections and bleeding occur very rarely following spontaneous, surgical, and medical abortions, including following Mifeprex use. Before prescribing Mifeprex, inform the patient about the risk of these serious events and discuss Medication Guide and Patient Agreement. Ensure that patient knows whom to call and what to do, including going to the ER if none of provided contacts are reachable, if she experiences sustained fever, severe abdominal pain, prolonged heavy bleeding, or syncope. **W/P:** Vaginal bleeding lasts for average 9-16 days. Infection and sepsis, including rare cases of fatal septic shock. Conduct follow-up visit 14 days after initial dose to confirm pregnancy termination. Preventive measures required to prevent rhesus immunization. Patients should review medication guide and patient agreement prior to procedure. Caution with women >35 yrs who smoke ≥10 cigarettes daily. Risk of fetal malformation if treatment fails. May cause decreases in Hgb, Hct, and RBCs. Very rare cases of fatal septic shock reported. **Contra:** Ectopic pregnancy, undiagnosed adnexal mass, IUD in place, chronic adrenal failure, concurrent long-term corticosteroid therapy, hemorrhagic disorders, concurrent anticoagulant therapy, inherited porphyrias, prostaglandin hypersensitivity. Patients who do not have access to medical facilities or who are unable to understand the treatment or comply with regimen. **P/N:** Not for use in pregnancy or nursing.	Abdominal pain, uterine cramping, N/V, headache, diarrhea, dizziness, fatigue, back pain, uterine hemorrhage, fever, viral infections, vaginitis.

†Bold entries denote special dental considerations.
BB = black box warning; **W/P** = warnings/precautions; **Contra** = contraindications; **P/N** = pregnancy category rating and nursing considerations.

NAME	FORM/ STRENGTH	DOSAGE	WARNINGS/PRECAUTIONS & CONTRAINDICATIONS	ADVERSE EFFECTS†
CONTRACEPTIVES, ORAL				
Desogestrel/Ethinyl Estradiol (Apri, Cyclessa, Desogen, Kariva, Mircette, Ortho-Cept, Velivet); **Drospirenone/ Ethinyl Estradiol** (Yasmin, YAZ); **Ethinyl Estradiol/ Ethynodiol Diacetate** (Demulen, Zovia); **Ethinyl Estradiol/Ferrous Fumarate/ Norethindrone** (Ovcon-35 Fe); **Ethinyl Estradiol/ Ferrous Fumarate/ Norethindrone Acetate** (Junel 1.5/30, Junel 1/20, Junel Fe 1.5/30, Junel Fe 1/20, Loestrin, Loestrin 1.5/30, Loestrin 1/20, Loestrin Fe 1.5/30, Loestrin Fe 1/20, Microgestin Fe 1.5/30, Microgestin Fe 1/20); **Ethinyl Estradiol/Levonorgestrel** (Alesse, Aviane, Enpresse, Lessina, Levora, Lybrel, Nordette-28, Portia, Seasonale, Seasonique, Trivora); **Ethinyl Estradiol/Norethindrone** (Balziva, Brevicon, Modicon, Necon 0.5/35, Necon 1/35, Necon 10/11, Norinyl 1/35, Nortrel 0.5/35, Nortrel 1/35, Nortrel 7/7/7, Ortho-Novum 1/35, Ortho-Novum 10/11, Ortho-Novum 7/7/7, Ovcon-35, Ovcon-50, Tri-Norinyl); **Ethinyl Estradiol/Norethindrone Acetate** (Estrostep Fe); **Ethinyl Estradiol/Norgestimate** (MonoNessa, Ortho-Cyclen, Ortho Tri-Cyclen, Ortho Tri-Cyclen Lo, Sprintec, Tri-Previfem, Tri-Sprintec); **Ethinyl Estradiol/Norgestrel** (Cryselle, Lo/Ovral, Low-Ogestrel); **Mestranol/Norethindrone** (Brevicon, Necon 1/50, Norinyl 1/50, Ortho-Novum 1/50); **Norethindrone** (Camila, Errin, Micronor, Nor-QD)	See manufacturer's package insert for specific brand information.	See manufacturer's package insert for specific brand information.	**W/P: [ALL]** Cigarette smoking increases risk of serious cardiovascular side effects. Risk increases with age (especially >35 yrs) and heavy smoking. Increased risk of MI, vascular disease, thromboembolism, stroke and gallbladder disease. Retinal thrombosis, hepatic neoplasia, carcinoma of breast and reproductive organs reported. May cause glucose intolerance. May increase BP, elevate LDL levels, or cause other lipid changes, fluid retention, breakthrough bleeding, and spotting. May cause or exacerbate migraine. May develop visual changes with contact lenses. Increased risk of MI with HTN, hyperlipidemia, certain inherited or acquired thrombophilias, obesity, and diabetes. D/C if jaundice, significant depression or ophthalmic irregularities develop. Perform annual physical exam. Not for use before menarche or with uncontrolled HTN. May affect certain endocrine, LFTs and blood components. **[Seasonale]** Weigh benefit of fewer planned menses against inconvenience of increased intermenstrual bleeding or spotting. **[Yasmin, YAZ]** Monitor K^+ levels during first cycle with conditions predisposing to hyperkalemia. **Contra: [ALL]:** Thrombophlebitis, DVT or thromboembolic disorders, pregnancy, cerebrovascular or coronary artery disease, undiagnosed abnormal genital bleeding, cholestatic jaundice of pregnancy or jaundice with prior pill use, hepatic adenomas or carcinomas, breast cancer, or other estrogen-dependent neoplasia. **[Alesse, Triphasil, Lo/Ovral]** Thrombophlebitis, DVT or thromboembolic disorders, pregnancy, cerebrovascular or coronary artery disease, undiagnosed abnormal genital bleeding, cholestatic jaundice of pregnancy or jaundice with prior pill use, hepatic adenomas or carcinomas, active liver disease (as long as liver function has not returned to normal). **[Ortho-Cyclen, Ortho Tri-Cyclen]** Migraine with focal aura, acute or chronic hepatocellular disease. **[Ortho Tri-Cyclen Lo]** Valvular heart disease with complications, severe HTN, diabetes with vascular involvement, headaches with focal neurological symptoms, major surgery with prolonged immobilization. **[Yasmin, Yaz]** Renal or adrenal insufficiency, hepatic dysfunction, liver tumor, active liver disease, heavy smoking (>15 cigarettes daily) and >35 yrs.	N/V, breakthrough bleeding, spotting, amenorrhea, migraine, depression, vaginal candidiasis, edema, weight changes.

Table 20.1. PRESCRIBING INFORMATION FOR ENDOCRINE/HORMONAL AND BONE METABOLISM DRUGS *(cont.)*

NAME	FORM/ STRENGTH	DOSAGE	WARNINGS/PRECAUTIONS & CONTRAINDICATIONS	ADVERSE EFFECTS†
ENDOMETRIOSIS AGENTS				
Danazol	**Cap:** 50mg, 100mg, 200mg	***Adults:* Endometriosis: Moderate-to-Severe Disease/Infertility: Initial:** 400mg bid. **Titrate:** Gradual downward titration to maintain amenorrhea. **Mild Disease: Initial:** 100-200mg bid. Start during menstruation. Continue for 3-6 months, up to 9 months if needed. **Fibrocystic Breast Disease:** 50-200mg bid, may use up to 6 months. Start during menstruation. **Hereditary Angioedema: Initial:** 200mg bid-tid. After favorable response, decrease by 50% or less at intervals of 1-3 months or longer if frequency of attacks before treatment dictates. May increase daily dose by up to 200mg if attack reoccurs.	**W/P:** Thromboembolism, thrombotic, thrombophlebitic events, benign intracranial HTN reported. Peliosis hepatitis, benign hepatic adenoma reported with long-term use. Alteration of lipoproteins may be marked; consider potential impact on the risk of atherosclerosis and coronary artery disease. Hepatic dysfunction reported; monitor LFTs. Exclude breast carcinoma before therapy for fibrocystic breast disease. Monitor for androgenic effects. Caution with epilepsy, migraine, and cardiac or renal dysfunction due to risk of fluid retention. Exacerbation of porphyria. Use nonhormonal method of contraception during therapy. **Contra:** Undiagnosed abnormal genital bleeding, pregnancy, nursing, porphyria, and markedly impaired hepatic, renal, or cardiac function. **P/N:** Category X, not for use in nursing.	Weight gain, acne, hirsutism, edema, hair loss, menstrual disturbances, hepatic dysfunction, flushing, vaginal dryness, breast size reduction, semen volume abnormality.
ESTROGEN				
Conjugated Estrogens (Cenestin, Enjuvia, Premarin); **Esterified Estrogens** (Menest); **Estradiol** (Alora, Climara, Divigel, Elestrin, Esclim, Estrace, Estraderm, Estrasorb, Estring, EstroGel, Evamist, Gynodiol, Vagifem, Vivelle, Vivelle-Dot); **Estradiol Acetate** (Femring, Femtrace); **Estradiol Cypionate** (Depo-Estradiol); **Estradiol Valerate** (Delestrogen); **Estropipate** (Ogen, Ortho-Est)	See manufacturer's package insert for specific brand information.	See manufacturer's package insert for specific brand information.	**BB:** Estrogens increase the risk of endometrial cancer. Estrogens, with or without progestins, should not be used for the prevention of CVD or dementia. Increased risks of MI, stroke, invasive breast cancer, PE, and DVT in postmenopausal women (50-79 yrs of age) reported. Increased risk of developing probable dementia in postmenopausal women ≥65 yrs of age reported. **W/P:** May increase risk of cardiovascular events (eg, MI, stroke), venous thrombosis, and PE; d/c immediately if any occur or suspected. May increase risk of breast/endometrial cancer, dementia and gallbladder disease. May lead to severe hypercalcemia with breast cancer and bone metastases; monitor and d/c if hypercalcemia occurs. Retinal vascular thrombosis reported; monitor and d/c if papilledema or retinal vascular lesions occur. Consider addition of a progestin if no hysterectomy. May elevate BP; monitor at regular intervals. May cause elevations of plasma triglycerides with preexisting hypertriglyceridemia. Caution with history of cholestatic jaundice associated with past estrogen use or with pregnancy; d/c with recurrence. May lead to increased TBG levels; monitor thyroid function. May cause fluid retention; caution with cardiac/renal dysfunction. Caution with severe hypocalcemia. May increase risk of ovarian cancer. May exacerbate endometriosis, asthma, DM, epilepsy, migraine, porphyria, SLE, and hepatic hemangiomas; use with caution. **Contra:** Pregnancy, undiagnosed abnormal genital bleeding, breast cancer unless being treated for metastatic disease, estrogen-dependent neoplasia, thrombophlebitis, or thromboembolic disorders. **P/N:** Category X, caution in nursing.	Altered vaginal bleeding, vaginal candidiasis, breast tenderness/enlargement, N/V, melasma, headache, weight changes, edema, altered libido.

†Bold entries denote special dental considerations.
BB = black box warning; **W/P** = warnings/precautions; **Contra** = contraindications; **P/N** = pregnancy category rating and nursing considerations.

NAME	FORM/ STRENGTH	DOSAGE	WARNINGS/PRECAUTIONS & CONTRAINDICATIONS	ADVERSE EFFECTS†
ESTROGEN COMBINATIONS				
Conjugated Estrogens/Medroxyprogesterone Acetate (Premphase, Prempro); **Drospirenone/Estradiol** (Angeliq); **Esterified Estrogens/Methyltestosterone** (Estratest, Estratest H.S.); **Estradiol/Levonorgestrel** (Climara Pro); **Estradiol/Norethindrone** (Activella) **Estradiol/Norethindrone Acetate** (CombiPatch); **Estradiol/Norgestimate** (Prefest); **Ethinyl Estradiol/Norethindrone Acetate** (femhrt)	See manufacturer's package insert for specific brand information.	See manufacturer's package insert for specific brand information.	**BB:** Estrogens increase the risk of endometrial cancer. Estrogens, with or without progestins, should not be used for the prevention of CVD or dementia. Increased risks of MI, stroke, invasive breast cancer, PE, and DVT in postmenopausal women (50-79 yrs of age) reported. Increased risk of developing probable dementia in postmenopausal women ≥65 yrs of age reported. **W/P:** May increase risk of cardiovascular events (eg, MI, stroke), venous thrombosis, and PE; d/c immediately if any occur or suspected. May increase risk of breast/endometrial cancer, dementia and gallbladder disease. May lead to severe hypercalcemia with breast cancer and bone metastases; monitor and d/c if hypercalcemia occurs. Retinal vascular thrombosis reported; monitor and d/c if papilledema or retinal vascular lesions occur. Consider addition of a progestin if no hysterectomy. May elevate BP; monitor at regular intervals. May cause elevations of plasma triglycerides with preexisting hypertriglyceridemia. Caution with history of cholestatic jaundice associated with past estrogen use or with pregnancy; d/c with recurrence. May lead to increased TBG levels; monitor thyroid function. May cause fluid retention; caution with cardiac/renal dysfunction. Caution with severe hypocalcemia. May increase risk of ovarian cancer. May exacerbate endometriosis, asthma, DM, epilepsy, migraine, porphyria, SLE, and hepatic hemangiomas; use with caution. **Contra:** Pregnancy, undiagnosed abnormal genital bleeding, breast cancer unless being treated for metastatic disease, estrogen-dependent neoplasia, thrombophlebitis, or thromboembolic disorders. **P/N:** Category X, caution in nursing.	Abdominal pain, dysmenorrhea, vaginal moniliasis, breast pain, nausea, arthralgia, headache, depression, back pain, infection, pain, vaginal hemorrhage, and vaginitis.
FERTILITY AGENTS				
Cetrorelix Acetate (Cetrotide)	**Inj:** 0.25mg, 3mg	***Adults:*** **Multiple-Dose Regimen:** 0.25mg SQ qd; start on Day 5 (am or pm) or Day 6 (am). Continue until HCG administration. **Single-Dose Regimen:** 3mg SQ single dose when estradiol level indicates appropriate stimulation response, usually on Day 7. If hCG not given within 4 days, then give 0.25mg SQ qd until day of hCG administration.	**W/P:** Exclude pregnancy before initiating therapy. **Contra:** Pregnancy, nursing, hypersensitivity to extrinsic peptide hormones or mannitol, severe renal impairment. **P/N:** Category X, not for use in nursing.	Ovarian hyperstimulation syndrome, nausea, headache.
Choriogonadotropin alfa (Ovidrel)	**Inj:** 250mcg/ 0.5mL	***Adults:*** 250mcg SQ 1 day following the last dose of follicle stimulating agent. Withhold if excessive ovarian response.	**W/P:** Ovarian hyperstimulation syndrome (OHSS), multiple births, and elevated ALTs reported. Potential for arterial thromboembolism. Withhold hCG if ovarian enlargement or OHSS occurs. Administer when adequate follicular development indicated by serum estradiol and vaginal ultrasonography occurs. **Contra:** Primary ovarian failure, uncontrolled thyroid or adrenal function, uncontrolled organic intracranial lesion	Injection-site pain/ bruising, abdominal pain, N/V.

Table 20.1. PRESCRIBING INFORMATION FOR ENDOCRINE/HORMONAL AND BONE METABOLISM DRUGS *(cont.)*

NAME	FORM/ STRENGTH	DOSAGE	WARNINGS/PRECAUTIONS & CONTRAINDICATIONS	ADVERSE EFFECTS†
FERTILITY AGENTS *(cont.)*				
Choriogonadotropin alfa (Ovidrel) *(cont.)*			(eg, pituitary tumor), abnormal uterine bleeding of undetermined origin, ovarian cyst or enlargement of undetermined origin, sex hormone-dependent tumors of reproductive tract and accessory organs, pregnancy. **P/N:** Category X, caution in nursing.	
Chorionic Gonadotropin (Novarel, Pregnyl)	**Inj:** 10,000 U	***Adults:*** **Hypogonadism:** 500-1000 U IM 3x/week (TIW) for 3 weeks, then twice weekly for 3 weeks; or 4000 U IM TIW for 6-9 months, then reduce to 2000 U TIW for 3 months. **Ovulation Induction:** 5000-10,000 U IM 1 day after last dose of menotropins. ***Pediatrics:*** **≥4 yrs: Cryptorchidism:** 4000 U IM TIW for 3 weeks; or 5000 U IM every second day for 4 doses; or 15 doses of 500-1000 U over 6 weeks; or 500 U TIW for 4-6 weeks (if treatment fails, give 1000 U/injection starting 1 month later). Initiate therapy between 4-9 yrs. **Hypogonadism:** 500-1000 U IM TIW for 3 weeks, then twice weekly for 3 weeks; or 4000 U IM TIW for 6-9 months, then reduce to 2000 U TIW for 3 months.	**W/P:** Potential ovarian hyperstimulation, enlargement or rupture of ovarian cysts, multiple births, and arterial thromboembolism with infertility treatment. D/C if precocious puberty occurs in cryptorchidism patients. Caution with cardiac or renal disease, epilepsy, migraine, asthma. Not effective treatment for obesity. **Contra:** Precocious puberty, prostatic carcinoma or other androgen-dependent neoplasms, pregnancy. **P/N:** (Novarel) Category C, caution in nursing; (Pregnyl) Safety in pregnancy and nursing not known.	Headache, irritability, restlessness, depression, fatigue, edema, precocious puberty, gynecomastia, injection-site pain.
Clomiphene Citrate (Clomid, Serophene)	**Tab:** (Clomid) 50mg*: (Serophene) 50mg	***Adults:*** **Initial:** 50mg/day for 5 days. Start any time if no recent uterine bleeding. If progestin-induced bleeding is intended, or if spontaneous uterine bleeding occurs, start on the 5th day of the cycle. If ovulation does not occur, increase to 100mg qd for 5 days, 30 days after the first course. **Max:** 100mg qd for 5 days and 3 courses of therapy.	**W/P:** Increased incidence of visual symptoms with increasing total dose or therapy duration; d/c treatment and perform complete ophthalmological evaluation. Ovarian hyperstimulation syndrome reported; monitor for abdominal pain, N/V, diarrhea, weight gain. Increased chance of multiple pregnancy. Perform pelvic exam before initiating therapy and before each course. Prolonged use may increase risk of borderline/invasive ovarian tumor. **Contra:** Pregnancy, liver disease or history of liver dysfunction, abnormal uterine bleeding of undetermined origin, ovarian cysts or enlargement not due to polycystic ovarian syndrome, uncontrolled thyroid or adrenal dysfunction, organic intracranial lesion (eg, pituitary tumor). **P/N:** Category X, caution in nursing.	Ovarian enlargement, vasomotor flushes, N/V, breast discomfort, abdominal-pelvic discomfort/distention/bloating, visual symptoms, headache, abnormal uterine bleeding.
Follitropin Alfa (Gonal-F)	**Inj:** 75 IU, 450 IU, 300 IU/0.5mL, 450 IU/0.75mL, 900 IU/1.5mL	***Adults:*** Individualize dose. **Oligo-Anovulation: Initial:** 75 IU/day SQ. **Titrate:** Increase up to 37.5 IU/day after 14 days and further increase after 7 days if needed. Give hCG 5000 U 1 day after last dose. Do not exceed 35 days of therapy unless an E2 rise indicates imminent follicular development. **Max:** 300 IU/day. **ART: Initial:** 150 IU/day SQ on cycle Day 2 or 3 (early follicular phase). If gonadotropins suppressed, initiate at 225 IU/day. **Titrate:** Adjust after 5 days if needed, then at intervals no less than 3-5 days and not exceeding 75-150 IU/adjustment. **Max:** 450 IU/day. Once follicular development is evident, give hCG 5000-10,000 U. **Hypogonadotropic Hypogonadism:** Pretreat with hCG 1000-2250 U 2-3x/	**W/P:** Ovarian enlargement may occur; monitor ovarian response. Ovarian hyperstimulation syndrome, multiple births, serious pulmonary and vascular complications reported. Avoid hCG if ovaries abnormally enlarged last day of therapy. Monitor follicular maturation by measuring estradiol levels and through ultrasonography. **Contra:** (Men, Women) High FSH levels indicating gonadal failure, uncontrolled thyroid or adrenal dysfunction, sex hormone dependent tumors of the reproductive tract and accessory organs, organic intracranial lesions (eg, pituitary tumor). (Women) Abnormal uterine bleeding of undetermined origin, ovarian cyst or enlargement, pregnancy. **P/N:** Category X, not for use in nursing.	(Women) Intermenstrual bleeding, breast pain, ovarian hyperstimulation, abdominal pain, nausea, diarrhea, flatulence, headache, ovarian cysts, pain, upper respiratory tract infection. (Men) Breast pain, acne, gynecomastia, injection-site pain, fatigue.

†Bold entries denote special dental considerations.
BB = black box warning; **W/P** = warnings/precautions; **Contra** = contraindications; **P/N** = pregnancy category rating and nursing considerations.

NAME	FORM/ STRENGTH	DOSAGE	WARNINGS/PRECAUTIONS & CONTRAINDICATIONS	ADVERSE EFFECTS†
Follitropin Alfa (Gonal-F) *(cont.)*		week to achieve normal serum testosterone levels. When normal, give 150 IU SQ and hCG 1000 U 3x/week. **Max:** 300 IU 3x/week.		
Follitropin Beta (Follistim AQ, Follistim AQ Cartridge)	**Cartridge:** 150 IU, 300 IU, 600 IU, 900 IU. **Inj:** 75 IU, 150 IU	***Adults:*** **Ovulation Induction:** (Cartridge) 75 IU for 7 days. **Titrate:** Increase by 25-50 IU at weekly intervals. **Max:** 175 IU daily. (Inj) 75 IU for 14 days. **Titrate:** Increase by 37.5 IU weekly. Administer hCG 5000-10,000 U when preovulatory conditions are equivalent to or greater than a normal individual. **ART:** Initial 150 to 225 IU for 5 days (cartridge) or 4 days (inj). **Titrate:** Adjust based upon ovarian response. Administer hCG 5000-10,000 U when a sufficient number of follicles of adequate size are present.	**W/P:** Exclude primary ovarian failure. Ovarian enlargement may occur; use the lowest effective dose and monitor ovarian response. Ovarian hyperstimulation syndrome (OHSS), multiple births, serious pulmonary and vascular complications reported. Avoid hCG if ovaries abnormally enlarged last day of therapy. Monitor follicular maturation by measuring estradiol levels and through sonographic visualization. **Contra:** High FSH level indicating primary ovarian failure, uncontrolled thyroid or adrenal dysfunction, pregnancy, heavy or irregular vaginal bleeding of undetermined origin, ovarian cysts or enlargement not due to polycystic ovary syndrome; or tumor of the ovary, breast, uterus, hypothalamus or pituitary gland. Hypersensitivity to streptomycin or neomycin and to recombinant hFSH products. **P/N:** Category X, not for use in nursing.	Abdominal pain, flatulence, nausea, breast pain, injection-site reaction, enlarged abdomen, back pain, constipation, headache, ovarian pain, OHSS, sinusitis, upper respiratory tract infection.
Ganirelix Acetate	**Inj:** 250mcg/ 0.5mL	***Adults:*** 250mcg SQ qd during the mid-to-late follicular phase. Continue until hCG administration.	**W/P:** Exclude pregnancy before initiate therapy. Contains natural rubber latex. **Contra:** Pregnancy. **P/N:** Category X, not for use in nursing.	Abdominal pain (gynecological), fetal death, headache, ovarian hyperstimulation syndrome.
Lutropin alfa (Luveris)	**Inj:** 75 IU	***Adults:*** **Initial:** 75 IU with 75-150 IU of Gonal-F qd SQ as two separate injections. Give hCG 1 day after last dose. Do not exceed 14 days of therapy unless signs of imminent follicular development. Do not exceed 225 IU/ day of Gonal-F.	**W/P:** Ovarian enlargement may occur; monitor ovarian response. Ovarian hyperstimulation syndrome (OHSS), multiple births, serious pulmonary and vascular complications reported. Do not administer hCG dose if evidence of OHSS. Monitor follicular maturation through ultrasonography and serum estradiol levels. **Contra:** Primary ovarian failure, uncontrolled thyroid or adrenal dysfunction, uncontrolled organic intracranial lesion (eg, pituitary tumor), abnormal uterine bleeding of undetermined origin, ovarian cyst or enlargement of undetermined origin, sex hormone–dependent tumors of the reproductive tract and accessory organs, and pregnancy. **P/N:** Category X, caution in nursing.	Headache, nausea, ovarian hyperstimulation, breast pain (female), abdominal pain, ovarian cyst, flatulence, injection-site reaction, dysmenorrhea, ovarian disorder, diarrhea, constipation, pain, fatigue, upper respiratory tract infection.
Menotropins (Menopur)	**Inj:** (FSH-LH) 75 IU-75 IU	***Adults:*** **Initial:** 225 IU SQ. **Titrate:** Adjust subsequent dosing to individual response at intervals no less than every 2 days and not exceeding 150 IU/adjustment. **Max:** 450 IU/day. Dosing >20 days not recommended. If adequate response, administer hCG. Withhold hCG if ovaries abnormally enlarged last day of therapy.	**W/P:** Ovarian hyperstimulation syndrome (OHSS) with or without pulmonary or vascular complications. Mild to moderate uncomplicated ovarian enlargement with abdominal distention and/or abdominal pain may occur. Reports of serious pulmonary conditions (eg, atelectasis, acute respiratory distress syndrome) and thromboembolic events (intravascular thrombosis, embolism, venous thrombophlebitis, pulmonary embolism, pulmonary infarction, cerebral vascular occlusion, arterial occlusion) which may lead to death. Potential risk of multiple births. **Contra:** High FSH level indicating primary ovarian failure; uncontrolled thyroid and	Headache, abdominal pain, injection-site reaction, N/V, abdominal cramps, abdominal fullness, OHSS, respiratory disorder.

Table 20.1. PRESCRIBING INFORMATION FOR ENDOCRINE/HORMONAL AND BONE METABOLISM DRUGS *(cont.)*

NAME	FORM/ STRENGTH	DOSAGE	WARNINGS/PRECAUTIONS & CONTRAINDICATIONS	ADVERSE EFFECTS†
FERTILITY AGENTS *(cont.)*				
Menotropins (Menopur) *(cont.)*			adrenal dysfunction; organic intracranial lesion (pituitary tumor); sex hormone–dependent tumor of the reproductive tract and accessory organs; abnormal uterine bleeding of undetermined origin; ovarian cysts or enlargement not due to polycystic ovary syndrome; pregnant women. **P/N:** Category X, caution in nursing.	
Menotropins (Repronex)	**Inj:** (FSH-LH) 75 IU-75 IU	***Adults:*** **Oligo-anovulation:** Individualize dose. **Initial:** 150 IU SQ/IM qd for 5 days. Adjust subsequent dose to individual response at intervals no less than every 2 days and not exceeding 75-150 IU/adjustment. **Max:** 450 IU/day. Dosing >12 days is not recommended. If adequate response, give 5000-10,000 U hCG. May repeat course if inadequate response. **Assisted Reproductive Technology: Initial:** 225 IU SQ/IM. Adjust subsequent dose to individual response at intervals no less than every 2 days and not exceeding 75-150 IU/adjustment. **Max:** 450 IU/day. Dosing >12 days is not recommended. If adequate response, give 5000-10,000 U hCG.	**W/P:** Exclude primary ovarian failure. Ovarian enlargement may occur; monitor ovarian response. Ovarian hyperstimulation syndrome (OHSS), hypersensitivity/anaphylactic reactions, multiple pregnancies, serious pulmonary and vascular complications reported. Avoid hCG if ovaries abnormally enlarged last day of therapy. Monitor follicular maturation by measuring estradiol levels and through ultrasonography. **Contra:** High FSH levels indicating primary ovarian failure, uncontrolled thyroid or adrenal dysfunction, organic intracranial lesions (eg, pituitary tumor), any cause of infertility other than anovulation (unless candidate for in vitro fertilization), abnormal bleeding of undetermined origin, ovarian cysts or enlargement not due to polycystic ovary syndrome, pregnancy. **P/N:** Category X, caution in nursing.	Pulmonary and vascular complications, OHSS, hemoperitoneum, adnexal torsion, ovarian enlargement, ovarian cysts, abdominal pain, GI symptoms, injection-site reactions, rash.
Progesterone (Crinone, Prochieve)	**Gel:** (Crinone, Prochieve) 4% [45mg, 6[s]], (Crinone, Prochieve) 8% [90mg, 6[s], 18[s]]	***Adults:*** **ART:** 90mg of 8% intravaginally qd if require progesterone supplementation. 90mg of 8% intravaginally bid with partial or complete ovarian failure requiring progesterone replacement. If pregnancy occurs, continue until placental autonomy is achieved, up to 10-12 weeks. **Secondary Amenorrhea:** 4% intravaginally every other day up to 6 doses. If fails, 8% intravaginally every other day up to 6 doses.	**W/P:** D/C if signs of thrombotic disorders develop. Include pap smear in pretreatment exam. Caution with depression, DM, epilepsy, migraine, asthma, cardiac or renal dysfunction. **Contra:** Undiagnosed vaginal bleeding, liver dysfunction, malignancy of breast or genital organs, missed abortion, thrombophlebitis, thromboembolic disorders, history of hormone-associated thrombophlebitis or thromboembolic disorders. **P/N:** Safety in pregnancy or nursing not known.	Bloating, abdominal pain/cramps, depression, headache, nausea, vaginal discharge, fatigue, genital pruritus.
Progesterone (Endometrin)	**Vaginal Insert:** 100mg [21[s]]	***Adults:*** 100mg vaginally bid or tid starting at oocyte retrieval and continuing for up to 10 weeks.	**W/P:** D/C if signs of MI, cerebrovascular disorders, thromboembolism, thrombophlebitis, or retinal thrombosis develop. Caution with history of depression. **Contra:** Known missed abortion or ectopic pregnancy, liver disease, known or suspected breast cancer. Active arterial or venous thromboembolism or severe thrombophlebitis, or a history of these events. **P/N:** Safety in pregnancy and nursing not known.	Postoocyte-retrieval pain, abdominal pain, N/V, ovarian hyperstimulation syndrome, abdominal distention, headache, uterine spasm, vaginal bleeding.
Urofollitropin (Bravelle)	**Inj:** 75 IU	***Adults:*** **Ovulation Induction: Initial:** 150 IU SQ/IM qd for 1st 5 days. Adjust subsequent dose to individual response at intervals no less than every 2 days and not exceeding 75-150 IU/adjustment. **Max:** 450 IU/day. Dosing >12 days is not recommended. If adequate response, give 5000-10,000 U hCG 1 day following last dose. May repeat course if inadequate follicle development or ovulation without pregnancy occurs.	**W/P:** Exclude primary ovarian failure. Ovarian enlargement may occur; monitor ovarian response. Ovarian hyperstimulation syndrome (OHSS), multiple births, hypersensitivity/anaphylactic reactions, serious pulmonary and vascular complications reported. Avoid hCG if ovaries are abnormally enlarged on last day of therapy. Monitor follicle growth and maturation with estradiol levels and ultrasonography. **Contra:** High	OHSS, vaginal hemorrhage, pelvic pain, nausea, headache, pain, UTI, respiratory disorder, hot flashes, abdominal enlargement or pain.

†Bold entries denote special dental considerations.
BB = black box warning; **W/P** = warnings/precautions; **Contra** = contraindications; **P/N** = pregnancy category rating and nursing considerations.

NAME	FORM/ STRENGTH	DOSAGE	WARNINGS/PRECAUTIONS & CONTRAINDICATIONS	ADVERSE EFFECTS†
Urofollitropin (Bravelle) *(cont.)*		**ART:** 225 IU SQ qd for 1st 5 days. Adjust subsequent dose to individual response at intervals no less than every 2 days and not exceeding 75-150 IU/ adjustment. **Max:** 450 IU/day. Dosing >12 days is not recommended. If adequate follicular development, give 5000-10,000 U hCG to induce final follicular maturation in preparation for oocyte retrieval.	FSH levels indicating primary ovarian failure, uncontrolled thyroid or adrenal dysfunction, organic intracranial lesions (eg, pituitary tumor), any cause of infertility other than anovulation, abnormal bleeding of undetermined origin, ovarian cysts or enlargement not due to polycystic ovary syndrome, pregnancy. **P/N:** Category X, not for use in nursing.	
HYPOGLYCEMIC AGENTS				
INSULINS				
Insulin Aspart (Novolog)	**Inj:** 100 U/mL; **PenFill:** 100 U/mL; **Prefilled:** 100 U/mL	***Adults/Pediatrics:* ≥4 yrs:** Individualize dose. Inject SQ within 5-10 min before a meal. Draw first when mixing with NPH human insulin; inject immediately. Do not mix with crystalline zinc insulins, animal source insulins, or other manufacturer insulins. (External Pump) Do not use or mix with any other insulin or diluent in pump.	**W/P:** Any change of insulin should be made cautiously. Changes in strength, manufacturer, type or method of manufacture may result in the need for a change in dosage. Hypoglycemia may occur with taking too much insulin, missing or delaying meals, exercising or working more than usual, diseases of adrenal, pituitary, or thyroid glands, or progression of kidney or liver disease. May cause hypokalemia. Dosage adjustments may be needed with hepatic or renal dysfunction, during any infection, illness (especially with diarrhea or vomiting) or pregnancy. A longer-acting insulin is usually required to maintain adequate glucose control. Infusion sets and the insulin in the infusion sets should be changed q48h or sooner. Do not use in quick-release infusion sets or cartridge adapters. **Contra:** Hypoglycemia. **P/N:** Category B, caution in nursing.	Hypoglycemia, hypokalemia, lipodystrophy, hypersensitivity reaction, injection-site reactions, pruritus, rash.
Insulin Aspart/ Insulin Aspart Protamine (Novolog Mix 70/30)	(Insulin Aspart Protamine-Insulin Aspart) **Inj:** 70 U-30 U/mL; **PenFill:** 70 U-30 U/mL; **Prefilled:** 70 U-30 U/mL	***Adults:*** Individualize dose. For SQ inj only. Inject SQ bid within 15 min before breakfast and dinner. Do not mix with other insulins or use in insulin pumps.	**W/P:** Any change of insulin should be made cautiously. Changes in strength, manufacturer, type or method of manufacture may result in the need for a change in dosage. Hypoglycemia and hypokalemia may occur; caution with fasting and autonomic neuropathy. Illness, stress, change in meals and exercise may change insulin requirements. Smoking, temperature, and exercise affect insulin absorption. Caution with liver or kidney disease. Administration of insulin SQ can result in lipoatrophy. **Contra:** Hypoglycemia. **P/N:** Category C, safety in nursing not known.	Hypoglycemia, hypokalemia, lipodystrophy, hypersensitivity reaction, injection-site reactions, pruritus, rash.
Insulin Detemir, rDNA origin (Levemir)	**Inj:** 100 U/mL [3mL, 10mL]	***Adults/Pediatrics:*** Individualize dose. Administer SQ qd or bid. **Once Daily Dosing:** Administer with evening meal or bedtime. **Twice Daily Dosing:** Administer evening dose with evening meal, at bedtime, or 12 hrs after morning dose. **Type 1/Type 2 Diabetes on Basal-Bolus Treatment or Patients Only on Basal Insulin:** Change on a unit-to-unit basis. ***Adults:* Insulin-Naive with Type 2 Diabetes Inadequately Controlled on Oral Antidiabetics: Initial:** 0.1-0.2 U/kg in evening or 10 U qd or bid.	**W/P:** Monitor glucose; may cause hypoglycemia. Not for use in an insulin infusion pump. Should not be diluted or mixed with any other insulin preparations. May cause lipodystrophy or hypersensitivity. Dose adjustment may be needed in renal or hepatic impairment and during intercurrent conditions such as illness, emotional disturbances, or other stresses. **P/N:** Category C, caution in nursing.	Allergic reactions, injection-site reactions, lipodystrophy, pruritus, rash, hypoglycemia, weight gain.

Table 20.1. PRESCRIBING INFORMATION FOR ENDOCRINE/HORMONAL AND BONE METABOLISM DRUGS *(cont.)*

NAME	FORM/ STRENGTH	DOSAGE	WARNINGS/PRECAUTIONS & CONTRAINDICATIONS	ADVERSE EFFECTS†
HYPOGLYCEMIC AGENTS *(cont.)*				
INSULINS *(cont.)*				
Insulin Glargine, Human (Lantus)	**Inj:** 100 U/mL; (OptiClik): 100 U/mL	***Adults/Pediatrics:*** **≥6 yrs:** Individualize dose. For SQ injection only. Administer qd at same time each day. Insulin naive patients on oral antidiabetic drugs, start with 10 U qd. Switching from once-daily NPH or Ultralente does not require initial dose change. Switching from bid NPH, reduce initial dose by 20%. **Maint:** 2-100 U/day.	**W/P:** Human insulin differs from animal source insulin. Any change of insulin should be made cautiously. Changes in strength, manufacturer, type or method of manufacture may result in the need for a change in dosage. Hypoglycemia may occur with taking too much insulin, missing or delaying meals, exercising or working more than usual. An infection or illness (especially with diarrhea or vomiting) may change insulin requirements. Administration of insulin SQ can result in lipodystrophy. Not for IV use. Do not mix with other insulins. May cause sodium retention and edema. Caution in patients with renal and hepatic dysfunction. **P/N:** Category C, caution in nursing.	Hypoglycemia, allergic reactions, injection-site reactions, lipodystrophy, pruritus, rash.
Insulin Glulisine, rDNA (Apidra)	**Inj:** 100 U/mL	***Adults/Pediatrics:*** **≥4 yr:** Individualize dose. Inject SQ within 15 min before a meal or within 20 min after starting a meal. Rotate inj site (abdomen, thigh, or deltoid).	**W/P:** Hypoglycemia and hypokalemia may occur; monitor glucose and potassium levels. Rapid onset and short duration of action; follow dosage directions. Adjust dose if change in physical activity or usual meal plan. Longer-acting insulin or insulin infusion pump may be required to maintain glucose control. When used in an external pump for SQ infusion, do not dilute or mix with any other insulin. Caution when changing insulin strength, manufacturer, type, or species. Concomitant antidiabetic therapy may need adjustment. As with other insulin therapy hypoglycemic reactions and local/systemic allergic reactions may occur. May be given IV under proper medical supervision. Caution in renal/hepatic impairment. **Contra:** Episodes of hypoglycemia. **P/N:** Category C, caution in nursing.	Allergic reactions, injection-site reactions, lipodystrophy, pruritus, rash, hypoglycemia.
Insulin Human, rDNA origin/ Insulin, Human (Isophane/Regular) (Humulin 50/50, Humulin 70/30) OTC	(Isophane-Regular) **Inj:** (Humulin 70/30) 70 U-30 U/mL, (Humulin 50/50) 50 U-50 U/mL	***Adults/Pediatrics:*** Individualize dose. Administer SQ.	**W/P:** Human insulin differs from animal source insulin. Make any change of insulin cautiously. Changes in strength, manufacturer, type, or method of manufacture may result in the need for a change in dosage. Hypoglycemia may occur with too much insulin, missing or delaying meals, exercising, or working more than usual. Infection or illness (especially with diarrhea or vomiting) may change insulin requirements. Administration of insulin SQ can result in lipoatrophy. **P/N:** Pregnancy category is not known.	Hypoglycemia, sweating, dizziness, palpitation, tremor, hunger, restlessness, lightheadedness, inability to concentrate, headache, injection-site reaction, allergic reaction.
Insulin Human, rDNA origin/ Insulin, Human (Isophane/Regular) (Novolin 70/30) OTC	(Isophane/Regular) **Inj:** 70 U-30 U/mL; **PenFill:** 70 U-30 U/mL; **Prefilled:** 70 U-30 U/mL	***Adults/Pediatrics:*** Individualize dose. Administer SQ.	**W/P:** Human insulin differs from animal source insulin. Any change of insulin should be made cautiously. Changes in strength, manufacturer, type or method of manufacture may result in the need for a change in dosage. Hypoglycemia may occur with taking too much insulin, missing or delaying meals, exercising or working more than usual. An infection or illness (especially with diarrhea or vomiting) may change insulin	Hypoglycemia, sweating, dizziness, palpitation, tremor, hunger, restlessness, lightheadedness, inability to concentrate, headache, injection-site reaction, allergic reaction.

†Bold entries denote special dental considerations.
BB = black box warning; **W/P** = warnings/precautions; **Contra** = contraindications; **P/N** = pregnancy category rating and nursing considerations.

NAME	FORM/ STRENGTH	DOSAGE	WARNINGS/PRECAUTIONS & CONTRAINDICATIONS	ADVERSE EFFECTS†
Insulin Human, rDNA origin/ Insulin, Human (Isophane/Regular) (Novolin 70/30) OTC *(cont.)*			requirements. Caution with diseases of adrenal, pituitary, or thyroid glands, or progression of kidney or liver disease. Administration of insulin SQ can result in lipoatrophy. **P/N:** Pregnancy category is not known.	
Insulin Human, rDNA origin/ Insulin, Human Isophane/Insulin, Human Regular (Humulin, Humulin N, Humulin R) OTC	**Inj:** 100 U/mL (Humulin N, Humulin R), 500 U/mL (Humulin R U-500); **Pen:** 100 U/mL (Humulin N)	***Adults/Pediatrics:*** Individualize dose.	**W/P:** Human insulin differs from animal source insulin. Any change of insulin should be made cautiously. Changes in strength, manufacturer, type or method of manufacture may result in the need for a change in dosage. Hypoglycemia may occur with taking too much insulin, missing or delaying meals, exercising or working more than usual. An infection or illness (especially with diarrhea or vomiting) may change insulin requirements. Administration of insulin SQ can result in lipoatrophy. **Contra:** Hypoglycemia. **P/N:** Pregnancy category is not known.	Hypoglycemia, sweating, dizziness, palpitation, tremor, hunger, restlessness, lightheadedness, inability to concentrate, headache, injection-site reaction, allergic reaction.
Insulin Human, rDNA origin/ Insulin, Human Isophane/Insulin, Human Regular (Novolin, Novolin N, Novolin R) OTC	**Inj:** 100 U/mL (Novolin N, Novolin R); **PenFill:** 100 U/mL (Novolin N, Novolin R); **Prefilled:** 100 U/mL (Novolin N, Novolin R)	***Adults/Pediatrics:*** Individualize dose.	**W/P:** Human insulin differs from animal source insulin. Any change in insulin should be made cautiously. Changes in strength, manufacturer, type or method of manufacture may result in the need for a change in dosage. Hypoglycemia may occur with taking too much insulin, missing or delaying meals, exercising or working more than usual. An infection or illness (especially if accompanied by diarrhea or vomiting) may change insulin requirements. Administration of insulin SQ can result in lipoatrophy. Novolin R is not recommended for use in insulin pumps. **P/N:** Pregnancy category is not known.	Hypoglycemia, sweating, dizziness, palpitations, tremor, hunger, restlessness, lightheadedness, inability to concentrate, headache, injection-site reaction, allergic reaction.
Insulin Lispro (Humalog)	**Cartridge:** 100 U/mL; **Inj:** 100 U/mL; **Pen:** 100 U/mL	***Adults/Pediatrics:* ≥3 yrs:** Individualize dose. Inject SQ within 15 min before or immediately after a meal. May use with external insulin pump; do not dilute or mix with other insulins when used with pump.	**W/P:** Any change of insulin should be made cautiously. Changes in strength, manufacturer, type or method of manufacture may result in the need for a change in dosage. Hypoglycemia may occur with taking too much insulin, missing or delaying meals, exercising or working more than usual. An infection or illness (especially with diarrhea or vomiting) may change insulin requirements. With Type 1 DM a longer-acting insulin is usually required to maintain glucose control; not required with Type 2 DM if regimen includes sulfonylureas. May be diluted with sterile diluent. Caution with potassium-lowering drugs or drugs sensitive to serum potassium levels. **Contra:** Hypoglycemia. **P/N:** Category B, caution in nursing.	Hypoglycemia, hypokalemia, allergic reactions, injection-site reaction, lipodystrophy, pruritus, rash.
Insulin Lispro/ Insulin Lispro Protamine (Humalog Mix 75/25)	(Insulin Lispro Protamine, Human-Insulin Lispro, Human) **Inj:** 75 U-25 U/mL; **Pen:** 75 U-25 U/mL	***Adults:*** Individualize dose. Inject SQ within 15 min before a meal. May need to reduce/adjust dose with renal/hepatic impairment.	**W/P:** Any change of insulin should be made cautiously. Changes in strength, manufacturer, type or method of manufacture may result in the need for a change in dosage. Hypoglycemia may occur with taking too much insulin, missing or delaying meals, exercising or working more than usual. An infection or illness (especially with diarrhea or vomiting) may change insulin requirements. **Contra:** Hypoglycemia. **P/N:** Category B, caution in nursing.	Hypoglycemia, hypokalemia, allergic reactions, injection-site reaction, lipodystrophy, pruritus, rash.

Table 20.1. PRESCRIBING INFORMATION FOR ENDOCRINE/HORMONAL AND BONE METABOLISM DRUGS *(cont.)*

NAME	FORM/ STRENGTH	DOSAGE	WARNINGS/PRECAUTIONS & CONTRAINDICATIONS	ADVERSE EFFECTS†
HYPOGLYCEMIC AGENTS *(cont.)*				
ORAL DIABETIC AGENTS				
Acarbose (Precose)	**Tab:** 25mg, 50mg, 100mg	***Adults:*** **Initial:** 25mg tid with first bite of each main meal. **To Minimize GI Effects:** 25mg qd, increase gradually to 25mg tid. **Titrate:** After reaching 25mg tid, may increase at 4- to 8-week intervals. **Maint:** 50-100mg tid. **Max:** **≤60kg:** 50mg tid. **>60kg:** 100mg tid. If no further reduction in postprandial or A1C with 100mg tid, consider reducing dose.	**W/P:** Avoid with significant renal dysfunction (SrCr >2mg/dL). May need to d/c and give insulin with stress (eg, fever, trauma). Dose-related elevated serum transaminase levels reported. Monitor serum transaminases every 3 months for first year then periodically. Reduce dose or d/c if elevated serum transaminases persist. Use glucose (dextrose) instead of sucrose (sugar cane) to treat mild to moderate hypoglycemia. **Contra:** Diabetic ketoacidosis, cirrhosis, inflammatory bowel disease, colonic ulceration, partial or predisposition to intestinal obstruction, chronic intestinal disease with marked disorders of digestion or absorption, and conditions that may deteriorate from increased intestinal gas formation. **P/N:** Category B, not for use in nursing.	Transient flatulence, diarrhea, abdominal pain.
Chlorpropamide (Diabinese)	**Tab:** 100mg*, 250mg*	***Adults:*** **Initial:** 250mg qd. **Titrate:** After 5-7 days, adjust by 50-125mg/day every 3-5 days for control. **Maint:** 100-500mg qd. **Max:** 750mg qd. **Elderly/ Debilitated/Malnourished/Renal or Hepatic Dysfunction: Initial:** 100-125mg qd. **Maint:** Conservative dosing. Take with breakfast. Divide dose with GI intolerance. If <40 U/day insulin, d/c therapy. If ≥40 U/day insulin, decrease dose by 50% and start chlorpropamide therapy. Adjust insulin dose depending on response.	**W/P:** Increased risk of cardiovascular mortality. Hypoglycemia risk especially with renal/hepatic insufficiency, elderly, debilitated, malnourished, and adrenal/ pituitary insufficiency. Loss of blood glucose control when exposed to stress (fever, trauma, infection or surgery); d/c therapy and start insulin. Secondary failure can occur over a period of time. **Contra:** Diabetic ketoacidosis and Type 1 diabetes. **P/N:** Category C, not for use in nursing.	Hypoglycemia, cholestatic jaundice, diarrhea, N/V, anorexia, pruritus, photosensitivity reactions, skin eruptions, blood dyscrasias, hepatic porphyria, disulfiram-like reactions.
Glimepiride (Amaryl)	**Tab:** 1mg*, 2mg*, 4mg*	***Adults:*** **Initial:** 1-2mg qd with breakfast or first main meal. **Titrate:** After 2mg, may increase by up to 2mg every 1-2 weeks. **Maint:** 1-4mg qd. **Max:** 8mg qd. **Amaryl/Metformin:** Add metformin to 8mg qd for better glucose control. **Amaryl/Insulin Therapy:** If FBG >150mg/ dL on 8mg qd, add low-dose insulin; increase insulin weekly as needed. **Renal Insufficiency: Initial:** 1mg qd. **Elderly/Debilitated/Malnourished/ Hepatic Insufficiency:** Dose conservatively to avoid hypoglycemia.	**W/P:** Increased cardiovascular mortality. Hypoglycemia risk if debilitated, malnourished, or with adrenal, pituitary, renal, or hepatic insufficiency. Hypoglycemia may be masked in elderly. May lose blood glucose control with stress. Secondary failure may occur. D/C if skin reactions persist or worsen. **Contra:** Diabetic ketoacidosis. **P/N:** Category C, not for use in nursing.	Dizziness, nausea, asthenia, headache, hypoglycemia.
Glimepiride/ Pioglitazone HCl (Duetact)	**Tab:** (Pioglitazone-Glimepiride) 30mg-2mg, 30mg-4mg	***Adults:*** Base recommended starting dose on current regimen of pioglitazone and/or sulfonylurea. Give with first meal of day. **Current Glimepiride Monotherapy or Prior Therapy of Pioglitazone plus Glimepiride Separately: Initial:** 30mg-2mg or 30mg-4mg qd. **Current Pioglitazone or Different Sulfonylurea Monotherapy or Combination of Both: Initial:** 30mg-2mg qd. Adjust dose based on response. **Max:** Once daily at any strength. **Elderly/Debilitated/ Malnourished/Renal or Hepatic Insufficiency (ALT ≤2.5x ULN): Initial:** 1mg glimepiride prior to prescribing Duetact. **Systolic Dysfunction: Initial:** 15-30mg of pioglitazone; titrate carefully to lowest Duetact dose.	**BB:** Thiazolidinediones may cause or exacerbate CHF in some patients. Duetact is not recommended in patients with symptomatic heart failure. **W/P:** (Glimepiride) Increased CV mortality. Hypoglycemia risk if debilitated, malnourished, or with adrenal, pituitary, renal or hepatic insufficiency. Hypoglycemia may be masked in elderly. May lose blood glucose control with stress. Secondary failure may occur. D/C if skin reactions persist or worsen. (Pioglitazone) May cause fluid retention and exacerbation/initiation of heart failure; d/c if cardiac status deteriorates. Avoid if NYHA Class III or IV cardiac status. Not for use in Type 1 DM or diabetic ketoacidosis treatment. Caution with	Hypoglycemia, upper respiratory tract infection, increased weight, lower limb edema/ pain, headache, UTI, diarrhea, nausea, new onset or worsening diabetic macular edema with decreased visual acuity.

*Scored. †Bold entries denote special dental considerations.
BB = black box warning; **W/P** = warnings/precautions; **Contra** = contraindications; **P/N** = pregnancy category rating and nursing considerations.

NAME	FORM/ STRENGTH	DOSAGE	WARNINGS/PRECAUTIONS & CONTRAINDICATIONS	ADVERSE EFFECTS†
Glimepiride/ Pioglitazone HCl (Duetact) *(cont.)*			edema dose-related weight gain reported. Ovulation in premenopausal anovulatory patient may occur; risk of pregnancy with inadequate contraception. May decrease Hgb and Hct. Avoid with active liver disease, if ALT levels >2.5x ULN, or if jaundice occurred. Check LFTs before therapy, every 2 months for 1 yr, and periodically thereafter, or if hepatic dysfunction symptoms occur. D/C if ALT >3x ULN on therapy. Macular edema and fractures reported. **Contra:** Established NYHA Class III or IV heart failure, diabetic ketoacidosis. **P/N:** Category C, not for use in nursing.	
Glimepiride/ Rosiglitazone Maleate (Avandaryl)	**Tab:** (Rosiglitazone-Glimepiride) 4mg-1mg, 4mg-2mg, 4mg-4mg, 8mg-2mg, 8mg-4mg	***Adults:*** **Initial:** 4mg-1mg qd with first meal of day. **With Sulfonylurea or Thiazolidinedione: Initial:** 4mg-2mg qd. **Switching From Prior Combination Therapy:** Same dose of each component already being taken. **Prior Thiazolidinedione Monotherapy:** Titrate dose. After 1-2 weeks with inadequate control, increase glimepiride component in no more than 2mg increments at 1- to 2-week intervals. **Max:** 8mg-4mg qd. **Prior Sulfonylurea Monotherapy:** May take 2-3 months for full effect of rosiglitazone; do not exceed 8mg of rosiglitazone daily. **Titrate:** May increase glimepiride component. **Elderly/Debilitated/Malnourished/ Renal, Hepatic or Adrenal Insufficiency: Initial:** 4mg-1mg qd. Titrate carefully.	**BB:** Thiazolidinediones may cause or exacerbate CHF in some patients. Avandaryl is not recommended in patients with symptomatic heart failure. Meta-analysis of studies has shown rosiglitazone to be associated with an increased risk of myocardial ischemic events. **W/P:** Should not be used in patients with Type 1 diabetes or for the treatment of diabetic ketoacidois. (Glimepiride) Increased cardiovascular mortality. Hypoglycemia risk if debilitated, malnourished, or with adrenal, pituitary, renal or hepatic insufficiency. Hypoglycemia may be masked in elderly. May lose blood glucose control with stress. Secondary failure may occur. D/C if skin reactions persist or worsen. (Rosiglitazone) May cause fluid retention and exacerbation/initiation of heart failure; d/c if cardiac status deteriorates. Increased risk of CV events with NYHA Class I and II heart failure. Initiation not recommended for patients experiencing an acute coronary event and d/c during this acute phase. Caution with edema. May cause macular edema. Dose-related weight gain reported. Ovulation in premenopausal anovulatory patient may occur; risk of pregnancy with inadequate contraception. May decrease Hgb and Hct. Avoid with active liver disease, if ALT levels >2.5x ULN, or if jaundice occurred with rosiglitazone. Check LFTs before therapy, every 2 months for 1 yr, and periodically thereafter, or if hepatic dysfunction symptoms occur. D/C if ALT >3x ULN on therapy. Increased incidence of bone fracture was noted in female patients. Combination use with insulin not recommended. **Contra:** Established NYHA Class III or IV heart failure. **P/N:** Category C, not for use in nursing.	Upper respiratory tract infection, injury, headache, hypoglycemia, anemia, edema.
Glipizide (Glipizide ER, Glucotrol, Glucotrol XL)	**Tab:** (Glipizide) 2.5mg, 5mg, 10mg; (Glucotrol) 5mg*, 10mg* ; **Tab, Extended-Release:** (XL) 2.5mg, 5mg, 10mg	***Adults:*** (Tab,ER) Do not chew, divide, or crush. **Initial:** 5mg qd with breakfast. Use lower doses if sensitive to hypoglycemics. **Usual:** 5-10mg qd. **Max:** 20mg/day. **Combination Therapy: Initial:** 5mg qd. (Tab) **Initial:** 5mg qd 30 min before breakfast. **Geriatric/Hepatic Impairment: Initial:** 2.5mg qd. **Titrate:** Increase by 2.5-5mg after several days. **Max:** 40mg/day. Divide	**W/P:** Increased risk of hypoglycemia with the elderly, debilitated, malnourished, renal and hepatic disease, adrenal or pituitary insufficiency. Increased risk of cardiovascular mortality. Loss of blood glucose control when exposed to stress (fever, trauma, infection, or surgery); d/c therapy and start insulin. Secondary failure can occur over a period of time. (Tab,ER) GI disease will reduce	Hypoglycemia, GI disturbances, allergic skin reactions, hematologic disturbances, disulfiram-like reactions, hyponatremia, SIADH, dizziness, drowsiness, headache.

Table 20.1. PRESCRIBING INFORMATION FOR ENDOCRINE/HORMONAL AND BONE METABOLISM DRUGS *(cont.)*

NAME	FORM/ STRENGTH	DOSAGE	WARNINGS/PRECAUTIONS & CONTRAINDICATIONS	ADVERSE EFFECTS†
HYPOGLYCEMIC AGENTS *(cont.)*				
ORAL DIABETIC AGENTS *(cont.)*				
Glipizide (Glipizide ER, Glucotrol, Glucotrol XL) *(cont.)*		doses >15mg and give 30 min before a meal. (Tab/Tab,ER) **Switch From Insulin: If on ≤20 U/day:** Stop insulin; start Tab,ER or Tab 5mg qd. **If on >20 U/day:** Reduce insulin dose by 50% and add Tab,ER or Tab 5mg qd. Further insulin reductions depend on response. **Elderly/Debilitated/Malnourished/ Renal or Hepatic Impairment:** Dose conservatively.	retention time of the drug. Caution with preexisting severe GI narrowing. **Contra:** Diabetic ketoacidosis. **P/N:** Category C, not for use in nursing.	
Glipizide/ Metformin HCl (Metaglip)	**Tab:** (Glipizide-Metformin) 2.5mg-250mg, 2.5mg-500mg, 5mg-500mg	***Adults:*** **Inadequate Glycemic Control on Diet/Exercise Alone: Initial:** 2.5mg-250mg qd. If FBG 280-320mg/dL, give 2.5mg-500mg bid. **Titrate:** Increase by 1 tab/day every 2 weeks. **Max:** 10mg-1g/day or 10mg-2g/day given in divided doses. **Inadequate Glycemic Control on Sulfonylurea or Metformin: Initial:** 2.5mg-500mg or 5mg-500mg bid (with morning and evening meals). Starting dose should not exceed daily dose of metformin or glipizide already being taken. **Titrate:** Increase by no more than 5mg-500mg/day. **Max:** 20mg-2g/ day. **Elderly/Debilitated/Malnourished:** Do not titrate to max dose. Take with meals.	**W/P:** Lactic acidosis reported (rare); increased risk with renal dysfunction, increased age, DM, CHF, and other conditions with risk of hypoperfusion and hypoxemia. Avoid use in patients ≥80 yrs unless renal function is normal. Increased risk of cardiovascular mortality. Increased risk of hypoglycemia in elderly, debilitated/malnourished, adrenal or pituitary insufficiency, or alcohol intoxication. D/C in hypoxic states (eg, CHF, shock, acute MI) and prior to surgical procedures (due to restricted food intake). Avoid in renal/hepatic impairment. May decrease serum vitamin B_{12} levels. Impaired renal and/or hepatic function may slow glipizide excretion. Withhold treatment with any condition associated with dehydration or sepsis. Monitor renal function. **Contra:** Renal disease/dysfunction (SrCr ≥1.5mg/dL [males], ≥1.4mg/dL [females], abnormal CrCl), metabolic acidosis, diabetic ketoacidosis. D/C temporarily (48 hrs) for radiologic studies with intravascular iodinated contrast materials. **P/N:** Category C, not for use in pregnancy or nursing.	Upper respiratory tract infection, HTN, headache, diarrhea, dizziness, musculoskeletal pain, N/V, abdominal pain.
Glyburide (DiaBeta, Glynase PresTab, Micronase)	**Tab:** (DiaBeta, Micronase) 1.25mg*, 2.5mg*, 5mg*; (Glynase PresTab) 1.5mg*, 3mg*, 6mg*	***Adults:*** (DiaBeta, Micronase) **Initial:** 2.5-5mg qd with breakfast or first main meal; give 1.25mg if sensitive to hypoglycemia. **Titrate:** Increase by no more than 2.5mg/day at weekly intervals. **Maint:** 1.25-20mg given qd or in divided doses. **Max:** 20mg/ day. May give bid with >10mg/day. **Renal or Hepatic Disease/Elderly/ Debilitated/Malnourished/Adrenal or Pituitary Insufficiency: Initial:** 1.25mg qd. **Transfer From Other Oral Antidiabetic Agents: Initial:** 2.5-5mg/ day. **Switch From Insulin: If <20 U/day:** 2.5-5mg qd. **If 20-40 U/day:** 5mg qd. **If >40 U/day:** Decrease dose by 50% and give 5mg qd. **Titrate:** Progressive withdrawal of insulin, and increase by 1.25-2.5mg/day every 2-10 days. **Concomitant Metformin:** Add glyburide gradually to max dose of metformin monotherapy after 4 weeks if needed. (Glynase PresTab) **Initial:** 1.5-3mg qd	**W/P:** Increased risk of cardiovascular mortality. Risk of hypoglycemia, especially with renal and hepatic disease, elderly, debilitated, malnourished, and adrenal or pituitary insufficiency. Loss of blood glucose control when exposed to stress (eg, fever, trauma, infection or surgery); d/c therapy and start insulin. Secondary failure can occur over a period of time. D/C if cholestatic jaundice or hepatitis occur. Hematologic reactions and hyponatremia reported. (Glynase PresTab) Retitrate when transferring from other glyburide products. **Contra:** Diabetic ketoacidosis, and as sole therapy of Type 1 DM. **P/N:** Category B, not for use in nursing.	Hypoglycemia, nausea, epigastric fullness, heartburn, allergic skin reactions, disulfiram-like reactions (rarely), hyponatremia, liver function abnormalities, photosensitivity reactions.

*Scored. †Bold entries denote special dental considerations.
BB = black box warning; **W/P** = warnings/precautions; **Contra** = contraindications; **P/N** = pregnancy category rating and nursing considerations.

NAME	FORM/ STRENGTH	DOSAGE	WARNINGS/PRECAUTIONS & CONTRAINDICATIONS	ADVERSE EFFECTS†
Glyburide (DiaBeta, Glynase PresTab, Micronase) *(cont.)*		with breakfast or first main meal. **Renal/Hepatic Disease/Elderly/ Debilitated/Malnourished/Adrenal or Pituitary Insufficiency: Initial:** 0.75mg qd. **Titrate:** Increase by no more than 1.5mg/day at weekly intervals. **Maint:** 0.75-12mg qd or in divided doses. **Max:** 12mg/day given qd or bid. **Transfer from Other Sulfonylureas:** Starting dose should not exceed 3mg/ day. **Switch from Insulin: If <20 U/ day:** Substitute with 1.5-3mg qd. **If 20-40 U/day:** Give 3mg qd. **If >40 U/ day:** Decrease insulin dose by 50% and give 3mg qd. **Titrate:** Progressive withdrawal of insulin and increase by 0.75-1.5mg every 2-10 days.		
Glyburide/ Metformin HCl (Glucovance)	**Tab:** (Glyburide-Metformin) 1.25mg-250mg, 2.5mg-500mg, 5mg-500mg	***Adults:*** Take with meals. **Inadequate Glycemic Control on Diet/Exercise Alone: Initial:** 1.25mg-250mg qd. If A1C >9% or FPG >200mg/dL, give 1.25mg-250mg bid (with morning and evening meals). **Titrate:** Increase by 1.25mg-250mg/day every 2 weeks. Do not use 5mg-500mg tab for initial therapy. **Inadequate Glycemic Control on Sulfonylurea or Metformin: Initial:** 2.5mg-500mg or 5mg-500mg bid. Starting dose should not exceed daily doses of glyburide (or sulfonylurea equivalent) or metformin already being taken. **Titrate:** Increase by no more than 5mg-500mg/day. **Max:** 20mg-2000mg/day. **With Concomitant TZD:** Initiate and titrate TZD as recommended. If hypoglycemia occurs, reduce glyburide component. **Elderly/ Debilitated/Malnourished:** Conservative dosing; do not titrate to max.	**W/P:** Lactic acidosis reported (rare); increased risk with renal dysfunction, increased age, DM, CHF, and other conditions with risk of hypoperfusion and hypoxemia. Avoid use in patients ≥80 yrs unless renal function is normal. Increased risk of cardiovascular mortality. Increased risk of hypoglycemia in elderly, debilitated/malnourished, adrenal or pituitary insufficiency, or alcohol intoxication. D/C in hypoxic states (eg, CHF, shock, acute MI), loss of blood glucose control due to stress (give insulin), acidosis and prior to surgical procedures (due to restricted food intake). Monitor renal function and for ketoacidosis and metabolic acidosis. Avoid in renal/hepatic impairment. May decrease serum vitamin B_{12} levels. When used with a TZD, monitor LFTs and for weight gain. Withhold treatment with any condition associated with hypoxemia, dehydration, or sepsis. **Contra:** Renal disease or dysfunction (SrCr ≥1.5mg/dL [males], ≥1.4mg/dL [females], or abnormal CrCl), metabolic acidosis, including diabetic ketoacidosis. D/C temporarily (48 hrs) for radiologic studies with intravascular iodinated contrast materials. **P/N:** Category B, not for use in pregnancy or nursing.	Hypoglycemia, N/V, abdominal pain, upper respiratory infection, headache, dizziness, diarrhea.
Metformin HCl (Fortamet)	**Tab, Extended-Release:** 500mg, 1000mg	***Adults:* ≥17 yrs:** Take with evening meal. **Initial:** 500-1000mg qd. **With Insulin: Initial:** 500mg qd. **Titrate:** May increase by 500mg/week. **Max:** 2500mg/day. Decrease insulin dose by 10-25% if FPG <120mg/dL. **Elderly/ Debilitated/Malnourished:** Conservative dosing; do not titrate to max.	**W/P:** Lactic acidosis (rare) reported; may occur with pathophysiologic conditions, including DM, hypoperfusion, and hypoxemia. Increased risk with renal insufficiency (both intrinsic renal disease and renal hyperfusion), CHF, and patient's age. Avoid use in patients ≥80 yrs unless renal function is not reduced. Should be promptly withheld with hypoxemia, dehydration, or sepsis. Caution against excessive alcohol intake. Diabetic patient with metabolic acidosis lacking evidence of ketoacidosis (ketonuria and ketonemia) may be suspected. Immediately d/c with lactic acidosis; prompt hemodialysis is recommended and remove the accumulated metformin. Caution using concomitant medications that may affect renal function, or result in significant hemodynamic change, or	Infection, diarrhea, nausea, accidental injury, headache, dyspepsia, rhinitis.

Table 20.1. PRESCRIBING INFORMATION FOR ENDOCRINE/HORMONAL AND BONE METABOLISM DRUGS *(cont.)*

NAME	FORM/ STRENGTH	DOSAGE	WARNINGS/PRECAUTIONS & CONTRAINDICATIONS	ADVERSE EFFECTS†
HYPOGLYCEMIC AGENTS *(cont.)*				
ORAL DIABETIC AGENTS *(cont.)*				
Metformin HCl (Fortamet) *(cont.)*			interfere with the disposition of metformin (eg, cationic drugs eliminated by renal tubular secretion). Temporarily d/c prior to surgery (due to restricted food intake) and procedures requiring intravascular iodinated contrast materials. D/C in hypoxic states (eg, shock, CHF, acute MI). Avoid in patients with hepatic impairment. May decrease vitamin B_{12} levels. Increased risk of hypoglycemia in elderly, debilitated/malnourished, adrenal or pituitary insufficiency, or alcohol intoxication. If loss of glycemic control occurs due to stress, temporarily withhold metformin and administer insulin. Reinstitute metformin after acute episode is resolved. **Contra:** Renal disease/dysfunction (SrCr ≥1.5mg/dL [males], ≥1.4mg/dL [females], or abnormal CrCl), acute or chronic metabolic acidosis, including diabetic ketoacidosis. D/C temporarily (48 hrs) for radiologic studies with intravascular iodinated contrast materials. **P/N:** Category B, not for use in pregnancy or nursing.	
Metformin HCl (Glucophage, Glucophage XR, Riomet)	**Sol:** (Riomet) 500mg/5mL; **Tab:** 500mg, 850mg, 1000mg*; **Tab, Extended-Release:** 500mg, 750mg	***Adults:*** (Sol, Tab) **Initial:** 500mg bid or 850mg qd with meals. **Titrate:** Increase by 500mg/week, or 850mg every 2 weeks, or may increase from 500mg bid to 850mg bid after 2 weeks. **Max:** 2550mg/day. Give in 3 divided doses with meals if dose is >2g/day. (Tab, Extended-Release) **Initial: ≥17 yrs:** 500mg qd with evening meal. **Titrate:** Increase by 500mg/week. **Max:** 2000mg/day. **With Insulin: Initial:** 500mg qd. **Titrate:** Increase by 500mg/week. **Max:** 2000mg/day. Decrease insulin dose by 10-25% when FPG <120mg/dL. Swallow whole; do not crush or chew. **Elderly/Debilitated/ Malnourished:** Conservative dosing; do not titrate to max. ***Pediatrics:* 10-16 yrs:** (Sol, Tab) **Initial:** 500mg bid with meals. **Titrate:** Increase by 500mg/week. **Max:** 2000mg/day.	**W/P:** Lactic acidosis reported (rare); increased risk with renal dysfunction, increased age, DM, CHF, and other conditions with risk of hypoperfusion and hypoxemia. Avoid use in patients ≥80 yrs unless renal function is normal. Monitor renal function and for ketoacidosis and metabolic acidosis. Avoid in renal/hepatic impairment. D/C in hypoxic states (eg, CHF, shock, acute MI), loss of blood glucose control due to stress (give insulin), acidosis, dehydration, sepsis. Temporarily d/c prior to surgery (due to restricted food intake) and procedures requiring intravascular iodinated contrast materials. May decrease serum vitamin B_{12} levels. Increased risk of hypoglycemia in elderly, debilitated/malnourished, adrenal or pituitary insufficiency, or alcohol intoxication. Monitor renal function. **Contra:** Renal disease/dysfunction (SrCr ≥1.5mg/dL [males], ≥1.4mg/dL [females], or abnormal CrCl), CHF, metabolic acidosis, diabetic ketoacidosis. D/C temporarily (48 hrs) for radiologic studies with intravascular iodinated contrast materials. **P/N:** Category B, not for use in nursing.	Lactic acidosis, diarrhea, N/V, flatulence, abdominal discomfort, abnormal stools, hypoglycemia, myalgia, dizziness, dyspnea, nail disorder, rash, sweating, **taste disorder,** chest discomfort, chills, flu syndrome, palpitations, asthenia, indigestion, headache.
Metformin HCl (Glumetza)	**Tab, Extended-Release:** 500mg, 1000mg	***Adults:* ≥18 yrs:** Take with evening meal. **Initial:** 1000mg qd. **With Insulin: Initial:** 500mg qd. **Titrate:** May increase by 500mg/week. **Max:** 2000mg/day. Decrease insulin dose by 10-25% if FPG <120mg/dL. **Elderly/Debilitated/ Malnourished:** Conservative dosing; do not titrate to max. Swallow whole; do not crush or chew.	**W/P:** Lactic acidosis reported (rare); increased risk with renal dysfunction, increased age, DM, CHF, and other conditions with risk of hypoperfusion and hypoxemia. Avoid use in patients ≥80 yrs unless renal function is normal. Monitor renal function and for ketoacidosis and metabolic acidosis. Avoid in renal/hepatic impairment. D/C in hypoxic states (eg, CHF, shock, acute MI), loss of blood glucose control due to stress	Hypoglycemia, diarrhea, nausea.

*Scored. †Bold entries denote special dental considerations.
BB = black box warning; **W/P** = warnings/precautions; **Contra** = contraindications; **P/N** = pregnancy category rating and nursing considerations.

NAME	FORM/ STRENGTH	DOSAGE	WARNINGS/PRECAUTIONS & CONTRAINDICATIONS	ADVERSE EFFECTS†
Metformin HCl (Glumetza) *(cont.)*			(give insulin), acidosis, dehydration, sepsis. Temporarily d/c prior to surgery (due to restricted food/fluid intake) or procedures requiring intravascular iodinated contrast materials. May decrease serum vitamin B_{12} levels. Increased risk of hypoglycemia in elderly, debilitated/malnourished, adrenal or pituitary insufficiency, or alcohol intoxication. **Contra:** Renal disease or dysfunction (SrCr ≥1.5mg/dL [males], ≥1.4mg/dL [females], or abnormal CrCl), CHF, metabolic acidosis, including diabetic ketoacidosis. D/C temporarily (48 hrs) for radiologic studies with intravascular iodinated contrast materials. **P/N:** Category B, not for use in nursing.	
Metformin HCl/ Pioglitazone HCl (Actoplus Met)	**Tab:** (Pioglitazone-Metformin) 15mg-500mg, 15mg-850mg	***Adults:*** Individualize dose. **Prior Pioglitazone/Metformin:** Base on current regimen. **Prior Metformin Monotherapy or Pioglitazone Monotherapy: Initial:** 15mg-500mg or 15mg-850mg qd-bid. **Titrate:** Gradually increase after assessing adequacy of therapeutic response. **Max:** (Pioglitazone) 45mg, (Metformin) 2550mg. **Elderly/Debilitated/Malnourished:** Conservative dosing; do not titrate to max dose.	**BB:** Thiazolidinediones may cause or exacerbate CHF in some patients. Actoplus Met is not recommended in patients with symptomatic heart failure. **W/P:** (Metformin) Lactic acidosis reported (rare); increased risk with renal dysfunction, increased age, DM, CHF, and other conditions with risk of hypoperfusion and hypoxemia. Avoid in patients ≥80 yrs unless normal renal function. Monitor renal function and for ketoacidosis and metabolic acidosis. Avoid in renal/hepatic impairment. D/C in hypoxic states (eg, CHF, shock, acute MI), loss of blood glucose control due to stress (give insulin), acidosis, dehydration, sepsis. Temporarily d/c prior to surgery (due to restricted food intake) and procedures requiring IV iodinated contrast materials. May decrease serum B_{12} levels. Increased risk of hypoglycemia in elderly, debilitated/malnourished, adrenal or pituitary insufficiency, or alcohol intoxication. Alcohol known to potentiate effect of metformin on lactate metabolism. (Pioglitazone) May cause fluid retention and exacerbation/initiation of heart failure; d/c if cardiac status deteriorates. Avoid if NYHA Class III of IV cardiac status. Use lowest approved dose if systolic heart failure (NYHA Class II). Not for use in Type 1 diabetes or for diabetic ketoacidosis treatment. Caution with edema. Dose-related wt gain reported. Ovulation in premenopausal anovulatory patients may occur; risk of pregnancy with inadequate contraception. May decrease Hgb and Hct. Avoid with active liver disease, if ALT levels >2.5x ULN. D/C if jaundice occurs or ALT >3x ULN on therapy. Macular edema reported. **Contra:** Established NYHA Class III or IV heart failure, renal disease or dysfunction (eg, SrCr ≥1.5mg/dL [males], ≥1.4mg/dL [females], or abnormal CrCl) and metabolic acidosis, including diabetic ketoacidosis. Temporarily d/c in patients undergoing radiologic studies involving intravascular iodinated contrast materials. **P/N:** Category C, not for use in nursing.	Upper respiratory tract infection, diarrhea, nausea, edema, headache, UTI, sinusitis, dizziness, weight increase, new onset or worsening diabetic macular edema.

Table 20.1. PRESCRIBING INFORMATION FOR ENDOCRINE/HORMONAL AND BONE METABOLISM DRUGS *(cont.)*

NAME	FORM/ STRENGTH	DOSAGE	WARNINGS/PRECAUTIONS & CONTRAINDICATIONS	ADVERSE EFFECTS†
HYPOGLYCEMIC AGENTS *(cont.)*				
ORAL DIABETIC AGENTS *(cont.)*				
Metformin HCl/ Repaglinide (Prandimet)	**Tab:** (Repaglinide-Metformin) 1mg-500mg, 2mg-500mg	***Adults:*** Individualize dose. Administer 2-3 times a day up to 4mg-1000mg/ meal. **Max Daily Dose:** 10mg of repaglinide-2500mg of metformin. **Patient Inadequately Controlled on Metformin Monotherapy: Initial:** 1mg-500mg bid with meals. **Titrate:** Gradually escalate dose to reduce risk of hypoglycemia. **Patient Inadequately Controlled with Meglitinide Monotherapy: Initial:** 500mg of metformin bid. **Titrate:** Gradually escalate dose to reduce GI side effects. **Concomitant Use of Repaglinide/Metformin:** Initiate at the dose of repaglinide and metformin HCl similar to (not exceeding) the current doses. Titrate to maximum daily dose as necessary.	**BB:** Lactic acidosis can occur due to metformin accumulation. If suspected, d/c drug and hospitalize patient. **W/P:** Lactic acidosis reported (rare), increased risk with sepsis, dehydration, excess alcohol intake, hepatic impairment, renal impairment, and acute congestive heart failure. Assess renal function prior to initiation and annually thereafter. Avoid in hepatic impairment and excess alcohol intake. D/C in hypoxic states (eg, acute CHF, shock, acute MI), prior to surgical procedures, procedures requiring use of intravascular iodinated contrast materials, and ketoacidosis. May cause vitamin B_{12} deficiency and hypoglycemia. **Contra:** Renal impairment (SrCr ≥1.5mg/dL [males], ≥1.4mg/dL [females], or abnormal CrCl). Acute or chronic metabolic acidosis, including diabetic ketoacidosis. Patients receiving both gemfibrozil and itraconazole. **P/N:** Category C, not for use in nursing.	Hypoglycemia, headache, diarrhea, nausea, upper respiratory tract infection.
Metformin HCl/ Rosiglitazone Maleate (Avandamet)	**Tab:** (Rosiglitazone-Metformin) 2mg-500mg, 4mg-500mg, 2mg-1000mg, 4mg-1000mg	***Adults:*** **Prior Metformin Therapy of 1000mg/day: Initial:** 2mg-500mg tab bid. **Prior Metformin Therapy of 2000mg/day: Initial:** 2mg-1000mg tab bid. **Prior Rosiglitazone Therapy of 4mg/day: Initial:** 2mg-500mg tab bid. **Prior Rosiglitazone Therapy of 8mg/day:** 4mg-500mg tab bid. **Titrate:** May increase by increments of 4mg rosiglitazone and/or 500mg metformin. **Max:** 8mg-2000mg/day. **Drug-Naive Patients: Initial:** 2mg-500mg qd-bid. **If A1C >11% and FPG >270mg/dL: Initial:** 2mg-500mg bid. **Titrate:** After 4 weeks, may increase by increments of 2mg-500mg per day. **Max:** 8mg-2000mg per day. **Elderly/Debilitated/ Malnourished:** Conservative dosing; do not titrate to max dose. Take with meals.	**BB:** Thiazolidinediones may cause or exacerbate CHF in some patients. Avandamet is not recommended in patients with symptomatic heart failure. Meta-analysis of studies showed rosiglitazone to be associated with an increased risk of myocardial ischemic events. Lactic acidosis may occur due to metformin accumulation. **W/P:** Lactic acidosis reported; increased risk with renal dysfunction, increased age, DM, CHF, and other conditions with risk of hypoperfusion and hypoxemia. Avoid use in patients ≥80 yrs unless renal function is normal. Monitor renal function and for ketoacidosis and metabolic acidosis. D/C in hypoxic states (eg, CHF, shock, acute MI), loss of blood glucose control due to stress, acidosis and prior to surgical procedures (due to restricted food intake). May decrease serum vitamin B_{12} levels. Increased risk of hypoglycemia with concomitant use with other hypoglycemic agents, elderly, debilitated/malnourished, adrenal or pituitary insufficiency, or alcohol intoxication. May cause fluid retention and exacerbation/initiation of heart failure; d/c if cardiac status deteriorates. Initiation not recommended in patients experiencing an acute coronary event. Avoid with NYHA Class III or IV cardiac status. Not for use in Type 1 diabetes or for diabetic ketoacidosis treatment. Caution with edema. Dose-related weight gain reported. Ovulation in premenopausal anovulatory patients may occur; risk of pregnancy with inadequate contraception. May decrease Hgb and Hct. Avoid with active liver disease, if ALT levels >2.5x ULN, or if jaundice occurred with troglitazone. Check LFTs before therapy, every 2 months for 1 year, and	Upper respiratory tract infection, headache, back pain, hyperglycemia, fatigue, sinusitis, diarrhea, viral infection, arthralgia, anemia, dyspepsia, dizziness, abdominal pain, N/V.

†Bold entries denote special dental considerations.
BB = black box warning; **W/P** = warnings/precautions; **Contra** = contraindications; **P/N** = pregnancy category rating and nursing considerations.

NAME	FORM/ STRENGTH	DOSAGE	WARNINGS/PRECAUTIONS & CONTRAINDICATIONS	ADVERSE EFFECTS†
Metformin HCl/ Rosiglitazone Maleate (Avandamet) *(cont.)*			periodically thereafter, or if hepatic dysfunction symptoms occur. D/C if ALT >3x ULN on therapy. Not for use with insulin. Increased incidence of bone fracture was noted in female patients. **Contra:** Established NYHA Class III or IV heart failure, renal disease/dysfunction (SrCr ≥1.5mg/dL [males], ≥1.4mg/dL [females], or abnormal CrCl), metabolic acidosis, including diabetic ketoacidosis. D/C temporarily (48 hrs) for radiologic studies with intravascular iodinated contrast materials. **P/N:** Category C, not for use in nursing.	
Metformin HCl/ Sitagliptin (Janumet)	**Tab:** (Sitagliptin-Metformin) 50mg-500mg, 50mg-1000mg	***Adults:*** Individualize dosing. **Patient Not Controlled on Metformin Monotherapy: Initial:** 100mg/day (50mg bid) of sitagliptin + metformin dose. **Patient on Metformin 850mg BID: Initial:** 50mg-1000mg tab bid. **Patient Not Controlled on Sitagliptin Monotherapy: Initial:** 50mg-500mg tab bid. **Titrate:** Gradual increase to 50mg-1000mg tab bid. **Max:** 100mg of sitagliptin and 2000mg of metformin. Take with meals.	**BB:** Lactic acidosis may occur due to metformin accumulation. If acidosis suspected, d/c drug and hospitalize patient immediately. **W/P:** Lactic acidosis reported (rare), increased risk with renal dysfunction. Assess renal function prior to initiation and during treatment; caution in elderly. Avoid in renal/hepatic impairment. May decrease vitamin B_{12} levels; monitor hematologic parameters. May cause hypoglycemia in elderly, debilitated/malnourished, adrenal or pituitary insufficiency, or alcohol intoxication. D/C in hypoxic states (eg, CHF, shock, acute MI), prior to surgical procedures (due to restricted food and fluid intake), and procedures requiring use of intravascular iodinated contrast materials. **Contra:** Renal disease (SrCr ≥1.5mg/dL [males], ≥1.4mg/dL [females], or abnormal CrCl), metabolic acidosis, including diabetic ketoacidosis. D/C for 48 hrs in patients undergoing radiologic studies with intravascular iodinated contrast materials. **P/N:** Category B, caution in nursing.	(Metformin) Diarrhea, N/V, flatulence, abdominal discomfort, indigestion, asthenia, headache. (Sitagliptin) **Nasopharyngitis.**
Miglitol (Glyset)	**Tab:** 25mg, 50mg, 100mg	***Adults:*** **Initial:** 25mg tid. May give 25mg qd (to minimize GI side effects) and gradually increase to tid. **Titrate:** After 4-8 weeks, increase to 50mg tid. **Maint:** 50mg tid. After 3 months may increase to 100mg tid if needed. **Max:** 100mg tid. Take with first bite of each main meal.	**W/P:** Use glucose (dextrose) not sucrose (cane sugar) to treat mild-moderate hypoglycemia. Temporary insulin therapy may be necessary at times of stress such as fever, trauma, infection, or surgery. Not recommended with renal impairment (SrCr >2mg/dL). **Contra:** Ketoacidosis, inflammatory bowel disease, colonic ulceration, partial intestinal obstruction or if predisposed to intestinal obstruction. Chronic intestinal diseases with digestion or absorption disorders/conditions may deteriorate with increased gas formation in the intestine. **P/N:** Category B, not for use in nursing.	Flatulence, diarrhea, abdominal pain, skin rash, decreased serum iron.
Nateglinide (Starlix)	**Tab:** 60mg, 120mg	***Adults:*** **Initial/Maint:** 120mg tid before meals (with or without metformin or TZD). Take 1-30 min before meals. May use 60mg tid (with or without metformin or TZD) in patients near goal A1C. Skip dose if meal is skipped.	**W/P:** Caution in moderate to severe hepatic impairment. Transient loss of glucose control with trauma, surgery, fever, and infection; may need insulin therapy. Secondary failure may occur in prolonged therapy. Hypoglycemia risk in elderly, debilitated, malnourished, strenuous exercise, and with adrenal or pituitary insufficiency. Autonomic neuropathy may mask hypoglycemia. **Contra:** Type 1 diabetes, diabetic ketoacidosis. **P/N:** Category C, not for use in nursing.	Upper respiratory infection, flu symptoms, dizziness, arthropathy, diarrhea, hypoglycemia, back pain, jaundice, cholestatic hepatitis, elevated liver enzymes.

Table 20.1. PRESCRIBING INFORMATION FOR ENDOCRINE/HORMONAL AND BONE METABOLISM DRUGS *(cont.)*

NAME	FORM/ STRENGTH	DOSAGE	WARNINGS/PRECAUTIONS & CONTRAINDICATIONS	ADVERSE EFFECTS†
HYPOGLYCEMIC AGENTS *(cont.)*				
ORAL DIABETIC AGENTS *(cont.)*				
Pioglitazone HCl (Actos)	**Tab:** 15mg, 30mg, 45mg	***Adults:*** **Monotherapy: Initial:** 15-30mg qd. **Max:** 45mg/day. **Combination Therapy: Initial:** 15-30mg qd. **Max:** 30mg/day. Decrease insulin dose by 10-25% if hypoglycemia occurs or if plasma glucose is <100mg/dL. Decrease sulfonylurea dose with hypoglycemia also.	**BB:** Thiazolidinediones may cause or exacerbate CHF in some patients. Pioglitazone is not recommended in patients with symptomatic heart failure. **W/P:** May cause fluid retention and exacerbation/initiation of heart failure; d/c if cardiac status deteriorates. Avoid if NYHA Class III or IV cardiac status. Use lowest approved dose if systolic heart failure (NYHA Class II). Not for use in Type 1 diabetes or for diabetic ketoacidosis treatment. Caution with edema. Dose-related weight gain reported. Ovulation in premenopausal anovulatory patients may occur; risk of pregnancy with inadequate contraception. May decrease Hgb and Hct. Avoid with active liver disease, if ALT levels >2.5x ULN, or if jaundice occurred with troglitazone. Check LFTs before therapy, every 2 months for 1 yr, and periodically thereafter, or if hepatic dysfunction symptoms occur. D/C if jaundice occurs or ALT >3x ULN on therapy. Macular edema reported. Increased incidence of bone fracture was noted in female patients. **Contra:** Established NYHA Class III or IV heart failure. **P/N:** Category C, not for use in nursing.	Upper respiratory tract infection, myalgia, **tooth disorder,** headache, sinusitis, **pharyngitis,** transient CPK level elevations, CHF, weight gain, aggravated DM, edema, dyspnea, new onset or worsening of diabetic macular edema.
Repaglinide (Prandin)	**Tab:** 0.5mg, 1mg, 2mg	***Adults:*** Take within 15-30 min before meals. Skip dose if skipping meal and add dose if adding meal. **Initial: Treatment-Naive or A1C <8%:** 0.5mg with each meal. **Previous Oral Therapy/ Combination Therapy and A1C ≥8%:** 1-2mg with each meal. **Titrate:** May double preprandial dose up to 4mg (bid-qid) at no less than 1 week intervals. **Maint:** 0.5-4mg with meals. **Max:** 16mg/day. If hypoglycemia with combination metformin or TZD occurs, reduce repaglinide dose. **Renal Dysfunction:** CrCl 20-40mg/dL: **Initial:** 0.5mg with each meal; titrate carefully. **Hepatic Dysfunction:** Increase intervals between dose adjustments.	**W/P:** Hypoglycemia risk especially with renal/hepatic insufficiency, elderly, malnourished and adrenal/pituitary insufficiency. Loss of blood glucose control when exposed to stress (fever, trauma, infection or surgery); d/c therapy and start insulin. Secondary failure can occur over a period of time. Caution with hepatic and renal dysfunction. Not indicated for use in combination with NPH insulin. **Contra:** Diabetic ketoacidosis and type 1 diabetes. **P/N:** Category C, not for use in nursing.	Hypoglycemia, cardiovascular effects, respiratory infections, URI, bronchitis, sinusitis, rhinitis, paresthesia, N/V, diarrhea, constipation, dyspepsia, arthralgia, back pain, headache, chest pain.
Rosiglitazone Maleate (Avandia)	**Tab:** 2mg, 4mg, 8mg	***Adults:*** **≥18 yrs: Initial:** 2mg bid or 4mg qd. **Titrate:** May increase after 8-12 weeks to 8mg daily as monotherapy or in combination with metformin, sulfonylurea, or sulfonylurea plus metformin. **Max:** 8mg/day.	**BB:** Thiazolidinediones may cause or exacerbate CHF in some patients. Rosiglitazone is not recommended in patients with symptomatic heart failure. Studies have shown rosiglitazone to be associated with an increased risk of myocardial ischemic events, such as angina or MI. **W/P:** May cause fluid retention and exacerbation/initiation of heart failure; d/c if cardiac status deteriorates. Increased risk of CV events with NYHA Class I or II cardiac status; avoid with NYHA Class III or IV cardiac status. An increased risk of myocardial ischemic events have been observed. CHF and MI during coadministration with insulin. Coadministration with insulin or nitrates is not recommended. Not for use in Type 1 diabetes or diabetic ketoacidosis	Upper respiratory tract infection, injury, headache, back pain, hyperglycemia, fatigue, sinusitis, anemia, edema.

*Scored. †Bold entries denote special dental considerations.
BB = black box warning; **W/P** = warnings/precautions; **Contra** = contraindications; **P/N** = pregnancy category rating and nursing considerations.

NAME	FORM/ STRENGTH	DOSAGE	WARNINGS/PRECAUTIONS & CONTRAINDICATIONS	ADVERSE EFFECTS†
Rosiglitazone Maleate (Avandia) *(cont.)*			treatment. Caution with edema. Macular edema reported. Dose-related weight gain and anemia reported. Avoid with active liver disease, if ALT levels >2.5x ULN, or if jaundice occurred with troglitazone. Check LFTs before therapy, every 2 months for 1 year, and periodically thereafter, or if hepatic dysfunction symptoms occur. D/C if ALT >3x ULN on therapy. Increased incidence of bone fracture in female patients. May decrease Hgb and Hct. Risk for hypoglycemia. Monitor blood glucose and A1C measurements. Ovulation in premenopausal anovulatory patients may occur; risk of pregnancy with inadequate contraception. **Contra:** Established NYHA Class III or IV heart failure. **P/N:** Category C, not for use in pregnancy or nursing.	
Sitagliptin Phosphate (Januvia)	**Tab:** 25mg, 50mg, 100mg	***Adults:*** 100mg qd. **CrCl ≥30 to <50mL/min:** 50mg qd. **CrCl: <30mL/min:** 25mg qd.	**W/P:** Assess renal function prior to initiation of treatment. Cause hypoglycemia when used in combination with a sulfonylurea. Anaphylaxis, angioedema, and exfoliative skin conditions reported. **Contra:** Anaphylaxis or angioedema. **P/N:** Category B, caution in nursing.	(Monotherapy/Combination therapy) Upper respiratory tract infection, **nasopharyngitis,** headache. (Combination therapy) hypoglycemia.
Tolazamide	**Tab:** 100mg*, 250mg*, 500mg*	***Adults:*** **Elderly/Malnourished/FBG <200mg/dL: Initial:** 100mg qd. **FBG >200mg/dL: Initial:** 250mg qd. Adjust weekly by 100-250mg if needed. **Max:** 1000mg/day. **Conversion From Insulin:** If insulin dose <20 U/day, replace with 100mg qd. If insulin dose <40 U/day but >20 U/day, replace with 250mg qd. If insulin dose >40 U/day, decrease insulin dose by 50% and give 250mg qd. Adjust dose weekly. **Renal/Hepatic Dysfunction:** Conservative dosing. Give with breakfast or first main meal. May give doses >500mg/day bid.	**W/P:** Increased risk of cardiovascular mortality. Hypoglycemia risk especially with renal/hepatic insufficiency, elderly, debilitated, malnourished, and adrenal/pituitary insufficiency. Loss of blood glucose control when exposed to stress (fever, trauma, infection or surgery); d/c therapy and start insulin. Secondary failure can occur over a period of time. **Contra:** Diabetic ketoacidosis; Type 1 diabetes (as sole therapy). **P/N:** Category C, not for use in nursing.	Hypoglycemia, GI disturbances, photosensitivity reactions, allergic reactions, blood dyscrasias, cholestatic jaundice (rare), disulfiram-like reactions (rare), hepatic porphyria, hyponatremia/SIADH.
Tolbutamide	**Tab:** 500mg*	***Adults:*** **Initial:** 1-2g qd. **Titrate:** Increase or decrease based on patient response. **Maint:** 0.25-3g qd. **Max:** 3g qd. **Elderly/Debiliated/Malnourished/Renal or Hepatic Dysfunction: Initial/Maint:** Conservative dosing. Take in am or divided doses (for GI intolerance). **Concomitant Insulin Therapy: Insulin Dose ≤20 U/day:** d/c insulin therapy and begin tolbutamide therapy. **Insulin Dose 20-40 U/day:** Reduce insulin by 30-50% and adjust based on tolbutamide response. **Insulin dose ≥40 U/day:** Reduce insulin by 20% on first day and adjust based on tolbutamide response.	**W/P:** Increased risk of cardiovascular mortality. Hypoglycemia risk especially with renal/hepatic insufficiencey, elderly, debilitated, malnourished, and adrenal/pituitary insufficiency. Loss of blood glucose control when exposed to stress (fever, trauma, infection or surgery); d/c therapy and start insulin. Secondary failure can occur over period of time. **Contra:** Diabetic ketoacidosis; Type 1 diabetes (as sole therapy). **P/N:** Category C, not for use in nursing.	Hypoglycemia, GI disturbances, headache, allergic skin reactions, photosensitivity reactions, blood dyscrasias, cholestatic jaundice (rare), disulfiram-like reactions (rare), hepatic porphyria, hyponatremia/SIADH, **taste disturbance.**
PITUITARY HORMONES				
Cabergoline (Dostinex)	**Tab:** 0.5mg*	***Adults:*** **Initial:** 0.25mg twice weekly. **Titrate:** May increase by 0.25mg twice weekly at 4-week intervals. **Max:** 1mg twice weekly. D/C after maintaining a normal serum prolactin level for 6 months. Efficacy >24 months not established.	**W/P:** Initial doses >1mg may produce orthostatic hypotension. Caution with hepatic impairment. Avoid with pregnancy-induced HTN (eg, preeclampsia, eclampsia). Not for inhibition/suppression of postpartum lactation. Use caution with respiratory or cardiac disorders linked to fibrotic tissue as risk of valvulopathy/fibrosis is possible;	Nausea, constipation, abdominal pain, headache, dizziness, postural hypotension, fatigue, somnolence, depression, asthenia.

Table 20.1. PRESCRIBING INFORMATION FOR ENDOCRINE/HORMONAL AND BONE METABOLISM DRUGS *(cont.)*

NAME	FORM/ STRENGTH	DOSAGE	WARNINGS/PRECAUTIONS & CONTRAINDICATIONS	ADVERSE EFFECTS†
PITUITARY HORMONES *(cont.)*				
Cabergoline (Dostinex)			patient should be informed to notify physician if he/she develops cough. **Contra:** Uncontrolled HTN, hypersensitivity to ergot derivatives. **P/N:** Category B, not for use in nursing.	
Desmopressin Acetate (DDAVP, DDAVP Nasal Spray, DDAVP Rhinal Tube)	**Inj:** 4mcg/mL; **Nasal Spray:** 10mcg/inh [5mL]; **Tab:** 0.1mg*, 0.2mg*; **Rhinal Tube:** 0.01% [2.5mL]	***Adults:*** **Diabetes Insipidus:** (Tab) **Initial:** 0.05mg bid. **Titrate:** May increase/decrease by 0.1-1.2mg/day given bid-tid. **Maint:** 0.1-0.8mg/day in divided doses. (Spray/Tube) **Usual:** 0.1-4mL/day given qd-tid. (Inj) 0.5-1mL/day IV/SQ given bid. **Hemophilia A/von Willebrand's Disease:** (Inj) 0.3mcg/kg IV over 15-30 min. Add 50mL diluent. If used pre-op, give 30 min before procedure. ***Pediatrics:*** **Diabetes Insipidus:** (Tab) **≥4 yrs: Initial:** 0.05mg bid. **Titrate:** May increase/decrease by 0.1-1.2mg/day given bid-tid. **Maint:** 0.1-0.8mg/day in divided doses. (Spray/Tube) **3 months to 12 yrs: Usual:** 0.05-0.3mL/day given qd-bid. (Inj) **≥12 yrs:** 0.5-1mL/day IV/SQ given bid. **Hemophilia A/von Willebrand's Disease:** (Inj) **≥3 months:** 0.3mcg/kg IV over 15-30 min. Add 50mL diluent (>10kg) or 10mL diluent (≤10kg). If used pre-op, give 30 min before procedure.	**W/P:** Mucosal changes with nasal forms may occur; d/c until resolved. Decrease fluid intake in pediatrics and elderly to decrease risk of water intoxication and hyponatremia; monitor osmolality. Caution with coronary artery insufficiency, hypertensive cardiovascular disease, fluid and electrolyte imbalance (eg, cystic fibrosis). Anaphylaxis reported with IV use. Caution with IV use if history of thrombus formation. For diabetes insipidus, dosage must be adjusted according to diurnal pattern of response; estimate response by adequate duration of sleep and adequate, not excessive, water turnover. **Contra:** Moderate-to-severe renal impairment (CrCL<50mL/min), hyponatremia, or history of hyponatremia. **P/N:** Category B, caution in nursing.	**Inj:** Headache, nausea, abdominal cramps, vulval pain, injection-site reactions, facial flushing, BP changes. **Spray:** Headache, dizziness, rhinitis, nausea, nasal congestion, **sore throat,** cough, respiratory infection, epistaxis. **Tab:** Nausea, flushing, abdominal cramps, headache, increased SGOT, water intoxication, hyponatremia.
Histrelin Acetate (Supprelin LA)	**Implant:** 50mg	***Pediatrics:*** **≥2 yrs:** 50mg every 12 months. Inject SQ into inner aspect of upper arm. Remove after 12 months of therapy.	**W/P:** Transient increase in estradiol in females and testosterone in both sexes with initial therapy. Proper surgical technique is critical during implant insertion and removal. Monitor LH, FSH, and estradiol or testosterone at 1 month postimplantation, then every 6 months. Assess height and bone age every 6-12 months. **Contra:** Women who are or may become pregnant. **P/N:** Category X, not for use in nursing.	Implant-site reactions, wound infection, dysmenorrhea, epistaxis, erythema, gynecomastia, headache, weight increase.
Somatropin (Genotropin, Genotropin MiniQuick)	**Inj:** 1.5mg, 5.8mg, 13.8mg; **Inj, MiniQuick:** 0.2mg, 0.4mg, 0.6mg, 0.8mg, 1mg, 1.2mg, 1.4mg, 1.6mg, 1.8mg, 2mg	***Adults:*** Individualize dose. **GHD: Initial:** Up to 0.04mg/kg/week. **Titrate:** May increase at 4- to 8-week intervals. **Max:** 0.08mg/kg/week. Divide dose into 6-7 SQ injections. Elderly patients should receive a lower starting dose. ***Pediatrics:*** Individualize dose. **GHD:** 0.16-0.24mg/kg/week. **PWS:** 0.24mg/kg/week. **SGA:** 0.48mg/kg/week. **TS:** 0.33mg/kg/week. Divide doses into 6-7 SQ injections.	**W/P:** In PWS, evaluate for upper airway obstruction prior to initiation; monitor weight, for sleep apnea, signs of upper airway obstruction (eg, suspend therapy with onset of or increased snoring), respiratory infections (treat early and aggressively if occur). Monitor GHD secondary to intracranial lesion for progression/recurrence. Monitor gait, glucose intolerance because insulin sensitivity is decreased, for malignant transformation of skin lesions, scoliosis progression, intracranial HTN (perform fundoscopic exam at start and periodically). Caution with DM, endocrine disorders, hypopituitarism, and Turner syndrome. Tissue atrophy may occur (rotate injection site). **Contra:** Evidence of neoplastic activity. Pediatrics with closed epiphyses. Patients with diabetic retinopathy or active malignancy. Acute critical illness due to complications after open heart or abdominal surgery, multiple accidental trauma, or with acute respiratory failure. Patients with PWS who are severely obese or have severe respiratory impairment. **P/N:** Category B, caution in nursing.	Peripheral swelling/edema, arthralgia, pain/stiffness in extremities, myalgia, upper respiratory infection, paresthesia.

†Bold entries denote special dental considerations.
BB = black box warning; **W/P** = warnings/precautions; **Contra** = contraindications; **P/N** = pregnancy category rating and nursing considerations.

NAME	FORM/ STRENGTH	DOSAGE	WARNINGS/PRECAUTIONS & CONTRAINDICATIONS	ADVERSE EFFECTS†
Somatropin (Humatrope)	**Inj:** 5mg, 6mg, 12mg, 24mg	***Adults:*** **GHD:** Up to 0.006mg/kg SQ qd. **Titrate:** Increase by individual requirements. **Max:** 0.0125mg/kg/day. **Alternative Dose: Initial:** 0.2mg/day (range, 0.15-0.30mg/day). **Titrate:** Increase gradually every 1-2 months to individual requirement. **Max:** 0.1-0.2mg/day. ***Pediatrics:*** **GHD:** 0.18mg/kg weekly SQ/IM. **Max:** 0.3mg/kg weekly in equally divided doses given either on 3 alternate days, 6 times per week, or daily. **Turner Syndrome:** Up to 0.375mg/kg SQ weekly equally divided, given either daily or on 3 alternate days. **Idiopathic Short Stature:** Up to 0.37mg/kg SQ weekly given 6 to 7 times per week equally divided. **SHOX Deficiency:** 0.35mg/kg SQ weekly given daily in equally divided doses.	**W/P:** If sensitivity to diluent occurs reconstitute with bacteriostatic (contains benzyl alcohol; avoid in newborns) or sterile water for injection. Monitor GHD secondary to intracranial lesion for progression/recurrence. Monitor gait, glucose intolerance, for malignant transformation of skin lesions, scoliosis progression, intracranial HTN (perform fundoscopic exam at start and periodically). Caution with DM, endocrine disorders, hypopituitarism. With Turner syndrome monitor for otic or cardiovascular disorders, autoimmune thyroid disease. Caution with endocrine disorders, monitor for otic and cardiovascular disorder. **Contra:** Pediatrics with closed epiphyses. Proliferative or preproliferative diabetic retinopathy. Active malignancy. Hypersensitivity to Metacresol or glycerin. Acute critical illness due to complications after open heart or abdominal surgery, multiple accidental trauma or acute respiratory failure. Prader-Willi syndrome who are severely obese or have severe respiratory impairment. **P/N:** Category C, caution in nursing.	Injection-site pain, headache, edema, myalgia, pain, rhinitis. (Adults) Arthralgia, paresthesia, HTN, back pain. (Pediatrics) Flu-syndrome, AST/ALT increases, **pharyngitis,** gastritis, respiratory disorder.
Somatropin (Norditropin, Norditropin Nordiflex)	**Inj:** (Norditropin [cartridge] and Norditropin Nordiflex [prefilled pen]) 5mg/1.5mL, 15mg/1.5mL, 10mg/1.5mL	***Adults:*** **Initial:** No more than 0.004mg/kg/day. Increase to no more than 0.016mg/kg/day after 6 weeks. ***Pediatrics:*** **Growth Hormone Deficiency:** 0.024-0.034mg/kg SQ 6-7x/week. **Noonan Syndrome:** Dose up to 0.066mg/kg/day. **Turner Syndrome/SGA:** Dose up to 0.067mg/kg/day. **<4 yrs (SGA): Initial:** 0.033mg/kg/day. Titrate dose over time as needed.	**W/P:** Monitor for recurrence or progression of underlying disease in growth hormone deficiency secondary to intracranial lesions. Hypothyroidism reported. May develop slipped capital epiphyses. Intracranial HTN with papilledema, visual changes, headache, N/V reported. Progression of scoliosis may occur in rapid growth. Monitor for any form of malignant skin lesion prior to and during therapy. May decrease insulin sensitivity; monitor blood sugar. Dose-dependent/transient fluid retention may occur. Increased occurrence of otitis media in patients with Turner syndrome. Monitor closely for cardiovascular disorders (eg, stroke, aortic aneurysm/dissection, hypertension). **Contra:** Presence of active neoplasia; acute critical illness due to complications following open heart or abdominal surgery, multiple accidental trauma or acute respiratory failure; proliferative or preproliferative diabetic retinopathy; closed epiphyses; and Prader-Willi syndrome with severe obesity or severe respiratory impairment. **P/N:** Category C, caution in nursing.	(Pediatrics) Headache, injection-site reaction, localized muscle pain, rash, weakness, mild hyperglycemia, glucosuria, arthralgia, leukemia. (Adults) Edema, arthralgia, myalgia, infection, parasthesia, skeletal pain, headache, bronchitis.
Somatropin (Nutropin, Nutropin AQ)	**Inj:** 5mg, 10mg, (AQ) 5mg/mL	***Adults:*** **GHD: Initial:** Up to 0.006mg/kg/day SQ. **Max: <35 yrs:** 0.025mg/kg/day. **≥35 yrs:** 0.0125mg/kg/day. Alternatively may use 0.2mg/day (range: 0.15-0.30mg/day). Increase every 1-2 months by increments of 0.1-0.2mg/day. ***Pediatrics:*** **GHD: Usual:** 0.3mg/kg/week divided into daily SQ doses. **Pubertal Patients:** Up to 0.7mg/kg/week divided into daily SQ doses. **CRI:** 0.35mg/kg/week divided into daily SQ doses. Continue until renal transplantation. **Hemodialysis:** Give qhs or 3 to 4 hrs postdialysis. **Chronic Cycling**	**W/P:** Caution with epiphyseal closure in adults treated with GH-replacement therapy in childhood. Recurrence/progression reported with intracranial lesions. Renal osteodystrophy may occur with growth failure secondary to renal impairment. Scoliosis and slipped capital femoral epiphysis may develop in rapid growth. Caution with Turner syndrome and ISS. Intracranial hypertension with papilledema, visual changes, headache, N/V has been reported. Funduscopic exam should be done before and during treatment. Monitor for malignant	Antibodies to the protein, leukemia, transient peripheral edema, arthralgia, carpal tunnel syndrome, malignant transformations, gynecomastia, pancreatitis.

Table 20.1. PRESCRIBING INFORMATION FOR ENDOCRINE/HORMONAL AND BONE METABOLISM DRUGS *(cont.)*

NAME	FORM/ STRENGTH	DOSAGE	WARNINGS/PRECAUTIONS & CONTRAINDICATIONS	ADVERSE EFFECTS†
PITUITARY HORMONES *(cont.)*				
Somatropin (Nutropin, Nutropin AQ) *(cont.)*		**Peritoneal Dialysis:** Give in am after dialysis. **Chronic Ambulatory Peritoneal Dialysis:** Give qhs during overnight exchange. **Turner Syndrome:** Up to 0.375mg/kg/week SQ in divided doses 3-7x/week. **ISS:** 0.3mg/kg/week divided into daily SQ doses.	transformation of skin lesions. Injecting SQ in same site over long period of time may cause tissue atrophy. May decrease insulin sensitivity; monitor blood sugar. **Contra:** Acute critical illness after serious surgeries (eg, open heart or abdominal surgery, accidental trauma, acute respiratory failure), closed epiphyses in pediatrics, active proliferative or severe non-proliferative diabetic retinopathy, active neoplasia, evidence of recurrence or progression of an intracranial tumor. Prader-Willi syndrome (unless also diagnosed with GH deficiency) with severe obesity or respiratory impairment. **P/N:** Category C, caution in nursing.	
Somatropin (Omnitrope)	**Inj:** 1.5mg, 5.8mg	***Adults:*** Individualize dose. **GHD:** ≤0.04mg/kg/week. May increase at 4- to 8-week intervals. **Max:** 0.08mg/kg/week. Divide dose into daily SQ injections (give preferably in the evening). ***Pediatrics:*** Individualize dose. **GHD:** 0.16-0.24mg/kg/week. Divide dose into daily SQ injections (give preferably in the evening).	**W/P:** Contains benzyl alcohol; avoid use in newborns. Patients with GHD secondary to an intracranial lesion should be monitored closely for progression or recurrence of underlying disease process. Monitor closely for any malignant transformation of skin lesions, scoliosis progression, or gait abnormalities. Monitor closely with DM, glucose intolerance, hypopituitarism. Intracranial HTN reported. Funduscopic exam recomended at initiation, and periodically during course of therapy. **Contra:** Evidence of neoplastic activity. Pediatrics with fused epiphyses. Acute critical illness due to complications after open heart or abdominal surgery, multiple accidental trauma, or with acute respiratory failure. Patients with Prader-Willi syndrome who are severely obese or have severe respiratory impairment. **P/N:** Category B, caution in nursing.	Hypothyroidism, elevated A1C, eosinophilia, hematoma, headache, hypertriglyceridemia, leg pain.
Somatropin (Saizen)	**Inj:** 4mg, 5mg, 8.8mg	***Adults:*** **Initial:** ≤0.005mg/kg/day SQ. **Titrate:** May increase after 4 weeks to ≤0.01mg/kg/day depending on patient tolerance. **Without Consideration of Body Weight: Initial:** 0.2mg/day (0.15-0.3mg/day) SQ. **Titrate:** May increase by increments of 0.1-0.2mg/day every 1-2 months. Consider dose reduction in elderly. ***Pediatrics:*** Individualize dose. **Usual:** 0.06mg/kg IM/SQ 3x/week. If epiphyses are fused, d/c therapy.	**W/P:** Benzyl alcohol associated with toxicity in newborns; if sensitivity occurs, may reconstitute with SWFI. Insulin resistance reported; use caution with DM or family history of DM. Hypothyroidism may occur; bone maturation should be carefully followed. Increased incidence of slipped capital femoral epiphysis may develop with endocrine disorders; monitor for limping or hip/knee pain. Intracranial hypertension (IH) reported; d/c treatment if papilledema observed. Patients with Turner syndrome, chronic renal insufficiency or Prader-Willi syndrome may have increased risk for IH. If idiopathic IH confirmed, may restart therapy at lower dose after signs/symptoms resolve. Alternate injection sites to reduce development of tissue atrophy. Monitor for any malignant transformation of skin lesions. **Contra:** Acute critical illness due to complications following open heart or abdominal surgery, accidental trauma or acute respiratory failure. Active proliferative or severe non-proliferative diabetic	Arthalgia, headache, influenza-like symptoms, peripheral edema, back pain, myalgia, rhinitis, dizziness, upper respiratory tract infection, paraesthesia, hypoaesthesia, insomnia, nausea, generalized edema, depression.

†Bold entries denote special dental considerations.
BB = black box warning; **W/P** = warnings/precautions; **Contra** = contraindications; **P/N** = pregnancy category rating and nursing considerations.

NAME	FORM/ STRENGTH	DOSAGE	WARNINGS/PRECAUTIONS & CONTRAINDICATIONS	ADVERSE EFFECTS†
Somatropin (Saizen) *(cont.)*			retinopathy. Active malignancy, or evidence of progression or recurrence of intracranial tumor. Prader-Willi syndrome when severely obese or have severe respiratory impairment, and in pediatric patients with closed epiphyses. Avoid reconstitution with bacteriostatic water if sensitive to benzyl alcohol. **P/N:** Category B, caution in nursing.	
Somatropin (Serostim)	**Inj:** 4mg, 5mg, 6mg, 8.8mg	***Adults:*** **>55kg:** 6mg SQ qhs. **45-55kg:** 5mg SQ qhs. **35-44kg:** 4mg SQ qhs. **<35kg:** 0.1mg/kg SQ qhs. **Dose Reductions Due to Side Effects:** Reduce total daily dose or number of doses/week. Rotate injection sites. Re-evaluate for infection if weight loss continues after 2 weeks of therapy.	**W/P:** Monitor malnutrition, malabsorption and hypogonadism; may contribute to catabolism. Maintain nucleoside analogue therapy throughout treatment. Carpal tunnel syndrome reported. Perform periodic funduscopic exams. **Contra:** Acute critical illness due to complications after open heart or abdominal surgery, accidental trauma, acute respiratory failure. **P/N:** Category B, caution in nursing.	Musculoskeletal discomfort, increased tissue turgor, edema, arthralgia, extremity pain, hypoesthesia, myalgia, hyperglycemia, arthrosis, diarrhea, headache, paraesthesia, insomnia, upper respiratory tract infection.
Somatropin (Tev-Tropin)	**Inj:** 5mg	***Pediatrics:*** 0.1mg/kg (0.3 IU/kg) SQ 3x week.	**W/P:** Reports of fatalities in pediatric patients with PWS. In PWS, evaluate for upper airway obstruction prior to initiation; monitor weight, for sleep apnea, signs of upper airway obstruction (eg, suspend therapy with onset of or increased snoring), respiratory infections (treat early and aggressively if occur). Monitor GHD secondary to intracranial lesion for progression/ recurrence; glucose intolerance; hypothyroidism; intracranial hypertension (perform fundoscopic exam at start and periodically). Slipped capital femoral epiphysis may occur. Monitor for malignant transformation of any skin lesion. When injected SQ in same site over long period of time, may cause tissue atrophy; rotate injection site. **Contra:** PWS with severe obesity or severe respiratory impairment. Growth failure due to PWS. Acute critical illness due to complications following open heart or abdominal surgery, multiple accidental traumas, acute respiratory failure; closed epiphyses; progression of an underlying intracranial lesion; active neoplasia, benzyl alcohol sensitivity. **P/N:** Category C, caution with nursing.	Headaches, injection-site reactions (pain, bruise), leukemia.
Somatropin (Valtropin)	**Inj:** 5mg	***Adults:*** Individualize dose. **Initial:** 0.33mg/day SQ 6 days a week. Dosage may be increased to individual patient requirement to maximum of 0.66mg/ day after 4 weeks. **Alternative Dosing:** 0.2mg/day (range: 0.15-0.3mg/ day). May increase gradually every 1-2 months by 0.1-0.2mg/day based on individual patient requirements. ***Pediatrics:*** Individualize dose. Divide weekly dose into equal amounts given either daily or 6 days a week by SQ injection. **GHD:** 0.17-0.3mg/kg of body weight/week. **Turner Syndrome:** Up to 0.375mg/kg of body weight/week.	**W/P:** Known sensitivity to supplied diluent (metacresol). Caution in pediatric patients with Prader-Willi syndrome with one or more risk factors (severe obesity, history of upper airway destruction or sleep apnea, or unidentified respiratory infection). May decrease insulin sensitivity. Patients with GHD secondary to intracranial lesion should be monitered closely for progression or recurrence of underlying disease process. Intracranial HTN reported. Monitor closely with DM, glucose intolerance, hypopituitarism. Fundoscopic exam recommended at initiation and periodically during course	Headache, pyrexia, **cough,** respiratory tract infection, diarrhea, vomiting, pharyngitis.

Table 20.1. PRESCRIBING INFORMATION FOR ENDOCRINE/HORMONAL AND BONE METABOLISM DRUGS *(cont.)*

NAME	FORM/ STRENGTH	DOSAGE	WARNINGS/PRECAUTIONS & CONTRAINDICATIONS	ADVERSE EFFECTS†
PITUITARY HORMONES *(cont.)*				
Somatropin (Valtropin) *(cont.)*			of therapy. Monitor carefully for any malignant transformation of skin lesions. **Contra:** Pediatrics with closed epiphyses. Active proliferative and severe nonproliferative diabetic retinopathy. Presence of active malignancy. Acute critical illness due to complications following open heart surgery, abdominal surgery, or multiple accidental trauma, or those with acute respiratory failure. Patients with Prader-Willi syndrome who are severely obese or have severe respiratory impairment. **P/N:** Category B, caution in nursing.	
Somatropin (Zorbtive)	**Inj:** 8.8mg	***Adults:*** 0.1mg/kg qd SQ for 4 weeks. **Max:** 8mg qd. Rotate injection site.	**W/P:** Associated with acute pancreatitis. New onset impaired glucose intolerance, new onset Type 2 DM, exacerbation of preexisting DM, ketoacidosis, diabetic coma reported; closely monitor with risk factors for glucose intolerance. Perform funduscopic evaluations periodically. Increased tissue turgor, musculoskeletal discomfort, and carpal tunnel syndrome may occur. **Contra:** Acute critical illness due to complications following open heart or abdominal surgery, multiple accidental trauma, or acute respiratory failure; active neoplasia (either newly diagnosed or recurrent); benzyl alcohol sensitivity. **P/N:** Category B, caution in nursing.	Peripheral/facial edema, chest/back pain, fever, flu-like disorder, malaise, flatulence, abdominal pain, N/V, viral infection, dizziness, headache, rash.
PROGESTINS				
Medroxyprogesterone Acetate (Provera)	**Tab:** 2.5mg*, 5mg*, 10mg*	***Adults:* Secondary Amenorrhea:** 5-10mg qd for 5-10 days. **Abnormal Uterine Bleeding:** 5-10mg qd for 5-10 days beginning on Day 16 or Day 21 of cycle. **Endometrial Hyperplasia:** 5-10mg qd for 12-14 consecutive days per month beginning on Day 1 or Day 16 of cycle.	**BB:** Not for use for prevention of cardiovascular disease or dementia. Increased risk of MI, stroke, invasive breast cancer, pulmonary emboli, and DVT in postmenopausal women (50-79 yrs) reported. Increased risk of developing probable dementia in postmenopausal women (≥65 yrs of age) reported. **W/P:** D/C if develop thrombotic disorders, papilledema, or retinal vascular lesions. D/C pending exam if sudden onset of proptosis, sudden partial or complete loss of vision, diplopia, or migraine. Include pap smear in pretreatment exam. Caution with depression, DM, and conditions aggravated by fluid retention (eg, epilepsy, migraine, asthma, cardiac, renal dysfunction). Increased risk of endometrial and ovarian cancer reported. **Contra:** Thrombophlebitis, thromboembolic disorders, cerebral apoplexy, liver dysfunction, malignancy of breast or genital organs, undiagnosed vaginal bleeding, missed abortion, pregnancy, as a diagnostic test for pregnancy. **P/N:** Category X, not for use in nursing.	Abnormal uterine bleeding, breast tenderness, galactorrhea, urticaria, pruritus, edema, rash, thromboembolic phenomena, menstrual changes, change in weight, cervical changes, cholestatic jaundice, depression, insomnia, nausea, somnolence.
Norethindrone Acetate (Aygestin)	**Tab:** 5mg*	***Adults:*** Assume interval between menses is 28 days. **Secondary Amenorrhea/ Abnormal Uterine Bleeding:** 2.5-10mg qd for 5-10 days during second half of menstrual cycle. **Endometriosis: Initial:** 5mg qd for 2 weeks. **Titrate:** Increase by 2.5mg qd every 2 weeks up to	**W/P:** D/C with migraine, vision loss, proptosis, diplopia, papilledema, or retinal vascular lesions. May cause thrombophlebitis, pulmonary embolism, and fluid retention. Caution with epilepsy, migraine, psychic depression, asthma, cardiac or renal dysfunction,	Breakthrough bleeding, spotting, change in menstrual flow, amenorrhea, edema, weight changes, cervical changes, cholestatic

*Scored. †Bold entries denote special dental considerations.
BB = black box warning; **W/P** = warnings/precautions; **Contra** = contraindications; **P/N** = pregnancy category rating and nursing considerations.

NAME	FORM/ STRENGTH	DOSAGE	WARNINGS/PRECAUTIONS & CONTRAINDICATIONS	ADVERSE EFFECTS†
Norethindrone Acetate (Aygestin) *(cont.)*		15mg/day. Continue for 6-9 months or until breakthrough bleeding demands temporary termination.	depression, DM, and hyperlipidemia. May mask onset of climacteric. Not for use during the first trimester of pregnancy; risk to the fetus. **Contra:** Pregnancy, thrombophlebitis, thromboembolic disorders, cerebral apoplexy, liver impairment, breast carcinoma, undiagnosed vaginal bleeding, missed abortion, use as a pregnancy diagnostic test. **P/N:** Category X, safety in nursing is not known.	jaundice, rash, melasma, chloasma, depression.
Progesterone (Prometrium)	**Cap:** 100mg, 200mg	***Adults:*** **Prevention of Endometrial Hyperplasia:** 200mg qpm for 12 days sequentially per 28 day cycle. **Secondary Amenorrhea:** 400mg qhs for 10 days.	**BB:** Progestins and estrogens should not be used for the prevention of cardiovascular disease. Increased risks of MI, stroke, invasive breast cancer, pulmonary emboli, DVT, and development of probable dementia in postmenopausal women. **W/P:** D/C if thrombotic disorders, papilledema, or retinal vascular lesions develop. D/C pending exam if sudden onset of proptosis, sudden partial or complete loss of vision, diplopia, or migraine. Include pap smear in pretreatment exam. Caution with depression, DM, and conditions aggravated by fluid retention (eg, epilepsy, migraine, asthma, cardiac/renal dysfunction). **Contra:** Peanut allergy, undiagnosed abnormal genital bleeding, breast cancer, DVT, PE, thromboembolic disorders (stroke, myocardial infarction), liver dysfunction or disease, pregnancy. **P/N:** Category B, caution in nursing.	Dizziness, headache, breast pain, nausea, diarrhea, dizziness, abdominal pain and distension, emotional lability, upper respiratory infection.
THYROID AGENTS				
ANTITHYROID HORMONES				
Methimazole (Tapazole)	**Tab:** 5mg*, 10mg*	***Adults:*** **Initial: Mild Hyperthyroidism:** 5mg q8h. **Moderately Severe Hyperthyroidism:** 30-40mg/day, in divided doses q8h. **Severe Hyperthyroidism:** 20mg q8h. **Maint:** 5-15mg/day. ***Pediatrics:*** **Initial:** 0.4mg/kg/day, in divided doses q8h. **Maint:** 1/2 of initial dose.	**W/P:** Can cause fetal harm. Agranulocytosis, leukopenia, thrombocytopenia, aplastic anemia may occur; monitor bone marrow function. D/C with agranulocytosis, aplastic anemia, or exfoliative dermatitis. D/C with liver abnormality (eg, hepatitis) including transaminases >3x ULN. Monitor thyroid function periodically. May cause hypoprothrombinemia and bleeding; monitor PT. **Contra:** Nursing mothers. **P/N:** Category D, contraindicated in nursing.	Rash, urticaria, N/V, arthralgia, paresthesia, myalgia, neuritis, vertigo, edema, **altered taste,** hair loss, lymphadenopathy, lupuslike syndrome, insulin autoimmune syndrome.
Propylthiouracil	**Tab:** 50mg	***Adults:*** **Initial:** 300mg/day in 3 divided doses, q8h. **Severe Hyperthyroidism/ Very Large Goiters: Initial:** 400mg/day in 3 divided doses; may give up to 600-900mg/day if needed. **Maint:** 100-150mg/day. ***Pediatrics:*** **6-10 yrs: Initial:** 50-150mg/day. **≥10 yrs: Initial:** 150-300mg/day. **Maint:** Determine by patient response.	**W/P:** D/C with agranulocytosis, aplastic anemia, hepatitis, fever, or exfoliative dermatitis. Rare reports of severe hepatic reactions exist. D/C with significant hepatic abnormality, including transaminases >3x ULN. Caution with pregnancy, may cause fetal harm. Monitor PT and TFTs. **Contra:** Nursing mothers. **P/N:** Category D, contraindicated in nursing.	Agranulocytosis, granulopenia, thrombocytopenia, aplastic anemia, drug fever, hepatitis, periarteritis, hypoprothrombinemia, skin rash, urticaria, N/V, epigastric distress, arthralgia, paresthesias.
THYROID HORMONES				
Levothyroxine Sodium (Levothroid)	**Tab:** 25mcg*, 50mcg*, 75mcg*, 88mcg*, 100mcg*, 112mcg*,	***Adults:*** **Hypothyroidism: Usual:** 100-200mcg/day. **Endocrine/Cardiovascular Complications: Initial:** 50mcg/day. **Titrate:** Increase by 50mcg/day every 2-4 weeks until euthyroid. **Hypothyroid with Angina: Initial:** 25mcg/day. **Titrate:**	**W/P:** Do not use in the treatment of obesity; larger doses in euthyroid patients can cause serious or even life threatening toxicity. Caution with cardiovascular disease, HTN. May aggravate diabetes mellitus or insipidus and adrenal cortical	Lactose hypersensitivity, transient partial hair loss in children.

Table 20.1. PRESCRIBING INFORMATION FOR ENDOCRINE/HORMONAL AND BONE METABOLISM DRUGS *(cont.)*

NAME	FORM/ STRENGTH	DOSAGE	WARNINGS/PRECAUTIONS & CONTRAINDICATIONS	ADVERSE EFFECTS†
THYROID AGENTS *(cont.)*				
THYROID HORMONES *(cont.)*				
Levothyroxine Sodium (Levothroid) *(cont.)*	125mcg*, 137mcg*, 150mcg*, 175mcg*, 200mcg*, 300mcg*	Increase by 25-50mcg every 2-4 weeks until euthyroid. ***Pediatrics:*** **Hypothyroidism: >12 yrs: Usual:** 100-200mcg/day. **6-12 yrs:** 4-5mcg/kg/day. **1-5 yrs:** 5-6mcg/kg/day. **6-12 months:** 6-8mcg/kg/day. **0-6 months:** 10-15mcg/kg/day. May crush tab and sprinkle over food (applesauce) or mix with 5-10mL water, formula (non-soy), or breast milk.	insufficiency. Excessive doses in infants may produce craniosynostosis. Add glucocorticoid with myxedema coma. **Contra:** Untreated thyrotoxicosis, acute MI, and uncorrected adrenal insufficiency. **P/N:** Category A, caution in nursing.	
Levothyroxine Sodium (Levoxyl, Synthroid, Unithroid)	**Tab:** (Levoxyl) 25mcg*, 50mcg*, 75mcg*, 88mcg*, 100mcg*, 112mcg*, 125mcg*, 137mcg*, 150mcg*, 175mcg*, 200mcg*; (Synthroid) 25mcg*, 50mcg*, 75mcg*, 88mcg*, 100mcg*, 112mcg*, 125mcg*, 137mcg*, 150mcg*, 175mcg*, 200mcg*, 300mcg*; (Unithroid) 25mcg*, 50mcg*, 75mcg*, 88mcg*, 100mcg*, 112mcg*, 125mcg*, 150mcg*, 175mcg*, 200mcg*, 300mcg*	***Adults:*** Take in am at least 0.5-1hr before food. **Hypothyroid: Usual:** 1.7mcg/kg/day. >200mcg/day (seldom). **>50 yrs/<50 yrs with Cardiac Disease: Initial:** 25-50mcg/day. **Titrate:** Increase by 12.5-25mcg/day every 6-8 weeks until euthyroid. **Elderly with Cardiac Disease: Initial:** 12.5-25mcg/day. **Titrate:** Increase by 12.5-25mcg/day every 4-6 weeks until euthyroid. **Severe Hypothyroidism: Initial:** 12.5-25mcg/day. **Titrate:** Increase by 25mcg/day every 2-4 weeks until euthyroid. **Pregnancy:** May increase dose requirements. **Subclinical Hypothyroidism:** Lower doses required. ***Pediatrics:*** Take in am at least 0.5-1hr before food. **Hypothyroidism: 0-3 months:** 10-15mcg/kg/day. **3-6 months:** 8-10mcg/kg/day. **6-12 months:** 6-8mcg/kg/day. **1-5 yrs:** 5-6mcg/kg/day. **6-12 yrs:** 4-5mcg/kg/day. **>12 yrs:** 2-3mcg/kg/day. **Growth/Puberty Complete:** 1.7mcg/kg/day. **Cardiac Risk: Initial:** Use lower dose. **Titrate:** Increase dose every 4-6 weeks until euthyroid. **Infants with Serum T_4 <5mcg/dL: Initial:** 50mcg/day. **Chronic/Severe Hypothyroidism: Children: Initial:** 25mcg/day. **Titrate:** Increase by 25mcg/day every 2-4 weeks until desired effect. **Minimize Hyperactivity in Older Children: Initial:** Give one-fourth of full replacement dose. **Titrate:** Increase by same amount weekly until full dose achieved. May crush tab and mix with 5-10mL water.	**W/P:** Do not use in the treatment of obesity; larger doses in euthyroid patients can cause serious or even life threatening toxicity. Caution with cardiovascular disease, CAD, adrenal insufficiency, and the elderly with risk of occult cardiac disease. Carefully titrate dose to avoid over or under treatment. Decreased bone mineral density with long term use. Caution with nontoxic diffuse goiter or nodular thyroid disease. With adrenal insufficiency supplement with glucocorticoids before therapy. **Contra:** Untreated thyrotoxicosis, acute MI, and uncorrected adrenal insufficiency. **P/N:** Category A, caution in nursing.	Pseudotumor cerebri in children reported. Seizures (rare), hypersensitivity reactions, dysphagia, craniosynostosis in infants, choking, gagging, hyperthyroidism (increased appetite, weight loss, heat intolerance, hyperactivity, tremors, palpitations, tachycardia, diarrhea, vomiting, hair loss).
Liothyronine Sodium (Cytomel)	**Tab:** 5mcg, 25mcg*, 50mcg*	***Adults:*** **Mild Hypothyroidism: Initial:** 25mcg qd. **Titrate:** May increase by up to 25mcg qd every 1-2 weeks. **Maint:** 25-75mcg qd. **Myxedema: Initial:** 5mcg qd. **Titrate:** May increase by 5-10mcg qd every 1-2 weeks up to 25mcg qd, then increase by 5-25mcg qd every 1-2 weeks. **Maint:** 50-100mcg/day. **Goiter: Initial:** 5mcg/day. **Titrate:** May increase by 5-10mcg qd every 1-2 weeks up to 25mcg qd, then by 12.5-25mcg qd every 1-2 weeks. **Maint:** 75mcg qd. **Elderly/Coronary Artery Disease: Initial:** 5mcg qd. **Titrate:** Increase by no more than 5mcg qd every 2 weeks. **Thyroid Suppression Therapy:** 75-100mcg qd for 7 days. Radioactive iodine uptake is determined before and after administration of hormone. ***Pediatrics:*** **Congenital**	**W/P:** Do not use in the treatment of obesity; larger doses in euthyroid patients can cause serious or even life threatening toxicity. Caution with angina pectoris and elderly; use lower doses. Rule out hypogonadism and nephrosis prior to therapy. With prolonged and severe hypothyroidism supplement with adrenocortical steroids. May aggravate diabetes mellitus or insipidus and adrenal cortical insufficiency. Add glucocorticoid with myxedema coma. Excessive doses may cause craniosynostosis in infants. **Contra:** Uncorrected adrenal cortical insufficiency and untreated thyrotoxicosis. **P/N:** Category A, caution in nursing.	Allergic skin reactions (rare).

*Scored. †Bold entries denote special dental considerations.
BB = black box warning; **W/P** = warnings/precautions; **Contra** = contraindications; **P/N** = pregnancy category rating and nursing considerations.

NAME	FORM/ STRENGTH	DOSAGE	WARNINGS/PRECAUTIONS & CONTRAINDICATIONS	ADVERSE EFFECTS†
Liothyronine Sodium (Cytomel) *(cont.)*		**Hypothyroidism: Initial:** 5mcg qd. **Titrate:** Increase by 5mcg qd every 3-4 days until desired response. **Maint: <1 yr:** 20mcg qd. **1-3 yrs:** 50mcg qd. **>3 yrs:** 25-75mcg/day.		
Liotrix (Thyrolar)	(T3-T4) **Tab:** (1/4) 3.1mcg-12.5mcg, (1/2) 6.25mcg-25mcg, (1) 12.5mcg-50mcg, (2) 25mcg-100mcg, (3) 37.5mcg-150mcg	***Adults:*** **Hypothyroidism: Usual:** 12.5mcg-50mcg to 25mcg-100mcg qd. **Elderly/Coronary Artery Disease: Initial:** 6.25mcg-25mcg qd. **Chronic Myxedema:** 3.1mcg-12.5mcg qd. **Titrate:** Increase by 3.1mcg-12.5mcg/d q 2-3 weeks. Reduce dose if angina occurs. **Myxedema Coma:** 400mcg IV levothyroxine sodium (100mcg/mL rapidly) followed by 100-200mcg/day IV. Switch to PO when stable. **Thyroid Suppression:** 1.56mg/kg/d levothyroxine (T4) for 7-10 days. ***Pediatrics:*** **Hypothyroidism: >12 yrs:** 18.75mcg-75mcg qd. **6-12 yrs:** 12.5mcg-50mcg to 18.75mcg-75mcg qd. **1-5 yrs:** 9.35mcg-37.5mcg to 12.5mcg-50mcg qd. **6-12 months:** 6.25mcg-25mcg to 9.35mcg-37.5mcg qd. **0-6 months:** 3.1mcg-12.5mcg to 6.25mcg-25mcg qd.	**W/P:** Do not use in the treatment of obesity; larger doses in euthyroid patients can cause serious or even life-threatening toxicity. Caution with angina pectoris and elderly; use lower doses. May aggravate diabetes mellitus or insipidus and adrenal cortical insufficiency. Excessive doses may cause craniosynostosis. Extreme caution with long-standing myxedema especially with cardiovascular impairment. **Contra:** Untreated thyrotoxicosis, uncorrected adrenal cortical insufficiency. **P/N:** Category A, caution in nursing.	
Thyroid (Armour Thyroid)	**Tab:** 15mg, 30mg, 60mg, 90mg, 120mg, 180mg, 240mg, 300mg	***Adults:*** **Hypothyroidism: Initial:** 30mg qd. **Titrate:** Increase by 15mg q2-3 weeks. **Myxedema with Cardiovascular Disorder:** 15mg qd. **Maint:** 60-120mg/day. **Thyroid Cancer:** Higher doses than replacement therapy are required. **Myxedema Coma: Levothyroxine Sodium: Initial:** 400mcg IV then 100-200mcg/day IV. Continue with oral therapy when stabilized. **Thyroid Suppression:** 1.56mg/kg/day for 7-10 days. **Elderly: Initial:** Use lower dose (eg, 15-30mg qd). ***Pediatrics:*** **Hypothyroidism: 0-6 months:** 4.8-6mg/kg/day; **6-12 months:** 3.6-4.8mg/kg/day; **1-5 yrs:** 3-3.6mg/kg/day; **6-12 yrs:** 2.4-3mg/kg/day; **>12 yrs:** 1.2-1.8mg/kg/day.	**W/P:** Do not use in the treatment of obesity; larger doses in euthyroid patients can cause serious or even life-threatening toxicity. Caution with cardiovascular disease, DM, diabetes insipidus, elderly, and adrenal cortical insufficiency. **Contra:** Untreated thyrotoxicosis; uncorrected adrenal cortical insufficiency. **P/N:** Category A, caution in nursing.	
MISCELLANEOUS METABOLIC AGENTS				
Alglucosidase Alfa (Myozyme)	**Inj:** 50 mg	***Adults/Pediatrics:*** 20 mg/kg IV every 2 weeks. Administer over 4 hrs.	**BB:** Risk of hypersensitivity reactions. Life-threatening anaphylactic reactions, including anaphylactic shock observed during infusion. Appropriate medical support should be readily available when administered. **W/P:** See Black Box Warning. Risk of cardiac arrhythmia, sudden cardiac death during general anesthesia for central venous catheter placement, and acute cardiorespiratory failure. Infusion reactions observed. Caution with acutely ill patients. **P/N:** Category B, caution in nursing.	Pyrexia, cough, respiratory distress/failure, pneumonia, otitis media, upper respiratory tract infection, gastroenteritis, pharyngitis, diarrhea, vomiting, rash, decreased oxygen saturation, anemia, **oral candidiasis.**
Aminoglutethimide (Cytadren)	**Tab:** 250mg*	***Adults:*** **Initial:** 250mg PO q6h. **Titrate:** May increase by 250mg/day q1-2 wks. **Max:** 2000mg. D/C if skin rash persists for >5-8 days or becomes severe. If glucocorticoid replacement therapy is needed, give 20-30mg of hydrocortisone PO in the morning.	**W/P:** May cause adrenocortical hypofunction, especially under conditions of stress; monitor closely. May suppress aldosterone production by the adrenal cortex and may cause orthostatic or persistent hypotension; monitor BP. May cause fetal harm. Therapy should be initiated in a hospital. May impair mental/physical abilities. **P/N:** Category D, not for use in nursing.	Drowsiness, morbilliform skin rash, nausea, anorexia, dizziness.

Table 20.1. PRESCRIBING INFORMATION FOR ENDOCRINE/HORMONAL AND BONE METABOLISM DRUGS *(cont.)*

NAME	FORM/ STRENGTH	DOSAGE	WARNINGS/PRECAUTIONS & CONTRAINDICATIONS	ADVERSE EFFECTS†
MISCELLANEOUS METABOLIC AGENTS *(cont.)*				
Calcitriol (Rocaltrol)	**Cap:** 0.25mcg, 0.5mcg; **Sol:** 1mcg/mL [15mL]	***Adults/Pediatrics:*** **≥3 yrs: Predialysis: Initial:** 0.25mcg/day. **Max:** 0.5mcg/day. **<3yrs: Initial:** 10-15ng/kg/day. **≥6 yrs: Hypoparathyroidism: Initial:** 0.25mcg/day every am. **Titrate:** May increase at 2- to 4-week intervals to 0.5-2mcg/day. **1-5 yrs: Initial:** 0.25mcg/day every am. **Titrate:** May increase at 2- to 4-week intervals up to 0.75mcg/day. **Elderly:** Start at low end of dosing range. **Dialysis: Initial:** 0.25mcg/day. **Titrate:** May increase by 0.25mcg/day every 4-8 weeks to 0.5-1mcg/day. Monitor serum calcium levels twice weekly during titration. Normal to slightly reduced serum calcium, give 0.25mcg every other day. D/C with hypercalcemia; when calcium levels return to normal continue therapy and decrease dose by 0.25 mcg.	**W/P:** Use non-aluminum phosphate binders and low phosphate diet to control serum phosphate. Chronic hypercalcemia can cause calcification of soft tissues. Monitor calcium levels twice a week initially. Avoid dehydration. Monitor SrCr. Maintain adequate calcium intake of at least 600mg/day. Caution in elderly. If treatment switched from ergocalciferol, may take several months for ergocalciferol level to decrease to baseline. May increase inorganic phosphate levels; ectopic calcification reported with renal failure. Monitor phosphorus, magnesium, alkaline phosphatase, and 24-hour urine periodically. **Contra:** Hypercalcemia or vitamin D toxicity. **P/N:** Category C, not for use in nursing.	Weakness, N/V, **dry mouth,** constipation, muscle and bone pain, **metallic taste,** polyuria, polydipsia, weight loss, pancreatitis, photophobia, pruritus, decreased libido.
Cinacalcet HCl (Sensipar)	**Tab:** 30mg, 60mg, 90mg	***Adults:*** Take with food. Swallow whole. Secondary **Hyperparathyroidism: Initial:** 30mg qd. **Titrate:** Increase no more frequently than every 2-4 weeks through sequential doses of 60, 90, 120, and 180mg qd to target iPTH of 150-300pg/mL. **Parathyroid Carcinoma: Initial:** 30mg bid. **Titrate:** Increase every 2-4 weeks through sequential doses of 30mg bid, 60mg bid, 90mg bid, and 90mg tid-qid prn to normalize serum Ca levels. Adjust based on serum Ca levels (see PI). May be used alone or in combination with vitamin D sterols and/or phosphate binders.	**W/P:** Monitor closely for hypocalcemia, especially with history of seizure disorder. Do not initiate with serum Ca <8.4mg/dL. Measure serum Ca and phosphorus within 1 week and iPTH 1-4 weeks after initiation or dose adjustment. After maintenance dose reached, measure serum Ca and phosphorus monthly and iPTH every 1-3 months. Adynamic bone disease may develop with iPTH levels <100pg/mL; reduce dose or d/c therapy if iPTH <150pg/mL. Caution with moderate/severe hepatic impairment. **P/N:** Category C, not for use in nursing.	N/V, diarrhea, myalgia, dizziness, HTN, asthenia, anorexia, chest pain (noncardiac), access infection.
Conivaptan HCl (Vaprisol)	**Inj:** 5mg/mL	***Adults:*** IV use only. Use large veins and change infusion site every 24 hrs. **Loading Dose:** 20mg IV over 30 min. Follow with 20mg continuous IV over 24 hrs. Following initial day of treatment, administer for an additional 1-3 days in continuous infusion of 20mg/day. **Titrate:** May increase to 40mg/day if needed. **Max:** 40mg/day. Total duration of infusion should not exceed 4 days.	**W/P:** Safety in CHF not established. Monitor sodium concentration and neurologic status during administration; d/c if rapid rise in serum sodium. Caution with hepatic or renal impairment. Rotate infusion site every 24 hrs. **Contra:** Hypovolemic hyponatremia. Concurrent potent CYP3A4 inhibitors (eg, ketoconazole, itraconazole, clarithromycin, ritonavir, and indinavir). **P/N:** Category C, caution in nursing.	Infusion-site reactions, erythema/pain/phlebitis at infusion site, anemia, constipation, diarrhea, dry mouth, N/V, peripheral edema, pyrexia, thirst, hypokalemia, headache, cardiac failure, atrial dyrthythmias, and sepsis.
Doxercalciferol (Hectorol)	**Cap:** 0.5mcg, 2.5mcg; **Inj:** 2mcg/mL [2mL]	***Adults:*** (Cap) **Dialysis: Initial:** 10mcg 3x/week (TIW) approximately qod at dialysis. **Titrate:** Adjust to obtain iPTH of 150-300 pg/mL. May increase by 2.5mcg at 8-week intervals if iPTH is not lowered by 50% and fails to reach target range. **Max:** 20mcg TIW (60mcg/week). Suspend therapy if iPTH <100pg/mL; restart after 1 week with dose at least 2.5mcg lower than last dose. **Hypercalcemia/Hyperphosphatemia/Ca x P product >55mg²/dL²:** Decrease or suspend therapy and/or adjust dose of phosphate binders; if suspended, restart at a dose at least 2.5mcg lower. **Predialysis: Initial:** 1mcg qd. **Titrate:** May increase by	**W/P:** Acute hypercalcemia may exacerbate arrythmias, seizures. Use oral Ca-based or non-aluminum containing antacids to control serum phosphate. Chronic hypercalcemia can cause calcification of soft tissues. Risk of hypercalcemia and hyperphospatemia. Maintain serum calcium times serum phosphorus at <55mg²/dL² in patients with chronic kidney disease. Avoid with recent history of hypercalcemia, hyperphosphatemia, or vitamin D toxicity. Caution with hepatic dysfunction. Monitor iPTH, serum calcium, and serum phosphorus initially then weekly during dose titration. Oversuppression of iPTH can cause adynamic bone syndrome. **Contra:**	Headache, malaise, bradycardia, NV, edema, dizziness, dyspnea, pruritus, abscess, anorexia, constipation, dyspepsia, arthralgia, weight increase, sleep disorder.

*Scored. †Bold entries denote special dental considerations.
BB = black box warning; **W/P** = warnings/precautions; **Contra** = contraindications; **P/N** = pregnancy category rating and nursing considerations.

NAME	FORM/ STRENGTH	DOSAGE	WARNINGS/PRECAUTIONS & CONTRAINDICATIONS	ADVERSE EFFECTS†
Doxercalciferol (Hectorol) *(cont.)*		0.5mcg at 2-week intervals to achieve target iPTH range. **Max:** 3.5mcg qd. **Hypercalcemia/Hyperphosphatemia/ Ca x P product >55mg²/dL²:** Decrease or suspend therapy and/or adjust dose of phosphate binders; if suspended, restart at a dose at least 0.5mcg lower. (Inj) **Initial:** 4mcg bolus TIW at the end of dialysis. **Titrate:** Adjust to obtain iPTH of 150-300pg/mL. May increase at 8-week intervals by 1-2mcg if iPTH is not lowered by 50% and fails to reach target range. **Max:** 18mcg/week. Suspend therapy if iPTH <100pg/mL; restart after 1 week with a dose at least 1mcg lower than last dose. **Hypercalcemia/Hyperphosphatemia/ Ca x P product >55mg²/dL²:** Decrease or suspend therapy and/or adjust dose of phosphate binders; if suspended, restart at a dose at least 1mcg lower.	Tendency to develop hypercalcemia or vitamin D toxicity. **P/N:** Category B, not for use in nursing.	
Ergocalciferol (Drisdol)	**Cap:** 1.25mg (50,000 IU vitamin D)	***Adults:*** **Vitamin D–Resistant Rickets:** 12,000-500,000 IU qd. **Hypoparathyroidism:** 50,000-200,000 IU qd given concomitantly with calcium lactate 4g six times/day. Individualize dosage.	**W/P:** Avoid in infants with idiopathic hypercalcemia. Monitor serum calcium and phosphorous levels every 2 weeks or more frequently if necessary. X-rays of bones should be taken every month until condition is corrected and stabilized. IV calcium, parathyroid hormone, and/or dihydrotachysterol may be needed when treating hypoparathyroidism. Maintain normal serum phosphorous levels when treating hyperphosphatemia to prevent metastatic calcification. Maintain adequate dietary calcium. Contains FD&C Yellow No. 5 (tartrazine). Protect from light. **Contra:** Hypercalcemia, malabsorption syndrome, abnormal sensitivity to the toxic effects of vitamin D, hypervitaminosis D. **P/N:** Category C, caution in nursing.	Anemia, anorexia, constipation, nausea, bone demineralization, stiffness, weakness, calcification of soft tissues, impaired renal function, polyuria, nocturia, polydipsia, hypercalciuria, azotemia, HTN, nephrocalcinosis.
Exenatide (Byetta)	**Inj:** 5mcg/ dose, 10mcg/ dose [60-dose prefilled pen]	***Adults:*** 5mcg SQ bid, 60 min before am and pm meals. **Titrate:** May increase to 10mcg bid after 1 month. Reduction of sulfonylurea dose may be considered to reduce risk of hypoglycemia.	**W/P:** Not a substitute for insulin. Avoid with type 1 DM, treatment of diabetic ketoacidosis, ESRD, severe renal impairment (CrCl <30mL/min), or severe GI disease. Acute pancreatitis reported. Increased incidence of hypoglycemia with sulfonylureas. Observe for signs and symptoms of hypersensitivity reactions; patients with abdominal pain should be investigated. When used with thiazolidinediones possible CP and/or chronic hypersensitivity pneumonitis. **P/N:** Category C, caution in nursing.	N/V, diarrhea, feeling jittery, dizziness, headache, **dyspepsia,** injection-site reactions; dysgeusia, somnolence, generalized pruritus and/or urticaria, macular or papular rash, angioedema, rare reports of anaphylactic reaction, abdominal pain, hypoglycemia.
Glucagon	**Inj:** 1mg	***Adults/Pediatrics:*** **Severe Hypoglycemia: ≥20kg:** 1mg (1 U) SQ/IM/IV. **<20kg:** 0.5mg (0.5 U) or 20-30mcg/kg. May give another dose after 15 min if patient does not respond, but IV glucose would be a better alternative. Use immediately after reconstitution; discard unused portion. After patient responds give supplemental carbohydrate. **Diagnostic Aid: Duodenum/ Small Bowel:** 0.25-0.5mg (0.25-0.5 U) IV, or 1mg (1 U) IM, or 2mg (2 U) IV/IM before procedure. **Stomach:** 0.5mg (0.5 U) IV or 2mg (2 U) IM before procedure. **Colon:** 2mg (2 U) IM 10 min before procedure.	**W/P:** Caution with history suggestive of insulinoma and/or pheochromocytoma. Glucagon can cause pheochromocytoma tumor to release catecholamines, which may result in a sudden and marked increase in BP. Effective in treating hypoglycemia only if sufficient liver glycogen is present. Glucagon is not effective in states of starvation, adrenal insufficiency, or chronic hypoglycemia; use glucose to treat instead. **Contra:** Pheochromocytoma. **P/N:** Category B, caution in nursing.	N/V, allergic reactions, urticaria, respiratory distress, hypotension.

Table 20.1. PRESCRIBING INFORMATION FOR ENDOCRINE/HORMONAL AND BONE METABOLISM DRUGS *(cont.)*

NAME	FORM/ STRENGTH	DOSAGE	WARNINGS/PRECAUTIONS & CONTRAINDICATIONS	ADVERSE EFFECTS†
MISCELLANEOUS METABOLIC AGENTS *(cont.)*				
Lanreotide (Somatuline Depot)	**Inj:** 60mg, 90mg, 120mg	***Adults:*** **Initial:** 90mg deep SQ at 4-week intervals for 3 months. **Titrate:** Adjust dose based on IGF and GH levels. **GH >1 to ≤2.5ng/mL, IGF-1 Normal and Controlled Clinical Symptoms:** 90mg every 4 weeks. **GH >2.5ng/mL, IGF-1 Elevated and/ or Clinical Symptoms Uncontrolled:** 120mg every 4 weeks. **GH ≤1ng/mL, IGF-1 Normal and Clinical Symptoms Controlled:** 60mg every 4 weeks. **Moderate-to-Severe Renal/Hepatic Impairment: Initial:** 60mg deep SQ at 4 week intervals for 3 months.	**W/P:** May reduce gallbladder motility and lead to gallstone formation; monitor periodically. Hypo- and/or hyperglycemia may occur; monitor glucose levels. Decreased thyroid function reported. May decrease HR; caution with bradycardia. **P/N:** Category C, caution in nursing.	Diarrhea, abdominal pain, N/V, constipation, flatulence, loose stools, cholethiasis, injection-site reactions.
Leuprolide Acetate (Lupron Depot-Ped, Lupron Pediatric)	**Inj:** 5mg/mL, (Depot) 7.5mg, 11.25mg, 15mg	***Pediatrics:*** **Initial:** 50mcg/kg/d as single SQ dose or (depot) 0.3mg/ kg every 4 weeks (minimum 7.5mg) as single IM dose. **Depot Start Dose: ≤25kg:** 7.5mg; **>25-37.5kg:** 11.25mg; **>37.5kg:** 15mg. **Titrate:** Increase by 10 mcg/kg/day SQ or (depot) 3.75mg IM every 4 weeks if downregulation not achieved. **Maint:** Dose that produces adequate downregulation. Verify adequate downregulation with significant weight increase.	**W/P:** Monitor hormonal effects after 1-2 months of therapy. Measure bone age every 6-12 months. Increase in clinical signs and symptoms may occur in early phase of therapy due to rise in gonadotropins and sex steroids. D/C before age 11 in females and age 12 in males. **Contra:** Pregnancy. **P/N:** Category X, not for use in nursing.	Initial exacerbation of signs and symptoms, injection-site reactions, pain, acne/seborrhea, rash, urogenital bleeding/discharge, vaginitis.
Levocarnitine (Carnitor, Carnitor SF)	**Inj:** 200mg/mL; **Sol:** 100mg/ mL [118mL]; **Tab:** 330mg; **Sol:** (Carnitor SF) 100mg/mL [118mL]	***Adults:*** (Inj) **Usual:** 50mg/kg/day IV bolus or infusion. **Max:** 300mg/kg/day. **Severe Metabolic Crisis: LD:** 50mg/ kg, then 50mg/kg over the next 24 hrs given q3-4h, and never less than q6h by infusion or IV injection. **ESRD: Initial:** 10-20mg/kg bolus into venous return line after dialysis. Adjust dose based on trough (predialysis) levocarnitine levels. Can make downward dose adjustments the third or fourth week of therapy. (Tab) 990mg PO bid-tid. (Sol) **Initial:** 1g/day. **Usual:** 1-3g/day per 50kg. Take after meals. May dissolve solution in fluids/liquid foods; drink slowly. ***Pediatrics:*** (Inj) **Usual:** 50mg/kg/day IV bolus or infusion. **Max:** 300mg/kg/day. **Severe Metabolic Crisis: LD:** 50mg/ kg, then 50mg/kg over the next 24 hrs given q3-4h, and never less than q6h by infusion or IV injection. **ESRD: Initial:** 10-20mg/kg bolus into venous return line after dialysis. Adjust dose based on trough (predialysis) levocarnitine levels. Can make downward dose adjustments the third or fourth week of therapy. (Sol/Tab) **Infants/Children: Initial:** 50mg/kg/day. **Maint:** 50-100mg/kg/ day in divided doses. **Max:** 3g/day. Take after meals. May dissolve solution in fluids/liquid foods; drink slowly.	**W/P:** Avoid long term, high oral dose therapy with severely compromised renal function or ESRD with dialysis. Monitor carnitine levels periodically. **P/N:** Category B, not for use in nursing.	N/V, abdominal cramps, diarrhea, gastritis, seizures.
Nafarelin Acetate (Synarel)	**Spray:** 200mcg/ inh [8mL]	(Endometriosis) ***Adults:*** **≥18 yrs:** 1 spray (200mcg) into one nostril qam and 1 spray into other nostril qpm. Initiate therapy between days 2-4 of menstrual cycle. Increase to 1 spray per nostril qam and qpm after 2 months (800mcg/day) if amenorrhea has not occurred. Treat for 6 months. (CPP) ***Pediatrics:*** **Usual:** 2 sprays (400mcg) per nostril qam and qpm. **Total Daily Dose:** 1600mcg. Increase to 3 sprays	**W/P:** (Endometriosis) Ovarian cysts reported in adult women. Caution if risk factors for decreased bone mineral content present. Avoid sneezing during or after administration. Use nonhormonal methods of contraception. (CPP) Determine diagnosis before initiating therapy. Monitor regularly. Assess growth and bone age velocity within 3-6 months of initiation. Avoid sneezing during or after administration. **Contra:** Pregnancy,	(Endometriosis) Hot flashes, decreased libido, vaginal dryness, headache, emotional lability, myalgia, acne, nasal irritation, reduced breast size, insomnia, edema, seborrhea, weight gain, depression,

†Bold entries denote special dental considerations.
BB = black box warning; **W/P** = warnings/precautions; **Contra** = contraindications; **P/N** = pregnancy category rating and nursing considerations.

NAME	FORM/ STRENGTH	DOSAGE	WARNINGS/PRECAUTIONS & CONTRAINDICATIONS	ADVERSE EFFECTS†
Nafarelin Acetate (Synarel) *(cont.)*		into alternating nostrils tid (1800mcg daily) if needed 30 seconds should elapse between sprays. Continue until resumption of puberty is desired.	women who may become pregnant, nursing, undiagnosed abnormal vaginal bleeding. **P/N:** Category X, not for use in nursing.	hirsutism. (CPP) Acne, breast enlargement, vaginal bleeding, emotional lability, transient increase in pubic hair, rhinitis, body odor, seborrhea, white or brownish vaginal discharge.
Octreotide Acetate (Sandostatin, Sandostatin LAR)	**Inj:** (Sandostatin) 50mcg/mL, 100mcg/mL, 200mcg/mL, 500mcg/mL, 1000mcg/mL; **Inj, Depot:** (Sandostatin LAR) 10mg, 20mg, 30mg	***Adults:*** (Inj) Give SQ/IV. **Acromegaly: Initial:** 50mcg tid. **Titrate:** Adjust dose based on IGF-I levels every 2 weeks. **Usual:** 100mcg tid. **Max:** 500mcg tid. Reduce dose if no additional benefit with dose increase. Reevaluate IGF-I or growth hormone levels every 6 months. Withdraw yearly for 4 weeks to assess disease activity after irradiation. **Carcinoid Tumors: Initial:** 100-600mcg/day given bid-qid (mean dose 300mcg/day) for 2 weeks. **Max:** 750mcg/day. **VIPomas: Initial:** 200-300mcg/day (range 150-750mcg) given bid-qid for 2 weeks. **Max:** 450mcg/day. (Inj, Depot) Administer intragluteally. **Acromegaly: Initial:** 20mg IM every 4 weeks for 3 months. **Titrate:** If GH ≤2.5ng/mL, IGF-1 normal, and clinical symptoms controlled then maintain dose. If GH >2.5, IGF-1 elevated, and/or clinical symptoms uncontrolled then increase to 30mg every 4 weeks. If GH ≤1, IGF-1 normal, and clinical symptoms controlled then reduce to 10mg every 4 weeks. **Max:** 40mg every 4 weeks. Withdraw yearly for 8 weeks to assess disease activity after pituitary irradiation. **Carcinoid Tumors/VIPomas: Initial:** 20mg IM every 4 weeks for 2 months. Continue with Sandostatin injection SQ for at least 2 weeks. **Titrate:** If symptoms not controlled, increase to 30mg every 4 weeks. If symptoms controlled at 20mg, reduce to 10mg. **Max:** 30mg every 4 weeks. For exacerbation of symptoms, give Sandostatin injection SQ for at least 2 weeks. Patients must be considered responders and tolerate the injection before switching to the depot. **Renal Failure Requiring Dialysis:** Reduce dose.	**W/P:** May inhibit gallbladder contractility and decrease bile secretions; increased risk of gallstones. May alter balance between insulin, glucagon and growth hormone and lead to hypoglycemia or hyperglycemia. Hypothyroidism may result due to TSH suppression; monitor thyroid function at baseline and periodically. Cardiac conduction and other cardiovascular abnormalities may occur. Monitor zinc levels periodically with TPNs. Pancreatitis reported. Depressed vitamin B_{12} levels and abnormal Schilling's test reported. May need dose adjustment in renal failure. **P/N:** Category B, caution in nursing.	Gallbladder and cardiac abnormalities, diarrhea, N/V, abdominal discomfort, flatulence, constipation, hypo- and hyperglycemia, injection-site pain, upper respiratory infection, flu-like symptoms, fatigue, dizziness, headache, malaise, fever.
Paricalcitol (Zemplar Oral, Zemplar IV)	**Cap:** 1mcg, 2mcg, 4mcg; **Inj:** 2mcg/mL, 5mcg/mL	***Adults:*** (Cap) **Initial: Baseline iPTH Level ≤500pg/mL:** 1mcg qd or 2mcg tiw. **Baseline iPTH Level >500pg/mL:** 2mcg qd or 4mcg tiw. May need dose adjustment based on iPTH level relative to baseline (see PI). ***Adults/Pediatrics:* ≥5 yrs:** (Inj) **Initial:** 0.04-0.1mcg/kg bolus no more frequently than every other day during dialysis. **Max:** 0.24mcg/kg (16.8mcg). **Titrate:** May increase by 2-4mcg at 2- to 4-week intervals. Monitor serum Ca and phosphorus more frequently during dose adjustments. Reduce or interrupt dose if elevated Ca level or Ca x P product >75, may reinitiate at lower dose once normalized. May need dose decrease as PTH levels decrease (see PI).	**W/P:** Overdose may cause progressive hypercalcemia. Should supplement with calcium and restrict phosphorus. May need phosphate-binding compounds to control serum phosphorus levels. Avoid concomitant phosphate or vitamin D–related compounds. **Contra:** Vitamin D toxicity, hypercalcemia. **P/N:** Category C, caution in nursing.	Pain, allergic reactions, headache, infection, hypotension, HTN, diarrhea, N/V, constipation, edema, arthritis, dizziness, vertigo, rhinitis, rash.

Table 20.1. PRESCRIBING INFORMATION FOR ENDOCRINE/HORMONAL AND BONE METABOLISM DRUGS *(cont.)*

NAME	FORM/ STRENGTH	DOSAGE	WARNINGS/PRECAUTIONS & CONTRAINDICATIONS	ADVERSE EFFECTS†
MISCELLANEOUS METABOLIC AGENTS *(cont.)*				
Pegvisomant (Somavert)	**Inj:** 10mg, 15mg, 20mg	***Adults:*** **LD:** 40mg SQ. **Maint:** 10mg SQ qd. **Titrate:** Adjust dose by 5mg increments/decrements, based on IGF-I levels, every 4-6 weeks. **Max:** 30mg/day. **LFTs ≥3x/<5x ULN (without symptoms of liver dysfunction):** Monitor LFTs weekly. **LFTs ≥5x ULN/ Transaminase Elevations ≥3x ULN:** D/C immediately and evaluate. Do not initiate if baseline LFTs >3x ULN until cause is determined.	**W/P:** May expand and cause serious complications of tumors that secrete GH; monitor with periodic imaging scans of the sella turcica. May increase glucose tolerance and risk of hypoglycemia in diabetics. May result in functional GH deficiency. AST/ALT elevations reported; obtain baseline ALT, AST, TBIL, and ALP levels prior to initiation. Monitor LFTs monthly for first 6 months, quarterly for next 6 months, then biannually; monitor more frequently if elevations occur. D/C if liver injury confirmed. Monitor IGF-I levels 4-6 weeks after initiation or dose adjustments; every 6 months after levels are normalized. Interferes with the measurement of serum GH levels by commercially available GH assays; do not adjust dosage based on serum GH levels. **P/N:** Category B; caution in nursing.	Infection, abnormal LFTs, pain, injection-site reactions, back pain, diarrhea, nausea, flu syndrome, chest pain, dizziness, paresthesia, HTN, sinusitis, peripheral edema.
Pramlintide Acetate (Symlin, SymlinPen)	**Inj:** 600mcg/ mL [5mL]; **Pen injector:** 1000mcg/mL [1.5mL, 2.7mL]	***Adults:*** Before initiating therapy reduce insulin dose by 50%. Monitor blood glucose frequently. Adjust insulin dose once target dose of pramlintide is maintained. **Type 2 DM: Initial:** 60mcg SQ immediately prior to meals. **Titrate:** 120mcg as tolerated. **Type 1 DM: Initial:** 15mcg SQ immediately prior to meals. **Titrate:** Increase by 15mcg increments to 30mcg or 60mcg as tolerated.	**BB:** Use with insulin. Risk of insulin-induced severe hypoglycemia, particularly with Type 1 DM. Severe hypoglycemia usually occurs within 3 hrs of injection. Serious injuries may occur if severe hypoglycemia occurs while operating a motor vehicle, heavy machinery, or other high-risk activities. Appropriate patient selection, careful patient instruction, and insulin dose adjustments are necessary to reduce this risk. **W/P:** Do not mix with insulin; administer as separate injections. **Contra:** Confirmed diagnosis of gastroparesis; hypoglycemia unawareness. **P/N:** Category C, caution in nursing.	N/V, headache, anorexia, abdominal pain, fatigue, dizziness, **cough, pharyngitis.**
Sapropterin Dihydrochloride (Kuvan)	**Tab:** 100mg	***Adults:*** **Initial:** 10mg/kg/day qd. **Titrate:** Adjust dose within the range of 5-20mg/kg/day. **Max:** 20mg/kg/day. Take with food.	**W/P:** Monitor blood Phe levels during treatment. Active management of dietary Phe intake is required to ensure Phe control and nutritional balance. Caution in patients with hepatic impairment. Monitor for allergic reactions. **P/N:** Category C, caution in nursing.	Headache, diarrhea, abdominal pain, upper respiratory tract infection, **pharyngolaryngeal pain,** N/V.

†Bold entries denote special dental considerations.
BB = black box warning; **W/P** = warnings/precautions; **Contra** = contraindications; **P/N** = pregnancy category rating and nursing considerations.

Table 20.2. DRUG INTERACTIONS FOR ENDOCRINE/HORMONAL AND BONE METABOLISM DRUGS

ANDROGENS

Fluoxymesterone (Halotestin) CIII	
Anticoagulants, oral	May increase sensitivity to oral anticoagulants (eg, warfarin).
Insulin	May decrease blood glucose and insulin requirements in diabetic patients.
Oxyphenbutazone	May increase levels of oxyphenbutazone.
Methyltestosterone (Testred) CIII	
Anticoagulants, oral	May increase sensitivity to oral anticoagulants (eg, warfarin).
Insulin	May decrease blood glucose and insulin requirements in diabetic patients.
Oxyphenbutazone	May increase levels of oxyphenbutazone.
Oxandrolone (Oxandrin) CIII	
ACTH	May increase fluid retention with ACTH; caution with cardiac or hepatic disease.
Anticoagulants, oral	May increase sensitivity to oral anticoagulants (eg, warfarin).
Corticosteroids	May increase fluid retention with corticosteroids; caution with cardiac or hepatic disease.
Hypoglycemics, oral	May inhibit metabolism of oral hypoglycemics.
Testosterone (Androderm, Androgel, Striant, Testim) CIII	
ACTH	May increase fluid retention with ACTH; caution with cardiac or hepatic disease.
Anticoagulants, oral	May increase sensitivity to oral anticoagulants (eg, warfarin).
Corticosteroids	May increase fluid retention with corticosteroids; caution with cardiac or hepatic disease.
Hypoglycemics, oral	May inhibit metabolism of oral hypoglycemics.
Insulin	May decrease blood glucose and insulin requirements in diabetic patients.
Ointments	Pretreatment with ointments may reduce testosterone absorption (Androderm).
Oxyphenbutazone	May increase levels of oxyphenbutazone.
Propranolol	May increase clearance of propranolol.
Testosterone Cypionate (Depo-Testosterone) CIII	
Anticoagulants, oral	May increase sensitivity to oral anticoagulants (eg, warfarin).
Insulin	May decrease blood glucose and insulin requirements in diabetic patients.
Oxyphenbutazone	May increase levels of oxyphenbutazone.
Testosterone Enanthate (Delatestryl) CIII	
ACTH	May increase fluid retention with ACTH; caution with cardiac or hepatic disease.
Anticoagulants, oral	May increase sensitivity to oral anticoagulants (eg, warfarin).
Corticosteroids	May increase fluid retention with corticosteroids; caution with cardiac or hepatic disease.
Insulin	May decrease blood glucose and insulin requirements in diabetic patients.
Oxyphenbutazone	May increase levels of oxyphenbutazone.

Table 20.2. DRUG INTERACTIONS FOR ENDOCRINE/HORMONAL AND BONE METABOLISM DRUGS *(cont.)*

BONE METABOLISM AGENTS	
Alendronate Sodium (Fosamax)	
Antacids	Antacids and other oral medications may interfere with absorption; dose at least 1/2 hour after alendronate.
Aspirin (ASA)	Concomitant use of aspirin and daily doses of alendronate >10 mg may increase upper GI adverse events.
Calcium supplements	Calcium supplements and other oral medications may interfere with absorption; dose at least 1/2 hour after alendronate.
NSAIDs	Caution with NSAIDS due to possible GI irritation.
Ranitidine	Intravenous ranitidine may increase bioavailability of alendronate.
Alendronate Sodium/Cholecalciferol (Fosamax Plus D)	
Antacids	Antacids may interfere with absorption; dose at least 1/2 hour after alendronate.
Anticonvulsants	May increase the catabolism of vitamin D; consider additional vitamin D supplementation.
Aspirin (ASA)	Concomitant use of aspirin and daily doses of alendronate >10 mg may increase upper GI adverse events.
Bile acid sequestrants	May decrease the absorption of vitamin D; consider additional vitamin D supplementation.
Calcium supplements	Calcium supplements may interfere with absorption; dose at least 1/2 hour after alendronate.
Cations, oral drugs containing multivalent	Oral medications containing multivalent cations may interfere with absorption; dose at least 1/2 hour after alendronate.
Cimetidine	May increase the catabolism of vitamin D; consider additional vitamin D supplementation.
Mineral oil	May decrease the absorption of vitamin D; consider additional vitamin D supplementation.
NSAIDs	Caution with NSAIDS due to possible GI irritation.
Olestra	May decrease the absorption of vitamin D; consider additional vitamin D supplementation.
Orlistat	May decrease the absorption of vitamin D; consider additional vitamin D supplementation.
Thiazides	May decrease the absorption of vitamin D; consider additional vitamin D supplementation.
Calcium Carbonate/Risedronate Sodium (Actonel with Calcium)	
Antacids	Antacids may interfere with absorption; dose at least 1/2 hour after risedronate.
Calcium supplements	Calcium supplements may interfere with absorption; dose at least 1/2 hour after risedronate.

BONE METABOLISM AGENTS *(cont.)*

Calcium Carbonate/Risedronate Sodium (Actonel with Calcium) *(cont.)*	
Cations, oral drugs containing multivalent	Oral medications containing multivalent cations may interfere with absorption; dose at least 1/2 hour after risedronate.
Fluoroquinolones	Calcium may decrease the absorption of fluoroquinolones (eg, ciprofloxacin, moxifloxacin, ofloxacin).
Glucocorticoids	Glucocorticoids may decrease absorption of calcium.
Iron	May interfere with absorption of iron; iron and calcium should be taken at different times of the day.
Levothyroxine	Calcium may decrease the absorption of levothyroxine.
Tetracyclines	Calcium may decrease the absorption of tetracyclines (eg, doxycycline, minocycline, tetracycline).
Thiazides	May decrease the urinary excretion of calcium.
Vitamin D	Vitamin D and its analogues (eg, calcitriol, doxercalciferol, paricalcitol) may increase the absorption of calcium.
Estradiol (Menostar)	
CYP3A4 inducers	CYP3A4 inducers (eg, St. John's wort, phenobarbital, carbamazepine, rifampin) may decrease levels.
CYP3A4 inhibitors	CYP3A4 inhibitors (eg, erythromycin, clarithromycin, ketoconazole, itraconazole, ritonavir, grapefruit juice) may increase levels.
Thyroid HRT	Patients taking estradiol may require increased doses of thyroid hormone replacement therapy.
Etidronate Disodium (Didronel)	
Antacids, aluminum- and magnesium-containing	Antacids containing aluminum or magnesium may decrease absorption; separate dose by 2 hours.
Calcium Supplements	Calcium supplements may interfere with absorption; dose at least 1/2 hour after etidronate.
Cations, oral drugs containing multivalent	Oral medications containing multivalent cations (eg, vitamins with mineral supplements, iron) may interfere with absorption; separate dose by 2 hours.
Warfarin	May increase prothrombin time of patients on warfarin.
Ibandronate Sodium (Boniva)	
Antacids	Antacids may interfere with absorption; dose at least 1 hour after ibandronate.
Calcium supplements	Calcium supplements may interfere with absorption; dose at least 1 hour after ibandronate.
Cations, oral drugs containing multivalent	Oral medications containing multivalent cations may interfere with absorption; dose at least 1hour after ibandronate.
Pamidronate Disodium (Aredia)	
Nephrotoxic agents	Caution with nephrotoxic agents.
Thalidomide	May increase the risk of renal dysfunction when in combination with thalidomide in multiple myeloma patients.

Table 20.2. DRUG INTERACTIONS FOR ENDOCRINE/HORMONAL AND BONE METABOLISM DRUGS *(cont.)*

BONE METABOLISM AGENTS *(cont.)*	
Raloxifene HCl (Evista)	
Cholestyramine	Avoid concomitant use with anion exchange resins; cholestyramine decreases absorption.
Estrogens, systemic	Avoid concomitant use with other systemic estrogens.
Protein-bound drugs	Caution with highly protein-bound drugs (eg, diazepam, diazoxide, lidocaine, NSAIDs).
Warfarin	May increase prothrombin time of patients on warfarin or warfarin derivatives.
Risedronate Sodium (Actonel)	
Antacids	Antacids may interfere with absorption; dose at least 1/2 hour after risedronate.
Calcium supplements	Calcium supplements may interfere with absorption; dose at least 1/2 hour after risedronate.
Cations, oral drugs containing multivalent	Oral medications containing multivalent cations may interfere with absorption; dose at least 1/2 hour after risedronate.
Teriparatide (Forteo)	
Digoxin	Caution with digoxin.
Tiludronate Disodium (Skelid)	
Antacids, aluminum- and magnesium-containing	Antacids containing aluminum or magnesium may decrease bioavailability by 60%.
Aspirin	Aspirin may decrease bioavailability by 50% when taken 2 hours after tiludronate.
Calcium supplements	Calcium supplements may decrease bioavailability by 80%.
Indomethacin	Indomethacin may increase bioavailability two- to fourfold.
Zoledronic Acid (Reclast)	
Aminoglycosides	Caution with aminoglycosides; may have an additive effect to lower serum calcium for prolonged periods.
Loop diuretics	Caution when used in combination with loop diuretics; may increase the risk of hypocalcemia.
Nephrotoxic drugs	Caution with nephrotoxic drugs (eg, NSAIDs).
CONTRACEPTIVES, MISCELLANEOUS	
Diaphragm (Ortho Diaphragm Kits)	
Cold cream lubricants	Avoid concomitant use.
Mineral oil lubricants	Avoid concomitant use.
Petroleum Jelly	Avoid concomitant use.
Vaginal preparations	Some vaginal drugs or lubricating agents may damage the diaphragm.
Vegetable oil lubricants	Avoid concomitant use.
Ethinyl Estradiol/Etonogestrel (NuvaRing)	
Acetaminophen	Acetaminophen may increase levels of ethinyl estradiol; may reduce levels of acetaminophen.

CONTRACEPTIVES, MISCELLANEOUS *(cont.)*

Ethinyl Estradiol/Etonogestrel (NuvaRing) *(cont.)*	
Antibiotics	Antibiotics may reduce the efficacy of hormonal contraceptives.
Anticonvulsants	Anticonvulsants may reduce the efficacy of hormonal contraceptives.
Antifungals	Antifungals may reduce the efficacy of hormonal contraceptives.
Ascorbic acid (vitamin C)	Ascorbic acid may increase levels of ethinyl estradiol.
Atorvastatin	Atorvastatin may increase levels of ethinyl estradiol.
Barbiturates	Barbiturates may reduce the efficacy of hormonal contraceptives.
Clofibric acid	May increase clearance of clofibric acid.
Cyclosporine	May increase levels of cyclosporine.
CYP3A4 inhibitors	CYP3A4 inhibitors (eg, itraconazole, ketoconazole) may increase levels of ethinyl estradiol.
Miconazole nitrate, vaginal	Vaginal miconazole nitrate may increase levels of both etonogestrel and ethinyl estradiol by up to 40%.
Morphine	May increase clearance of morphine.
Prednisolone	May increase levels of prednisolone.
Protease inhibitors (PIs), anti-HIV	Anti-HIV PIs may alter the safety and efficacy of hormonal contraceptives; refer to the label of the individual PI.
Salicylic acid	May increase clearance of salicylic acid.
St. John's wort	May reduce the efficacy of contraceptive steroids.
Temazepam	May increase clearance of temazepam.
Theophylline	May increase levels of theophylline.
Ethinyl Estradiol/Norelgestromin (Ortho Evra)	
Acetaminophen	Acetaminophen may increase levels of ethinyl estradiol; may reduce levels of acetaminophen.
Antibiotics	Antibiotics may reduce the efficacy of hormonal contraceptives.
Anticonvulsants	Anticonvulsants may reduce the efficacy of hormonal contraceptives.
Antifungals	Antifungals may reduce the efficacy of hormonal contraceptives.
Ascorbic acid (vitamin C)	Ascorbic acid may increase levels of ethinyl estradiol.
Atorvastatin	Atorvastatin may increase levels of ethinyl estradiol.
Barbiturates	Barbiturates may reduce the efficacy of hormonal contraceptives.
Clofibric acid	May increase clearance of clofibric acid.
Cyclosporine	May increase levels of cyclosporine.
CYP3A4 inducers	CYP3A4 inducers may reduce the efficacy of hormonal contraceptives.
CYP3A4 inhibitors	CYP3A4 inhibitors (eg, itraconazole, ketoconazole) may increase levels of ethinyl estradiol.
Lamotrigine	May decrease levels of lamotrigine due to the induction of glucuronidation; dose adjustment of lamotrigine may be necessary.

Table 20.2. DRUG INTERACTIONS FOR ENDOCRINE/HORMONAL AND BONE METABOLISM DRUGS *(cont.)*

CONTRACEPTIVES, MISCELLANEOUS *(cont.)*	
Ethinyl Estradiol/Norelgestromin (Ortho Evra) *(cont.)*	
Miconazole nitrate, vaginal	Vaginal miconazole nitrate may increase levels of both etonogestrel and ethinyl estradiol by up to 40%.
Morphine	May increase clearance of morphine.
Prednisolone	May increase levels of prednisolone.
Protease inhibitors, anti-HIV	Anti-HIV PIs may alter the safety and efficacy of hormonal contraceptives; refer to the label of the individual PI.
Salicylic acid	May increase clearance of salicylic acid.
St. John's wort	May reduce the efficacy of contraceptive steroids.
Temazepam	May increase clearance of temazepam.
Theophylline	May increase levels of theophylline.
Levonorgestrel (Jadelle, Norplant II)	
Anticonvulsants	Anticonvulsants (eg, phenytoin, phenobarbital, carbamazepine, oxcarbazepine) may reduce the efficacy of hormonal contraceptives.
Barbiturates	Barbiturates may reduce the efficacy of hormonal contraceptives.
Rifampin	Rifampin may reduce the efficacy of hormonal contraceptives.
Levonorgestrel (Mirena)	
CYP450 inducers	Inducers of CYP450 may decrease levels.
Levonorgestrel (Plan B)	
Anticonvulsants	Anticonvulsants (eg, phenytoin, phenobarbital, carbamazepine, oxcarbazepine) may reduce the efficacy of hormonal contraceptives.
Rifampicin	Rifampicin may reduce the efficacy of hormonal contraceptives.
St. John's wort	May reduce the efficacy of contraceptive steroids.
Medroxyprogesterone Acetate (Depo-Provera Contraceptive, depo-subQ provera 104)	
Aminoglutethimide	Aminoglutethimide may decrease levels.
Mifepristone (Mifeprex)	
CYP3A4 inducers	CYP3A4 inducers (eg, St. John's wort, phenytoin, phenobarbital, carbamazepine, rifampin, dexamethasone) may decrease levels.
CYP3A4 inhibitors	CYP3A4 inhibitors (eg, erythromycin, ketoconazole, itraconazole, grapefruit juice) may increase levels.

CONTRACEPTIVES, ORAL

Desogestrel/Ethinyl Estradiol (Apri, Cyclessa, Desogen, Kariva, Mircette, Ortho-Cept, Velivet); **Drospirenone/Ethinyl Estradiol** (Yasmin, YAZ); **Ethinyl Estradiol/Ethynodiol Diacetate** (Demulen, Zovia); **Ethinyl Estradiol/Ferrous Fumarate/Norethindrone** (Ovcon-35 Fe); **Ethinyl Estradiol/Ferrous Fumarate/Norethindrone Acetate** (Junel 1.5/30, Junel 1/20, Junel Fe 1.5/30, Junel Fe 1/20, Loestrin, Loestrin 1.5/30, Loestrin 1/20, Loestrin Fe 1.5/30, Loestrin Fe 1/20, Microgestin Fe 1.5/30, Microgestin Fe 1/20); **Ethinyl Estradiol/Levonorgestrel** (Alesse, Aviane, Enpresse, Lessina, Levora, Lybrel, Nordette-28, Portia, Seasonale, Seasonique, Triphasil, Trivora); **Ethinyl Estradiol/Norethindrone** (Balziva, Brevicon, Modicon, Necon 0.5/35, Necon 1/35, Necon 10/11, Norinyl 1/35, Nortrel 0.5/35, Nortrel 1/35, Nortrel 7/7/7, Ortho-Novum 1/35, Ortho-Novum 10/11, Ortho-Novum 7/7/7, Ovcon-35, Ovcon-50, Tri-Norinyl); **Ethinyl Estradiol/Norethindrone Acetate** (Estrostep Fe); **Ethinyl Estradiol/Norgestimate** (MonoNessa, Ortho-Cyclen, Ortho Tri-Cyclen, Ortho Tri-Cyclen Lo, Sprintec, Tri-Previfem, Tri-Sprintec); **Ethinyl Estradiol/Norgestrel** (Cryselle, Lo/Ovral, Low-Ogestrel); **Mestranol/Norethindrone** (Brevicon, Necon 1/50, Norinyl 1/50, Ortho-Novum 1/50); **Norethindrone** (Camila, Errin, Micronor, Nor-QD)

Acetaminophen	Acetaminophen may increase levels of ethinyl estradiol; may reduce levels of acetaminophen.
Antibiotics	Antibiotics (eg, rifampin, ampicillin, tetracyclines) may reduce the efficacy of hormonal contraceptives.
Anticonvulsants	Anticonvulsants (eg, phenytoin, carbamazepine, felbamate, oxcarbazepine, topiramate) may reduce the efficacy of hormonal contraceptives.
Antifungals	Antifungals (eg, griseofulvin) may reduce the efficacy of hormonal contraceptives.
Ascorbic acid (vitamin C)	Ascorbic acid may increase levels of ethinyl estradiol.
Atorvastatin	Atorvastatin may increase levels of ethinyl estradiol.
Barbiturates	Barbiturates may reduce the efficacy of hormonal contraceptives.
Bosentan	Bosentan may reduce the efficacy of hormonal contraceptives.
Clofibric acid	May increase clearance of clofibric acid.
Cyclosporine	May increase levels of cyclosporine.
CYP2C9 substrates/inhibitors	CYP2C9 substrates and inhibitors (eg, ibuprofen, piroxicam, naproxen, phenytoin, fluconazole, diclofenac, tolbutamide, glipizide, celecoxib sulfamethoxazole, isoniazid, torsemide, irbesartan, losartan, valsartan) may inhibit the metabolism of desogestrel to its active metabolite etonogestrel.
CYP3A4 inhibitors	CYP3A4 inhibitors (eg, itraconazole, ketoconazole, indinavir, fluconazole, troleandomycin) may increase levels of ethinyl estradiol.
Lamotrigine	May decrease levels of lamotrigine due to the induction of glucuronidation; dose adjustment of lamotrigine may be necessary.
Morphine	May increase clearance of morphine.
Phenylbutazone	Phenylbutazone may reduce the efficacy of hormonal contraceptives.
Prednisolone	May increase levels of prednisolone.
Protease inhibitors, anti-HIV	Anti-HIV PIs may alter the safety and efficacy of hormonal contraceptives; refer to the label of the individual PI.
Salicylic acid	May increase clearance of salicylic acid.

Table 20.2. DRUG INTERACTIONS FOR ENDOCRINE/HORMONAL AND BONE METABOLISM DRUGS *(cont.)*

CONTRACEPTIVES, ORAL *(cont.)*

Desogestrel/Ethinyl Estradiol (Apri, Cyclessa, Desogen, Kariva, Mircette, Ortho-Cept, Velivet); **Drospirenone/Ethinyl Estradiol** (Yasmin, YAZ); **Ethinyl Estradiol/Ethynodiol Diacetate** (Demulen, Zovia); **Ethinyl Estradiol/Ferrous Fumarate/Norethindrone** (Ovcon-35 Fe); **Ethinyl Estradiol/Ferrous Fumarate/Norethindrone Acetate** (Junel 1.5/30, Junel 1/20, Junel Fe 1.5/30, Junel Fe 1/20, Loestrin, Loestrin 1.5/30, Loestrin 1/20, Loestrin Fe 1.5/30, Loestrin Fe 1/20, Microgestin Fe 1.5/30, Microgestin Fe 1/20); **Ethinyl Estradiol/Levonorgestrel** (Alesse, Aviane, Enpresse, Lessina, Levora, Lybrel, Nordette-28, Portia, Seasonale, Seasonique, Triphasil, Trivora); **Ethinyl Estradiol/Norethindrone** (Balziva, Brevicon, Modicon, Necon 0.5/35, Necon 1/35, Necon 10/11, Norinyl 1/35, Nortrel 0.5/35, Nortrel 1/35, Nortrel 7/7/7, Ortho-Novum 1/35, Ortho-Novum 10/11, Ortho-Novum 7/7/7, Ovcon-35, Ovcon-50, Tri-Norinyl); **Ethinyl Estradiol/Norethindrone Acetate** (Estrostep Fe); **Ethinyl Estradiol/Norgestimate** (MonoNessa, Ortho-Cyclen, Ortho Tri-Cyclen, Ortho Tri-Cyclen Lo, Sprintec, Tri-Previfem, Tri-Sprintec); **Ethinyl Estradiol/Norgestrel** (Cryselle, Lo/Ovral, Low-Ogestrel); **Mestranol/Norethindrone** (Brevicon, Necon 1/50, Norinyl 1/50, Ortho-Novum 1/50); **Norethindrone** (Camila, Errin, Micronor, Nor-QD) *(cont.)*	
St. John's wort	St. John's wort may induce hepatic enzymes and reduce the efficacy of contraceptive steroids.
Temazepam	May increase clearance of temazepam.
Theophylline	May increase levels of theophylline.
Troleandomycin	Troleandomycin may increase the risk of intrahepatic cholestasis.

ENDOMETRIOSIS AGENTS

Danazol	
Carbamazepine	May increase levels of carbamazepine.
Warfarin	Prolongation of prothrombin time occurs in patients stabilized on warfarin.

ESTROGENS

Conjugated Estrogens (Cenestin, Enjuvia, Premarin, Premarin Vaginal), **Esterified Estrogens** (Menest), **Estradiol** (Alora, Climara, Divigel, Elestrin, Esclim, Estrace, Estraderm, Estrasorb, Estring, EstroGel, Evamist, Gynodiol, Vagifem, Vivelle, Vivelle-Dot), **Estradiol Acetate** (Femring, Femtrace), **Estradiol Cypionate** (Depo-Estradiol), **Estradiol Valerate** (Delestrogen), **Estropipate** (Ogen, Ortho-Est)	
CYP3A4 inducers	CYP3A4 inducers (eg, St. John's wort, phenobarbital, carbamazepine, rifampin) may decrease levels, which may decrease therapeutic effects and/or change uterine bleeding profile.
CYP3A4 inhibitors	CYP3A4 inhibitors (eg, erythromycin, clarithromycin, ketoconazole, itraconazole, ritonavir, grapefruit juice) may increase levels, which may result in side effects.

ESTROGEN COMBINATIONS

Conjugated Estrogens/Medroxyprogesterone Acetate (Premphase, Prempro)	
Aminoglutethimide	Concomitant aminoglutethimide may significantly depress the bioavailability of medroxyprogesterone.
CYP3A4 inducers	CYP3A4 inducers (eg, St. John's wort, phenobarbital, carbamazepine, rifampin) may decrease levels, which may decrease therapeutic effects and/or change uterine bleeding profile.

ESTROGEN COMBINATIONS *(cont.)*

Conjugated Estrogens/Medroxyprogesterone Acetate (Premphase, Prempro) *(cont.)*	
CYP3A4 inhibitors	CYP3A4 inhibitors (eg, erythromycin, clarithromycin, ketoconazole, itraconazole, ritonavir, grapefruit juice) may increase levels, which may result in side effects.
Drospirenone/Estradiol (Angeliq)	
ACE inhibitors	Concomitant use increases the risk for hyperkalemia.
Angiotensin II receptor blockers (ARBs)	Concomitant use increases the risk for hyperkalemia.
CYP3A4 inducers	CYP3A4 inducers (eg, St. John's wort, phenobarbital, carbamazepine, rifampin) may decrease levels, which may decrease therapeutic effects and/or change uterine bleeding profile.
CYP3A4 inhibitors	CYP3A4 inhibitors (eg, erythromycin, clarithromycin, ketoconazole, itraconazole, ritonavir, grapefruit juice) may increase levels, which may result in side effects.
Heparin	Concomitant use increases the risk for hyperkalemia.
K^+-sparing diuretics	Concomitant use increases the risk for hyperkalemia.
K^+-supplements	Concomitant use increases the risk for hyperkalemia.
NSAIDs	Concomitant use increases the risk for hyperkalemia.
Esterified Estrogens/Methyltestosterone (Estratest, Estratest H.S.)	
Anticoagulants, oral	May decrease the anticoagulant requirement for patients on oral anticoagulants.
CYP3A4 inducers	CYP3A4 inducers (eg, St. John's wort, phenobarbital, carbamazepine, rifampin) may decrease levels, which may decrease therapeutic effects and/or change uterine bleeding profile.
CYP3A4 inhibitors	CYP3A4 inhibitors (eg, erythromycin, clarithromycin, ketoconazole, itraconazole, ritonavir, grapefruit juice) may increase levels, which may result in side effects.
Insulin	May decrease blood glucose and thus decrease insulin requirements.
Oxyphenbutazone	May increase levels of oxyphenbutazone
Estradiol/Levonorgestrel (Climara Pro)	
CYP2C inducers	CYP2C inducers may decrease levels, which may decrease therapeutic effects and/or change uterine bleeding profile.
CYP2C inhibitors	CYP2C inhibitors may increase levels, which may result in side effects.
CYP2E inducers	CYP2E inducers may decrease levels, which may decrease therapeutic effects and/or change uterine bleeding profile.
CYP2E inhibitors	CYP2E inhibitors may increase levels, which may result in side effects.
CYP3A4 inducers	CYP3A4 inducers (eg, St. John's wort, phenobarbital, carbamazepine, rifampin) may decrease levels, which may decrease therapeutic effects and/or change uterine bleeding profile.
CYP3A4 inhibitors	CYP3A4 inhibitors (eg, erythromycin, clarithromycin, ketoconazole, itraconazole, ritonavir, grapefruit juice) may increase levels, which may result in side effects.

Table 20.2. DRUG INTERACTIONS FOR ENDOCRINE/HORMONAL AND BONE METABOLISM DRUGS *(cont.)*

ESTROGEN COMBINATIONS *(cont.)*

Estradiol/Norethindrone (Activella); **Estradiol/Norethindrone Acetate** (CombiPatch); **Estradiol/Norgestimate** (Prefest)	
CYP3A4 inducers	CYP3A4 inducers (eg, St. John's wort, phenobarbital, carbamazepine, rifampin) may decrease levels, which may decrease therapeutic effects and/or change uterine bleeding profile.
CYP3A4 inhibitors	CYP3A4 inhibitors (eg, erythromycin, clarithromycin, ketoconazole, itraconazole, ritonavir, grapefruit juice) may increase levels, which may result in side effects.
Ethinyl Estradiol/Norethindrone Acetate (Femhrt)	
Acetaminophen (APAP)	APAP may increase levels of ethinyl estradiol; may decrease levels of APAP.
Anticoagulants	Estrogens may diminish the effectiveness of anticoagulants.
Antihypertensives	Estrogens may diminish the effectiveness of antihypertensives.
Ascorbic acid (vitamin C)	May increase levels of ethinyl estradiol.
Atorvastatin	Coadministration increases the AUC of ethinyl estradiol by 20%.
Clofibric acid	Ethinyl estradiol increases the clearance of clofibric acid.
Cyclosporine	Ethinyl estradiol may inhibit the metabolism of cyclosporine, leading to increased levels.
CYP3A4 inducers	CYP3A4 inducers (eg, St. John's wort, phenobarbital, carbamazepine, rifampin) may decrease levels, which may decrease therapeutic effects and/or change uterine bleeding profile.
Hypoglycemic agents	Estrogens may diminish the effectiveness of hypoglycemic agents.
Morphine	Ethinyl estradiol increases the clearance of morphine.
Prednisolone	Ethinyl estradiol may inhibit the metabolism of prednisolone, leading to increased levels.
Salicylic acid	Ethinyl estradiol increases the clearance of salicylic acid.
Temazepam	Ethinyl estradiol increases the clearance of temazepam.
Theophylline	Ethinyl estradiol may inhibit the metabolism of theophylline, leading to increased levels.
Troglitazone	Coadministration reduces the plasma concentration of ethinyl estradiol by 30%.

FERTILITY AGENTS

Progesterone (Endometrin)	
CYP3A4 inducers	CYP3A4 inducers (eg, St. John's wort, phenobarbital, carbamazepine, rifampin) may decrease levels.
Vaginal products	Avoid use with other vaginal products (eg, antifungals) due to a possible alteration in absorption.

HYPOGLYCEMIC AGENTS

Insulins

Insulin Aspart (Novolog), **Insulin Aspart/Insulin Aspart Protamine** (Novolog Mix 50/50, Novolog Mix 70/30), **Insulin Glulisine, rDNA** (Apidra)	
ACE inhibitors	Glucose-lowering effects are potentiated when administered concomitantly.
Alcohol	Alcohol may potentiate or weaken glucose-lowering effects of insulin.
Antipsychotics, atypical	Glucose-lowering effects are weakened when administered concomitantly with atypical antipsychotics (eg, olanzapine and clozapine).
β-Blockers	β-Blockers may potentiate or weaken glucose-lowering effects of insulin and mask or reduce the symptoms of hypoglycemia.
Clonidine	Clonidine may potentiate or weaken glucose-lowering effects of insulin and mask or reduce the symptoms of hypoglycemia.
Corticosteroids	Glucose-lowering effects are weakened when administered concomitantly with corticosteroids.
Danazol	Glucose-lowering effects are weakened when administered concomitantly with danazol.
Diazoxide	Glucose-lowering effects are weakened when administered concomitantly with diazoxide.
Disopyramide	Glucose-lowering effects are potentiated when administered concomitantly with disopyramide.
Diuretics	Glucose-lowering effects are weakened when administered concomitantly with diuretics.
Estrogens	Glucose-lowering effects are weakened when administered concomitantly with estrogens.
Fibrates	Glucose-lowering effects are potentiated when administered concomitantly with fibrates.
Fluoxetine	Glucose-lowering effects are potentiated when administered concomitantly with fluoxetine.
Glucagon	Glucose-lowering effects are weakened when administered concomitantly with glucagon.
Guanethidine	Guanethidine masks or reduces the symptoms of hypoglycemia.
Hypoglycemic agents	Glucose-lowering effects are potentiated when administered concomitantly with other hypoglycemic agents.
Isoniazid	Glucose-lowering effects are weakened when administered concomitantly with isoniazid.
K^+-lowering drugs	Caution with K^+-lowering drugs or drugs sensitive to serum K^+ levels.
Lithium	Lithium salts may potentiate or weaken glucose-lowering effects of insulin.
MAOIs	Glucose-lowering effects are potentiated when administered concomitantly with MAOIs.
Pentamidine	May cause hypoglycemia followed by hyperglycemia.

Table 20.2. DRUG INTERACTIONS FOR ENDOCRINE/HORMONAL AND BONE METABOLISM DRUGS *(cont.)*

HYPOGLYCEMIC AGENTS *(cont.)*

Insulins

Insulin Aspart (Novolog), **Insulin Aspart/Insulin Aspart Protamine** (Novolog Mix 50/50, Novolog Mix 70/30), **Insulin Glulisine, rDNA** (Apidra) *(cont.)*	
Phenothiazine derivatives	Glucose-lowering effects are weakened when administered concomitantly with phenothiazine derivatives.
Progestins	Glucose-lowering effects are weakened when administered concomitantly with progestins.
Propoxyphene	Glucose-lowering effects are potentiated when administered concomitantly with propoxyphene.
Protease inhibitors (PIs)	Glucose-lowering effects are weakened when administered concomitantly with PIs.
Reserpine	Reserpine masks or reduces the symptoms of hypoglycemia.
Salicylates	Glucose-lowering effects are potentiated when administered concomitantly with salicylates.
Somatostatin	Glucose-lowering effects are potentiated when administered concomitantly with somatostatin analog.
Somatropin	Glucose-lowering effects are weakened when administered concomitantly with somatropin.
Sulfonamide antibiotics	Glucose-lowering effects are potentiated when administered concomitantly with sulfonamide antibiotics.
Sympathomimetics	Glucose-lowering effects are weakened when administered concomitantly with sympathomimetic agents (eg, epinephrine, albuterol, terbutaline).
Thyroid hormones	Glucose-lowering effects are weakened when administered concomitantly with thyroid hormones.
Insulin Detemir, rDNA origin (Levemir), **Insulin Glargine, Human** (Lantus)	
ACE inhibitors	Glucose-lowering effects are potentiated when administered concomitantly with ACE inhibitors.
Alcohol	Alcohol may potentiate or weaken glucose-lowering effects of insulin.
Antipsychotics, atypical	Glucose-lowering effects are weakened when administered concomitantly with atypical antipsychotics (eg, olanzapine and clozapine).
β-Blockers	β-Blockers may potentiate or weaken glucose-lowering effects of insulin and mask or reduce the symptoms of hypoglycemia.
Clonidine	Clonidine may potentiate or weaken glucose-lowering effects of insulin and mask or reduce the symptoms of hypoglycemia.
Corticosteroids	Glucose-lowering effects are weakened when administered concomitantly with corticosteroids.
Danazol	Glucose-lowering effects are weakened when administered concomitantly with danazol.
Diazoxide	Glucose-lowering effects are weakened when administered concomitantly with diazoxide.

HYPOGLYCEMIC AGENTS *(cont.)*

Insulins

Insulin Detemir, rDNA origin (Levemir), **Insulin Glargine, Human** (Lantus) *(cont.)*	
Disopyramide	Glucose-lowering effects are potentiated when administered concomitantly with disopyramide.
Diuretics	Glucose-lowering effects are weakened when administered concomitantly with diuretics.
Estrogens	Glucose-lowering effects are weakened when administered concomitantly with estrogens.
Fibrates	Glucose-lowering effects are potentiated when administered concomitantly with fibrates.
Fluoxetine	Glucose-lowering effects are potentiated when administered concomitantly with fluoxetine.
Glucagon	Glucose-lowering effects are weakened when administered concomitantly with glucagon.
Guanethidine	Guanethidine masks or reduces the symptoms of hypoglycemia.
Hypoglycemic agents	Glucose-lowering effects are potentiated when administered concomitantly with other hypoglycemic agents.
Isoniazid	Glucose-lowering effects are weakened when administered concomitantly with isoniazid.
Lithium	Lithium salts may potentiate or weaken glucose-lowering effects of insulin.
MAOIs	Glucose-lowering effects are potentiated when administered concomitantly with MAOIs.
Pentamidine	May cause hypoglycemia followed by hyperglycemia.
Phenothiazine derivatives	Glucose-lowering effects are weakened when administered concomitantly with phenothiazine derivatives.
Progestins	Glucose-lowering effects are weakened when administered concomitantly with progestins.
Propoxyphene	Glucose-lowering effects are potentiated when administered concomitantly with propoxyphene.
Protease inhibitors	Glucose-lowering effects are weakened when administered concomitantly with protease inhibitors.
Reserpine	Reserpine masks or reduces the symptoms of hypoglycemia.
Salicylates	Glucose-lowering effects are potentiated when administered concomitantly with salicylates.
Somatostatin	Glucose-lowering effects are potentiated when administered concomitantly with somatostatin analog.
Somatropin	Glucose-lowering effects are weakened when administered concomitantly with somatropin.
Sulfonamide antibiotics	Glucose-lowering effects are potentiated when administered concomitantly with sulfonamide antibiotics.

Table 20.2. DRUG INTERACTIONS FOR ENDOCRINE/HORMONAL AND BONE METABOLISM DRUGS *(cont.)*

HYPOGLYCEMIC AGENTS *(cont.)*

Insulins

Insulin Detemir, rDNA origin (Levemir), **Insulin Glargine, Human** (Lantus) *(cont.)*	
Sympathomimetics	Glucose-lowering effects are weakened when administered concomitantly with sympathomimetic agents (eg, epinephrine, albuterol, terbutaline).
Thyroid hormones	Glucose-lowering effects are weakened when administered concomitantly with thyroid hormones.
Insulin, Human (rDNA origin) (Humulin, Novolin); **Insulin, Human (rDNA origin) Isophane** (Humulin N, Novolin N); **Insulin, Regular Human (rDNA origin)** (Humulin R, Novolin R)	
Alcohol	Alcohol may potentiate or weaken glucose-lowering effects of insulin.
Atypical Antipsychotics	Glucose-lowering effects are weakened when administered concomitantly with atypical antipsychotics (eg, olanzapine and clozapine).
β-Blockers	β-Blockers mask or reduce the symptoms of hypoglycemia.
Corticosteroids	Glucose-lowering effects are weakened when administered concomitantly with corticosteroids.
Estrogens	Glucose-lowering effects are weakened when administered concomitantly with estrogens.
Hypoglycemic agents	Glucose-lowering effects are potentiated when administered concomitantly with other hypoglycemic agents.
Progestins	Glucose-lowering effects are weakened when administered concomitantly with progestins.
Salicylates	Glucose-lowering effects are potentiated when administered concomitantly with salicylates.
Sulfonamide antibiotics	Glucose-lowering effects are potentiated when administered concomitantly with sulfonamide antibiotics.
Thyroid hormones	Glucose-lowering effects are weakened when administered concomitantly with thyroid hormones.
Insulin Lispro (Humalog); **Insulin Lispro/Insulin Lispro Protamine** (Humalog Mix 75/25)	
ACE inhibitors	Glucose-lowering effects are potentiated when administered concomitantly with ACE inhibitors.
Alcohol	Alcohol may potentiate or weaken glucose-lowering effects of insulin.
Angiotensin II receptor blockers (ARBs)	Glucose-lowering effects are potentiated when administered concomitantly with ARBs.
β-Blockers	β-Blockers mask or reduce the symptoms of hypoglycemia.
Corticosteroids	Glucose-lowering effects are weakened when administered concomitantly with corticosteroids.
Estrogens	Glucose-lowering effects are weakened when administered concomitantly with estrogens.
Hypoglycemic agents	Glucose-lowering effects are potentiated when administered concomitantly with other hypoglycemic agents.
Isoniazid	Glucose-lowering effects are weakened when administered concomitantly with isoniazid.

HYPOGLYCEMIC AGENTS *(cont.)*

Insulins

Insulin Lispro (Humalog); **Insulin Lispro/Insulin Lispro Protamine** (Humalog Mix 75/25) *(cont.)*	
K^+-lowering drugs	Caution with K^+-lowering drugs or drugs sensitive to serum K^+ levels.
Niacin	Glucose-lowering effects are weakened when administered concomitantly with niacin.
Octreotide	Glucose-lowering effects are potentiated when administered concomitantly with octreotide.
Phenothiazine derivatives	Glucose-lowering effects are weakened when administered concomitantly with phenothiazine derivatives.
Progestins	Glucose-lowering effects are weakened when administered concomitantly with progestins.
Salicylates	Glucose-lowering effects are potentiated when administered concomitantly with salicylates.
Sulfonamide antibiotics	Glucose-lowering effects are potentiated when administered concomitantly with sulfonamide antibiotics.
Thyroid hormones	Glucose-lowering effects are weakened when administered concomitantly with thyroid hormones.

Oral Diabetic Agents

Acarbose (Precose)	
Adsorbents, intestinal	Intestinal adsorbents (eg, charcoal) may reduce the effects of acarbose; avoid concomitant use
Calcium channel blockers (CCBs)	Concomitant use may lead to hyperglycemia and loss of glucose control; monitor closely during concomitant therapy and discontinuation.
Contraceptives, oral	Concomitant use may lead to hyperglycemia and loss of glucose control; monitor closely during concomitant therapy and discontinuation.
Corticosteroids	Concomitant use may lead to hyperglycemia and loss of glucose control; monitor closely during concomitant therapy and discontinuation.
Digoxin	Acarbose alters the bioavailability of digoxin; may require dose adjustment of digoxin.
Diuretics	Concomitant use may lead to hyperglycemia and loss of glucose control; monitor closely during concomitant therapy and discontinuation.
Enzymes, digestive	Digestive enzymes containing carbohydrate-splitting enzymes (eg, amylase, pancreatin) may reduce the effects of acarbose; avoid concomitant use
Estrogens	Concomitant use may lead to hyperglycemia and loss of glucose control; monitor closely during concomitant therapy and discontinuation.
Insulin	Concomitant use with insulin may lead to hypoglycemia.
Isoniazid	Concomitant use may lead to hyperglycemia and loss of glucose control; monitor closely during concomitant therapy and discontinuation.
Nicotinic acid	Concomitant use may lead to hyperglycemia and loss of glucose control; monitor closely during concomitant therapy and discontinuation.

Table 20.2. DRUG INTERACTIONS FOR ENDOCRINE/HORMONAL AND BONE METABOLISM DRUGS *(cont.)*

HYPOGLYCEMIC AGENTS *(cont.)*

ORAL DIABETIC AGENTS

Acarbose (Precose) *(cont.)*	
Phenothiazines	Concomitant use may lead to hyperglycemia and loss of glucose control; monitor closely during concomitant therapy and discontinuation.
Phenytoin	Concomitant use may lead to hyperglycemia and loss of glucose control; monitor closely during concomitant therapy and discontinuation.
Sulfonylureas	Concomitant use with sulfonylureas may lead to hypoglycemia.
Sympathomimetics	Concomitant use may lead to hyperglycemia and loss of glucose control; monitor closely during concomitant therapy and discontinuation.
Thyroid products	Concomitant use may lead to hyperglycemia and loss of glucose control; monitor closely during concomitant therapy and discontinuation.
Chlorpropamide (Diabinese)	
Alcohol	Alcohol may produce a disulfiram-like reaction.
Barbiturates	Caution with barbiturates; chlorpropamide may prolong their action.
β-Blockers	The hypoglycemic action of sulfonylureas may be potentiated by β-blockers.
Calcium channel blockers (CCBs)	Concomitant use may lead to hyperglycemia and loss of glucose control; monitor closely during concomitant therapy and discontinuation.
Chloramphenicol	The hypoglycemic action of sulfonylureas may be potentiated by chloramphenicol.
Contraceptives, oral	Concomitant use may lead to hyperglycemia and loss of glucose control; monitor closely during concomitant therapy and discontinuation.
Corticosteroids	Concomitant use may lead to hyperglycemia and loss of glucose control; monitor closely during concomitant therapy and discontinuation.
Coumarins	The hypoglycemic action of sulfonylureas may be potentiated by coumarins.
Diuretics	Concomitant use may lead to hyperglycemia and loss of glucose control; monitor closely during concomitant therapy and discontinuation.
Estrogens	Concomitant use may lead to hyperglycemia and loss of glucose control; monitor closely during concomitant therapy and discontinuation.
Insulin	Concomitant use with insulin may lead to hypoglycemia.
Isoniazid	Concomitant use may lead to hyperglycemia and loss of glucose control; monitor closely during concomitant therapy and discontinuation.
Miconazole	Concomitant use with miconazole may lead to severe hypoglycemia.
Nicotinic acid	Concomitant use may lead to hyperglycemia and loss of glucose control; monitor closely during concomitant therapy and discontinuation.
NSAIDs	The hypoglycemic action of sulfonylureas may be potentiated by NSAIDs.
Phenothiazines	Concomitant use may lead to hyperglycemia and loss of glucose control; monitor closely during concomitant therapy and discontinuation.
Phenytoin	Concomitant use may lead to hyperglycemia and loss of glucose control; monitor closely during concomitant therapy and discontinuation.

HYPOGLYCEMIC AGENTS *(cont.)*

Oral Diabetic Agents

Chlorpropamide (Diabinese) *(cont.)*	
Probenecid	The hypoglycemic action of sulfonylureas may be potentiated by probenecid.
Protein-bound drugs	The hypoglycemic action of sulfonylureas may be potentiated by highly protein-bound drugs.
Salicylates	The hypoglycemic action of sulfonylureas may be potentiated by salicylates.
Sulfonamides	The hypoglycemic action of sulfonylureas may be potentiated by sulfonamides.
Sympathomimetics	Concomitant use may lead to hyperglycemia and loss of glucose control; monitor closely during concomitant therapy and discontinuation.
Thyroid products	Concomitant use may lead to hyperglycemia and loss of glucose control; monitor closely during concomitant therapy and discontinuation.
Glimepiride (Amaryl)	
β-Blockers	The hypoglycemic action of sulfonylureas may be potentiated by β-blockers. β-Blockers mask or reduce the symptoms of hypoglycemia.
Chloramphenicol	The hypoglycemic action of sulfonylureas may be potentiated by chloramphenicol.
Clarithromycin	The hypoglycemic action of sulfonylureas may be potentiated by clarithromycin.
Contraceptives, oral	Concomitant use may lead to hyperglycemia and loss of glucose control; monitor closely during concomitant therapy and discontinuation.
Corticosteroids	Concomitant use may lead to hyperglycemia and loss of glucose control; monitor closely during concomitant therapy and discontinuation.
Coumarins	The hypoglycemic action of sulfonylureas may be potentiated by coumarins.
CYP2C9 inducers	CYP2C9 inducers (eg, rifampicin) may decrease levels of glimepiride.
CYP2C9 inhibitors	CYP2C9 inhibitors (eg, fluconazole) may increase levels of glimepiride.
Disopyramide	The hypoglycemic action of sulfonylureas may be potentiated by disopyramide.
Diuretics	Concomitant use may lead to hyperglycemia and loss of glucose control; monitor closely during concomitant therapy and discontinuation.
Fluoxetine	The hypoglycemic action of sulfonylureas may be potentiated by fluoxetine.
Insulin	Concomitant use with insulin may lead to hypoglycemia.
Isoniazid	Concomitant use may lead to hyperglycemia and loss of glucose control; monitor closely during concomitant therapy and discontinuation.
MAOIs	The hypoglycemic action of sulfonylureas may be potentiated by MAOIs.
Metformin	Concomitant use with metformin may lead to hypoglycemia.
Miconazole	Concomitant use with miconazole may lead to severe hypoglycemia.
Nicotinic acid	Concomitant use may lead to hyperglycemia and loss of glucose control; monitor closely during concomitant therapy and discontinuation.
Phenothiazines	Concomitant use may lead to hyperglycemia and loss of glucose control; monitor closely during concomitant therapy and discontinuation.

Table 20.2. DRUG INTERACTIONS FOR ENDOCRINE/HORMONAL AND BONE METABOLISM DRUGS *(cont.)*

HYPOGLYCEMIC AGENTS *(cont.)*

Oral Diabetic Agents

Glimepiride (Amaryl) *(cont.)*	
Phenytoin	Concomitant use may lead to hyperglycemia and loss of glucose control; monitor closely during concomitant therapy and discontinuation.
Probenecid	The hypoglycemic action of sulfonylureas may be potentiated by probenecid.
Protein-bound drugs	The hypoglycemic action of sulfonylureas may be potentiated by highly protein-bound drugs.
Quinolones	The hypoglycemic action of sulfonylureas may be potentiated by quinolones.
Salicylates	The hypoglycemic action of sulfonylureas may be potentiated by salicylates.
Sympathomimetics	Concomitant use may lead to hyperglycemia and loss of glucose control; monitor closely during concomitant therapy and discontinuation.
Glimepiride/Pioglitazone HCl (Duetact)	
	Refer to the interactions of each drug.
Glimepiride/Rosiglitazone Maleate (Avandaryl)	
	Refer to the interactions of each drug.
Glipizide (Glipizide ER, Glucotrol, Glucotrol XL)	
Azoles	The hypoglycemic action of sulfonylureas may be potentiated by some azoles (eg, fluconazole).
β-Blockers	The hypoglycemic action of sulfonylureas may be potentiated by β-blockers. β-Blockers mask or reduce the symptoms of hypoglycemia.
Calcium channel blockers (CCBs)	Concomitant use may lead to hyperglycemia and loss of glucose control; monitor closely during concomitant therapy and discontinuation.
Chloramphenicol	The hypoglycemic action of sulfonylureas may be potentiated by chloramphenicol.
Contraceptives, oral	Concomitant use may lead to hyperglycemia and loss of glucose control; monitor closely during concomitant therapy and discontinuation.
Corticosteroids	Concomitant use may lead to hyperglycemia and loss of glucose control; monitor closely during concomitant therapy and discontinuation.
Coumarins	The hypoglycemic action of sulfonylureas may be potentiated by coumarins.
Diuretics	Concomitant use may lead to hyperglycemia and loss of glucose control; monitor closely during concomitant therapy and discontinuation.
Estrogens	Concomitant use may lead to hyperglycemia and loss of glucose control; monitor closely during concomitant therapy and discontinuation.
Fluconazole	Concomitant use of fluconazole and glipizide lead to a mean percentage increase of the glipizide AUC of 56.9%.
Insulin	Concomitant use with insulin may lead to hypoglycemia.
Isoniazid	Concomitant use may lead to hyperglycemia and loss of glucose control; monitor closely during concomitant therapy and discontinuation.
MAOIs	The hypoglycemic action of sulfonylureas may be potentiated by MAOIs.

HYPOGLYCEMIC AGENTS *(cont.)*

Oral Diabetic Agents

Glipizide (Glipizide ER, Glucotrol, Glucotrol XL) *(cont.)*	
Miconazole	Concomitant use with miconazole may lead to severe hypoglycemia.
Nicotinic acid	Concomitant use may lead to hyperglycemia and loss of glucose control; monitor closely during concomitant therapy and discontinuation.
NSAIDs	The hypoglycemic action of sulfonylureas may be potentiated by NSAIDs.
Phenothiazines	Concomitant use may lead to hyperglycemia and loss of glucose control; monitor closely during concomitant therapy and discontinuation.
Phenytoin	Concomitant use may lead to hyperglycemia and loss of glucose control; monitor closely during concomitant therapy and discontinuation.
Probenecid	The hypoglycemic action of sulfonylureas may be potentiated by probenecid.
Protein-bound drugs	The hypoglycemic action of sulfonylureas may be potentiated by highly protein-bound drugs.
Salicylates	The hypoglycemic action of sulfonylureas may be potentiated by salicylates.
Sulfonamides	The hypoglycemic action of sulfonylureas may be potentiated by sulfonamides.
Sympathomimetics	Concomitant use may lead to hyperglycemia and loss of glucose control; monitor closely during concomitant therapy and discontinuation.
Thyroid products	Concomitant use may lead to hyperglycemia and loss of glucose control; monitor closely during concomitant therapy and discontinuation.
Glipizide/Metformin HCl (Metaglip)	
	Refer to the interactions of each drug.
Glyburide (DiaBeta, Glynase PresTab, Micronase)	
Alcohol	The hypoglycemic action of sulfonylureas may be potentiated by alcohol. Although it is rare, alcohol may produce a disulfiram-like reaction.
β-Blockers	The hypoglycemic action of sulfonylureas may be potentiated by β-blockers. β-Blockers mask or reduce the symptoms of hypoglycemia.
Calcium channel blockers (CCBs)	Concomitant use may lead to hyperglycemia and loss of glucose control; monitor closely during concomitant therapy and discontinuation.
Chloramphenicol	The hypoglycemic action of sulfonylureas may be potentiated by chloramphenicol.
Contraceptives, oral	Concomitant use may lead to hyperglycemia and loss of glucose control; monitor closely during concomitant therapy and discontinuation.
Corticosteroids	Concomitant use may lead to hyperglycemia and loss of glucose control; monitor closely during concomitant therapy and discontinuation.
Coumarins	The hypoglycemic action of sulfonylureas may be potentiated by coumarins; sulfonylureas may potentiate or weaken the effects of coumarin derivatives.
Diuretics	Concomitant use may lead to hyperglycemia and loss of glucose control; monitor closely during concomitant therapy and discontinuation.
Estrogens	Concomitant use may lead to hyperglycemia and loss of glucose control; monitor closely during concomitant therapy and discontinuation.

Table 20.2. DRUG INTERACTIONS FOR ENDOCRINE/HORMONAL AND BONE METABOLISM DRUGS *(cont.)*

HYPOGLYCEMIC AGENTS *(cont.)*

Oral Diabetic Agents

Glyburide (DiaBeta, Glynase PresTab, Micronase) *(cont.)*	
Fluoroquinolones	The hypoglycemic action of sulfonylureas may be potentiated by fluoroquinolones (eg, ciprofloxacin).
Isoniazid	Concomitant use may lead to hyperglycemia and loss of glucose control; monitor closely during concomitant therapy and discontinuation.
MAOIs	The hypoglycemic action of sulfonylureas may be potentiated by MAOIs.
Miconazole	Concomitant use with miconazole may lead to severe hypoglycemia.
Nicotinic acid	Concomitant use may lead to hyperglycemia and loss of glucose control; monitor closely during concomitant therapy and discontinuation.
NSAIDs	The hypoglycemic action of sulfonylureas may be potentiated by NSAIDs.
Phenothiazines	Concomitant use may lead to hyperglycemia and loss of glucose control; monitor closely during concomitant therapy and discontinuation.
Phenytoin	Concomitant use may lead to hyperglycemia and loss of glucose control; monitor closely during concomitant therapy and discontinuation.
Probenecid	The hypoglycemic action of sulfonylureas may be potentiated by probenecid.
Protein-bound drugs	The hypoglycemic action of sulfonylureas may be potentiated by highly protein-bound drugs.
Salicylates	The hypoglycemic action of sulfonylureas may be potentiated by salicylates.
Sulfonamides	The hypoglycemic action of sulfonylureas may be potentiated by sulfonamides.
Sympathomimetics	Concomitant use may lead to hyperglycemia and loss of glucose control; monitor closely during concomitant therapy and discontinuation.
Thyroid products	Concomitant use may lead to hyperglycemia and loss of glucose control; monitor closely during concomitant therapy and discontinuation.
Glyburide/Metformin HCl (Glucovance)	
	Refer to the interactions of each drug.
Metformin HCl (Fortamet, Glucophage, Glucophage XR, Glumetza, Riomet)	
Alcohol	Alcohol increases the risk for lactic acidosis; avoid acute or chronic ingestion of excessive amounts of alcohol. The hypoglycemic action of metformin may be potentiated by alcohol.
Cationic drugs	Cationic drugs (eg, amiloride, digoxin, morphine, procainamide, quinidine, quinine, ranitidine, triamterene, trimethoprim, vancomycin) may potentially increase metformin levels by competing for common renal tubular transport systems.
Calcium channel blockers (CCBs)	Concomitant use may lead to hyperglycemia and loss of glucose control; monitor closely during concomitant therapy and discontinuation.
Cimetidine	Cimetidine increases metformin levels by competing for common renal tubular transport systems.
Contraceptives, oral	Concomitant use may lead to hyperglycemia and loss of glucose control; monitor closely during concomitant therapy and discontinuation.

HYPOGLYCEMIC AGENTS *(cont.)*

Oral Diabetic Agents

Metformin HCl (Fortamet, Glucophage, Glucophage XR, Glumetza, Riomet) *(cont.)*	
Corticosteroids	Concomitant use may lead to hyperglycemia and loss of glucose control; monitor closely during concomitant therapy and discontinuation.
Diuretics	Concomitant use may lead to hyperglycemia and loss of glucose control; monitor closely during concomitant therapy and discontinuation.
Estrogens	Concomitant use may lead to hyperglycemia and loss of glucose control; monitor closely during concomitant therapy and discontinuation.
Furosemide	Furosemide decreases levels of metformin; metformin decreases levels of furosemide.
Isoniazid	Concomitant use may lead to hyperglycemia and loss of glucose control; monitor closely during concomitant therapy and discontinuation.
Nicotinic acid	Concomitant use may lead to hyperglycemia and loss of glucose control; monitor closely during concomitant therapy and discontinuation.
Nifedipine	Nifedipine enhances the absorption of metformin and increases levels.
Phenothiazines	Concomitant use may lead to hyperglycemia and loss of glucose control; monitor closely during concomitant therapy and discontinuation.
Phenytoin	Concomitant use may lead to hyperglycemia and loss of glucose control; monitor closely during concomitant therapy and discontinuation.
Sympathomimetics	Concomitant use may lead to hyperglycemia and loss of glucose control; monitor closely during concomitant therapy and discontinuation.
Thyroid products	Concomitant use may lead to hyperglycemia and loss of glucose control; monitor closely during concomitant therapy and discontinuation.
Metformin HCl/Pioglitazone HCl (Actoplus Met)	
	Refer to the interactions of each drug.
Metformin HCl/Repaglinide (Prandimet)	
	Refer to the interactions of each drug.
Metformin HCl/Rosiglitazone Maleate (Avandamet)	
	Refer to the interactions of each drug.
Metformin HCl/Sitagliptin (Janumet)	
	Refer to the interactions of each drug.
Miglitol (Glyset)	
Adsorbents, intestinal	Intestinal adsorbents (eg, charcoal) may reduce the effects of miglitol; avoid concomitant use.
Enzymes, digestive	Digestive enzymes containing carbohydrate-splitting enzymes (eg, amylase, pancreatin) may reduce the effects of miglitol; avoid concomitant use.
Propranolol	Miglitol may significantly reduce the bioavailability of propranolol by 40%.
Ranitidine	Miglitol may significantly reduce the bioavailability of ranitidine by 60%.

Table 20.2. DRUG INTERACTIONS FOR ENDOCRINE/HORMONAL AND BONE METABOLISM DRUGS *(cont.)*

HYPOGLYCEMIC AGENTS *(cont.)*

Oral Diabetic Agents

Nateglinide (Starlix)	
β-Blockers	The hypoglycemic action of nateglinide may be potentiated by β-blockers. β-Blockers mask or reduce the symptoms of hypoglycemia.
Corticosteroids	Concomitant use may lead to hyperglycemia and loss of glucose control; monitor closely during concomitant therapy and discontinuation.
CYP2C9 substrates	Nateglinide is an inhibitor of CYP2C9 and may increase the concentrations of drugs metabolized by this enzyme (eg, tolbutamide).
MAOIs	The hypoglycemic action of nateglinide may be potentiated by MAOIs.
NSAIDs	The hypoglycemic action of nateglinide may be potentiated by NSAIDs.
Protein-bound drugs	Caution with highly protein-bound drugs.
Salicylates	The hypoglycemic action of nateglinide may be potentiated by salicylates.
Sympathomimetics	Concomitant use may lead to hyperglycemia and loss of glucose control; monitor closely during concomitant therapy and discontinuation.
Thiazides	Concomitant use may lead to hyperglycemia and loss of glucose control; monitor closely during concomitant therapy and discontinuation.
Thyroid products	Concomitant use may lead to hyperglycemia and loss of glucose control; monitor closely during concomitant therapy and discontinuation.
Pioglitazone HCl (Actos)	
CYP2C8 inducers	CYP2C8 inducers (eg, rifampin) may significantly decrease the AUC of pioglitazone.
CYP2C8 inhibitors	CYP2C8 inhibitors (eg, gemfibrozil) may significantly increase the AUC of pioglitazone.
Ethinyl estradiol/norethindrone	Coadministration with an oral contraceptive containing ethinyl estradiol and norethindrone led to a decrease in AUC and C_{max} of ethinyl estradiol. The significance of this interaction is unknown.
Hypoglycemic agents	Glucose-lowering effects are potentiated when administered concomitantly with other hypoglycemic agents.
Insulin	Glucose-lowering effects are potentiated when administered concomitantly with insulin.
Midazolam	Coadministration with midazolam led to a decrease in AUC and C_{max} of midazolam.
Repaglinide (Prandin)	
β-Blockers	The hypoglycemic action of repaglinide may be potentiated by β-blockers. β-Blockers mask or reduce the symptoms of hypoglycemia.
Calcium channel blockers (CCBs)	Use of calcium channel blockers tends to lead to hyperglycemia and may lead to a loss of glucose control; monitor closely during concomitant therapy and discontinuation.
Chloramphenicol	The hypoglycemic action of repaglinide may be potentiated by chloramphenicol.

HYPOGLYCEMIC AGENTS *(cont.)*

Oral Diabetic Agents

Repaglinide (Prandin) *(cont.)*	
Contraceptives, oral	Concomitant use may lead to hyperglycemia and loss of glucose control; monitor closely during concomitant therapy and discontinuation.
Corticosteroids	Concomitant use may lead to hyperglycemia and loss of glucose control; monitor closely during concomitant therapy and discontinuation.
Coumarins	The hypoglycemic action of repaglinide may be potentiated by coumarins.
Cyclosporine	The hypoglycemic action of repaglinide may be potentiated by cyclosporine.
CYP2C8 inducers	CYP2C8 inducers (eg, rifampin, barbiturates, carbamazepine) may decrease levels.
CYP2C8 inhibitors	CYP2C8 inhibitors (eg, trimethoprim, gemfibrozil, montelukast) may increase levels.
CYP3A4 inducers	CYP3A4 inducers (eg, St. John's wort, phenobarbital, carbamazepine, rifampin) may decrease levels.
CYP3A4 inhibitors	CYP3A4 inhibitors (eg, erythromycin, clarithromycin, ketoconazole, itraconazole, ritonavir, grapefruit juice) may increase levels.
Diuretics	Concomitant use may lead to hyperglycemia and loss of glucose control; monitor closely during concomitant therapy and discontinuation.
Estrogens	Concomitant use may lead to hyperglycemia and loss of glucose control; monitor closely during concomitant therapy and discontinuation.
Ethinyl estradiol/Levonorgestrel	Concomitant use may lead to hyperglycemia and loss of glucose control; monitor closely during concomitant therapy and discontinuation.
Gemfibrozil	Avoid use with gemfibrozil, which significantly increases exposure to repaglinide. The combination of gemfibrozil and itraconazole significantly increases levels and should be avoided.
Isoniazid	Concomitant use may lead to hyperglycemia and loss of glucose control; monitor closely during concomitant therapy and discontinuation.
Itraconazole	Concomitant use with itraconazole increases exposure to repaglinide. The combination of gemfibrozil and itraconazole significantly increases levels and should be avoided.
MAOIs	The hypoglycemic action of repaglinide may be potentiated by MAOIs.
Nicotinic acid	Concomitant use may lead to hyperglycemia and loss of glucose control; monitor closely during concomitant therapy and discontinuation.
NSAIDs	The hypoglycemic action of repaglinide may be potentiated by NSAIDs.
OATP1B1 inhibitors	OATP1B1 inhibitors (eg, cyclosporine) may have the potential to increase levels.
Phenothiazines	Concomitant use may lead to hyperglycemia and loss of glucose control; monitor closely during concomitant therapy and discontinuation.
Phenytoin	Concomitant use may lead to hyperglycemia and loss of glucose control; monitor closely during concomitant therapy and discontinuation.

Table 20.2. DRUG INTERACTIONS FOR ENDOCRINE/HORMONAL AND BONE METABOLISM DRUGS *(cont.)*

HYPOGLYCEMIC AGENTS *(cont.)*

Oral Diabetic Agents

Repaglinide (Prandin) *(cont.)*	
Probenecid	The hypoglycemic action of repaglinide may be potentiated by probenecid.
Protein-bound drugs	The hypoglycemic action of repaglinide may be potentiated by highly protein-bound drugs.
Salicylates	The hypoglycemic action of repaglinide may be potentiated by salicylates.
Simvastatin	Concomitant use with simvastatin increases the levels of repaglinide.
Sulfonamides	The hypoglycemic action of repaglinide may be potentiated by sulfonamides.
Sympathomimetics	Concomitant use may lead to hyperglycemia and loss of glucose control; monitor closely during concomitant therapy and discontinuation.
Thyroid products	Concomitant use may lead to hyperglycemia and loss of glucose control; monitor closely during concomitant therapy and discontinuation.
Rosiglitazone Maleate (Avandia)	
CYP2C8 inducers	CYP2C8 inducers (eg, rifampin) may significantly decrease the AUC of rosiglitazone.
CYP2C8 inhibitors	CYP2C8 inhibitors (eg, gemfibrozil) may significantly increase the AUC of rosiglitazone.
Hypoglycemic agents	Glucose-lowering effects are potentiated when administered concomitantly with other hypoglycemic agents.
Insulin	Concomitant use with insulin may lead to hypoglycemia.
Sitagliptin Phosphate (Januvia)	
Digoxin	Sitagliptin may slightly increase digoxin levels; monitor appropriately.
Sulfonylureas	Glucose-lowering effects are potentiated when administered concomitantly with sulfonylureas; consider dose reduction of concomitant sulfonylureas.
Tolazamide	
Alcohol	The hypoglycemic action of sulfonylureas may be potentiated by alcohol.
β-Blockers	The hypoglycemic action of sulfonylureas may be potentiated by β-blockers. β-blockers mask or reduce the symptoms of hypoglycemia.
Calcium channel blockers (CCBs)	Concomitant use may lead to hyperglycemia and loss of glucose control; monitor closely during concomitant therapy and discontinuation.
Chloramphenicol	The hypoglycemic action of sulfonylureas may be potentiated by chloramphenicol.
Contraceptives, oral	Concomitant use may lead to hyperglycemia and loss of glucose control; monitor closely during concomitant therapy and discontinuation.
Corticosteroids	Concomitant use may lead to hyperglycemia and loss of glucose control; monitor closely during concomitant therapy and discontinuation.
Coumarins	The hypoglycemic action of sulfonylureas may be potentiated by coumarins.
Diuretics	Concomitant use may lead to hyperglycemia and loss of glucose control; monitor closely during concomitant therapy and discontinuation.

HYPOGLYCEMIC AGENTS *(cont.)*

ORAL DIABETIC AGENTS

Tolazamide *(cont.)*	
Estrogens	Concomitant use may lead to hyperglycemia and loss of glucose control; monitor closely during concomitant therapy and discontinuation.
Isoniazid	Concomitant use may lead to hyperglycemia and loss of glucose control; monitor closely during concomitant therapy and discontinuation.
MAOIs	The hypoglycemic action of sulfonylureas may be potentiated by MAOIs.
Miconazole	Concomitant use with miconazole may lead to severe hypoglycemia.
Nicotinic acid	Concomitant use may lead to hyperglycemia and loss of glucose control; monitor closely during concomitant therapy and discontinuation.
NSAIDs	The hypoglycemic action of sulfonylureas may be potentiated by NSAIDs.
Phenothiazines	Concomitant use may lead to hyperglycemia and loss of glucose control; monitor closely during concomitant therapy and discontinuation.
Phenytoin	Concomitant use may lead to hyperglycemia and loss of glucose control; monitor closely during concomitant therapy and discontinuation.
Probenecid	The hypoglycemic action of sulfonylureas may be potentiated by probenecid.
Protein-bound drugs	The hypoglycemic action of sulfonylureas may be potentiated by highly protein-bound drugs.
Salicylates	The hypoglycemic action of sulfonylureas may be potentiated by salicylates.
Sulfonamides	The hypoglycemic action of sulfonylureas may be potentiated by sulfonamides.
Sympathomimetics	Concomitant use may lead to hyperglycemia and loss of glucose control; monitor closely during concomitant therapy and discontinuation.
Thyroid products	Concomitant use may lead to hyperglycemia and loss of glucose control; monitor closely during concomitant therapy and discontinuation.
Tolbutamide	
Alcohol	The hypoglycemic action of sulfonylureas may be potentiated by alcohol.
β-Blockers	The hypoglycemic action of sulfonylureas may be potentiated by β-blockers. β-Blockers mask or reduce the symptoms of hypoglycemia.
CCBs	Concomitant use may lead to hyperglycemia and loss of glucose control; monitor closely during concomitant therapy and discontinuation.
Chloramphenicol	The hypoglycemic action of sulfonylureas may be potentiated by chloramphenicol.
Contraceptives, oral	Concomitant use may lead to hyperglycemia and loss of glucose control; monitor closely during concomitant therapy and discontinuation.
Corticosteroids	Concomitant use may lead to hyperglycemia and loss of glucose control; monitor closely during concomitant therapy and discontinuation.
Coumarins	The hypoglycemic action of sulfonylureas may be potentiated by coumarins.
Diuretics	Concomitant use may lead to hyperglycemia and loss of glucose control; monitor closely during concomitant therapy and discontinuation.

Table 20.2. DRUG INTERACTIONS FOR ENDOCRINE/HORMONAL AND BONE METABOLISM DRUGS *(cont.)*

HYPOGLYCEMIC AGENTS *(cont.)*

Oral Diabetic Agents

Tolbutamide *(cont.)*	
Estrogens	Concomitant use may lead to hyperglycemia and loss of glucose control; monitor closely during concomitant therapy and discontinuation.
Isoniazid	Concomitant use may lead to hyperglycemia and loss of glucose control; monitor closely during concomitant therapy and discontinuation.
MAOIs	The hypoglycemic action of sulfonylureas may be potentiated by MAOIs.
Miconazole	Concomitant use with miconazole may lead to severe hypoglycemia.
Nicotinic acid	Concomitant use may lead to hyperglycemia and loss of glucose control; monitor closely during concomitant therapy and discontinuation.
NSAIDs	The hypoglycemic action of sulfonylureas may be potentiated by NSAIDs.
Phenothiazines	Concomitant use may lead to hyperglycemia and loss of glucose control; monitor closely during concomitant therapy and discontinuation.
Phenytoin	Concomitant use may lead to hyperglycemia and loss of glucose control; monitor closely during concomitant therapy and discontinuation.
Probenecid	The hypoglycemic action of sulfonylureas may be potentiated by probenecid.
Protein-bound drugs	The hypoglycemic action of sulfonylureas may be potentiated by highly protein-bound drugs.
Salicylates	The hypoglycemic action of sulfonylureas may be potentiated by salicylates.
Sulfonamides	The hypoglycemic action of sulfonylureas may be potentiated by sulfonamides.
Sympathomimetics	Concomitant use may lead to hyperglycemia and loss of glucose control; monitor closely during concomitant therapy and discontinuation.
Thyroid products	Concomitant use may lead to hyperglycemia and loss of glucose control; monitor closely during concomitant therapy and discontinuation.

PITUITARY HORMONES

Cabergoline (Dostinex)	
Antihypertensive agents	Caution with other drugs that lower blood pressure.
D_2-antagonists	Avoid with D_2-antagonists (eg, phenothiazines, butyrophenones, thioxanthines, metoclopramide).
Desmopressin Acetate (DDAVP, DDAVP Nasal Spray, DDAVP Rhinal Tube)	
Carbamazepine	Caution with drugs that may increase the risk of water intoxication with hyponatremia.
Chlorpromazine	Caution with drugs that may increase the risk of water intoxication with hyponatremia.
Lamotrigine	Caution with drugs that may increase the risk of water intoxication with hyponatremia.
NSAIDs	Caution with drugs that may increase the risk of water intoxication with hyponatremia.

PITUITARY HORMONES *(cont.)*

Desmopressin Acetate (DDAVP, DDAVP Nasal Spray, DDAVP Rhinal Tube) *(cont.)*	
Opiate analgesics	Caution with drugs that may increase the risk of water intoxication with hyponatremia.
SSRIs	Caution with drugs that may increase the risk of water intoxication with hyponatremia.
Tricyclic antidepressants	Caution with drugs that may increase the risk of water intoxication with hyponatremia.
Vasopressors	Caution with other pressor agents.
Somatropin (Genotropin, Genotropin MiniQuick, Humatrope, Norditropin, Norditropin Nordiflex, Nutropin, Nutropin AQ, Omnitrope, Saizen, Serostim, Tev-Tropin, Valtropin, Zorbtive)	
CYP450 substrates	Somatropin may potentiate the clearance of CYP450 substrates (eg, corticosteroids, sex steroids, anticonvulsants, cyclosporine).
Estrogens, oral	Concomitant use of oral estrogen may necessitate an increase in the dose of somatropin.
Glucocorticoids	Glucocorticoid therapy may attenuate the growth-promoting effects of somatropin.
Hypoglycemics, oral	Somatropin may decrease insulin sensitivity; monitor glucose levels and adjust the dose of concomitant oral hypoglycemics as necessary.
Insulin	Somatropin may decrease insulin sensitivity; monitor glucose levels and adjust insulin dose as necessary.

PROGESTINS

Medroxyprogesterone Acetate (Provera)	
Estrogens	Concomitant use of a progestin and an estrogen may result in an exacerbation of asthma, DM, epilepsy, migraine, porphyria, SLE, hypertriglyceridemia, and hepatic hemangiomas. Caution in patients with hypocalcemia, cardiac or renal dysfunction, and a history of cholestatic jaundice due to prior estrogen use or pregnancy.
Progesterone (Prometrium)	
CYP3A4 inhibitors	CYP3A4 inhibitors (eg, erythromycin, clarithromycin, ketoconazole, itraconazole, ritonavir, grapefruit juice) may increase levels, which may result in side effects.

THYROID AGENTS

Antithyroid Hormones

Methimazole (Tapazole)	
Anticoagulants, oral	Thyroid hormones may increase catabolism of vitamin K-dependent clotting factors, increasing anticoagulant activity of oral anticoagulants; monitor PT and adjust dose accordingly.
Agranulocytosis, drugs associated with	Caution with other drugs that cause agranulocytosis (eg, clozapine).

Table 20.2. DRUG INTERACTIONS FOR ENDOCRINE/HORMONAL AND BONE METABOLISM DRUGS *(cont.)*

THYROID AGENTS *(cont.)*

ANTITHYROID HORMONES

Methimazole (Tapazole) *(cont.)*	
β-Blockers	A dose reduction of β-blockers may be needed when a hyperthyroid patient becomes euthyroid.
Digoxin	A dose reduction of digoxin may be needed when a hyperthyroid patient becomes euthyroid.
Theophylline	A dose reduction of theophylline may be needed when a hyperthyroid patient becomes euthyroid.
Propylthiouracil	
Anticoagulants, oral	Thyroid hormones may increase catabolism of vitamin K-dependent clotting factors, increasing the anticoagulant activity of oral anticoagulants; monitor PT and adjust dose accordingly.
Agranulocytosis, drugs associated with	Caution with other drugs that cause agranulocytosis (eg, clozapine).
β-Blockers	A dose reduction of β-blockers may be needed when a hyperthyroid patient becomes euthyroid.
Digoxin	A dose reduction of digoxin may be needed when a hyperthyroid patient becomes euthyroid.
Theophylline	A dose reduction of theophylline may be needed when a hyperthyroid patient becomes euthyroid.

THYROID HORMONES

Levothyroxine Sodium (Levothroid, Levoxyl, Synthroid, Unithroid)	
5-Fluorouracil	5-Fluorouracil may increase serum TBG concentrations.
6-Mercaptopurine	6-Mercaptopurine is associated with alterations in the levels of thyroid hormone/TSH.
Aminoglutethimide	Long-term aminoglutethimide therapy may minimally decrease T_4 and T_3 levels and increase TSH.
Amiodarone	Use of amiodarone may decrease thyroid hormone secretion and result in hypothyroidism. Amiodarone may also induce hyperthyroidism by causing thyroiditis. Amiodarone decreases the peripheral conversion of T_4 to T_3, leading to decreased T_3 levels.
Anabolic steroids	Anabolic steroids may decrease serum TBG concentrations.
Androgens	Androgens may decrease serum TBG concentrations.
Antacids, aluminum- and magnesium-containing	Concurrent use of aluminum- and magnesium-containing antacids may prevent or delay the absorption of levothyroxine; separate administration by ≥4 hrs.
Anticoagulants, oral	Thyroid hormones may increase catabolism of vitamin K-dependent clotting factors, increasing the anticoagulant activity of oral anticoagulants; monitor PT and adjust dose accordingly.
Asparaginase	Asparaginase may decrease serum TBG concentrations.
β-Blockers	β-Blockers (eg, propranolol >160 mg/day) decrease the peripheral conversion of T_4 to T_3, leading to decreased T_3 levels.

THYROID AGENTS *(cont.)*

Thyroid Hormones

Levothyroxine Sodium (Levothroid, Levoxyl, Synthroid, Unithroid) *(cont.)*	
Bile acid sequestrants	Concurrent use of bile acid sequestrants (eg, cholestyramine, colestipol) may prevent or delay the absorption of levothyroxine; separate administration by ≥4 hrs.
Calcium carbonate	Calcium carbonate may form an insoluble chelate with levothyroxine; separate administration by ≥4 hrs.
Carbamazepine	Carbamazepine may induce the hepatic metabolism of levothyroxine.
Cation exchange resins	Concurrent use of cation exchange resins (eg, sodium polystyrene sulfonate) may prevent or delay the absorption of levothyroxine; separate administration by ≥4 hrs.
Chloral hydrate	Chloral hydrate is associated with alterations in the levels of thyroid hormone/TSH.
Clofibrate	Clofibrate may increase serum TBG concentrations.
Diazepam	Diazepam is associated with alterations in the levels of thyroid hormone/TSH.
Digoxin	Concomitant use may lead to reduced levels or therapeutic effects of digoxin.
Dopamine agonists	Use of dopamine or dopamine agonists may result in a transient reduction in TSH secretion.
Estrogens, oral	Estrogens (eg, estrogen-containing oral contraceptives) may increase serum TBG concentrations.
Ethionamide	Ethionamide is associated with alterations in the levels of thyroid hormone/TSH.
Ferrous sulfate	Ferrous sulfate may form an insoluble chelate with levothyroxine; separate administration by ≥4 hrs.
Furosemide	Furosemide (>80 mg IV) may displace levothyroxine from its protein-binding site.
Glucocorticoids	Use of glucocorticoids may result in a transient reduction in TSH secretion. Glucocorticoids may decrease serum TBG concentrations. Glucocorticoids (dexamethasone ≥4 mg/day) decrease the peripheral conversion of T_4 to T_3, leading to decreased T_3 levels.
Growth hormones	Excessive use of thyroid hormones with growth hormones (eg, somatrem, somatropin) may accelerate epiphyseal closure.
Heparin	Heparin may displace levothyroxine from its protein-binding site.
Heroin	Heroin may increase serum TBG concentrations.
Hydantoins	Hydantoins (eg, phenytoin) may displace levothyroxine from its protein-binding site. Hydantoins may induce the hepatic metabolism of levothyroxine.
Hypoglycemic agents	Addition of levothyroxine to hypoglycemic therapy may result in increased hypoglycemic agent requirements.
Insulin	Addition of levothyroxine to insulin therapy may result in increased insulin requirements.

Table 20.2. DRUG INTERACTIONS FOR ENDOCRINE/HORMONAL AND BONE METABOLISM DRUGS *(cont.)*

THYROID AGENTS *(cont.)*

Thyroid Hormones

Levothyroxine Sodium (Levothroid, Levoxyl, Synthroid, Unithroid) *(cont.)*	
Interferon-α	Interferon-α has been associated with the development of antithyroid microsomal antibodies in 20% of patients and some have transient hypothyroidism, hyperthyroidism, or both.
Interleukin-2	Interleukin-2 has been associated with transient painless thyroiditis in 20% of patients.
Iodide	Use of iodide (including iodine-containing radiographic contrast agents) may decrease thyroid hormone secretion, resulting in hypothyroidism. The use of iodide may also lead to hyperthyroidism, which may develop over several weeks and persist for several months after d/c.
Ketamine	Caution with ketamine; concurrent use may produce marked hypertension and tachycardia.
Lithium	Long-term lithium therapy can result in goiter in up to 50% of patients, and either subclinical or overt hypothyroidism in up to 20% of patients.
Lovastatin	Lovastatin is associated with alterations in the levels of thyroid hormone/TSH.
Methadone	Methadone may increase serum TBG concentrations.
Methimazole	Use of methimazole may decrease thyroid hormone secretion, which may result in hypothyroidism.
Theophylline	Decreased theophylline clearance may occur in hypothyroid patients.
Metoclopramide	Metoclopramide is associated with alterations in the levels of thyroid hormone/TSH.
Mitotane	Mitotane may increase serum TBG concentrations.
Nicotinic acid, slow-release	Slow-release nicotinic acid may decrease serum TBG concentrations.
Nitroprusside	Nitroprusside is associated with alterations in the levels of thyroid hormone/TSH.
NSAIDs	NSAIDs (eg, fenamates, phenylbutazone) may displace levothyroxine from its protein-binding site.
Octreotide	Use of octreotide may result in a transient reduction in TSH secretion.
Para-aminosalicylate sodium	Para-aminosalicylate sodium is associated with alterations in the levels of thyroid hormone/TSH.
Perphenazine	Perphenazine is associated with alterations in the levels of thyroid hormone/TSH.
Phenobarbital	Phenobarbital may induce the hepatic metabolism of levothyroxine.
Propylthiouracil	Use of propylthiouracil may decrease thyroid hormone secretion, which may result in hypothyroidism. Propylthiouracil decreases the peripheral conversion of T_4 to T_3, leading to decreased T_3 levels.
Radiographic agents	Levothyroxine may reduce the uptake of ^{123}I, ^{131}I, and ^{99m}Tc.
Resorcinol	Excessive topical use of resorcinol is associated with alterations in the levels of thyroid hormone/TSH.

THYROID AGENTS *(cont.)*

Thyroid Hormones

Levothyroxine Sodium (Levothroid, Levoxyl, Synthroid, Unithroid) *(cont.)*	
Salicylates	Salicylates (>2 g/day) may displace levothyroxine from its protein-binding site.
Sertraline	Administration of sertraline in patients stabilized on levothyroxine may result in increased levothyroxine requirements.
Simethicone	Concurrent use of simethicone may prevent or delay the absorption of levothyroxine; separate administration by ≥4 hrs.
Sucralfate	Concurrent use of sucralfate may prevent or delay the absorption of levothyroxine; separate administration by ≥4 hrs.
Sulfonamides	Use of sulfonamides may decrease thyroid hormone secretion, which may result in hypothyroidism.
Sympathomimetics	Concomitant use may increase the effects of both drugs.
Tamoxifen	Tamoxifen may increase serum TBG concentrations.
TCAs	Concomitant use of levothyroxine and TCAs (eg, amitriptyline) may increase the therapeutic and toxic effects of both drugs.
Tetracyclic antidepressants	Concomitant use of levothyroxine and tetracyclic antidepressants (eg, maprotiline) may increase the therapeutic and toxic effects of both drugs.
Thiazides	Thiazide diuretics are associated with alterations in the levels of thyroid hormone/TSH.
Tolbutamide	Use of tolbutamide may decrease thyroid hormone secretion, which may result in hypothyroidism.
Liothyronine Sodium (Cytomel)	
Anticoagulants, oral	Thyroid hormones may increase catabolism of vitamin K-dependent clotting factors, increasing the anticoagulant activity of oral anticoagulants; monitor PT and adjust dose accordingly.
Cholestyramine	Concurrent use of cholestyramine may prevent or delay the absorption of liothyronine; separate administration by ≥4 hrs.
Digoxin	Thyroid preparations may potentiate digoxin toxicity; concomitant use of liothyronine and digoxin may lead to reduced levels or reduced therapeutic effects of digoxin.
Estrogens, oral	Estrogens (eg, estrogen-containing oral contraceptives) may increase serum TBG concentrations.
Hypoglycemic agents	Addition of liothyronine to hypoglycemic therapy may result in increased hypoglycemic agent requirements.
Insulin	Addition of liothyronine to insulin therapy may result in increased insulin requirements.
Ketamine	Caution with ketamine; concurrent use may produce marked hypertension and tachycardia.
Sympathomimetic amines	Larger doses of liothyronine may produce serious or even life-threatening manifestations of toxicity, particularly when given in association with sympathomimetic amines such as those used for their anorectic effects.

Table 20.2. DRUG INTERACTIONS FOR ENDOCRINE/HORMONAL AND BONE METABOLISM DRUGS *(cont.)*

THYROID AGENTS *(cont.)*

Thyroid Hormones

Liothyronine Sodium (Cytomel) *(cont.)*	
TCAs	Concomitant use of liothyronine and TCAs (eg, amitriptyline) may increase the therapeutic and toxic effects of both drugs.
Vasopressors	Caution with vasopressors; thyroxine increases the adrenergic effect of catecholamines (eg, epinephrine, norepinephrine).
Radiographic agents	Liothyronine may reduce the uptake of ^{123}I, ^{131}I, and ^{99m}Tc.
Liotrix (Thyrolar)	
Anticoagulants, oral	Thyroid hormones may increase catabolism of vitamin K-dependent clotting factors, increasing the anticoagulant activity of oral anticoagulants; monitor PT and adjust dose accordingly.
Bile acid sequestrants	Concurrent use of bile acid sequestrants (eg, cholestyramine, colestipol) may prevent or delay the absorption of liotrix; separate administration by ≥4 hrs.
Estrogens, oral	Estrogens (eg, estrogen-containing oral contraceptives) may increase serum TBG concentrations.
Hypoglycemic agents	Addition of liotrix to hypoglycemic therapy may result in increased hypoglycemic agent requirements.
Insulin	Addition of liotrix to insulin therapy may result in increased insulin requirements.
Sympathomimetic amines	Larger doses of liotrix may produce serious or even life-threatening manifestations of toxicity, particularly when given with sympathomimetic amines such as those used for their anorectic effects.
Thyroid (Armour Thyroid)	
Anticoagulants, oral	Thyroid hormones may increase catabolism of vitamin K-dependent clotting factors, increasing the anticoagulant activity of oral anticoagulants; monitor PT and adjust dose accordingly.
Bile acid sequestrants	Concurrent use of bile acid sequestrants (eg, cholestyramine, colestipol) may prevent or delay the absorption of thyroid; separate administration by ≥4 hrs.
Estrogens, oral	Estrogens (eg, estrogen-containing oral contraceptives) may increase serum TBG concentrations.
Hypoglycemic agents	Addition of thyroid to hypoglycemic therapy may result in increased hypoglycemic agent requirements.
Insulin	Addition of thyroid to insulin therapy may result in increased insulin requirements.
Sympathomimetic amines	Larger doses of thyroid may produce serious or even life-threatening manifestations of toxicity, particularly when given with sympathomimetic amines such as those used for their anorectic effects.

MISCELLANEOUS METABOLIC AGENTS

Aminoglutethimide (Cytadren)	
Alcohol	Alcohol may potentiate effects.

MISCELLANEOUS METABOLIC AGENTS *(cont.)*

Aminoglutethimide (Cytadren) *(cont.)*	
Coumarin	Aminoglutethimide diminishes the effects of coumarin.
Dexamethasone	Aminoglutethimide potentiates the metabolism of dexamethasone; if glucocorticoid replacement is needed, hydrocortisone should be prescribed.
Warfarin	Aminoglutethimide diminishes the effects of warfarin.
Calcitriol (Rocaltrol)	
Calcium-containing preparations	Changes in diet or uncontrolled intake of calcium preparations can cause hypercalcemia.
Cholestyramine	Cholestyramine reduces the intestinal absorption of calcitriol.
Corticosteroids	Corticosteroids antagonize the effects of calcitriol.
Digoxin	Caution with digoxin; hypercalcemia may precipitate arrhythmias.
Ketoconazole	Ketoconazole may inhibit the metabolism of calcitriol.
Magnesium-containing preparations	Hypermagnesemia may occur with magnesium-containing preparations (eg, antacids).
Phenobarbital	Phenobarbital may potentiate the metabolism of calcitriol; may be necessary to increase the dose of calcitriol.
Phenytoin	Phenytoin may potentiate the metabolism of calcitriol; may be necessary to increase the dose of calcitriol.
Phosphate-binding agents	Adjust dose of phosphate-binding agents based on serum phosphate levels.
Thiazide diuretics	Caution with thiazides due to the increased risk of hypercalcemia.
Vitamin D	Avoid vitamin D products and derivatives during therapy.
Cinacalcet HCl (Sensipar)	
Amitriptyline	Cinacalcet increases levels of amitriptyline and its active metabolite (nortriptyline) by approximately 20% in CYP2D6 extensive metabolizers.
CYP2D6 substrates	Cinacalcet is a potent inhibitor of CYP2D6 and may increase the concentrations of drugs metabolized by this enzyme (eg, flecainide, vinblastine, thioridazine, most TCAs); dose adjustment of concomitant drugs may be required.
CYP3A4 inhibitors	CYP3A4 inhibitors (eg, erythromycin, ketoconazole, itraconazole) may increase levels, which may result in side effects; may require dose adjustment or discontinuation of cinacalcet.
CYP3A4 substrates	Cinacalcet is a potent inhibitor of CYP3A4 and may increase the concentrations of drugs metabolized by this enzyme (eg, statins, etc.). Dose adjustment or d/c of concomitant drugs may be required; allow a wash-out period prior to reinitiation.
Desipramine	Cinacalcet increases the exposure of desipramine by 3.6-fold in CYP2D6 extensive metabolizers.
Conivaptan HCl (Vaprisol)	
CYP3A4 inhibitors	CYP3A4 inhibitors (eg, erythromycin, ketoconazole, itraconazole, grapefruit juice) may increase levels.

Table 20.2. DRUG INTERACTIONS FOR ENDOCRINE/HORMONAL AND BONE METABOLISM DRUGS *(cont.)*

MISCELLANEOUS METABOLIC AGENTS *(cont.)*

Conivaptan HCl (Vaprisol) *(cont.)*	
CYP3A4 substrates	Conivaptan is a potent inhibitor of CYP3A4 and may increase the concentrations of drugs metabolized by this enzyme (eg, statins, etc.). Dose adjustment or d/c of concomitant drugs may be required; allow a wash-out period prior to reinitiation.
HMG-CoA reductase inhibitors (statins)	Two cases of rhabdomyolysis occurred in patients who were also receiving a CYP3A4-metabolized statin.
Digoxin	May increase levels of digoxin.
Doxercalciferol (Hectorol)	
Cholestyramine	Cholestyramine reduces the intestinal absorption of doxercalciferol.
CYP450 inhibitors	CYP450 inhibitors (eg, ketoconazole, erythromycin) may prevent the formation of an active metabolite.
Digoxin	Caution with digoxin; hypercalcemia may precipitate arrhythmias.
Enzyme inducers	Enzyme inducers (eg, glutethimide and phenobarbital) may affect metabolism; consider adjusting dose.
Magnesium-containing preparations	Hypermagnesemia may occur with magnesium-containing preparations (eg, antacids).
Vitamin D	Avoid vitamin D products and derivatives during therapy.
Ergocalciferol (Drisdol)	
Mineral oil	Mineral oil reduces the intestinal absorption of ergocalciferol.
Thiazide diuretics	Caution with thiazides due to the increased risk of hypercalcemia.
Exenatide (Byetta)	
GI absorption-dependent drugs	Caution with drugs that require rapid GI absorption.
Threshold concentration-dependent drugs	Drugs dependent on threshold concentrations for efficacy (eg, contraceptives, antibiotics) should be taken 1 hr before.
Warfarin	Caution with concomitant use of warfarin; may lead to increased INR and possible bleeding.
Lanreotide (Somatuline Depot)	
Bradycardia-inducing drugs	Lanreotide may have an additive effect on the reduction of heart rate when given concomitantly with bradycardia-inducing drugs (eg, β-blockers).
Bromocriptine	Lanreotide may increase the availability of bromocriptine.
Cyclosporine	May decrease the bioavailability of cyclosporine; may require dose adjustment.
CYP3A4 substrates	Lanreotide is an inhibitor of CYP3A4 and may increase the concentrations of drugs metabolized by this enzyme; caution with drugs metabolized by CYP3A4 with a narrow therapeutic index (eg, quinidine, terfenadine). Consider dose adjustment of concomitant drugs.
GI absorption-dependent drugs	Lanreotide may reduce the GI absorption of concomitant drugs.
Hypoglycemic agents	Lanreotide inhibits the secretion of insulin and glucagon; monitor glucose levels and adjust hypoglycemic therapy.
Insulin	Lanreotide inhibits the secretion of insulin and glucagon; monitor glucose levels and adjust insulin therapy.

MISCELLANEOUS METABOLIC AGENTS *(cont.)*

Nafarelin Acetate (Synarel)	
Decongestants, topical	Avoid topical decongestants within 2 hrs after dosing.
Octreotide Acetate (Sandostatin, Sandostatin LAR)	
Bradycardia-inducing drugs	Octreotide may have an additive effect on the reduction of heart rate when given concomitantly with bradycardia-inducing drugs (eg, β-blockers).
Bromocriptine	May increase the availability of bromocriptine.
Cyclosporine	May decrease the levels of cyclosporine, resulting in transplant rejection; may require dose adjustment.
CYP3A4 substrates	Octreotide is an inhibitor of CYP3A4 and may increase the concentrations of drugs metabolized by this enzyme; caution with drugs metabolized by CYP3A4 with a narrow therapeutic index (eg, quinidine, terfenadine). Consider dose adjustment of concomitant drugs.
GI absorption-dependent drugs	Octreotide may reduce the GI absorption of concomitant drugs.
Hypoglycemic agents	Octreotide inhibits the secretion of insulin and glucagon; monitor glucose levels and adjust hypoglycemic therapy.
Insulin	Octreotide inhibits the secretion of insulin and glucagon; monitor glucose levels and adjust insulin therapy.
Paricalcitol (Zemplar IV, Zemplar Oral)	
Aluminum-containing preparations	Avoid excessive use of aluminum-containing preparations to control phosphorus levels in patients with chronic kidney disease.
CYP3A4 inhibitors, potent	CYP3A4 inhibitors (eg, atazanavir, clarithromycin, indinavir, itraconazole, ketoconazole, nefazodone, nelfinavir, ritonavir, saquinavir, telithromycin, voriconazole) may increase levels, which may result in side effects; may require dose adjustment or discontinuation of paricalcitol.
Cholestyramine	Cholestyramine reduces the intestinal absorption of paricalcitol (Zemplar Oral).
Digoxin	Caution with digoxin; hypercalcemia may precipitate arrhythmias.
Pegvisomant (Somavert)	
Hypoglycemic agents	Hypoglycemic agents may require dose reduction after initiation of pegvisomant.
Insulin	Insulin may require dose reduction after initiation of pegvisomant.
Opioids	Concomitant opioids may increase dosage requirements of pegvisomant.
Pramlintide Acetate (Symlin, SymlinPen)	
ACE inhibitors	Glucose-lowering effects are potentiated when administered concomitantly with ACE inhibitors.
β-Blockers	β-Blockers mask or reduce the symptoms of hypoglycemia.
Clonidine	Clonidine masks or reduces the symptoms of hypoglycemia.
Disopyramide	Glucose-lowering effects are potentiated when administered concomitantly with disopyramide.
Drugs, oral	Pramlintide has the potential to delay the absorption of concomitantly administered oral medications; administer drugs whose effectiveness is determined by rapid onset (eg, analgesics) at least 1 hr prior to or 2 hrs after pramlintide.

Table 20.2. DRUG INTERACTIONS FOR ENDOCRINE/HORMONAL AND BONE METABOLISM DRUGS *(cont.)*

MISCELLANEOUS METABOLIC AGENTS *(cont.)*	
Pramlintide Acetate (Symlin, SymlinPen) *(cont.)*	
Fibrates	Glucose-lowering effects are potentiated when used with fibrates.
GI absorption, drugs slowing	Avoid concomitant use with drugs that slow the intestinal absorption of nutrients (eg, alpha-glucosidase inhibitors).
GI motility, drugs altering	Avoid concomitant use with drugs that alter GI motility (eg, anticholinergics).
Guanethidine	Guanethidine masks or reduces the symptoms of hypoglycemia.
Hypoglycemic agents	Glucose-lowering effects are potentiated when used with other hypoglycemics.
MAOIs	Glucose-lowering effects are potentiated when used with MAOIs.
Pentoxifylline	Glucose-lowering effects are potentiated when used with pentoxifylline.
Propoxyphene	Glucose-lowering effects are potentiated when used with propoxyphene.
Reserpine	Reserpine masks or reduces the symptoms of hypoglycemia.
Salicylates	Glucose-lowering effects are potentiated when used with salicylates.
Sulfonamide antibiotics	Glucose-lowering effects are potentiated when used with sulfonamide antibiotics.
Sapropterin Dihydrochloride (Kuvan)	
Levodopa	Caution with levodopa; concomitant administration has resulted in exacerbation of convulsions, overstimulation, or irritability.
Methotrexate	Caution with drugs that inhibit folate metabolism (eg, methotrexate).
PDE-5 inhibitors	Caution with PDE-5 inhibitors (eg, sildenafil, tadalafil, vardenafil); both may induce vasorelaxation.

Table 20.3. SIGNS OF HYPO- AND HYPERGLYCEMIA

HYPOGLYCEMIA	HYPERGLYCEMIA
Anxiety	Xerostomia
Blood pressure normal or increased	Blood pressure normal or decreased
Breath normal in odor	Smell of acetone on breath
Breathing may be stertorous but at normal depth and rate	Breathing is deep and fast
Confusion, inability to concentrate	Warm and dry skin
Cool and moist skin	Loss of appetite
Hunger	Normal or depressed reflexes
Hyperactive reflexes	Lethargy
Lethargy	Gradual onset of symptoms
Rapid onset of symptoms	Rapid, normal, or thready pulse
Rapid pulse	
Tired, weak	
Unsteadiness	
Vision problems	

Chapter 21

Drugs Used for Connective Tissue Disorders and Oral Mucosal Diseases

Eric T. Stoopler, D.M.D.; Martin S. Greenberg, D.D.S.

This chapter describes the major drugs used to manage connective tissue diseases as well as the drugs used to treat diseases of the oral mucosa. Dentists have a major responsibility for the diagnosis and management of diseases affecting the oral mucosa; therefore, this chapter emphasizes the clinical application of these drugs. The section devoted to connective tissue disorders highlights the effect of this group of drugs on oral health and the precautions necessary when providing dental treatment for patients receiving drug therapy for this group of diseases.

CONNECTIVE TISSUE DISORDER DRUGS

The connective tissue diseases are a group of disorders with a prominent feature of tissue damage caused by the patient's own immune system. These diseases are often classified as autoimmune and the cause of tissue damage is complex and multifactorial. The major connective tissue diseases include lupus erythematosus, rheumatoid arthritis, scleroderma (systemic sclerosis), dermatomyositis, mixed connective tissue disease, and Sjögren's syndrome.

See **Tables 21.1** and **21.2** for general information on connective tissue disorder drugs.

Lupus Erythematosus Drugs

Lupus erythematosus is caused by the formation of autoantibodies to nuclear components, particularly DNA. Tissue damage may result directly from autoantibodies or, more commonly, from immune complexes composed of antigen, antibody, and complement, which cause an inflammatory reaction involving skin, mucosa, internal organs (particularly the kidneys and brain), or joints.

Discoid lupus is confined to the skin and mucosa and causes skin lesions with scales that project into hair follicles (follicular plugging). Typical oral lesions of discoid lupus appear as a mixture of inflammation, atrophy, ulceration, and keratosis. The lesions easily may be confused with lichen planus or, occasionally, leukoplakia. Systemic lupus is a multisystem disease with a strong genetic component that most commonly affects women in their childbearing years. Patients with systemic lupus have skin and mucosal lesions, as well as renal, central nervous, cardiovascular, and hematologic systemic manifestations. Patients with systemic lupus may have discoid lupus-type oral lesions or nonspecific ulcers caused by vasculitis. Dentists should be suspicious of the possibility of systemic lupus when a woman between the ages of 20 and 40 years develops oral lesions with associated symptoms, such as joint pains or skin lesions.

The lesions of discoid lupus often respond to use of topical and intralesional glucocorticoids (see **Chapter 5** for a discussion of those drugs). Patients with discoid lupus that does not respond to this therapy may be placed on systemic therapy with antimalarial agents such as hydroxychloroquine. Patients with mild-to-moderate manifestations of lupus are treated symptomatically for joint pains and skin or mucosal lesions. Patients with serious organ involvement, such as kidney or central nervous system manifestations, are treated with systemic glucocorticoids alone or glucocorticoids in combination with immunosuppressive drugs such as azathioprine or cyclophosphamide. Mycophenolate mofetil has been used in combination with glucocorticoids to treat discoid lupus lesions that are refractory to conventional therapies, although this use is not FDA-approved. Methotrexate has been shown to be beneficial in treating SLE arthritis; however, multiple complications may occur secondary to use, including thrombocytopenia, neutropenia, acute renal failure, and mucositis. The most promising class of drugs to treat SLE are biologics, such as rituximab, a monoclonal antibody that targets the CD20 receptor protein on the surfaces of B cells. Further open clinical trials are required for these agents prior to FDA approval for treatment of SLE.

Rheumatoid Arthritis Drugs

Rheumatoid arthritis (RA) is a systemic inflammatory disease whose chief manifestation is destruction of the synovial membrane that spreads to the joint cartilage. Susceptibility to the disease has a strong hereditary basis, and an infectious etiology is suspected but not proved. RA chiefly manifests itself as symmetrical swelling and pain of the joints in people between the ages of 30 and 50 years. RA is a systemic disease; therefore, generalized manifestations such as weakness, fatigue, and subcutaneous nodules are also common.

A form of RA, Felty's syndrome, affects the blood, causing anemia and a decrease in white blood cells and platelets. Dentists treating patients who have this syndrome must be aware of the potential for infection and bleeding. Involvement of the temporomandibular joints is common, but it is a major problem for only a small percentage of patients.

Dentists treating patients with RA must be aware of the drugs prescribed and their possible effect on dental treatment. The major classes of drugs used to treat RA include the following:

- nonsteroidal anti-inflammatory drugs (NSAIDs), which can increase bleeding after surgery
- gold sodium thiomalate, which can cause oral ulcers, decreased white blood cells, and decreased platelets; patients receiving systemic gold should receive periodic hematologic evaluations, and dentists performing surgical procedures on such patients should obtain the results of recent laboratory tests
- penicillamine, which may cause decreased white blood cells and platelets, drug-induced pemphigus with oral lesions, or nephrotic syndrome; patients must have periodic hematologic evaluation; loss of taste has also been reported
- systemic glucocorticoids (see **Chapter 5**)
- immunosuppressive drugs (see **Chapter 23**)
- tumor necrosis factor (TNF) inhibitors, which may increase the risk of infection when used in combination with immunosuppressive agents and may cause reactivation of latent tuberculosis (TB); patients must have periodic hematologic evaluations; status of TB must be determined prior to dental treatment and elective treatment should be deferred if active; patients should be monitored for TB-associated oral lesions.
- biologics that target specific cellular types in the treatment of RA, such as rituximab and abatacept. Rituximab may

cause decreased cell counts and reactivation of hepatitis B; therefore, baseline and periodic hematologic evaluations are recommended. Severe mucocutaneous reactions have been reported as side effects of rituximab, such as paraneoplastic pemphigus, lichenoid dermatitis, Stevens-Johnson syndrome, and toxic epidermal necrolysis. Evaluate and monitor patients using rituximab for presence of oral lesions.

Scleroderma Drugs

Patients with scleroderma (systemic sclerosis) develop fibrosis of the skin and internal organs owing to the overproduction of collagen. Tightening of the skin, especially around the face and hands, is a characteristic of the disease. Raynaud's phenomenon, ischemia, and blanching of the fingers caused by vasoconstriction are common. Patients with this form of scleroderma may develop fibrosis of the heart, kidney or lung, and dentists treating these patients should consult with the managing physician regarding the extent of organ involvement before performing dental treatment.

Drugs frequently used to treat scleroderma include:

- penicillamine (see Rheumatoid Arthritis above)
- systemic glucocorticoids (see **Chapter 5**)
- immunosuppressive drugs (see **Chapter 23**)

Calcium channel blockers such as nifedipine are used to manage Raynaud's phenomenon (refer to **Chapter 14** for more information on calcium channel blockers). These drugs may cause gingival enlargement that can be minimized by good oral hygiene. Newer agents that are used in the management of scleroderma-associated pulmonary arterial hypertension (PAH) are prostacyclin analogues, including epoprostenol. This agent can inhibit platelet aggregation; therefore, dentists may anticipate increased bleeding when treating patients using this medication.

Dermatomyositis Drugs

Patients with dermatomyositis have skin lesions and muscle weakness. The term "polymyositis" is used when patients have only muscle involvement. The disease may occur alone or in association with an underlying malignancy or another connective-tissue disease. Oral involvement may include weakness of the palatal muscles and oral mucosal lesions.

Treatment of dermatomyositis includes use of high doses of systemic glucocorticoids (**Chapter 5**) and cytotoxic immunosuppressive drugs (**Chapter 23**).

Mixed Connective Tissue Disease Drugs

Patients with mixed connective tissue disease (MCTD) have signs and symptoms that overlap more than one connective tissue disease. MCTD is considered a separate disorder as patients have a distinct laboratory finding of high levels of autoantibodies to nuclear ribonucleoprotein. The drugs taken by patients with MCTD are determined by the particular overlap syndrome; they are the same drugs described above for use with lupus, RA, scleroderma, and dermatomyositis.

Sjögren's Syndrome Agents

Sjögren's syndrome (SS) is an autoimmune disease that primarily affects the lacrimal and salivary glands, but also may be associated with other connective tissue diseases or lymphoma. Primary SS, which occurs primarily in women (at a 9:1 ratio), causes destruction of salivary and lacrimal gland tissue and leads to severe xerostomia and dry eyes. Oral manifestations include an increased incidence of dental caries and candidiasis owing to a decrease in both the detergent and the antibacterial properties of saliva. Patients with SS also have difficulty wearing dentures. People with secondary SS have dry eyes and mouth in association with any one of the connective tissue diseases described above, most frequently RA.

A major concern of clinicians managing patients who have SS is the high incidence of lymphoma in people with this condition. The diagnosis of SS is made by testing for salivary and lacrimal gland function and abnormal serologic findings and detection of inflammatory foci in biopsy specimens of minor salivary glands.

The medical management of xerostomia in patients with SS includes use of topical rinses, such as artificial saliva substitutes, and systemic medications to increase salivary flow. Pilocarpine 5 mg taken four times daily increases salivary flow for patients who still have functional salivary gland tissue. The most common side effects of pilocarpine include sweating and gastrointestinal symptoms. Pilocarpine should not be used for patients with asthma, chronic bronchitis, narrow-angle glaucoma, or chronic obstructive pulmonary disease. Use the drug with caution in patients with severe cardiovascular disease.

Cevimeline 30 mg three times a day has been shown to increase salivary output in patients with SS. The most common side effects of cevimeline include nausea and sweating; however, these symptoms are mild compared to similar adverse reactions induced by pilocarpine. See **Chapter 8** for further information on xerostomia and agents used to treat it.

Special Dental Considerations

Drug Interactions of Dental Interest

Many of the drugs taken by patients receiving treatment for a connective tissue disease may have a profound effect on both oral disease and the safety of dental treatment. Treating a patient with a connective tissue disease requires taking a careful drug history and understanding the potential side effects of the drugs the patient is taking and how they may affect the safety of dental treatment. Many of the drugs described in this chapter affect the hematologic and immune systems and, therefore, increase the risk of both infection and bleeding. Long-term glucocorticoid or immunosuppressive drug therapy, for example, may require significant modification of the dental treatment plan. Dentists may be consulted to treat oral and dental complications of connective tissue diseases, such as oral mucosal lesions in patients who have lupus or xerostomia in patients who have SS. Knowledge of the use of topical and intralesional glucocorticoids for patients with lupus and systemic medications for patients with SS, such as pilocarpine and cevimeline, can be an important component of good medical therapy.

Lupus

Dentists should be aware of a disorder called "drug-induced lupus," which occurs when patients develop symptoms and signs of lupus triggered by drug therapy. Drugs most frequently associated with drug-induced lupus include hydralazine, procainamide, penicillamine D, and oral contraceptives. Dentists should also be aware that drug therapy may exacerbate systemic lupus. Antibiotics such as penicillin and sulfonamides, as well as NSAIDs, have been reported to cause lupus flare-ups. Dentists should check with the treating medical specialist before prescribing these drugs for patients with lupus. Use NSAIDs with caution for patients treated with methotrexate due to the potential of significant methotrexate toxicity.

Scleroderma

Scleroderma of the face results in a progressive decrease in oral opening that leads to difficulty with both oral home care and dental treatment. Difficulty with proper oral hygiene increases the risk of dental caries, especially when scleroderma is complicated by xerostomia as a result of secondary SS. Patients using epoprostenol for scleroderma-associated PAH should avoid analgesics such as NSAIDs and aspirin due to further inhibitory effects on platelet aggregation.

Sjögren's syndrome

Patients with SS systemic manifestations may be receiving therapy with antimalarial drugs such as hydroxychloroquine, particularly when there is joint involvement. Systemic glucocorticoids and/or immunosuppressive drugs also are used to manage severe systemic manifestations of SS. Patients receiving antimalarial therapy should be closely monitored for the development of blood dyscrasias, including neutropenia and agranulocytosis. Patients receiving antimalarials may develop dark pigmentation of the skin and mucosa and may ask their dentist about the cause of a pigmented area discovered on the oral mucosa.

Laboratory Value Alterations

Many drugs used to treat connective tissue diseases—such as immunosuppressive drugs, methotrexate, rituximab, gold sodium thiomalate, and penicillamine—may cause bone marrow suppression. Patients taking these drugs should have a hematologic evaluation, including a white blood cell and platelet count, before undergoing dental and oral surgical procedures.

Adverse Effects, Precautions, and Contraindications

Table 21.1 lists adverse effects related to connective tissue disorder drugs.

Pharmacology

Cevimeline. Cevimeline is a parasympathetic agonist that is specific for M3 muscarinic receptors, the major receptor subtype found on salivary-gland tissue. As compared to pilocarpine, onset of increased salivation may be later; however, duration of action is generally longer and the adverse effects are milder.

Gold sodium thiomalate. The mechanism that makes this drug an effective anti-inflammatory agent for patients with RA is unknown. It is effective in reducing synovitis in patients with active joint inflammation.

Hydroxychloroquine. This is an antimalarial drug that also is effective in the treatment of discoid and SLE. The mechanism of action in patients with lupus is not understood.

Immunosuppressive drugs. Azathioprine is an immunosuppressive drug used to prevent graft rejection in organ transplant patients. It also is effective for the management of some autoimmune and connective tissue diseases owing to its effect on lymphocyte response and delayed hypersensitivity.

Cyclophosphamide is used in cancer chemotherapy, which also suppresses the immune response and therefore is useful in the management of autoimmune and connective tissue diseases, such as pemphigus and SLE.

Mycophenolate mofetil is a potent immunosuppressive agent and was originally approved to prevent rejection of kidney transplants. Currently, mycophenolate mofetil is also being used to treat discoid lupus erythematosus, pemphigus, and mucous membrane pemphigoid, although these uses are not FDA-approved.

Tumor necrosis factor (TNF) inhibitors decrease the amount of circulating TNF-α, an inflammatory cytokine that is present in increased concentrations in patients with RA. Etanercept is a receptor protein that prevents TNF-α from attaching to its cellular receptors and neutralizes its inflammatory behavior. Infliximab is a monoclonal antibody that binds to TNF-α, rendering it inactive. It may also promote lysis of TNF-producing cells. Both medications have demonstrated efficacy in managing symptoms associated with RA.

Nonsteroidal anti-inflammatory drugs. Pharmacological information on these drugs is provided in **Chapter 3**.

Penicillamine. This drug decreases the level of rheumatoid factor related to immunoglobulin M. It also depresses the activity of T-lymphocytes.

Rituximab. This drug is a chimeric monoclonal antibody that targets and destroys B cells expressing the cell surface antigen CD20. It was initially approved for the treatment of non-Hodgkin's lymphoma.

Abatacept. This drug blocks the costimulatory pathway for activation of T cells, which plays a fundamental role in the immunopathology of RA.

ORAL MUCOSAL DISEASE DRUGS

This portion of the chapter will discuss the therapy for the major oral mucosal diseases not covered in other chapters.

Erythema Multiforme Drugs

Erythema multiforme (EM) is an acute inflammatory disease that may affect the mucosa, the skin, or both. EM that involves multiple sites—including the mouth, conjunctiva, skin, and genitals—is called Stevens-Johnson syndrome. Toxic epidermal necrolysis is a severe, life-threatening form of EM in which large areas of skin peel away, leaving the patient susceptible to fluid and electrolyte imbalance as well as secondary infection. EM may be caused by drug reactions or reactions to microorganisms. Drugs that most commonly cause EM include sulfonamides, oxicam NSAIDs (such as piroxicam), allopurinol, and anticonvulsant drugs such as phenytoin and carbamazepine. Antiretroviral drugs such as protease inhibitors and reverse transcriptase inhibitors may also cause difficult-to-diagnose EM in HIV patients.

Use of genotyping to detect patients susceptible to severe EM reactions to certain medications is being developed and presently recommended for Asians prior to taking carbamazepine.

Herpes simplex virus (HSV) is the microorganism most commonly responsible for triggering episodes of EM, and recurrent herpes infections are believed to be the most common cause of recurrent episodes of EM. Mycoplasma and chlamydia infections also trigger cases of EM.

The oral lesions associated with EM can be extensive and cause severe ulceration of the lips and intraoral mucosa. Patients may have oral lesions as the sole or chief manifestation of EM. Extensive oral lesions are frequently present as part of generalized EM.

The management of mild cases of oral EM includes supportive care with topical anesthetic agents, such as viscous lidocaine. Severe cases of EM in adults frequently are treated with a short course of systemic glucocorticoids. The use of glucocorticoids to treat EM has been controversial, but studies have demonstrated both relief of symptoms and shortened healing times with few significant side effects when the drug is administered to adults. Children treated with glucocorticoids for EM have a higher incidence of side effects, particularly gastrointestinal bleeding or secondary infection. Patients with recurrent episodes of EM caused by HSV benefit from prophylaxis with antiherpes drugs, such as acyclovir or valacyclovir. Severe cases of recurrent EM not related to HSV may respond to therapy with dapsone or azathioprine.

Patients with severe stomatitis resulting from EM or other causes may obtain temporary relief with the use of topical anesthetic agents such as viscous lidocaine.

Lichen Planus Drugs

Lichen planus (LP) is a chronic mucocutaneous disease that affects the skin, mucosal surfaces, or both. LP is the most common cause of chronic oral mucosal lesions affecting an estimated 1.2 % of the population. LP oral lesions can present as reticular white lines, white plaques, areas of desquamation, or ulcers. LP is also the most common cause of desquamative gingivitis. When LP is characterized by ulceration, desquamation, or blisters, it is called ulcerative or erosive LP. The etiology of the disease is unknown, but LP is divided into idiopathic and lichenoid reactions. Patients with idiopathic LP have no identifiable underlying trigger for the disease, whereas patients with lichenoid reactions have an underlying cause such as drug therapy, contact allergy, or a systemic disease such as hepatitis C. The lesions of idiopathic LP and lichenoid reactions cannot be reliably distinguished either clinically or histologically; therefore, dentists or dental specialists who manage patients with oral LP should obtain a thorough history to rule out a possible underlying cause, particularly in severe cases of erosive LP. The drugs most commonly associated with LP include angiotensin-converting enzyme (ACE) inhibitors such as captopril, β-blockers, and NSAIDs. Allergic reactions to dental materials (such as amalgam or gold) that are directly in contact with the lesions also have been reported as a cause of LP. Flavoring agents such as peppermint and cinnamon are another potential cause of oral lichenoid reactions.

Proper management of oral LP includes an attempt to identify an underlying cause, such as a lichenoid drug reaction or systemic disease such as SLE, which has similar appearing lesions, and then to control symptomatic lesions with topical or, occasionally, systemic agents. Topical glucocorticoids are the most effective agents for a majority of patients with lesions symptomatic of erosive LP. The effectiveness of topical glucocorticoids when managing desquamative gingival lesions can be improved by fabrication of a soft splint or mouthguard that covers the gingiva and holds the glucocorticoid in place more effectively. In severe cases, the topical glucocorticoid may be supplemented with intralesional glucocorticoid injections. Plaque-like lesions of LP, which require therapy, have been successfully managed with the use of topical retinoids such as tretinoin. Cyclosporine, an immunosuppressive drug used to prevent graft rejection in organ transplant patients, has been used topically to treat oral LP. The usefulness of this therapy is limited because it is significantly more expensive than the use of topical glucocorticoids. The topical calcineurin inhibitors, tacrolimus and pimecrolimus, are nonsteroidal topical immunomodulators that inhibit production of inflammatory cytokines and are effective in the treatment of erosive LP that is refractory to topical glucocorticoid treatment. Prior to prescribing these medications patients must be counseled that the long-term safety of topical calcineurin inhibitors has not been established, and there is a concern about potential risk since rare cases of skin malignancy and lymphoma have been reported.

Inform patients starting therapy for LP that LP is a chronic disease that may last for many years and that treatment is designed to control symptomatic lesions, not cure the disease. Data strongly suggest that patients with oral LP have an increased risk of developing oral cancer; therefore, patients with LP should be adequately counseled and evaluated periodically for the presence of suspicious lesions.

Mucous Membrane Pemphigoid Drugs

Mucous membrane pemphigoid (MMP) is a chronic subepithelial autoimmune disease caused by autoantibodies directed toward proteins in the basement membrane zone of the epithelium, which work in conjunction with and complement neutrophils to cause a separation of the epidermis from the dermis. The oral mucosa is the most common site of involvement in MMP, and desquamation of the gingiva is the most common oral manifestation. Involvement of the conjunctiva may lead to visual impairment and blindness, and in some cases the genital, tracheal, and esophageal mucosa also may be affected. Diagnosis is made by biopsy of lesions that should be studied by means of both routine histology and direct immunofluorescence. Some patients with pemphigoid may have an increased risk of an underlying malignancy and therefore a thorough evaluation by a family physician or internist is indicated after initial diagnosis.

Oral lesions of MMP initially are treated with potent topical glucocorticoids, which can be more effective when held in place with occlusive dental splints if gingival or palatal lesions are involved. Intralesional glucocorticoids can be used when extensive localized lesions do not respond to topical glucocorticoids alone. Systemic therapy may be necessary to control severe cases of MMP. Systemic therapy found effective in some cases includes dapsone, a tetracycline such as doxycycline or minocycline, and in severe cases of resistant disease immunosuppressive drugs (such as azathioprine and mycophenolate mofetil) and systemic glucocorticoids may be required. These drugs may have serious side effects and should be prescribed only by a dental or medical specialist trained in managing patients who are taking these drugs.

Pemphigus Vulgaris Drugs

Pemphigus vulgaris (PV) is an autoimmune disease caused by antibodies directed against the glucoprotein adhesion molecules that bind epithelial cells, causing separation of the cells (called "acantholysis") that results in intraepithelial blister formation. PV may occur alone or in association with other autoimmune diseases, such as myasthenia gravis. The blistering and peeling of the skin and mucosa are potentially fatal if not treated. The oral mucosa is the initial site of involvement in 60% of cases and 80% to 90% of patients with PV develop oral lesions during the course of the disease. PV is frequently diagnosed by biopsy of oral lesions using both routine histology and direct immunofluorescence. Most cases of PV are of unknown origin, but a minority of cases is caused by a reaction to drugs, particularly penicillamine or captopril. Paraneoplastic pemphigus is a form of PV triggered by neoplasms, such as lymphomas.

Systemic glucocorticoid therapy is the mainstay of treatment of PV. Adjuvant therapy with immunosuppressive drugs such as azathioprine allows the clinician to use lower doses of systemic glucocorticoids, which reduces the risk of serious side effects. Mycophenolate mofetil, described earlier in this chapter, has a lower incidence of hepatotoxicity and nephrotoxicity compared with other immunosuppressive agents, and is used in the treatment of PV.

Recurrent Aphthous Stomatitis Drugs

Recurrent aphthous stomatitis (RAS) is a disease of unknown etiology, but it is well established that the tendency to develop RAS is inherited. RAS affects approximately 15% of the population and is a common complaint of dental patients. The disease is characterized by recurring oral ulcers with no signs or symptoms of disease involving other mucosal or skin surfaces and no evidence of involvement of other organ systems. Dentists managing patients with recurring oral ulcers should eliminate the possibility of other serious disorders that can cause recurring oral ulcers, such as connective tissue disease, blood dyscrasias, or HIV infection, by obtaining a thorough history and performing a careful examination. In severe or atypical cases such as recurring ulcers beginning in adulthood, laboratory tests may be necessary to eliminate the possibility of underlying systemic disease. RAS is divided into minor and major forms. Patients with the minor form experience ulcers that are <1 cm in diameter and heal in 10 to 14 days. The major form of RAS is less common and causes ulcers that are >1 cm in diameter, take weeks to months to heal, and cause scarring.

The mainstay of treatment for RAS is the use of topical glucocorticoids. High-potency glucocorticoids such as fluocinonide placed directly on the lesion shorten the healing time of the lesion and increase patient comfort in a majority of cases, but do not prevent the formation of new lesions. Less potent glucocorticoids appear to have little effect. Other topical preparations that can decrease the healing time of RAS include amlexanox paste (Aphthasol) and topical tetracycline mouthrinses. The latter therapy may cause candidiasis or allergic reactions.

Patients with severe major aphthae may not experience adequate relief from topical preparations. Systemic drugs that have been reported to be effective in reducing the number of ulcers in some cases of major RAS include colchicine, pentoxifylline, and dapsone. Pentoxifylline is a methylxanthine related to caffeine, which is used chiefly to treat peripheral vascular disease because of its effect on the flexibility of red blood cells. Because it also has an effect on leukocytes, it appears useful for a number of inflammatory diseases. There have been several reports and uncontrolled trials of the successful use of pentoxifylline for the treatment of severe aphthous stomatitis.

Thalidomide has been shown to reduce the incidence and severity of RAS in both HIV and non-HIV patients, but it must be used with extreme caution in women of childbearing years owing to its potential for causing severe life-threatening and deforming birth defects. Clinicians prescribing thalidomide must be registered with the System for Thalidomide Education and Prescribing Safety (STEPS) prescriber registry, and patients receiving the drug must be carefully counseled regarding proper use of birth control methods during treatment with this drug. Other side effects of thalidomide include peripheral neuropathy, drowsiness, and gastrointestinal disturbances.

See **Tables 21.1** and **21.2** for general information on oral mucosal disease drugs.

Special Dental Considerations

Topical glucocorticoids. Treatment with topical glucocorticoids is common for patients with inflammatory diseases involving the oral mucosa. Topical glucocorticoids are largely synthetic derivatives of hydrocortisone with an 11-β-hydroxyl group required for anti-inflammatory action. The topical glucocorticoids are effective anti-inflammatory agents; these agents' effectiveness results from a combination of activities, including increased vasoconstriction, decreased migration of leukocytes, decreased complement activity, and decreased fibroblast proliferation.

Long-term repeated use of topical glucocorticoids may cause resistance to the anti-inflammatory effects owing to tachyphylaxis, which primarily results from a decreased ability to cause vasoconstriction. Discontinuing the use of the drug for three to four days restores the normal response. Vasoconstriction is an important part of the action of topical glucocorticoids, and the potency of these drugs is established by an assay that measures vasoconstriction.

Topical glucocorticoids are grouped according to their potency. Examples of drugs in each group are as follows:

- Group 1: ultra high potency—betamethasone dipropionate 0.05%, clobetasol 0.05%
- Group 2: high potency—fluocinonide 0.05%, desoximetasone 0.25%, 0.05%
- Group 3: medium potency—betamethasone dipropionate 0.05%, triamcinolone acetonide 0.5%
- Group 4: lower potency—triamcinolone acetonide, fluocinolone acetonide

The effect of topical glucocorticoids on the desquamative lesions of LP may be enhanced by the use of soft occlusive dental splints that fit over the teeth and hold the glucocorticoid onto the attached gingiva, increasing contact of the glucocorticoid and preventing the medication from being washed away by saliva. The most frequent complication of the long-term use of topical glucocorticoids when treating chronic oral mucosal lesions such as LP or MMP is oral candidiasis. The incidence of candidiasis can be decreased by the concomitant use of topical antifungal agents such as nystatin suspension or clotrimazole troches. Dentists prescribing prolonged use of topical glucocorticoids must carefully instruct patients regarding safe use in the mouth, warn about overuse, and periodically monitor patients who are using these medications for extensive oral lesions. Long-term use of high-potency topical steroids should be done cautiously in patients with diabetes.

Intralesional glucocorticoids. Patients with chronic, severe lesions of LP, MMP, or major RAS that do not respond to topical glucocorticoids may be helped by the use of intralesional glucocorticoids. Glucocorticoids developed for intralesional use such as triamcinolone hexacetonide 5 mg/cc are useful in managing resistant lesions in patients with major aphthae, LP, or MMP.

Systemic glucocorticoids. Many clinicians recommend a short course of systemic glucocorticoids for the management of EM. Use of systemic glucocorticoids in the management of chronic oral mucosal disease should be rare and for short periods to manage acute, severe exacerbations of diseases such as LP and major RAS.

Topical immunomodulators. Tacrolimus and pimecrolimus are calcineurin inhibitors—drugs that prevent the formation of numerous cytokines—that are critical in the development of inflammatory skin disorders. Originally developed as systemic drugs to prevent transplant rejection, the topical formulations of tacrolimus or pimecrolimus are primarily used for treatment of atopic dermatitis (eczema). They are also effective for treatment of erosive LP that is refractory to topical glucocorticoid therapy. Topical tacrolimus ointment is currently available in concentrations of 0.03% and 0.1%, with the latter formulation demonstrating greater clinical results when used to treat erosive LP. Pimecrolimus is available in a 1% cream formulation.

Retinoids. Retinoids include vitamin A and its synthetic analogues. Systemic retinoids such as isotretinoin (13-cis-retinoic acid) and etretinate have been shown to promote healing of premalignant oral leukoplakias in a significant number of cases and to reduce the incidence of second cancers in patients with a history of head and neck malignancies. Systemic retinoids have the potential for inducing serious side effects, such as severe birth defects; benign intracranial hypertension (pseudotumor cerebri); an increase in plasma triglycerides, high-density lipoproteins and cholesterol; and liver toxicity. Patients taking systemic retinoids may also develop mucocutaneous signs such as cheilitis and conjunctivitis. Topical retinoids have been used to treat oral mucosal leukoplakia and LP. The white plaques or reticulated lesions of LP have been reversed with the use of topical tretinoin. Mucosal irritation may result from use of topical retinoids.

Dapsone. Dapsone, a synthetic sulfone, was used initially to treat leprosy and malaria. In the 1950s, the drug's anti-inflammatory properties became known, and it was used to successfully treat a number of inflammatory disorders, particularly those with neutrophil-rich infiltrates such as dermatitis herpetiformis. In oral medicine, dapsone is used most frequently to treat mucous membrane pemphigoid; however, according to some controlled studies, it also has been used in severe refractory cases of major aphthous ulcers, pemphigus, and LP. Side effects of dapsone are common, and the drug should be prescribed by a clinician experienced in its use. The most common side effects are hemolytic anemia and methemoglobinemia, and most patients receiving the drug will demonstrate a decrease in hemoglobin. The use of dapsone is contraindicated in patients with glucose-6-phosphate dehydrogenase (G6PD) deficiency. Before prescribing dapsone, the clinician must screen the patient for this deficiency.

Thalidomide. This drug, which originally was prescribed for the treatment of nausea in pregnant women, was banned in the U.S. because it causes severe birth defects and fetal death. The drug was approved for limited use in 1998 for the treatment of erythema nodosum leprosum, but it also has been shown to be beneficial in the management of severe minor and major recurrent aphthous ulcers in some patients, including some patients with HIV infection. The drug may be prescribed to pregnant women only by specially registered (see above) physicians or dentists who have received formal education on the risk of fetal abnormalities. Use of thalidomide for recurrent aphthous stomatitis should be reserved for patients with severe intractable forms of the disease who have not responded to other less toxic forms of therapy. In addition to birth defects, the side effects of thalidomide include peripheral neuropathy, constipation, drowsiness, and neutropenia.

Adverse Effects, Precautions, and Contraindications

Table 21.1 lists adverse effects related to oral mucosal disease drugs.

Pharmacology

Colchicine. Colchicine, indicated for gouty arthritis, is used to reduce the number of ulcers in RAS. It suppresses white blood cell function by interfering on the cellular level with microtubule formation, inhibiting lysosomal degranulation and increasing the level of cyclic AMP. This decreases both the chemotactic and the phagocytic activity of neutrophils.

Cyclosporine. Cyclosporine is an immunosuppressive drug used to prevent graft rejection in organ transplant patients. It has a potent effect on the response of T-lymphocytes and cell-mediated immunity. It also has been used to treat connective tissue and autoimmune diseases.

Dapsone. Dapsone is a sulfone that has been used for its antibacterial properties for more than 50 years. It continues to be used to treat leprosy, malaria, and Pneumocystis carinii infections in people with HIV infection. The anti-inflammatory properties of dapsone are unrelated to its antibacterial actions, but diseases that respond favorably to the drug are associated with significant neutrophil infiltration. There is evidence that dapsone suppresses neutrophil function by interfering with the myeloperoxidase-H2O2-halide cytotoxic function of neutrophils, as well as inhibiting the synthesis of prostaglandins by neutrophils.

Retinoids. This class of drugs has a major effect on cellular growth and cell differentiation. The use of these drugs can reverse keratinization and premalignant changes. There also is evidence that retinoids have anti-inflammatory properties.

Tacrolimus/Pimecrolimus. The major adverse reaction associated with topical tacrolimus ointment and pimecrolimus cream is burning at the site of application. The FDA has issued an alert that use of topical tacrolimus ointment and pimecrolimus cream for treatment of atopic dermatitis in pediatric patients may increase the risk of developing cancer; further clinical studies are needed to substantiate this advisory.

Thalidomide. This drug was marketed as a nonaddictive sedative until its severe teratogenic properties became known and its use was discontinued. More recently, it has been used for its immune-modulating effects and its angiogenesis-inhibiting properties, which are believed to result from suppression of TNF-α and inhibition of leukocyte migration.

Viscous lidocaine. Pharmacological information on this drug is provided in **Chapter 1**.

SUGGESTED READING

Akintoye SO, Greenberg MS. Recurrent aphthous stomatitis. *Dent Clin North Am.* 2005;49:31-47.

Atkinson JC, Imanguli MM, Challacombe S. Immunologic diseases. In: Greenberg MS, Glick M, Ship J, eds. *Burket's Oral Medicine*, 11th ed. Ontario: BC Decker; 2008:435-460.

Beck LA. The efficacy and safety of tacrolimus ointment: A clinical review. *J Am Acad Dermatol.* 2005;53:S165-170.

Eisen D. The clinical features, malignant potential, and systemic associations of oral lichen planus: a study of 723 patients. *J Am Acad Dermatol.* 2002;476:207-214.

King JK, Hahn BH. Systemic lupus erythematosus: modern strategies for management: a moving target. *Best Pract Res Clin Rheumatol.* 2007; 21:971-987.

Manadan AM, Block JA. Rheumatoid arthritis: beyond tumor necrosis factor-α antagonists, B-cell depletion, and T-cell blockade. *Am J Ther.* 2008;15: 53-58.

McCartan BE, Healy CM. The reported prevalence of oral lichen planus: a review and critique. *J Oral Pathol Med.* 2008;37:447-453.

Williams PM, Conklin RJ. Erythema multiforme: A review and contrast from Stevens-Johnson syndrome/toxic epidermal necrolysis. *Dent Clin North Am.* 2005;49:67-76.

Woo SB, Greenberg MS. Ulcerative, vesicular, and bullous lesions. In: Greenberg MS, Glick M, Ship J, eds. *Burket's Oral Medicine,* 11th ed. Ontario: BC Decker; 2008:41-75.

Table 21.1. PRESCRIBING INFORMATION FOR DRUGS USED FOR CONNECTIVE TISSUE DISORDERS AND ORAL MUCOSAL DISEASES

NAME	FORM/ STRENGTH	DOSAGE	WARNINGS/PRECAUTIONS & CONTRAINDICATIONS	ADVERSE EFFECTS†
ANALGESIC, TOPICAL				
Lidocaine HCl (Xylocaine Viscous)	**Sol:** 2% [100mL, 450mL]	***Adults:* Irritated/Inflamed Mucous Membranes: Usual:** 15mL undiluted. **(Mouth)** Swish and spit out. **(Pharynx)** Gargle and may swallow. Do not administer in <3 hour intervals. **Max:** 8 doses/24hr; **(Single Dose)** 4.5mg/kg or total of 300mg. ***Pediatrics:* >3 yrs: Max:** Determine by age and weight. ***Infants:* <3 yrs:** Apply 1.25mL with cotton-tipped applicator to immediate area. Do not administer in <3 hour intervals. **Max:** 8 doses/24hr.	**W/P:** Reduce dose in elderly, debilitated, acutely ill and children. Caution with heart block, severe shock, and known drug sensitivities. Excessive dosage or too frequent administration may result in high plasma levels and serious adverse effects requiring resuscitative measures. Extreme caution if mucosa traumatized; risk of rapid systemic absorption. Overdose reported in pediatrics due to inappropriate dosing. **P/N:** Category B, caution in nursing.	Lightheadedness, nervousness, confusion, euphoria, dizziness, drowsiness, blurred vision, tremors, convulsions, respiratory depression, bradycardia, hypotension, urticaria, edema, anaphylactoid reactions.
ANTIBIOTIC				
Dapsone	**Tab:** 25mg*, 100mg*	***Adults/Pediatrics:* Dermatitis Herpetiformis: Initial:** 50mg/day. **Usual:** 50-300mg/day, may increase dose prn. Reduce to minimum maintenance dose. **Leprosy:** Give with one or more antileprosy drugs. **Maint:** 100mg/day.	**W/P:** Agranulocytosis, aplastic anemia, and other blood dyscrasias reported. CBC weekly for the first month, monthly for 6 months and semiannually thereafter. D/C if significant reduction in leukocytes, platelets, or hemopoiesis occurs. Treat severe anemia prior to therapy. D/C if sensitivity occurs. Caution in those with G6PD deficiency, methemoglobin reductase deficiency, or hemoglobin M. Toxic hepatitis and cholestatic jaundice reported. Monitor LFT's. **P/N:** Category C, not for use in nursing.	Hemolysis, peripheral neuropathy, N/V, abdominal pain, pancreatitis, vertigo, blurred vision, tinnitus, insomnia, fever, headache, psychosis, phototoxicity, pulmonary eosinophilia, tachycardia, albuminuria, renal papillary necrosis, male infertility.
ANTI-INFLAMMATORY AGENT				
Amlexanox (Aphthasol) OTC	**Paste:** 5% [5g]	***Adults:*** Begin at 1st sign of aphthous ulcer. Apply 1/4 inch qid, pc and qhs, following oral hygiene. Use until ulcer heals. Re-evaluate if healing or pain reduction has not occurred after 10 days of use.	**W/P:** Wash hands immediately after applying paste. D/C if rash or contact mucositis occurs. Re-evaluate if healing or pain reduction has not occurred after 10 days. Avoid eyes. **P/N:** Category B; caution in nursing.	Transient pain, stinging, burning.
ANTIMALARIAL AGENT				
Hydroxychloroquine Sulfate (Plaquenil)	**Tab:** 200mg (200mg tab= 155mg base)	***Adults:* Malaria: Suppression:** 400mg weekly. Begin 2 weeks before exposure and continue for 8 weeks after leaving endemic area. Give 400mg q6h for two doses if therapy is not started before exposure. **Acute Attack:** 800mg, then 400mg 6-8 hrs later, then 400mg for 2 more days. **RA: Initial:** 400-600mg qd with food or milk; increase until optimum response. **Maint:** After 4-12 weeks, 200-400mg qd with food or milk. **Lupus Erythematosus: Initial:** 400mg qd-bid for several weeks or months depending on response. **Maint:** 200-400mg/day. ***Pediatrics:* Malaria: Suppression:** 5mg base/kg weekly, max 400mg/dose. Begin 2 weeks before exposure and continue for 8 weeks after leaving endemic area. **Acute Attack:** 10mg base/kg, max 800mg/dose; then 5mg base/kg, max 400mg/dose at 6, 24 and 48 hrs after 1st dose. **Total Dose:** 25mg base/kg in 3 days.	**BB:** Be familiar with complete prescribing information before prescribing hydroxychloroquine. **W/P:** Caution with hepatic disease, G6PD deficiency, alcoholism, psoriasis, and porphyria. Perform baseline and periodic (3 months) ophthalmologic exams and blood cell counts with prolonged therapy. Test periodically for muscle weakness. D/C if blood disorders occur. Avoid if possible in pregnancy. D/C after 6 months if no improvement in RA. **Contra:** Long term therapy in children or if retinal/visual field changes due to 4-aminoquinoline compounds. **P/N:** Safety in pregnancy and nursing not known.	Headache, dizziness, diarrhea, loss of appetite, muscle weakness, nausea, abdominal cramps, bleaching of hair, dermatitis, ocular toxicity, visual field defects.

*Scored. †Bold entries denote special dental considerations.
BB = black box warning; **W/P** = warnings/precautions; **Contra** = contraindications; **P/N** = pregnancy category rating and nursing considerations.

Table 21.1. PRESCRIBING INFORMATION FOR DRUGS USED FOR CONNECTIVE TISSUE DISORDERS AND ORAL MUCOSAL DISEASES *(cont.)*

NAME	FORM/ STRENGTH	DOSAGE	WARNINGS/PRECAUTIONS & CONTRAINDICATIONS	ADVERSE EFFECTS†
ARTHRITIS AGENTS, NONANALGESIC				
Abatacept (Orencia)	**Inj:** 250mg	***Adults:* RA: Initial: <60kg:** 500mg; **60-100kg:** 750mg; **>100kg:** 1g IV over 30 min. **Maint:** Give at 2 and 4 weeks after initial infusion, then every 4 weeks thereafter. ***Pediatrics:* JA: 6-17 yrs: >75 kg:** Follow adult dosing regimen. **Max:** 1000mg; **<75kg: Initial:** 10mg/kg IV over 30 min. **Maint:** Give at 2 and 4 weeks after initial infusion, then every 4 weeks thereafter.	**W/P:** Increased risk of infections and serious infections with concomitant TNF-antagonist therapy; concurrent use not recommended. Anaphylaxis or anaphylactoid reactions reported. Caution with history of recurrent infections; d/c if serious infections develop. Screen for latent TB prior to initiation. Avoid live vaccines. Caution with COPD. Concurrent use with anakinra is not recommended. Cases of lung cancer and lymphoma reported. Screening for viral hepatitis is recommended before initiation of therapy. Juvenile idiopathic arthritis patients should be brought up to date with all immunizations prior to therapy. **P/N:** Category C, not for use in nursing.	Headache, **nasopharyngitis,** dizziness, cough, back pain, HTN, dyspepsia, UTI, rash, pain in extremities.
Auranofin (Ridaura)	**Cap:** 3mg	***Adults:* RA: Usual:** 6mg qd or 3mg bid. If response not adequate after 6 months, increase to 3mg tid. If inadequate response with 9mg/day after 3 months, d/c. **Max:** 9mg/day. **Transferring from Injectable Gold:** D/C injectable agent and start with 6mg qd.	**BB:** May cause gold toxicity. **W/P:** Gold toxicity manifests as a falling Hgb, leukopenia <4000 WBC/mm³, granulocytes <1500/mm³, decrease in platelets <150,000/mm³, proteinuria, hematuria, pruritus, rash, stomatitis, or persistent diarrhea. Thrombocytopenia and proteinuria reported. Caution in renal/hepatic disease, inflammatory bowel disease, skin rash or a history of bone marrow depression. GI reactions, dermatitis, stomatitis, nephrotic syndrome and blood dyscrasias reported. **Contra:** History of gold induced disorders: anaphylactic reactions, necrotizing enterocolitis, pulmonary fibrosis, exfoliative dermatitis, bone marrow aplasia or severe hematologic disorders. **P/N:** Category C, not for use in nursing.	Diarrhea, nausea, constipation, anorexia, flatulence, dyspepsia, rash, conjunctivitis, exfoliative dermatitis, anemia, proteinuria, hematuria, elevated liver enzymes.
Etanercept (Enbrel)	**Inj:** (MDV) 25mg, (Syringe) 50mg/mL	***Adults:* ≥18 yrs: RA/PA/AS:** 50mg SQ per week, given as one SQ injection. May continue MTX, glucocorticoids, salicylates, NSAIDs or analgesics. **Psoriasis: Initial:** 50mg SQ twice weekly given 3 or 4 days apart for 3 months. May begin with 25-50mg/week. **Maint:** 50mg/week. ***Pediatrics:* 2-17 yrs: JIA:** 0.8mg/kg/week. **Max:** 50mg/week.	**BB:** Serious infections, including bacterial sepsis and TB, reported; d/c if severe infection develops. Evaluate for TB risk factors and test for latent TB infection prior to initiation. **W/P:** May cause autoimmune antibodies. Avoid with active infections. Monitor closely if new infection develops. Caution with pre-existing or recent onset CNS demyelinating disorders. Rare cases of pancytopenia including aplastic anemia reported; d/c if significant hematologic abnormalities occur. May cause reactivation of hepatitis B virus; evaluate prior to therapy initiation. Caution in patients with heart failure; monitor closely. JRA patients should be brought up to date with current immunization guidelines prior to initiating therapy. D/C temporarily with significant varicella virus exposure and consider prophylaxis. Avoid with Wegener's granulomatosis. Needle cap on prefilled syringe and autoinjector contains dry natural rubber; caution with latex allergy. **Contra:** Sepsis. **P/N:** Category B, not for use in nursing.	(Adults/Pediatrics) Injection-site reactions, infections, headache. (Pediatrics) Varicella, gastroenteritis, depression, cutaneous ulcer, esophagitis.

*Scored. †Bold entries denote special dental considerations.
BB = black box warning; **W/P** = warnings/precautions; **Contra** = contraindications; **P/N** = pregnancy category rating and nursing considerations.

NAME	FORM/ STRENGTH	DOSAGE	WARNINGS/PRECAUTIONS & CONTRAINDICATIONS	ADVERSE EFFECTS†
Infliximab (Remicade)	**Inj:** 100mg	***Adults:*** **RA (Combo with MTX):** 3mg/kg as IV infusion; repeat at 2 and 6 weeks. **Maint:** 3mg/kg every 8 weeks. **Incomplete Response:** May increase to 10mg/kg or give every 4 weeks. **CD/Fistulizing CD: Induction Regimen:** 5mg/kg IV at 0, 2, and 6 weeks. **Maint:** 5mg/kg every 8 weeks. For patients who respond then lose their response, may increase to 10mg/kg. May d/c therapy if no response by Week 14. **AS:** 5mg/kg as IV infusion; repeat at 2 and 6 weeks. **Maint:** 5mg/kg every 6 weeks. **PA:** 5mg/kg as IV infusion; repeat at 2 and 6 weeks. **Maint:** 5mg/kg every 8 weeks. May be used with or without MTX. **UC:** 5mg/kg at 0, 2, and 6 weeks. **Maint:** 5mg/kg every 8 weeks. **Plaque Psoriasis:** 5mg/kg IV infusion; repeat at 2 and 6 weeks. **Maint:** 5mg/kg every 8 weeks. ***Pediatrics:*** **≥6 yrs: CD: Induction Regimen:** 5mg/kg IV at 0, 2, and 6 weeks. **Maint:** 5mg/kg every 8 weeks.	**BB:** Increased risk for developing serious infections that may lead to hospitalization or death. Should be discontinued if patient develops serious infection or sepsis. Reports of TB, invasive fungal infections and other opportunistic infections. Evaluate for latent TB and treat if necessary prior to initiation of therapy. Hepatosplenic T-cell lymphoma reported in adolescent and young adult males patients with Crohn's disease or ulcerative colitis. **W/P:** Leukopenia, neutropenia, thrombocytopenia and pancytopenia reported. Serious infections, including sepsis and pneumonia, reported. Avoid with active infection. Monitor for signs of infection during and after therapy; d/c if serious infection develops. Caution in patients who have resided in areas where histoplasmosis or coccidioidomycosis are endemic. Hypersensitivity reactions reported. Caution with optic neuritis, chronic and recurrent infections, CNS demyelinating disease (eg, MS) and seizure disorder. May result in autoantibody formation; d/c if lupus-like syndrome develops. Monitor closely and d/c if new or worsening symptoms of heart failure appear. Lymphoma reported; caution with malignancies. Severe hepatic reactions, including acute liver failure, jaundice, hepatitis and cholestasis reported rarely. Caution in elderly. **Contra:** Hypersensitivity to murine proteins. Moderate or severe CHF (NYHA Class III/IV) with doses >5mg/kg. **P/N:** Category B, not for use in nursing.	Nausea, infections, infusion reactions, headache, sinusitis, **pharyngitis,** coughing, abdominal pain, diarrhea, bronchitis, dyspepsia, fatigue, rhinitis, pain, arthralgia, hepatotoxicity.
Methotrexate (Rheumatrex)	**Inj:** (Generic) (Methotrexate Sodium) 25mg/mL, 1g; **Tab:** (Generic) (Methotrexate) 2.5mg*; **Tab:** (Rheumatrex) (Methotrexate) 2.5mg* [Dose Pack 15mg, 4 x 6 tabs; 12.5mg, 4 x 5 tabs; 10mg, 4 x 4 tabs; 7.5mg, 4 x 3 tabs; 5mg, 4 x 2 tabs]	***Adults:*** **Choriocarcinoma/Trophoblastic Disease:** 15-30mg qd PO/IM for 5 days. May repeat 3-5 times as required with rest period of ≥1 week. **Leukemia: Induction:** 3.3mg/m^2 with prednisone 60mg/m^2 qd. **Remission Maintenance:** 15mg/m^2 PO/IM twice weekly or 2.5mg/kg IV every 14 days. **Burkitt's Tumor: Stages I-II:** 10-25mg/day PO for 4-8 days. Administer several courses with rest periods of 7-10 days in between. **Lymphosarcoma: Stage III:** 0.625-2.5mg/kg/day with other antitumor agents. **Mycosis Fungoides:** 5-50mg once weekly. If poor response, give 15-37.5mg twice weekly. Adjust dose based on response and hematologic monitoring. **Osteosarcoma: Initial:** 12g/m^2 IV, increase to 15g/m^2 if peak serum levels of 1000 micromolar not reached at end of infusion. **Meningeal Leukemia:** Dilute preservative free MTX to 1mg/mL. Give 12mg intrathecally at 2- to 5-day intervals. **Psoriasis: Initial:** 10-25mg PO/IM/IV weekly until response or use divided oral dose schedule, 2.5mg at 12 hr intervals for 3 doses. **Titrate:** Increase gradually until optimal response. **Maint:** Reduce	**BB:** Should only be used by physicians whose knowledge and experience includes the use of antimetabolite therapy. Only for life-threatening neoplastic diseases, or with severe, recalcitrant, disabling disease not adequately responsive to other forms of therapy. Fetal death/congenital anomalies reported. Elimination reduced with impaired renal function, ascites, or pleural effusions; monitor carefully. Severe, sometimes fatal, bone marrow suppression and GI toxicity reported with concomitant NSAIDs. May cause hepatotoxicity, fibrosis, and cirrhosis (usually after prolonged use). Lung disease, malignant melanomas, and potentially fatal opportunistic infections may occur. Interrupt therapy if diarrhea or ulcerative colitis occur. May induce tumor lysis syndrome. Severe, occasionally fatal, skin reactions reported. Concomitant radiotherapy may increase risk of soft tissue necrosis and osteonecrosis. **W/P:** Monitor closely; toxicity may be related to dose and frequency of administration. When reactions do occur, doses should be reduced or d/c and corrective measures should be taken. Avoid pregnancy	Ulcerative stomatitis, leukopenia, nausea, abdominal distress, malaise, fatigue, chills, fever, dizziness, decreased resistance to infection, anemia, photosensitivity, rash, pruritus, hepatotoxicity.

Table 21.1. PRESCRIBING INFORMATION FOR DRUGS USED FOR CONNECTIVE TISSUE DISORDERS AND ORAL MUCOSAL DISEASES *(cont.)*

NAME	FORM/ STRENGTH	DOSAGE	WARNINGS/PRECAUTIONS & CONTRAINDICATIONS	ADVERSE EFFECTS†
ARTHRITIS AGENTS, NONANALGESIC *(cont.)*				
Methotrexate (Rheumatrex) *(cont.)*		to lowest effective dose. **Max:** 30mg/week. **RA: Initial:** 7.5mg PO once weekly, or 2.5mg q12h for 3 doses given as a course once weekly. **Titrate:** Gradual increase. **Max:** 20mg weekly. After response, reduce dose to lowest effective amount of drug. ***Pediatrics:*** **Meningeal Leukemia:** Dilute preservative free MTX to 1mg/mL. **<1 yr:** 6mg. **1 yr:** 8mg. **2 yrs:** 10mg. **≥3yrs:** 12mg. Give intrathecally at 2-5 day intervals. **JRA: 2-16 yrs: Initial:** 10mg/m² once weekly. Adjust dose gradually to achieve optimal response.	if either partner is receiving therapy. Avoid intrathecal administration or high-dose therapy. Injection contains benzyl alcohol; avoid use in neonates (<1 month), may cause gasping syndrome. **Contra:** Pregnant women with psoriasis or RA (should be used in treatment of pregnant women with neoplastic diseases only when potential benefit outweighs risk), nursing mothers. Psoriasis or RA patients with alcoholism, alcoholic liver disease, chronic liver disease, immunodeficiency syndromes, and pre-existing blood dyscrasias (eg, bone marrow hypoplasia, leukopenia, thrombocytopenia, significant anemia). **P/N:** Category X, contraindicated in nursing.	
Rituximab (Rituxan)	**Inj:** 10mg/mL [10mL, 50mL]	***Adults:*** **Administer only as IV infusion. Relapsed or Refractory, Low-Grade or Follicular, CD20-Positive, B-cell NHL:** 375mg/m² IV once weekly for 4 or 8 doses. **Retreatment for Relapsed or Refractory, Low-Grade or Follicular, CD20-Positive, B-cell NHL:** 375mg/m² IV once weekly for 4 doses. **Previously Untreated, Follicular, CD20-Positive, B-cell NHL:** 375mg/m² IV on Day 1 of each CVP chemotherapy cycle for up to 8 doses. **Nonprogressing, Low-Grade, CD20-Positive, B-cell NHL:** Following completion of 6-8 cycles of CVP chemotherapy, 375mg/m² IV once weekly for 4 doses at 6-month intervals to maximum of 16 doses. **Diffuse Large B-cell NHL:** 375mg/m² IV given on Day 1 of each chemotherapy cycle for up to 8 infusions. **RA:** Give with methotrexate. Administer two 1000mg IV infusions separated by 2 weeks. Give methylprednisolone 100mg IV (or equivalent) 30 min prior to each infusion to reduce incidence and severity of infusion reactions. Do not administer as IV push or bolus. For dosing as a component of Zevalin® (ibritumomab tiuxetan) please refer to PI.	**BB:** Serious, sometimes fatal, infusion reactions reported. Acute renal failure reported in the setting of tumor lysis syndrome (TLS) following treatment of non-Hodgkin's lymphoma. Severe mucocutaneous reactions reported. JC virus infection resulting in progressive multifocal leukoencephalopathy (PML) reported. **W/P:** May premedicate patients with an antihistamine and acetaminophen prior to dosing. Interrupt if severe reaction develops; may resume at a 50% rate reduction when symptoms subside. Rapid reduction in tumor volume followed by acute renal failure, hyperkalemia, hypocalcemia, hyperuricemia, or hyperphosphatemia, can occur withinin 12-24 hours after first infusion. D/C if severe mucocutaneous reaction occurs. Consider the diagnosis of PML in patients presenting with new-onset neurologic manifestations; d/c and consider reduction or discontinuation of concomitant chemotherapy or immunosuppressive therapy. HBV reactivation with fulminant hepatitis, hepatic failure, and death reported; d/c if viral hepatitis develops. Additional serious viral infections, either new, reactivated, or exacerbated, reported. Hypersensitivity reactions may respond to infusion rate adjustment and medical management. D/C if serious arrhythmias occur. Use caution with pre-existing cardiac conditions. Use with extreme caution in combination with cisplatin; renal failure may occur. Severe renal toxicity reported; d/c if SCr rises or oliguria occurs. Monitor CBC and platelets regularly; more frequently with cytopenias. Abdominal pain, bowel obstruction and perforation reported. Not recommended in patients with RA who have not had prior inadequate response to one or more TNF-antagonists. **P/N:** Category C, safety not known in nursing.	Fever, chills, infection, asthenia, nausea, lymphopenia, leukopenia, neutropenia, headache, abdominal pain, night sweats, rash, pruritus, pain.

*Scored. †Bold entries denote special dental considerations.
BB = black box warning; **W/P** = warnings/precautions; **Contra** = contraindications; **P/N** = pregnancy category rating and nursing considerations.

NAME	FORM/ STRENGTH	DOSAGE	WARNINGS/PRECAUTIONS & CONTRAINDICATIONS	ADVERSE EFFECTS†
CHELATING AGENT				
Penicillamine (Cuprimine, Depen)	**Cap:** (Cuprimine): 250mg; **Tab:** (Depen) 250mg*	***Adults:*** **Wilson's Disease:** Determine dosage by 24-hr urinary copper excretion. **Maint:** 0.75-1.5g/day for 3 months. **Max:** Up to 2g/day, based on serum free copper. **Cystinuria: Initial:** 250mg qd. **Usual:** 250mg-1g qid. **RA: Initial:** 125-250mg/day. **Titrate:** May increase by 125-250mg/day every 1-3 months. If needed after 2-3 months, increase by 250mg/day every 2-3 months. D/C if no improvement after 3-4 months at dose of 1-1.5g/day. **Maint:** 500-750mg/day. **Max:** 1.5g/day. Give on empty stomach, 1 hr before or 2 hrs after meals, and 1 hr apart from any other drug, food or milk. Supplemental pyridoxine 25mg/day recommended. ***Pediatrics:*** **Cystinuria:** 30 mg/kg/day given qid.	**BB:** Supervise closely due to toxicity, special dosage considerations and therapeutic benefits. **W/P:** Aplastic anemia, agranulocytosis, drug fever, thrombocytopenia, Goodpasture's syndrome, myasthenia gravis, pemphigus foliaceus/ vulgaris, obliterative bronchiolitis, proteinuria, hematuria allergic reactions (eg, rash), positive antinuclear antibody (ANA) test and hypogeusia reported. Perform routine urinalysis, CBC with differentials, Hgb and platelet count twice weekly for 1st month, every 2 weeks for next 5 months, then monthly. Do not use with concurrent gold therapy, antimalarial or cytotoxic drugs, oxyphenbutazone or phenylbutazone. Caution with patients allergic to penicillin. Iron deficiency may occur. Patients with Wilson's disease, rheumatoid arthritis or cystinuria should be given a daily supplement of pyridoxine. Dosage should be reduced to 250 mg/day when surgery is contemplated. **Contra:** Pregnancy (except for treatment of Wilson's disease or certain cases of cystinuria), nursing, RA patients with renal insufficiency, history of penicillamine-related aplastic anemia or agranulocytosis. **P/N:** Category D, not for use in nursing.	Rash, urticaria, anorexia, epigastric pain, N/V, diarrhea, leukopenia, thrombocytopenia, proteinuria, taste perversion, proteinuria
GOUT AGENTS				
Allopurinol (Zyloprim)	**Tab:** 100mg*, 300mg*	***Adults:*** **Gout: Initial:** 100mg/day. **Titrate:** Increase by 100mg/week until serum uric acid level is ≤6mg/dL. **Mild Gout: Usual:** 200-300mg/day. **Moderately Severe Gout: Usual:** 400-600mg/ day. **Max:** 800mg/day. **Recurrent Calcium Oxalate Stones: Usual:** 200-300mg/day. **Prevention of Uric Acid Nephropathy with Chemotherapy: Usual:** 600-800mg/day for 2-3 days with high fluid intake. **CrCl 10-20mL/ min:** 200mg/day. **CrCl <10mL/min: Max:** 100mg/day. **CrCl <3mL/min:** Also increase dosing intervals. Take after meals. Divide dose if >300mg. ***Pediatrics:*** **Hyperuricemia with Malignancies: 6-10 yrs:** 300mg/day. **<6 yrs:** 150mg/day. Evaluate response after 48 hrs. Take after meals.	**W/P:** D/C if skin rash occurs. Severe hypersensitivity reactions, hepatotoxicity, and bone marrow depression reported. Monitor LFTs during early stages of therapy with liver disease. Caution with activities that require alertness. Caution with renal impairment. Renal failure reported with hyperuricemia secondary to neoplastic diseases. Fluid intake should yield ≥2L of urinary output/day. Maintain neutral or slightly alkaline urine. Acute gout attacks increase during early stages of therapy; give colchicine. **P/N:** Category C, caution in nursing.	Acute gout attacks, rash, diarrhea, SGOT/SGPT increase, alkaline phosphatase increase, nausea.
Colchicine	**Tab:** 0.5mg, 0.6mg	***Adults:*** **Gouty Arthritis: Acute Treatment: Initial:** 1-1.2mg, followed by 0.5-0.6mg q1h, or 1-1.2mg q2h or 0.5-0.6mg q2-3h until pain relief, GI discomfort or diarrhea ensues. **Usual:** 4-8mg/attack. Wait 3 days before retreatment. **Prophylaxis: <1 attack/ yr:** 0.5-0.6mg/day given 3-4x/week. **>1 attack/yr:** 0.5-0.6mg qd. **Severe Cases:** 2-3 tabs of 0.5mg or 0.6mg daily. **Surgical Gout Prophylaxis:** 0.5-0.6mg tid 3 days before and 3 days after surgery.	**W/P:** Caution in elderly, debilitated, or with GI, renal, hepatic, cardiac, and hematologic disorders. D/C if nausea, vomiting, or diarrhea occurs. Monitor blood counts periodically with long-term therapy. May adversely affect spermatogenesis. Elevates SGOT and alkaline phosphatase. May cause false-positive for urine RBC and Hgb. **Contra:** Serious GI, renal, hepatic or cardiac disorders, and blood dyscrasias. **P/N:** Category C, caution in nursing.	Bone marrow depression, peripheral neuritis, purpura, myopathy, alopecia, dermatoses, reversible azoospermia, N/V, diarrhea.

Table 21.1. PRESCRIBING INFORMATION FOR DRUGS USED FOR CONNECTIVE TISSUE DISORDERS AND ORAL MUCOSAL DISEASES *(cont.)*

NAME	FORM/ STRENGTH	DOSAGE	WARNINGS/PRECAUTIONS & CONTRAINDICATIONS	ADVERSE EFFECTS†
GOUT AGENTS *(cont.)*				
Colchicine/ Probenecid	**Tab:** (Colchicine-Probenecid) 0.5mg-500mg	***Adults:* Gouty Arthritis: Acute Gout: Initial:** 1 tab qd for 1 week, then 1 tab bid. **Titrate:** May increase by 1 tab/day every 4 weeks. **Max:** 4 tabs/day. May reduce dose by 1 tab every 6 months if acute attacks have been absent ≥6 months. Decrease dose with gastric intolerance. **Renal Impairment:** May need to increase dose. May not be effective if CrCl ≤30mL/min.	**W/P:** Exacerbation of gout may occur. Use APAP if analgesic needed. Severe allergic reaction and anaphylaxis reported (rare). D/C if hypersensitivity occurs. Caution with peptic ulcer. Monitor for glycosuria. Determine benefit/risk ratio with long-term therapy. Maintain liberal fluid intake and alkalization of urine. **Contra:** Blood dyscrasias, uric acid kidney stones, children <2 yrs and pregnancy. Do not use in acute gout attack. **P/N:** Contraindicated in pregnancy; safety in nursing not known.	Headache, dizziness, hepatic necrosis, N/V, anorexia, **sore gums,** uric acid stones, renal colic, anaphylaxis, fever, pruritus, blood dyscrasias, peripheral neuritis, muscular weakness, abdominal pain, diarrhea, alopecia, dermatitis.
Probenecid	**Tab:** 500mg	***Adults:* Gout: Initial:** 250mg bid for 1 week. **Titrate:** May increase by 500mg every 4 weeks. **Maint:** 500mg bid. **Max:** 2g/day. May reduce by 500mg every 6 months if acute attack has been absent ≥6 months and serum urate levels are normal. **Renal Impairment: Usual:** 1g/day. **Adjunct Antibiotic Therapy:** 500mg qid. **Elderly/Renal Impairment:** Reduce dose. Decrease dose with gastric intolerance. May not be effective if CrCl ≤30mL/min. ***Pediatrics:* 2-14 yrs: Adjunct Antibiotic Therapy: Initial:** 25mg/kg. **Maint:** 10mg/kg qid. **≥50kg:** 500mg qid.	**W/P:** Initiate therapy when acute gout attack subsides. Exacerbation of gout may occur; treat with colchicine. Use APAP if analgesic needed. Severe allergic reactions and anaphylaxis reported. D/C if hypersensitivity occurs. Caution with peptic ulcer. Monitor for glycosuria. Maintain liberal fluid intake and alkalization of urine. **Contra:** Blood dyscrasias, uric acid kidney stones and children <2 yrs. Do not use in acute gout attack. **P/N:** Safety in pregnancy and nursing is not known.	Headache, acute gouty arthritis, dizziness, hepatic necrosis, N/V, anorexia, **sore gums,** nephrotic syndrome, uric acid stones, renal colic, costovertebral pain, urinary frequency, anaphylaxis, fever, urticaria, pruritus, blood dyscrasias, dermatitis, alopecia, flushing.
IMMUNOMODULATORS				
Azathioprine (Azasan)	**Tab:** 25mg*, 50mg*, 75mg*, 100mg*	***Adults:* Renal Homotransplantation: Initial:** 3-5mg/kg/day, start at time of transplant. **Maint:** 1-3mg/kg/day. **RA: Initial:** 1mg/kg/day given qd-bid. **Titrate:** Increase by 0.5mg/kg/day after 6-8 weeks, then at 4-week intervals. **Max:** 2.5mg/kg/day. **Maint:** Lowest effective dose. Decrease by 0.5mg/kg/day or 25mg/day every 4 weeks. If no response by Week 12, then consider refractory. **Renal Dysfunction:** Lower dose.	**BB:** Increased risk of neoplasia with chronic therapy. Mutagenic potential and possible hematological toxicities. **W/P:** Dose-related leukopenia, thrombocytopenia, macrocytic anemia, and severe bone marrow suppression may occur. Monitor CBCs, including platelets, weekly during the 1st month, twice monthly for the 2nd and 3rd months, then monthly or more frequently if dose/therapy changes. TPMT testing cannot substitute for CBC monitoring. Monitor for infections. **Contra:** Pregnancy in RA treatment. Previous treatment of RA with alkylating agents (eg, cyclophosphamide, chlorambucil, melphalan) may increase risk of neoplasia. **P/N:** Category D, not for use in nursing.	Leukopenia, thrombocytopenia, infections, N/V, hepatotoxicity.
Cyclosporine (Gengraf)	**Cap:** 25mg, 100mg	***Adults:* Newly Transplanted Patients: Initial:** May be given 4-12 hrs prior to transplantation or be given postoperatively. Dose varies depending on the transplanted organ and other immunosuppressive agents included in immunosuppressive protocol. **Renal Transplant:** 9±3 mg/kg/day. **Liver Transplant:** 8±4 mg/kg/day. **Heart Transplant:** 7±3 mg/kg/day. Adjunct therapy with adrenal corticosteroid recommended. **Prednisone taper: 1st 4 days:** 2mg/kg/day. **Taper to: Week 1:** 1mg/kg/day. **Week 2:** 0.6mg/kg/day. **Month 1:** 0.3mg/kg/day. **Month 2 onwards:** 0.15mg/kg/day. **Conversion**	**BB:** Only physicians with experience in the management of systemic immunosuppresive therapy for indicated disease may prescribe cyclosporine. Increase in degree of immunosuppression may increase susceptibility to infection and possible development of neoplasia (eg, lymphoma). Cyclosporine may be co-administered with other immunosuppressive agents in kidney, liver, and heart transplant patients. Monitor cyclosporine blood concentrations in transplant and rheumatoid arthritis (RA) patients to avoid toxicity. Dose adjustments should be made to minimize possible organ rejection in transplant	Renal dysfunction, HTN, cramps, hirsutism, acne, tremor, convulsions, **gum hyperplasia,** diarrhea.

*Scored. †Bold entries denote special dental considerations.
BB = black box warning; **W/P** = warnings/precautions; **Contra** = contraindications; **P/N** = pregnancy category rating and nursing considerations.

NAME	FORM/ STRENGTH	DOSAGE	WARNINGS/PRECAUTIONS & CONTRAINDICATIONS	ADVERSE EFFECTS†
Cyclsporine (Gengraf) *(cont.)*		**from Sandimmune:** Start with same daily dose as was previously with Sandimmune, (1:1 dose conversion). Should be adjusted to attain pre-conversion cyclosporine blood trough levels. **Transplant Patients with Poor Sandimmune Absorption:** May be titrated individually based on cyclosporine levels. **RA: Initial:** 2.5mg/kg/day. **Titrate:** May be increased by 0.5-0.75mg/kg/day after 8 weeks and again after 12 weeks to maximum of 4mg/kg/day. **Max:** 4mg/kg/day. D/C if no clinical response after 16 weeks of therapy, uncontrolled abnormalities, or severe abnormality. Reduce dose by 25-50% if adverse events such as HTN, elevated SrCr, or clinically significant laboratory abnormalities occur. **Psoriasis: Initial:** 2.5mg/kg/day for 4 weeks. If no significant clinical improvement occurs, may increase dosage at 2 weeks interval. **Titrate:** May increase approximately 0.5mg/kg/day to a maximum of 4mg/kg/day based on clinical response. **Max:** 4mg/kg/day. All daily dose recommendations should be given bid.	patients. Increased risk of developing skin malignancies in psoriasis patients previously treated with PUVA, MTX, or other immunosuppressive agents, UVB, coal tar, or radiation therapy. Cyclosporine may cause systemic hypertension (HTN) and nephrotoxicity. Monitor renal function for renal dysfunction, including structural kidney damage, during therapy. Gengraf and Sandimmune are not bioequivalent and cannot be used interchangeably without physician supervision. **W/P:** May cause hepatotoxicity and nephrotoxicity. Elevated SrCr and BUN levels reported. Evaluate before initiating dose adjustments in transplant patients. Reversibility of arteriolopathy reported after stopping cyclosporine or lowering dosage. May develop syndrome of thrombocytopenia and microangiopathic hemolytic anemia; may result in graft failure. Significant hyperkalemia and hyperuricemia reported, potassium-sparing diuretics should be avoided. Encephalopathy has been described in postmarketing reports. Increased risk for development of lymphomas and malignancies of the skin. Caution in elderly. Consider the risks and benefits before treatment for psoriasis patients. Patients with increased risk (abnormal renal function, uncontrolled HTN, or malignancies) should not receive cyclosporine. Cyclosporine is reported to cause convulsions with high dose methylprednisolone. May increase the risk of development of lymphomas and other malignancies. **Contra:** Renal function abnormality, uncontrolled HTN or malignancies in RA or psoriasis patients. Concomitant PUVA or UVB therapy, methotrexate or other immunosuppressive agents, coal tar or radiation therapy in psoriasis patients. **P/N:** Category C, not for use in nursing.	
Cyclosporine (Neoral)	**Cap:** 25mg, 100mg; **Sol:** 100mg/mL [50mL]	***Adults:*** **Transplant:** Give initial oral dose 4-12 hrs before transplant or post-op. Dose bid. **Initial: Renal Transplant:** 9±3mg/kg/day. **Liver Transplant:** 8±4mg/kg/day. **Heart Transplant:** 7±3mg/kg/day. Give with corticosteroids initially. **Conversion from Sandimmune:** 1:1 dose conversion. Adjust to trough levels. Monitor every 4-7 days. **RA: Initial:** 1.25mg/kg bid. **Titrate:** May increase by 0.5-0.75mg/kg/day after 8 weeks, again after 12 weeks. **Max:** 4mg/kg/day. D/C if no benefit by week 16. **Psoriasis: Initial:** 1.25mg/kg bid for 4 weeks. **Titrate:** May increase by 0.5mg/kg/day every 2 weeks. **Max:** 4mg/kg/day. Decrease dose by 25-50% to control adverse events. Take at the same time every day. Dilute sol in orange or apple juice that is room temp.	**BB:** Increased susceptibility to infection and development of neoplasia, HTN, nephrotoxicity. Monitor blood levels to avoid toxicity. Neoral is not bioequivalent to Sandimmune. Risk of skin malignancies if previously treated with PUVA, UVB, coal tar, radiation, MTX, or other immunosuppressives. **W/P:** Risk of hepatotoxicity and nephrotoxicity. Caution in elderly. Hyperkalemia, hyperuricemia, thrombocytopenia, microangiopathic hemolytic anemia and encephalopathy reported in transplant patients. Monitor SrCr after initiation or increase NSAID dose in RA. Monitor CBC, uric acid, K^+, lipids, magnesium, SrCr and BP every 2 weeks during 1st 3 months, then monthly if stable in RA. Monitor LFTs repeatedly. **Contra:** Abnormal renal function, uncontrolled HTN, malignancies. PUVA or UVB therapy, MTX, other immunosuppressants, coal tar, or radiation in psoriasis patients. **P/N:** Category C, not for use in nursing.	Renal dysfunction, HTN, hirsutism, muscle cramps, acne, tremor, headache, **gingival hyperplasia**, diarrhea, nausea, vomiting, paresthesia, flushing, dyspepsia, hypertrichosis, stomatitis, hypomagnesemia.

Table 21.1. PRESCRIBING INFORMATION FOR DRUGS USED FOR CONNECTIVE TISSUE DISORDERS AND ORAL MUCOSAL DISEASES *(cont.)*

NAME	FORM/ STRENGTH	DOSAGE	WARNINGS/PRECAUTIONS & CONTRAINDICATIONS	ADVERSE EFFECTS†
IMMUNOMODULATORS *(cont.)*				
Cyclosporine (Sandimmune)	**Cap:** 25mg, 100mg; **Inj:** 50mg/mL; **Sol:** 100mg/mL [50mL]	***Adults/Pediatrics:*** **≥ 6 months: Transplant Rejection: Initial: PO:** 15mg/kg single dose 4-12 hrs before transplant; continue same dose qd for 1-2 weeks. **Usual:** Taper by 5% per week until 5-10mg/kg/day. May mix oral solution with milk, chocolate milk, or orange juice. **IV:** 1/3 PO dose. **Initial:** 5-6mg/kg/day single dose; begin 4 to 12 hrs prior to transplantation. **Maint:** Continue single daily dose until PO forms are tolerated. Due to risk of anaphylaxis, only use injection if unable to take oral agents.	**BB:** Give with adrenal corticosteroids but not with other immunosuppressives. Increased susceptibility to infection and development of lymphoma. Sandimmune and Neoral are not bioequivalent. Monitor blood levels to avoid toxicity. **W/P:** May cause hepatotoxicity and nephrotoxicity. Convulsions, elevated SrCr and BUN levels reported. Thrombocytopenia and microangiopathic hemolytic anemia may develop. Monitor for hyperkalemia and hyperuricemia. Increases risk for development of lymphomas and other malignancies. Observe for 30 min after start of infusion and frequently thereafter. Caution with malabsorption. **Contra:** Hypersensitivity to Cremophor EL (polyoxyethylated castor oil). **P/N:** Category C, not for use in nursing.	Renal dysfunction, tremor, hirsutism, HTN, **gum hyperplasia,** glomerular capillary thrombosis, cramps, acne, convulsions, headache, diarrhea, hepatotoxity, abdominal discomfort, paresthesia, flushing.
Mycophenolate Mofetil (CellCept)	**Cap:** 250mg; **Inj:** 500mg; **Sus:** 200mg/mL [175mL]; **Tab:** 500mg	***Adults:*** **Renal Transplant:** 1g IV/PO bid. **Cardiac Transplant:** 1.5g IV/PO bid. **Hepatic Transplant:** 1g IV bid or 1.5g PO bid. Start PO as soon as possible after transplant. Start IV within 24 hrs after transplant; can continue for up to 14 days. Switch to oral when tolerated. Give on an empty stomach. ***Pediatrics:*** **3 months-18 yrs: Renal Transplant:** (Sus) 600mg/m^2 PO bid. **Max:** 2g/day (10 mL/day). (Cap) **BSA 1.25m^2 to 1.5m^2:** 750mg PO bid. (Cap/Tab) **BSA >1.5m^2:** 1g bid.	**BB:** Immunosuppression may lead to increased susceptibility to infection and possible development of lymphoma. Female users of childbearing potential must use contraception. Mycophenolate mofetil use during pregnancy associated with increased risk of pregnancy loss and congenital malformations. **W/P:** Risk of lymphomas and other malignancies, especially of the skin. Avoid sunlight to decrease risk of skin cancer. May cause fetal harm during pregnancy. Must have negative serum/urine pregnancy test within 1 week before therapy. Two reliable forms of contraception required before and during therapy, and 6 weeks following discontinuation. Monitor for bone marrow suppression. Risk of GI ulceration, hemorrhage and perforation; caution with active digestive system disease. Caution with delayed renal graft function post-transplant. Oral suspension contains phenylalanine; caution with phenylketonurics. Monitor CBC weekly during the 1st month, twice monthly for the 2nd and 3rd months, and then monthly through 1st year. Avoid with rare hereditary deficiency of hypoxanthine-guanine phosphoribosyltransferase (eg, Lesch-Nyhan and Kelley-Seegmiller syndrome). Increased susceptibility infections/sepsis. **Contra:** (Inj) Hypersensitivity to Polysorbate 80 (TWEEN). **P/N:** Category D, not for use in nursing.	Infections, diarrhea, leukopenia, sepsis, vomiting, GI bleeding, pain, abdominal pain, fever, headache, asthenia, chest pain, back pain, anemia, thrombocytopenia.
Thalidomide (Thalomid)	**Cap:** 50mg, 100mg, 200mg	***Adults/Pediatrics:*** **≥12 yrs: Acute Erythema Nodosum Leprosum (ENL): Initial:** 100-300mg qhs with water at least 1 hr after evening meal. **<50kg:** Start therapy at lower end of dosing range. **Severe Cutaneous ENL: Initial:** 400mg qhs or in divided doses with water at least 1 hr after meal(s). Use with corticosteroids in moderate to severe neuritis with severe ENL. Taper steroid when neuritis is ameliorated.	**BB:** Severe, life-threatening human birth defects if taken during pregnancy. Women of childbearing potential should have a pregnancy test before starting therapy, then weekly for first month, and monthly thereafter. Males must use latex condoms during sexual contact with females of childbearing potential. Effective contraception must be used 4 weeks before, during and 4 weeks after therapy. Only prescribers and pharmacists	Drowsiness, somnolence, peripheral neuropathy, dizziness, orthostatic hypotension, neutropenia, increased HIV viral load, rash, constipation, hypocalcemia, thrombosis/embolism, dyspnea.

†Bold entries denote special dental considerations.
BB = black box warning; **W/P** = warnings/precautions; **Contra** = contraindications; **P/N** = pregnancy category rating and nursing considerations.

NAME	FORM/ STRENGTH	DOSAGE	WARNINGS/PRECAUTIONS & CONTRAINDICATIONS	ADVERSE EFFECTS†
Thalidomide (Thalomid) *(cont.)*		Duration of therapy is usually 2 weeks. **Taper Dose:** Decrease by 50mg every 2-4 weeks. **Maintenance Therapy for Prevention/Suppression of ENL Recurrence:** Use minimum dose to control reaction. **Taper Dose:** Every 3-6 months, attempt to decrease dose by 50mg every 2-4 weeks. **Multiple Myeloma:** 200mg qhs at least 1 hr after evening meal. Give with dexamethasone in 28-day treatment cycles.	registered with the S.T.E.P.S.® distribution program can prescribe and dispense. The use of thalidomide in multiple myeloma results in an increased risk of venous thromboembolic events (eg, DVT, PE). **W/P:** If hypersensitivity reaction occurs such as rash, fever or tachycardia; d/c drug. Stevens-Johnson syndrome and toxic epidermal necrolysis reported. May cause severe birth defects. Drowsiness and somnolence reported; caution when operating machinery. May cause neuropathy; monitor for symptoms. If symptoms of neuropathy arise, d/c immediately. Do not initiate if ANC <750/mm^3. Measure viral load of HIV patients after 1st and 3rd month of therapy and every 3 months thereafter. **Contra:** Women of childbearing potential unless alternative therapies are considered inappropriate and if precautions are taken to avoid pregnancy. Sexually mature males unless they comply with the S.T.E.P.S.® program and mandatory contraceptive measures. **P/N:** Category X, not for use in nursing.	
IMMUNOMODULATORS, TOPICAL				
Pimecrolimus (Elidel)	**Cre:** 1% [30g, 60g, 100g]	***Adults/Pediatrics:* ≥2 yrs:** Apply bid. Re-evaluate if symptoms persist after 6 weeks.	**W/P:** Increased risk of varicella zoster infection, herpes simplex virus infection or eczema herpeticum. Lymphadenopathy reported; d/c if unknown etiology of lymphadenopathy or acute mononucleosis presents. Skin papilloma or warts reported; consider discontinuation if worsening or unresponsive skin papilloma. Minimize or avoid natural or artificial sunlight exposure. Avoid with Netherton's syndrome, areas of active cutaneous viral infections, or occlusive dressings. Long-term safety has not been established. Rare cases of malignancy (eg, skin and lymphoma) reported with topical calcineurin inhibitors; therefore, continuous long-term use should be avoided and application limited to areas of involvement. Not indicated for use in children <2 yrs. **P/N:** Category C, not for use in nursing.	Application-site burning, headache, nasopharyngitis, influenza, **pharyngitis,** viral infection, pyrexia, **cough,** skin discoloration.
Tacrolimus (Protopic)	**Oint:** 0.03%, 0.1% [30g, 60g, 100g]	***Adults/Pediatrics:* ≥16 yrs:** (0.03% or 0.1%) Apply thin layer bid. Rub in gently. Stop use when signs and symptoms resolve. ***Pediatrics:* 2-15 yrs:** (0.03%) Apply thin layer bid. Rub in gently. Stop use when signs and symptoms resolve.	**W/P:** Do not use with occlusive dressings. Increased risk of varicella zoster, herpes simplex, or eczema herpeticum. Lymphadenopathy reported; monitor closely. D/C if unknown etiology of lymphadenopathy or presence of acute infectious mononucleosis. Avoid in Netherton's syndrome. Minimize or avoid exposure to natural or artificial sunlight. Long-term safety not established. Rare cases of malignancy (eg, skin, lymphoma) reported with topical calcineurin inhibitors; therefore, continuous long-term use should be avoided and application limited to areas of involvement. Should not use in immunocompromised adults and children. Caution in patients predisposed to renal impairment. **P/N:** Category C, not for use in nursing.	Skin burning, pruritus, flu-like symptoms, allergic reaction, skin erythema, headache, skin infection, fever, herpes simplex, rhinitis.

Table 21.1. PRESCRIBING INFORMATION FOR DRUGS USED FOR CONNECTIVE TISSUE DISORDERS AND ORAL MUCOSAL DISEASES *(cont.)*

NAME	FORM/ STRENGTH	DOSAGE	WARNINGS/PRECAUTIONS & CONTRAINDICATIONS	ADVERSE EFFECTS†
RETINOID				
Isotretinoin (Accutane)	**Cap:** 10mg, 20mg, 40mg	***Adults/Pediatrics:*** **≥12 yrs: Acne: Initial/Usual:** 0.5-1mg/kg/day given bid for 15-20 weeks. **Max:** 2mg/kg/day (for very serious cases). Adjust for side effects and disease response. May d/c if nodule count reduced by >70% prior to completion. Repeat only if necessary after 2 months off drug. Take with food.	**BB:** Not for use by females who are or may become pregnant, or if breastfeeding. Birth defects have been documented. Increased risk of spontaneous abortion, and premature births reported. Approved for marketing only under special restricted distribution program called iPLEDGE™. Must have 2 negative pregnancy tests. Repeat pregnancy test monthly. Use 2 forms of contraception at least 1 month prior, during, and 1 month following discontinuation. Must fill written prescriptions within 7 days; refills require new prescriptions. May dispense maximum of 1 month supply. Prescriber, dispensing pharmacy, and patient must be registered with iPLEDGE. **W/P:** Acute pancreatitis, impaired hearing, anaphylactic reactions, inflammatory bowel disease, elevated TG and LFTs, hepatotoxicity, premature epiphyseal closure, and hyperostosis reported. May cause depression, psychosis, aggressive and/or violent behaviors, rarely suicidal ideation/attempts and suicide; may need further evaluation after discontinuation. May cause decreased night vision, and corneal opacities. Associated with pseudotumor cerebri. Check lipids before therapy, and then at intervals until response established (within 4 weeks). D/C if significant decrease in WBC, hearing or visual impairment, abdominal pain, rectal bleeding, or severe diarrhea occurs. Monitor LFTs before therapy, weekly or biweekly until response established. May develop musculoskeletal symptoms. Avoid prolonged UV rays or sunlight, and donating blood up to 1 month after discontinuing therapy. Caution with genetic predisposition for age-related osteoporosis, history of childhood osteoporosis, osteomalacia, other bone metabolism disorders (eg, anorexia nervosa). Spontaneous osteoporosis, osteopenia, bone fractures, and delayed fracture healing reported; caution in sports with repetitive impact. Use 2 forms of effective contraception for 1 month. Female patients of childbearing potential must fill and pick up the prescription within 7 days of the date of specimen collection for the pregnancy test. Must only be dispensed in no more than 30-day supply and with a Medication Guide. **Contra:** Pregnancy, paraben sensitivity (preservative in gelatin cap). **P/N:** Category X, not for use in nursing.	**Cheilitis,** dry skin and mucous membranes, conjunctivitis, blood dyscrasias, epistaxis, decreased HDL, elevated cholesterol and TG, elevated blood sugar, arthralgias, back pain, hearing/ vision impairment, rash, photosensitivity reactions, psychiatric disorders, abnormal menses, cardiovascular disorders.
MISCELLANEOUS CARDIOVASCULAR AGENTS				
Epoprostenol (Flolan)	**Inj:** 0.5mg, 1.5mg	***Adults:*** **PAH/PAH with Scleroderma: Initial:** 2ng/kg/min IV chronic infusion. **Titrate:** Increase by 2ng/kg/min every 15 min until no further increases are clinically warranted. May use a lower initial infusion rate if not tolerated.	**W/P:** Abrupt withdrawal or large dose reductions may result in symptoms associated with rebound pulmonary HTN (eg, dyspnea, dizziness, and asthenia); avoid abrupt withdrawal. Unless contraindicated, administer anticoagulant therapy to reduce risk of pulmonary	Flushing, headache, N/V, hypotension, anxiety, nervousness, agitation, chest pain, dizziness, bradycardia, abdominal pain.

†Bold entries denote special dental considerations.
BB = black box warning; **W/P** = warnings/precautions; **Contra** = contraindications; **P/N** = pregnancy category rating and nursing considerations.

NAME	FORM/ STRENGTH	DOSAGE	WARNINGS/PRECAUTIONS & CONTRAINDICATIONS	ADVERSE EFFECTS†
Epoprostenol (Flolan) *(cont.)*			thromboembolism or systemic embolism through a patent foramen ovale. Monitor standing and supine BP and HR for several hours after dose adjustments. **Contra:** Chronic use in CHF due to left ventricular systolic dysfunction, chronic therapy in patients who develop pulmonary edema during dose initiation. **P/N:** Category B, caution in nursing.	
Pentoxifylline (Trental)	**Tab:** 400mg	***Adults:*** **Intermittent Claudication:** 400mg tid with meals for at least 8 weeks. Reduce to 400mg bid if digestive and CNS side effects occur; d/c if side effects persist.	**W/P:** Monitor Hgb and Hct with risk factors complicated by hemorrhage (eg, recent surgery, peptic ulceration, cerebral/retinal bleeding). Occasional reports of angina, hypotension, and arrhythmia in patients with concurrent coronary artery and cerebrovascular diseases. **P/N:** Category C, not for use in nursing.	Bloating, dyspepsia, N/V, dizziness, headache.
MISCELLANEOUS DENTAL/PERIODONTAL AGENTS				
Cevimeline HCl (Evoxac)	**Cap:** 30mg	***Adults:*** **Dry Mouth in Sjogren's Syndrome:** 30mg tid.	**W/P:** May alter cardiac conduction and/or HR; caution with angina or MI. Potential to increase airway resistance, bronchial smooth muscle tone, and bronchial secretions; caution with controlled asthma, chronic bronchitis or COPD. Toxicity characterized by exaggerated parasympathomimetic effects (eg, headache, visual disturbance, lacrimation, sweating, respiratory distress, GI spasm, N/V, cardiac abnormalities, mental confusion, tremors). Caution with history of nephrolithiasis, cholelithiasis. Ophthalmic formulations decrease visual acuity; caution while night driving or hazardous activities in reduced lighting. Risk of cholecystitis. **Contra:** Uncontrolled asthma, when miosis is undesirable (eg, acute iritis, narrow-angle glaucoma). **P/N:** Category C, caution in nursing.	Excessive sweating, nausea, rhinitis, diarrhea, cough, sinusitis, upper respiratory infection.
Pilocarpine (Salagen)	**Tab:** 5mg, 7.5mg	***Adults:*** **Cancer Patients: Initial:** 5mg tid. **Usual:** 15-30mg/day for 12 weeks. **Max:** 10mg/dose. **Sjogren's Syndrome: Usual:** 5mg qid for 6 weeks.	**W/P:** Caution with significant cardiovascular disease, night driving, performing hazardous activities in reduced lighting, cholelithiasis, biliary tract disease, controlled asthma, chronic bronchitis, or COPD requiring pharmacotherapy. Monitor for toxicity and dehydration. May cause renal colic. Possible dose-related CNS effects. **Contra:** Uncontrolled asthma, when miosis is undesirable (eg, acute iritis, narrow-angle glaucoma). **P/N:** Category C, not for use in nursing.	

Table 21.2. DRUG INTERACTIONS FOR DRUGS USED FOR CONNECTIVE TISSUE DISORDERS AND ORAL MUCOSAL DISEASES

ANTIBIOTIC	
Dapsone	
Folic acid antagonists	Folic acid antagonists (eg, pyrimethamine) may increase hematologic reactions.
Rifampin	Rifampin may accelerate metabolism of dapsone.
Trimethoprim	Dapsone may increase levels of trimethoprim; trimethoprim may increase levels of dapsone.
ANTIMALARIAL AGENT	
Hydroxychloroquine Sulfate (Plaquenil)	
Hepatotoxic drugs	Caution with hepatotoxic drugs.
ARTHRITIS AGENTS, NONANALGESIC	
Abatacept (Orencia)	
Biologic RA therapy	Concomitant use with other biologic RA therapy (eg, anakinra) is not recommeneded.
Blood glucose monitors	May cause falsely elevated blood glucose readings on the day of infusion.
TNF antagonists	Concomitant use is not recommeneded due to increased risk of infection with no apparent benefit.
Vaccines, live	Live vaccines should be avoided during treatment and for 3 months following discontinuation.
Auranofin (Ridaura)	
Phenytoin	May increase phenytoin levels.
Etanercept (Enbrel)	
Anakinra	Concomitant use with anakinra may increase the risk of serious infections and neutropenia.
Cyclophosphamide	Concomitant use with cyclophosphamide is not recommended.
Sulfasalazine	Concomitant use with sulfasalazine may lead to a mild decrease in neutrophil count.
Vaccines, live	Live vaccines should be avoided.
Infliximab (Remicade)	
6-Mercaptopurine	Hepatosplenic T-cell lymphomas (HSTCL) have been reported in patients treated with etanercept and azathioprine or 6-mercaptopurine.
Anakinra	Concomitant use with anakinra may increase the risk of serious infections and neutropenia.
Azathioprine	Hepatosplenic T-cell lymphomas (HSTCL) have been reported in patients treated with etanercept and azathioprine or 6-mercaptopurine.
Vaccines, live	Live vaccines should be avoided.
Methotrexate (Rheumatrex)	
Folic acid	May decrease response to MTX.
GI flora, drugs altering	May decrease intestinal absorption or disrupt enterohepatic recirculation.

Table 21.2. DRUG INTERACTIONS FOR DRUGS USED FOR CONNECTIVE TISSUE DISORDERS AND ORAL MUCOSAL DISEASES *(cont.)*

ARTHRITIS AGENTS, NONANALGESIC *(cont.)*	
Methotrexate (Rheumatrex) *(cont.)*	
Hepatotoxic drugs	Caution with hepatotoxic drugs (eg, azathioprine, retinoids, sulfasalazine).
NSAIDs	Concomitant use of some NSAIDs with high-dose MTX may cause severe (sometimes fatal) bone marrow suppression, aplastic anemia, and GI toxicity. Caution should be used when NSAIDs and salicylates are administered concomitantly with lower doses of MTX. These drugs may increase and prolong levels and enhance MTX toxicity.
Penicillins	May reduce the renal clearance of MTX; concomitant use should be carefully monitored.
Probenecid	Caution with probenecid; renal tubular transport is diminished.
Protein bound, drugs highly	Caution with highly protein-bound drugs (eg, salicylates, phenylbutazone, phenytoin, sulfonamides) which may increase toxicity.
Radiation therapy	Radiotherapy may increase the risk of soft tissue necrosis and osteonecrosis.
Theophylline	May decrease clearance of theophylline.
TMP-SMX	TMP-SMX has been rarely reported to increase bone marrow suppression.
Vaccines, live	Live vaccines should be avoided.
Rituximab (Rituxan)	
Biologic RA therapy	Monitor closely for signs of infection if biologic agents are used concomitantly.
Cisplatin	Concomitant use of cisplatin may potentiate renal toxicity.
DMARDs	Monitor closely for signs of infection if DMARDs are used concomitantly.
CHELATING AGENT	
Penicillamine (Cuprimine, Depen)	
Antacids	Space dosing of antacids by at least 1 hour.
Antimalarial agents	Hematologic and renal adverse reactions increase with antimalarial agents.
Cytotoxic agents	Hematologic and renal adverse reactions increase with cytotoxic agents.
Gold therapy	Hematologic and renal adverse reactions increase with gold therapy.
Iron, oral	Orally administered iron reduces the effect of penicillamine; separate dose by 2 hours.
Mineral supplements	Avoid the use of mineral supplements, which may block the response to penicillamine.
Oxyphenbutazone	Hematologic and renal adverse reactions increase with oxyphenbutazone.
Phenylbutazone	Hematologic and renal adverse reactions increase with phenylbutazone.
Zinc	Space dosing of zinc by at least 1 hour.
GOUT AGENTS	
Allopurinol (Zyloprim)	
Amoxicillin	An increase in the frequency of skin rash has been reported in patients taking amoxicillin.

GOUT AGENTS *(cont.)*

Allopurinol (Zyloprim) *(cont.)*	
Ampicillin	An increase in the frequency of skin rash has been reported in patients taking ampicillin.
Azathioprine	Reduce dose of azathioprine to approximately 1/3 to 1/4 of usual dose; base further dose adjustments on therapeutic response and the appearance of toxic effects.
Chlorpropamide	May prolong the half-life of chlorpropamide by competing for excretion by the renal tubules.
Cyclophosphamide	Enhances bone marrow suppression by cyclophosphamide in patients with neoplastic disease (except leukemia).
Cyclosporine	May increase levels of cyclosporine; monitor effects and consider dose adjustment.
Cytotoxic agents	Enhances bone marrow suppression by cytotoxic agents in patients with neoplastic disease (except leukemia).
Dicumarol	Prolongs the half-life of dicumarol.
Mercaptopurine	Reduce dose of mercaptopurine to approximately 1/3 to 1/4 of usual dose; base further dose adjustments on therapeutic response and the appearance of toxic effects.
Sulfinpyrazone	Caution with sulfinpyrazone
Thiazides	Increased toxicity with thiazide diuretics; monitor renal function.
Uricosuric agents	Uricosuric agents may decrease effects; the use of uricosuric agents and allopurinol both together and separately may result in the formation of kidney stones.
Colchicine	
Acidifying agents	Acidifying agents inhibit the effects of colchicine.
Alkalinizing agents	Alkalinizing agents potentiate the effects of colchicine.
CNS depressants	Colchicine potentiates the effects of CNS depressants.
Sympathomimetics	Colchicine potentiates the effects of sympathomimetics.
Colchicine/Probenecid	
	Refer to the interactions under each individual drug entry.
Probenecid	
Acetaminophen (APAP)	Increases the half-life of APAP.
β-Lactams	Probenecid increases plasma levels of penicillin and other ß-lactams; psychic disturbances reported.
Indomethacin	Increases the half-life of indomethacin.
Ketoprofen	Increases the half-life of ketoprofen.
Lorazepam	Increases the half-life of lorazepam.
Meclofenamate	Increases the half-life of meclofenamate.
Methotrexate (MTX)	Increases plasma levels of MTX.

Table 21.2. DRUG INTERACTIONS FOR DRUGS USED FOR CONNECTIVE TISSUE DISORDERS AND ORAL MUCOSAL DISEASES *(cont.)*

GOUT AGENTS *(cont.)*	
Probenecid *(cont.)*	
Naproxen	Increases the half-life of naproxen.
Pyrazinamide	Pyrazinamide antagonizes the uricosuric effects of probenecid.
Rifampin	Increases the half-life of rifampin.
Salicylates	Salicylates antagonize the uricosuric effects of probenecid.
Sulfonylureas	May prolong or enhance the action of oral sulfonylureas and thereby increase the risk of hypoglycemia.
Sulindac	Increases the levels of sulindac; sulindac slightly reduces the uricosuric effects of probenecid.
Theophylline	Falsely high plasma levels of theophylline have been reported when taken with probenecid.
Thiopental	Patients on probenecid reportedly require significantly less thiopental for induction of anesthesia.
IMMUNOMODULATORS	
Azathioprine (Azasan)	
ACE inhibitors	ACE inhibitors may induce anemia and severe leukopenia.
Allopurinol	Allopurinol inhibits the inactivation of azathioprine; reduce dose of azathioprine to 1/3 to 1/4 of the normal dose.
Aminosalicylate derivatives	Caution with aminosalicylate derivatives (eg, sulfasalazine, mesalamine, olsalazine); aminosalicylates inhibit the TPMT enzyme.
Leukocyte production, drugs affecting	Drugs affecting leukocyte production (eg, cotrimoxazole) may exaggerate leukopenia.
Warfarin	May inhibit the anticoagulant effect of warfarin.
Cyclosporine (Gengraf, Neoral, Sandimmune)	
ACE inhibitors	Caution with ACE inhibitors due to potential hyperkalemia.
Allopurinol	Allopurinol may increase levels; proper dose adjustment should be made.
Amiodarone	Amiodarone may increase levels; proper dose adjustment should be made.
Amphotericin B	Concomitant use of amphotericin B may potentiate renal dysfunction.
Angiotensin II receptor blockers	Caution with angiotensin II receptor blockers due to potential hyperkalemia.
Azapropazon	Concomitant use of azapropazon may potentiate renal dysfunction.
Azithromycin	Azithromycin may increase levels; proper dose adjustment should be made.
Bromocriptine	Bromocriptine may increase levels; proper dose adjustment should be made.
Carbamazepine	Carbamazepine may decrease levels; proper dose adjustment should be made.
Cimetidine	Concomitant use of cimetidine may potentiate renal dysfunction.
Ciprofloxacin	Concomitant use of ciprofloxacin may potentiate renal dysfunction.
Clarithromycin	Clarithromycin may increase levels; proper dose adjustment should be made.

IMMUNOMODULATORS *(cont.)*

Cyclosporine (Gengraf, Neoral, Sandimmune) *(cont.)*	
Colchicine	Concomitant use of colchicine may potentiate renal dysfunction. Colchicine may increase levels; proper dose adjustment should be made. Cyclosporine may reduce the clearance of colchicine, enhancing its toxic effects (eg, myopathy, neuropathy).
Contraceptives, oral	Oral contraceptives may increase levels; proper dose adjustment should be made.
Danazol	Danazol may increase levels; proper dose adjustment should be made.
Diclofenac	Increases the levels of diclofenac; concomitant use of diclofenac may potentiate renal dysfunction.
Digoxin	May reduce the clearance of digoxin, leading to toxicity.
Diltiazem	Diltiazem may increase levels; proper dose adjustment should be made.
Diuretics, potassium-sparing	Should not be used with K^+-sparing diuretics because hyperkalemia can occur.
Erythromycin	Erythromycin may increase levels; proper dose adjustment should be made.
Fibric acid derivatives	Concomitant use of fibric acid derivatives (eg, bezafibrate, fenofibrate) may potentiate renal dysfunction.
Fluconazole	Fluconazole may increase levels; proper dose adjustment should be made.
Gentamicin	Concomitant use of gentamicin may potentiate renal dysfunction.
Grapefruit	Grapefruit may increase levels and should be avoided.
HMG-CoA reductase inhibitors (statins)	May reduce the clearance of statins. Cases of myotoxicity (eg, muscle pain and weakness, myositis, rhabdomyolysis) reported with concomitant administration with lovastatin, simvastatin, atorvastatin, pravastatin, fluvastatin (rare).
Imatinib	Imatinib may increase levels; proper dose adjustment should be made.
Immunosuppressants	Concomitant use of immunosuppressants in psoriasis patients should be avoided.
Itraconazole	Itraconazole may increase levels; proper dose adjustment should be made.
Ketoconazole	Concomitant use of ketoconazole may potentiate renal dysfunction. Ketoconazole may increase levels; proper dose adjustment should be made.
Melphalan	Concomitant use of melphalan may potentiate renal dysfunction.
Methotrexate (MTX)	Inhibits the metabolism of MTX.
Methylprednisolone	Methylprednisolone may increase levels; proper dose adjustment should be made. Convulsions have been reported with high-dose methylprednisolone.
Metoclopramide	Metoclopramide may increase levels; proper dose adjustment should be made.
Nafcillin	Nafcillin may decrease levels; proper dose adjustment should be made.
Naproxen	Concomitant use of naproxen may potentiate renal dysfunction.
Nicardipine	Nicardipine may increase levels; proper dose adjustment should be made.
Nifedipine	Frequent gingivial hyperplasia has been reported with nifedipine.

Table 21.2. DRUG INTERACTIONS FOR DRUGS USED FOR CONNECTIVE TISSUE DISORDERS AND ORAL MUCOSAL DISEASES *(cont.)*

IMMUNOMODULATORS *(cont.)*

Cyclosporine (Gengraf, Neoral, Sandimmune) *(cont.)*	
NSAIDs	Concomitant use of NSAIDs may potentiate renal dysfunction.
Octreotide	Octreotide may decrease levels; proper dose adjustment should be made.
Orlistat	Orlistat may decrease the absorption of cyclosporine.
Phenobarbital	Phenobarbital may decrease levels; proper dose adjustment should be made.
Phenytoin	Phenytoin may decrease levels; proper dose adjustment should be made.
Prednisolone	May reduce the clearance of prednisolone.
Protease inhibitors	Caution with protease inhibitors; concomitant use may lead to an increase in cyclosporine levels.
Quinupristin/dalfopristin	Quinupristin/dalfopristin may increase levels; proper dose adjustment should be made.
Radiation therapy	Concomitant use of radiation therapy (eg, PUVA, UVB) in psoriasis patients should be avoided.
Ranitidine	Concomitant use of ranitidine may potentiate renal dysfunction.
Rifabutin	Caution with rifabutin; concomitant use may lead to a decrease in cyclosporine levels.
Rifampin	Rifampin may decrease levels; proper dose adjustment should be made.
Sirolimus	Concomitant use of sirolimus may lead to an increase in SCr; cyclosporine significantly increases levels of sirolimus.
St. John's wort	St. John's wort significantly decreases cyclosporine levels.
Sulfinpyrazone	Sulfinpyrazone may decrease levels; proper dose adjustment should be made.
Sulindac	Concomitant use of sulindac may potentiate renal dysfunction.
Tacrolimus	Concomitant use of tacrolimus may potentiate renal dysfunction.
Terbinafine	Terbinafine may decrease levels; proper dose adjustment should be made.
Ticlopidine	Ticlopidine may decrease levels; proper dose adjustment should be made.
TMP-SMX	Concomitant use of trimethoprim-sulfamethoxazole may potentiate renal dysfunction.
Tobramycin	Concomitant use of tobramycin may potentiate renal dysfunction.
Vaccines, live	Live vaccines should be avoided.
Vancomycin	Concomitant use of vancomycin may potentiate renal dysfunction.
Verapamil	Verapamil may increase levels; proper dose adjustment should be made.
Mycophenolate Mofetil (CellCept)	
Acyclovir	Concomitant use may lead to an increase in both mycophenolate mofetil and acyclovir levels.
Antacids, aluminum- and magnesium-containing	Antacids containing aluminum or magnesium hydroxides may decrease levels; separate administration.
Azathioprine	Avoid concomitant use due to possible additive bone marrow suppression.

IMMUNOMODULATORS *(cont.)*

Mycophenolate Mofetil (CellCept) *(cont.)*	
Cholestyramine	Drugs that interfere with enterohepatic recirculation (eg, cholestyramine) reduce efficacy. Concomitant use is not recommended.
Contraceptives, oral	Caution with oral contraceptives; additional birth control methods should be considered.
Ganciclovir	Concomitant use may lead to an increase in both mycophenolate mofetil and ganciclovir levels.
Immunosuppressants	Efficacy/safety with other immunosuppressive agents not determined.
Metronidazole	The combination of norfloxacin and metronidazole may decrease levels of mycophenolate mofetil; metronidazole given alone has no interaction.
Norfloxacin	The combination of norfloxacin and metronidazole may decrease levels of mycophenolate mofetil; norfloxacin given alone has no interaction.
Phosphate binders, calcium-free	Calcium-free phosphate binders (eg, sevelamer) may decrease absorption; administer 2 hours after mycophenolate mofetil dose.
Probenecid	May increase levels with probenecid.
Rifampin	May decrease levels; concomitant use should be avoided unless benefits outweigh risks.
Tubular secretion, drugs inhibiting	Drugs that inhibit tubular secretion (eg, probenecid) may increase levels.
Vaccines, live attenuated	Live attenuated vaccines should be avoided.
Valacyclovir	Concomitant use may lead to an increase in both mycophenolate mofetil and valacyclovir levels.
Valganciclovir	Concomitant use may lead to an increase in both mycophenolate mofetil and valganciclovir levels.
Thalidomide (Thalomid)	
Alcohol	May enhance sedative activity of alcohol.
Barbiturates	May enhance sedative activity of barbiturates.
Chlorpromazine	May enhance sedative activity of chlorpromazine.
Peripheral neuropathy, drugs causing	Caution with drugs associated with peripheral neuropathy.
Reserpine	May enhance sedative activity of reserpine.

IMMUNOMODULATORS, TOPICAL

Pimecrolimus (Elidel)	
CYP3A4 inhibitors	Caution with CYP3A4 inhibitors (eg, erythromycin, itraconazole, ketoconazole, fluconazole, CCBs, cimetidine) in widespread and/or erythrodermic disease.
Tacrolimus (Protopic)	
CYP3A4 inhibitors	Caution with CYP3A4 inhibitors (eg, erythromycin, itraconazole, ketoconazole, fluconazole, CCBs, cimetidine) in widespread and/or erythrodermic disease.

Table 21.2. DRUG INTERACTIONS FOR DRUGS USED FOR CONNECTIVE TISSUE DISORDERS AND ORAL MUCOSAL DISEASES *(cont.)*

IMMUNOMODULATORS, TOPICAL *(cont.)*	
Tacrolimus (Protopic) *(cont.)*	
Immunosuppressants	Concomitant use of systemic immunosuppressants in transplant patients increases the risk for lymphoma.
RETINOID	
Isotretinoin (Accutane)	
Alcohol	Limit alcohol consumption.
Contraceptives	Pregnancy reported with oral and injectable/implantable contraceptives. Avoid pregnancy with isotretinoin.
Corticosteroids	Caution with drugs that cause drug-induced osteoporosis/osteomalacia and affect vitamin D metabolism (eg, corticosteroids).
Phenytoin	Caution with drugs that cause drug-induced osteoporosis/osteomalacia and affect vitamin D metabolism (eg, phenytoin).
St. John's wort	Avoid St. John's wort with concomitant oral contraceptives due to pregnancy risk during treatment with isotretinoin. Avoid pregnancy with isotretinoin.
Tetracyclines	Avoid use with tetracyclines; increased incidence of pseudotumor cerebri.
Vitamin A	Avoid vitamin A.
MISCELLANEOUS CARDIOVASCULAR AGENTS	
Epoprostenol (Flolan)	
Anticoagulants	May increase risk of bleeding with anticoagulants.
Antihypertensives	Potentiates blood pressure reduction with antihypertensives.
Antiplatelets	May increase risk of bleeding with antiplatelets.
Diuretics	Potentiates blood pressure reduction with diuretics.
Vasodilators	Potentiates blood pressure reduction with other vasodilators.
Pentoxifylline (Trental)	
Antihypertensives	May increase effects of antihypertensives.
Theophylline	May increase theophylline levels; risk of theophylline toxicity.
Warfarin	Increased risk of bleeding; monitor PT/INR more frequently.
MISCELLANEOUS DENTAL/PERIODONTAL AGENTS	
Cevimeline HCl (Evoxac)	
Antimuscarinics	May interfere with the desired effects of antimuscarinics.
β-Blockers	Caution with β-blockers due to possible conduction disturbances.
CYP2D6 inhibitors	CYP2D6 inhibitors may increase cevimeline levels.
CYP3A3 inhibitors	CYP3A3 inhibitors may increase cevimeline levels.
CYP3A4 inhibitors	CYP3A4 inhibitors (eg, erythromycin, clarithromycin, indinavir, ritonavir) may increase cevimeline levels.

MISCELLANEOUS DENTAL/PERIODONTAL AGENTS *(cont.)*

Cevimeline HCl (Evoxac) *(cont.)*	
Parasympathomimetics	May enhance effects of parasympathomimetics.
Pilocarpine (Salagen)	
Anticholinergics	May antagonize anticholinergic agents.
β-Adrenergic antagonists	Caution with β-adrenergic antagonists.
Parasympathomimetics	Possible additive effects with parasympathomimetics.

Chapter 22

Skeletal Muscle Relaxants

Lida Radfar D.D.S., M.S.; Lakshmanan Suresh, D.D.S., M.S.

Skeletal muscle relaxants have a myriad of indications in dentistry. They may be used to reduce facial pain from muscle spasms associated with temporomandibular disorders and trismus after dental or oral surgical procedures. In addition, centrally acting muscle relaxants such as benzodiazepines are commonly used as antianxiety agents for patients undergoing dental procedures.

Muscle relaxants are divided into two major therapeutic groups: neuromuscular blockers and spasmolytics. Neuromuscular blockers are peripherally acting agents used primarily in combination with general anesthetics to induce muscle relaxation and, thus, provide an optimal surgical working condition. Spasmolytics are centrally acting agents used to reduce spasticity in a variety of neurologic conditions such as cerebral palsy, inflammation, and multiple sclerosis. Drugs within this class of muscle relaxants also are commonly used for antianxiety effects and to induce amnesia. The skeletal muscles are innervated by large myelinated nerve fibers that originate in the large motor neurons of the spinal cord. The nerve ending joins the muscle at the neuromuscular junction. When the action potential in the nerve reaches the nerve terminal, a neurotransmitter is released. In the case of skeletal muscle, the neurotransmitter is acetylcholine. Acetylcholine is released into the synaptic cleft, which allows it to bind to its receptor on the muscle membrane. This binding results in a conformational change that increases the permeability of the muscle terminal to potassium and sodium ions, leading to skeletal muscle contraction. The released acetylcholine is removed from the end plate by diffusion and rapid enzymatic destruction by acetylcholinesterase.

NEUROMUSCULAR BLOCKERS

Neuromuscular blocking agents are used to produce paralysis and are structurally similar to acetylcholine. These drugs can be divided into depolarizing and nondepolarizing agents. Neuromuscular blocking agents are potentially hazardous medications and should be administered only by highly trained clinicians in a setting where respiratory and cardiovascular resuscitation are immediately available; therefore, they are not used routinely in the dental office.

This chapter provides a summary of neuromuscular blocking agents; however, these drugs are to be used only by clinicians trained in sedation and general anesthesia. Those administering any kind of general anesthetic or sedative should be well-versed in the drug's applications and contraindications. This text is not intended to be comprehensive in terms of information on sedative/general anesthetic agents. General prescribing information for these drugs can be found in **Appendix L**; for more specific details, consult anesthesia texts.

Depolarizing Neuromuscular Blockers

Succinylcholine is an example of a depolarizing neuromuscular blocker and is the only one used clinically. It provides rapid induction of paralysis to facilitate intubation of the trachea during induction of anesthesia. The most common use of succinylcholine in dental practice is to break a laryngospasm that occurs in a patient undergoing conscious sedation. The intravenous dose of succinylcholine to treat laryngospasm is 0.2 mg to 0.5mg/kg. If intravenous access is unavailable, 2 mg/kg to 5mg/kg can be given sublingually or intramuscularly. Neuromuscular blocking agents are administered parenterally.

See **Tables 22.1** and **22.2** for general information on succinylcholine.

Special Dental Considerations

The sustained depolarization produced by initial administration of succinylcholine is manifested initially by transient generalized skeletal muscle contractions known as fasciculations. Various degrees of increased muscle tension in the masseter muscles may develop with succinylcholine, especially in pediatric patients. In extreme cases, trismus can occur and make it difficult to open the mouth for intubation of the trachea. Patients who develop trismus with succinylcholine administration are prone to developing malignant hyperthermia.

Head, neck, abdomen, and back myalgia can occur postoperatively owing to muscle fasciculation associated with depolarization.

Succinylcholine is a general anesthetic agent and should be used only by clinicians trained in sedation and general anesthesia.

Drug interactions of dental interest

Succinylcholine causes paralysis and does not have anesthetic or analgesic effects. Therefore, ensure that not only paralysis but also adequate anesthesia has been achieved before performing procedures.

No interactions/contraindications are reported regarding the use of succinylcholine with general anesthetic for dental procedures performed in a surgical setting.

Laboratory value alterations

- Hyperkalemia sufficient to cause cardiac arrest may follow administration of succinylcholine; patients at risk include those with denervation of skeletal muscle, major burns, multiple trauma, or upper motor neuron injury.

Pharmacology

Succinylcholine is an example of a depolarizing neuromuscular blocker and is the only one used clinically. It binds to the acetylcholine receptor and causes a prolonged depolarization of the postsynaptic membrane. This initial depolarization causes muscle contraction, which is seen clinically as muscle fasciculations throughout the patient's body. The duration of these initial contractions is short. The sustained depolarization of the postsynaptic membrane does not allow the function of acetylcholine to take place, because a depolarized membrane cannot respond to the release of acetylcholine.

These agents are metabolized by plasma cholinesterase, an enzyme found in the bloodstream but not in the synaptic cleft. Therefore, the duration of a depolarizing muscle relaxant is related to the rate of diffusion from the neuromuscular junction. In rare cases, a patient may have an atypical plasma cholinesterase that is not as effective in metabolizing the drug. In such patients, the action of a depolarizing agent may be significantly prolonged. The function of a patient's plasma cholinesterase activity can be evaluated according to his or her dibucaine number. Dibucaine is an amide local anesthetic that reduces the function of normal cholinesterase to a greater degree than it diminishes atypical cholinesterase. This number reflects the quality, but not the quantity, of plasma cholinesterase. Any dentist administering a drug metabolized by plasma cholinesterase to a patient with a suspected history of plasma cholinesterase deficiency should obtain a dibucaine number to assess the quality of the patient's plasma cholinesterase enzyme system.

Adverse Effects, Precautions, and Contraindications

Succinylcholine mimics acetylcholine at the cardiac postganglionic muscarinic receptors and induces cardiac dysrhythmias. Cardiac dysrhythmias including sinus bradycardia, junctional rhythm, and sinus arrest have occurred after administration of succinylcholine.

Many medications used for general anesthesia are potential triggers for malignant hyperthermia, and clinicians should be aware of this potentially fatal hypermetabolism of skeletal muscle.

Transient increases in ocular pressure are seen 2 to 4 minutes after injection of succinylcholine. Theoretically, succinylcholine may contribute to extrusion of intraocular contents in patients with open eye injuries.

Fasciculations induced by succinylcholine lead to unpredictable increases in gastric pressure and may cause gastric fluid to pass into the esophagus and pharynx, thus resulting in pulmonary aspiration.

Table 22.1 presents adverse effects and precautions/contraindications associated with succinylcholine.

Nondepolarizing Neuromuscular Blockers

Nondepolarizing neuromuscular blockers act through competitive inhibition of acetylcholine. They are useful for prolonged muscle relaxation in the operating room and intensive care units due to their long duration of action. Nondepolarizing neuromuscular blockers are categorized based on the duration of action as long-acting, intermediate-acting, and short-acting. Examples include gallamine, atracurium, and vecuronium. The use of these drugs is primarily limited to muscle relaxation for general anesthesia.

Special Dental Considerations

Drug interactions of dental interest

No special consideration or drug intersections/contraindications are reported regarding the use of nondepolarizing neuromuscular blockers with general anesthetic for dental procedures. Nondepolarizing neuromuscular blockers have limited ability to cross lipid membrane barriers. Therefore, this class of drugs does not affect the fetus.

Pharmacology

Nondepolarizing neuromuscular blockers have a structure similar to that of acetylcholine, which enables them to bind at the same receptor as that neurotransmitter. When the majority of acetylcholine receptors are bound by neuromuscular blockers, acetylcholine can no longer bind to the receptor. This mechanism produces the profound muscle relaxation characteristic of this class of skeletal muscle relaxants. The use of these drugs is primarily limited to muscle relaxation for general anesthesia.

The majority of nondepolarizing drugs are eliminated through renal excretion; however, some also undergo metabolism in the liver, ester hydrolysis or Hoffman elimination. Regardless of how these agents are metabolized, their duration of action is determined primarily by how rapidly they are redistributed to the peripheral tissues.

Adverse Effects, Precautions, and Contraindications

Nondepolarizing neuromuscular blockers cause cardiovascular effects; take into consideration these agents' specific cardiovascular manifestations when selecting the appropriate one for a patient. These cardiac effects usually are transient and vary because of these agents' interactions with other medications. Many drugs used in anesthetic practice can trigger malignant hyperthermia; consider this when obtaining the patient's medical history before beginning treatment. Skeletal muscle fasciculations do not occur with onset of action of nondepolarizing neuromuscular blocking agents.

This category of medications is highly ionized at physiologic pH and has limited lipid solubility, resulting in a small volume of distribution primarily in the extracellular fluid. They have limited ability to cross lipid membrane barriers. Therefore, this class of drugs has few central nervous system effects and minimal oral and renal absorption; it also does not affect the fetus.

SPASMOLYTICS

Spasmolytics are drugs that eliminate muscular spasms. The primary use of spasmolytics in the dental office is to relieve anxiety, postprocedural trismus, and muscle spasms of the head and neck, including temporomandibular disorders. These agents often are used in conjunction with heat, physical therapy, rest, and analgesics. Some of these agents have anxiolytic properties that may help reduce muscle tension.

Spasmolytics may be used to manage spasticity owing to systemic disease. Spasticity refers to abnormalities of regulation of skeletal muscle tone that result from lesions in the central nervous system (CNS). The most effective agents for control of spasticity include two that act directly on the CNS (benzodiazepines and baclofen) and one that acts directly on skeletal muscle (dantrolene).

Tables 22.1 and **22.2** present general information on spasmolytics.

Benzodiazepines

More than 2,000 benzodiazepines have been synthesized. Among these, several are recommended as spasmolytics: chlordiazepoxide, clonazepam, diazepam, lorazepam, and midazolam. Although benzodiazepines exert similar clinical effects, differences in their pharmacokinetic properties have led to varying therapeutic applications. Chlordiazepoxide and diazepam are considered the prototypic drugs of their class.

Benzodiazepines have sedative-hypnotic, muscle relaxant, anxiolytic and anticonvulsant effects. The antianxiety effects of this class of drugs make them an excellent choice for preoperative oral sedation in the fearful dental patient.

Most benzodiazepines reduce sleep latency and reduce the number of awakenings. They can be used for insomnia, but prescribing for this purpose should be done only by a clinician who is an expert in sleep disorders. Prolonged use of benzodiazepines for insomnia can have serious detrimental effects on the sleep cycle. When administered intravenously, diazepam can be used to break status epilepticus in patients who suffer from grand mal seizures.

Chlordiazepoxide. Chlordiazepoxide is the original prototype for the benzodiazepines. It has been demonstrated to have sedative, anxiolytic, and weak analgesic properties. Chlordiazepoxide is used for treatment of anxiety disorders, short-term anxiety, and preoperative anxiety. It is not recommended for the management of stress associated with everyday life. Paradoxical reactions, including excitement and rage, have been reported, especially in psychiatric patients and hyperactive pediatric patients.

Clonazepam. General medical use of clonazepam includes use for treatment of seizures and panic disorders. In dentistry, it has been used for treatment of acute myofascial pain and burning mouth syndrome. No formal recommendations of dosage have been made for its use in this area, and it is usually given in doses similar to those used for panic disorders.

Diazepam. Diazepam is useful as an anxiolytic and as a spasmolytic. When administered intravenously, diazepam can be used to break status epilepticus in patients who suffer from grand mal seizures.

Lorazepam. Lorazepam produces excellent amnesia. Unfortunately, its peak onset can occur as long as 2 to 4 hours after oral administration. Its long duration and slow onset make it impractical as an oral sedative for outpatient procedures.

Midazolam. Midazolam is a rapid-onset, short-acting benzodiazepine that is commonly used intravenously for conscious sedation in an outpatient environment. It has good anxiolytic and amnesic effects, making it an excellent choice for IV sedation.

Special Dental Considerations

Benzodiazepines in general do not have any adverse interactions with dental materials. No special precautions are required for local anesthetic administration in conjunction with their use. Xerostomia is a common side effect that reverses itself when use of the medication is discontinued.

Drug interactions of dental interest

CNS depressants (eg, alcohol, barbiturates, opioids) may enhance sedation and respiratory depression.

Patients with convulsant disorders may experience an increase in grand mal seizure activity with benzodiazepines; therefore, an increase in their standard anticonvulsant medication may be indicated.

Theophylline may antagonize the sedative effects of midazolam. Cimetidine may increase midazolam's serum concentrations.

Laboratory value alterations

- Isolated reports of benzodiazepine-associated neutropenia and jaundice exist, so periodic blood counts and liver function tests are recommended during long-term benzodiazepine therapy.

Pharmacology

The action of benzodiazepines is the result of potentiating the neural inhibition that is mediated by γ-aminobutyric acid (GABA) resulting in relaxation of skeletal muscles.

Benzodiazepines are metabolized by the cytochrome P450 system in the liver and then are excreted by the kidney. The rate of elimination depends on the drug's half-life. The duration of action of specific benzodiazepines ranges from short to very long.

Benzodiazepines with long half-lives accumulate during repeated dosages and even with a single dose. This is of particular concern in elderly people, in whom half-life may be increased two- to fourfold. Several benzodiazepines, such as diazepam (see below), produce active metabolites when they are metabolized. Metabolites of lorazepam and oxazepam are inactive and, therefore, make these drugs safer than diazepam for patients with liver disease.

Chlordiazepoxide. Chlordiazepoxide's mechanism of action is not known. Animal studies suggest that it acts on the limbic system of the brain (which is involved with emotional response).

Clonazepam. The mechanism of action of clonazepam is not fully understood. Its proposed pharmacologic effects are related to its ability to increase GABA activity. Peak concentrations of clonazepam are reached 1 to 4 hours after oral administration. The elimination half-life is about 30 to 40 hours.

Diazepam. The metabolism of diazepam warrants special attention. Diazepam is metabolized into desmethyldiazepam, an active metabolite. Desmethyldiazepam can re-enter the bloodstream through the enterohepatic circulation and produce delayed-onset sedation. Therefore, even after the initial effects of diazepam have disappeared, the patient must not engage in any potentially dangerous activity for 24 hours. Diazepam is known to act on the limbic system and induce a calming effect. The peak onset of diazepam occurs 30 to 60 minutes after oral administration.

Lorazepam. Lorazepam acts on the CNS, resulting in a tranquilizing effect. IM onset of hypnosis is 20 to 30 minutes. Duration of action is 6 to 8 hours.

Midazolam. Midazolam is a short-acting, water-soluble benzodiazepine that depresses the CNS.

Adverse Effects, Precautions, and Contraindications

Benzodiazepines may cause varying degrees of lightheadedness, motor incoordination, ataxia, impaired psychomotor and mental function, confusion, amnesia, dry mouth, and bitter taste. Other side effects include headache, blurred vision, vertigo, nausea, vomiting, epigastric distress, joint pain, chest pain, and incontinence. Anticonvulsant benzodiazepines can increase the frequency of seizures in patients with epilepsy. Benzodiazepines can have paradoxical effects such as nightmares, restlessness, hallucinations, paranoia, depression, unusual uninhibited behavior, and occasional suicidal ideation. When the drug is administered in oral doses at the intended time of sleep, weakness and other previously mentioned side effects may not be noticed. It is considered undesirable if the drug was administered at bedtime and side effects persist during waking hours.

Benzodiazepines have a low incidence of abuse and dependence; however, the possibility must not be overlooked. Mild dependence may occur in patients who have taken benzodiazepines for a prolonged period. Tolerance to benzodiazepines can develop.

Benzodiazepines slightly reduce alveolar ventilation in preanesthetic doses. This group of drugs may cause CO_2 narcosis in patients with chronic obstructive pulmonary disease (COPD). Apnea can occur when benzodiazepines are given during general anesthesia or in combination with opioids. Cases have been reported in which respiratory distress has occurred when patients have combined benzodiazepines with other CNS depressants such as alcohol. Warn patients of potentially serious interactions with ethanol. Because their cognitive and motor function may be impaired, advise patients not to drive or participate in other potentially dangerous activities. Long-acting benzodiazepines have been associated with falls in elderly people and should be avoided in this patient population.

A specific benzodiazepine should be avoided if a patient has a known hypersensitivity to it. It should be noted that a cross-sensitivity between various benzodiazepines may exist. Administer benzodiazepines with caution to patients with liver disease or impaired renal function. They should not be used in patients who have CNS or respiratory depression or who are comatose. Do not administer benzodiazepines to pregnant or nursing women. An increased risk of congenital malformations is associated with the use of tranquilizers during the first trimester of pregnancy. Patients with narrow-angle glaucoma should not receive benzodiazapines.

Clonazepam. Clonazepam should not be used in patients with a history of adverse reactions to benzodiazepines. Administer with caution to patients with liver disease or impaired renal function. Clonazepam may increase the incidence or precipitate the onset of grand mal seizures. It has not been shown to interfere with the pharmacokinetics of phenytoin, carbamazepine, or phenobarbital. Valproic acid administered concomitantly with clonazepam may produce absence status.

Hypersalivation has been reported with the use of clonazepam; consider this when selecting a medication for a patient who has difficulty controlling salivary flow. However, xerostomia is a more common complaint.

Diazepam. Diazepam should not be given to any patient with acute narrow-angle or open-angle glaucoma. Take precautions when it is administered to patients with a history of seizure disorders, COPD, or liver failure.

Midazolam. Theophylline may antagonize the sedative effects of midazolam. Cimetidine may increase serum concentrations. CNS depressants increase sedation and respiratory depression.

Benzodiazepine Antagonist: Flumazenil

Flumazenil is a benzodiazepine antagonist that binds to the GABA/benzodiazepine receptor in the CNS. This antagonist has been shown to reverse the effects of sedation, amnesia, and respiratory depression in humans. If a benzodiazepine overdose is observed, flumazenil can be administered IV to reverse the effects of the benzodiazepine. Onset of reversal will occur in 1 to 2 minutes, with peak reversal occurring 6 to 10 minutes after administration. If a long-acting benzodiazepine has been given, the patient should be re-evaluated about every 20 to 30 minutes to see if repeat doses of flumazenil are necessary.

Special Dental Considerations

Drug interactions of dental interest

CNS depressants (eg, alcohol, barbiturates, opioids), if used concurrently, may enhance sedation and respiratory depression.

Adverse Effects, Precautions, and Contraindications

Side effects of the benzodiazepine antagonists include dizziness, drowsiness, somnolence, confusion, and respiratory depression. Cardiovascular effects include palpitations, chest pain, and syncope. Patients may also experience anorexia, xerostomia, vomiting, and diarrhea.

Other Spasmolytics

Baclofen. Baclofen, a derivative of the inhibitory neurotransmitter GABA, functions as a GABA agonist in the brain as well as in the spinal cord. Baclofen may reduce substance P and, therefore, pain; it also may function as a spasmolytic. It is most effective for spasticity associated with multiple sclerosis and traumatic spinal cord lesions. In dentistry, it can be used for temporomandibular dystonia and is helpful in some cases of trigeminal neuralgia.

Baclofen is especially helpful in alleviating the spasticity of multiple sclerosis and spinal cord injury when administered intrathecally. Baclofen is as effective as, but much less sedating than, diazepam in reducing spasticity. It also does not reduce general muscle strength, as happens with other spasmolytics such as dantrolene.

Dantrolene. Dantrolene is indicated for spasticity secondary to upper motor neuron disease (eg, multiple sclerosis, stroke, cerebral palsy) and is not indicated for spasms caused by rheumatic disorders. Treatment for chronic spasticity requires gradual titration until the patient experiences maximum effect. Dantrolene also is used for the management of malignant hyperthermia. This is a rare, dominantly inherited syndrome that is precipitated by the use of inhalation anesthetics or neuromuscular blocking agents. Vigorous muscle contraction occurs, leading to a rapid and dangerous rise in body temperature, renal failure, and rhabdomyolysis. Dantrolene is administered IV immediately during an attack, or it may be administered prophylactically to patients who are susceptible to this syndrome.

Metaxalone. This drug is indicated as an adjunct to rest and physical therapy for the treatment of acute painful musculoskeletal conditions.

Tizanidine. This drug is used for the management of spasticity associated with multiple sclerosis and spinal cord injury. Tizanidine has a short-acting duration and administration should be reserved for daily activities when relief of spasticity is most important.

Special Dental Considerations

Baclofen. No information has been reported indicating the need for special precaution when baclofen is used with local anesthetics and vasoconstrictors.

Dantrolene. The safety of long-term use of dantrolene in humans has not been established.

Metaxalone. Patients with liver damage should undergo liver function tests before surgical procedures.

Tizanidine. Tizanidine has been associated with visual hallucinations or delusions. Before beginning dental treatment, assess the psychological status of a patient taking tizanidine.

Drug interactions of dental interest

Baclofen. Lithium decreases the effect of baclofen. Benzodiazepines, antihypertensive agents, and opioid analgesics increase baclofen's effect. Increased toxicity is noted when baclofen is administered concomitantly with CNS depressants, alcohol, and monoamine oxidase inhibitors. Increased short-term memory loss is noted when baclofen is taken with tricyclic antidepressants.

Dantrolene. Hepatotoxicity has occurred more frequently in women >35 years of age who are receiving estrogen therapy while taking dantrolene. The exact interaction is unclear, and caution must be exercised when estrogen and dantrolene are given together.

Cardiovascular collapse has been reported on rare occasion in patients taking both dantrolene and verapamil; therefore, this combination is not recommended. Dantrolene potentiates vecuronium-induced neuromuscular blocking.

Increased toxicity also occurs with concomitant administration of CNS depressants (sedation), MAO inhibitors, phenothiazines, clindamycin (which increase neuromuscular blockade), verapamil (associated with hyperkalemia and cardiac depression), warfarin, clofibrate, and tolbutamide.

Metaxalone. No drug interactions are reported. However, this drug is a possible CNS depressant and, therefore, it is suggested that prescribing clinicians follow the precautions for CNS depressant drugs.

Tizanidine. It has been shown that tizanidine and CNS depressants have an additive effect. The effects of tizanidine may be additive when it is taken with other muscle relaxants and sedatives. Oral contraceptives reduce the clearance of tizanidine by approximately 50%. Tizanidine interacts with antihypertensives and may increase levels of antihypertensive drugs.

Laboratory value alterations

- Obtain liver function tests on a regular basis to monitor for hepatotoxicity with dantrolene.
- Leukopenia, thrombocytopenia, and aplastic anemia also have been reported with dantrolene; monitor patients for hematologic abnormalities.

Special patients

Dantrolene. Dantrolene's safety in women who are pregnant or may become pregnant has not been established. Its long-term side effects in the pediatric population <5 years of age have not been established.

Pharmacology

Baclofen. Baclofen is rapidly absorbed and has a half-life of 3 to 4 hours.

Dantrolene. Dantrolene acts directly on the skeletal muscle by reducing the amount of calcium released from the sarcoplasmic reticulum.

Metaxalone. The mechanism of action for metaxalone is not known at this time, but it is believed it may be due to general CNS depression. It has been established that no direct action takes place at the contractile mechanism of the striated muscle, motor end plate, or nerve fiber.

Tizanidine. Tizanidine hydrochloride is an agonist at the α_2-adrenergic receptor site and, therefore, increases the presynaptic inhibition of motor neurons.

Adverse Effects, Precautions, and Contraindications

Baclofen. Side effects include dizziness, drowsiness, somnolence, confusion, and respiratory depression. Cardiovascular effects include palpitations, chest pain, and syncope. Patients taking baclofen may experience anorexia, xerostomia, vomiting, and diarrhea.

Dantrolene. Dantrolene has a serious side effect of hepatotoxicity; therefore, monitor hepatic function after this drug is administered. Active hepatic disease, such as hepatitis and cirrhosis, is a contraindication for use of dantrolene. Discontinue long-term use if clear benefits are not evident. Used with caution in patients with impaired pulmonary and cardiac function resulting from myocardial disease. Cardiovascular side effects may include pleural effusion with pericarditis.

Other side effects include weakness, confusion, lightheadedness, drowsiness, severe diarrhea, abdominal cramps, urinary retention, erectile dysfunction, blurred vision, and fatigue. These side effects usually are temporary and can be reduced by using a small initial dose and slowly increasing the dose until the optimal amount is reached. Diarrhea can be severe and require discontinuation of use of dantrolene.

Caution patients against driving or participating in potentially hazardous activities while taking dantrolene.

Photosensitivity has been associated with dantrolene; caution patients taking it to avoid sun exposure.

Taste changes have been noted with dantrolene.

No information has been reported indicating the need for special precautions when dantrolene is used concomitantly with local anesthetics and vasoconstrictors.

Metaxalone. Adverse reactions have included leukopenia and hemolytic anemia. Metaxalone has been associated with false-positive results in Benedict's test. Use with caution in patients with impaired liver and kidney function. It is contraindicated for use with patients who have severe damage and in those with a history of drug-induced, hemolytic, or other anemias.

Tizanidine. Adverse reactions have included orthostatic hypotension, liver damage, hallucinations, and psychotic-like symptoms. Use tizanidine with caution in patients who have liver or kidney damage. Caution patients that limited clinical trials exist with regard to duration of use and use of higher dosages to reduce muscle tone.

Tizanidine should never be used with other α_2-adrenergic agonists.

Spasmolytics for Acute Local Spasm

Many spasmolytic drugs are indicated for the treatment of temporary relief of muscle spasm caused by trauma. Cyclobenzaprine is considered the prototype of this group of drugs. It is structurally related to the tricyclic antidepressants and has similar properties. It is believed to act at the brainstem. Other drugs in this category include carisoprodol, chlorzoxazone, methocarbamol, and orphenadrine. These medications are not helpful in the treatment of muscle spasm that is caused by spinal cord injury, CNS disease, or systemic disease.

Carisoprodol. Carisoprodol is used for acute skeletal muscle pain in conjunction with rest, physical therapy, and other measures used to manage acute skeletal muscle spasm.

Chlorzoxazone. Chlorzoxazone is indicated as an adjunct to rest, physical therapy, and other measures for the relief of acute, painful musculoskeletal conditions.

Cyclobenzaprine. Cyclobenzaprine relieves muscle spasm of local origin without interfering with muscle function. It is used as an adjunct to rest and physical therapy for relief of acute painful muscle spasms.

Methocarbamol. Methocarbamol is recommended as an adjunct to rest, physical therapy, and other measures to manage acute skeletal muscle spasm.

Orphenadrine. Orphenadrine is used with rest and physical therapy for the treatment of acute skeletal muscle spasms. It is intended for short-term use only, and no studies of its long-term efficacy and safety have been published.

Special Dental Considerations

No complications have been reported with dental treatment of patients taking spasmolytics used for acute local spasm.

Cyclobenzaprine. It is recommended that cyclobenzaprine be used only for short periods (up to 2 weeks), as research demonstrating its effectiveness and safety for prolonged use has not been conducted. This is not likely to be an issue, as the drug is indicated for the treatment of acute painful muscle spasm of short duration.

Drug interactions of dental interest

Cyclobenzaprine. Cyclobenzaprine is closely related to tricyclic antidepressants; it also may interact with monoamine oxidase inhibitors and potentially can lead to hyperpyretic crisis, convulsions, and death. It should not be used concomitantly with, or within 14 days of use of, MAO inhibitors. Use with caution in patients taking anticholinergic medications.

Laboratory value alterations

- **Chlorzoxazone:** Liver enzyme changes may occur with use, suggesting hepatic toxicity. Therefore, consider monitoring the patient's liver function.
- **Cyclobenzaprine:** This drug is indicated for short-term use and significant laboratory value changes are not expected. Thrombocytopenia and leukopenia have been reported only rarely, and no causal relationship has been established.
- **Methocarbamol:** This drug may cause inaccurate results in screening tests for 5-hydroxyin-doleacetic acid and vanillylmandelic. Inform the patient's physician when prescribing methocarbamol.

Special patients

Carisoprodol. No reports have been published of studies testing this drug's effect on pregnant or nursing women; therefore, it is suggested that use of carisoprodol be avoided in such patients. The drug is not recommended for use in children.

Chlorzoxazone. No reports have been published of studies testing this drug's effect on pregnant or nursing women; therefore, it is suggested that use of chlorzoxazone be avoided in such patients. There are no established guidelines for its use in children, so it should not be administered to pediatric patients.

Cyclobenzaprine. Animal studies have not demonstrated that cyclobenzaprine poses a risk to the fetus or affects fertility. It has not been determined if this drug is excreted in breast milk; therefore, it should be used cautiously in nursing women.

Methocarbamol. Methocarbamol's safety in pregnant and lactating women has not been established, and it is not known if methocarbamol is excreted in breast milk. Safety in children <12 years has not been established.

Orphenadrine. No studies have been conducted testing orphenadrine's safety in pregnant and nursing women. Neither have pediatric safety and efficacy studies been performed. Use with caution in patients with coronary insufficiency, cardiac decompensation, tachycardia, palpitations, and dysrhythmia.

Pharmacology

Carisoprodol. Carisoprodol is centrally acting and blocks interneuronal activity in the spinal cord. Its onset is rapid and lasts 6 hours. Its exact mechanism of action is not clear, but it is known that carisoprodol does not directly act on skeletal muscle.

Chlorzoxazone. Chlorzoxazone acts primarily at the spinal cord and the subcortical areas of the brain, where it inhibits multisynaptic reflex arcs involved in producing skeletal muscle spasm of varying etiology. Its exact mode of action has not been identified. This drug does not directly relax tense skeletal muscles. Peak blood levels of chlorzoxazone are detected 1 to 2 hours after oral administration.

Cyclobenzaprine. Cyclobenzaprine primarily acts within the CNS at the brainstem, as opposed to the spinal cord levels. It does not act at the neuromuscular junction or directly on skeletal muscle.

Methocarbamol. The drug's mechanism of action has not been determined, but it may be linked to the drug's CNS depressive abilities.

Orphenadrine. The mode of action of orphenadrine is not clear, but it may be related to its analgesic action. Orphenadrine has mild anticholinergic activity and analgesic properties. It does not directly relax skeletal muscles.

Adverse Effects, Precautions, and Contraindications

Table 22.1 presents adverse effects and precautions/contraindications associated with spasmolytics.

Carisoprodol. Carisoprodol is metabolized by the liver and secreted by the kidneys and should be used with caution in patients with impaired liver or kidney function. Other adverse reactions may include drowsiness, malaise, dizziness, lightheadedness, epigastric distress, tachycardia, postural hypotension, facial flushing and, occasionally, idiosyncratic reaction. Seizure threshold may be lowered in patients with convulsive disorders. Patients should be advised of CNS effects and avoid driving and drinking alcohol.

Chlorzoxazone. Cardiovascular side effects include tachycardia and chest pain. Syncope, depression, dizziness, lightheadedness, headaches, trembling, hiccups, and shortness of breath have been reported. Angioedema is a noted side effect. Serious and potentially fatal hepatotoxity has been reported with the use of this drug. The mechanism of this is not known, and factors predisposing patients to hepatotoxity have not been identified. Instruct patients to report early signs of toxicity such as dark urine, anorexia, or upper-right-quadrant pain. Monitor liver enzymes if this drug is administered on a long-term basis. Other adverse reactions may include drowsiness, malaise, lightheadedness and, occasionally, overstimulation. Idiosyncratic reactions have been manifested as severe muscle weakness, confusion, and ataxia. Patients may note a discoloration of the urine as a result of a phenolic metabolite of chlorzoxazone. This discoloration has no clinical significance.

Cyclobenzaprine. Cyclobenzaprine's potential side effects include drowsiness, malaise, tachycardia, and dysrhythmia. Cyclobenzaprine may enhance the effects of alcohol, barbiturates, and other CNS depressants. Use cyclobenzaprine with caution in patients who have a history of urinary retention, closed-angle glaucoma, and increased intraocular pressure. It is contraindicated in patients who are taking MAO inhibitors or who have hyperthyroidism, congestive heart failure, or dysrhythmias. This drug has no reported interactions with dental materials. No information has been reported indicating the need for special precautions with concomitant use of local anesthetics/vasoconstrictors. Patients may experience xerostomia while taking cyclobenzaprine.

Methocarbamol. Methocarbamol has CNS depressant effects. Patients taking CNS depressants should be cautioned not to combine methocarbamol with alcohol or other CNS depressants. Renal impairment has occurred on rare occasions as a side effect of methocarbamol use. Light-headedness, dizziness, drowsiness, nausea, blurred vision, headache and fever are common side effects. The drug should be used with caution in patients with renal disease, hepatic disease, seizure disorders, myasthenia gravis, and addictive personality.

Orphenadrine. As with all spasmolytic agents, orphenadrine may cause light-headedness, drowsiness and syncope. This medication contains sodium bisulfate and may cause severe allergic reactions in patients with sulfite sensitivity. Sulfite sensitivity is seen more frequently in asthmatic patients. On rare occasions, aplastic anemia has been reported with orphenadrine use. It has mild anticholinergic effects, which may result in dry mouth and constipation. Other side effects include urinary retention, tachycardia, palpitations, blurred vision, dilation of pupils, or gastric irritation. This drug can cause increased ocular tension and is contraindicated in patients with glaucoma. Orphenadrine also is contraindicated in people with pyloric or duodenal obstruction, prostate hypertrophy, obstruction of the bladder, cardiospasm, and myasthenia gravis.

SUGGESTED READING

Beebe FA, Barkin RL, Barkin S. A clinical and pharmacologic review of skeletal muscle relaxants for musculoskeletal conditions. *Am J Ther*. 2005;12:151-171.

Drug Facts and Comparisons. 60th ed. St. Louis, MO. Facts and Comparisons; 2006.

Neidle EA, Yagiela JA. *Pharmacology and Therapeutics for Dentistry*. 4th ed. Philadelphia: C.V. Mosby Co.; 1998.

Physicians' Desk Reference®. 63rd ed. Montvale, NJ: Physicians' Desk Reference Inc; 2009.

Table 22.1. PRESCRIBING INFORMATION FOR SKELETAL MUSCLE RELAXANTS

NAME	FORM/ STRENGTH	DOSAGE	WARNINGS/PRECAUTIONS & CONTRAINDICATIONS	ADVERSE EFFECTS†
ALPHA$_2$-ADRENERGIC AGONIST (CENTRALLY ACTING)				
Tizanidine HCl (Zanaflex)	**Cap:** 2mg, 4mg, 6mg; **Tab:** 4mg	***Adults:*** **Initial:** 4mg single dose q6-8h. **Titrate:** Increase by 2-4mg. **Usual:** 8mg single dose q6-8h. **Max:** 3 doses/24h or 36mg/day.	**W/P:** May prolong QT interval. May cause liver damage; monitor baseline LFTs and at 1, 3, and 6 months. Retinal degeneration and corneal opacities reported. Caution with renal impairment or elderly. May cause hypotension, caution with antihypertensives; avoid ciprofloxacin and fluvoxamine. Use with extreme caution in patients with hepatic impairment. May cause sedation and hallucinations. Avoid concomitant use with oral contraceptives. When discontinuing, taper dose to avoid withdrawal and rebound HTN, tachycardia, and hypertonia. **Contra:** Concomitant use with fluvoxamine, ciprofloxacin, or potent inhibitors of CYP1A2. **P/N:** Category C, caution in nursing.	**Dry mouth,** somnolence, asthenia, dizziness, UTI, urinary frequency, flu-like syndrome, rhinitis.
GABA ANALOG				
Baclofen (Kemstro)	**Tab:** (Generic) 10mg, 20mg; **Tab, Disintegrating (ODT):** (Kemstro) 10mg, 20mg	***Adults/Pediatrics:*** **≥12 yrs: Initial:** 5mg tid for 3 days. **Titrate:** May increase dose by 5mg tid every 3 days. **Usual:** 40-80mg/day. **Max:** 80 mg/day (20mg qid). **Renal Impairment:** Reduce dose.	**W/P:** Caution with psychosis, schizophrenia, confusional states; may exacerbate conditions. Caution with bladder sphincter hypertonia, peptic ulceration, seizures, elderly, cerebrovascular disorder, respiratory failure, hepatic or renal failure. Abnormal AST, alkaline phosphatase, and blood glucose reported. Caution when used to maintain locomotion or to obtain increased function. Decreased alertness with operating machinery. Has not significantly benefited stroke patients. Avoid abrupt discontinuation; reduce dose slowly over 1-2 weeks. **P/N:** Category C, caution in nursing.	Drowsiness, dizziness, weakness, fatigue, confusion, daytime sedation, headache, insomnia, hypotension, nausea, constipation, urinary frequency.
MUSCULAR ANALGESICS (CENTRALLY ACTING)				
Chlorzoxazone (Parafon Forte DSC)	**Tab:** 500mg	***Adults:*** **Usual:** 500mg tid-qid. **Titrate:** May increase to 750mg tid-qid.	**W/P:** Serious (including fatal) hepatocellular toxicity reported. D/C if signs of hepatotoxicity develop. Caution with history of drug allergies. Concomitant use of alcohol or other CNS depressants may have an additive effect. **P/N:** Safety in pregnancy and nursing not known.	Drowsiness, dizziness, malaise, lightheadedness, overstimulation.
Metaxalone (Skelaxin)	**Tab:** 800mg	***Adults/Pediatrics:*** **>12 yrs:** 800mg tid-qid.	**W/P:** May enhance the effects of alcohol and other CNS depressants. Caution with preexisting liver damage. Monitor hepatic function. False-positive Benedict's test reported. **Contra:** Tendency for drug-induced, hemolytic, and other anemias. Significant renal or hepatic impairment. **P/N:** Not for use in pregnancy or nursing.	N/V, GI upset, drowsiness, dizziness, headache, nervousness, leukopenia, hemolytic anemia, jaundice.

†Bold entries denote special dental considerations.
BB = black box warning; **W/P** = warnings/precautions; **Contra** = contraindications; **P/N** = pregnancy category rating and nursing considerations.

Table 22.1. PRESCRIBING INFORMATION FOR SKELETAL MUSCLE RELAXANTS *(cont.)*

NAME	FORM/ STRENGTH	DOSAGE	WARNINGS/PRECAUTIONS & CONTRAINDICATIONS	ADVERSE EFFECTS†
MUSCULAR ANALGESICS (CENTRALLY ACTING) *(cont.)*				
Methocarbamol (Robaxin, Robaxin Injection, Robaxin-750)	**Inj:** 100mg/mL [10mL]; **Tab:** 500mg, 750mg	***Adults:*** **(PO) Initial:** (500mg tab) 1500mg qid for 2-3 days. **Maint:** 1000mg qid. **Initial:** (750mg tab) 1500mg qid for 2-3 days. **Maint:** 750mg q4h or 1500mg tid. **Max:** 6g/d for 2-3 days; 8g/d if severe. **(Inj) Moderate Symptoms:** 10mL IV/IM. **IV Max Rate:** 3mL undiluted drug/min. **IM Max:** 5mL into each gluteal region. **Severe/Post-Op Condition: Max:** 20-30mL/day up to 3 consecutive days. If feasible, continue with PO. **Tetanus:** 10-20mL up to 30mL. May repeat q6h until NG tube can be inserted. Continue with crushed tabs. **Max:** 24g/day PO. ***Pediatrics:*** **Tetanus: Initial:** 15mg/kg or 500mg/m^2. Repeat q6h prn. **Max:** 1.8g/m^2 for 3 consecutive days. Administer by injection into tubing or IV infusion.	**W/P:** May impair mental/physical abilities required for operating machinery or driving a motor vehicle. May cause color interference in certain screening tests for 5-hydroxy-indoleacetic acid (5-HIAA) and vanillylmandelic acid (VMA). Caution in epilepsy with the injection. Injection rate should not exceed 3mL/min. Avoid extravasation with injection. Avoid use of injection particularly during early pregnancy. **Contra:** (Inj) Renal pathology with injection due to propylene glycol content. **P/N:** Category C, caution in nursing.	Lightheadedness, dizziness, drowsiness, nausea, urticaria, pruritus, rash, conjunctivitis, nasal congestion, blurred vision, headache, fever, seizures, syncope, flushing.
Orphenadrine Citrate	**Inj:** 30mg/mL [2mL]; **Tab, Extended-Release:** 100mg	***Adults:*** **(Tab)** 100mg bid, in the am and pm. **(Inj)** 60mg IM/IV q12h.	**W/P:** Caution with tachycardia, cardiac decompensation, coronary insufficiency, cardiac arrhythmias. Monitor blood, urine, and LFTs periodically with prolonged use. Injection contains sodium bisulfite. **Contra:** Glaucoma, pyloric or duodenal obstruction, stenosing peptic ulcers, prostatic hypertrophy, bladder neck obstruction, cardiospasm, myasthenia gravis. **P/N:** Category C, safety in nursing not known.	**Dry mouth,** tachycardia, palpitation, urinary hesitancy/retention, blurred vision, pupil dilation, increased ocular tension, weakness, dizziness, constipation.
Orphenadrine Citrate/Aspirin/ Caffeine (Norgesic, Norgesic Forte)	**Tab:** (Orphenadrine-ASA-Caffeine) 25mg-385mg-30mg; **Tab:** (Forte) 50mg-770mg-60mg	***Adults:*** 1-2 tabs tid-qid. **(Forte)** 0.5-1 tab tid-qid.	**W/P:** Reye's Syndrome may develop with chickenpox, influenza, or flu symptoms. Extreme caution with peptic ulcers and coagulation abnormalities. Monitor blood, urine, and LFT's periodically with prolonged use. **Contra:** Glaucoma, pyloric or duodenal obstruction, achalasia, prostatic hypertrophy, bladder neck obstruction, myasthenia gravis. **P/N:** Safety in pregnancy and nursing not known.	Tachycardia, urinary hesitancy/retention, **dry mouth,** blurred vision, increased intraocular tension, N/V, headache, dizziness, constipation, drowsiness, urticaria, GI hemorrhage.
PURIFIED NEUROTOXIN COMPLEX				
Botulinum Toxin Type A (Botox)	**Inj:** 100 U	***Adults/Pediatrics:*** **≥16 yrs: Cervical Dystonia: Average Dose:** 236 U divided among affected muscles. Adjust to individual response. **Max:** 100 U total dose in sternocleidomastoid muscles. **≥12 yrs: Strabismus: Initial: Vertical Muscle and Horizontal Strabismus <20 Prism Diopters:** 1.25-2.5 U in any muscle. **Horizontal Strabismus of 20-50 Prism Diopters:** 2.5-5 U in any one muscle. **Persistent VI Nerve Palsy Lasting ≥1 Month:** 1.25-2.5 U into medial rectus muscle. Increase dose by twofold if previous dose results in incomplete paralysis. **Max:** 25 U/muscle. Reassess 7-14 after each injection. **Blepharospasm: Initial:** 1.25-2.5 U into medial and lateral pretarsal orbicularis oculi of the upper lid and into lateral pretarsal orbicularis oculi of the lower lid. **Max:** 200 U/30 day. **Primary Axillary Hyperhidrosis:** 50 units per axilla.	**W/P:** Do not exceed dosing recommendations. Caution with peripheral motor neuropathic diseases (eg, amyotrophic lateral sclerosis, motor neuropathy), neuromuscular junctional disorders (eg, myasthenia gravis, Lambert-Eaton syndrome), increased risk of dysphagia and respiratory compromise. Contains albumin. Have epinephrine available if anaphylactic reaction occurs. Caution with inflammation at injection site, excessive weakness or atrophy in target muscles. Injection of orbicularis muscle may reduce blinking. Caution to resume activities gradually. Retrobulbular hemorrhages compromising retinal circulation reported; have instruments to decompress orbit accessible. Increased risk of dysphagia in patients with smaller neck muscle mass and those with bilateral injections into sternocleidomastoid muscle; limit dose. Caution in elderly. Weakness of hand muscles and blepharoptosis with hyperhidrosis and facial hyperhidrosis may occur, respectively. **Contra:** Presence of infection at proposed injection site. **P/N:** Category C, caution in nursing.	(Cervical Dystonia) Dysphagia, upper respiratory infection, neck pain, headache; (Blepharospasm) ptosis, keratitis, eye dryness; (Strabismus) ptosis, vertical deviation; (Primary Axillary Hyperhidrosis) injection-site pain and hemorrhage, infection, **pharyngitis,** flu syndrome, headache, fever, neck/back pain, pruritus, anxiety.

†Bold entries denote special dental considerations.
BB = black box warning; **W/P** = warnings/precautions; **Contra** = contraindications; **P/N** = pregnancy category rating and nursing considerations.

NAME	FORM/ STRENGTH	DOSAGE	WARNINGS/PRECAUTIONS & CONTRAINDICATIONS	ADVERSE EFFECTS†
Botulinum Toxin Type B (Myobloc)	**Inj:** 2500 U/0.5mL, 5000 U/mL, 10,000 U/2mL	***Adults:* Cervical Dystonia: Initial:** 2500-5000 U divided among affected muscles with history of tolerating the toxin. Use lower dose without history of tolerance. Adjust dose to response.	**W/P:** Do not exceed dosing recommendations. Caution with peripheral motor neuropathic diseases (eg, amyotrophic lateral sclerosis, motor neuropathy), neuromuscular junctional disorders (eg, myasthenia gravis, Lambert-Eaton syndrome); increased risk of dysphagia and respiratory compromise. Contains albumin. Treatment-naive patients should be initiated at lower doses. **P/N:** Category C, caution in nursing.	**Dry mouth,** dysphagia, dyspepsia, injection-site pain, infection, pain.
SKELETAL MUSCLE RELAXANTS (CENTRALLY ACTING)				
Carisoprodol (Soma)	**Tab:** 250mg, 350mg	***Adults:* ≤65 yrs/*Pediatrics* ≥16 yrs:** 250-350mg qid for 2-3 weeks.	**W/P:** May have sedative properties. Taking alcohol or other CNS depressants may have an additive effect. Cases of drug abuse, dependence, and withdrawal reported. Caution in addiction-prone patients. First-dose idiosyncratic reactions reported (rare). Occasionally within period of first to fourth dose, allergic reactions have occured. Rare reports of seizures in postmarketing surveillance. Caution with liver or renal dysfunction. Seizures reported. **Contra:** Acute intermittent porphyria and hypersensitivity to a carbamate. **P/N:** Category C, caution in nursing.	Drowsiness, dizziness, headache, N/V, tachycardia, postural hypotension, agitation, irritability, insomnia, seizures.
Carisoprodol/ Aspirin (Soma Compound)	**Tab:** (Carisoprodol-ASA) 200mg-325mg	***Adults/Pediatrics:* ≥16 yrs:** 1-2 tabs qid. **Max:** 2 tabs qid for 2-3 weeks.	**W/P:** First-dose idiosyncratic reactions reported (rare). Caution with liver or renal dysfunction, elderly, peptic ulcer, gastritis, addiction-prone patients, and anticoagulant therapy. Carisoprodol may have sedative properties and may impair physical/mental abilities. Increased risk of seizures reported. **Contra:** Acute intermittent porphyria, bleeding disorders, aspirin-induced asthma. **P/N:** Category D, caution in nursing.	Drowsiness, dizziness, vertigo, ataxia, N/V, gastritis, occult bleeding, postural hypotension, leukopenia, pancytopenia, constipation, diarrhea.
Carisoprodol/ Codeine Phosphate/ Aspirin (Soma Compound Codeine) CIII	**Tab:** (Carisoprodol-Codeine-Aspirin) 200mg-16mg-325mg	***Adults/Pediatrics:* ≥16 yrs:** 1-2 tabs qid. **Max:** 2 tabs qid for 2-3 weeks.	**W/P:** First-dose idiosyncratic reactions reported (rare). Contains sodium metabisulfate; may cause allergic type reactions. Caution with liver or renal dysfunction, elderly, peptic ulcer, gastritis, addiction-prone patients, and anticoagulant therapy. Caution in individuals who are ultra-rapid metabolizers of codeine. May have sedative properties. Withdrawal symptoms reported with abrupt discontinuation after long-term use. May cause respiratory depression, GI obstruction, and hypotension. Opioid-associated respiratory depression may increase with increased intracranial pressure, COPD, restrictive lung disease, and decreased respiratory drive. Psychological and/or physical dependence may occur. **Contra:** Acute intermittent porphyria, bleeding disorders, aspirin-induced asthma. **P/N:** Category D, caution in nursing.	Drowsiness, dizziness, vertigo, ataxia, NV, gastritis, occult bleeding, constipation, diarrhea, miosis, allergic-skin rash, postural hypotension.

Table 22.1. PRESCRIBING INFORMATION FOR SKELETAL MUSCLE RELAXANTS *(cont.)*

NAME	FORM/ STRENGTH	DOSAGE	WARNINGS/PRECAUTIONS & CONTRAINDICATIONS	ADVERSE EFFECTS†
SKELETAL MUSCLE RELAXANTS (CENTRALLY ACTING) *(cont.)*				
Cyclobenzaprine HCl (Amrix)	**Cap, Extended-Release:** 15mg, 30mg	***Adults:*** **Usual:** 15mg qd. **Titrate:** May increase to 30mg qd if needed. Use for longer than 2-3 weeks not recommended.	**W/P:** Avoid in hepatic impairment and elderly patients. Caution with history of urinary retention, angle-closure glaucoma, increased IOP, and use of anticholinergic medication. May impair mental and/or physical performance. **Contra:** MAOI use during or within 14 days. Hyperpyretic crisis seizures and deaths associated with concomitant use of cyclobenzaprine (or stucturally similar to TCAs) and MAOIs reported. Acute recovery phase of MI, arrhythmias, heart block conduction disturbances, CHF, hyperthyroidism. **P/N:** Category B, caution in nursing.	Drowsiness, **dry mouth,** dizziness, somnolence, headache.
Cyclobenzaprine HCl (Flexeril)	**Tab:** 5mg, 10mg	***Adults/Pediatrics:*** **≥15 yrs: Usual:** 5mg tid. **Titrate:** May increase to 10mg tid. **Mild Hepatic Dysfunction/Elderly: Initial:** 5mg qd, then slowly increase. **Moderate/Severe Hepatic Dysfunction:** Avoid use. Treatment should not exceed 2-3 weeks.	**W/P:** Caution with history of urinary retention, angle-closure glaucoma, increased IOP, hepatic dysfunction. Caution in elderly due to increased risk of CNS effects. May produce arrhythmias, sinus tachycardia, and conduction time prolongation. May impair mental/physical abilities. May enhance effect of barbiturates, alcohol, and other CNS depressants. **Contra:** Acute recovery phase of MI, arrhythmias, heart block or conduction disturbances, CHF, hyperthyroidism, MAOI use during or within 14 days. **P/N:** Category B, caution in nursing.	Drowsiness, **dry mouth,** headache, fatigue.
SKELETAL MUSCLE RELAXANTS (DIRECT-ACTING)				
Dantrolene Sodium (Dantrium IV)	**Inj:** 20mg	***Adults/Pediatrics:*** **Malignant Hyperthermia: Initial:** Minimum 1mg/kg IV push. Continue until symptoms subside or max cumulative dose 10mg/kg. **Pre-Op Malignant Hyperthermia Prophylaxis:** 2.5mg/kg 1.25 hrs before anesthesia and infuse over 1 hr. May need additional therapy during anesthesia/surgery if symptoms arise. **Post-Op Prophylaxis: Initial:** 1mg/kg or more as clinical situation dictates.	**W/P:** Use with supportive therapies to treat malignant hyperthermia. Take steps to prevent extravasation. Fatal and nonfatal hepatic disorders reported. Do not operate automobile or engage hazardous activity for 48 hrs after therapy. Caution at meals on day of administration because difficulty in swallowing/choking reported. Monitor vital signs if given preoperatively. **P/N:** Category C, safety in nursing not known.	Loss of grip strength, weakness in legs, drowsiness, dizziness, pulmonary edema, thrombophlebitis, urticaria, erythema.
Dantrolene Sodium (Dantrium)	**Cap:** 25mg, 50mg, 100mg	***Adults:*** **Chronic Spasticity: Initial:** 25mg qd for 7 days. **Titrate:** Increase to 25mg tid for 7 days, then 50mg tid for 7 days, then 100mg tid. **Max:** 100mg qid. If no further benefit at next higher dose, decrease to previous lower dose. **Malignant Hyperthermia: Pre-Op:** 4-8mg/kg/day given tid-qid for 1-2 days before surgery, with last dose given 3-4 hrs before surgery. **Post-Op Following Malignant Hyperthermia Crisis:** 4-8mg/kg/day given qid for 1-3 days. ***Pediatrics:*** **≥5 yrs: Chronic Spasticity: Initial:** 0.5mg/kg qd for 7 days. **Titrate:** Increase to 0.5mg/kg tid for 7 days, then 1mg/kg tid for 7 days, then 2mg/kg tid. **Max:** 100mg qid. If no further benefit at next higher dose, decrease to previous lower dose.	**BB:** Associated with hepatotoxicity; monitor hepatic function. Discontinue if no benefit after 45 days. **W/P:** Monitor LFTs at baseline, then periodically. Increased risk of hepatocellular disease in females and patients >35 yrs. Caution with pulmonary, cardiac, and liver dysfunction. Photosensitivity reaction may occur; limit sunlight exposure. **Contra:** Active hepatic disease, where spasticity is utilized to sustain upright posture and balance in locomotion, when spasticity is utilized to obtain or maintain increased function. **P/N:** Category C, not for use in nursing.	Drowsiness, dizziness, weakness, malaise, fatigue, diarrhea, hepatitis, tachycardia, aplastic anemia, thrombocytopenia, depression, seizure.

†Bold entries denote special dental considerations.
BB = black box warning; **W/P** = warnings/precautions; **Contra** = contraindications; **P/N** = pregnancy category rating and nursing considerations.

NAME	FORM/ STRENGTH	DOSAGE	WARNINGS/PRECAUTIONS & CONTRAINDICATIONS	ADVERSE EFFECTS†
SKELETAL MUSCLE RELAXANT (DEPOLARIZING)				
Succinylcholine Chloride (Anectine)	**Inj:** 20mg/mL	***Adults:* Short Surgical Procedure: Average Dose:** 0.6mg/kg IV. **Range:** 0.3-1.1mg/kg IV. Blockade develops in 1 min, may persist up to 2 min. **Long Surgical Procedure:** 2.5-4.3mg/min IV; or 0.3-1.1mg/kg initial IV inj, then 0.04-0.07mg/kg IV at appropriate intervals. **Adults/Older Children/Infants: (if vein not accessible): IM:** Up to 3-4mg/kg IM. **Max:** 150mg/total dose. Effect observed in 2-3 min. ***Pediatrics:* Procedure to Secure Airway: Infants/Small Children:** 2mg/kg IV. **Older Children/ Adolescents:** 1mg/kg IV.	**BB:** Rare reports of acute rhabdomyolysis with hyperkalemia followed by ventricular dysrhythmias, cardiac arrest, and death in children with undiagnosed skeletal muscle myopathy. Reserve in children for emergency intubation where securing airway is necessary. **W/P:** Avoid administration before unconsciousness has been induced. May induce arrhythmias or cardiac arrest in electrolyte abnormalities or massive digitalis toxicity. Caution with chronic abdominal infection, subarachnoid hemorrhage, conditions causing degeneration of central and peripheral nervous system, fractures, muscle spasms, reduced plasma cholinesterase activity, and acute phase of injury following major burns, multiple trauma, extensive skeletal muscle denervation, upper motor neuron injury. Malignant hyperthermia reported. Higher incidence of bradycardia progressing to asystole with second dose. May increase IOP, intracranial or intragastric pressure. With prolonged therapy, Phase I block will progress to Phase II block associated with prolonged respiratory paralysis and weakness. Confirm Phase II block before therapy. Hypokalemia or hypocalcemia prolong neuromuscular blockade. **Contra:** Personal or familial history of malignant hyperthermia, skeletal muscle myopathies. Acute phase of injury following major burns, multiple trauma, extensive skeletal muscle denervation, upper motor neuron injury. **P/N:** Category C, caution in nursing.	Respiratory depression, cardiac arrest, malignant hyperthermia, arrhythmia, bradycardia, tachycardia, HTN, hypotension, hyperkalemia, increased IOP, muscle fasciculation, **jaw rigidity,** post-op muscle pains.
SKELETAL MUSCLE RELAXANTS (NONDEPOLARIZING)				
Atracurium Besylate	**Inj:** 10mg/mL	***Adults:* ICU:** 11-13mcg/kg/min IV. **Following Succinylcholine: Initial:** 0.3-0.4mg/kg IV. ***Adults/Pediatrics:* >2 yrs: Initial:** 0.4-0.5mg/kg IV bolus. **Prolonged Procedure: Maint:** 0.08-0.1mg/kg at regular intervals to meet needs; give after first dose. **Operating Room Infusion: Initial:** 0.3-0.5mg/kg IV bolus. **Maint:** 9-10mcg/kg/min initial infusion to counteract recovery from bolus followed by 5-9mcg/kg/min. **Isoflurane/Enflurane at Steady State:** Reduce dose by 1/3. **≥1 month: Significant Cardiovascular Disease/ Histamine-Release Sensitive Patients: Initial:** 0.3-0.4mg/kg IV slowly or in divided doses. **1 month-2 yrs (under halothane): Initial:** 0.3-0.4mg/kg IV bolus. **Maint:** Slightly greater frequency than adults.	**W/P:** Avoid IM administration or administration before unconsciousness has been induced. Use with adequate anesthesia. The 10mL vial contains benzyl alcohol. May release histamines; caution in those where substantial histamine release would be hazardous (eg, severe cardiovascular disease) or if at a greater risk of histamine release (eg, anaphylactoid reactions, asthma). Use peripheral nerve stimulators to assess neuromuscular block in myasthenia gravis, Eaton-Lambert syndrome, other neuromuscular diseases, severe electrolyte disorders, elderly, carcinomatosis. Malignant hyperthermia (rare) reported. Resistance may develop in burn patients; increase dose. Monitor neuromuscular transmission of ICU patients continuously with a nerve stimulator. **P/N:** Category C, caution in nursing.	Allergic reactions, inadequate/ prolonged block, hypotension, vasodilation (flushing), tachycardia, bradycardia, dyspnea, bronchospasm, **laryngospasm,** rash, urticaria, injection-site pain.

Table 22.1. PRESCRIBING INFORMATION FOR SKELETAL MUSCLE RELAXANTS *(cont.)*

NAME	FORM/ STRENGTH	DOSAGE	WARNINGS/PRECAUTIONS & CONTRAINDICATIONS	ADVERSE EFFECTS†
SKELETAL MUSCLE RELAXANTS (NONDEPOLARIZING) *(cont.)*				
Cisatracurium Besylate (Nimbex)	**Inj:** 2mg/mL, 10mg/mL	***Adults:*** **ICU:** 3mcg/kg/min IV; dose requirements may increase/decrease with time. ***Adults/Pediatrics:* >12 yrs: Initial:** 0.15mg/kg (3 x ED95) or 0.20mg/kg (4 x ED95) IV. **Serious Cardiovascular Disease:** Up to 8 x ED95. **Maint/Prolonged Surgical Procedures:** 0.03mg/kg IV (for 20 min blockade) 40-50 min after initial 0.15mg/kg, and 50-60 min after initial 0.20mg/kg. **2-12 yrs: Initial:** 0.10-0.15mg/kg over 5-10 seconds during halothane or opioid anesthesia. **1-23 months: Initial:** 0.15mg/kg over 5-10 sec during halothane or opioid anesthesia. **≥2 yrs: Operating Room Infusion:** After initial bolus dose, give 3mcg/kg/min to counteract recovery from bolus, then 1-2mcg/kg/min.	**W/P:** Avoid administration before unconsciousness has been induced. Use in facility with resuscitation and life support, and have antagonist available. Monitor neuromuscular function with peripheral nerve stimulator during administration. Multidose vials contain benzyl alcohol. Not for rapid sequence endotracheal intubation. May have profound effect with neuromuscular diseases (eg, myasthenia gravis, carcinomatosis); monitor neuromuscular function with peripheral nerve stimulator. Resistance may develop in burn victims; consider increasing dose. Resistance with hemiparesis or paraparesis. Acid-base and/or serum electrolyte abnormalities may potentiate or antagonize effect. Monitor for malignant hyperthermia. **Contra:** Hypersensitivity to bisbenzylisoquinolinium agents and benzyl alcohol. **P/N:** Category B, caution in nursing.	Bradycardia, hypotension, flushing, bronchospasm, rash, muscle weakness, myopathy, prolonged/inadequate neuromuscular blockade.
Pancuronium Bromide	**Inj:** 1mg/mL, 2mg/mL	***Adults/Pediatrics:*** Individualize dose. **Initial:** 0.04-0.1mg/kg IV. Late incremental doses of 0.01mg/kg may be used. **Skeletal Muscle Relaxation For Endotracheal Intubation:** 0.06-0.1mg/kg bolus. **Neonates:** Use test dose of 0.02mg/kg.	**BB:** Administer by adequately trained individuals familiar with actions, characteristics, and hazards. **W/P:** May have profound effect in myasthenia gravis or myasthenic (Eaton-Lambert) syndrome; use small test dose and monitor closely. Contains benzyl alcohol; caution in neonates. Use peripheral nerve stimulator to monitor neuromuscular blocking effect. Caution with preexisting pulmonary, hepatic, or renal disease. Conditions associated with slower circulation time in cardiovascular disease, old age, and edematous states may delay onset time; dosage should not be increased. Possible slower onset, higher total dosage, and prolongation of neuromuscular blockade with hepatic and/or biliary tract disease. In ICU, long-term use may be associated with prolonged paralysis and/or skeletal muscle weakness; monitor closely. Severe obesity and neuromuscular disease may pose airway or ventilatory problems. Electrolyte imbalances may alter neuromuscular blockade. **P/N:** Category C, safety in nursing not known.	Skeletal muscle weakness and paralysis, **salivation,** rash.

†Bold entries denote special dental considerations.
BB = black box warning; **W/P** = warnings/precautions; **Contra** = contraindications; **P/N** = pregnancy category rating and nursing considerations.

NAME	FORM/ STRENGTH	DOSAGE	WARNINGS/PRECAUTIONS & CONTRAINDICATIONS	ADVERSE EFFECTS†
Rocuronium Bromide (Zemuron)	**Inj:** 10mg/mL	***Adults:*** Individualize dose. **Rapid Sequence Intubation:** 0.6-1.2mg/kg; **Tracheal Intubation: Initial:** 0.6mg/kg. **Maint:** 0.1, 0.15, or 0.2mg/kg. **Continuous Infusion: Initial:** 10-12mcg/kg/min. **Range:** 4-16mcg/kg/min. ***Pediatrics:*** **3 months-14 yrs:** Individualize dose. **Initial:** 0.6mg/kg. A lower dose of 0.45mg/kg may be used depending on age and anesthetic technique. Not recommended for rapid sequence intubation.	**W/P:** Employ peripheral nerve stimulator to monitor drug response. Appropriate anethesia or sedation is necessary. May have profound effects with myasthenia gravis or myasthenic (Eaton-Lambert) syndrome; use small test dose and monitor closely. Do not mix with alkaline solutions (eg, barbiturate solutions) in the same syringe or administer simultaneously during IV infusion through the same needle. Anaphylactic reactions reported. Tolerance may develop during chronic administration. Not recommended for rapid sequence induction in Cesarean section. Caution with clinically significant hepatic disease. Conditions associated with slower circulation time (eg, cardiovascular disease or advanced age) may delay onset time. Electrolyte imbalances may enhance neuromuscular blockade. **P/N:** Category C, safety in nursing not known.	Arrhythmia, abnormal ECG, tachycardia, N/V, asthma, hiccup, rash, injection-site edema, pruritus.
Vecuronium Bromide	**Inj:** 10mg, 20mg	***Adults/Pediatrics:*** **10-17 yrs:** Individualize dose. **Initial:** 0.08-0.1mg/kg IV bolus. **Maint:** 0.01-0.015mg/kg IV within 25-40 min of initial dose. Administer subsequent doses at 12-15 min intervals under balanced anesthesia and slightly longer with inhalation agents. **Max:** 0.15-0.28mg/kg. **Prior Succinylcholine:** Reduce dose to 0.04-0.06mg/kg with inhalation anesthesia and 0.05-0.06mg/kg with balanced anesthesia. **Continuous Infusion: Initial:** 1mcg/kg/min administered 20-40 min after intubating dose of 80-100mcg/kg. Administer infusion after evidence of recovery from bolus. Adjust infusion rate to maintain 90% suppression of twitch response. **Maint:** 0.8-1.2mcg/kg/min. **Concurrent Steady-State Enflurane/Isoflurane:** Reduce rate 25-60%, 45-60 min after intubating dose. **1-10 yrs:** May require a slightly higher initial dose and may also require supplementation slightly more often than adults.	**BB:** Administer by adequately trained individuals familiar with actions, characteristics, and hazards. **W/P:** May have profound effect in myasthenia gravis or myasthenic (Eaton-Lambert) syndrome; use small test dose and monitor closely. Prolongation of neuromuscular blockade may occur in anephric patients; consider lower initial dose. Conditions associated with slower circulation time in cardiovascular disease, old age, and edematous states may delay onset time; dosage should not be increased. Prolonged recovery time reported with cirrhosis or cholestasis. In ICU, long-term use may be associated with prolonged paralysis and/or skeletal muscle weakness. Monitor neuromuscular transmission of ICU patients continuously with a nerve stimulator. Severe obesity and neuromuscular disease may pose airway or ventilatory problems. Electrolyte imbalances may alter neuromuscular blockade. **P/N:** Category C, safety in nursing not known.	Skeletal muscle weakness and paralysis.

Table 22.2. DRUG INTERACTIONS FOR SKELETAL MUSCLE RELAXANTS

$ALPHA_2$-ADRENERGIC AGONIST (CENTRALLY ACTING)

Tizanidine HCl (Zanaflex)	
Acetaminophen	May delay T_{max} of acetaminophen.
Alcohol	May increase plasma levels with alcohol. Additive CNS depressant effects with coadministration.
Antihypertensives	Additive hypotensive effects with other antihypertensives. Avoid concomitant α_2-adrenergic agonists (eg, clonidine).
Contraceptives, oral	May decrease clearance with coadministration of oral contraceptives.
CYP1A2 inhibitors	Avoid use with potent inhibitors of CYP1A2 (eg, fluvoxamine, ciprofloxacin); may decrease clearance and increase plasma levels.

GABA ANALOG

Baclofen (Kemstro)	
Antidiabetic agents	May increase blood glucose and require dosage adjustment of antidiabetic agents.
Antihypertensives	May potentiate antihypertensive effect.
Carbidopa/levodopa therapy	Mental confusion, hallucinations, and agitation with levodopa/carbidopa therapy.
CNS depressants	Additive effects with other CNS depressants, including alcohol.
Magnesium sulfate	Synergistic effects with magnesium sulfate and other neuromuscular blockers.
MAOI	May increase CNS depressant effects of MAOIs.
Neuromuscular blockers	Synergistic effects with magnesium sulfate and other neuromuscular blockers.
TCAs	May be potentiated by TCAs.

MUSCULAR ANALGESICS (CENTRALLY ACTING)

Chlorzoxazone (Parafon Forte DSC)	
CNS depressants	Additive effects with other CNS depressants, including alcohol.
Metaxalone (Skelaxin)	
Barbiturates	Additive effects with barbiturates.
CNS depressants	Additive effects with other CNS depressants, including alcohol.
Methocarbamol (Robaxin, Robaxin Injection, Robaxin-750)	
CNS depressants	Additive CNS depressant effects with other CNS depressants, including alcohol.
Pyridostigmine bromide	May inhibit effect of pyridostigmine bromide; caution in patients with myasthenia gravis receiving anticholinergics.
Orphenadrine Citrate	
Propoxyphene	Confusion, anxiety, and tremors reported with propoxyphene.
Orphenadrine Citrate/Aspirin/Caffeine (Norgesic, Norgesic Forte)	
Propoxyphene	Confusion, anxiety, and tremors reported with propoxyphene.

Table 22.2. DRUG INTERACTIONS FOR SKELETAL MUSCLE RELAXANTS *(cont.)*

PURIFIED NEUROTOXIN COMPLEX

Botulinum Toxin Type A (Botox)	
Aminoglycosides	Interfere with neuromuscular transmission; may potentiate effect of toxin.
Botulinum neurotoxin serotypes	Neuromuscular paralysis may be exacerbated by coadministration or overlapping administration of different botulinum toxin serotypes.
Neuromuscular transmission, agents interfering with	May potentiate effect of toxin with agents that interfere with neuromuscular transmission (eg, curare-like compounds).
Botulinum Toxin Type B (Myobloc)	
Aminoglycosides	Interfere with neuromuscular transmission; may potentiate effect of toxin.
Botulinum neurotoxin serotypes	Neuromuscular paralysis may be exacerbated by coadministration or overlapping administration of different botulinum toxin serotypes.
Neuromuscular transmission, agents interfering with	May potentiate effect of toxin with agents that interfere with neuromuscular transmission (eg, curare-like compounds).

SKELETAL MUSCLE RELAXANTS (CENTRALLY ACTING)

Carisoprodol (Soma)	
Benzodiazepines	Additive sedative effects with benzodiazepines.
CNS depressants	Additive sedative effects with other CNS depressants, including alcohol.
CYP2C19 inducers	May decrease plasma levels and increase levels of active metabolite with concomitant CYP2C19 inducers (eg, rifampin, St. John's wort).
CYP2C19 inhibitors	May increase plasma levels and decrease levels of active metabolite with concomitant CYP2C19 inhibitors (eg, omeprazole, fluvoxamine).
Meprobamate	Avoid concomitant use of meprobamate.
Opioids	Additive sedative effects with opioids.
TCAs	Additive sedative effects with TCAs.
Carisoprodol/Aspirin (Soma Compound)	
Ammonium chloride	May increase plasma levels of salicylates with coadministration.
Antacids	May decrease plasma levels of salicylates with concomitant use.
Anticoagulants, oral	May increase risk of bleeding with oral anticoagulants.
Antidiabetic agents, oral	May increase risk of hypoglycemia with antidiabetic agents.
CNS depressants	Additive effects with other CNS depressants, including alcohol.
Corticosteroids	May decrease plasma levels of salicylates with coadministration.
Ethyl alcohol	May increase aspirin-induced fecal blood loss reported with coadministration.
Methotrexate	May enhance methotrexate toxicity with coadministration.
Psychotropic agents	Additive effects with psychotropic agents.
Uricosuric agents	May reduce uricosuric effect of probenecid and sulfinpyrazone; renal excretion of salicylate may be reduced.

SKELETAL MUSCLE RELAXANTS (CENTRALLY ACTING) *(cont.)*

Carisoprodol/Aspirin/Codeine Phosphate (Soma Compound/Codeine) CIII	
Ammonium chloride	May increase plasma levels of salicylates with coadministration.
Antacids	May decrease plasma levels of salicylates with concomitant use.
Anticoagulants, oral	May increase risk of bleeding with oral anticoagulants.
Antidiabetic agents, oral	May increase risk of hypoglycemia with antidiabetic agents.
CNS depressants	Additive effects with other CNS depressants, including alcohol.
Corticosteroids	May decrease plasma levels of salicylates with coadministration.
Ethyl alcohol	May increase aspirin-induced fecal blood loss reported with coadministration.
Methotrexate	May enhance methotrexate toxicity with coadministration.
Psychotropic agents	Additive effects with psychotropic agents.
Uricosuric agents	May reduce uricosuric effect of probenecid and sulfinpyrazone; renal excretion of salicylate may be reduced.
Cyclobenzaprine HCl (Amrix, Flexeril)	
Anticholinergic agents	Caution with anticholinergic agents.
Barbiturates	Additive effects with barbiturates.
CNS depressants	Additive effects with other CNS depressants, including alcohol.
Guanethidine	May block antihypertensive action of guanethidine and similar compounds.
MAOIs	Life-threatening reaction with MAOIs; avoid coadministration or use within 14 days.
Tramadol	May increase seizure risk with tramadol.

SKELETAL MUSCLE RELAXANT (DIRECT-ACTING)

Dantrolene Sodium (Dantrium, Dantrium IV)	
CCBs	Avoid CCBs (eg, verapamil) with IV dantrolene; rare possibility of cardiovascular collapse.
Clofibrate	May decrease binding to plasma proteins with clofibrate (IV only).
CNS depressants	May potentiate adverse effects with sedatives and tranquilizing agents; caution with coadministration.
Estrogen therapy	May increase risk of hepatotoxicity in women >35 years on estrogen therapy; caution with coadministration (oral only).
Hepatic enzymes inducers	May increase metabolism with drugs known to induce hepatic enzymes.
Tolbutamide	May increase binding to plasma proteins with tolbutamide (IV only).
Vecuronium	May potentiate vecuronium-induced neuromuscular block.
Warfarin	May decrease binding to plasma proteins with warfarin (IV only).

Table 22.2. DRUG INTERACTIONS FOR SKELETAL MUSCLE RELAXANTS *(cont.)*

SKELETAL MUSCLE RELAXANT (DEPOLARIZING)

Succinylcholine Chloride (Anectine)	
Anesthetics, volatile	May increase risk of malignant hyperthermia with coadministration of volatile anesthetics.
Antibiotics, nonpenicillin	Effects may be enhanced with certain nonpenicillin antibiotics.
Aprotinin	Effects may be enhanced with aprotinin.
β-blockers	Effects may be enhanced with β-adrenergic blockers.
Chloroquine	Effects may be enhanced with chloroquine.
Cholinesterase inhibitors	Effects may be enhanced with drugs that reduce plasma cholinesterase activity (eg, chronically administered oral contraceptives, glucocorticoids, certain MAOIs) or inhibit plasma cholinesterase.
Desflurane	Effects may be enhanced with desflurane.
Diethylether	Effects may be enhanced with diethylether.
Isoflurane	Effects may be enhanced with isoflurane.
Lidocaine	Effects may be enhanced with lidocaine.
Lithium carbonate	Effects may be enhanced with lithium carbonate.
Magnesium salts	Effects may be enhanced with magnesium salts.
Metoclopramide	Effects may be enhanced with metoclopramide.
Neuromuscular blockers	Possibility of synergistic/antagonistic effect with other neuromuscular blockers during same procedure.
Oxytocin	Effects may be enhanced with oxytocin.
Procainamide	Effects may be enhanced with procainamide.
Promazine	Effects may be enhanced with promazine.
Quinidine	Effects may be enhanced with quinidine.
Quinine	Effects may be enhanced with quinine.
Terbutaline	Effects may be enhanced with terbutaline.
Trimethaphan	Effects may be enhanced with trimethaphan.

SKELETAL MUSCLE RELAXANTS (NONDEPOLARIZING)

Atracurium Besylate	
Alkaline solutions	Do not mix with alkaline solutions (eg, barbiturate solutions).
Antibiotics	Effects may be enhanced with certain antibiotics (eg, aminoglycosides, polymyxins).
Enflurane	Effects may be enhanced with enflurane.
Halothane	Effects may be enhanced with halothane.
Isoflurane	Effects may be enhanced with isoflurane.
Lithium	Effects may be enhanced with lithium.
Magnesium salts	Effects may be enhanced with magnesium salts.

SKELETAL MUSCLE RELAXANTS (NONDEPOLARIZING) *(cont.)*

Atracurium Besylate *(cont.)*	
Muscle relaxants	Possibility of synergistic or antagonistic effect with other muscle relaxants.
Procainamide	Effects may be enhanced with procainamide.
Quinidine	Effects may be enhanced with quinidine.
Succinylcholine	Avoid administration until recovery from succinylcholine has been observed.
Cisatracurium Besylate (Nimbex)	
Alkaline solutions	May not be compatible with alkaline solutions with a pH >8.5 (eg, barbiturate solutions).
Anesthetics, local	Effects may be enhanced with local anesthetics.
Antibiotics	Effects may be enhanced with certain antibiotics (eg, aminoglycosides, tetracyclines, bacitracin, polymyxins, lincomycin, clindamycin, colistin, sodium colistemethate).
Carbamazepine	Resistance reported with chronic carbamazepine; infusion rate requirements may be higher.
Enflurane with nitrous oxide/oxygen	May prolong duration of action and decrease required infusion rate with enflurane with nitrous oxide/oxygen.
Isoflurane with nitrous oxide/oxygen	May prolong duration of action and decrease required infusion rate with isoflurane with nitrous oxide/oxygen.
Lithium	Effects may be enhanced with lithium.
Magnesium salts	Effects may be enhanced with magnesium salts.
Phenytoin	Resistance reported with chronic phenytoin; infusion rate requirements may be higher.
Procainamide	Effects may be enhanced with procainamide.
Quinidine	Effects may be enhanced with quinidine.
Pancuronium Bromide	
Alkaline solutions	May not be compatible with alkaline solutions (eg, barbiturate solutions such as thiopental).
Anesthetics, volatile	Effects may be enhanced with volatile inhalational anesthetics (eg, enflurane, isoflurane, halothane).
Antibiotics	May enhance and prolong neuromuscular blockade with certain antibiotics (eg, aminoglycosides, tetracyclines, bacitracin, polymyxin B, colistin, sodium colistemethate).
Magnesium salts	Effects may be enhanced with magnesium salts.
Neuromuscular blockers, nondepolarizing	Avoid use with other nondepolarizing neuromuscular blockers (eg, vecuronium, atracurium, d-tubocurarine, metocurine, and gallamine); may manifest synergistic effects.
Quinidine	Recurrent paralysis reported with quinidine injection during recovery from use of other muscle relaxants.
Succinylcholine	Avoid administration until recovery from succinylcholine has been observed.

Table 22.2. DRUG INTERACTIONS FOR SKELETAL MUSCLE RELAXANTS *(cont.)*

SKELETAL MUSCLE RELAXANTS (NONDEPOLARIZING) *(cont.)*

Rocuronium Bromide (Zemuron)	
Anesthetics, local	May increase the duration of neuromuscular block and decrease infusion requirements of neuromuscular blocking agents.
Anesthetics, volatile	Effects may be enhanced with volatile inhalational anesthetics (eg, enflurane, isoflurane, halothane).
Antibiotics	May enhance and prolong neuromuscular blockade with certain antibiotics (eg, aminoglycosides, vancomycin, tetracyclines, bacitracin, polymyxins, colistin, sodium colistemethate).
Anticonvulsants	Resistance reported with chronic anticonvulsants (eg, carbamazepine, phenytoin); may require higher rate of infusion.
Magnesium salts	Effects may be enhanced with magnesium salts.
Neuromuscular blockers, nondepolarizing	Caution with other nondepolarizing neuromuscular blocking agents; may manifest additive effects.
Procainamide	May increase the duration of neuromuscular block and decrease infusion requirements of neuromuscular blocking agents.
Quinidine	Recurrent paralysis reported with quinidine injection during recovery from use of other muscle relaxants.
Succinylcholine	Avoid administration until recovery from succinylcholine has been observed.
Vecuronium Bromide	
Anesthetics, volatile	Effects may be enhanced with volatile inhalational anesthetics (eg, enflurane, isoflurane, halothane).
Antibiotics	Effects may be enhanced with certain antibiotics (eg, aminoglycosides, tetracyclines, bacitracin, polymyxin B, colistin, sodium colistemethate).
Magnesium salts	Effects may be enhanced with magnesium salts.
Neuromuscular blockers, nondepolarizing	Caution with other nondepolarizing neuromuscular blocking agents (eg, vecuronium, atracurium, d-tubocurarine, metocurine, and gallamine); may manifest additive effects.
Quinidine	Recurrent paralysis reported with quinidine injection during recovery from use of other muscle relaxants.
Succinylcholine	Avoid administration until recovery from succinylcholine has been observed.

Chapter 23

Drugs for Neoplastic Disorders

Sol Silverman Jr., D.D.S., M.A.; Alan M. Kramer, M.D.

More than 1.4 million new cases of cancer are diagnosed in the United States each year. In spite of improvements in surgical techniques and radiation therapy, only about half of these people will survive their disease. To diminish this high rate of mortality, chemotherapeutic drugs have become an increasingly important part of treatment regimens. These agents are used as single agents or in combination with other treatments. The intent of using these agents for many neoplasms is cure; however, they are more often used for palliation; to gain partial control over the growths and thus prolong life; or as adjuvants to improve response rates in radiation and surgical approaches. Additionally, highly cytotoxic levels of chemotherapeutic drugs are being used increasingly for persistent and recurrent cancers followed by rescue with bone-marrow and stem-cell transplantations. Use of targeted therapy is increasing to improve survival rates as well as limit toxicity (see "Biologic Agents" later in this chapter).

The medications used for neoplastic disorders can create cytotoxicity-induced immunosuppression, which can lead to significant symptoms and affect survival. Because the oral mucosae and microbial flora are extremely sensitive to immunosuppression, maintaining optimal oral and dental health becomes a key factor in patient management and outcomes.

Many agents are used to attack neoplastic cells through a variety of biochemical processes. They have efficacies for both solid and hematopoietic cancers. Response rates depend on the type of neoplasm, the combination of antineoplastic drugs, and the patient's physical status and tolerance. Because these agents are detoxified either in the liver or kidneys, these organs must be functional.

For oral and pharyngeal malignancies, these agents are used primarily as adjuvants to radiation, with the aim of improving responses to radiation. By far the best results for control of nasopharyngeal carcinomas have been achieved by the combination of radiation therapy and chemotherapy. However, in such cases, chemotherapy also accentuates the adverse effects of radiation.

The choice of drug(s) and dosage regimen(s) depends on response rates derived from multi-institutional and group cooperative studies. The toxic side effects of these agents, as well as response rates, are the factors that limit their application. These effects often limit dental procedures required for optimal oral health and create oral problems that lead to dysfunction and pain and require professional help (see "Guidelines for Dental Care of Patients Undergoing Chronic or Periodic Drug Treatment for Neoplastic Disorders" on the next page). Adverse side effects vary from patient to patient. Management by altering treatment, prescribing medications, or instituting empirical procedures depends on the severity of symptoms and the effects of patient outcomes.

ANTINEOPLASTIC DRUGS

Alkylating Agents

Alkylating agents are the oldest and most widely used class of anticancer drugs, being the major components of the combination chemotherapy regimens for disseminated solid tumors and for high-dose/stem-cell-support treatment regimens. Aklyating agents interfere with DNA synthesis by causing cross-linking, which can lead to cell death via several pathways. Examples of alkylating agents are cyclophosphamide, cisplatin, and nitrogen mustard.

Antibiotics

Antibiotics are a class of cytotoxic agents naturally derived from microbial fermentation broths that include bacteria, fungi,

Guidelines for Dental Care of Patients Undergoing Chronic or Periodic Drug Treatment for Neoplastic Disorders

Dental, clinical, and radiographic evaluation

- Dental caries, periapical lesions, periodontal disease, bone abnormalities
- Oral mucosal lesions

Consultation with primary care physician/oncologist

- Tumor site, type, stage
- Prognosis
- Medication(s)
- Other systemic diseases
- Suggested premedications
- Past treatment, next treatment

Dental treatment plan

- Immediate: Remove all sources of infection to prevent pain and bacteremia
- Long-term: Promote optimal function and esthetics and prevent infections

Optimal oral hygiene

- Pretreatment prophylaxis
- Initiation of fluoride applications
- Mouthrinses as tolerated (such as nonalcohol chlorhexidine)
- Home care instructions
- Orient patient to the side effects of treatment (such as mucositis) and hygiene modifications (such as soft brushes)

Limitations of treatment

- Infection risk: Leukopenia when white blood cell counts are <1,500 mm^3 (if procedure necessary, use antibiotics)
- Bleeding risk: Thrombocytopenia when platelet count is <100,000 mm^3 (extractions, cutting, invasive procedures)
- Candidiasis (yeast overgrowth): Use of topical/systemic antifungal drugs
- Herpes simplex virus reactivation: Use of systemic antiviral drugs
- Hyposalivation: Use of moisturizing agents and sialogogues
- Mucositis: Use of moisturizing agents, sialogogues, antimicrobial agents, and anti-inflammatory agents

and related organisms. Their mechanisms involve intercalation with DNA base pairs, thereby interfering with DNA synthesis. Examples of antibiotics are bleomycin and doxorubicin.

Antimetabolites

Antimetabolites are one of the more diversified and best characterized types of the chemotherapeutic agents in use. Both RNA and DNA syntheses are interrupted by competitive inhibition of purine and pyrimidine nucleosides and of folic acid. Examples are hydroxyurea, 5-fluorouracil, cytarabine, gemcitabine, and methotrexate (see **Chapter 21** for prescribing information for methotrexate).

Biologic agents

Targeted Therapy in Head and Neck Cancer

Targeted therapy implies a new method to treat cancer, exploiting unique molecular targets highly expressed in cancer cells. Small molecules and monoclonal antibodies are used to target receptors involved with tumorgenesis.

Epidermal growth factor-receptor (EGF-R) is one such target highly expressed in squamous cell carcinoma of the head and neck. Cetuximab (IMC-C225, Ertbitux) is a monoclonal antibody directed at the EGF-binding domain on the outer portion of the cell membrane. It has been shown to reduce cellular growth and to potentiate chemotherapy (cisplatin, taxanes) as well as radiotherapy in preclinical Models. Cetuximab has gone through Phase I, II, and III testing with both chemotherapy and radiotherapy and has been FDA-approved for use with radiotherapy and in platinum-refractory disease in patients with head and neck cancer. More recently, based on a large randomized trial for patients with recurrent or advanced head and neck cancer, cetuximab combined with platinum-fluorouracil chemotherapy improved overall survival compared to non-cetuximab arms, and as such, has become a new standard of care. Toxicity was tolerable (mostly skin rashes).

The internal domain of the EGF-R contains tyrosine kinase, which has also been targeted in an effort to block cell growth. Erlotinib (Tarceva, OSI-774) is one such tyrosine kinase inhibitor that has gone through clinical testing. Response rate remains modest for patients with head and neck cancer, but stable disease can be observed in 30% to 40% of patients for up to six months.

The side effect profile that accompanies all the EGF-R targeted therapies remains consistent, usually in the form of tolerable skin rashes and mild diarrhea.

The future of targeted therapy remains in finding additional targets that exploit unique pathways to cancer growth. Combination targeted therapy with and without radiotherapy and chemotherapy is the challenge for the future.

Other examples of biologic agents that produce antitumor effects include interferons, interleukin-2, tumor vaccines, and retinoids.

Hormonal Agents

Hormonal agents are used in the hormonally responsive cancers, such as breast, prostate, and endometrial carcinomas. As a group they have both cytostatic and cytocidal activity, which is largely mediated by secondary messengers via cytoplasmic and nuclear receptors. Examples of hormonal agents are tamoxifen, prednisone, androgens and estrogens, letrozole, and flutamide.

Miscellaneous Antineoplastic Agents

There are other miscellaneous antineoplastic agents. Taxanes are novel agents that promote the formation of microtubules and stabilize them by preventing depolymerization. Examples are paclitaxel and docetaxel, which are used in breast, lung, and ovarian cancers.

Topoisomerase I inhibitors are a group of agents derived from cantothecin. They kill cancer cells by inhibiting the production of the enzyme topoisomerase I, which is essential to DNA replication. Examples are topotecan and irinotecan, used in refractory colon and ovarian cancers.

Vinca alkaloids are part of a group of agents that interfere with microtubule assembly, thereby inhibiting the mitosis phase of the cell cycle. Examples are vinblastine, vincristine, and a new agent, vinorelbine. These agents are used in patients with lymphomas, Kaposi's sarcoma, lung cancer, and breast cancer.

Agents Under Investigation

Researchers have studied the use of vitamin A analogues (for example, 13-cis retinoic acid [Accutane]), as well as the use of antioxidants beta carotene or vitamin A ester, combined with vitamins C (ascorbic acid) and E (alpha tocopherol). Daily ingestion may help control precancerous oral lesions (leukoplakia). While antioxidant vitamins have no evident clinical adverse side effects, 13-cis retinoic acid may cause skin dryness, pruritus, rash, angular cheilitis, photosensitivity, and an increase in blood triglycerides. Optimal dosages and combinations have not yet been established and are presently not recommended. Clinical trials with COX-2 (cyclooxygenase) inhibitors have been discontinued because of the associated risk for cardiovascular disease. **Table 23.1** provides general information on selected antineoplastic drugs.

Special Dental Considerations

The patient's response to chemotherapeutic agents, many of which suppress white blood cells and platelets, influences the timing and types of dental procedures. The dentist's main concern before providing care to a patient receiving chemotherapy relates to adequate numbers of white blood cells (because of concerns about infection) and blood platelets (because of concerns about excessive bleeding). The marrow suppression usually is cyclical, and there are periods during which the risks of infection and bleeding are minimal.

Before undertaking any dental procedure involving a patient with cancer, contact the patient's primary care physician or oncologist regarding the need for any premedication. This includes the use of antibiotics to protect against bacteremias.

Because many medications used by dental clinicians to control oral complaints (signs and symptoms) may put an extra burden on a patient's ability to detoxify drugs, the dentist should notify the physician before using such medications. It is important to coordinate medical and dental treatment to minimize complications for the patient.

Careful clinical and radiographic examination followed by any indicated corrective procedure are essential to minimize subsequent complications of dental pain, abscesses, poor hygiene, and periodontal disease that may occur during cancer therapy. This is an important step in prevention, because dental infections that occur when the patient is temporarily compromised while undergoing chemotherapy can create critical problems in patient care and recovery.

Nausea and vomiting often complicate patient progress because of poor hygiene, inadequate food and liquid intake, pain and discomfort, malaise, and depression. However, it is essential that patients maintain optimal oral hygiene by using appropriate brushing and flossing techniques as well as mouthrinses. If mouthrinses that contain alcohol cause discomfort, then blander mouthrinses (such as baking soda rinses) should be used. Alcohol-free mouthrinses are available, eg, chlorhexidine (prescription) and Biotene (OTC). Some reports have stated that a daily rinse with chlorhexidine may reduce the risk of developing candidiasis and mucositis. Because of frequent instances of gingival sensitivity, soft toothbrushes or even gelfoam-type applicators are needed to apply a baking soda slurry or a flavor-free toothpaste (eg, Biotene toothpaste) that also contains fluoride and an enzyme system to help control oral flora proliferation.

ORAL CONDITIONS ASSOCIATED WITH CANCER THERAPY

Mucositis

Mucositis, or stomatitis, is a complex pathologic process of inflammation and ulceration probably caused by a combination of suppression of epithelial growth, mucosal erosion, abnormal connective tissue cytokine signaling, and bacterial overgrowth. It is a common manifestation of induced leukopenia. The oral mucosal reaction usually is associated with pain, which interferes with nutrition and hydration. This can significantly alter a patient's course of recovery and become a major complaint and therapeutic problem.

Mucositis is best managed by maintaining optimal oral hygiene and waiting for the critical white blood cell recovery. During this period, controlling pain with medication is important for maintaining the patient's comfort and nutritional intake. Antibiotics, antifungal drugs, and antiviral agents are often necessary. These medications are administered by the medical team. Short-course glucocorticoid therapy (such as 40 mg to 80 mg of prednisone daily as needed) is often helpful in reducing inflammation and discomfort. If tolerated, topical corticosteroids may be helpful (eg, elixir of dexamethasone 5 mg/5 mL). Fluocinonide (Lidex) ointment 0.05% as a gel or mixed with equal parts Orabase B can be administered topically for possible relief. Sometimes a mild mouthwash made up of anti-inflammatory, antifungal, and antihistamine solutions is helpful. Administration of granulocyte-stimulating factors may help accelerate white blood cell proliferation and recovery. Studies have indicated that some mouthrinses may help prevent or accelerate the recovery from mucositis, eg, L-glutamine, an amino acid associated with healing; and benzydamine, a nonsteroidal analgesic. Palifermin, an epithelial growth agent administered intravenously, has shown efficacy, as well as amifostine (Ethyol), an organic thiophosphate cytoprotective agent, administered intravenously or subcutaneously.

When utilizing bone marrow/stem cell transplantation to aid recovery from cytotoxic therapy and immunosuppression, graft-versus-host disease can mimic mucositis and cause considerable chronic discomfort. Management is similar to approaches for mucositis.

Xerostomia

Because many antineoplastic drugs affect the salivary glands and suppress saliva production, subsequent oral dryness can be bothersome and interfere with eating, speech, and hygiene. If hyposalivation is prolonged, it can also cause dental caries and promote candidiasis.

Fortunately, this hyposalivation is almost always transient. Therefore, conservative approaches are usually sufficient. These approaches include sucking on ice chips, taking frequent sips of water, sucking on sugarless candy, chewing sugarless gum and using saliva substitutes that provide temporary lubrication. More severe or longer-lasting xerostomia can be palliated by the use of systemic sialogogues (such as pilocarpine 5 mg tid or qid; bethanechol 25 mg to 50 mg tid or qid; or cevimeline 30 mg tid. See **Chapter 8**).

Topical lubricants, eg, Gelclair gel (prescription) or Oral*balance* liquid or gel (OTC) may be of some help. Nonalcohol Biotene mouthwash (OTC) contains ingredients (glucose oxidase, lactoperoxidase, lysozyme, and lactoferrin) that help control the oral microbial flora and are soothing.

Taste

Some agents used to control neoplastic growth affect the sensitive taste buds. Use of these agents often forms the basis for patients' complaints of altered food tastes (dysgeusia), or a "bad taste in the mouth." In some patients, this may even cause food aversion and further complicate their maintenance of adequate caloric intake. This complaint usually is a transient, direct response to a drug or combination of drugs.

Infections

Bone-marrow suppression is a common response to many antineoplastic drugs. This response often will reduce a normal white blood cell count of >4,000 cells/mm^3 to <2,000, and sometimes even to zero. The ensuing leukopenia lowers a patient's ability to control the proliferation of microorganisms.

Overgrowth of bacteria, viruses, and fungi that stems from drug-induced leukopenia can complicate patient care and the course of the disease. The main concern with bacterial overgrowth is the possibility of bacteremia, fevers of unknown origin, and patient morbidity and mortality.

Reactivation of the herpes simplex virus commonly occurs in the patient who is immunocompromised. The diagnosis is based on clinical suspicion combined with smears or cultures. Because of the acute nature of the viral infection, diagnosis and treatment are combined by instituting an antiviral drug along with the selected diagnostic technique.

Fungal overgrowth is usually caused by leukopenia, xerostomia, and poor hygiene. The organism is candidal, most often *Candida albicans.* Different species of the organism may have implications regarding responses to antifungal drugs. As with bacteria and foci of infection, the possibility of candidemia exists.

Identifying a causative agent of the infection is important. The medical team will prescribe the appropriate medications. It is important to rule out dental sources by examining the teeth, gingival, and mucosal surfaces.

Bleeding

Bleeding may be the result of a reduction of blood platelets, which occurs along with the marrow suppression and leukopenia. As platelet levels decrease to <100,000/mm^3, the patient's risk of experiencing hemorrhage, either spontaneous or in response to trauma, increases. Therefore, it is important that the clinician have knowledge of a patient's blood status before beginning dental procedures. Bleeding in addition to marrow suppression often results in anemia. This in turn contributes to patient malaise and weakness.

Osteonecrosis

Bisphosphonates, such as zoledronic acid or pamidronate, are widely used by medical oncologists as a preventive measure in malignancies that have a predilection for bone metastases and osteoporosis. It is estimated that up to 15% of patients treated with bisphosphonates given intravenously will develop associated osteonecrosis of the mandible or maxilla, most commonly following an invasive dental procedure, eg, extraction. There is no reproducibly effective curative treatment. Conservative supportive measures, utilizing antibiotics and analgesic agents, or smoothing sharp bone spicules, are helpful. Surgery, hyperbaric oxygen, and discontinuing the bisphosphonate have not been effective in controlling the problem.

Dental anomalies

In children, antineoplastic drug therapy may result in various dental anomalies. When a drug is given during tooth development, it may result in delayed eruption, noneruption, malformations of crowns and/or roots, and discolorations of the crown. While the clinical features and the patient's history can be fairly conclusive as to the cause of such conditions, the differential diagnosis still must include genetic dental dysplasia, hypoparathyroidism, and adverse influences of excess fluoride and broad-spectrum antibiotics.

Drug Interactions of Dental Interest

Because combinations of drugs, dosage ranges, and patient profiles and responses differ so greatly, it is necessary to maintain contact with the patient's physician to determine palliation and therapeutic dosages, expected side effects, and potential drug interactions. Interactions, if they do occur, are most commonly related to detoxification and elimination of drug products, resulting in high and potentially toxic drug levels in the blood. In turn, the blood levels required for effective pharmacologic response are balanced against potential adverse side effects.

Table 23.2 lists drug interactions related to antineoplastic drugs.

Significant Laboratory Value Alterations

- Values for leukocytes in leukopenia: <2,000 cells/mm^3 as opposed to the normal values, 5,000/mm^3 to 10,000 cells/mm^3.
- Values for platelets in thrombocytopenia: <50,000 platelets/mm^3 as opposed to the normal values, 150,000/mm^3 to 350,000 platelets/mm^3.

Special Patients

Pregnant and nursing women

Chemotherapy is contraindicated in pregnant and nursing women.

Pediatric, geriatric, and other special patients

In children, depending on the type of tumor and the patient's age and size, neoplastic drugs might affect tooth development.

In some geriatric patients and patients with disabilities, the dental treatment plan depends on the patient's overall prognosis, the type of tumor, the patient's medical status (in terms of general well-being), and the patient's ability to comply with protocols and self-care regimens.

Adverse Effects, Precautions, and Contraindications

Table 23.1 lists adverse effects related to antineoplastic drugs.

The following precautions and contraindications apply to all antineoplastic agents: concerns of myelosuppression, hepatotoxicity, nephrotoxicity, ototoxicity, and gastrointestinal upset. All antineoplastic drugs are classified in pregnancy risk category D.

Pharmacology

In general, aklylating agents, intercalators, and antibiotics damage or disrupt DNA, block activity of topoisomerases or alter resistance gene nucleotide binding site (RNBS) structure. Antimetabolites block or decrease synthesis of both RNA and DNA. Steroids interfere with transcription, while plant alkaloids disrupt mitosis. Biologic agents stimulate natural host defense mechanisms. Taxanes are considered spindle poisons, but unlike the vinca alkaloids, the taxanes allow microtubular assembly to occur and block disassociations.

SUGGESTED READING

Adaji AA, Dy GK. Systemic cancer therapy: Evolution over the last 60 years. *Cancer*. 2008; 113 (7 suppl):1857-87.

Antonadou D, Pepelassi M, Synodinou M, et al. Prophylactic use of amifostine to prevent radiochemotherapy-induced mucositis and xerostomia in head-and-neck cancer. *Int J Radiat Oncol Biol Phys*. 2002;52:739-747.

Bonner JA, Harari PM, Giralt J, et al. Radiotherapy plus cetuximab for squamous-cell carcinoma of the head and neck. *N Engl J Med*. 2006;354:567-578.

Cognetti DM, Weber RS, Lai SY. Head and neck cancer. An evolving treatment paradigm. *Cancer*. 2008; 113 (7 suppl):1911-32.

Edwards BJ, Hellstein JW, Jacobsen PL, et al. Updated recommendations for managing the care of patients receiving oral bisphosphonate therapy. *JADA*. 2008; 139:1674-77.

Elting LS, Keefe DM, Sonis ST, et al. Patient-reported measurements of oral mucositis in head and neck cancer patients treated with radiotherapy with or without chemotherapy. *Cancer*. 2008; 113:2704-13.

Frohling S, Dohner H. Chromosomal abnormalities in cancer. *N Engl J Med*. 2008; 359:722-34.

Haddad RI, Shin DM. Recent advances in head and neck cancer. *N Engl J Med*. 2008; 359:1143-54.

Hesketh PJ. Chemotherapy-induced nausea and vomiting. *N Engl J Med*. 2008; 358:2482-92.

Imanguli MM, Pavletic SZ, Guadagnini J-P, et al. Chronic graft versus host disease of oral mucosa: Review of available therapies. *Oral Surg Oral Med Oral Pathol Oral Radiol Endod*. 2006;101:177-185.

Jemal A, Siegel R, Ward E, et al. Cancer statistics, 2009. *CA—Cancer J Clin*. 2009;59:225-249.

Jensen SB, Mouridsen HT, Bergmann OJ, et al. Oral mucosal lesions, microbial changes, and taste disturbances induced by adjuvant chemotherapy in breast cancer patients. *Oral Surg Oral Med Oral Pathol OralRadiol Endod*. 2008; 139:1674-77.

Langer CJ. Targeted therapy in head and neck cancer. *Cancer*. 2008; 2635-45.

McNeil C. Human papillomavirus and oral cancer: Looking toward the clinic. *JNCI*. 2008; 100:840-41.

Migliorati CA, Chopra S, Kaltman SS. Dental management of patients with a history of bisphosphonate therapy: clinical dilemma. *CDA J*. 2008; 36:769-74.

Physicians' Desk Reference®. 63rd ed. Montvale, NJ: Physicians' Desk Reference Inc.; 2009.

Saba NF, Khuri FR, Shin DM. Targeting the epidermal growth factor receptor. *Oncology*. 2006;20:153-161.

Tsao AS, Kim ES, Hong WK. Chemoprevention of cancer. *CA Cancer J Clin*. 2004;54:150-180.

Vermorken JB, Mesia R, Rivera A et al. Platinum-based chemotherapy plus cetuximab in head and neck cancer. *N Engl J Med* 2008; 359:1116-27.

Table 23.1. PRESCRIBING INFORMATION FOR ANTINEOPLASTIC DRUGS

NAME	FORM/ STRENGTH	DOSAGE	WARNINGS/PRECAUTIONS & CONTRAINDICATIONS	ADVERSE EFFECTS†
ACTINOMYCIN ANTIBIOTIC				
Dactinomycin (Cosmegen)	**Inj:** 0.5mg	***Adults/Pediatrics:* >6-12 months: Wilms' Tumor/Childhood Rhabdomyosarcoma/Ewing's Sarcoma:** 15mcg/kg IV daily for 5 days. **Testicular Cancer:** 1000mcg/m² IV on Day 1 of combination therapy. **Gestational Trophoblastic Neoplasia: Monotherapy:** 12mcg/kg IV daily for 5 days. **Combination Therapy:** 500mcg/m² IV on Days 1 and 2. **Solid Malignancies:** 50mcg/kg IV for lower extremity or pelvis. 35mcg/kg IV for upper extremity. May need lower dose with obese patients, or with previous chemotherapy or radiation use. Dose intensity per 2-week cycle should not exceed 15mcg/kg/day or 400-600mcg/m² daily for 5 days. Calculate dose for obese or edematous patients based on BSA. **Elderly:** Start at low end of dosing range.	**BB:** Administer only under supervision of physician experienced in the use of cancer chemotherapeutic agents. Drug is highly toxic; handle and administer with care. Avoid inhalation of dust or vapors and contact with skin or mucous membranes. Avoid exposure during pregnancy. Extremely corrosive to soft tissue. Severe damage to soft tissue will occur with extravasation during IV use. **W/P:** Monitor renal, hepatic, and bone marrow functions frequently. Can cause fetal harm during pregnancy. Possible anaphylactoid reactions. If stomatitis, diarrhea, or severe hematopoietic depression occurs; d/c until recovery. Caution in elderly; increased risk of myelosuppression. Veno-occlusive disease (primarily hepatic) reported. Not for oral administration. **Contra:** At or about the time of infection with chickenpox or herpes zoster. **P/N:** Category D, not for use in nursing.	N/V, fatigue, lethargy, fever, **cheilitis,** esophagitis, abdominal pain, liver toxicity, anemia, blood dyscrasias, skin eruptions, acne, alopecia.
ADRENAL CYTOTOXIC AGENT				
Mitotane (Lysodren)	**Tab:** 500mg*	***Adults:* Adrenal Cancer: Initial:** 2-6g/day given tid-qid. **Titrate:** Increase up to 9-10g/day. If severe side effects occur, reduce to max tolerated dose (MTD). MTD varies from 2-16g/day.	**BB:** Temporarily d/c immediately following shock or severe trauma and administer exogenous steroids. **W/P:** Caution with liver disease other than metastatic lesions from the adrenal cortex. Surgically remove all possible tumor tissues from large metastatic masses before administration. Perform behavioral and neurological assessments at regular intervals when continuous treatment >2 yrs. Monitor for signs of adrenal insufficiency and institute steroid replacement where appropriate. May impair mental/physical abilities. Prolonged use may lead to brain damage and impairment of function. **P/N:** Category C, not for use in nursing.	GI disturbances, depression, lethargy, somnolence, dizziness, vertigo, skin toxicity.
ALKYLATING AGENTS				
Bendamustine HCl (Treanda)	**Inj:** 100mg	***Adults:* CLL:** 100mg/m² IV over 30 min on Days 1 and 2, of a 28-day cycle. **Max:** 6 cycles. Delay treatment for Grade 4 hematologic toxicity or clinically significant ≥Grade 2 non-hematologic toxicity. **≥Grade 3 Hematologic Toxicity:** Reduce dose to 50mg/m² on Days 1 and 2 of each cycle; if ≥Grade 3 toxicity recurs, reduce dose to 25mg/m² on Days 1 and 2. **≥Grade 3 Non-Hematologic Toxicity:** Reduce dose to 50mg/m² on Days 1 and 2 of each cycle. Consider dose re-escalation in subsequent cycles. **NHL:** 120mg/m² IV over 60 mins on Days 1 and 2 of a 21-day cycle. **Max:** 8 cycles. Delay treatment for Grade 4 hematologic toxicity or clinically significant ≥Grade 2 non-hematologic toxicity. **Grade 4 Hematologic Toxicity:** Reduce dose to 90mg/m² on days 1 and 2 of each	**W/P:** Myelosuppression reported; monitor leukocytes, platelets, Hgb and neutrophils closely. Infection, including pneumonia and sepsis, reported. May cause infusion reactions; monitor clinically and consider d/c with Grade 3 or 4 infusion reactions. May cause tumor lysis syndrome; use preventative measures. Skin reactions reported; if severe or progressive, withhold or d/c treatment. Pre-malignant and malignant diseases (eg, myelodysplastic syndrome, myeloproliferative disorders, acute myeloid leukemia, bronchial carcinoma) reported. Caution with mild hepatic impairment or mild/moderate renal impairment. Avoid with moderate/severe hepatic impairment or CrCl <40mL/min. **Contra:** Hypersensitivity to mannitol. **P/N:** Category D, not for use in nursing.	Neutropenia, thrombocytopenia, anemia, leukopenia, pyrexia, N/V, diarrhea, fatigue, asthenia, chills, hypersensitivity, rash, hyperuricemia, nasopharyngitis.

*Scored †Bold entries denote special dental considerations.
BB = black box warning; **W/P** = warnings/precautions; **Contra** = contraindications; **P/N** = pregnancy category rating and nursing considerations.

Table 23.1. PRESCRIBING INFORMATION FOR ANTINEOPLASTIC DRUGS *(cont.)*

NAME	FORM/ STRENGTH	DOSAGE	WARNINGS/PRECAUTIONS & CONTRAINDICATIONS	ADVERSE EFFECTS†
ALKYLATING AGENTS *(cont.)*				
Bendamustine HCl (Treanda) *(cont.)*		cycle; if grade 4 toxicity recurs, reduce dose to 60mg/m² in days 1 and 2 of each cycle. **≥Grade 3 Non-Hematologic Toxicity:** Reduce dose to 90mg/m² on days 1 and 2 of each cycle; if ≥Grade 3 toxicity recurs, reduce dose to 60mg/m² on days 1 and 2 of each cycle.		
Busulfan (Myleran)	**Tab:** 2mg*	***Adults/Pediatrics:*** **CML:** 60mcg/kg/day or 1.8mg/m²/day. **Range:** 4-8mg/day. Reserve dose >4mg/day for the most compelling symptoms.	**BB:** Do not use unless CML diagnosis is established. May induce severe bone marrow hypoplasia; reduce dose or d/c if unusual depression of bone marrow function occurs. **W/P:** Induction of bone marrow failure resulting in severe pancytopenia reported. Bronchopulmonary dysplasia with pulmonary fibrosis, cellular dysplasia, malignant tumors, acute leukemias, hepatic veno-occlusive disease reported. Ovarian suppression and amenorrhea with menopausal symptoms have occurred. Cardiac tamponade in patients with thalassemia and seizures reported. Caution with compromised bone marrow reserve from prior irradiation/chemotherapy. Seizures reported. **Contra:** Lack of definitive diagnosis of CML. **P/N:** Category D, not for use in nursing.	Myelosuppression, pulmonary fibrosis, cardiac tamponade, hyperpigmentation, weakness, fatigue, weight loss, N/V, melanoderma, hyperuricemia, myasthenia gravis, hepatic veno-occlusive disease.
Temozolomide (Temodar)	**Cap:** 5mg, 20mg, 100mg, 140mg, 180mg, 250mg	***Adults:*** Adjust according to nadir neutrophil and platelet counts of previous cycle and at time of initiating next cycle. **Glioblastoma Multiforme:** 75mg/m² qd for 42 days with focal radiotherapy. **Maint: Cycle 1 (28 days):** 150mg/m² qd for 5 days. **Cycle 2-6 (28 days):** If Cycle 1 toxicity Grade ≤2, ANC ≥1.5 x 10⁹/L and platelets ≥100 x 10⁹/L, increase to 200mg/m²/day for 5 consecutive days per 28-day cycle. Do not increase dose in subsequent cycles if dose not escalated at Cycle 2. **Anaplastic Astrocytoma: Initial:** 150mg/m² qd for 5 consecutive days per 28-day cycle. If ANC ≥1.5 x 10⁹/L and platelets ≥100 x 10⁹/L for both the nadir and Day 29 (Day 1 of next cycle), may increase to 200mg/m²/day for 5 consecutive days per 28-day cycle. Start next cycle when ANC >1.5 x 10⁹/L and platelets >100 x 10⁹/L . If ANC <1 x 10⁹/L or platelets <50 x 10⁹/L during any cycle, reduce next cycle by 50mg/m², but not <100mg/m². Swallow whole with water.	**W/P:** Before therapy, must have ANC ≥1.5 x 10⁹/L and platelets ≥100 x 10⁹/L. Myelosuppression may occur; obtain CBC on Day 22 (21 days after 1st dose) or within 48 hrs of that day, repeat weekly until ANC >1.5 x 10⁹/L and platelets >100 x 10⁹/L. Greater risk of myelosuppression in women and elderly. May cause fetal harm during pregnancy. Very rare cases of myelodysplastic syndrome and secondary malignancies, including myeloid leukemia, have been observed. Do not open capsules. Caution in elderly or severe renal/hepatic impairment. **Contra:** Hypersensitivity to DTIC (dacarbazine). **P/N:** Category D, not for use in nursing.	Anorexia, alopecia, headache, fatigue, myelosuppression (thrombocytopenia, neutropenia), N/V, convulsions, hemiparesis, asthenia, fever, peripheral edema, constipation, dizziness, diarrhea.
ANTHRACYCLINES				
Daunorubicin Citrate Liposome (DaunoXome)	**Inj:** 2mg/mL	***Adults:*** **Kaposi's Sarcoma:** 40mg/m² IV infusion; repeat every 2 weeks until evidence of progressive disease or until other complications of HIV preclude continuation.	**BB:** Monitor for cardiac toxicity. Severe myelosuppression may occur. Reduce dose with hepatic dysfunction. A triad of back pain, flushing and chest tightness reported during 1st 5 minutes of infusion; resume infusion at slower rate. Administer only under supervision of a physician experienced in the use of antineoplastic agents. **W/P:** Primary toxicity is myelosuppression; careful	Myelosuppression, alopecia, cardiomyopathy with CHF, N/V, fatigue, fever, diarrhea, cough, dyspnea, abdominal pain, anorexia, rigors, back pain, increased sweating, rhinitis, neuropathy.

*Scored. †Bold entries denote special dental considerations.
BB = black box warning; **W/P** = warnings/precautions; **Contra** = contraindications; **P/N** = pregnancy category rating and nursing considerations.

NAME	FORM/ STRENGTH	DOSAGE	WARNINGS/PRECAUTIONS & CONTRAINDICATIONS	ADVERSE EFFECTS†
Daunorubicin Citrate Liposome (DaunoXome) *(cont.)*			hematologic monitoring (prior to each dose) required. Evaluate cardiac function before each course and determine left ventricular ejection fraction (LVEF) at total cumulative dose of 320mg/m², and every 160mg/m² thereafter. Monitor LVEF at cumulative doses prior to therapy and every 160mg/m² in those with prior anthracycline therapy, pre-existing cardiac disease or previous radiotherapy. Avoid extravasation. Can cause fetal harm during pregnancy. **P/N:** Category D, safety in nursing not known.	
Daunorubicin HCl (Cerubidine)	**Inj:** 20mg	***Adults:* ANLL: Combination Therapy: <60 yrs:** 45mg/m²/day IV on Days 1, 2, 3 of 1st course and on Days 1, 2 of subsequent courses. **≥60 yrs:** 30mg/m²/day IV on Days 1, 2, 3 of 1st course and on Days 1, 2 of subsequent courses. **ALL: Combination Therapy:** 45mg/m²/day IV on Days 1, 2, 3. **Renal Impairment:** If SCr >3mg/dL, reduce dose by 50%. **Hepatic Impairment:** If serum bilirubin 1.2-3mg/dL, reduce dose by 25%. If >3mg/dL, reduce dose by 50%. ***Pediatrics:* ALL: Combination Therapy:** 25mg/m² IV on Day 1 every week. If complete remission not obtained after 4 courses, may give additional 1-2 courses. If <2 yrs or <0.5m² BSA, calculate dose based on weight (1mg/kg) instead of BSA.	**BB:** Avoid IM/SQ route. Severe local tissue necrosis with extravasation. Myocardial toxicity may occur during or after terminate therapy; increased risk if cumulative dose >400-550mg/m² in adults, >300mg/m² in pediatrics >2 yrs, or >10mg/m² in pediatrics <2 yrs. Severe myelosuppression may occur. Reduce dose with impaired hepatic or renal function. **W/P:** Avoid if pre-existing drug-induced bone-marrow suppression occurs unless benefit warrants the risk. May cause fetal harm during pregnancy. May impart red color to urine. Monitor blood uric acid levels. Determine CBC frequently. Evaluate cardiac, renal and hepatic function before each course. **P/N:** Category D, not for use in nursing.	Cardiotoxicity, myelosuppression, alopecia, N/V, diarrhea, abdominal pain, hyperuricemia, mucositis (3-7 days after therapy).
Doxorubicin HCl	**Inj:** (2mg/mL) 10mg, 20mg, 50mg	***Adults/Pediatrics:* Monotherapy:** 60-75mg/m² IV every 21 days. Use the lower dose with inadequate bone marrow reserves due to old age, prior therapy, or neoplastic marrow infiltration. **Concomitant Chemotherapy:** 40-60mg/m² IV every 21-28 days. **Hyperbilirubinemia:** Reduce dose by 50% if 1.2-3mg/dL; reduce dose by 75% if 3.1-5mg/dL.	**BB:** Severe local tissue necrosis will occur if extravasation occurs. Do not give IM/SQ route. Myocardial toxicity may occur during or after therapy. Increased risk of CHF with high cumulative doses, previous anthracycline/anthracenedione therapy, pre-existing heart disease, radiotherapy to mediastinal/pericardial area, concomitant cardiotoxic drugs. Increased risk of delayed cardiotoxicity in pediatrics. Secondary acute myelogenous leukemia reported. Reduce dose in hepatic impairment. Severe myelosuppression may occur. **W/P:** Irreversible myocardial toxicity may occur. Bone marrow depression and arrhythmias reported. Enhanced toxicity with hepatic impairment; evaluate hepatic function before dosing. Imparts a red coloration to urine for 1-2 days after administration. May induce tumor lysis syndrome and hyperuricemia with rapidly growing tumors. Periodically monitor CBC, hepatic function and radionuclide left ventricular ejection fraction. May cause prepubertal growth failure and gonadal impairment. **Contra:** Marked myelosuppression induced by previous treatment with other antitumor agents or radiotherapy. Previous therapy with complete cumulative doses of doxorubicin, daunorubicin, idarubicin or other anthracyclines and anthracenes. **P/N:** Category D, not for use in nursing.	Myelosuppression, cardiotoxicity, alopecia, N/V, mucositis, ulceration and necrosis of colon, fever, chills, urticaria, phlebosclerosis, facial flushing.

Table 23.1. PRESCRIBING INFORMATION FOR ANTINEOPLASTIC DRUGS *(cont.)*

NAME	FORM/ STRENGTH	DOSAGE	WARNINGS/PRECAUTIONS & CONTRAINDICATIONS	ADVERSE EFFECTS†
ANTHRACYCLINES *(cont.)*				
Doxorubicin HCl Liposome (Doxil)	**Inj:** 2mg/mL	***Adults:*** Administer as IV infusion at initial rate of 1mg/min to minimize risk of infusion-related reactions; if no reactions, may increase rate to complete infusion over 1 hr. **Ovarian Cancer:** 50mg/m² IV every 4 weeks for minimum of 4 courses. **Kaposi's Sarcoma:** 20mg/m² IV once every 3 weeks. **Multiple Myeloma:** Give bortezomib 1.3mg/m² IV bolus on Days 1, 4, 8, and 11, every 3 weeks. Give doxorubicin 30mg/m² IV on Day 4 following bortezomib. May treat for up to 8 cycles depending on disease progression or unaccepable toxicity. **Hepatic Dysfunction:** If serum bilirubin 1.2-3mg/dL, give 50% of normal dose. If serum bilirubin >3mg/dL, give 25% of normal dose. Adjust dose based on toxicities (see PI).	**BB:** Myocardial damage may lead to CHF when cumulative dose approaches 550mg/m². May lead to cardiac toxicity, consider prior use of anthracyclines or anthracenediones in cumulative dose calculations. Cardiac toxicity may occur at lower cumulative doses with prior mediastinal irradiation or concurrent cardiotoxic agents (eg, cyclophosphamide). Acute infusion-associated reactions reported. Severe myelosuppression, myocardial toxicity may occur. Reduce dose with impaired hepatic function. Severe side effects reported with accidental substitution for doxorubicin HCl; do not substitute on mg per mg basis. **W/P:** Monitor cardiac function. Cardiac toxicity may occur after d/c. Recall of skin reaction due to radiotherapy reported. Myelosuppression may occur; obtain CBCs, including platelets frequently and at a minimum before each dose. Secondary AML reported with anthracyclines. Evaluate hepatic function before therapy. Avoid extravasation. Can cause fetal harm. Hand-foot syndrome and acute infusion-related reactions reported. **Contra:** Nursing mothers. **P/N:** Category D, not for use in nursing.	Neutropenia, leukopenia, anemia, thromobocytopenia, stomatitis, fever, anorexia, fatigue, N/V, asthenia, rash, alopecia, diarrhea, constipation, hand-foot syndrome.
Epirubicin HCl (Ellence)	**Inj:** 2mg/mL [25mL, 100mL]	***Adults:*** **Initial:** 100-120mg/m² IV infusion, repeat at 3-4 week cycles. May give total dose on Day 1 of each cycle or divide equally on Days 1 and 8. **Bone Marrow Dysfunction: Initial:** 75-90mg/m². **Hepatic Dysfunction: Bilirubin 1.2-3mg/dL or AST 2-4X ULN:** Give 1/2 of initial dose. **Bilirubin >3mg/dL or AST 4X ULN:** Give 1/4 of initial dose. **Severe Renal Dysfunction: Serum Creatinine >5mg/dL:** Lower dose. Give prophylactic therapy with TMP-SMX or fluoroquinolone with 120mg/m² regimen. Consider pretreatment with antiemetics. Adjust dose after 1st treatment cycle based on hematologic and nonhematologic toxicities (see PI).	**BB:** Severe local tissue necrosis with extravasation. Not for IM/SQ administration. Risk of myocardial toxicity, severe myelosuppression. Secondary acute myelogenous leukemia reported. Reduce dose with hepatic dysfunction. **W/P:** Increased risk of cardiotoxicity with active or dormant cardiovascular disease. Use extreme caution if exceeding cumulative dose of 900mg/m². Resolve acute toxicities from other cytotoxic agents prior to initiation. Monitor CBC, total bilirubin, AST, SCr and cardiac function before and during each cycle. May induce hyperuricemia. Potential for tumor lysis syndrome. Thrombophlebitis, thromboembolic phenomena reported. **Contra:** Baseline neutrophils <1500 cells/mm³, severe myocardial insufficiency, recent MI, severe arrhythmias, previous anthracycline therapy with maximum cumulative dose, anthracenedione hypersensitivity, severe hepatic dysfunction. **P/N:** Category D, not for use in nursing.	Hematologic abnormalities, amenorrhea, hot flashes, lethargy, fever, GI disturbances, infection, conjunctivitis/keratitis, alopecia, local toxicity, rash/itch, skin changes.
Idarubicin HCl (Idamycin PFS)	**Inj:** 1mg/mL	***Adults:*** **Induction:** 12mg/m² qd over 10-15 min IV qd for 3 days. Administer cytarabine 100mg/m² qd IV infusion for 7 days, or cytarabine 25mg/m² IV bolus followed by 200mg/m² qd IV infusion for 5 days. May give 2nd course if unequivocal evidence of leukemia after 1st course. If severe mucositis, delay 2nd course until recovery, then administer at 25% dose reduction. **Hepatic/Renal Dysfunction:** Reduce dose. Avoid if bilirubin >5mg%.	**BB:** Administer as freely flowing IV infusion. Severe local tissue necrosis with extravasation. Can cause myocardial toxicity and severe myelosuppression. Reduce dose with hepatic or renal dysfunction. Administer only under supervision of a physician experienced in leukemia chemotherapy and in a facility able to monitor drug tolerance and toxicity, and respond to severe hemorrhagic conditions and/or overwhelming infection. **W/P:** Avoid use with pre-	Severe myelosuppression, infection, N/V, alopecia, abdominal pain/diarrhea, hemorrhage, mucositis, rash, urticaria, bullous erythrodermatous rash of palms/soles of feet, fever, headache, cardiac toxicity (CHF,

†Bold entries denote special dental considerations.
BB = black box warning; **W/P** = warnings/precautions; **Contra** = contraindications; **P/N** = pregnancy category rating and nursing considerations.

NAME	FORM/ STRENGTH	DOSAGE	WARNINGS/PRECAUTIONS & CONTRAINDICATIONS	ADVERSE EFFECTS†
Idarubicin HCl (Idamycin PFS) *(cont.)*			existing bone marrow suppression induced by drug therapy or radiotherapy unless benefit warrants the risk. Monitor CBC, LFTs, and renal function tests frequently. Caution with pre-existing heart disease. Monitor cardiac function during therapy; cardiomyopathy associated with decreased left ventricular ejection fraction. Increased risk of myocardial toxicity with anemia, bone marrow depression, infections, leukemic pericarditis and/or myocarditis. May induce hyperuricemia secondary to rapid lysis of leukemic cells. Should prevent hyperuricemia and control systemic infection before starting therapy. D/C if extravasation occurs; can cause local tissue necrosis. **P/N:** Category D, not for use in nursing.	arrhythmia), pulmonary effects, mental status effects.
Valrubicin (Valstar)	**Inj:** 40mg/mL	***Adults:*** **Bladder Cancer:** 800mg intravesically once weekly for 6 weeks. Delay administration for at least 2 weeks after transurethral resection and/or fulguration.	**W/P:** Avoid in patients with a perforated bladder or to those in whom the integrity of the bladder mucosa has been compromised. Caution with with severe irritable bladder symptoms. Bladder spasm and spontaneous discharge of the intravesical instillate may occur; clamping of urinary catheter is not advised and, if performed, should be executed under medical supervision and with caution. **Contra:** Concurrent UTI, small bladder capacity (unable to tolerate a 75mL instillation). Hypersensitivity to anthracyclines or Cremophor® EL (polyoxyethyleneglycol triricinoleate). **P/N:** Category C, not for use in nursing.	(Local bladder symptoms) urinary frequency, dysuria, urinary urgency, bladder spasm, hematuria, bladder pain, urinary incontinence, cystitis, nocturia, local burning symptoms, urethral pain. (Systemic symptoms) UTI, nausea, abdominal pain.
ANTIESTROGENS				
Tamoxifen Citrate (Soltamox Sol)	**Sol:** 10mg/5mL; **Tab:** 10mg, 20mg	***Adults:*** **Breast Cancer Treatment:** 20-40mg qd. Divide dosages >20mg into AM and PM doses. **Breast Cancer Risk Reduction/DCIS:** 20mg qd for 5 yrs.	**BB:** For women with ductal carcinoma in situ (DCIS) and women at high risk for breast cancer. Fatal uterine malignancies (eg, endometrial adenocarcinoma, uterine sarcoma), stroke, and PE reported with use in risk reduction setting. Discuss benefits/risks of events with this patient population. Benefits of tamoxifen outweigh risks in women already diagnosed with breast cancer. **W/P:** Hypercalcemia reported in patients with bone metastases. Increased incidence of uterine malignancies (eg, endometrial cancer, uterine sarcoma) and endometrial changes including hyperplasia and polyps reported. Increased incidence of thromboembolic events (eg, DVT, PE). Malignant and non-malignant effects on the liver and ocular disturbances reported. Leukopenia, anemia, thrombocytopenia, neutropenia, pancytopenia reported. Promptly evaluate abnormal vaginal bleeding if receiving or previously received tamoxifen. Patients receiving or previously received tamoxifen should have annual gynecological exam. Do not become pregnant within 2 months of therapy. May cause fetal harm during pregnancy. Does not cause infertility even with menstrual irregularity. **Contra:** Reduction in breast cancer incidence in	(Females) Hot flashes, increased bone and tumor pain, vaginal discharge, irregular menses; (males) loss of libido, impotence.

Table 23.1. PRESCRIBING INFORMATION FOR ANTINEOPLASTIC DRUGS *(cont.)*

NAME	FORM/ STRENGTH	DOSAGE	WARNINGS/PRECAUTIONS & CONTRAINDICATIONS	ADVERSE EFFECTS†
ANTIESTROGENS *(cont.)*				
Tamoxifen Citrate (Soltamox Sol) *(cont.)*			high risk women and women with DCIS who require coumarin-type anticoagulant therapy or have a history of DVT, PE. **P/N:** Category D, not for use in nursing.	
ANTIFOLATES				
Pemetrexed Disodium (Alimta)	**Inj:** 100mg, 500mg	***Adults:*** **Premedication: Dexamethasone:** 4mg PO bid on day before, day of, and day after pemetrexed. **Folic Acid:** At least 5 daily doses (350-1000mcg) during 7 days prior to pemetrexed. Continue for 21 days after last pemetrexed dose. **Vitamin B_{12}:** 1000mcg IM once during week preceding first pemetrexed dose and every 3 cycles thereafter. **Treatment: Mesothelioma/NSCLC:** 500mg/m² IV over 10 min on Day 1 of each 21-day cycle with cisplatin 75mg/m² infused over 2 hrs beginning 30 min after pemetrexed. **NSCLC/Single Agent:** 500mg/m² IV over 10 minutes on day 1 of each 21 cycle. Refer to PI for dose adjustments for hematologic, nonhematologic and neurotoxicities.	**W/P:** Avoid use if CrCl <45mL/min. May suppress bone marrow function. With pleural effusions, ascites, consider draining prior to therapy. Monitor CBCs, for nadir and recovery before each dose and on Days 8 and 15 of each cycle. Do not begin new cycle unless ANC ≥1500 cells/mm³, platelets ≥100,000 cells/mm³, CrCl ≥45mL/min. **P/N:** Category D, not for use in nursing.	N/V, fatigue, dyspnea, hematologic effects, constipation, chest pain, anorexia, fever, infection, stomatitis, **pharyngitis,** rash/desquamation.
ANTIMETABOLITES				
Clofarabine (Clolar)	**Inj:** 1mg/mL	***Pediatrics:*** **1-21 yrs: ALL:** 52mg/m² IV over 2 hours daily for 5 consecutive days. Treatment cycles are repeated following recovery or return to baseline organ function, approximately 2-6 weeks. Continuous IV fluids throughout 5 days of clofarabine therapy is recommended. The use of prophylactic steroids (eg, 100mg/m² hydrocortisone on Days 1-3) may be of benefit in preventing signs and symptoms of systemic inflammatory response syndrome (SIRS) or capillary leak. If patient develops signs and symptoms of SIRS or capillary leak, d/c clofarabine therapy and appropriate supportive measures should be provided. Close monitoring of renal and hepatic function is required. If substantial increases in creatine or bilirubin occur, d/c clofarabine therapy.	**W/P:** Suppression of bone marrow function should be anticipated. Increased risk of infection, including severe sepsis is possible. Monitor for signs and symptoms of tumor lysis syndrome, as well as cytokine release that could develop into SIRS/capillary leak syndrome and organ dysfunction. D/C immediately if SIRS or capillary leak syndrome develop. Severe bone marrow suppression (eg, neutropenia, anemia, thrombocytopenia) have been observed. Dehydration may occur due to vomiting and diarrhea. D/C clofarabine if patient develops hypotension. Since clofarabine is excreted primarily by the kidneys, drugs with known renal toxicity should be avoided during the 5 days of administration. Since the liver is a known target of clofarabine, concomitant use of medications known to induce hepatic toxicity should be avoided. Patients taking medications known to affect BP or cardiac function should be closely monitored during administration. **P/N:** Category D, not for use in nursing.	N/V, diarrhea, anemia, leukopenia, thrombocytopenia, neutropenia, febrile neutropenia, and infection.
Cytarabine	**Inj:** 100mg, 500mg, 1g, 2g	***Adults/Pediatrics:*** **ANLL: Induction:** 100mg/m²/day continuous infusion or 100mg/m² IV q12h for Days 1-7. **Meningeal Leukemia:** Give intrathecally. **Range:** 5-75mg/m² given qd to every 4 days. **Usual:** 30mg/m² every 4 days until CSF normal, followed by 1 additional treatment.	**BB:** Associated with bone marrow suppression, N/V, oral ulceration, hepatic dysfunction, diarrhea and abdominal pain. For induction therapy, treat in a facility able to monitor drug tolerance and toxicity. **W/P:** Caution with pre-existing drug-induced bone marrow suppression, hepatic or renal dysfunction. Perform	Anorexia, N/V, diarrhea, anal/**oral inflammation or ulceration,** hepatic dysfunction, fever, rash, thrombophlebitis, bleeding (all sites).

†Bold entries denote special dental considerations.
BB = black box warning; **W/P** = warnings/precautions; **Contra** = contraindications; **P/N** = pregnancy category rating and nursing considerations.

NAME	FORM/ STRENGTH	DOSAGE	WARNINGS/PRECAUTIONS & CONTRAINDICATIONS	ADVERSE EFFECTS†
Cytarabine *(cont.)*			leukocyte and platelet counts daily during induction therapy. Monitor bone marrow, hepatic and renal functions, platelets and leukocytes frequently. Sudden respiratory distress, cardiomyopathy, alopecia reported with high dose therapy. Severe and fatal CNS, GI and pulmonary toxicity reported. Contains benzyl alcohol; fatal "Gasping Syndrome" in premature infants reported. Acute pancreatitis, hyperuricemia reported. **P/N:** Category D, not for use in nursing.	
Cytarabine Liposome (DepoCyt)	**Inj:** 10mg/mL	***Adults:*** **Lymphomatous Meningitis: Induction:** 50mg intrathecally every 14 days for 2 doses (weeks 1 and 3). **Consolidation:** 50mg intrathecally every 14 days for 3 doses (weeks 5, 7, 9) followed by 1 additional dose at week 13. **Maint:** 50mg intrathecally every 28 days for 4 doses (weeks 17, 21, 25, 29). Reduce to 25mg if drug-related neurotoxicity develops. D/C if toxicity persists.	**BB:** Chemical arachnoiditis (eg, N/V, headache, fever), a common adverse event, can be fatal if untreated. Treat concurrently with dexamethasone to reduce incidence and severity. **W/P:** Intrathecal use of free cytarabine may cause myelopathy and other neurotoxicity. CSF blockage may increase free cytarabine levels and increase risk of neurotoxicity. Can cause fetal harm during pregnancy. Monitor for neurotoxicity. Anaphylactic reactions with IV-free cytarabine. Transient elevations of CSF protein and WBC reported. Monitor hematopoietic system carefully. **Contra:** Active meningeal infection. **P/N:** Category D, not for use in nursing.	Chemical arachnoiditis (headache, fever, back pain, N/V), confusion, somnolence, abnormal gait, peripheral edema, neutropenia, thrombocytopenia, urinary incontinence, convulsions, weakness.
Floxuridine (FUDR)	**Inj:** 0.5g	***Adults:*** **GI Carcinoma Metastatic to Liver:** 0.1-0.6mg/kg/day continuous arterial infusion. Use higher dose (0.4-0.6mg) for hepatic artery infusion. Continue therapy until adverse reactions appear and resume when reactions subside. Maintain on therapy as long as response continues.	**BB:** Hospitalize for 1st course of therapy due to possible severe toxic reactions. **W/P:** Highly toxic drug with narrow margin of safety. Extreme caution in poor risk patients with renal or hepatic dysfunction, history of high-dose pelvic irradiation, or previous use of alkylating agents. Not intended as an adjuvant to surgery. D/C promptly if myocardial ischemia, stomatitis or esophagopharyngitis, leukopenia, intractable vomiting, diarrhea, GI ulceration and bleeding, thrombocytopenia, or if hemorrhage from any site occur. May cause fetal harm during pregnancy. Carefully monitor WBCs and platelets. **Contra:** Poor nutritional state, depressed bone marrow function, potentially serious infections. **P/N:** Category D, not for use in nursing.	N/V, diarrhea, enteritis, stomatitis, localized erythema, anemia, leukopenia, thrombocytopenia, LFT elevation, alopecia.
Fludarabine Phosphate (Fludara)	**Inj:** 50mg	***Adults:*** **B-Cell CLL:** 25mg/m² over 30 min qd for 5 days. Repeat course every 28 days. Administer 3 additional courses after achievement of maximum response. May decrease or delay dose based on hematologic or nonhematologic toxicity. Consider delaying or d/c if neurotoxicity occurs. **CrCl 30-70mL/min:** Reduce dose by 20%. **CrCl <30mL/min:** Not recommended.	**BB:** Can severely suppress bone marrow function. High doses associated with severe neurologic effects (eg, blindness, coma, death). Autoimmune hemolytic anemia reported. Monitor closely for hemolysis. High incidence of fatal pulmonary toxicity with pentostatin. **W/P:** Severe bone marrow suppression reported. Predisposition to increased toxicity with advanced age, renal insufficiency, and bone marrow impairment; monitor for toxicity. Caution with renal insufficiency. Tumor lysis syndrome associated with large tumor burdens. Monitor hematologic profile regularly. Can cause fetal harm during pregnancy. Use irradiated blood products if transfusion required. **P/N:** Category D, not for use in nursing.	Myelosuppression, fever, chills, infection, N/V, malaise, fatigue, anorexia, weakness, serious opportunistic infections.

Table 23.1. PRESCRIBING INFORMATION FOR ANTINEOPLASTIC DRUGS *(cont.)*

NAME	FORM/ STRENGTH	DOSAGE	WARNINGS/PRECAUTIONS & CONTRAINDICATIONS	ADVERSE EFFECTS†
ANTIMETABOLITES *(cont.)*				
Fluorouracil‡	**Inj:** 50mg/mL [10mL, 50mL, 100mL]	***Adults:* Breast, Colon, Gastric, Pancreatic, Rectal Cancers:** 12mg/kg IV qd for 4 days. **Max:** 800mg/day. If no toxicity, give 6mg/kg IV on 6th, 8th, 10th, and 12th days. Skip Days 5, 7, 9, and 11. **Inadequate Nutritional State:** 6mg/kg IV for 3 days. If no toxicity, give 3mg/kg IV on 5th, 7th, and 9th days. **Max:** 400mg/day. Skip Days 4, 6, and 8. **Maint (Use Schedule 1 or Schedule 2): Schedule 1:** If no toxicity, repeat 1st course every 30 days after last day of previous course. **Schedule 2:** When toxic signs from initial course subside, give 10-15mg/kg/week IV single dose; do not exceed 1g/week.	**BB:** Hospitalize patient during initial therapy due to possible severe toxic reactions. **W/P:** Extreme caution in poor risk patients with history of high-dose irradiation, previous use of alkylating agents, hepatic/renal dysfunction, widespread bone marrow involvement by metastatic tumors. Dipyrimidine dehydrogenase deficiency prolongs 5-FU clearance; can cause severe toxicity. May cause fetal harm in pregnancy. Other therapy interfering with nutrition or depressing bone marrow function increases toxicity. D/C with stomatitis, esophagopharyngitis, leukopenia, intractable vomiting, diarrhea, GI ulceration or bleeding, thrombocytopenia or hemorrhage from any site. Palmar-plantar erythrodysesthesia syndrome (hand-foot syndrome) reported. Perform WBC with differential before each dose. Narrow margin of safety; monitor patients very closely. **Contra:** Poor nutritional state, depressed bone marrow function, potentially serious infection. **P/N:** Category D, not for use in nursing.	Stomatitis, **esophagopharyngitis,** diarrhea, anorexia, nausea, emesis, leukopenia, alopecia, dermatitis.
ANTIMICROTUBULE AGENTS				
Docetaxel (Taxotere)	**Inj:** 20mg/ 0.5mL, 80mg/2mL	***Adults:*** Premedicate with oral corticosteroids. Adjust dose based on febrile neutropenia, neutrophil count, cutaneous reactions, peripheral neuropathy, neurosensory signs/symptoms or GI toxicities (see PI). **Breast Cancer:** 60-100mg/m^2 IV over 1 hr every 3 weeks. **Adjuvant Treatment Operable Node-Positive Breast CA:** 75mg/m^2 1 hr after doxorubicin 50mg/m^2 and cyclophosphamide 500mg/m^2 every 3 weeks for 6 courses. **NSCLC:** 75mg/m^2 IV over 1 hr every 3 weeks. **Prostate Cancer:** 75mg/m^2 every 3 weeks over 1 hr with prednisone 5mg bid. **Gastric Adenocarcinoma:** Premedicate with antiemetics and appropriate hydration. 75mg/m^2 IV over 1 hr, followed by cisplatin 75mg/m^2 IV over 1-3 hrs (both on Day 1 only), followed by fluorouracil 750mg/m^2/day IV over 24 hrs for 5 days, starting at end of cisplatin infusion. Repeat treatment every 3 weeks. **SCCHN: Induction followed by Radiotherapy:** 75mg/m^2 IV over 1 hr, followed by cisplatin 75mg/m^2 IV over 1 hr, on Day 1, followed by fluorouracil as a continuous IV infusion at 750mg/m^2/day for 5 days. Administer every 3 weeks for 4 cycles. **Induction followed by Chemoradiotherapy:** 75mg/m^2 IV over 1 hr on Day 1, followed by cisplatin 100mg/m^2 IV over 30 min to 3 hrs, followed by fluorouracil 1000mg/m^2/day as a continuous IV infusion from Day 1 to Day 4. Administer every 3 weeks for 3 cycles.	**BB:** Increased treatment-related mortality reported with hepatic dysfunction, high-dose therapy, and in non-small cell lung carcinoma previously treated with platinum-based chemotherapy with docetaxel 100mg/m^2. Avoid if neutrophils <1500 cells/mm^3, bilirubin >ULN, or SGOT/SGPT >1.5x ULN with alkaline phosphatase >2.5x ULN. Severe hypersensitivity reactions reported. Severe fluid retention may occur despite dexamethasone. **W/P:** Toxic deaths, febrile neutropenia, neutropenia, localized erythema of extremities with edema and desquamation, severe neurosensory symptoms, severe asthenia reported. Monitor for hypersensitivity reactions. Can cause fetal harm. Caution in elderly. Monitor CBC frequently; avoid subsequent cycles until neutrophils recover to >1500 cells/mm^3 and platelets recover to >100,000 cells/mm^3. **Contra:** Neutrophils <1500 cells/mm^3, hypersensitivity to polysorbate 80. **P/N:** Category D, not for use in nursing.	Arthralgia, myalgia, alopecia, stomatitis, N/V, diarrhea, nail changes, cutaneous/ neurosensory reactions, fluid retention, hypersensitivity reaction, leukopenia, thrombocytopenia, anemia, neutropenia, fever.

†Bold entries denote special dental considerations.
‡Used as single or combination agent for head and neck cancer.
BB = black box warning; **W/P** = warnings/precautions; **Contra** = contraindications; **P/N** = pregnancy category rating and nursing considerations.

NAME	FORM/ STRENGTH	DOSAGE	WARNINGS/PRECAUTIONS & CONTRAINDICATIONS	ADVERSE EFFECTS†
Ixabepilone (Ixempra)	**Inj:** 15mg, 45mg	***Adults:* Breast Cancer:** 40mg/m^2 IV infusion over 3 hrs every 3 weeks. Adjust dose based on toxicities (see PI). Premedicate with H_1-antagonist (eg, diphenhydramine 50mg PO) and H_2-antagonist (eg, ranitidine 150-300mg PO) approximately 1 hr before infusion. Also premedicate with corticosteroid (eg, dexamethasone 20mg, IV 30 min before infusion or PO 60 min before infusion) if prior hypersensitivity reaction to ixabepilone. **Hepatic Impairment: Monotherapy: Mild: AST and ALT ≤2.5x ULN and Bilirubin ≤1x ULN:** 40mg/m^2. **AST or ALT ≤10x ULN and Bilirubin ≤1x ULN:** 32mg/m^2. **Moderate (AST and ALT ≤10x ULN and Bilirubin >1.5 to ≤3x ULN):** 20-30mg/m^2. **Strong CYP3A4 Inhibitors:** Avoid or reduce dose to 20mg/m^2.	**BB:** Contraindicated in combination with capecitabine in patients with AST/ALT ≥2.5x ULN or bilirubin >1x ULN due to increased toxicity and neutropenia-related death. **W/P:** Peripheral neuropathy may occur; monitor for symptoms and manage by dose adjustment and delays. Myelosuppression, primarily neutropenia, may occur and is dose-dependent; monitor with frequent peripheral blood cell counts and adjust dose as needed. Hypersensitivity reactions may occur; premedicate all patients with H_1- and H_2-antagonists 1 hr before treatment. Caution with history of cardiac disease. Consider d/c of therapy if cardiac ischemia or impaired cardiac function develops. Avoid monotherapy if AST or ALT >10x ULN or bilirubin >3x ULN and use caution if AST or ALT >5x ULN. **Contra:** Baseline neutrophil count <1500 cells/mm^3 or platelet count <100,000 cells/mm^3. In combination with capecitabine, AST or ALT >2.5x ULN or bilirubin >1x ULN. History of severe (CTC Grade 3/4) hypersensitivity reaction to Cremophor® EL or derivatives (eg, polyoxyethylated castor oil). **P/N:** Category D, not for use in nursing.	Peripheral neuropathy, fatigue/asthenia, myalgia/arthralgia, alopecia, N/V, stomatitis/mucositis, diarrhea, musculoskeletal pain, palmar-plantar erythrodysesthesia (hand-foot) syndrome, anorexia, abdominal pain, nail disorder, constipation, neutropenia, leukopenia, anemia, thrombocytopenia.
Paclitaxel (Taxol)	**Inj:** 6mg/mL	***Adults:* (IV) Ovarian Carcinoma: Previously Untreated:** 175mg/m^2 over 3 hrs or 135mg/m^2 over 24 hrs every 3 weeks followed by cisplatin. **Previous Treatment:** 135mg/m^2 or 175mg/m^2 over 3 hrs every 3 weeks. **Breast Cancer:** 175mg/m^2 over 3 hrs every 3 weeks for 4 courses. **NSCLC:** 135mg/m^2 over 24 hrs every 3 weeks followed by cisplatin. **Kaposi's Sarcoma:** 135mg/m^2 over 3 hrs every 3 weeks or 100mg/m^2 over 3 hrs every 2 weeks. Reduce dose of subsequent courses by 20% if neutrophils <500 cells/mm^3 for ≥1 week or severe peripheral neuropathy occurs. Premedicated prior to administration to prevent severe hypersensitivity reactions; dexamethasone 20mg PO 12 and 6 hrs before, diphenhydramine 50mg IV 30-60 min prior, and cimetidine 300mg or ranitidine 50mg IV 30-60 min before.	**BB:** Anaphylaxis, severe hypersensitivity reactions reported. Pretreat with corticosteroids, diphenhydramine and H_2-antagonists. Do not rechallenge if severe hypersensitivity reaction occurs. Monitor CBC frequently. **W/P:** Severe conduction abnormalities, injection site reactions, peripheral neuropathy (more common in elderly) reported. Bone marrow suppression is dose dependent, dose limiting, and more common in elderly. Can cause fetal harm. Hypotension, bradycardia and HTN may occur during administration. Toxicity enhanced with elevated liver enzymes. Contains dehydrated alcohol. **Contra:** Hypersensitivity to drugs formulated in Cremophor® EL (eg, cyclosporine for injection concentrate, teniposide for injection concentrate), solid tumor patients with baseline neutrophils <1500 cells/mm^3, AIDS-related Kaposi's sarcoma patients with baseline neutrophils <1000 cells/mm^3. **P/N:** Category D, not for use in nursing.	Neutropenia, leukopenia, thrombocytopenia, anemia, infections, bleeding, bradycardia, hypotension, peripheral neuropathy, myalgia/arthralgia, N/V, diarrhea, mucositis, alopecia.
Paclitaxel Protein-bound Particles (Abraxane)	**Inj:** 100mg	***Adults:* Breast Cancer:** 260mg/m^2 IV over 30 min every 3 weeks. **Severe neutropenia (neutrophil <500 cells/mm^3 for week or longer) or severe sensory neuropathy (Grade 3 or 4):** Hold dose until neutrophil >1500 cells/mm^3 or sensory neuropathy resolves to Grade 1 or 2. Reduce subsequent courses to 220mg/m^2, if recurrence reduce subsequent courses to 180mg/m^2.	**BB:** Do not administer to patients with metastatic breast cancer who have baseline neutrophil counts of <1,500 cells/mm^3. Perform peripheral blood cell counts on all patients to monitor occurence of bone marrow suppression, primarily neutropenia. Should only be administered under the supervision of a physician experienced in the use of cancer chemotherapeutic agents. Do not substitute for or with other paclitaxel	Neutropenia, infectious episodes, anemia, hypotension, ECG abnormalities, dyspnea, cough, sensory neuropathy, ocular/visual disturbances, arthralgia, myalgia, NV, asthenia, abnormal LFT.

Table 23.1. PRESCRIBING INFORMATION FOR ANTINEOPLASTIC DRUGS *(cont.)*

NAME	FORM/ STRENGTH	DOSAGE	WARNINGS/PRECAUTIONS & CONTRAINDICATIONS	ADVERSE EFFECTS†
ANTIMICROTUBULE AGENTS *(cont.)*				
Paclitaxel Protein-bound Particles (Abraxane) *(cont.)*			formulations. **W/P:** Perform frequent blood counts to monitor for bone marrow suppression. Men should be advised to not father a child while receiving treatment. Remote risk for transmission of viral diseases; theoretical risk for transmission of Creutzfeldt-Jacob disease. Sensory neuropathy occurs frequently. Reports of injection site reactions. **Contra:** Patients with baseline neutrophil counts of <1,500 cells/mm^3. **P/N:** Category D, not for use in nursing.	
AROMATASE INACTIVATOR				
Exemestane (Aromasin)	**Tab:** 25mg	***Adults:* Breast Cancer: Early/ Advanced:** 25mg qd after a meal. Continue in the absence of recurrence of contralateral breast cancer until completion of 5 yrs of adjuvant endocrine therapy in postmenopausal women with early breast cancer treated with 2-3 yrs of tamoxifen. Continue until tumor progression is evident. **Concomitant Potent CYP3A4 Inducers (eg, rifampicin, phenytoin):** 50mg qd after a meal.	**W/P:** Fetal harm in pregnancy. Avoid in premenopausal women. **P/N:** Category D, caution in nursing.	Fatigue, N/V, hot flushes, pain, depression, insomnia, anxiety, dyspnea, dizziness, headache, increased sweating, edema, HTN, anorexia.
AROMATASE INHIBITOR (NONSTEROIDAL)				
Anastrozole (Arimidex)	**Tab:** 1mg	***Adults:* Breast Cancer:** 1mg qd. Continue until tumor progression with advanced breast cancer.	**W/P:** May cause fetal harm during pregnancy. Avoid in premenopausal women. May cause reduction in bone mineral density. May elevate serum cholesterol. **P/N:** Category D, caution in nursing.	Joint disorders, mood disturbances, **pharyngitis,** depression, HTN, osteoporosis, peripheral edema, bone fractures, asthenia, headache, hot flushes, dyspnea, N/V, cough, pain, edema.
ATTENUATED LIVE BCG CULTURES				
BCG Live (TheraCys, Tice BCG)	**Inj:** (TheraCys) 81mg, (Tice BCG) 50mg	***Adults:* Bladder Cancer:** (81mg) Begin 7-14 days after biopsy or resection. **Induction:** 81mg intravesically weekly for 6 weeks. **Maint:** 81mg at 3, 6, 12, 18, and 24 months. Avoid fluids for 4 hrs before treatment. Empty badder before administration. Retain in bladder for 2 hrs, then void. During the 1st 15 min following instillation, patient should lie prone. (50mg) Allow 7-14 days after biopsy before initiating therapy. Administer 1 vial (50mg) intravesically weekly for 6 weeks; may repeat schedule once if tumor remission not achieved. Then, continue monthly for 6-12 months. Retain in bladder for 2 hrs, then void. During bladder retention, reposition patient every 15 min to maximize bladder surface exposure.	**BB:** Contains live, attenuated mycobacteria. Potential risk for transmission; prepare, handle, and dispose of as a biohazard material. Nosocomial infections reported in immunosuppressed. Fatal reactions reported with intravesical BCG. **W/P:** Not a vaccine for prevention of cancer. Risk of infectious complications; avoid with actively bleeding urinary mucosa; delay treatment for ≥1 week after TUR, biopsy, traumatic catheterization, or gross hematuria. Possible increased risk of severe local reactions with small bladder capacity. May cause tuberculin sensitivity. BCG infection of aneurysms and prosthetic devices (eg, arterial grafts, cardiac devices, artificial joints) reported. Stopper of vial contains natural rubber latex which may cause allergic	Malaise, fever, chills, crapms/pain, uveitis, conjunctivitis, iritis, keratitis, granulomatous choreoretinitis, myalgia, arthritis, arthralgia, N/V, urinary symptoms, skin rash.

†Bold entries denote special dental considerations.
BB = black box warning; **W/P** = warnings/precautions; **Contra** = contraindications; **P/N** = pregnancy category rating and nursing considerations.

NAME	FORM/ STRENGTH	DOSAGE	WARNINGS/PRECAUTIONS & CONTRAINDICATIONS	ADVERSE EFFECTS†
BCG Live (TheraCys, Tice BCG) *(cont.)*			reactions. Evaluate for serious infectious complication if fever ≥101.3°F, or acute localized inflammation (eg, epididymitis, prostatitis, orchitis) persists >2-3 days. Febrile episodes with flu-like symptoms >72 hrs, fever ≥103°F, systemic manifestations increasing in intensity with repeated instillations, or persistent abnormal LFTs suggest systemic BCG infection and may require antitubercu-lous therapy. D/C if fever persists or if acute febrile illness consistent with BCG infection occur. Administer ≥2 antimy-cobacterials while diagnostic evaluation is conducted. Sensitive to INH, rifampin and ethambutol; not sensitive to pyra-zinamide. Caution with groups at risk of HIV. Not recommended for stage TaG1 papillary tumors, unless judged to be at high risk of tumor recurrence. Persons with immunologic deficiency should not handle agent. **Contra:** Immunocompro-mised patients, congenital or acquired immune deficiency patients (eg, AIDS, cancer, immunosuppressives), concur-rent febrile illness, UTI, gross hematuria, active TB. Wait 7-14 days after biopsy, TUR or traumatic catheterization. **P/N:** Category C, not for use in nursing.	
BIOLOGICAL RESPONSE MODIFIER				
Aldesleukin (Proleukin)	**Inj:** 22MIU/vial	***Adults:* Metastatic RCC or Melanoma:** 600,000 IU/kg IV q8h. **Max:** 14 doses. After 9-day rest period, repeat for 14 doses. **Max:** 28 doses/course. **Retreat-ment:** Evaluate response after 4 weeks of course completion. Give additional courses if tumor shrinks. Separate courses by at least 7 weeks. Hold dose or interrupt therapy if toxicity occurs.	**BB:** Caution with history of cardiac or pulmonary disease. Associated with capillary leak syndrome and impaired neutrophil function. Increased risk of infection. Withhold treatment with moderate to severe lethargy or somno-lence. **W/P:** May exacerbate or cause autoimmune/inflammatory disorders. May exacerbate Crohn's disease, scleroderma, thyroiditis, inflammatory arthritis, DM, oculo-bulbar myasthenia gravis, crescentic IgA glomerulonephri-tis, cholecystitis, cerebral vasculitis, Stevens-Johnson syndrome and bullous pemphigoid reported. Confirm negative CNS metastases before treatment. Neu-rologic impairments reported without CNS metastases. Caution with history of seizures. May cause reduced kidney and hepatic function. **Contra:** See Black Box Warning. Abnormal thallium stress test, abnormal pulmonary function tests or organ allografts. Do not retreat if previous treatment caused sustained ventricular tachycardia, chest pain with ECG changes showing angina or MI, un-responsive cardiac arrythymias, cardiac tamponade, intubation >72 hrs, renal failure requiring dialysis >72 hrs, coma >48 hrs, uncontrollable seizures, bowel ischemia/perforation and GI bleeding requiring surgery. **P/N:** Category C, not for use in nursing.	Chills, fever, malaise, infection, hypotension, abdominal pain, tachycardia, vasodi-lation, arrhythmia, diarrhea, N/V, stomatitis, anorexia, anemia, bilirubi-nemia, edema, wt gain, confusion, dyspnea.

Table 23.1. PRESCRIBING INFORMATION FOR ANTINEOPLASTIC DRUGS *(cont.)*

NAME	FORM/ STRENGTH	DOSAGE	WARNINGS/PRECAUTIONS & CONTRAINDICATIONS	ADVERSE EFFECTS†
CHLORINATED PURINE NUCLEOSIDE ANALOG				
Cladribine (Leustatin)	**Inj:** 1mg/mL	***Adults:* Hairy Cell Leukemia:** 0.09mg/kg/day continuous IV infusion for 7 days given as a single course. Delay or d/c if neurotoxicity or renal toxicity occurs.	**BB:** Anticipate reversible and dose dependent suppression of bone-marrow function. Serious neurological toxicity and acute nephrotoxicity reported with high doses (4-9x recommended dose). Acute nephrotoxicity observed especially with other nephrotoxic therapies. **W/P:** Periodically monitor peripheral blood counts, especially during 1st 4-8 weeks post-treatment. Fever reported in 1st month of therapy. Benzyl alcohol is in the diluent for 7-day infusion; associated with fatal "Gasping Syndrome" in premature infants. Can cause fetal harm during pregnancy. Caution with renal or hepatic insufficiency or with severe bone-marrow impairment. Assess renal and hepatic function periodically. Monitor for hematologic and non-hematologic toxicity. **P/N:** Category D, not for use in nursing.	Bone-marrow suppression, neutropenia, fever, infection, fatigue, N/V, rash, headache, injection site reactions, decreased appetite.
CYCLOPHOSPHAMIDE ANALOG				
Ifosfamide (Ifex, Ifex/Mesnex)	**Inj** (Ifosfamide): 1g, 3g; (Ifosfamide-Mesna) 1g-1g; 3g-1g	***Adults:* Testicular Cancer:** 1.2g/m²/day slow IV infusion over a minimum of 30 min for 5 consecutive days. Repeat treatment every 3 weeks or after recovery from hematologic toxicity (platelets ≥100,000/µL, WBC ≥4000/µL). Give with extensive hydration (eg, 2L fluid/day) and protector (eg, mesna) to prevent bladder toxicity/hemorrhagic cystitis.	**BB:** Risk of urotoxic side effects, especially hemorrhagic cystitis and CNS toxicities (eg, confusion, coma); may require d/c of therapy. Severe myelosuppression reported. Administer only under supervision of a physician experienced in the use of antineoplastic agents. **W/P:** Hemorrhagic cystitis reported; obtain urinalysis before each dose. Withhold dose until complete resolution of microscopic hematuria. Monitor WBCs, platelets, Hgb before each dose and at appropriate intervals. Avoid with WBC <2000/µL and/or platelets <50,000/µL. D/C if somnolence, confusion, hallucinations and/or coma occur. Caution with impaired renal function, compromised bone marrow reserve, prior radiation therapy. May interfere with normal wound healing. **Contra:** Severely depressed bone marrow function. **P/N:** Category D, not for use in nursing.	Myelosuppression, alopecia, N/V, hematuria, CNS toxicity, infection, renal impairment, liver dysfunction, increased liver enzymes/bilirubin.
CYTOTOXIC GLYCOPEPTIDE ANTIBIOTIC				
Bleomycin Sulfate (Blenoxane)	**Inj:** 15 U, 30 U	***Adults:* Squamous Cell Carcinoma/Non-Hodgkin's Lymphoma/Testicular Carcinoma:** 0.25-0.5U/kg IV/IM/SQ weekly or twice weekly. For lymphoma patients, give ≤2U for the 1st two doses; continue with regular dosage schedule if no acute reaction occurs. **Hodgkin's Disease:** 0.25-0.5U/kg IV/IM/SQ weekly or twice weekly. **Maint:** After 50% response, give 1U/day or 5U weekly IV/IM. **Malignant Pleural Effusion:** 60U as a single dose bolus intrapleural injection. **Renal Insufficiency: CrCl 40-50:** 70% of dose. **CrCl 30-40:** 60% of dose. **CrCl 20-30:** 55% of dose. **CrCl 10-20:** 45% of dose. **CrCl 5-10:** 40% of dose.	**BB:** Pulmonary fibrosis is the most severe toxicity reported (usually presents as pneumonitis occasionally progressing to pulmonary fibrosis); higher occurrence in elderly and if receiving >400 units total dose. A severe idiosyncratic reaction including hypotension, mental confusion, fever, chills, and wheezing reported in lymphoma patients. Administer only under supervision of a physician experienced in the use of antineoplastic agents. **W/P:** Extreme caution with significant renal impairment or compromised pulmonary function. Pulmonary toxicity (dose and age related) may occur; frequent radiographs are recommended. Monitor for severe	Pneumonitis, erythema, rash, striae, vesiculation, hyperpigmentation, skin tenderness, hyperkeratosis, nail changes, alopecia, pruritus, stomatitis, pulmonary toxicity.

†Bold entries denote special dental considerations.
BB = black box warning; **W/P** = warnings/precautions; **Contra** = contraindications; **P/N** = pregnancy category rating and nursing considerations.

NAME	FORM/ STRENGTH	DOSAGE	WARNINGS/PRECAUTIONS & CONTRAINDICATIONS	ADVERSE EFFECTS†
Bleomycin Sulfate (Blenoxane) *(cont.)*			idiosyncratic reactions, especially after 1st and 2nd doses. Renal and hepatic toxicity reported. Can cause fetal harm during pregnancy. Risk of pulmonary toxicity with total dose >400 U. Caution with dose selection in elderly. **P/N:** Category D, not for use in nursing.	
DEOXYGUANOSINE ANALOGUE				
Nelarabine (Arranon)	**Inj:** 5mg/mL	***Adults:*** **T-Cell ALL or Lymphoblastic Lymphoma:** 1500mg/m² IV over 2 hrs on days 1, 3, and 5 repeated every 21 days. **CrCl <50ml/min:** Insufficient data to support dose recommendation. ***Pediatrics:*** 650mg/m²/day IV over 1 hr daily for 5 consecutive days. Repeat every 21 days. **CrCl <50ml/min:** Insufficient data to support dose recommendation.	**BB:** Severe neurologic events reported; close monitoring is strongly recommended. D/C for neurologic events of NCI Common Toxicity Criteria ≥ grade 2. **W/P:** Leukopenia, thrombocytopenia, anemia, neutropenia/febrile neutropenia reported; regularly monitor CBC including platelets. Intravenous hydration recommended for management of hyperuricemia with risk of tumor lysis syndrome; may also consider allopurinol. Avoid administration of live vaccines. Closely monitor toxicities with severe renal impairment (eg, CrCl <30mL/min) and/or severe hepatic impairment (eg, bilirubin >3mg/dL); increased risk of adverse reactions. **P/N:** Category D, not for use in nursing.	See BB Warning, W/P. (Adults) fatigue, N/V, diarrhea, constipation, cough, dyspnea, dizziness, pyrexia, blurred vision. (Pediatrics) headache, increased transaminases, decreased blood potassium, decreased/ increased blood albumin, vomiting.
DNA FRAGMENTATION AGENT				
Arsenic Trioxide (Trisenox)	**Inj:** 1mg/mL	***Adults/Pediatrics:*** **Acute Promyelocytic Leukemia: ≥5 yrs: Induction:** 0.15mg/kg IV qd until bone marrow remission. **Max:** 60 doses. **Consolidation:** 0.15mg/kg IV qd for 25 doses over 5 weeks. Begin 3-6 weeks after complete induction therapy.	**BB:** Administer under supervision of a physician experienced in the management of acute leukemia. Acute promyelocytic leukemia (APL) differentiation syndrome reported. Can cause QT interval prolongation and complete AV block. Monitor ECG, serum electrolytes and creatinine before and during therapy. **W/P:** Hyperleukocytosis, QT interval prolongation, torsades de pointes and complete AV block reported. Caution with renal failure. Monitor electrolyte, hematologic and coagulation profiles at least twice weekly and more frequently in unstable patients during induction. Obtain ECG weekly and more frequently for unstable patients. May cause fetal harm; avoid pregnancy. **P/N:** Category D, not for use in nursing.	Fatigue, pyrexia, edema, chest pain, injection site pain, N/V, abdominal pain, constipation, hypokalemia, hypomagnesemia, hyperglycemia, increased ALT, headache, insomnia, dyspnea.
DNA METHYLTRANSFERASE INHIBITOR				
Decitabine (Dacogen)	**Inj:** 50mg	***Adults:*** **Myelodysplastic Syndromes: Initial:** 15mg/m² IV over 3 hrs q8h for 3 days. Repeat cycle every 6 weeks. Treat for ≥4 cycles. Adjust dose based on hematology lab values, renal function and serum electrolytes.	**W/P:** May cause fetal harm. Avoid pregnancy in women of childbearing potential. Men should be advised not to father a child while receiving treatment and for 2 months afterwards. Neutropenia and thrombocytopenia may occur; monitor CBC and platelets periodically (at minimum, before each cycle). Caution with renal and hepatic dysfunction. Avoid with SrCr >2mg/dL, transaminase >2x normal or serum bilirubin >1.5mg/dL. **P/N:** Category D, not for use in nursing.	Neutropenia, thrombocytopenia, anemia, fatigue, pyrexia, nausea, cough, petechiae, constipation, diarrhea, hyperglycemia, febrile neutropenia, leukopenia, headache, insomnia.

Table 23.1. PRESCRIBING INFORMATION FOR ANTINEOPLASTIC DRUGS *(cont.)*

NAME	FORM/ STRENGTH	DOSAGE	WARNINGS/PRECAUTIONS & CONTRAINDICATIONS	ADVERSE EFFECTS†
DNA SYNTHESIS INHIBITORS				
Mitomycin (Mutamycin)	**Inj:** 5mg, 20mg, 40mg	***Adults:* Gastric or Pancreatic Cancer: Usual: (after full hematological recovery):** 20mg/m² IV single dose q6-8 weeks. **Dosage Adjustments: Leukocytes 2000-2999/mm³, Platelets 25,000-74,999/mm³:** Give 70% of prior dose. Leukocytes <2000/mm³, Platelets <25,000/mm³: Give 50% of prior dose. No repeat dosage should be given until leukocyte count has returned to 4000/mm³ and platelet count to 100,000/mm³.	**BB:** Bone marrow suppression (eg, thrombocytopenia, leukopenia) may occur. Hemolytic Uremic Syndrome (HUS) reported, mostly with high doses (≥60mg). Blood product transfusion may exacerbate HUS. Administer only under supervision of a physician experienced in the use of antineoplastic agents. **W/P:** See Black Box Warning. Monitor platelets, WBCs, differential and Hgb repeatedly during therapy and for at least 8 weeks after. May cause renal toxicity, avoid if SrCr >1.7mg %. Bladder fibrosis/contraction reported with intravesical administration. **Contra:** Thrombocytopenia, coagulation disorder, increased bleeding tendency due to other causes. **P/N:** Safety in pregnancy unknown, not for use in nursing.	Bone marrow toxicity, integument and mucous membrane toxicity (eg, cellulitis, stomatitis, alopecia, skin necrosis), renal/pulmonary cardiac toxicity, fever, anorexia, N/V.
Streptozocin (Zanosar)	**Inj:** 1g	***Adults:* Pancreatic Cancer: Daily Schedule:** 500mg/m² IV daily for 5 days every 6 weeks until maximum benefit or treatment-limiting toxicity occurs. **Weekly Schedule:** 1g/m² IV at 1 week intervals for 1st two doses. **Titrate:** May increase dose for subsequent courses if response not achieved. **Max:** 1.5g/m²/dose. **Significant Renal Toxicity:** Reduce dose or d/c. Administer IV by rapid injection or short/prolonged infusion.	**BB:** Associated with dose-related renal toxicity, N/V, liver dysfunction, diarrhea and hematological changes. Mutagenic. **W/P:** Monitor renal function before and after each course of therapy. Obtain urinalysis, BUN, SCr, electrolytes and CrCl prior to, at least weekly during, and 4 weeks after drug is given. May cause extravasation. Monitor CBCs and LFTs at least weekly. Caution in elderly. May impair mental/physical activities. **P/N:** Category D, not for use in nursing.	N/V, diarrhea, hepatic and renal toxicity, glucose tolerance abnormality.
EPIDERMAL GROWTH FACTOR RECEPTOR (EGFR) ANTAGONIST				
Cetuximab‡ (Erbitux)	**Inj:** 2mg/mL	***Adults:*** Premedication with H_1-antagonist (eg, diphenhydramine 50mg) IV 30-60 min prior to 1st dose is recommended. **Colorectal Cancer: LD:** 400mg/m² IV infusion over 120 min. **Maint:** 250mg/m² IV infusion over 60 min once weekly. **Max Infusion Rate:** 10mg/min. **SCCHN: Combination Therapy: Initial:** 400mg/m² IV over 120 min 1 week prior to initiation of a course of radiation treatment. **Maint:** 250mg/m² over 60 min weekly for duration of radiation therapy. **Max Infusion Rate:** 10mg/min. **Recurrent/Metastatic SCCHN: Monotherapy: Initial:** 400mg/m². **Maint:** 250mg/m² until disease progression or unacceptable toxicity. **Mild-Moderate (Grade 1 or 2) Infusion Reactions:** Reduce rate by 50%. **Severe (Grade 3 or 4) Infusion Reactions:** D/C. **Development of Severe Acneform Rash:** Delay infusion 1-2 weeks for 1st three occurrences. **1st Occurrence:** If improvement, continue at 250mg/m². **2nd Occurrence:** If improvement, reduce dose to 200mg/m². **3rd Occurrence:** If improvement, reduce dose to 150mg/m². **4th Occurrence/No Improvement After Delaying Therapy:** D/C therapy.	**BB:** Severe infusion reactions have occurred; immediately interrupt and permanently d/c infusion if these reactions occur. Cardiopulmonary arrest and/or sudden death have occurred with squamous cell carcinoma of the head and neck treated with radiation therapy and cetuximab; closely monitor serum electrolytes during and after therapy. **W/P:** Infusion reactions reported; observe closely for 1 hr following infusion. Permanently d/c therapy if serious infusion reactions develop. Dermatologic (eg, acneform rash, skin drying/fissuring, paronychial inflammation, infectious sequelae) or pulmonary toxicities may occur. D/C if interstitial lung disease confirmed. Adjust dose in cases of severe acneform rash. Apply sunscreen and limit sun exposure. Caution with hypersensitivity to murine proteins. Potential for immunogenicity. Caution with radiation therapy and cisplatin therapy. Monitor for hypomagnesemia, hypocalcemia, and hypokalemia during and for at least 8 weeks following completion of therapy. **P/N:** Category C, not for use in nursing.	Acneform rash, mucositis, asthenia/malaise, diarrhea, N/V, abdominal pain, fatigue, fever, constipation, infusion reactions, dermatologic toxicities, infection, headache, anorexia, dyspnea, insomnia.

†Bold entries denote special dental considerations.
‡Used as single or combination agent for head and neck cancer.
BB = black box warning; **W/P** = warnings/precautions; **Contra** = contraindications; **P/N** = pregnancy category rating and nursing considerations.

NAME	FORM/ STRENGTH	DOSAGE	WARNINGS/PRECAUTIONS & CONTRAINDICATIONS	ADVERSE EFFECTS†
EPIDERMAL GROWTH FACTOR RECEPTOR (EGFR) TYROSINE KINASE INHIBITOR				
Erlotinib (Tarceva)	**Tab:** 25mg, 100mg, 150mg	***Adults:* NSCLC:** 150mg at least 1 hr before or 2 hrs after ingestion of food. **Pancreatic Cancer:** 100mg at least 1 hr before or 2 hrs after ingestion of food, in combination with gemcitabine. Continue until disease progression or unacceptable toxicity. **Acute Onset of New or Progressive Pulmonary Symptoms:** D/C therapy. **Severe Diarrhea/Severe Skin Reactions:** May require dose reduction or temporary interruption of therapy. **Strong CYP3A4 Inhibitors:** Consider dose reduction. When dose reduction is necessary, reduce dose in 50mg decrements.	**W/P:** Serious interstitial lung disease (ILD), including fatalities, reported; d/c if ILD diagnosed. May increase risk of MI and cerebrovascular accident. Asymptomatic increases in liver transaminases observed. Consider dose reduction or interruption if changes in liver function are severe. Elevations in INR and infrequent reports of bleeding reported. Monitor closely with concomitant anticoagulants. Cases of acute renal failure and renal insufficiency with or without hypokalemia reported. Caution in patients at risk of dehydration; monitor renal function and serum electrolytes periodically. May cause fetal harm; avoid pregnancy. May cause MI/ischemia. **P/N:** Category D, not for use in nursing.	Rash, diarrhea, anorexia, fatigue, dyspnea, cough, N/V, infection, edema, pyrexia, constipation, abdominal pain, decreased weight, bone pain.
ESTRADIOL/NORNITROGEN MUSTARD				
Estramustine Phosphate Sodium (Emcyt)	**Cap:** 140mg	***Adults:* Prostate Cancer: Usual:** 14mg/kg/day given tid-qid. Take with water at least 1 hr before or 2 hrs after meals.	**W/P:** Increased risk of thrombosis and MI. Caution with CVD, CAD, metabolic bone disease associated with hypercalcemia, hepatic or renal dysfunction, or with history of thrombophlebitis, thrombosis, or thromboembolic disorders. May decrease glucose tolerance. HTN may occur; monitor BP periodically. May exacerbate pre-existing peripheral edema or CHF. Allergic reactions, angioedema reported. Gynecomastia, impotence may occur. **Contra:** Active thrombophlebitis, thromboembolic disorders; except when the tumor mass is causing the thromboembolic phenomenon and therapy benefits outweigh risks. **P/N:** Safety in pregnancy and nursing not known.	Edema, dyspnea, leg cramps, nausea, diarrhea, GI upset, breast tenderness/enlargement, increased hepatic enzymes.
ESTROGEN RECEPTOR ANTAGONIST				
Fulvestrant (Faslodex)	**Inj:** 50mg/mL [2.5mL, 5mL]	***Adults:* Metastatic Breast Cancer:** 250mg IM into buttock once monthly as either a single 5mL injection or two concurrent 2.5mL injections. Administer slowly.	**W/P:** May cause fetal harm during pregnancy; women of childbearing age should be advised not to become pregnant and pregnancy should be ruled out prior to initiating therapy. Avoid in patients with bleeding diatheses or thrombocytopenia. Safety and efficacy have not been studied in patients with moderate or severe hepatic impairment. **Contra:** Pregnancy. **P/N:** Category D, not for use in nursing.	N/V, constipation, diarrhea, abdominal pain, headache, back pain, vasodilatation (hot flushes), **pharyngitis,** injection-site reactions, asthenia, pain, dyspnea, increased cough.
FLUOROPYRIMIDINE CARBAMATE				
Capecitabine (Xeloda)	**Tab:** 150mg, 500mg	***Adults:*** Take with water within 30 min after meals. **Metastatic Breast Cancer: Usual/Concomitantly w/Docetaxel:** 1250mg/m² bid for 2 weeks, then 1 week off. Give as 3-week cycles. **Adjuvant treatment of Dukes' C Colon Cancer:** 3-week cycles for a total of 8 cycles (24 weeks). **CrCl 30-50mL/min:** Reduce to 75% of starting dose. Interrupt and/or reduce dose if toxicity occurs. Readjust according to adverse effects (see PI for details).	**BB:** Altered coagulation parameters and/or bleeding, including death, reported with coumarin-derivative anticoagulants (eg, warfarin). Monitor PT/INR frequently to adjust anticoagulant dose. **W/P:** Reduce dose with moderate renal dysfunction. Carefully monitor for adverse events with mild to moderate renal dysfunction. Carefully monitor with severe diarrhea fluid/electrolyte balance; may need dose adjustment. Patients ≥80 yrs may experience increased Grade 3	Diarrhea, hand and foot syndrome, pyrexia, anemia, N/V, fatigue, dermatitis, neutropenia, thrombocytopenia, stomatitis, anorexia, hyperbilirubinemia, abdominal pain, paresthesia.

Table 23.1. PRESCRIBING INFORMATION FOR ANTINEOPLASTIC DRUGS *(cont.)*

NAME	FORM/ STRENGTH	DOSAGE	WARNINGS/PRECAUTIONS & CONTRAINDICATIONS	ADVERSE EFFECTS†
FLUOROPYRIMIDINE CARBAMATE *(cont.)*				
Capecitabine (Xeloda) *(cont.)*			and 4 adverse events (see full prescribing info). Possible fetal harm with pregnancy. Monitor for hand-and-foot syndrome. Cardiotoxicity reported; more common with history of CAD. Carefully monitor with mild to moderate hepatic dysfunction due to hepatic metastases. Hyperbilirubinemia, neutropenia, thrombocytopenia, and decrease in hemoglobin reported. **Contra:** Hypersensitivity to 5-FU, dihydropyrimidine dehydrogenase (DPD) deficiency, severe renal impairment (CrCl <30mL/min). **P/N:** Category D, not for use in nursing.	
FUSION PROTEIN				
Denileukin Diftitox (Ontak)	**Inj:** 150mcg/mL	***Adults:*** **T-Cell Lymphoma: Treatment Cycle:** 9 or 18mcg/kg/day IV over 30-60 min for 5 consecutive days, every 21 days for 8 cycles. Withhold administration if serum albumin <3g/dL.	**BB:** Serious and fatal infusion reactions, capillary leak syndrome, loss of visual acuity and color vision reported. Stop and permanently D/C for serious infusion reactions. Administer in a facility equipped and staffed for cardiopulmonary resuscitation. **W/P:** Capillary leak syndrome reported; caution with pre-existing cardiovascular disease. Pre-existing low serum albumin may increase risk of syndrome; monitor weight, edema, BP, and serum albumin levels. Monitor for infection. Test malignant cells for CD25 expression prior to therapy. Perform CBC, blood chemistry panel, liver and renal function, and serum albumin prior to and weekly during therapy. Hypoalbuminemia reported; delay therapy until serum albumin ≥3g/dL. Loss of visual acuity, usually with loss of color vision, with or without retinal pigment mottling reported. **P/N:** Category C, not for use in nursing.	Pyrexia, rigors, fatigue, asthenia, hypotension, N/V, pain, headache, anorexia, diarrhea, hypoalbuminemia, anemia, myalgia, dizziness, dyspnea, cough, rash, infusion-associated reactions.
HEAVY-METAL PLATINUM COMPLEX				
Cisplatin‡ (Platinol-AQ)	**Inj:** 50mg, 100mg	***Adults:*** **Testicular Tumor:** 20mg/m² IV qd for 5 days per cycle. **Ovarian Tumor: Cyclophosphamide Combination Therapy:** 75-100mg/m² IV per cycle once every 4 weeks. **Monotherapy:** 100mg/m² IV per cycle once every 4 weeks. **Bladder Cancer:** 50-70mg/m² IV per cycle every 3-4 weeks. Pretreatment hydration with 1-2L of fluid 8-12 hrs before therapy, and maintain adequate hydration and urinary output for the 24 hrs after infusion. Hold repeat course until SCr <1.5mg/100mL, BUN <25mg/100mL, platelets ≥100,000/mm³, WBC ≥4000/mm³. Hold subsequent doses until audiometric analysis is within normal limits.	**BB:** Cumulative renal toxicity is severe. Myelosuppression and N/V are also dose-related toxicities. Ototoxicity is significant. Anaphylactic-like reactions reported. Avoid inadvertent confusion with carboplatin. Doses >100mg/m²/cycle once every 3-4 weeks are rarely used. **W/P:** Severe neuropathies reported with higher doses or greater frequency than recommended. Loss of motor function reported. Perform audiometric testing and measure SrCr, BUN, CrCl, magnesium, sodium, potassium, and calcium before each dose. Can cause fetal harm during pregnancy. Perform peripheral blood counts weekly, LFTs periodically, and neurologic exam regularly. Avoid aluminum containing IV sets; may cause precipitate. Caution in elderly. **Contra:** Renal impairment, myelosuppression, hearing impairment, allergy to platinum-containing compounds. **P/N:** Category D, not for use in nursing.	Nephrotoxicity, ototoxicity, vestibular toxicity, myelosuppression, Coombs' positive hemolytic anemia, immediate or delayed N/V, serum electrolyte disturbances, hyperuricemia, neurotoxicity, hepatotoxicity.

†Bold entries denote special dental considerations.
‡Used as single or combination agent for head and neck cancer.
BB = black box warning; **W/P** = warnings/precautions; **Contra** = contraindications; **P/N** = pregnancy category rating and nursing considerations.

NAME	FORM/ STRENGTH	DOSAGE	WARNINGS/PRECAUTIONS & CONTRAINDICATIONS	ADVERSE EFFECTS†
HISTONE DEACETYLASE INHIBITOR				
Vorinostat (Zolinza)	**Cap:** 100mg	**Adults: Cutaneous Manifestations of T-Cell Lymphoma** 400mg PO qd with food. **Intolerant to Therapy:** May reduce dose to 300mg PO qd with food. If necessary, may further reduce dose to 300mg PO qd with food for 5 consecutive days each week.	**W/P:** Pulmonary embolism and DVT reported; monitor for signs and symptoms. Dose-related thrombocytopenia and anemia may occur; consider dose modification or d/c. GI disturbances reported. Hyperglycemia observed; monitor glucose levels. QTc prolongation reported; monitor electrolytes and ECGs at baseline and periodically during treatment. Monitor CBC and chemistry tests every 2 weeks during first 2 months of therapy and monthly thereafter. **P/N:** Category D, not for use in nursing.	Diarrhea, fatigue, thrombocytopenia, anorexia, dysgeusia, decreased weight, muscle spasms, alopecia, **dry mouth,** increased SCr, chills, N/V, constipation, dizziness.
HYDRAZINE DERIVATIVE				
Procarbazine HCl (Matulane)	**Cap:** 50mg	***Adults:* Hodgkin's Disease:** 2-4mg/kg/day as single or divided doses for first week then increase to 4-6mg/kg/day until maximum response or WBC <4000/mm^3 or platelets <100,000/mm^3. **Maint:** 1-2mg/kg/day. **In MOPP:** 100mg/m^2 qd for 14 days. Adjust dose for combination regimens. ***Pediatrics:*** 50mg/m^2/day for first week then increase to 100mg/m^2/day until response is obtained or leukopenia or thrombocytopenia occurs. **Maint:** 50mg/m^2/day. Adjust dose for combination regimens.	**BB:** To be given only by or under supervision of experienced physician in use of potent antineoplastics. Proper monitoring with adequate clinical and laboratory facilities should be conducted. **W/P:** Toxicity may occur in renal or hepatic impairment. Wait one month or longer with prior use of bone marrow suppressing radiation or chemotherapy. D/C if CNS symptoms (eg, paresthesias, neuropathies, confusion), leukopenia, thrombocytopenia, hypersensitivity, stomatitis, diarrhea, hemorrhage or bleeding tendencies occur. Bone marrow depression often occurs 2-8 weeks after initiation. Monitor urinalysis, transaminases, LFTs weekly, hematologic status every 3-4 days. **Contra:** Inadequate marrow reserve. **P/N:** Category D, not for use in nursing.	Leukopenia, anemia, thrombopenia, N/V.
IgG4 KAPPA ANTIBODY/CALICHEAMICIN CONJUGATE				
Gemtuzumab Ozogamicin (Mylotarg)	**Inj:** 5mg	***Adults:* ≥60 yrs: AML:** 9mg/m^2 as 2 hr IV infusion, for 2 doses with 14 days between doses. Premedicate 1 hr prior with diphenhydramine 50mg and APAP 650-1000mg (may give additional APAP dose q4h for 2 doses as needed). Monitor vital signs during infusion and for 4 hrs after.	**BB:** Only use as monotherapy. Severe myelosuppression, severe hypersensitivity reactions (eg, anaphylaxis, pulmonary events, infusion related-reactions) can occur. Hepatotoxicity, including severe hepatic veno-occlusive disease (VOD) reported. **W/P:** Monitor CBC, LFTs and electrolytes. Monitor vital signs during infusion and 4 hrs after. Interrupt infusion if dyspnea or significant hypotension develops. Consider d/c if anaphylaxis, pulmonary edema or ARDS develops. Increased risk of severe VOD if used before or after hematopoietic stem-cell transplant, underlying hepatic disease or abnormal liver function, or with combination chemotherapy. Extra caution with hepatic impairment. Administer in appropriate facility. Tumor lysis syndrome may occur. Not for IV push or bolus use. **Contra:** Lactating mothers. **P/N:** Category D, not for use in nursing.	Chills, fever, N/V, headache, hypotension, HTN, hypoxia, dyspnea, hyperglycemia, antibody formation, myelosuppression, anemia, thrombocytopenia, sepsis, pneumonia, epistaxis, mucositis, hepatotoxicity, neutropenia.

Table 23.1. PRESCRIBING INFORMATION FOR ANTINEOPLASTIC DRUGS *(cont.)*

NAME	FORM/ STRENGTH	DOSAGE	WARNINGS/PRECAUTIONS & CONTRAINDICATIONS	ADVERSE EFFECTS†
KINASE INHIBITORS				
Lapatinib (Tykerb)	**Tab:** 250mg	***Adults:* Breast Cancer: Usual:** 1250mg qd on Days 1-21 continuously with capecitabine 2000mg/m²/day (administered orally in 2 doses 12 hrs apart) on Days 1-14 in a repeating 21-day cycle. Give at least 1 hr before or after a meal (however, give capecitabine with food). **≥Grade 2 LVEF:** D/C dose. If LVEF recovers and asymptomatic after 2 weeks, restart at 1000mg/day. **Hepatic Impairment (Child-Pugh Class C):** Consider dose reduction to 750mg/day. **Concomitant Strong CYP3A4 Inhibitors:** Avoid use. **Concomitant Strong CYP3A4 Inducers:** Avoid use and if must coadminister titrate gradually from 1250mg/day up to 4500mg/day based on tolerability. **≥Grade 2 NCI CTC Toxicity:** D/C or interrupt dose and restart with 1250mg/day when toxicity ≤Grade 1. Restart at 1000mg/day if toxicity recurs.	**BB:** Severe hepatotoxicity and deaths have been reported. **W/P:** Decreased left ventricular ejection fraction reported; confirm normal LVEF prior to therapy and evaluate during treatment. Reduce dose in patients with severe hepatic impairment. Severe diarrhea reported; manage with antidiarrheals, replace electrolytes. Prolongs the QT interval in some patients; consider ECG and electrolyte monitoring. Fetal harm may occur if administered to pregnant women; women should not become pregnant during therapy. Has been associated with interstitial lung disease and pneumonitis in monotherapy or in combination with other chemotherapies. **P/N:** Category D, not for use in nursing.	Diarrhea, N/V, stomatitis, dyspepsia, palmar-plantar erythrodysesthesia, rash, dry skin, mucosal inflammation, pain in extremity, back pain, dyspnea, insomnia.
Nilotinib (Tasigna)	**Cap:** 200mg	***Adults:* CML:** 400mg PO bid, approximately 12 hrs apart. Swallow whole with water. Avoid food for at least 2 hrs before and 1 hr after dosing. Adjust dose based on hematologic and non-hematologic toxicities, and drug interactions (see PI).	**BB:** Prolongs QT interval. Sudden deaths reported. Avoid with hypokalemia, hypomagnesemia or long QT syndrome. Correct hypokalemia or hypomagnesemia prior to administration and monitor periodically. Avoid drugs known to prolong the QT interval and strong CYP3A4 inhibitors. Avoid food 2 hrs before and 1 hr after taking dose. Caution with hepatic impairment. Monitor QTc at baseline, 7 days after initiation, and periodically thereafter, as well as following any dose adjustments. **W/P:** Myelosuppression associated with neutropenia, thrombocytopenia and anemia may occur; perform CBC every 2 weeks for first 2 months, then monthly. Myelosuppression may be reversed by reducing or withholding dose. May increase serum lipase; monitor periodically and use caution with history of pancreatitis. May elevate bilirubin, AST/ALT and alkaline phosphatase; monitor LFTs periodically. May cause hypophosphatemia, hypokalemia, hyperkalemia, hypocalcemia, hyponatremia; correct electrolyte abnormalities prior to initiation and monitor periodically during therapy. Caps contain lactose; avoid with rare hereditary problems of galactose intolerance, severe lactase deficiency or glucose-galactose malabsorption. **Contra:** Hypokalemia, hypomagnesemia or long QT syndrome. **P/N:** Category D, not for use in nursing.	Rash, pruritus, N/V, fatigue, headache, constipation, diarrhea, thrombocytopenia, neutropenia, leukopenia, pneumonia, intracranial hemorrhage, elevated lipase, pyrexia.
Temsirolimus (Torisel)	**Inj:** 25mg/mL	***Adults:* RCC:** 25mg infused over 30-60 min once a week. Hold if ANC <1,000/mm³, platelet count <75,000/mm³, or NCI CTCAE grade 3 or greater adverse reactions. Once toxicities resolve to grade 2 or less, restart with dose reduced by 5mg/week to a dose no lower than 15mg/week. **Concomitant**	**W/P:** Hypersensitivity reactions such as anaphylaxis, dyspnea, flushing and chest pain have been observed. Give H_1-antihistamine before starting infusion. Hyperglycemia, glucose intolerance and hyperlipemia may occur; monitor glucose and lipid profiles. Infections may result from immunosuppression.	Rash, asthenia, mucositis, nausea, edema, anorexia, anemia, hyperlipemia, hyperglycemia, hypertriglyceridemia, lymphopenia, leukopenia,

†Bold entries denote special dental considerations.
BB = black box warning; **W/P** = warnings/precautions; **Contra** = contraindications; **P/N** = pregnancy category rating and nursing considerations.

NAME	FORM/ STRENGTH	DOSAGE	WARNINGS/PRECAUTIONS & CONTRAINDICATIONS	ADVERSE EFFECTS†
Temsirolimus (Torisel) *(cont.)*		**Strong CYP3A4 Inhibitors:** Consider dose reduction to 12.5mg/week. If strong inhibitor is discontinued, allow wash-out period of about 1 week before dose adjustment. **Concomitant Strong CYP3A4 Inducers:** Consider dose increase to 50mg/week. If strong inducer is discontinued, return to dose used prior to initiation of strong inducer.	Monitor for interstitial lung disease (ILD); if ILD is suspected, d/c and consider use of corticosteroids and/or antibiotics. Bowel perforation may occur; monitor closely. Renal failure, sometimes fatal, reported; monitor renal function. May cause abnormal wound healing; caution during perioperative period. Caution with CNS tumors and/or anticoagulant therapy. Avoid live vaccines and close contact with those who have received live vaccines. Monitor CBC weekly and chemistry panel every 2 weeks. May cause fetal harm; avoid pregnancy during, and for 3 months after, therapy. **P/N:** Category D, not for use in nursing.	hypophosphatemia, thrombocytopenia, and elevated alkaline phosphatase, AST, SCr.
LUTEINIZING HORMONE–RELEASING HORMONE AGONISTS				
Histrelin Acetate (Vantas)	**Implant:** 50mg	***Adults:*** **Prostate Cancer:** 50mg every 12 months. Inject SQ into inner aspect of the upper arm. Refrain from wetting the inserted arm for 24 hours. Refrain from heavy lifting or strenuous exercise of the inserted arm for 7 days after implant insertion. Must remove after 12 months of therapy.	**W/P:** Transient increase in serum testosterone and worsening of symptoms of prostate cancer with initial therapy. Urethral obstruction and spinal cord compression reported. Anaphylactic reactions may occur. **Contra:** Women and pediatric patients. **P/N:** Category X, not for use in nursing.	Hot flushes, fatigue, implant site reaction, testicular atrophy, renal impairment, gynecomastia, constipation, erectile dysfunction.
Triptorelin Pamoate (Trelstar Depot, Trelstar LA)	**Inj:** (Depot) 3.75mg, (LA) 11.25mg	***Adults:*** **Prostate Cancer:** (Depot) 3.75mg IM every month or (LA) 11.25mg IM every 84 days.	**W/P:** Anaphylactic shock, angioedema, urethral obstruction, spinal cord compression, renal impairment reported. May worsen symptoms during 1st few weeks of treatment. Closely monitor patients with metastatic vertebral lesions and/or urinary tract obstruction during 1st few weeks of therapy. Monitor serum testosterone levels, PSA. **Contra:** Pregnancy. **P/N:** Category X, not for use in nursing.	Hot flushes, HTN, headache, skeletal pain, dysuria, leg edema, pain, impotence.
MONOCLONAL ANTIBODY				
Ibritumomab Tiuxetan (Zevalin)	**Inj:** 3.2mg/2mL	***Adults:*** **B-Cell NHL: Day 1:** Rituximab 250mg/m² IV single infusion. Within 4 hrs, give 5mCi of In-111 ibritumomab IV. Assess biodistribution by conducting 1st image at 2-24 hrs, 2nd image at 48-72 hrs, and optional 3rd image at 90-120 hrs. If biodistribution acceptable, **Day 7-9:** Rituximab 250mg/m² IV. Within 4 hrs, give Y-90 ibritumomab 0.4mCi/kg (or 0.3mCi/kg if platelets 100,000-149,000 cells/mm³). **Max:** Y-90 ibritumomab 32mCi.	**BB:** D/C if severe infusion reactions occurs. Severe and prolonged cytopenias reported; avoid if ≥25% lymphoma marrow involvement and/or impaired bone marrow reserve. Severe, some fatal, cutaneous and mucocutaneous reactions reported. Do not exceed max dose. Avoid patients with altered biodistribution. **W/P:** Use with rituximab. Contains albumin; remote risk of transmission of viral disease and CJD. Single course treatment only. Minimize radiation exposure during and after radiolabeling. Monitor CBC and platelets weekly until levels recover. Increased risk of hypersensitivity reactions with HAMA from prior murine protein use. Caution with transfusion. Secondary leukemia and mylodysplastic syndrome reported. Monitor closely for evidence of extravasation. Immediately terminate infusion if signs or symptoms of extravasation occured. **Contra:** Type I hypersensitivity or anaphylactic reactions to murine proteins or to any component of this product including rituximab, yttrium chloride, and indium chloride. **P/N:** Category D, not for use in nursing.	Neutropenia, thrombocytopenia, anemia, NV, abdominal pain, diarrhea, increased cough, dyspnea, dizziness, arthralgia, anorexia, anxiety, ecchymosis, infusion site erythema, ulceration following extravasation, radiation injury, tissue complications.

Table 23.1. PRESCRIBING INFORMATION FOR ANTINEOPLASTIC DRUGS *(cont.)*

NAME	FORM/ STRENGTH	DOSAGE	WARNINGS/PRECAUTIONS & CONTRAINDICATIONS	ADVERSE EFFECTS†
MONOCLONAL ANTIBODY/CD20-BLOCKER				
Iodine I 131 Tositumomab/ Tositumomab (Bexxar)	**Inj: For Dosimetric Dosing: Tositumomab:** 225mg [2 single-use vials], 35mg [1 single-use vial]; **Iodine I 131 Tositumomab:** 1 single-use vial. **For Therapeutic Dosing: Tositumomab:** 225mg [2 single-use vials], 35mg [1 single-use vial]; **Iodine I 131 Tositumomab:** 1 or 2 single-use vials.	***Adults:* CD20-positive, Follicular NHL: Premedication: Day 1:** Begin thyro-protective regimen of either SSKI (4 drops po tid), Lugol's sol (20 drops po tid), or potassium iodide (130mg po qd). Continue until 14 days post-therapeutic dose. **Day 0:** APAP 650mg and diphenhydramine 50mg. **Dosimetric Step: IV:** 450mg tositumomab over 60 min followed by 5mCi Iodine I 131 tositumomab (35mg) over 20 min. **Day 0 + Day 2, 3, or 4 + Day 6 or 7:** Whole body dosimetry and biodistribution. **Day 6 or 7:** Calculation of patient-specific activity of iodine I 131 tositumomab to deliver 75cGy total body irradiation or 65cGy if platelets ≥100,000 but <150,000 platelets/mm³. **Day 7 (up to Day 14):** Premedicate with APAP and diphenhydramine. **Therapeutic Step: IV:** Do not administer if biodistribution is altered. 450mg tositumomab over 60 min followed by prescribed therapeutic dose of iodine I 131 tositumomab (35mg) over 20 min.	**BB:** Hypersensitivity reactions, including anaphylaxis, and prolonged and severe cytopenias reported. Can cause fetal harm if given during pregnancy. Contains radioactive component. **W/P:** Obtain CBCs weekly for 10-12 weeks. Safety not established with >25% lymphoma marrow involvement, platelet <100,000 cells/mm³, or neutrophil count <1500 cells/mm³. Secondary malignancies reported. May cause hypothyroidism; monitor TSH prior to initiation and then annually. Thyroid blocking agents must be used; initiate at least 24 hrs before dosimetric dose and continue until 14 days after therapeutic dose. Caution with impaired renal function. Effective contraceptive methods should be used during, and for 12 months following treatment. Increased risk of serious allergic reactions if positive for human anti-murine antibodies (HAMA). **Contra:** Pregnant women. **P/N:** Category X, not for use in nursing.	Neutropenia, thrombocytopenia, anemia, asthenia, fever, infection, cough, pain, chills, headache, GI effects, myalgia, arthralgia, **pharyngitis,** dyspnea, rash.
Rituximab (Rituxan)	**Inj:** 10mg/mL [10mL, 50mL]	***Adults:*** Administer only as IV infusion. **Relapsed or Refractory, Low-Grade or Follicular, CD20-Positive, B-cell NHL:** 375mg/m² IV once weekly for 4 or 8 doses. **Retreatment for Relapsed or Refractory, Low-Grade or Follicular, CD20-Positive, B-cell NHL:** 375mg/m² IV once weekly for 4 doses. **Previously Untreated, Follicular, CD20-Positive, B-cell NHL:** 375mg/m² IV on Day 1 of each CVP chemotherapy cycle for up to 8 doses. **Nonprogressing, Low-Grade, CD20-Positive, B-cell NHL:** Following completion of 6-8 cycles of CVP chemotherapy, 375mg/m² IV once weekly for 4 doses at 6-month intervals to maximum of 16 doses. **Diffuse Large B-cell NHL:** 375mg/m² IV given on Day 1 of each chemotherapy cycle for up to 8 infusions. **RA:** Give with methotrexate. Administer two 1000mg IV infusions separated by 2 weeks. Give methylprednisolone 100mg IV (or equivalent) 30 min prior to each infusion to reduce incidence and severity of infusion reactions. Do not administer as IV push or bolus. For dosing as a component of Zevalin® (ibritumomab tiuxetan) please refer to PI.	**BB:** Serious, sometimes fatal, infusion reactions reported. Acute renal failure reported in the setting of tumor lysis syndrome (TLS) following treatment of non-Hodgkin's lymphoma. Severe mucocutaneous reactions reported. JC virus infection resulting in progressive multifocal leukoencephalopathy (PML) reported. **W/P:** Interrupt if severe reaction develops; may resume at a 50% rate reduction when symptoms subside. Consider the diagnosis of PML in patients presenting with new-onset neurologic manifestations; d/c and consider reduction or d/c of concomitant chemotherapy or immunosuppressive therapy. HBV reactivation with fulminant hepatitis, hepatic failure and death reported; d/c if viral hepatitis develops. Additional serious viral infections, either new, reactivated, or exacerbated, reported. Hypersensitivity reactions may respond to infusion rate adjustment and medical management. D/C if serious arrhythmias occur. Use caution with pre-existing cardiac conditions. Use with extreme caution in combination with cisplatin; renal failure may occur. Severe renal toxicity reported; d/c if SCr rises or oliguria occurs. Monitor CBC and platelets regularly; more frequently with cytopenias. Abdominal pain, bowel obstruction and perforation reported. **P/N:** Category C, not for use in nursing.	Fever, chills, infection, asthenia, nausea, lymphopenia, leukopenia, neutropenia, headache, abdominal pain, night sweats, rash, pruritus, pain.

†Bold entries denote special dental considerations.
BB = black box warning; **W/P** = warnings/precautions; **Contra** = contraindications; **P/N** = pregnancy category rating and nursing considerations.

NAME	FORM/ STRENGTH	DOSAGE	WARNINGS/PRECAUTIONS & CONTRAINDICATIONS	ADVERSE EFFECTS†
MONOCLONAL ANTIBODY/CD52-BLOCKER				
Alemtuzumab (Campath)	**Inj:** 30mg/mL	***Adults:* B-Cell CLL:** Administer as IV infusion over 2 hours. **Initial:** 3mg IV qd until tolerated, then increase to 10mg IV qd. Continue until tolerated, then increase to maint dose of 30mg (escalation to 30mg usually takes 3-7 days). **Maint:** 30mg/day IV 3x/week on alternate days up to 12 weeks. **Max:** 30mg single dose or 90mg/week. Refer to PI for dose modifications for neutropenia or thrombocytopenia.	**BB:** Cytopenias such as serious, including fatal, pancytopenia/marrow hypoplasia, autoimmune idiopathic thrombocytopenia, and autoimmune hemolytic anemia may occur; avoid single doses >30mg or cumulative doses >90mg/week. Serious, including fatal, infusion reactions can result; gradually escalate dose to prevent. Serious, including fatal, bacterial, viral, fungal, and protozoan infections can occur; administer prophylaxis against PCP and herpes virus infections. **W/P:** Premedicate with oral antihistamine, APAP to avoid infusion reactions. Monitor BP, hypotensive symptoms in ischemic heart disease, with antihypertensives. If serious infection occurs, withhold treatment until infection resolves. Monitor CBC, platelets weekly during therapy and CD4 counts after therapy. D/C for autoimmune or severe hematologic adverse reactions. Severe, including fatal, autoimmune anemia and thrombocytopenia, and prolonged myelosuppression reported. Hemolytic anemia, pure red cell aplasia, bone marrow aplasia, and hypoplasia reported. D/C for autoimmune cytopenias. Severe and prolonged lymphopenias with increased incidence of opportunistic infections reported. Administer PCP and herpes viral prophylaxis for a minimum of 2 months after completion or until CD4+ count is ≥200 cells/μL and monitor for CMV infection during and for at least 2 months after completion of treatment. **P/N:** Category C, not for use in nursing.	Cytopenias, infusion reactions, cytomegalovirus (CMV) and other infections, nausea, emesis, diarrhea, insomnia.
MONOCLONAL ANTIBODY/EGFR-BLOCKER				
Panitumumab (Vectibix)	**Inj:** 20mg/mL	***Adults:* Metastatic Colorectal Carcinoma:** 6mg/kg IV infusion over 60 min every 14 days. Infuse doses >1000mg over 90 min. Reduce infusion rate by 50% with mild or moderate (Grade 1 or 2) infusion reaction for duration of that infusion. Immediately and permanently d/c infusion with severe (Grade 3 or 4) infusion reactions. Withhold for dermatologic toxicities that are ≥Grade 3 or considered intolerable. If toxicity does not improve to ≤Grade 2 within 1 month, permanently d/c. If dermatologic toxicity improves to ≤Grade 2 and symptoms improve after withholding no more than 2 doses, treatment may be resumed at 50% of original dose. If toxicities recur, permanently d/c. If toxicities do not recur, subsequent doses may be increased by increments of 25% of original dose until recommended dose of 6mg/kg is reached.	**BB:** Dermatologic toxicities and severe infusion reactions reported; d/c if severe dermatologic or infusion reaction occurs. **W/P:** See Black Box Warning. Toxicity involving GI mucosa, eye, and nail reported. Pulmonary fibrosis reported; d/c with interstitial lung disease, pneumonitis, or lung infiltrates. Diarrhea may occur; incidence and severity may increase when used in combination with irinotecan. Use with leucovorin not recommended. Hypomagnesemia and hypocalcemia reported; monitor electrolytes during and for 8 weeks following therapy. Sunlight may exacerbate any skin reactions that may occur; use sunscreen and/or hats and limit sun exposure during therapy. Detection of EGFR protein expression is necessary for selection of appropriate patients. Avoid in combination with chemotherapy with or without bevacizumab. **P/N:** Category C, not for use in nursing.	Rash, hypomagnesemia, paronychia, fatigue, abdominal pain, N/V, diarrhea, constipation, erythema, acneiform dermatitis, pruritus, skin exfoliation, skin fissures, cough.

Table 23.1. PRESCRIBING INFORMATION FOR ANTINEOPLASTIC DRUGS *(cont.)*

NAME	FORM/ STRENGTH	DOSAGE	WARNINGS/PRECAUTIONS & CONTRAINDICATIONS	ADVERSE EFFECTS†
MONOCLONAL ANTIBODY/HER2-BLOCKER				
Trastuzumab (Herceptin)	**Inj:** 440mg	***Adults:* Adjuvant Treatment: During and Following Paclitaxel, Docetaxel, or Docetaxel/Carboplatin for 52 Weeks: IV infusion: Initial:** 4mg/kg over 90 min. **Maint:** 2mg/kg/week over 30 min for the first 12 weeks (paclitaxel or docetaxel) or 18 weeks (docetaxel/ carboplatin). **One Week Following the Last Weekly Dose:** 6mg/kg IV over 30-60 min q3 weeks. **Following Completion of Multimodality, Anthracycline-based Regimens: Initial:** 8mg/kg IV over 90 min. **Maint:** 6mg/kg over 30 min q3 weeks. **Metastatic Breast Cancer: IV Infusion: Alone or With Paclitaxel: Initial:** 4mg/kg over 90 min. **Maint:** 2mg/kg/week over 30 min until disease progression.	**BB:** May result in cardiac failure manifesting as CHF and decreased left ventricular ejection fraction (LVEF). Increased incidence/severity of left ventricular cardiac dysfunction in combination with anthracycline-containing regimens. Evaluate LVEF prior to and during therapy; d/c with significant decrease in left ventricular function or cardiomyopathy. Serious infusion reactions and pulmonary toxicity may result. Interrupt infusion if dyspnea or clinically significant hypotension develops. D/C with anaphylaxis, angioedema, interstitial pneumonitis, or acute respiratory distress syndrome. **W/P:** Left ventricular cardiac dysfunction, arrhythmias, HTN, disabling cardiac failure, cardiomyopathy, and cardiac death may occur. Obtain baseline cardiac assessment (eg, history, physical, LVEF). Monitor LVEF prior to initiation, every 3 months during, and every 6 months following completion for at least 2 yrs. Fatal pulmonary toxicity may result. May exacerbate chemotherapy-induced neutropenia. HER2 testing is necessary to detect HER2 protein overexpression, which is needed to select patients for trastuzumab therapy. May increase risk of neutropenia. May cause severe infusion reactions; interrupt infusion and d/c permanently. **P/N:** Category D, caution in nursing.	Pain, asthenia, fever, N/V, chills, headache, increased cough, diarrhea, abdominal pain, back pain, dyspnea, infection, rash, tachycardia, anemia, peripheral edema.
MULTIKINASE INHIBITORS				
Sorafenib (Nexavar)	**Tab:** 200mg	***Adults:* RCC or Hepatocellular Carcinoma:** 400mg bid without food (1 hr before or 2 hrs after eating). Continue until no clinical benefit or unacceptable toxicity. Temporary interruption or dose reduction to 400mg qd or qod may be necessary if serious adverse events suspected.	**W/P:** Risk of ischemia and/or infarction occured; temporary or permanent d/c may be necessary. Increased risk of bleeding may occur; consider d/c if bleeding necessitates medical intervention. HTN reported; monitor BP weekly during first 6 weeks and periodically thereafter. Hand-foot skin reaction and rash may occur; may require topical treatment, temporary treatment interruption, dose modification, or permanent d/c. D/C if GI perforation occurs. Temporary interruption of therapy recommended when undergoing surgical procedures. May cause fetal harm; women of childbearing potential should avoid becoming pregnant during therapy. Hepatic impairment may reduce plasma levels. Caution when co-administered with docetaxel and doxorubicin. **P/N:** Category D, not for use in nursing.	HTN, fatigue, weight loss, rash/desquamation, hand-foot skin reaction, alopecia, pruritus, diarrhea, N/V, anorexia, constipation, hemorrhage, dyspnea, abdominal pain, liver dysfunction, cardiac ischemia.
Sunitinib Malate (Sutent)	**Cap:** 12.5mg, 25mg, 50mg	***Adults:* GIST or RCC:** 50mg once daily; 4 weeks on, 2 weeks off. Dose increase/ reduction in 12.5mg increments is recommended. **Concomitant Strong CYP3A4 Inhibitors:** Consider dose reduction to minimum of 37.5mg	**W/P:** Cases of decreased left ventricular ejection fraction (LVEF) reported. Patients with cardiac risk factors should be carefully monitored for signs and symptoms of CHF; baseline and periodic evaluation of LVEF should be considered.	Fatigue, asthenia, diarrhea, NV, **mucositis/stomatitis,** dyspepsia, abdominal pain, HTN, rash,

†Bold entries denote special dental considerations.
BB = black box warning; **W/P** = warnings/precautions; **Contra** = contraindications; **P/N** = pregnancy category rating and nursing considerations.

NAME	FORM/ STRENGTH	DOSAGE	WARNINGS/PRECAUTIONS & CONTRAINDICATIONS	ADVERSE EFFECTS†
Sunitinib Malate (Sutent) *(cont.)*		daily. **Concomitant CYP3A4 Inducer:** Consider dose increase to maximum of 87.5mg daily.	D/C if clinical manifestations of CHF occur. Prolongation of QT interval and torsade de pointes observed; consider monitoring ECG and electrolytes (magnesium, potassium). Cases of hemorrhagic events reported. Serious, sometimes fatal GI complications including GI perforation have occurred with intra-abdominal malignancies. Cases of HTN reported; monitor for HTN and treat as needed with standard antihypertensive therapy. Temporary suspension recommended if severe HTN occurs. Adrenal toxicity reported; monitor for adrenal insufficiency with stress, trauma, or severe infection. Myelosuppression, hypothyroidism, increases in serum lipase/amylase, and pancreatitis reported. Monitor CBCs, platelet count, thyroid function, and serum chemistries beginning each treatment cycle. May cause fetal harm; avoid pregnancy. **P/N:** Category D, not for use in nursing.	hand-foot syndrome, skin discoloration, **altered taste,** anorexia, bleeding.
NITROGEN MUSTARD ALKYLATING AGENTS				
Chlorambucil (Leukeran)	**Tab:** 2mg	***Adults:*** **Usual:** 0.1-0.2mg/kg qd for 3-6 weeks. Adjust according to response; reduce with abrupt WBC decline. **Lymphocytic Infiltration of Bone Marrow/Hypoplastic Bone Marrow: Max:** 0.1mg/kg/day. Caution within 4 weeks of full course of radiation or chemotherapy.	**BB:** Risk of severe bone marrow suppression. Potentially carcinogenic, mutagenic, and teratogenic. Produces human infertility. **W/P:** Convulsions, infertility, leukemia and secondary malignancies observed. Shown to cause chromatid or chromosome damage and sterility. Skin rash progressing to erythema multiforme, toxic epidermal necrolysis, or Stevens-Johnson syndrome reported. Avoid becoming pregnant. Lymphopenia reported, usually returns to normal upon completion. Monitor Hgb, leukocyte count and differential, platelet counts weekly. Avoid live vaccines in the immunocompromised. **Contra:** Prior resistance to therapy. **P/N:** Category D, not for use in nursing.	Bone marrow suppression, N/V, diarrhea, tremors, muscular twitching, confusion, agitation, ataxia, urticaria, angioneurotic syndrome, pulmonary fibrosis, hepatotoxicity, jaundice.
Cyclophosphamide (Cytoxan)	**Inj (Lyophilized):** 500mg, 1g, 2g; **Tab:** 25mg, 50mg	***Adults:*** **Malignant Diseases (Without Hematologic Deficiency): Monotherapy: Initial:** 40-50mg/kg IV in divided doses over 2-5 days, or 10-15mg/kg IV given every 7-10 days, or 3-5mg/kg twice weekly. **Oral Dosing: Initial/Maint:** 1-5mg/kg/day PO. Adjust dose according to antitumor activity and/or leukopenia. May need to reduce dose when combined with other cytotoxic drugs. ***Pediatrics:*** **Malignant Diseases (Without Hematologic Deficiency): Monotherapy: Initial:** 40-50mg/kg IV in divided doses over 2-5 days, or 10-15mg/kg IV given every 7-10 days, or 3-5mg/kg twice weekly. **Oral Dosing: Initial/Maint:** 1-5mg/kg/day PO. Adjust dose according to antitumor activity and/or leukopenia. May need to reduce dose when combined with other cytotoxic drugs. **Nephrotic Syndrome:** 2.5-3mg/kg/day PO for 60-90 days.	**W/P:** Second malignancies, cardiac dysfunction, and hemorrhagic cystitis reported. May cause fetal harm in pregnancy. Serious, fatal infections may develop if severely immunosuppressed. Monitor for toxicity with leukopenia, thrombocytopenia, tumor cell infiltration of bone marrow, previous x-ray therapy or cytotoxic therapy, and impaired hepatic and/or renal function. Monitor hematologic profile for hematopoietic suppression. Examine urine for RBCs. Anaphylactic reactions reported. Possible cross-sensitivity with other alkylating agents. May cause sterility. May interfere with normal wound healing. Consider dose adjustment with adrenalectomy. **Contra:** Severely depressed bone marrow function. **P/N:** Category D, not for use in nursing.	Impairment of fertility, amenorrhea, N/V, anorexia, abdominal discomfort, diarrhea, alopecia, leukopenia, thrombocytopenia, hemorrhagic ureteritis, interstitial pneumonitis, malaise, asthenia, renal tubular necrosis.

Table 23.1. PRESCRIBING INFORMATION FOR ANTINEOPLASTIC DRUGS *(cont.)*

NAME	FORM/ STRENGTH	DOSAGE	WARNINGS/PRECAUTIONS & CONTRAINDICATIONS	ADVERSE EFFECTS†
NITROGEN MUSTARD ALKYLATING AGENTS *(cont.)*				
Melphalan HCl (Alkeran)	**Inj:** 50mg; **Tab:** 2mg	***Adults:*** (Inj) **Usual:** 16mg/m² IV at 2-week intervals for 4 doses. After recover from toxicity, resume at 4-week intervals. **Renal Impairment (BUN ≥30mg/dL):** Reduce dose up to 50%. (Tab) **Multiple Myeloma:** 6mg qd. Adjust weekly based on blood counts. After 2-3 weeks, d/c for up to 4 weeks and monitor blood counts. **Maint:** 2mg qd. **Epithelial Ovarian Cancer:** 0.2mg/kg qd for 5 days. Repeat every 4-5 weeks depending on hematologic tolerance.	**BB:** Severe bone marrow suppression resulting in bleeding or infection may occur. Potentially mutagenic and leukemogenic. **W/P:** Marked bone marrow suppression with excessive doses. Monitor platelets, Hgb, WBCs, and differential before therapy and each dose. Use blood counts for dosing to avoid toxicity. Do not readminister if hypersensitivity occurs. Secondary malignancies reported. Ovary function suppression (eg, amenorrhea) may occur in premenopausal women. Reversible and irreversible testicular suppression reported. Extreme caution with compromised bone marrow reserve or if marrow function recovering from previous cytotoxic therapy. Caution in renal dysfunction; reduce IV dose. (Tab) If leukocytes <3000 cells/mcL or platelets <100,000 cells/mcL; d/c until peripheral blood counts recover. Avoid live vaccines in the immunocompromised. **Contra:** Prior resistance to agent. **P/N:** Category D, not for use in nursing.	Bone marrow suppression, alopecia, hemolytic anemia, pulmonary fibrosis, interstitial pneumonitis, GI reactions (eg, N/V, diarrhea, **oral ulceration**), hepatic disorders (eg, abnormal LFTs, hepatitis, jaundice). (Inj) Hypersensitivity reactions (eg, urticaria, pruritus, edema, tachycardia).
NITROSOUREA ALKYLATING AGENTS				
Carmustine (BiCNU)	**Inj:** 100mg	***Adults:*** **Single Agent in Untreated Patients:** 150-200mg/m² IV every 6 weeks, as a single dose or divide into daily injections (75-100mg/m² for 2 days). Adjust subsequent doses according to hematologic response. If leukocytes 2000-2999 and platelets 25,000-74,999, give 70% of dose. If leukocytes <2000 and platelets <25,000, then give 50% of dose.	**BB:** Bone marrow suppression, thrombocytopenia, leukopenia reported. Monitor blood counts weekly for at least 6 weeks after dose. Base dose adjustments on nadir blood counts from prior dose. Pulmonary toxicity may be dose related (>1400 mg/m² at greater risk) and can occur years after treatment. Administer only under supervision of a physician experienced in the use of antineoplastic agents. **W/P:** Long-term use may be associated with secondary malignancies. Monitor hepatic/renal function. Conduct baseline and periodic pulmonary function tests during treatment. Caution in elderly; monitor renal function. **P/N:** Category D, not for use in nursing.	Delayed myelosuppression, pulmonary infiltrates/fibrosis, N/V, hepatic toxicity, azotemia, renal failure, neuroretinitis, chest pain, headache, allergic reaction, hypotension, tachycardia.
Lomustine (CeeNU)	**Cap:** 10mg, 40mg, 100mg	***Adults/Pediatrics:*** **Single Regimen/ Previously Untreated:** 130mg/m² PO single dose every 6 weeks. **Compromised Bone Marrow:** 100mg/m² PO single dose every 6 weeks. **Subsequent Doses:** Adjust according to hematologic response. **Leukocytes 2000-2999, platelets 25,000-74,999:** Give 70% of dose. **Leukocytes <2000, platelets <25,000:** Give 50% of dose.	**BB:** Bone-marrow suppression (eg, thrombocytopenia, leukopenia) may contribute to bleeding and infections in compromised patients. Monitor blood counts weekly for 6 weeks after each dose. Adjust dose based on nadir blood counts from prior dose. **W/P:** Pulmonary toxicity is dose-related. May develop secondary malignancies with long-term use. Monitor hepatic and renal function. Caution in elderly. **P/N:** Category D, not for use in nursing.	Delayed myleosuppression, pulmonary infiltrates/fibrosis, N/V, hepatotoxicity, azotemia, renal failure, **stomatitis,** alopecia, optic atrophy, visual disturbances, lethargy, ataxia.
NITROSOUREA ONCOLYTIC AGENT				
Polifeprosan 20 with Carmustine Implant (Gliadel Wafer)	**Implant Wafers:** 7.7mg [8[s]]	***Adults:*** **Glioblastoma Multiforme or Malignant Glioma:** Place 8 wafers in resection cavity if size and shape allows; if not, place maximum number of wafers allowed. **Max:** 8 wafers per surgical procedure.	**W/P:** Avoid communication between the surgical resection cavity and ventricular system. May cause CT and MRI enhancement due to edema and inflammation. Monitor closely for known complications of craniotomy. May cause fetal harm. Risk of possible cyst formation. **P/N:** Category D, not for use in nursing.	Fever, pain, abnormal healing, N/V, brain edema, confusion, somnolence, UTI, seizures, headache, intracranial infection.

†Bold entries denote special dental considerations.
BB = black box warning; **W/P** = warnings/precautions; **Contra** = contraindications; **P/N** = pregnancy category rating and nursing considerations.

NAME	FORM/ STRENGTH	DOSAGE	WARNINGS/PRECAUTIONS & CONTRAINDICATIONS	ADVERSE EFFECTS†
NONSTEROIDAL ANTIANDROGENS				
Bicalutamide (Casodex)	**Tab:** 50mg	***Adults:*** **Prostate Cancer:** 50mg qd at the same time each day. Initiate with LHRH analogue therapy.	**W/P:** Rare cases of death or hospitalization due to severe liver injury reported. Hepatitis and marked increases in liver enzymes leading to drug discontinuation have occurred. Caution with moderate-severe hepatic impairment; serum transaminase levels should be measured prior to starting treatment, at regular intervals for 1st four months, then periodically. Monitor PSA regularly to assess therapy. For patients who have objective progression of disease together with elevated PSA, a treatment-free period of antiandrogen, while continuing LHRH analogue, may be considered. Gynecomastia, breast pain reported with single agent. **Contra:** Women, pregnancy. **P/N:** Category X, caution in nursing.	Hot flushes, pain, back pain, asthenia, constipation, pelvic pain, infection, nausea, dyspnea, peripheral edema, diarrhea, hematuria, nocturia.
Flutamide	**Cap:** 125mg	***Adults:*** **Prostate Cancer:** 250mg q8h. **Max:** 750mg/day.	**BB:** Hepatic injury reported; d/c if jaundice occurs or if ALT >2x ULN. Monitor LFTs monthly for first 4 months and periodically thereafter. **W/P:** Monitor PSA regularly. Not for use in women. If disease progression is evident, d/c therapy and continue LHRH agonist. Monitor methemoglobin levels in G6PD deficiency, hemoglobin M disease, or smokers. **Contra:** Severe hepatic impairment. **P/N:** Category D, safety in nursing is not known.	Hot flashes, loss of libido, impotence, diarrhea, N/V, gynecomastia, other GI disturbances, anemia, edema, hepatitis, jaundice, skin rash.
Nilutamide (Nilandron)	**Tab:** 150mg	***Adults:*** **Prostate Cancer: Initial:** 300mg/day for 30 days. **Maint:** 150mg qd. Begin on the same day or the day after surgical castration.	**BB:** Interstitial pneumonitis reported. Perform routine chest X-ray and baseline pulmonary function test before therapy. D/C if symptoms occur. **W/P:** Hepatotoxicity, aplastic anemia reported. D/C if develop jaundice or ALT >2x ULN. Delay in adaptation to dark; caution with driving at night or in tunnels; wear tinted glasses to alleviate effect. Evaluate baseline hepatic enzymes before therapy, at regular intervals for 1st 4 months, and periodically thereafter. **Contra:** Severe hepatic impairment, respiratory insufficiency. **P/N:** Category C, safety in nursing not known	Hot flushes, decreased libido, abnormal vision, increased LFTs, dyspnea, GI effects, dry skin, sweating, dizziness, HTN, anemia, testicular atrophy, gynecomastia.
NONSTEROIDAL AROMATASE INHIBITOR				
Letrozole (Femara)	**Tab:** 2.5mg	***Adults:*** **Breast Cancer:** 2.5mg qd. Continue until tumor progression is evident. **Cirrhosis/Severe Liver Dysfunction:** 2.5mg qod.	**W/P:** May cause fetal harm in pregnancy. May elevate LFTs and total cholesterol. May decrease bone density; monitor bone mineral density. Reduce dose in cirrhosis and severe liver dysfunction. May cause fatigue and dizziness; caution when driving or using machinery. **Contra:** Women of premenopausal endocrine status. **P/N:** Category D, caution in nursing.	Bone pain, back pain, N/V, arthralgia, dyspnea, fatigue, chest pain, decreased weight, hot flushes, peripheral edema, HTN, constipation, diarrhea, musculoskeletal pain, insomnia, cough, alopecia.
NONSTEROIDAL TRIPHENYLETHYLENE DERIVATIVE				
Toremifene Citrate (Fareston)	**Tab:** 60mg	***Adults:*** **Breast Cancer: Usual:** 60mg qd. Treat until disease progression is evident.	**W/P:** Hypercalcemia and tumor flare reported with bone metastases. Endometrial hyperplasia reported. Avoid with history of thromboembolic diseases. Do not treat long-term in pre-existing endometrial hyperplasia. Leukopenia	Hot flashes, sweating, N/V, vaginal discharge, dizziness, edema, vaginal bleeding, cataracts, dry eyes, abnormal

Table 23.1. PRESCRIBING INFORMATION FOR ANTINEOPLASTIC DRUGS *(cont.)*

NAME	FORM/ STRENGTH	DOSAGE	WARNINGS/PRECAUTIONS & CONTRAINDICATIONS	ADVERSE EFFECTS†
NONSTEROIDAL TRIPHENYLETHYLENE DERIVATIVE *(cont.)*				
Toremifene Citrate (Fareston) *(cont.)*			and thrombocytopenia reported (rarely). May cause fetal harm with pregnancy. **P/N:** Category D, safety in nursing not known.	visual fields, elevated LFTs.
NUCLEOSIDE ANALOGUE ANTIMETABOLITE				
Gemcitabine HCl (Gemzar)	**Inj:** 200mg, 1g	***Adults:*** **Pancreatic Cancer:** 1000mg/m² IV weekly up to 7 weeks, then 1 week off. Give subsequent cycles as weekly infusions for 3 out of every 4 weeks. **Lung Cancer: 4-Week Cycle:** 1000mg/m² IV on Days 1, 8, and 15 of each 28-day cycle. Give cisplatin 100mg/m² IV on Day 1 after gemcitabine infusion. **3-Week Cycle:** 1250mg/m² on Days 1 and 8 of each 21-day cycle. Give cisplatin 100mg/m² IV on Day 1 after gemcitabine infusion. **Breast Cancer:** 1250mg/m² IV on Days 1 and 8 of each 21-day cycle. Give paclitaxel 175mg/m² IV on Day 1 before gemcitabine. **Ovarian Cancer:** 1000mg/m² IV on Days 1 and 8 of each 21-day cycle. Give carboplatin AUC 4 on Day 1 after gemcitabine. Adjust dose based on hematologic toxicity. Infuse IV over 30 min.	**W/P:** Increased toxicity with infusion time >60 min and more than once weekly dosing. Hemolytic-uremic syndrome, hepatotoxicity, pulmonary toxicity, renal failure, leukopenia, thrombocytopenia, and anemia reported. Myelosuppression is dose-limiting toxicity. D/C if severe lung toxicity occurs. Caution with significant renal or hepatic impairment. Pattern of tissue injury typically associated with radiation toxicity reported with concurrent and nonconcurrent use. Greater tendency for older women not to proceed to next cycle and to experience Grade 3/4 neutropenia and thrombocytopenia. Perform CBC, differential, and platelets before each dose. Decreased clearance in women and elderly. **P/N:** Category D, not for use in nursing.	Myelosuppression, N/V, diarrhea, **stomatitis,** elevated serum transaminases, proteinuria, hematuria, fever, rash, dyspnea, edema, flu syndrome, infection, alopecia, paresthesia.
ORGANOPLATINUM COMPLEX				
Oxaliplatin (Eloxatin)	**Inj:** 50mg, 100mg, 200mg	***Adults:*** **Advanced Colorectal Cancer: Day 1:** 85mg/m² IV with LV 200mg/m²; give over 120 min in separate bags using a Y-line; followed by 5-FU 400mg/m² bolus over 2-4 min, then 5-FU 600mg/m² as a 22 hr infusion. **Day 2:** LV 200mg/m² over 120 min; followed by 5-FU 400mg/m² bolus over 2-4 min, then 5-FU 600mg/m² as a 22 hr infusion. Repeat cycle every 2 weeks. **Persistent Grade 2 Neurosensory Events:** Reduce oxaliplatin to 65mg/m². **Grade 3 Neurosensory Events:** Consider d/c. **After Recovery From Grade 3/4 GI or Grade 4 Hematologic Toxicity:** Reduce oxaliplatin to 65mg/m² and 5-FU by 20%. **Adjuvant Therapy Stage III Colon Cancer:** Recommended cycle every 2 weeks for 6 months. **Persistent Grade 2 Neurosensory Events:** Reduce oxaliplatin to 75mg/m². **Persistent Grade 3 Neurosensory Events:** Consider d/c. **After Recovery From Grade 3/4 GI or Grade 3/4 Hematologic Toxicity:** Reduce oxaliplatin to 75mg/m² and 5-FU to 300mg/m² bolus and 500mg/m² 22 hr infusion.	**BB:** Anaphylactic-like reactions may occur within minutes of administration. **W/P:** Acute and persistent neuropathy reported. Cold may exacerbate acute neurological symptoms; avoid ice for mucositis prophylaxis. Potentially fatal pulmonary fibrosis reported. If unexplained respiratory symptoms develop, d/c until interstitial lung disease or pulmonary fibrosis is ruled out. Monitor WBC with differential, Hgb, platelets, and blood chemistries (including ALT, AST, bilirubin, creatinine) before each cycle. Caution with renal impairment. **Contra:** Hypersensitivity to platinum compounds. **P/N:** Category D, not for use in nursing.	Neuropathy, fatigue, nausea, neutropenia, emesis, diarrhea.
PLATINUM COORDINATION COMPOUND				
Carboplatin‡	**Inj:** 10mg/mL	***Adults:*** **Monotherapy:** 360mg/m² IV on Day 1 every 4 weeks. **Concomitant Cyclophosphamide:** 300mg/m² IV on Day 1 every 4 weeks for 6 cycles, with cyclophosphamide 600mg/m² IV on Day 1 every 4 weeks for 6 cycles. **Platelets >100,000 or Neutrophils**	**BB:** Bone marrow suppression, resulting in infection or bleeding reported. Anemia and anaphylactic-like reactions reported. **W/P:** Bone marrow suppression is dose-dependent and is the dose-limiting toxicity. May need transfusion for anemia. Bone marrow suppression increased	Blood dyscrasias, infection, bleeding, N/V, peripheral neuropathies, ototoxicity, central neurotoxicity, elevated LFTs/bilirubin/SCr,

*Scored. †Bold entries denote special dental considerations.
‡Used as single or combination agent for head and neck cancer.
BB = black box warning; **W/P** = warnings/precautions; **Contra** = contraindications; **P/N** = pregnancy category rating and nursing considerations.

NAME	FORM/ STRENGTH	DOSAGE	WARNINGS/PRECAUTIONS & CONTRAINDICATIONS	ADVERSE EFFECTS†
Carboplatin *(cont.)*		**>2000:** Give 125% of dose. **Platelets <50,000 or Neutrophils <500:** Give 75% of dose. **Renal Impairment: Initial: CrCl 41-59mL/min:** 250mg/m². **CrCl 16-40mL/min:** 200mg/m². Subsequent dose adjustments based on the degree of bone marrow suppression.	in patients who received prior therapy. Neurotoxicity increased if ≥65 yrs and previous cisplatin treatment. LFT abnormalities and temporary loss of vision with high doses. Emesis reported. **Contra:** Severe bone marrow depression, significant bleeding. History of severe allergic reactions to cisplatin, platinum-containing compounds, or mannitol. **P/N:** Category D, not for use in nursing.	electrolyte loss, allergic reactions, alopecia, mucositis.
PODOPHYLLOTOXIN DERIVATIVES				
Etoposide (Etopophos, VePesid)	**Cap:** 50mg; **Inj:** (Etopophos) 100mg, (VePesid) 20mg/mL	***Adults:*** (Inj) **Testicular Cancer: Range:** 50-100mg/m²/day IV on Days 1-5 to 100mg/m²/day on Days 1, 3, and 5. **SCLC: Range:** 35mg/m²/day IV for 4 days to 50mg/m²/day for 5 days. After adequate recovery from toxicity, repeat course for either therapy at 3-4 week intervals. (PO) **SCLC:** 2x the IV dose and round to nearest 50mg. **Renal Impairment: CrCl 15-50mL/min:** Use 75% of dose.	**BB:** Administer under supervision of qualified physician experienced in use of cancer chemotherapeutic agents. Severe myelosuppression with resulting infection or bleeding may occur. **W/P:** Observe for myelosuppression during and after therapy. Risk of anaphylactic reaction manifested by chills, fever, tachycardia, bronchospasm, dyspnea, and hypotension. Perform CBC before each dose, during, and after therapy. May cause fetal harm in pregnancy. Caution with low serum albumin. **P/N:** Category D, not for use in nursing.	Myelosuppression, leukopenia, thrombocytopenia, anemia, N/V, **stomatitis,** anaphylactic-like reactions, hypotension (after rapid IV use), alopecia, anorexia.
PROGESTERONE				
Megestrol Acetate	**Sus:** 40mg/mL [240mL]; **Tab:** 20mg*, 40mg*	***Adults:*** (Tab) **Breast Carcinoma:** 40mg qid for a minimum of 2 months. **Endometrial Carcinoma:** 40-320mg/day in divided doses for a minimum of 2 months. **Elderly:** Start at lower end of dosing range. (Sus) 400-800mg/day (10-20mL/day); shake well.	**W/P:** May cause fetal harm; avoid in pregnancy. May cause adrenal suppression; monitor for Cushing's syndrome or new onset/exacerbation of DM. Risk of adrenal suppression if taking or withdrawing from chronic therapy; monitor for hypotension, N/V, dizziness, weakness. Caution with history of thromboembolic diseases. **Contra:** Known or suspected pregnancy. **P/N:** Category D, not for use in nursing.	Heart failure, N/V, edema, break-through menstrual bleeding, dyspnea, glucose intolerance, alopecia, HTN, carpal tunnel syndrome, mood changes, hot flashes, malaise, weight gain.
PROGESTOGEN				
Medroxyprogesterone Acetate (Depo-Provera)	**Inj:** 400mg/mL [2.5mL]	***Adults:*** **Endometrial or Renal Carcinoma: Initial:** 400-1000mg IM weekly. **Maint:** 400mg/month if disease stabilizes and/or improves within a few weeks or months.	**W/P:** Avoid during first 4 months of pregnancy. May cause thromboembolic disorders, ocular disorders, fluid retention. Caution with depression, family history of breast cancer or patients with breast nodules. May mask the onset of climacteric. **Contra:** Pregnancy, undiagnosed vaginal bleeding, breast malignancy, thrombophlebitis, thromboembolic disorders, cerebral vascular disease, liver dysfunction. **P/N:** Safety in pregnancy and nursing not known.	Menstrual irregularities, nervousness, dizziness, edema, wt changes, cervical changes, cholestatic jaundice, breast tenderness, galactorrhea, rash, acne, alopecia, hirsutism, depression, pyrexia, fatigue, insomnia, nausea.
PROTEASOME INHIBITOR				
Bortezomib (Velcade)	**Inj:** 3.5mg	***Adults:*** **Multiple Myeloma or Mantle Cell Lymphoma: Initial:** 1.3mg/m²/dose IV bolus twice weekly for 2 weeks (Days 1, 4, 8, and 11) followed by a 10-day rest period (Days 12-21). At least 72 hrs should elapse between consecutive doses. **Grade 3 Non-Hematological/Grade 4 Hematological Toxicities (excluding neuropathy):** Withhold therapy until symptoms of toxcitiy resolve. Reinitiate at 25% reduced dose. **Peripheral Neuropathy:**	**W/P:** Avoid pregnancy. May cause or worsen peripheral neuropathy along with reports of severe sensory and motor peripheral neuropathy. Thrombocytopenia and neutropenia reported; monitor CBC and platelets frequently. May cause orthostatic/postural hypotension; caution with history of syncope or dehydration. May cause acute development or exacerbation of CHF and/or new onset of decreased left ventricular ejection fraction. Rare reports of acute diffuse in-	Asthenic disorders, diarrhea, N/V, constipation, peripheral neuropathy, pyrexia, thrombocytopenia, psychiatric disorders, anorexia/decreased appetite, paresthesia/dysesthesia, anemia, headache, cough, dyspnea.

Table 23.1. PRESCRIBING INFORMATION FOR ANTINEOPLASTIC DRUGS *(cont.)*

NAME	FORM/ STRENGTH	DOSAGE	WARNINGS/PRECAUTIONS & CONTRAINDICATIONS	ADVERSE EFFECTS†
PROTEASOME INHIBITOR *(cont.)*				
Bortezomib (Velcade) *(cont.)*		**Grade 1 with pain or Grade 2 (interfering with function but not activities of daily living):** Reduce dose to 1mg/m². **Grade 2 with pain or Grade 3 (interfering with activities of daily living):** Withhold dose until toxicity resolves. Reinitiate at 0.7mg/m² once weekly. **Grade 4 (permanent sensory loss interfering with function):** D/C therapy.	filtrative pulmonary disease of unknown etiology such as pneumonitis, interstitial pneumonia, lung infiltration and ARDS. May cause N/V, diarrhea, constipation; use of antiemetic and antidiarrheal medications may be necessary. Rare reports of Reversible Posterior Leukoencephalopathy syndrome. May cause tumor lysis syndrome. Hepatic impairment may decrease clearance. Closely monitor if CrCl <13mL/min or on hemodialysis. Patients on oral antidiabetic agents may require close monitoring of blood glucose levels. Monitor CBC frequently. Dosing adjustments not necessary for patients with renal impairment. Should be administered after dialysis procedure. **Contra:** Hypersensitivity to boron or mannitol. **P/N:** Category D, not for use in nursing.	
PROTEIN SYNTHESIS INHIBITOR				
Pegaspargase (Oncaspar)	**Inj:** 750 IU/mL [5mL]	***Adults:* ALL: Usual:** 2500 IU/m² IM or IV every 14 days. ***Pediatrics:* 1-9 yrs:** 2500 IU/m² IM on Day 3 of 4-Week induction phase and on Day 3 of each of two 8-Week delayed intensification phases.	**W/P:** May be a contact irritant. Avoid inhalation or contact with skin or mucous membranes. Serious allergic reaction, pancreatitis, or glucose intolerance can occur. Increased prothrombin time, partial thromboplastin time, and hypofibrinogenemia can occur; monitor coagulation parameters. May predispose to infections, bleeding, thrombosis. D/C in patients with serious thrombotic events including sagittal sinus thrombosis. **Contra:** Pancreatitis. History of pancreatitis, significant hemorrhagic events, or serious thrombosis with prior L-asparaginase therapy. **P/N:** Category C, not for use in nursing.	Allergic reactions (including anaphylaxis), CNS thrombosis, coagulopathy, elevated transaminases, hyperbilirubinemia, hyperglycemia, pancreatitis.
PROTEIN-TYROSINE KINASE INHIBITOR				
Imatinib Mesylate (Gleevec)	**Tab:** 100mg, 400mg	***Adults:* CML: Chronic Phase:** 400mg/d, may increase to 600mg qd. **Accelerated Phase/Blast Crisis:** 600mg/d, may increase to 400mg bid. **Relapsed/ Refractory Ph+ ALL:** 600mg/d. **MDS or MPD/ASM/HES and/or CEL:** 400mg/d. **ASM with eosinophilia/HES or CEL with FIP1L1-PDGFRα: Initial:** 100mg/d. **Titrate:** May increase up to 400mg/d in the absence of adverse reactions and insufficient response. **DFSP:** 800mg/d. **GIST (unresectable or metastatic/malignant):** 400mg/d. **Titrate:** May increase up to 800mg (as 400mg bid) if clear signs/symptoms of disease progression and in the absence of adverse reactions. **Severe Hepatic Impairment:** Reduce dose by 25%. **Co-administration with Strong CYP3A4 Inducers:** Increase dose by at least 50% and monitor carefully. **Hepatotoxicity/Non-Hematologic Adverse Reaction:** If bilirubin >3x ULN or transaminases >5x ULN,	**W/P:** Fluid retention/edema (eg, pleural effusion, pericardial effusion, pulmonary edema, ascites) reported; monitor weight. Anemia/neutropenia/ thrombocytopenia reported; monitor CBC weekly during 1st month, biweekly during 2nd month, and periodically thereafter. In pediatric patients, the most frequent toxicities observed were grade 3 and 4 cytopenias. May be hepatotoxic; monitor LFTs at baseline, then monthly or as needed. Avoid becoming pregnant. Interrupt treatment if severe non-hematologic adverse reaction develops (eg, severe hepatotoxicity, severe fluid retention); resume if appropriate. GI bleeds reported. Severe CHF and left ventricular dysfunction. Hypereosinophilic cardiac toxicity. Stevens-Johnson syndrome reported. Hypothyroidism reported; monitor thyroid stimulating hormone (TSH) levels. **P/N:** Category D, not for nursing.	N/V, fluid retention, neutropenia, thrombocytopenia, diarrhea, hemorrhage, pyrexia, rash, headache, fatigue, abdominal pain, elevated transaminases or bilirubin, edema, muscle cramps, musculoskeletal pain, flatulence, nasopharyngitis, insomnia, anemia, anorexia, rhinitis.

*Scored. †Bold entries denote special dental considerations.

BB = black box warning; **W/P** = warnings/precautions; **Contra** = contraindications; **P/N** = pregnancy category rating and nursing considerations.

NAME	FORM/ STRENGTH	DOSAGE	WARNINGS/PRECAUTIONS & CONTRAINDICATIONS	ADVERSE EFFECTS†
Imatinib Mesylate (Gleevec) *(cont.)*		hold drug until bilirubin <1.5x ULN and transaminases <2.5x ULN. Continue at reduced dose. **Neutropenia/Thrombocytopenia:** See PI for dosage adjustment. Take with food and plenty of water. ***Pediatrics:*** **CML: Newly Diagnosed:** 340mg/m²/d. **Chronic Phase:** 260mg/m²/day given qd or split into 2 doses (morning and evening). **Severe Hepatic Impairment:** Reduce dose by 25%. **Co-administration with Strong CYP3A4 Inducers:** Increase dose by at least 50% and monitor carefully. **Hepatotoxicity/Non-Hematologic Adverse Reaction:** If bilirubin >3x ULN or transaminases >5x ULN, hold drug until bilirubin <1.5x ULN and transaminases <2.5x ULN. **Continue at reduced dose. Neutropenia/Thrombocytopenia:** See PI for dosage adjustments. Take with food and plenty of water. See PI for further dosage adjustments.		
PURINE ANALOGS				
Mercaptopurine (Purinethol)	**Tab:** 50mg*	***Adults/Pediatrics:*** **ALL: Maint:** 1.5-2.5mg/kg/day as single dose. **Renal/Hepatic Impairment:** Reduce dose. **Concomitant Allopurinol:** Reduce mercaptopurine dose by 1/3-1/4 of usual dose. **TPMT Deficiency:** Consider dose reduction.	**W/P:** Risk of dose-related bone marrow suppression. Monitor weekly platelet counts, Hgb, Hct, total WBC with differential; increase frequency during induction phase. Monitor closely for life-threatening infection or bleeding. Risk of hepatotoxicity, anorexia, diarrhea, jaundice, and ascites (especially with >2.5mg/kg dose). Perform LFTs weekly initially, then monthly; monitor more frequently with hepatotoxic drugs or pre-existing liver disease. Increased sensitivity to myelosuppressive effects with thiopurine-S-methyltransferase (TPMT) gene deficiency; consider TPMT testing with evidence of severe toxicity. **Contra:** Lack of definitive diagnosis of ALL. Prior resistance to mercaptopurine or thioguanine. **P/N:** Category D, not for use in nursing.	Bone marrow toxicity, hepatotoxicity, hyperuricemia (reduce incidence by prehydration, urine alkalinization, prophylactic allopurinol), intestinal ulceration, rash, hyperpigmentation, alopecia, transient oligospermia.
Thioguanine	**Tab:** 40mg*	***Adults/Pediatrics:*** **Acute Nonlymphocytic Leukemias: Monotherapy:** 2mg/kg/day. After 4 weeks, may increase to 3mg/kg/day if no improvement and leukocyte or platelet depression. Usual therapy is with other agents in combination.	**W/P:** Dose-related bone-marrow suppression. Increased sensitivity to myelosuppression with thiopurine-S-methyltransferase (TPMT) deficiency. D/C temporarily at 1st sign of abnormally large fall in any formed elements of the blood. Withhold therapy with toxic hepatitis or biliary stasis. Monitor Hgb, Hct, platelets, WBCs, and differential frequently. Monitor LFTs weekly at start of therapy, monthly thereafter. **Contra:** Prior resistance to this drug. **P/N:** Category D, not for use in nursing.	Myelosuppression, hyperuricemia, hepatotoxicity, N/V, anorexia, **stomatitis.**
PURINE PRECURSOR ANALOG				
Dacarbazine (DTIC-Dome)	**Inj:** 200mg	***Adults:*** **Malignant Melanoma:** 2-4.5mg/kg/day for 10 days. May repeat every 4 weeks. **Alternate Dosage:** 250mg/m²/day IV for 5 days. May repeat every 3 weeks. **Hodgkin's Disease:** 150mg/m²/day for 5 days. May repeat every 4 weeks. **Alternate Dosage:** 375mg/m²/day on day 1. May repeat every 15 days.	**BB:** Hemopoietic toxicity and hepatotoxicity reported. **W/P:** Hematopoietic depression, anemia, anaphylactic reactions reported. Hepatotoxicity with hepatic vein thrombosis and hepatocellular necrosis may result in death. Extravasation may result in tissue damage and severe pain. **P/N:** Category C, safety in nursing not known.	N/V, anorexia, diarrhea, flu-like syndromes, alopecia, renal or hepatic dysfunction, rash.

Table 23.1. PRESCRIBING INFORMATION FOR ANTINEOPLASTIC DRUGS *(cont.)*

NAME	FORM/ STRENGTH	DOSAGE	WARNINGS/PRECAUTIONS & CONTRAINDICATIONS	ADVERSE EFFECTS†
PYRIMIDINE NUCLEOSIDE ANALOG				
Azacitidine (Vidaza)	**Inj:** 100mg	***Adults:* Myelodysplastic Syndromes: Initial:** 75mg/m² SQ or IV (administer over 10-40 min) daily for 7 days. Repeat cycle every 4 weeks. May increase to 100mg/m² after 2 cycles if no beneficial effect and no toxicity. Treat ≥4 cycles. Adjust dose based on hematology lab values, renal function, and serum electrolytes.	**W/P:** May cause fetal harm. Avoid pregnancy in women of childbearing potential. Neutropenia and thrombocytopenia may occur; monitor CBC periodically (at minimum, before each cycle). May cause hepatotoxicity; caution with liver disease. Renal abnormalities reported; reduce dose or hold for unexplained reductions in serum bicarbonate <20mEq/L or elevations of BUN or SrCr occur. Monitor for toxicity with renal impairment. **Contra:** Advanced malignant hepatic tumors. **P/N:** Category D, not for use in nursing.	(SQ) N/V, anemia, thrombocytopenia, pyrexia, leukopenia, diarrhea, fatigue, injection site erythema, constipation, neutropenia, ecchymosis, cough, dyspnea, weakness. (IV) Petechiae, rigors, weakness, hypokalemia.
RETINOID				
Tretinoin (Vesanoid)	**Cap:** 10mg	***Adults/Pediatrics:* ≥1 yr: Acute Promyelocytic Leukemia:** 45mg/m²/day in 2 divided doses. D/C 30 days after achieving complete remission or after 90 days of therapy, whichever occurs 1st.	**BB:** Administer under strict supervision of experienced physician and institution. Risk of retinoic acid-APL syndrome and leukocytosis. High risk of teratogenic effects. **W/P:** May cause abortion or fetal abnormalities. Females should use contraception during and 1 month after therapy. Confirm APL diagnosis. Pseudotumor cerebri reported, especially in pediatrics. Reversible hypercholesterolemia, hypertriglyceridemia reported. Elevated LFTs reported; d/c if >5x ULN. Monitor for signs of respiratory compromise or leukocytosis. Check hematologic profile, coagulation profile, LFTs, and cholesterol frequently. **Contra:** Sensitivity to parabens. **P/N:** Category D, not for use in nursing.	Malaise, shivering, hemorrhage, infections, peripheral edema, pain, chest discomfort, edema, disseminated intravascular coagulation, weight change, injection site reactions, dyspnea, pleural effusion, respiratory insufficiency, pneumonia.
RIBONUCLEOTIDE REDUCTASE INHIBITOR				
Hydroxyurea (Hydrea)	**Cap:** 500mg	***Adults:* Solid Tumors: Intermittent:** 80mg/kg single dose every 3rd day. **Continuous:** 20-30mg/kg qd. **Head and Neck Carcinoma:** 80mg/kg single dose every 3rd day. Start at least 7 days before irradiation. **Resistant CML:** 20-30mg/kg qd. **Elderly/Renal Impairment:** May need dose reduction.	**W/P:** Patients with previous irradiation therapy may have exacerbation of postirradiation erythema. Bone marrow suppression, erythrocytic abnormalities may occur. Correct severe anemia before initiating therapy. Caution with marked renal dysfunction. May develop secondary leukemia with long-term therapy for myeloproliferative disorders. Monitor CBC, bone marrow, hepatic and kidney function before therapy and repeatedly thereafter. Interrupt therapy if WBC <2500/mm³ or platelets <100,000/mm³. Cutaneous vasculitic toxicities reported (eg, vasculitic ulcerations, gangrene); d/c if cutaneous vasculitic ulcerations develop. **Contra:** Marked bone marrow depression (leukopenia, thrombocytopenia, or severe anemia). **P/N:** Category D, not for use in nursing.	Bone marrow depression (leukopenia, anemia, thrombocytopenia), GI effects (stomatitis, anorexia, N/V, diarrhea, constipation), and dermatological reactions (maculopapular rash, skin ulceration, dermatomyositis-like skin changes, peripheral and facial erythema), cutaneous vasculitic toxicities.
S-TRIAZINE DERIVATIVE				
Altretamine (Hexalen)	**Cap:** 50mg	***Adults:* Ovarian Cancer:** 260 mg/m²/day in 4 divided doses for 14 or 21 consecutive days in 28 day cycle. Take after meals and qhs. Temporarily d/c for ≥14 days and restart at 200 mg/m²/day if any of the following occur: GI intolerance unresponsive to symptomatic	**BB:** Monitor peripheral blood counts at least monthly, before each course of therapy, and as clinically indicated. Possible neurotoxicity; perform neurologic exam regularly. Administer only under supervision of a physician experienced in the use of antineoplastic agents. **W/P:**	N/V, peripheral neuropathy, CNS symptoms (mood disorders, consciousness disorders, ataxia, dizziness, vertigo),

†Bold entries denote special dental considerations.
BB = black box warning; **W/P** = warnings/precautions; **Contra** = contraindications; **P/N** = pregnancy category rating and nursing considerations.

NAME	FORM/ STRENGTH	DOSAGE	WARNINGS/PRECAUTIONS & CONTRAINDICATIONS	ADVERSE EFFECTS†
Altretamine (Hexalen) *(cont.)*		measures; WBC <2000/mm³ or granulocytes <1000/mm³; platelets <75,000/mm³; progressive neurotoxicity. Permanently d/c if neurological symptoms do not stabilize.	Can cause mild to moderate myelosuppression and neurotoxicity. Perform blood counts and neurologic exam before each course of therapy and adjust dose as indicated. **Contra:** Pre-existing severe bone marrow depression or severe neurologic toxicity. **P/N:** Category D, not for use in nursing.	leukopenia, thrombocytopenia, anemia, increased alkaline phosphatase.
SYNTHETIC GONADOTROPIN RELEASING HORMONE ANALOGS				
Goserelin Acetate (Zoladex 1-Month)	**Implant:** 3.6mg	***Adults:*** Inject SQ into anterior abdominal wall below navel line. **Advanced Prostate/Breast Cancers:** 3.6mg every 28 days. **Stage B2-C Prostate Cancer:** 3.6mg starting 8 weeks before radiotherapy then 10.8mg formulation 28 days after 1st injection or 3.6mg at 28-day intervals for 4 doses (2 before and 2 during radiotherapy). **Endometriosis:** 3.6mg every 28 days for up to 6 months. **Endometrial Thinning:** 3.6mg then surgery 4 weeks later, or 3.6mg for 2 doses (4 weeks apart) followed by surgery 2-4 weeks after 2nd dose.	**W/P:** Exclude pregnancy before initiating therapy. Premenopausal women should use nonhormonal contraception during and 12 weeks post-therapy. Worsening of symptoms of prostate and breast cancer with initial therapy. Ureteral obstruction and spinal cord compression reported with prostate cancer. Temporary increases in bone pain may occur. Ovarian cysts reported. Hypercalcemia reported in prostate and breast cancer patients with bone metastases. May increase cervical resistance. Hypersensitivity, antibody formation, and acute anaphylactic reactions may occur. **Contra:** Pregnancy, nursing. **P/N:** Category X (endometriosis and endometrial thinning), Category D (breast cancer), not for use in nursing.	(Males) Hot flashes, sexual dysfunction, decreased erections, lower urinary tract symptoms, lethargy, pain (worsened in the first 30 days), edema, URI, rash, sweating, diarrhea, nausea. (Females, Endometriosis Treatment) Hot flashes, vaginitis, emotional lability, decreased libido, sweating, depression, headache, acne, breast atrophy. (Breast Cancer Treatment) Hot flashes, tumor flare, edema, malaise/fatigue/ lethargy, N/V.
Goserelin Acetate (Zoladex 3-Month)	**Implant:** 10.8mg	***Adults:*** Inject SQ into anterior abdominal wall below navel line. **Advanced Prostate Cancer:** 10.8mg every 12 weeks. **Stage B2-C Prostate Cancer:** 3.6mg depot formulation 8 weeks before radiotherapy then 10.8mg 28 days after 1st injection.	**W/P:** Worsening of symptoms of prostate cancer with initial therapy. Ureteral obstruction and spinal cord compression reported. Temporary increase in bone pain may occur. Hypersensitivity, antibody formation, and acute anaphylactic reactions may occur. **Contra:** Pregnancy, 10.8mg implant is not indicated in women. **P/N:** Category X, not for use in nursing.	Hot flashes, sexual dysfunction, decreased erections, osteoporosis, pain, asthenia, gynecomastia.
Leuprolide Acetate (Eligard)	**Inj:** 7.5mg, 22.5mg, 30mg, 45mg	***Adults:*** 7.5mg SQ monthly, 22.5mg SQ every 3 months, 30mg SQ every 4 months, or 45mg SQ every 6 months. Rotate injection sites.	**W/P:** Transient worsening of symptoms or onset of new signs/symptoms may occur during 1st few weeks of therapy. Closely monitor patients with metastatic vertebral lesions and/or urinary tract obstruction during first few weeks of therapy. Urethral obstruction and spinal cord compression reported. Monitor serum testosterone, PSA. **Contra:** Women, pregnancy, pediatric patients. **P/N:** Category X, safety in nursing not known.	Hot flashes, pain/ burning/stinging/ erythema/bruising at injection site, malaise/fatigue, atrophy of testes, weakness, gynecomastia, myalgia, dizziness, decreased libido, rigors, lethargy, dyspepsia, scanty urination, limb pain, insomnia, breast soreness, clamminess, pituitary aplopexy, HTN.
Leuprolide Acetate (Lupron Depot, Lupron Depot 3-Month 22.5 mg, Lupron Depot 4-Month, Lupron Depot 7.5mg)	**Inj:** (1-month) 7.5mg, (3-month) 22.5mg, (4-month) 30mg	***Adults:*** 7.5mg IM as single dose monthly, 22.5mg IM single dose every 3 months, or 30mg IM single dose every 4 months. Rotate injection site.	**W/P:** Transient worsening of symptoms may occur during 1st few weeks of therapy. Closely monitor patients with metastatic vertebral lesions and/or urinary tract obstruction during 1st few weeks of therapy. Monitor serum testosterone, PSA. (7.5mg, 30mg) Temporary increase in bone pain. Ureteral obstruction and spinal cord compression	Injection site reactions, general pain, headache, hot flashes, sweating, edema, urinary disorders, dizziness/ vertigo, asthenia, GI disorders, impotence.

Table 23.1. PRESCRIBING INFORMATION FOR ANTINEOPLASTIC DRUGS *(cont.)*

NAME	FORM/ STRENGTH	DOSAGE	WARNINGS/PRECAUTIONS & CONTRAINDICATIONS	ADVERSE EFFECTS†
SYNTHETIC GONADOTROPIN RELEASING HORMONE ANALOGS *(cont.)*				
Leuprolide Acetate (Lupron Depot (Oncology), Lupron Depot 3-Month 22.5 mg, Lupron Depot 4-Month, Lupron Depot 7.5mg) *(cont.)*			reported; may initiate with SQ formulation for 1st 2 weeks to facilitate withdrawal if needed. **Contra:** Pregnancy. **P/N:** Category X, safety in nursing not known.	
Leuprolide Acetate (Lupron)	**Inj:** 5mg/mL	***Adults:*** 1mg SQ qd. Rotate injection sites.	**W/P:** Transient worsening of symptoms may occur during 1st few weeks of therapy. Closely monitor patients with metastatic vertebral lesions and/or urinary tract obstruction during 1st few weeks of therapy; may cause neurological problems or increase obstruction. Monitor serum testosterone, acid phosphatase levels. Contains benzyl alcohol. **Contra:** Pregnancy. **P/N:** Category X, not for use in nursing.	General pain, headache, hot flashes, urinary disorders, dizziness/vertigo, ECG changes/ischemia, peripheral edema, HTN, asthenia, constipation, anorexia, insomnia, myocardial infarction, diabetes, respiratory problems.
Leuprolide Acetate (Viadur)	**Implant:** 65mg	***Adults:*** Insert 1 implant SQ in upper arm every 12 months.	**W/P:** Transient worsening of symptoms may occur during 1st few weeks of therapy. Closely monitor patients with metastatic vertebral lesions and/or urinary tract obstruction during 1st few weeks of therapy. Monitor serum testosterone, PSA. Ureteral obstruction and spinal cord decompression reported. **Contra:** Women, pregnancy, pediatrics. **P/N:** Category X, safety in nursing not known.	Headache, asthenia, hot flashes, ecchymosis, peripheral edema, depression, sweating, gynecomastia, nocturia, urinary frequency, testis atrophy, breast pain, urinary retention/frquency, local bruising/ burning.
TOPOISOMERASE I INHIBITORS				
Irinotecan HCl (Camptosar)	**Inj:** 20mg/mL	***Adults:* Combination Therapy (5-FU/ LV, see PI for dosage):** 125mg/m² IV over 90 min on days 1, 8, 15, 22 for 6 weeks; or 180mg/m² IV over 90 min on days 1, 15, and 29 for 6 weeks. **Both regimens:** Begin next cycle on Day 43. **Single Therapy:** 125mg/m² IV over 90 min on days 1, 8, 15, 22 followed by a 2 week rest; or 350mg/m² IV over 90 min once every 3 weeks. Premedicate with antiemetics at least 30 min prior to therapy. Dose modifications for reduced UGT1A1 activity, neutropenia, diarrhea, and other toxicities: See PI. All dose modifications should be based on worst preceding toxicity.	**BB:** Early and/or late forms of diarrhea, severe myelosuppression may occur. Interrupt and reduce subsequent doses if severe diarrhea occurs. Carefully monitor with diarrhea; give fluid/electrolyte replacement if dehydrated or give antibiotics if ileus, fever, or severe neutropenia develops. **W/P:** Due to increased toxicity, avoid use of irinotecan with the "Mayo Clinic" regimen of 5-FU/LV (given 4-5 days every 4 weeks). Treat/prevent early diarrhea with atropine IV/SQ and late diarrhea (occurring >24 hrs after dose) with loperamide PO. If late diarrhea occurs, delay therapy until return of pretreatment bowel function for at least 24 hrs without antidiarrheals; decrease subsequent doses if late diarrhea is Grade 2, 3, or 4. Deaths due to sepsis reported following severe neutropenia. Temporarily hold therapy if neutropenic fever occurs or if neutrophils <1000/ mm³. Increased risk for neutropenia in patients homozygous for the UGT1A1 28 allele. Consider reduced initial dose. Heterozygous patients may also have increased risk. Hypersensitivity reactions, colitis, ileus, and renal impairment/ failure, thromboembolic events reported. May cause fetal harm during	N/V, diarrhea, abdominal pain, blood dyscrasias, asthenia, mucositis, anorexia, alopecia, fever, pain, constipation, infection, dyspnea, increased bilirubin.

†Bold entries denote special dental considerations.
BB = black box warning; **W/P** = warnings/precautions; **Contra** = contraindications; **P/N** = pregnancy category rating and nursing considerations.

NAME	FORM/ STRENGTH	DOSAGE	WARNINGS/PRECAUTIONS & CONTRAINDICATIONS	ADVERSE EFFECTS†
Irinotecan HCl (Camptosar) *(cont.)*			pregnancy. Monitor for extravasation at infusion site. Consider atropine for cholinergic symptoms. Caution with modestly elevated baseline bilirubin levels (eg, 1-2mg/dL), abnormal glucuronidation of bilirubin, hepatic insufficiency, elderly with comorbidities, previous pelvic/abdominal irradiation. Careful monitoring of WBC with differential, Hgb, and platelets is recommended before each dose. Avoid in severe bone marrow failure, and fructose intolerant patients. **P/N:** Category D, not for use in nursing.	
Topotecan (Hycamtin Capsules)	**Cap:** 0.25mg, 1mg	***Adults:*** 2.3mg/m²/day PO qd for 5 consecutive days repeated every 21 days. Round calculated dose to nearest 0.25mg and give minimum number of 1mg and 0.25mg caps. Do not treat with subsequent courses until neutrophils recover to >1000 cells/m³, platelets recover to >100,000 cells/mm³, and Hgb levels recover to ≥9g/dL. If severe neutropenia (neutrophils <500 cells/mm³ associated with fever or infection or lasting for ≥7 days), neutropenia (neutrophils 500-1,000 cells/mm³ lasting beyond Day 21 of treatment course), or if platelet count falls below 25,000 cells/mm³, reduce dose by 0.4mg/m²/day for subsequent courses. **Moderate Renal Impairment (CrCl 30-49mL/min):** 1.8mg/m²/day. **Severe Renal Impairment (CrCl <30mL/min):** Insufficient data. Swallow caps whole; do not chew, crush or divide. If patient vomits after taking dose, do not give replacement dose.	**BB:** Administer only to patients with baseline neutrophil counts of ≥1,500 cells/mm³ and platelet count ≥100,000 cells/mm³. Monitor blood cell counts. **W/P:** Neutropenia, pancytopenia, thrombocytopenia, and/or anemia may occur. Bone marrow suppression is dose-limiting toxicity; administer only to patients with adequate bone marrow reserves and monitor peripheral blood counts. Neutropenia may lead to neutropenia colitis. Diarrhea, including severe diarrhea requiring hospitalization, reported. **Contra:** Pregnancy, breastfeeding, severe bone marrow depression. **P/N:** Category D, contraindicated in nursing.	Anemia, leukopenia, neutropenia, thrombocytopenia, N/V, diarrhea, alopecia, fatigue, anorexia, asthenia, pyrexia.
Topotecan HCl (Hycamtin Injection)	**Inj:** 4mg	***Adults:*** **Ovarian Cancer and SCLC:** 1.5mg/m² IV qd over 30 min for 5 days, starting on Day 1 of 21-day course. Minimum of 4 courses recommended in absence of tumor progression. **Severe Neutropenia During Therapy:** Reduce dose by 0.25mg/m², or give G-CSF following subsequent course (before dose reduction) starting from Day 6 of the course (24 hrs after completion of topotecan administration). **Cervical Cancer:** 0.75mg/m² IV qd over 30 min on Days 1, 2, and 3; followed by cisplatin 50mg/m² IV on Day 1 of every 21-day course. **Severe Febrile Neutropenia (<1000 cells/mm³ & temperature of 38°C):** Reduce dose by 20% to 0.60mg/m² for subsequent courses (doses should be similarly reduced if platelet count falls below 10,000 cells/mm³) or give G-CSF following subsequent course (before dose reduction) starting from Day 4 of course (24 hrs after completion of topotecan administration); if febrile neutropenia occurs despite use of G-CSF, reduce dose by another 20% to 0.45mg/m² for subsequent courses. **Renal Impairment: CrCl 39-20mL/min:** 0.75mg/m². **CrCl <20mL/min:** Insufficient data.	**BB:** Do not give if baseline neutrophils <1500 cells/mm³. Monitor peripheral blood cell counts frequently due to risk of bone marrow suppression, primarily neutropenia. Administer only under supervision of a physician experienced in the use of antineoplastic agents. **W/P:** Bone marrow suppression (thrombocytopenia, anemia and primarily neutropenia) is dose-limiting toxicity. Baseline neutrophils ≥1500 cells/mm³ and platelets ≥100,000 cells/mm³ required. Neutrophils >1000 cells/mm³, platelets >100,000 cells/mm³, and HgB ≥9g/dL required before subsequent courses. May cause fetal harm during pregnancy. Neutropenia can lead to neutropenic colitis. **Contra:** Pregnancy, nursing, severe bone marrow depression. **P/N:** Category D, contraindicated in nursing.	Neutropenia, leukopenia, thrombocytopenia, anemia, sepsis/fever/infection, N/V, diarrhea, constipation, abdominal pain, anorexia, fatigue, pain, asthenia, alopecia.

Table 23.1. PRESCRIBING INFORMATION FOR ANTINEOPLASTIC DRUGS *(cont.)*

NAME	FORM/ STRENGTH	DOSAGE	WARNINGS/PRECAUTIONS & CONTRAINDICATIONS	ADVERSE EFFECTS†
TOPOISOMERASE II INHIBITOR				
Mitoxantrone (Novantrone)	**Inj:** 2mg/mL	***Adults:*** **Prostate Cancer:** 12-14mg/m²/day IV every 21 days. **ANLL: Induction:** 12mg/m²/day IV on days 1-3 and 100mg/m²/day IV of cytarabine on days 1-7. **Consolidation:** 12mg/m²/day on days 1-2 and cytarabine 100mg/m²/day on days 1-5. **MS:** 12mg/m²/day IV every 3 months.	**BB:** Severe local tissue damage with extravasation. Administer only as slow IV infusion; not for IM, SQ, intra-arterial, or intrathecal use. Should not be given to patients with baseline neutrophil count <1,500 cells/mm³. Cardiotoxicity can occur at any time and risk increases with cumulative dose; toxicity can occur during therapy or months to years after d/c. CHF may occur during or after termination of therapy. Secondary AML reported in MS and cancer patients treated with Novatrone. **W/P:** Can cause myelosuppression at any dose. Severe myelosuppression with high doses (leukemia); assure full hematologic recovery before consolidation therapy. Avoid with pre-existing myelosuppression. Increased risk of cardiac toxicity with prior anthracyclines or mediastinal radiotherapy, or with pre-existing cardiovascular disease. Irreversible CHF has been reported. Avoid in MS when baseline left ventricular ejection fraction <50%. Caution in hepatic impairment. Risk of hyperuricemia in leukemia; monitor serum uric acid levels. Obtain CBC, platelet count, and LFTs before each course. May cause blue-green urine and bluish sclera 24 hrs after administration. Perform pregnancy test in women with MS before each dose. Caution in elderly. **P/N:** Category D, not for use in nursing.	Nausea, alopecia, menstrual disorder, upper respiratory infection, UTI, **stomatitis,** arrhythmia, diarrhea, constipation, back pain, abnormal ECG, asthenia, headache, cardiac toxicity.
TYPE II TOPOISOMERASE INHIBITOR				
Teniposide (Vumon)	**Inj:** 10mg/mL [5mL]	***Pediatrics:*** 165mg/m² with cytarabine 300mg/m² IV twice weekly for 8-9 doses; or 250mg/m² with vincristine 1.5mg/m² IV weekly for 4-8 weeks and prednisone 40mg/m² PO for 28 days. **Down Syndrome: Initial:** Half usual dose. **Maint:** Increase based on degree of myelosuppression/mucositis.	**BB:** Cytotoxic. Severe myelosuppression, with resulting infection or bleeding, and/or hypersensitivity reactions may occur. **W/P:** Monitor CBC, hepatic and renal function before and during therapy. Avoid rapid IV infusion. May cause fetal harm. Dose-limiting bone marrow suppression. D/C if significant hypotension occurs. Hypersensitivity (HS) reactions manifested by chills, fever, urticaria, tachycardia, bronchospasm, dyspnea, HTN, and hypotension may occur. If re-treating patient with earlier HS reaction, pretreat with corticosteroid and antihistamine. Continuously observe for at least 60 minutes after starting infusion and frequently thereafter. Use gloves when handling or preparing solution. Reduce dose or d/c if severe reactions occur. **Contra:** Hypersensitivity to Cremophor EL (polyoxyethylated castor oil). **P/N:** Category D, not for use in nursing.	Myelosuppression, leukopenia, neutropenia, thrombocytopenia, anemia, mucositis, diarrhea, N/V, infection, alopecia, bleeding, hypersensitivity reactions, rash, fever.

†Bold entries denote special dental considerations.
BB = black box warning; **W/P** = warnings/precautions; **Contra** = contraindications; **P/N** = pregnancy category rating and nursing considerations.

NAME	FORM/ STRENGTH	DOSAGE	WARNINGS/PRECAUTIONS & CONTRAINDICATIONS	ADVERSE EFFECTS†
TYROSINE KINASE INHIBITOR				
Dasatinib (Sprycel)	**Tab:** 20mg, 50mg, 70mg	***Adults:*** **Chronic Phase CML:** 100mg qd. **Accelerated Phase CML/Myeloid or Lymphoid Blast Phase CML/Ph+ ALL:** 70mg bid. Swallow whole; do not crush. **Concomitant Strong CYP3A4 Inducers:** Consider dose increase. **Concomitant Strong CYP3A4 Inhibitors:** Consider dose decrease to 20mg daily. Refer to PI for dose modifications for neutropenia and thrombocytopenia.	**W/P:** Severe thrombocytopenia, neutropenia, and anemia reported; monitor CBC weekly for first 2 months, then monthly thereafter. Severe CNS hemorrhages including fatalities, GI hemorrhage, and other hemorrhage cases reported; caution in patients on medications that inhibit platelet function or anticoagulants. Pleural and pericardial effusion reported. Severe ascites, generalized edema, severe pulmonary edema reported. QT prolongation reported; caution in patients at risk (eg, hypokalemia or hypomagnesemia, congenital long QT syndrome, concomitant antiarrhythmics or other QT prolonging agents, cumulative high-dose anthracycline therapy); correct hypokalemia or hypomagnesemia prior to administration. Caution with hepatic impairment. Fetal harm may occur; avoid pregnancy. **P/N:** Category D, not for use in nursing.	Fluid retention events, diarrhea, N/V, headache, abdominal pain, bleeding events, pyrexia, pleural effusion, neutropenia, thrombocytopenia, dyspnea, anemia, skin rash, fatigue, myelosuppression, QT prolongation.
VASCULAR ENDOTHELIAL GROWTH FACTOR (VEGF) INHIBITOR				
Bevacizumab (Avastin)	**Inj:** 25mg/mL [4mL, 16mL]	***Adults:*** **Colon/Rectum Metastatic Carcinoma:** 5mg/kg (in combination with bolus IFL) or 10 mg/kg (in combination with FOLFOX4) given once every 14 days. **Lung Cancer:** 15mg/kg every 3 weeks. **Breast Cancer:** 10mg/kg every 2 weeks. Give as IV infusion over 90 min; if 1st infusion is well tolerated, give 2nd infusion over 60 min and subsequent doses over 30 min.	**BB:** Fatal pulmonary hemorrhage has occurred in patients with non-small cell lung cancer treated with chemotherapy and bevacizumab; avoid with recent hemoptysis. Avoid if GI perforation or wound dehiscence develops; may be fatal. **W/P:** D/C with nephrotic syndrome, serious hemorrhage, and arterial thromboembolic events. Increased risk of HTN; permanently d/c if hypertensive crisis or hypertensive encephalopathy occurs. Monitor BP every 2-3 weeks during treatment. Increased incidence/severity of proteinuria. Potential for immunogenicity. CHF and neutropenia reported. Avoid initiation of therapy for at least 28 days following major surgery; surgical incision must be fully healed prior to start of therapy. Suspend treatment prior to elective surgery. Reversible posterior leukoencephalopathy syndrome reported; d/c and treat HTN if present. Non-GI fistula formation reported. May impair fertility. **P/N:** Category C, not for use in nursing.	Asthenia, pain, abdominal pain, headache, HTN, diarrhea, N/V, anorexia, **stomatitis,** constipation, upper respiratory infection, epistaxis, dyspnea, exfoliative dermatitis.
VINCA ALKALOIDS				
Vinblastine Sulfate	**Inj:** 1mg/mL [10mL]	***Adults:*** Dose at intervals of ≥7 days. **1st Dose:** 3.7mg/m². **2nd Dose:** 5.5mg/m². **3rd Dose:** 7.4mg/m². **4th Dose:** 9.25mg/m². **5th Dose:** 11.1mg/m². **Max:** 18.5mg/m². Do not increase dose after that dose which reduces WBC to 3000 cells/mm³. **Maint:** Use dose of 1 increment smaller than this dose at weekly intervals. Reduce to 50% dose if direct serum bilirubin >3mg/100mL. Only dose if WBC ≥4000 cells/mm³. ***Pediatrics:*** **Letterer-Swine Disease as Single Agent: Initial:** 6.5mg/m². **Hodgkin's Disease in Combination Therapy: Initial:** 6mg/m². **Testicular Germ Cell Carcinoma in Combination Therapy: Initial:** 3mg/m².	**BB:** For IV use only; fatal if given intrathecally. Considerable irritation if leakage occurs into surrounding tissue. If this occurs, d/c and restart in another vein. Heat and hyaluronidase minimize discomfort and cellulitis. **W/P:** Avoid pregnancy. Acute shortness of breath, severe bronchospasm, aspermia, stomatitis, neurologic toxicity reported. Increased toxicity with hepatic insufficiency. Monitor for infection with WBC <2000 cells/mm³. Avoid with malignant-cell infiltration of bone marrow, or in older persons with cachexia or ulcerated skin. Small daily amounts for long periods is not advised. Avoid eye contamination. Monitor WBCs. May cause fetal	Leukopenia (granulocytopenia), anemia, thrombocytopenia, alopecia, constipation, anorexia, N/V, abdominal pain, diarrhea, HTN, paresthesis.

Table 23.1. PRESCRIBING INFORMATION FOR ANTINEOPLASTIC DRUGS *(cont.)*

NAME	FORM/ STRENGTH	DOSAGE	WARNINGS/PRECAUTIONS & CONTRAINDICATIONS	ADVERSE EFFECTS†
VINCA ALKALOIDS *(cont.)*				
Vinblastine Sulfate *(cont.)*			harm during pregnancy. Caution with ischemic cardiac disease. **Contra:** Significant granulocytopenia (unless result of disease being treated), bacterial infections. **P/N:** Category D, not for use in nursing.	
Vincristine Sulfate	**Inj:** 1mg/mL	***Adults:* Usual:** 1.4mg/m² IV at weekly intervals. **Bilirubin >3mg/dL:** 50% dose reduction. If given together with L-asparaginase, give 12-24 hrs before the enzyme. ***Pediatrics:* Usual:** 2mg/m² IV at weekly intervals. **≤10kg: Initial:** 0.05mg/kg IV once weekly. **Bilirubin >3mg/dL:** 50% dose reduction. If given together with L-asparaginase, give 12-24 hrs before the enzyme.	**BB:** Properly position IV needle or catheter before injection; considerable irritation with extravasation. Use hyaluronidase and heat to minimize discomfort and cellulitis with extravasation. Fatal with intrathecal use. For IV use only. **W/P:** Acute uric acid nephropathy may occur. May require additional agents with CNS leukemia. Neurotoxicity is dose-limiting toxicity. Perform CBC before each dose. Determine serum uric acid levels frequently during 1st 3-4 weeks. Acute shortness of breath, severe bronchospasm reported. Monitor with pre-existing neuromuscular disease. Avoid eye contamination. May cause fetal harm during pregnancy. **Contra:** Demyelinating form of Charcot-Marie-Tooth syndrome. **P/N:** Category D, not for use in nursing.	Alopecia, abdominal cramps, weight loss, N/V, diarrhea, constipation, paralytic ileus, HTN, hypotension, polyuria, dysuria, urinary retention, sensory impairment, paresthesia, neuritic pain, motor difficulties, rash, fever.
Vinorelbine Tartrate (Navelbine)	**Inj:** 10mg/mL	***Adults:* Single-Agent:** 30mg/m² IV weekly over 6-10 min. **With Cisplatin:** 25mg/m² weekly with cisplatin 100mg/m² every 4 weeks, or 30mg/m² weekly with cisplatin 120mg/m² on Days 1 and 29, then every 6 weeks. **Adjustments Based on Granulocytes:** If 1000-1499 cells/mm³ give 50% starting dose. If <1000 cells/mm³, hold dose and repeat count in 1 week. D/C if hold 3 consecutive weekly doses because granulocyte <1000 cells/mm³. If fever and/or sepsis occurs while granulocytopenic or if hold 2 consecutive weekly doses due to granulocytopenia; give 75% of the starting dose if granulocytes ≥1500 cells/mm³, and 37.5% of the starting dose if granulocytes 1000-1499 cells/mm³. **Hepatic Insufficiency:** (bilirubin 2.1-3mg/dL) 50% of starting dose or (bilirubin >3mg/dL) 25% of starting dose. If both hematologic toxicity and hepatic insufficiency, use lowest dose. **Neurotoxicity:** D/C if Grade ≥2 develops.	**BB:** For IV use only; fatal if given intrathecally. Severe granulocytopenia may occur; granulocyte counts should be ≥1000 cells/mm³ prior to administration. Use extreme caution to prevent extravasation (can cause local tissue necrosis); if this occurs, d/c and restart in another vein. Administer only under supervision of a physician experienced in the use of antineoplastic agents. **W/P:** Monitor for myleosuppression during and after therapy, and for infection and/or fever with developing severe granulocytopenia. Interstitial pulmonary changes, ARDS, acute shortness of breath and severe bronchospasm reported. Extreme caution with compromised bone marrow reserve due to prior irradiation or chemotherapy. Radiation recall reactions may occur. Monitor for new or worsening signs/symptoms of neuropathy. D/C if moderate or severe neurotoxicity develops. Avoid contact with skin, mucosa, and eyes. Avoid pregnancy. May cause severe constipation, paralytic ileus, intestinal obstruction, necrosis, and/or perforation. **Contra:** Pretreatment granulocytes <1000 cells/mm³. **P/N:** Category D, not for use in nursing.	Granulocytopenia, leukopenia, thrombocytopenia, anemia, asthenia, injection site reactions/pain, phlebitis, peripheral neuropathy, N/V, diarrhea, severe constipation, paralytic ileus, intestinal obstruction, necrosis, and/or perforation, dyspnea, alopecia, chest pain, fatigue.

†Bold entries denote special dental considerations.
BB = black box warning; **W/P** = warnings/precautions; **Contra** = contraindications; **P/N** = pregnancy category rating and nursing considerations.

Table 23.2. DRUG INTERACTIONS FOR ANTINEOPLASTIC DRUGS

ACTINOMYCIN ANTIBIOTIC	
Dactinomycin (Cosmegen)	
Radiation therapy	May cause or increase GI toxicity, bone marrow suppression, second primary tumors, erythema, and vesiculation with radiation. Avoid or use caution within 2 months of radiation in treatment of Wilm's tumor.
ADRENAL CYTOTOXIC AGENT	
Mitotane (Lysodren)	
Anticoagulants, coumarin	May increase metabolism of coumarin anticoagulants; may require dose increase of anticoagulant.
Hepatic enzyme induction, drugs susceptible to	Caution with drugs susceptible to hepatic enzyme induction.
ALKYLATING AGENTS	
Bendamustine HCl (Treanda)	
CYP1A2 inducers	CYP1A2 inducers (eg, omeprazole) may decrease plasma levels of bendamustine and increase plasma levels of active metabolites.
CYP1A2 inhibitors	CYP1A2 inhibitors (eg, ciprofloxacin, fluvoxamine) may increase plasma levels of bendamustine and decrease plasma levels of active metabolites.
Busulfan (Myleran)	
Alkylating agents	Coadministration with multiple alkylating agents may increase risk of hepatic veno-occlusive disease.
Cyclophosphamide	May decrease busulfan clearance; hepatic veno-occlusive disease reported with cyclophosphamide.
Cytotoxic agents	Additive pulmonary toxicity with other cytotoxic agents.
Itraconazole	Decreases busulfan clearance; possible busulfan toxicity with coadministration.
Myelosuppressive drugs	Additive myelosuppression with other myelosuppressive drugs.
Phenytoin	May increase clearance and decrease plasma levels of cyclophosphamide and busulfan when given with phenytoin.
Thioguanine	Concurrent use may cause portal hypertension and esophageal varices associated with abnormal LFTs; caution with continuous long-term therapy.
Temozolomide (Temodar)	
Valproic acid	Coadminstration with valproic acid may decrease clearance of temozolomide.
ANTHRACYCLINES	
Daunorubicin HCl (Cerubidine)	
Antineoplastic agents	Possible secondary leukemia with other antineoplastic agents.
Cyclophosphamide	May increase risk of cardiotoxicity with concomitant cyclophosphamide.
Doxorubicin	May increase risk of cardiotoxicity with previous doxorubicin therapy.

Table 23.2. DRUG INTERACTIONS FOR ANTINEOPLASTIC DRUGS *(cont.)*

ANTHRACYCLINES *(cont.)*	
Daunorubicin HCl (Cerubidine) *(cont.)*	
Hepatotoxic drugs	Hepatotoxic drugs (eg, high dose MTX) may impair liver function and increase the risk of toxicity.
Myelosuppressive agents	May require dose reduction with other myelosuppressive agents.
Radiation therapy	Possible secondary leukemia with radiation therapy.
Doxorubicin HCl	
6-mercaptopurine	May enhance 6-MP hepatotoxicity with coadministration.
Actinomycin-D	May cause acute "recall" pneumonitis in pediatric patients following local radiation therapy.
Anticancer therapies	May increase toxicities of other anticancer therapies with coadministration.
CCBs	Increases risk of doxorubicin cardiotoxicity when administered concomitantly with CCBs.
Cisplatin	Peripheral neurotoxicity, seizures, and coma reported when administered concomitantly with cisplatin.
Cyclophosphamide	May increase plasma levels of less active doxorubicin metabolite. May exacerbate cyclophosphamide-induced hemorrhagic cystitis. Acute myeloid leukemia reported.
Cyclosporine	Decreases clearance of doxorubicin and decreases metabolism of metabolite. May prolong and exacerbate hematologic toxicity. Seizures and coma reported.
Cytarabine	May cause necrotizing colitis manifested by typhlitis, bloody stools, and severe fatal infections.
Cytotoxic drugs	May increase doxorubicin toxicities (eg, hematologic and GI events) with other cytotoxic drugs.
Dexrazoxane	May decrease chemotherapeutic activity of chemotherapy regimen when initiated; later administration of dexrazoxane was not associated with this effect.
Paclitaxel	May increase risk of cardiotoxicity with coadministration of paclitaxel. Paclitaxel infused before doxorubicin may decrease doxorubicin clearance and increase neutropenic and stomatitis episodes.
Phenobarbital	Increases elimination of doxorubicin.
Phenytoin	May decrease plasma levels of phenytoin.
Progesterone	May increase risk of doxorubicin-induced neutropenia and thrombocytopenia with IV progesterone.
Radiation therapy	Radiation-induced toxicity to myocardium, mucosae, skin, and liver reported with concomitant use.
Streptozocin	May inhibit hepatic metabolism of doxorubicin.
Vaccines, live	Coadministration of live vaccines may be hazardous.
Vincristine	Seizures and coma reported with concomitant vincristine.

ANTHRACYCLINES *(cont.)*

Doxorubicin HCl Liposome (Doxil)	
6-mercaptopurine	May enhance 6-MP hepatotoxicity when coadministered.
Anticancer therapies	May increase toxicities of other anticancer therapies.
Bone marrow suppression, drugs causing	May increase severity of hematologic toxicity.
Cyclophosphamide	May increase risk of cardiotoxicity and exacerbate cyclophosphamide-induced hemorrhagic cystitis.
Radiation therapy	Radiation-induced toxicity to myocardium, mucosae, skin, and liver reported with concomitant therapy.
Epirubicin HCl (Ellence)	
Anthracyclines	May increase risk of cardiotoxicity with previous anthracycline therapy.
Antineoplastic agents, DNA-damaging	May increase risk of secondary leukemias.
Cardioactive drugs	Caution with cardioactive drugs that can cause heart failure (eg, calcium channel blockers); monitor cardiac function throughout treatment.
Cimetidine	Coadministraton with cimetidine may increase AUC of epirubicin and decrease its plasma clearance; avoid cimetidine.
Cyclophosphamide	Coadministration with cyclophosphamide may cause severe leukopenia, neutropenia, thrombocytopenia, and anemia.
Cytotoxic drugs	Additive toxicity, including hematologic and GI effects, with other cytotoxic drugs. May increase risk of secondary leukemias.
Fluorouracil	Coadministration with fluorouracil may cause severe leukopenia, neutropenia, thrombocytopenia, and anemia.
Hepatic function, drugs altering	Caution with agents that cause changes in hepatic function; may alter pharmacokinetics, efficacy, and toxicity of epirubicin.
Radiation therapy	May induce inflammatory recall reaction at irradiation site with previous radiation therapy.
Idarubicin HCl (Idamycin PFS)	
Anthracyclines	May increase risk of idarubicin-induced cardiotoxicity with previous anthracycline therapy.
Cardiotoxic agents	Coadministration with cardiotoxic agents may increase risk of idarubicin-induced cardiotoxicity.
Radiation therapy	May increase risk of idarubicin-induced cardiotoxicity with previous or concomitant radiation to the mediastinal-pericardial area.

ANTIESTROGEN

Tamoxifen Citrate	
Aminoglutethimide	Coadministration with aminoglutethamide may decrease plasma levels of tamoxifen.
Anastrozole	Avoid coadministration; may decrease plasma levels of anastrozole.

Table 23.2. DRUG INTERACTIONS FOR ANTINEOPLASTIC DRUGS *(cont.)*

ANTIESTROGEN *(cont.)*

Tamoxifen Citrate *(cont.)*	
Anticoagulants, coumarin	Coadministration with coumarin anticoagulants increases anticoagulant effect; monitor PT.
Bromocriptine	Coadministration with bromocriptine may increase plasma levels of tamoxifen.
Cytotoxic agents	Coadministration with cytotoxic agents may increase risk of thromboembolic events.
Letrozole	Coadministration with letrozole may decrease plasma levels of letrozole.
Medroxyprogesterone	Coadministration with medroxyprogesterone decreases plasma levels of tamoxifen metabolite.
Rifampin	Coadministration with rifampin may decrease plasma levels of tamoxifen.

ANTIFOLATE

Pemetrexed Disodium (Alimta)	
Ibuprofen	May decrease clearance of pemetrexed disodium; caution in mild to moderate renal insufficiency (CrCl 49-79mL/min).
Nephrotoxic drugs	Coadministration may delay clearance of pemetrexed disodium.
NSAIDs	Avoid NSAIDs with short elimination half-lives in patients with mild to moderate renal insufficiency for a period of 2 days before to 2 days following administration of pemetrexed disodium. Interrupt dosing of NSAIDs with longer half-lives for at least 5 days before to 2 days following administration of pemetrexed disodium.
Probenecid	Coadministration with tubularly secreted drugs (eg, probenecid) may delay clearance of pemetrexed disodium.

ANTIMETABOLITES

Clofarabine (Clolar)	
Cyclophosphamide	Coadministration with cyclophosphamide and etoposide may increase risk of hepatotoxicity following previous hematopoietic stem cell transplant.
Etoposide	Coadministration with cyclophosphamide and etoposide may increase risk of hepatotoxicity following previous hematopoietic stem cell transplant.
Cytarabine	
Cyclophosphamide	Cardiomyopathy and death reported following high-dose cytarabine therapy with cyclophosphamide.
Cytotoxic agents	May develop a diffuse interstitial pneumonitis with cytotoxic agents.
Daunorubicin	Coadministration with daunorubicin and L-asparaginase may cause peripheral motor and sensory neuropathies.
Digoxin	May decrease plasma levels and renal excretion of digoxin.
Fluorocytosine	May inhibit efficacy of fluorocytosine.
Gentamicin	Antagonizes susceptibility of gentamicin for *K.pneumoniae.*
L-asparaginase	Acute pancreatitis reported with prior L-asparaginase treatment.

ANTIMETABOLITES *(cont.)*

Cytarabine Liposome (DepoCyt)	
Cytotoxic agents, intrathecal	Concomitant use of intrathecally administered cytotoxic agents may enhance neurotoxicity.
Floxuridine	
Bone marrow suppression, therapies causing	May increase toxicity of floxuridine.
Fludarabine Phosphate (Fludara)	
Pentostatin	Avoid pentostatin due to the risk of severe pulmonary toxicity.
Fluorouracil	
Bone marrow suppression, therapies causing	May increase toxicity of fluorouracil.
Leucovorin	May enhance toxicity of fluorouracil with concomitant leucovorin.

ANTIMICROTUBULE AGENTS

Docetaxel (Taxotere)	
CYP3A4 pathway, drugs involved with	May affect the metabolism of docetaxel. Caution with agents that induce, inhibit, or are metabolized by CYP3A4 (eg, cyclosporine, erythromycin, ketoconazole, terfenadine).
Protease inhibitors	May inhibit the metabolism of docetaxel. Caution in patients receiving protease inhibitors (eg, ritonavir) which are inhibitors and substrates of CYP3A.
Ixabepilone (Ixempra)	
CYP3A4 inducers	May decrease plasma levels with CYP3A4 inducers (eg, dexamethasone, phenytoin, carbamazepine, rifampin, rifabutin, phenobarbital); agents with low enzyme induction potential should be considered with ixabepilone coadministration.
CYP3A4 inhibitors	May increase plasma levels with CYP3A4 inhibitors (eg, ketoconazole, erythromycin, fluconazole, verapamil); caution with coadministration.
Grapefruit or grapefruit juice	May increase plasma levels of ixabepilone; avoid coadministration.
St. John's Wort	May unpredictably decrease ixabepilone plasma levels; avoid coadministration.
Paclitaxel (Taxol)	
Cisplatin	May increase myelosuppression with coadministration; may be more profound if paclitaxel administered after cisplatin.
CYP2C8/ CYP3A4 inducers	Caution with concomitant CYP2C8 and CYP3A4 inducers (eg, rifampin, carbamazepine, phenytoin, efavirenz, nevirapine).
CYP2C8/ CYP3A4 inhibitors	Caution with concomitant CYP2C8 and CYP3A4 inhibitors (eg, erythromycin, fluoxetine, gemfibrozil).
CYP2C8/ CYP3A4 substrates	Caution with concomitant administration of CYP2C8 and CYP3A4 substrates.
Doxorubicin	May increase plasma levels of doxorubicin with coadministration.

Table 23.2. DRUG INTERACTIONS FOR ANTINEOPLASTIC DRUGS *(cont.)*

ANTIMICROTUBULE AGENTS *(cont.)*	
Paclitaxel Protein-Bound Particles (Abraxane)	
CYP2C8/ CYP3A4 inhibitors	Caution with concomitant administration of CYP2C8 and CYP3A4 inhibitors (eg, erythromycin, fluoxetine, gemfibrozil).
CYP2C8/ CYP3A4 substrates	Caution with concomitant administration of CYP2C8 and CYP3A4 substrates.
AROMATASE INACTIVATOR	
Exemestane (Aromasin)	
CYP3A4 inducers	CYP3A4 inducers (eg, rifampin, phenytoin, carbamazepine, phenobarbital, St. John's wort) may decrease plasma levels of exemestane; may require dose adjustment with potent CYP3A4 inducers.
Estrogen-containing agents	Avoid estrogen-containing agents; may interfere with the pharmacologic action of exemestane.
AROMATASE INHIBITOR (NON-STEROIDAL)	
Anastrozole (Arimidex)	
Estrogen-containing agents	Avoid estrogen-containing agents; may decrease the pharmacologic action of anastrozole.
Tamoxifen	Avoid tamoxifen; may decrease plasma levels of anastrozole.
ATTENUATED LIVE BCG CULTURE	
BCG Live (TheraCys, Tice BCG)	
Antimicrobials	May interfere with efficacy of BCG Live; postpone BCG therapy.
Antituberculosis drugs	Avoid antituberculosis drugs (eg, INH) to prevent or treat the local, irritative toxicities of BCG Live.
Bone marrow suppressants	Avoid concomitant bone marrow suppressants; may interfere with immune response.
Cancer therapy	Avoid concomitant cancer therapy (eg, cytotoxic drugs, radiation); may interfere with immune response.
Immunosuppressants	Avoid concomitant immunosuppressive therapy (eg, corticosteroids); may interfere with immune response.
BIOLOGICAL RESPONSE MODIFIER	
Aldesleukin (Proleukin)	
Antihypertensives	May potentiate hypotension with antihypertensives (eg, β-blockers).
Antineoplastic agents	Caution with other antineoplastic agents; may cause hypersensitivity reactions.
Cardiotoxic drugs	Coadministration may increase cardiac toxicity (eg, doxorubicin).
Glucocorticoids	May decrease antitumor effects; avoid concomitant use.
Hepatotoxic drugs	Coadministration may increase hepatic toxicity (eg, methotrexate, asparaginase).

BIOLOGICAL RESPONSE MODIFIER *(cont.)*

Aldesleukin (Proleukin) *(cont.)*	
Interferon alfa	Increased risk of myocardial infraction, myocarditis, ventricular hypokinesia, and severe rhabdomyolysis with coadministration.
Iodinated contrast media	May cause acute, atypical adverse reactions (eg, fever, chills, N/V, hypotension, edema) up to several months after therapy.
Myelotoxic drugs	Coadministration may increase toxicity to bone marrow (eg, cytotoxic chemotherapy).
Nephrotoxic drugs	Coadministration may increase renal toxicity (eg, aminoglycosides, indomethacin).
Psychotropics	May increase CNS effects with psychotropic agents (eg, narcotics, analgesics, antiemetics, sedatives, tranquilizers).

CHLORINATED PURINE NUCLEOSIDE ANALOG

Cladribine (Leustatin)	
Immunosuppressive drugs	Caution with other immunosuppressive drugs.
Myelosuppressive drugs	Caution with other myelosuppressive drugs.
Nephrotoxic drugs	May increase risk of acute nephrotoxicity with coadministration.

CYCLOPHOSPHAMIDE ANALOG

Ifosfamide (Ifex, Ifex/Mesnex)	
Cytotoxic drugs	Caution with other cytotoxic drugs; may increase risk of severe myelosuppression.

CYTOTOXIC GLYCOPEPTIDE ANTIBIOTIC

Bleomycin Sulfate (Blenoxane)	
G-CSF	Pulmonary toxicity reported with G-CSF (filgrastim) and other cytokines.
Nephrotoxic drugs	May decrease clearance and increase toxicity of bleomycin.

DEOXYGUANOSINE ANALOGUE

Nelarabine (Arranon)	
Adenosine deaminase inhibitors	Avoid coadministration with adenosine deaminase inhibitors (eg, pentostatin).

DNA FRAGMENTATION AGENT

Arsenic Trioxide (Trisenox)	
Electrolyte abnormalities, drugs causing	Caution with drugs that cause electrolyte abnormalities (eg, diuretics, amphotericin B).
QT interval, drugs prolonging	Caution with drugs that prolong the QT interval (eg, certain antiarrhythimcs, thioridazine).

Table 23.2. DRUG INTERACTIONS FOR ANTINEOPLASTIC DRUGS *(cont.)*

DNA SYNTHESIS INHIBITORS	
Mitomycin (Mutamycin)	
Chemotherapy	Adult respiratory distress syndrome reported with concomitant chemotherapy; monitor oxygen and fluid balance.
Vinca alkaloids	Acute shortness of breath and severe bronchospasm reported following administration of vinca alkaloids with previous or simultaneous mitomycin.
Streptozocin (Zanosar)	
Cytotoxic drugs	Additive toxicity with other cytotoxic drugs.
Doxorubicin	May prolong doxorubicin half-life and lead to severe bone marrow suppression; consider reducing doxorubicin dose.
Nephrotoxic drugs	Avoid other potential nephrotoxic drugs.
Phenytoin	May reduce streptozocin cytotoxicity with coadministration.
EPIDERMAL GROWTH FACTOR RECEPTOR TYROSINE KINASE INHIBITOR	
Erlotinib (Tarceva)	
Cigarette smoking	May decrease plasma levels of erlotinib; consider increasing dose of erlotinib if patient continues to smoke cigarettes; reduce dose back to starting dose upon cessation of smoking.
CYP3A4 inducers	May decrease plasma levels of erlotinib with CYP3A4 inducers (eg, rifampin, rifabutin, rifapentine, phenytoin, carbamazepine, phenobarbital, St. John's wort).
CYP3A4 inhibitors	May increase plasma levels of erlotinib with CYP3A4 inhibitors (eg, ketoconazole, atazanavir, clarithromycin, indinavir, itraconazole, nefazodone, nelfinavir, ritonavir, saquinavir, telithromycin, troleandomycin, voriconazole).
Grapefruit or grapefruit juice	May increase plasma levels of erlotinib; avoid coadministration.
pH-dependent drugs	May alter the solubility and reduce the bioavailability of erlotinib with drugs that alter gastric pH (eg, PPIs, H_2-blockers); consider antacids as alternate therapy, separated by several hours with erlotinib.
ESTRADIOL/NORNITROGEN MUSTARD	
Estramustine Phosphate Sodium (Emcyt)	
Calcium-rich foods or drugs	May impair absorption when coadministered with calcium-rich foods or drugs, including milk and milk products.
ESTROGEN RECEPTOR ANTAGONIST	
Fulvestrant (Faslodex)	
Anticoagulants	Avoid with anticoagulants.
FLUOROPYRIMIDINE CARBAMATE	
Capecitabine (Xeloda)	
Antacids, aluminum and magnesium	May increase plasma levels of capecitabine when coadministered with aluminum and magnesium antacids.

FLUOROPYRIMIDINE CARBAMATE *(cont.)*

Capecitabine (Xeloda) *(cont.)*	
Anticoagulants, coumarin	Altered coagulation parameters and/or bleeding reported with coumarin anticoagulants; monitor PT/INR frequently.
CYP2C9 substrates	Caution with CYP2C9 substrates.
Phenytoin	May increase plasma levels of phenytoin; consider phenytoin dose reduction.

HEAVY-METAL PLATINUM COMPLEX

Cisplatin (Platinol-AQ)	
Altretamine/pyridoxine	May adversely affect response duration with pyridoxine and altretamine.
Aminoglycosides	May potentiate cumulative nephrotoxicity; monitor for signs of toxicity prior to initiating therapy and at each subsequent course; cisplatin should not be given more than once every 3 to 4 weeks.
Anticonvulsants	Plasma levels of anticonvulsants may become subtherapeutic with cisplatin.

HISTONE DEACETYLASE INHIBITOR

Vorinostat (Zolinza)	
Anticoagulants, coumarin	Prolongation of PT and INR observed with coumarin anticoagulants; monitor closely.
Histone deacetylase inhibitors (HDAC)	Severe thrombocytopenia and GI bleeding reported with HDAC inhibitors (eg, valproic acid); monitor platelet count every 2 weeks for the first two months of therapy.

HYDRAZINE DERIVATIVE

Procarbazine HCl (Matulane)	
Alcohol	May cause disulfiram-type reaction with alcohol.
Antihistamines	May potentiate CNS depression; avoid concomitant use.
Barbiturates	May potentiate CNS depression; avoid concomitant use.
Hypotensives	May potentiate CNS depression; avoid concomitant use.
Narcotics	May potentiate CNS depression; avoid concomitant use.
Phenothiazines	May potentiate CNS depression; avoid concomitant use.
Sympathomimetics	Avoid sympathomimetics with procarbazine.
TCAs	Avoid TCAs with procarbazine.
Tyramine-containing drugs/foods	Avoid tyramine-containing drugs/foods (eg, wine, yogurt, ripe cheese, bananas) with procarbazine.

KINASE INHIBITORS

Lapatinib (Tykerb)	
CYP2C8 substrates	Caution with CYP2C8 substrates with a narrow therapeutic index.

Table 23.2. DRUG INTERACTIONS FOR ANTINEOPLASTIC DRUGS *(cont.)*

KINASE INHIBITORS *(cont.)*	
Lapatinib (Tykerb) *(cont.)*	
CYP3A4 inducers	May decrease plasma levels with CYP3A4 inducers (eg, carbamazepine, dexamethasone, phenytoin, rifampin, rifabutin, rifapentin, phenobarbital, St. John's wort); may require dose adjustment.
CYP3A4 inhibitors	May increase plasma levels with CYP3A4 inhibitors (eg, ketoconazole, itraconazole, clarithromycin, atazanavir, indinavir, nefazodone, nelfinavir, ritonavir, saquinavir, telithromycin, voriconazole); may require dose adjustment.
CYP3A4 substrates	Caution with CYP3A4 substrates with a narrow therapeutic index.
Grapefruit or grapefruit juice	May increase plasma levels of lapatinib; avoid coadministration.
P-glycoprotein inhibitors	May increase plasma levels of lapatinib; caution with coadministration.
P-glycoprotein substrate	May increase plasma levels of substrate drug; caution with coadministration.
Nilotinib (Tasigna)	
CYP2B6 substrates	May decrease plasma levels of CYP2B6 substrates.
CYP2C8 substrates	May increase or decrease plasma levels of CYP2C8 substrates; caution with drugs with a narrow therapeutic index.
CYP2C9 substrates	May increase or decrease plasma levels of CYP2C9 substrates; caution with drugs with a narrow therapeutic index.
CYP2D6 substrates	May increase plasma levels of CYP2D6 substrates; caution with drugs with a narrow therapeutic index.
CYP3A4 inducers	May decrease plasma levels of nilotinib. Avoid use of strong CYP3A4 inducers (eg, rifampin, dexamethasone, phenytoin, carbamazepine, rifabutin, rifapentin, phenobarbital).
CYP3A4 inhibitors	May increase plasma levels of nilotinib and prolong QT interval. Avoid use of strong CYP3A4 inhibitors (eg, ketoconazole, itraconazole, clarithromycin, atazanavir, indinavir, nefazodone, nelfinavir, ritonavir, saquinavir, telithromycin, voriconazole); may require dose adjustment.
CYP3A4 substrates	May increase plasma levels of CYP3A4 substrates; caution with drugs with a narrow therapeutic index.
Grapefruit or grapefruit juice	May increase plasma levels of nilotinib; avoid coadministration.
QT interval, drugs prolonging	Avoid or use caution with drugs known to prolong the QT interval.
P-glycoprotein inhibitors	May increase plasma levels of nilotinib; caution with coadministration.
P-glycoprotein substrates	May increase plasma levels of substrate drug; caution with coadministration.
St. John's wort	Avoid concomitant use of St. John's wort; may decrease plasma levels of nilotinib.
UGT1A1 enzyme substrates	May increase plasma levels of UGT1A1 substrates.
Warfarin	Avoid coadministration with warfarin, if possible.
Temsirolimus (Torisel)	
CYP3A4/5 inducers	May decrease plasma levels of primary metabolite (sirolimus) with strong inducers of CYP3A4/5 (eg, dexamethasone, carbamazepine, phenytoin, phenobarbital, rifampin, rifabutin, rifampacin); consider alternative if possible or dose increase should be considered.

KINASE INHIBITORS *(cont.)*

Temsirolimus (Torisel) *(cont.)*	
CYP3A4 inhibitors	May increase plasma levels of primary metabolite (sirolimus) with strong CYP3A4 inhibitors (eg, atazanavir, clarithromycin, indinavir, itraconazole, ketoconazole, nefazodone, nelfinavir, ritonavir, saquinavir, telithromycin); consider alternative if possible or dose reduction should be considered.
Sunitinib	Concomitant use with sunitinib may result in dose-limiting toxicity.
Vaccines, live	Avoid administration of live vaccines during temsirolimus treatment.

LUTEINIZING HORMONE RELEASING HORMONE AGONIST

Triptorelin Pamoate (Trelstar Depot, Trelstar LA)	
Hyperprolactinemic drugs	Avoid hyperprolactinemic drugs; may reduce the number of pituitary GnRH receptors.

MONOCLONAL ANTIBODY

Ibritumomab Tiuxetan (Zevalin)	
Anticoagulants	Increases risk of bleeding and hemorrhage with anticoagulants; avoid coadministration.
Antiplatelet agents	Increases risk of bleeding and hemorrhage with antiplatelet agents; avoid coadministration.
Vaccines, live	Avoid administration of live viral vaccines to patients recently treated with ibritumomab.

MONOCLONAL ANTIBODY/CD20-BLOCKERS

Iodine I 131 Tositumomab/Tositumomab (Bexxar)	
Anticoagulants	Increases risk of bleeding and hemorrhage with anticoagulants; monitor frequently for thrombocytopenia.
Antiplatelet agents	Increases risk of bleeding and hemorrhage with antiplatelet agents; monitor frequently for thrombocytopenia.
Rituximab (Rituxan)	
Biologic agents	Safety unknown with concomitant use; observe closely for signs of infection if biologic agents are coadministered.
Cisplatin	Renal toxicity reported with cisplatin.
DMARDs	Safety unknown with concomitant use; observe closely for signs of infection if DMARDs are coadministered.
Vaccines, live	Avoid administration of live virus vaccines with rituxan.

MONOCLONAL ANTIBODY/CD52-BLOCKER

Alemtuzumab (Campath)	
Vaccines, live	Avoid live viral vaccines if recently received alemtuzumab.

Table 23.2. DRUG INTERACTIONS FOR ANTINEOPLASTIC DRUGS *(cont.)*

MONOCLONAL ANTIBODY/HER2-BLOCKER	
Trastuzumab (Herceptin)	
Anthracyclines	Concomitant anthracyclines may increase incidence/severity of cardiac dysfunction.
Paclitaxel	May increase plasma levels of trastuzumab.
MULTIKINASE INHIBITORS	
Sorafenib (Nexavar)	
CYP2B6 substrates	May increase plasma levels of CYP2B6 substrates; coadminister with caution.
CYP2C8 substrates	May increase plasma levels of CYP2C8 substrates; coadminister with caution.
CYP3A4 inducers	May increase metabolism and decrease plasma levels with concomitant CYP3A4 inducers (eg, rifampin, St. John's wort, phenytoin, carbamazepine, dexamethasone).
Docetaxel	May increase plasma levels of docetaxel; coadminister with caution.
Doxorubicin	May increase plasma levels of doxorubicin; coadminister with caution.
Fluorouracil	May alter AUC of fluorouracil; coadminister with caution.
UGT1A1 substrates	May increase plasma levels of UGT1A1 substrates (eg, irinotecan).
UGT1A9 substrates	May increase plasma levels of UGT1A9 substrates.
Warfarin	Increased INR and infrequent bleeding reported; monitor PT, INR, and clinical bleeding episodes with coadministration.
Sunitinib Malate (Sutent)	
CYP3A4 inducers	May decrease plasma levels with concomitant CYP3A4 inducers (eg, dexamethasone, phenytoin, carbamazepine, rifampin, rifabutin, rifapentin, phenobarbital); consider dose increase.
CYP3A4 inhibitors	May increase plasma levels with concomitant strong CYP3A4 inhibitors (eg, ketoconazole, itraconazole, clarithromycin, atazanavir, indinavir, nefazodone, ritonavir, saquinavir, telithromycin, voriconazole); consider dose reduction.
Grapefruit or grapefruit juice	May increase plasma levels of sunitinib; avoid coadministration.
St. John's wort	May decrease plasma levels of sunitinib unpredictably; avoid coadministration.
NITROGEN MUSTARD ALKYLATING AGENTS	
Chlorambucil (Leukeran)	
Alkylating agents	Cross-hypersensitivity may occur with other alkylating agents.
Cyclophosphamide (Cytoxan)	
Anesthesia, general	Caution if cyclophosphamide administered within 10 days of general anesthesia.
Doxorubicin	May potentiate doxorubicin-induced cardiotoxicity.
Phenobarbital	May increase metabolism and leukopenic activity of cyclophosphamide with chronic high doses of phenobarbital.
Succinylcholine chloride	May potentiate the effect of succinylcholine chloride by marked and persistent inhibition of cholinesterase activity.

NITROGEN MUSTARD ALKYLATING AGENTS *(cont.)*

Melphalan HCl (Alkeran) (Inj)	
BCNU	May reduce the threshold for BCNU lung toxicity.
Cisplatin	May alter melphalan clearance by inducing renal dysfunction.
Cyclosporine	Severe renal failure reported with oral cyclosporine.
Nalidixic acid	Increased incidence of severe hemorrhagic necrotic enterocolitis reported in pediatrics.

NITROSOUREA ALKYLATING AGENT

Carmustine (BiCNU)	
Cimetidine	May increase myelotoxicity (eg, leukopenia, neutropenia) when coadministered with cimetidine.

NONSTEROIDAL ANTIANDROGENS

Bicalutamide (Casodex)	
Anticoagulants, coumarin	May displace coumarin anticoagulants from protein-binding site; monitor PT.
CYP3A4 substrates	May increase plasma levels of CYP3A4 substrates; caution with coadministration.
Flutamide (Flutamide)	
Coumadin	May increase PT with coadministration; monitor PT and adjust dose if necessary.
Nilutamide (Nilandron)	
Alcohol	Intolerance to alcohol, including facial flushes, malaise, and hypotension reported; avoid use if symptoms experienced.
Phenytoin	Coadministration may delay elimination and increase serum half-life leading to toxic levels; may require dose adjustment of phenytoin.
Theophylline	Coadministration may delay elimination and increase serum half-life leading to toxic levels; may require dose adjustment of theophylline.
Vitamin K antagonists	Coadministration may delay elimination and increase serum half-life leading to toxic levels; may require dose adjustment of vitamin K antagonists.

NONSTEROIDAL AROMATASE INHIBITOR

Letrozole (Femara)	
Tamoxifen	Coadministration may decrease plasma levels of letrozole; administer letrozole immediately after tamoxifen to avoid impairment in therapeutic effect.

NONSTEROIDAL TRIPHENYLETHYLENE DERIVATIVE

Toremifene Citrate (Fareston)	
Anticoagulants, coumarin	May increase PT with coadministration; monitor PT time with coadministration.
CYP3A4 inducers	May increase metabolism and decrease plasma levels with CYP3A4 inducers (eg, phenobarbital, phenytoin, carbamazepine).

Table 23.2. DRUG INTERACTIONS FOR ANTINEOPLASTIC DRUGS *(cont.)*

NONSTEROIDAL TRIPHENYLETHYLENE DERIVATIVE *(cont.)*	
Toremifene Citrate (Fareston) *(cont.)*	
CYP3A4/6 inhibitors	May inhibit metabolism of toremifene with CYP3A4/6 inhibitors (eg, ketoconazole, erythromycin).
Renal calcium excretion, drugs decreasing	May increase the risk of hypercalcemia with drugs that decrease renal calcium excretion (eg, thiazides).
NUCLEOSIDE ANALOGUE ANTIMETABOLITE	
Gemcitabine HCl (Gemzar)	
Cisplatin	Monitor SCr, potassium, calcium, and magnesium with cisplatin.
Hepatotoxic drugs	Serious hepatotoxicity reported with other hepatotoxic drugs.
ORGANOPLATINUM COMPLEX	
Oxaliplatin (Eloxatin)	
5-FU	May increase plasma levels of 5-FU.
Nephrotoxic drugs	May decrease clearance of oxaliplatin.
PLATINUM COORDINATION COMPOUND	
Carboplatin	
Aminoglycosides	Caution with coadministration; may increase renal and audiologic toxicity.
Nephrotoxic drugs	May potentiate renal adverse effects.
PODOPHYLLOTOXIN DERIVATIVE	
Etoposide (Etopophos, VePesid)	
Cyclosporine A	May decrease clearance and increase plasma levels of oral etoposide with high-dose cyclosporine A.
Phosphatase activity, drugs inhibiting	Caution with drugs known to inhibit phosphatase activities (eg, levamisole).
PROGESTOGEN	
Medroxyprogesterone Acetate (Depo-Provera)	
Aminoglutethimide	May decrease plasma levels of medroxyprogesterone.
Estrogen	Coadministration may cause adverse effects on carbohydrate and lipid metabolism. May decrease glucose tolerance; caution in diabetics.
PROTEASOME INHIBITOR	
Bortezomib (Velcade)	
Antidiabetic agents, oral	Hypoglycemia and hyperglycemia reported with concomitant use in diabetics; may require dose adjustment of antidiabetic medication.
Antihypertensive agents	May increase risk of hypotension with antihypertensive agents.

PROTEASOME INHIBITOR *(cont.)*

Bortezomib (Velcade) *(cont.)*	
CYP3A inhibitors	May increase plasma levels of bortezomib with potent CYP3A inhibitors (eg, ketoconazole, ritonavir).
CYP3A4 inducers/inhibitors	May alter plasma levels of bortezomib; monitor for toxicities or reduced efficacy.

PROTEIN SYNTHESIS INHIBITOR

Pegaspargase (Oncaspar)	
Anticoagulants	Caution with concomitant anticoagulants (eg, coumarin, heparin, dipyridamole, ASA); may potentiate increases in PT and PTT.

PROTEIN-TYROSINE KINASE INHIBITOR

Imatinib Mesylate (Gleevec)	
Acetaminophen	May inhibit metabolism and increase plasma levels of acetaminophen; caution with coadministration.
CYP2D6 substrates	May increase plasma levels of CYP2D6 substrates; caution is recommended.
CYP3A inducers	May increase clearance and decrease plasma levels with CYP3A inducers (eg, dexamethasone, carbamazepine, rifampin, phenytoin, phenobarbital); consider dose adjustment if coadministration required.
CYP3A inhibitors	May decrease metabolism and increase plasma levels with CYP3A inhibitors (eg, ketoconazole, itraconazole, clarithromycin, atazanavir, indinavir, nefazodone, nelfinavir, ritonavir, saquinavir, telithromycin, voriconazole).
CYP3A4 substrates	May increase plasma levels of CYP3A4 substrates (eg, triazolo-benzodiazepines, dihydropyridine calcium channel blockers, certain HMG-CoA reductase inhibitors); caution with CYP3A4 substrates with a narrow therapeutic index (eg, alfentanil, cyclosporine, diergotamine, ergotamine, fentanyl, pimozide, quinidine, sirolimus, tacrolimus).
Grapefruit or grapefruit juice	May increase plasma levels of imatinib; avoid coadministration.
Warfarin	Avoid coadministration with warfarin; LMWH or standard heparin recommended for anticoagulation in patients on imatinib.

PURINE ANALOGS

Mercaptopurine (Purinethol)	
Allopurinol	Decrease mercaptopurine 1/3 to 1/4 of the usual dose with concomitant allopurinol to avoid toxicity.
Myelosuppressive drugs	May potentiate myelosuppression; consider dose reduction of mercaptopurine with coadministration.
Thioguanine	Cross-resistance between thioguanine and mercaptopurine.
Thiopurine S-methyltransferase (TPMT) inhibitors	May potentiate bone marrow suppression with concomitant TPMT inhibitors such as aminosalicylate derivates (eg, olsalazine, mesalazine, sulphasalazine); caution with coadministration.

Table 23.2. DRUG INTERACTIONS FOR ANTINEOPLASTIC DRUGS *(cont.)*

PURINE ANALOGS *(cont.)*	
Mercaptopurine (Purinethol) *(cont.)*	
TMP-SMX	Increased bone marrow suppression reported with trimethoprim-sulfamethoxazole.
Warfarin	Inhibition of anticoagulant effect of warfarin reported with concomitant mercaptopurine.
Thioguanine	
Chemotherapeutic agents	Veno-occlusive liver disease reported with concomitant chemotherapeutic agents.
Mercaptopurine	Cross-resistance between mercaptopurine and thioguanine.
Myelosuppressive drugs	May potentiate myelosuppression; consider dose reduction of thioguanine with coadministration.
Thiopurine S-methyltransferase (TPMT) inhibitors	May potentiate bone marrow suppression with concomitant TPMT inhibitors such as aminosalicylate derivates (eg, olsalazine, mesalazine, sulphasalazine); caution with coadministration.
RETINOID	
Tretinoin (Vesanoid)	
Antifibrinolytic agents	Fatal thrombotic complications reported with antifibrinolytic agents (eg, tranexamic acid, aminocaproic acid, aprotinin).
CYP450 inducers	May decrease plasma levels of tretinoin with CYP450 inducers (eg, rifampicin, glucocorticoids, phenobarbital, pentobarbital).
CYP450 inhibitors	May increase plasma levels of tretinoin with CYP450 inhibitors (eg, ketoconazole, cimetidine, erythromycin, verapamil, diltiazem, cyclosporine).
Pseudotumor cerebri/intracranial HTN, drugs causing	May increase risk of pseudotumor cerebri/intracranial HTN with drugs known to cause pseudotumor cerebri/intracranial HTN (eg, tetracyclines).
Vitamin A	Avoid concomitant vitamin A; may aggravate symptoms of hypervitaminosis A.
RIBONUCLEOTIDE REDUCTASE INHIBITOR	
Hydroxyurea (Hydrea)	
Antiretroviral agents	Peripheral neuropathy, hepatotoxicity, and hepatic failure reported in HIV patients with concomitant antiretroviral agents and hydroxyurea. Fatal hepatic events reported with concomitant hydroxyurea, didanosine, and stavudine; avoid this combination. Fatal and nonfatal pancreatitis reported in HIV patients with concomitant didanosine.
Myelosuppressive agents	May increase risk of bone marrow depression with other myelosuppressive agents.
Radiation therapy	May increase risk of bone marrow depression with radiation therapy.
Uricosuric agents	Hydroxyurea may increase uric acid levels; may require dose adjustment of uricosuric agents.

S-TRIAZINE DERIVATIVE

Altretamine (Hexalen)	
Cimetidine	May increase altretamine half-life and toxicity with cimetidine.
Monoamine oxidase inhibitors (MAOI)	Severe orthostatic hypotension with concomitant MAOIs.
Pyridoxine	May adversely affect response duration; avoid concomitant pyridoxine.

SYNTHETIC GONADOTROPIN RELEASING HORMONE ANALOG

Goserelin Acetate (Zoladex 1-Month)	
Gonadotropins	Ovarian hyperstimulation syndrome reported with coadministration of other gonadotropins.

TOPOISOMERASE I INHIBITORS

Irinotecan HCl (Camptosar)	
Antineoplastic agents	May exacerbate adverse effects such as myelosuppression and diarrhea with other antineoplastic agents having similar adverse effects.
Atazanavir	May increase exposure to irinotecan and active metabolite with atazanavir (CYP3A4 and UGT1A1 inhibitor).
CYP3A4 inducers	May decrease exposure to irinotecan and active metabolite with CYP3A4 inducers (eg, rifampin, St. John's wort, anticonvulsants such as carbamazepine, phenytoin, and phenobarbital). Consider substituting non-enzyme-inducing anticonvulsants 2 weeks prior to irinotecan therapy. Avoid St. John's wort 2 weeks prior to the first cycle of irinotecan and during irinotecan therapy.
Dexamethasone	Possible hyperglycemia and lymphocytopenia with dexamethasone.
Diuretics	May potentiate dehydration; consider withholding diuretics during dosing with irinotecan and periods of acute vomiting and diarrhea.
Irradiation	Increases risk of myelosuppression with previous irradiation; avoid concomitant irradiation therapy.
Ketoconazole	May increase exposure to irinotecan and active metabolite with ketoconazole (strong CYP3A4 inhibitor). Avoid ketoconazole at least one week prior to starting irinotecan and during irinotecan therapy.
Laxatives	May worsen the incidence or severity of diarrhea.
Neuromuscular blocking agents	Coadministration may prolong neuromuscular blocking effects of suxamethonium. Neuromuscular blockade of non-depolarizing drugs may be antagonized.
Prochlorperazine	May increase risk of akathisia with concomitant prochlorperazine.
Topotecan (Hycamtin Capsules)	
P-glycoprotein inhibitors	May increase topotecan exposure with P-glycoprotein inhibitors (eg, cyclosporine A, elacridar, ketoconazole, ritonavir, saquinavir); avoid concomitant use.

Table 23.2. DRUG INTERACTIONS FOR ANTINEOPLASTIC DRUGS *(cont.)*

TOPOISOMERASE I INHIBITORS *(cont.)*	
Topotecan HCl (Hycamtin Injection)	
G-CSF	Coadministration may prolong the duration of neutropenia; avoid initiation of G-CSF until day 6 of therapy course, 24 hrs after treatment completion with topotecan.
Platinum agents	Sequence-dependent interaction on myelosuppression reported; may increase severity of myelosuppression with coadministration of cytotoxic agents cisplatin or carboplatin.
TOPOISOMERASE II INHIBITOR	
Mitoxantrone (Novantrone)	
Anthracyclines	May increase risk of cardiotoxicity with previous treatment with other anthracyclines.
Antineoplastic agents	Possible development of acute leukemia associated with concomitant antineoplastic agents.
Cardiotoxic drugs	May increase risk of cardiotoxicity with other cardiotoxic drugs.
Radiation therapy	May increase risk of cardiotoxicity with previous or concomitant radiotherapy to the mediastinal/pericardial area.
TYPE II TOPOISOMERASE INHIBITOR	
Teniposide (Vumon)	
Antiemetics	CNS depression and hypotension reported with antiemetics and high-dose teniposide.
Methotrexate	May increase clearance of methotrexate.
Sodium salicylate	May displace protein-bound teniposide; may potentiate toxicity.
Sulfamethizole	May displace protein-bound teniposide; may potentiate toxicity.
Tolbutamide	May displace protein-bound teniposide; may potentiate toxicity.
TYROSINE KINASE INHIBITOR	
Dasatinib (Sprycel)	
Antacids	May alter plasma levels of dasatinib with antacids. Avoid concomitant use or administer antacids at least 2 hours prior to or 2 hours after dose of dasatinib.
CYP3A4 inducers	May decrease plasma levels with CYP3A4 inducers (eg, dexamethasone, phenytoin, carbamazepine, rifampicin, phenobarbital, St. John's wort). Avoid with CYP3A4 inducers or may consider higher doses of dastinib with concomitant use.
CYP3A4 inhibitors	May increase plasma levels with CYP3A4 inhibitors (eg, ketoconazole, itraconazole, erythromycin, clarithromycin, ritonavir, atazanavir, indinavir, nefazodone, nelfinavir, saquinavir, telithromycin, grapefruit juice). Avoid with CYP3A4 inhibitors or consider dose reduction with concomitant use.

TYROSINE KINASE INHIBITOR *(cont.)*

Dasatinib (Sprycel) *(cont.)*	
CYP3A4 substrates	May increase plasma levels of CYP3A4 substrates; caution with CYP3A4 substrates with narrow therapeutic windows (eg, alfentanil, astemizole, terfenadine, cisapride, cyclosporine, fentanyl, pimozide, quinidine, sirolimus, tacrolimus, or ergot alkaloids such as ergotamine and dihydroergotamine).
H_2-antagonists	May decrease exposure to dasatinib with long-term suppression of gastric acid secretion by H_2-antagonists (eg, famotidine); avoid concomitant use.
PPIs	May decrease exposure to dasatinib with long-term suppression of gastric acid secretion by PPIs (eg, omeprazole); avoid concomitant use.

VASCULAR ENDOTHELIAL GROWTH FACTOR (VEGF) INHIBITOR

Bevacizumab (Avastin)	
Chemotherapy	May increase risk of arterial thromboembolic events (ATE) when coadministered with chemotherapy; permanently d/c bevacizumab if severe ATE develops.

VINCA ALKALOIDS

Vinblastine Sulfate	
CYP3A inhibitors	Caution with CYP3A inhibitors (eg, erythromycin); may cause earlier onset and/or increase severity of side effects.
Mitomycin C	May increase risk of acute shortness of breath and severe bronchospasm with mitomycin C.
Phenytoin	May decrease plasma levels of phenytoin; may increase seizure activity.
Vincristine Sulfate	
CYP3A inhibitors	Caution with CYP3A inhibitors (eg, itraconazole); may cause earlier onset and/or increase severity of neuromuscular side effects.
L-asparaginase	May reduce hepatic clearance of vincristine; administer vincristine 12-24 hours before L-asparaginase to minimize toxicity.
Mitomycin C	May increase risk of acute shortness of breath and severe bronchospasm with mitomycin C.
Neurotoxic agents	May increase neurologic side effects with other neurotoxic agents.
Phenytoin	May decrease plasma levels of phenytoin; may increase seizure activity.
Urinary retention, drugs causing	D/C drugs known to cause urinary retention for first few days following vincristine administration.
Vinorelbine Tartrate (Navelbine)	
Cisplatin	May increase occurrence of granulocytopenia with cisplatin.
CYP3A inhibitors	Caution with CYP3A inhibitors; may cause earlier onset and/or increase severity of side effects.
Mitomycin	Risk of acute pulmonary reactions with mitomycin.

Table 23.2. DRUG INTERACTIONS FOR ANTINEOPLASTIC DRUGS *(cont.)*

VINCA ALKALOIDS *(cont.)*	
Vinorelbine Tartrate (Navelbine) *(cont.)*	
Paclitaxel	Monitor for signs and symptoms of neuropathy with concomitant or sequential paclitaxel therapy.
Radiation therapy	Radiosensitizing effect may occur with prior or concomitant radiation therapy.

Section III.

Drug Issues in Dental Practice

Chapter 24

Oral Manifestations of Systemic Agents

B. Ellen Byrne, D.D.S., Ph.D.

Many commonly prescribed medications are capable of causing adverse oral drug reactions. The oral manifestations of drug therapy are often nonspecific and vary in significance. These undesirable effects can mimic many disease processes, such as erythema multiforme. They may also be very characteristic of a particular drug reaction (as in the case of phenytoin and gingival enlargement).

Oral Manifestations

Oral manifestations can be divided into several broad categories: abnormal hemostasis, altered host resistance, angioedema, coated tongue (black hairy tongue), dry socket, dysgeusia (altered taste), erythema multiforme, gingival enlargement, leukopenia and neutropenia, lichenoid lesions, movement disorders, salivary gland enlargement, sialorrhea (increased salivation), soft-tissue reactions, and xerostomia. Table 24 lists systemic drugs that are associated with these side effects, as well as other oropharyngeal manifestations.

Abnormal Hemostasis

Abnormal hemostasis is seen with drugs that interfere with platelet function or that decrease coagulation by depressing prothrombin synthesis in the liver. Patients using such medications require a bleeding profile before undergoing extensive dental procedures.

Altered Host Resistance

Altered host resistance occurs when the microflora of the mouth is altered, resulting in an overgrowth of organisms that are part of the normal oral flora. Bacterial, fungal, and viral superinfections all occur as a result of drug therapy. Broad-spectrum antibiotics and corticosteroids, as well as xerostomia, radiation, and side effects of cancer chemotherapy (and AIDS), can elicit episodes of oral candidiasis. Oropharyngeal candidiasis or thrush has been associated with the use of orally inhaled and oral systemic corticosteroids, while pharyngeal candidiasis has been associated with the use of nasally inhaled and oral systemic corticosteroids. Treatment includes elimination of the causative factor, if possible, combined with use of an antifungal agent, such as nystatin suspension, clotrimazole troche, or ketoconazole tablets. Various conditions such as diabetes, leukemia, lymphomas, and AIDS can also render a patient more susceptible to oral candidal infections.

Angioedema

Angioedema is the result of drug-induced hypersensitivity reactions and can be life-threatening when it involves the mucosal and submucosal layers of the upper aerodigestive tract. Mild angioedema is treated with antihistamines. In more severe cases where the airway is threatened, the emergency treatment is managed the same way as in the case of an anaphylactic reaction. It may occur at any time during treatment with a drug; however, many times it will follow the first dose of a drug.

Coated Tongue (Black Hairy Tongue)

The most common discoloration of the tongue is a condition known as black hairy tongue. This results from hypertrophy of the filiform papillae. This condition is asymptomatic. The color is usually black, but may be various shades of brown. The exact mechanism by which this condition is produced is unknown and there is no effective treatment for this condition.

Dry Socket

Dry socket, or alveolar osteitis, is the result of lysis of a fully formed blood clot before the clot is replaced with granulation tissue. The incidence of dry socket seems to be higher in patients who smoke and in female patients who take oral contraceptives. Dry socket can be minimized in patients taking oral contraceptives if extractions are performed during days 23-28 of the tablet cycle.

Dysgeusia

Dysgeusia is manifested in taste alterations; medication taste; unusual taste; bitter, peculiar, and metallic taste; taste perversion; and changes in taste and distaste for food. Xerostomia, malnutrition, neurological deficiencies, and olfactory deficiencies also can be responsible for taste changes. Although the operative mechanism is unclear, there is some evidence that medications alter taste by affecting trace metal ions, which interact with the cell membrane proteins of the taste pores. There is no treatment other than withdrawal of the drug.

Erythema Multiforme

Erythema multiforme is a syndrome consisting of symmetrical mucocutaneous lesions that have a predilection for the oral mucosa, hands, and feet. It presents initially as erythema, and vesicles and erosions develop within hours. Erythema multiforme usually has its onset from 1-3 weeks after the person begins taking the offending drug. Skin lesions can have concentric rings of erythema, producing the "target" or "bull's-eye" appearance that is associated with this condition. The lesions are normally self-limiting but will persist if the patient continues to take the offending drug. Oral lesions heal without scarring.

Gingival Enlargement

Gingival enlargement has been associated with numerous types of systemic drug therapy, and usually becomes apparent in the first 3 months after drug therapy begins. Clinically, the overgrowth starts as a diffuse swelling of the interdental papillae, which then coalesces for a nodular appearance. Many theories have been suggested to explain the overgrowth. The most attractive theory is that it is a direct effect of the drug or its metabolites on certain subpopulations of fibroblasts, which are capable of greater synthesis of protein and collagen. Many studies have shown a clear relationship between a patient's oral hygiene status and the extent of overgrowth. Also, mouth breathing and other local factors, such as crowding of teeth, significantly relate to the occurrence of gingival enlargement.

Leukopenia and Neutropenia

Many drugs can alter a patient's hematopoietic status. These effects can take the form of leukopenia, agranulocytosis, and neutropenia. These conditions can have a variety of effects in the mouth: increased infections, ulcerations, nonspecific inflammation, bleeding gingiva, and significant bleeding after a dental procedure. Treatment includes discontinuing use of the suspected offending drug and replacing it with a structurally dissimilar agent if continued therapy is indicated.

Lichenoid Lesions

Lichenoid lesions seen with systemic use of drugs differ from actual lichen planus in that the condition resolves when the patient discontinues taking the offending drug. Patients have pain after ulcerations have developed. Buccal mucosa and lateral borders of the tongue are most often involved, and characteristic white striations (Wickham's striae) usually occur.

Movement Disorders

Movement disorders in the muscles of facial expression and mastication can be brought on by systemic drug therapy. These side effects include pseudoparkinsonism (rigidity, bradykinesia, tremor), akathisia (restlessness), and involuntary dystonic movements such as tardive dyskinesia. Tardive dyskinesia is characterized by repetitive, involuntary movements, usually of the mouth and tongue, secondary to long-term neuroleptic drug treatment. This type of movement, once developed, cannot be controlled and is usually irreversible. Tardive dyskinesia occurs in approximately 20% of all patients who take neuroleptic medications regularly. These patients may find it difficult to communicate, eat, and use removable oral prostheses.

Osteonecrosis

Osteonecrosis of the jaw has been reported in cancer patients receiving IV bisphosphonate therapy. The majority of cases have been diagnosed after dental procedures such as tooth extraction. Less commonly, bisphosphonate-associated osteonecrosis of the jaw (BON) appears to occur spontaneously in patients taking these drugs. Rare cases of BON have also been reported in individuals taking orally administered nitrogen-containing bisphosphonates, used for the treatment of osteoporosis. See **Appendix N** for ADA recommendations on the dental management of patients on bisphosphonate therapy.

Typical signs and symptoms of osteonecrosis of the jaw include pain, soft-tissue swelling and infection, loosening of teeth, drainage, and exposed bone, which may occur spontaneously or, more commonly, at the site of previous tooth extraction. Some patients may present with atypical complaints, such as numbness, the feeling of a "heavy jaw," and various dysesthesias. Signs and symptoms that may occur before the development of clinical osteonecrosis include a sudden change in the health of periodontal or mucosal tissues, failure of the oral mucosa to heal, undiagnosed oral pain, loose teeth, or soft-tissue infection.

Salivary Gland Enlargement

Salivary gland problems can appear as salivary gland swelling or pain and can resemble mumps. Differential diagnosis must include salivary gland infections, obstructions, and neoplasms. The mechanism of salivary gland enlargement is unknown, and the treatment is discontinuing the use of the offending drug.

Sialorrhea

Any drug that works by increasing cholinergic stimulation by directly stimulating parasympathetic receptors (such as pilocarpine) or by inhibiting the action of cholinesterase (such as neostigmine) may cause sialorrhea or increased salivation.

Soft-Tissue Reactions

Soft-tissue problems include discoloration, ulcerations, stomatitis, and glossitis. Gingivitis is inflammation of the gingiva, while gingival enlargement is an overgrowth of fibrous gingival tissue.

Xerostomia

Xerostomia, defined as dry mouth or a decrease in salivation, is the most common adverse drug-related effect in the oral cavity. This effect may be exaggerated during prolonged drug use by elderly people and may be even more pronounced when several drugs causing dry mouth are taken simultaneously. Dry mouth can reduce or alter taste sensation as well as impair speech and impede swallowing. Possible nondrug causes of xerostomia include dehydration, salivary gland infection, neoplasm, obstruction, radiation to the mouth, diabetes mellitus, nutritional deficiencies, Sjögren's syndrome, and drugs that either stimulate sympathetic activity or depress parasympathetic activity.

SUGGESTED READING

Ackerman BH, Kasbekar N. Disturbances of taste and smell induced by drugs. *Pharmacotherapy*. 1997;17(3):482-496.

Doty RL, Philip S, Reddy K, et al. Influences of antihypertensives and antihyperlipidemic drugs on the senses of taste and smell: a review. *J Hypertens*. 2003;21:1805-1813.

Felder RS, Millar SB, Henry RH. Oral manifestations of drug therapy. *Spec Care Dentist*. 1988;8(3):119-124.

Femiano F, Lanza A, Buonaiuto C, et al. Oral manifestations of adverse drug reactions: guidelines. *JEADV*. 2008;22:681-691.

Lewis IK, Hanlon JT, Hobbins MJ, et al. Use of medications with potential oral adverse drug reactions in community-dwelling elderly. *Spec Care Dentist*. 1993;13(4):171-176.

Marx RE, Sawatari Y, Fortin M, Broumand V. Bisphosphonate-induced exposed bone (osteonecrosis/osteopetrosis) of the jaws: risk factors, recognition, prevention, and treatment. *J Oral Maxillofac Surg*. 2005;63:1567-1575.

Migliorati CA, Schubert MM, Peterson DE, et al. Bisphosphonate-associated osteonecrosis of mandibular and maxillary bone: an emerging oral complication of supportive cancer therapy. *Cancer*. Jul 1 2005;104(1):83-93.

Mott AE, Grushka M, Sessle BJ. Diagnosis and management of taste disorders and burning mouth syndrome. *Dent Clin North Am*. 1993;37(1):33-71.

Walton JG. Dental disorders. In: Davies DM, ed. *Textbook of Adverse Drug Reactions*. 4th ed. Oxford, England: Oxford University Press; 1991:205-229.

Zelickson BD, Rogers RS 3rd. Oral drug reactions. *Dermatol Clin*. 1987;5(4):695-708.

Table 24. ORAL MANIFESTATIONS OF SYSTEMIC AGENTS

Abscess, periodontal/peritonsillar

- Alefacept (Amevive)
- Arformoterol tartrate (Brovana)
- Aripiprazole (Abilify)
- Bicalutamide (Casodex)
- Cilostazol (Pletal)
- Clindamycin phosphate (Clindesse)
- Delavirdine mesylate (Rescriptor)
- Divalproex sodium (Depakote ER)
- Donepezil hydrochloride (Aricept)
- Doxorubicin hydrochloride liposome (Doxil)
- Fentanyl citrate (Actiq)
- Fluoxetine hydrochloride/Olanzapine (Symbyax)
- Gabapentin (Neurontin)
- Glatiramer acetate (Copaxone)
- Hydrochlorothiazide/Moexipril (Uniretic)
- Modafinil (Provigil)
- Oseltamivir phosphate (Tamiflu)
- Pantoprazole sodium (Protonix)
- Pregabalin (Lyrica)
- Ritonavir (Norvir)
- Rosuvastatin calcium (Crestor)
- Selegiline (Emsam)
- Tacrolimus (Protopic)
- Tiagabine hydrochloride (Gabitril)
- Valproate sodium (Depacon)
- Valproic acid (Depakene)

Aftertaste

- Disulfiram (Antabuse)
- Etoposide (Etopophos, Vepesid)
- Flunisolide (Nasarel)

Ageusia

- Acitretin (Soriatane)
- Alemtuzumab (Campath)
- Amitriptyline hydrochloride
- Amlodipine besylate/Atorvastatin (Caduet)
- Amoxicillin/Clarithromycin/Lansoprazole (PREVPAC)
- Aspirin/Dipyridamole (Aggrenox)
- Atorvastatin calcium (Lipitor)
- Atropine sulfate/Hyoscyamine sulfate/Phenobarbital/Scopolamine hydrobromide (Donnatal)
- Azelastine hydrochloride (Astelin, Astepro)
- Beclomethasone dipropionate monohydrate (Beconase AQ)
- Betaxolol hydrochloride (Kerlone)
- Capecitabine (Xeloda)
- Captopril (Capoten)
- Cefpodoxime proxetil (Vantin)
- Cetirizine hydrochloride (Zyrtec)
- Cetirizine hydrochloride/Pseudoephedrine hydrochloride (Zyrtec-D)
- Ciprofloxacin (Cipro, Cipro XR)
- Cisplatin (Platinol-AQ)
- Citalopram hydrobromide (Celexa)
- Clonazepam (Klonopin)
- Cyclobenzaprine hydrochloride (Flexeril)
- Diclofenac sodium/Misoprostol (Arthrotec)
- Dicyclomine hydrochloride (Bentyl)
- Doxorubicin hydrochloride liposome (Doxil)
- Esomeprazole (Nexium)
- Etidronate disodium (Didronel)
- Flunisolide (Aerobid, Aerobid-M)
- Fluoxetine hydrochloride (Prozac)
- Fluticasone propionate (Flonase)
- Fluvoxamine maleate (Luvox, Luvox CR)
- Gabapentin (Neurontin)
- Glatiramer acetate (Copaxone)
- Glycopyrrolate (Robinul)
- Interferon alfa-2b, recombinant (Intron A)
- Lamotrigine (Lamictal)
- Lansoprazole (Prevacid)
- Levofloxacin (Levaquin)
- Mirtazapine (Remeron)
- Moxifloxacin hydrochloride (Avelox)
- Paroxetine hydrochloride (Paxil, Paxil CR)
- Penicillamine (Cuprimine)
- Pilocarpine hydrochloride (Salagen)
- Pramipexole dihydrochloride (Mirapex)
- Pregabalin (Lyrica)
- Rifaximin (Xifaxan)
- Riluzole (Rilutek)
- Rimantadine hydrochloride (Flumadine)
- Ritonavir (Norvir)
- Rivastigmine tartrate (Exelon)
- sodium oxybate (Xyrem)
- Sulindac (Clinoril)
- Sunitinib malate (Sutent)
- Tamoxifen citrate
- Terbinafine hydrochloride (Lamisil)
- Tiagabine hydrochloride (Gabitril)
- Topiramate (Topamax)
- Valrubicin (Valstar)
- Venlafaxine hydrochloride (Effexor, Effexor XR)
- Voriconazole (Vfend)
- Zaleplon (Sonata)

Airway constriction

- Naratriptan hydrochloride (Amerge)

Table 24. ORAL MANIFESTATIONS OF SYSTEMIC AGENTS *(Cont.)*

Airway obstruction

Calfactant (Infasurf)
Candesartan cilexetil/Hydrochlorothiazide (Atacand HCT)
Captopril (Capoten)
Cetuximab (Erbitux)
Enalapril maleate (Vasotec)
Enalapril maleate/Hydrochlorothiazide (Vaseretic)
Enalaprilat
Eprosartan mesylate/Hydrochlorothiazide (Teveten HCT)
Hydrochlorothiazide/Irbesartan (Avalide)
Hydrochlorothiazide/Losartan potassium (Hyzaar)
Hydrochlorothiazide/Telmisartan (Micardis HCT)
Hydrochlorothiazide/Valsartan (Diovan HCT)
Levofloxacin (Levaquin)
Lisinopril (Prinivil, Zestril)
Lisinopril/Hydrochlorothiazide (Prinzide, Zestoretic)
Lorazepam (Ativan)
Midazolam hydrochloride
Muromonab-cd3 (Orthoclone OKT3)
Naratriptan hydrochloride (Amerge)
Ofloxacin (Floxin)
Propofol (Diprivan)
Ramipril (Altace)
Sevoflurane (Ultane)

Airway resistance

Pilocarpine hydrochloride (Salagen)

Angioedema, glottis

Aliskiren hemifumarate/Hydrochlorothiazide (Tekturna HCT)
Amlodipine besylate/Benazepril hydrochloride (Lotrel)
Benazepril hydrochloride (Lotensin)
Candesartan cilexetil/Hydrochlorothiazide (Atacand HCT)
Captopril (Capoten)
Enalapril maleate (Vasotec)
Enalapril maleate/Hydrochlorothiazide (Vaseretic)
Eprosartan mesylate/Hydrochlorothiazide (Teveten HCT)
Hydrochlorothiazide/Irbesartan (Avalide)
Hydrochlorothiazide/Lisinopril (Prinzide)
Hydrochlorothiazide/Losartan potassium (Hyzaar)
Hydrochlorothiazide/Telmisartan (Micardis HCT)
Hydrochlorothiazide/Valsartan (Diovan HCT)
Lisinopril (Prinivil)
Losartan potassium (Cozaar)
Perindopril erbumine (Aceon)
Ramipril (Altace)
Trandolapril (Mavik)
Trandolapril/Verapamil hydrochloride (Tarka)
Zolpidem tartrate (Ambien)

Angioedema, larynx

Aliskiren hemifumarate/Hydrochlorothiazide (Tekturna HCT)
Alteplase (Activase)
Benazepril hydrochloride (Lotensin)
Candesartan cilexetil/Hydrochlorothiazide (Atacand HCT)
Captopril (Capoten)
Enalapril maleate (Vasotec)
Enalapril maleate/Hydrochlorothiazide (Vaseretic)
Eprosartan mesylate/Hydrochlorothiazide (Teveten HCT)
Hydrochlorothiazide/Irbesartan (Avalide)
Hydrochlorothiazide/Lisinopril (Prinzide)
Hydrochlorothiazide/Losartan potassium (Hyzaar)
Hydrochlorothiazide/Telmisartan (Micardis HCT)
Hydrochlorothiazide/Valsartan (Diovan HCT)
Levofloxacin (Levaquin)
Lisinopril (Prinivil)
Perindopril erbumine (Aceon)
Ramipril (Altace)
Trandolapril (Mavik)
Zolpidem tartrate (Ambien)

Table 24. ORAL MANIFESTATIONS OF SYSTEMIC AGENTS *(Cont.)*

Angioedema, lips

- Albuterol sulfate/Ipratropium bromide (Combivent)
- Aliskiren hemifumarate/Hydrochlorothiazide (Tekturna HCT)
- Amlodipine besylate/Benazepril hydrochloride (Lotrel)
- Benazepril hydrochloride (Lotensin)
- Candesartan cilexetil/Hydrochlorothiazide (Atacand HCT)
- Captopril
- Enalapril maleate (Vasotec)
- Enalapril maleate/Hydrochlorothiazide (Vaseretic)
- Eprosartan mesylate/Hydrochlorothiazide (Teveten HCT)
- Hydrochlorothiazide/Irbesartan (Avalide)
- Hydrochlorothiazide/Lisinopril (Prinzide)
- Hydrochlorothiazide/Losartan potassium (Hyzaar)
- Hydrochlorothiazide/Telmisartan (Micardis HCT)
- Hydrochlorothiazide/Valsartan (Diovan HCT)
- Ipratropium bromide (Atrovent HFA)
- Irbesartan (Avapro)
- Lisinopril (Prinivil)
- Losartan potassium (Cozaar)
- Perindopril erbumine (Aceon)
- Ramipril (Altace)
- Tamsulosin hydrochloride (Flomax)
- Trandolapril (Mavik)

Angioedema, mucous membranes of the mouth

- Alteplase (Activase)
- Captopril

Angioedema, oropharyngeal

- Aliskiren Hemifumarate/Hydrochlorothiazide (Tekturna HCT)
- Hydrochlorothiazide/Irbesartan (Avalide)
- Hydrochlorothiazide/Lisinopril (Prinzide)
- Hydrochlorothiazide/Losartan potassium (Hyzaar)
- Irbesartan (Avapro)
- Losartan potassium (Cozaar)
- Nifedipine (Procardia, Procardia XL)

Angioedema, throat

- Ipratropium bromide (Atrovent)
- Levofloxacin (Levaquin)
- Omalizumab (Xolair)

Angioedema, tongue

- Albuterol sulfate/Ipratropium bromide (Combivent Inhalation Aerosol)
- Aliskiren (Tekturna)
- Aliskiren hemifumarate/Hydrochlorothiazide (Tekturna HCT)
- Amlodipine besylate/Benazepril hydrochloride (Lotrel)
- Benazepril hydrochloride (Lotensin)
- Candesartan cilexetil/Hydrochlorothiazide (Atacand HCT)
- Captopril (Capoten)
- Clonidine (Catapres-TTS)
- Enalapril maleate (Vasotec)
- Enalapril maleate/Hydrochlorothiazide (Vaseretic)
- Eprosartan mesylate/Hydrochlorothiazide (Teveten HCT)
- Hydrochlorothiazide/Irbesartan (Avalide)
- Hydrochlorothiazide/Lisinopril (Prinzide)
- Hydrochlorothiazide/Losartan potassium (Hyzaar)
- Hydrochlorothiazide/Telmisartan (Micardis HCT)
- Hydrochlorothiazide/Valsartan (Diovan HCT)
- Ipratropium bromide (Atrovent HFA)
- Irbesartan (Avapro)
- Levofloxacin (Levaquin)
- Lisinopril (Prinivil)
- Losartan potassium (Cozaar)
- Omalizumab (Xolair)
- Perindopril erbumine (Aceon)
- Ramipril (Altace)
- Tamsulosin hydrochloride (Flomax)
- Trandolapril (Mavik)
- Zolpidem tartrate (Ambien)

Table 24. ORAL MANIFESTATIONS OF SYSTEMIC AGENTS *(Cont.)*

Bleeding, dental

Acitretin (Soriatane)
Alteplase (Activase)
Amoxicillin/Clarithromycin/Lansoprazole (PREVPAC)
Amphotericin B, liposomal (AmBisome)
Aripiprazole (Abilify)
Aspirin/Dipyridamol (Aggrenox)
Atorvastatin calcium (Lipitor)
Bevacizumab (Avastin)
Bupropion hydrochloride (Wellbutrin SR, Wellbutrin XL, Zyban SR)
Cilostazol (Pletal)
Citalopram hydrobromide (Celexa)
Clofarabine (Clolar)
Cyclosporine (Gengraf, Neoral)
Decitabine (Dacogen)
Delavirdine mesylate (Rescriptor)
Divalproex sodium (Depakote, Depakote ER)
Doxorubicin hydrochloride liposome (Doxil)
Fentanyl citrate (Actiq)
Fluoxetine hydrochloride (Prozac)
Gabapentin (Neurontin)
Glatiramer acetate (Copaxone)
Indinavir sulfate (Crixivan)
Interferon alfa-2b, recombinant (Intron A)
Isotretinoin (Accutane)
Lamotrigine (Lamictal)
Lansoprazole (Prevacid)
Mechlorethamine hydrochloride (Mustargen)
Mirtazapine (Remeron)
Oxcarbazepine (Trileptal)
Pentosan polysulfate sodium (Elmiron)
Propafenone hydrochloride (Rythmol, Rythmol SR)
Quetiapine fumarate (Seroquel)
Riluzole (Rilutek)
Sunitinib malate (Sutent)
Topiramate (Topamax)
Venlafaxine hydrochloride (Effexor, Effexor XR)
Voriconazole (VFEND)
Warfarin sodium (Coumadin)
Zaleplon (Sonata)
Zidovudine (Retrovir)
Ziprasidone hydrochloride (Geodon)
Zonisamide (Zonegran)

Bleeding, gums

Amlodipine besylate/Atorvastatin calcium (Caduet)
Fluoxetine hydrochloride/Olanzapine (Symbyax)
Gemtuzumab ozogamicin (Mylotarg)
Lansoprazole (Prevacid)
Nifedipine (Procardia, Procardia XL)
Pentosan polysulfate sodium (Elmiron)

Bleeding, lip

Gabapentin (Neurontin)

Bleeding, mouth

Abciximab (ReoPro)
Cevimeline hydrochloride (Evoxac)
Interferon alfa-2b, recombinant (Intron A)

Bleeding, mucosal

Venlafaxine hydrochloride (Effexor, Effexor XR)
Sodium phosphate monobasic monohydrate/sodium phosphate dibasic anhydrous (Visicol)

Bleeding, oropharyngeal

Eptifibatide (Integrilin)
Tenecteplase (Tnkase)

Bleeding tendency, increased

Cilostazol (Pletal)
Montelukast sodium (Singulair)
Paroxetine hydrochloride (Paxil, Paxil CR)

Table 24. ORAL MANIFESTATIONS OF SYSTEMIC AGENTS *(Cont.)*

Bleeding time, prolongation

Acitretin (Soriatane)
Antihemophilic factor (recombinant) (Advate)
Aspirin (St. Joseph's Aspirin)
Clavulanate potassium/Ticarcllin disodium (Timentin)
Diclofenac (Flector, Voltaren, Voltaren-XR)
Diltiazem hydrochloride (Cardizem, Cardizem LA)
Divalproex sodium (Depakote, Depakote ER)
Fentanyl citrate (Actiq)
Gabapentin (Neurontin)
Hydrocodone bitartrate/Ibuprofen (Vicoprofen)
Ketorolac tromethamine (Acular)
Mefenamic acid (Ponstel)
Naproxen (EC-Naprosyn, Naprosyn, Anaprox, Anaprox DS)
Paroxetine hydrochloride (Paxil, Paxil CR)
Pentosan polysulfate sodium (Elmiron)
Piperacillin sodium/Tazobactam sodium (Zosyn)
Propafenone hydrochloride (Rythmol)
Sulindac (Clinoril)
Tolmetin sodium (Tolectin DS)
Venlafaxine hydrochloride (Effexor, Effexor XR)
Voriconazole (VFEND)

Buccoglossal syndrome

Aripiprazole (Abilify)
Fluoxetine hydrochloride (Prozac)
Fluoxetine hydrochloride/Olanzapine (Symbyax)
Olanzapine (Zyprexa, Zyprexa ZYDIS)
Quetiapine fumarate (Seroquel)
Venlafaxine hydrochloride (Effexor, Effexor XR)
Ziprasidone hydrochloride (Geodon)

Candidiasis, oral

Amoxicillin/Clavulanate potassium (Augmentin)
Amoxicillin/Clarithromycin/Lansoprazole (PREVPAC)
Anti-Thymocyte Globulin
Arformoterol tartrate (Brovana)
Aripiprazole (Abilify)
Arsenic trioxide (Trisenox)
Atovaquone (Mepron)
Azithromycin (Zithromax, Zmax)
Bortezomib (Velcade)
Budesonide (Pulmicort)
Budesonide/Formoterol fumarate dihydrate (Symbicort)
Capecitabine (Xeloda)
Cefazolin sodium
Cefditoren pivoxil (Spectracef)
Cefepime hydrochloride (Maxipime)
Cefpodoxime proxetil (Vantin)
Ceftazidime (Fortaz)
Ciclesonide (Alvesco)
Ciprofloxacin hydrochloride (Cipro, Cipro XR)
Clofarabine (Clolar)
Conivaptan hydrochloride (Vaprisol)
Dalfopristin/Quinupristin (Synercid)
Daptomycin (Cubicin)
Decitabine (Dacogen)
Delavirdine mesylate (Rescriptor)
Doripenem (Doribax)
Doxorubicin hydrochloride liposome (Doxil)
Ertapenem sodium (Invanz)
Fentanyl citrate (Actiq, Fentora)
Fluticasone propionate (Flovent Diskus, Flovent HFA)
Fluticasone propionate/Salmeterol xinafoate (Advair Diskus, Advair HFA)
Gabapentin (Neurontin)
Glatiramer acetate (Copaxone)
Griseofulvin (Gris-PEG)
Haemophilus b conjugate vaccine/Hepatitis b vaccine, recombinant (Comvax)
Hyoscyamine
Lansoprazole (Prevacid)
Leflunomide (Arava)
Linezolid (Zyvox)
Megestrol acetate (Megace ES)
Meropenem (Merrem)
Mometasone furoate (Asmanex, Nasonex)
Moxifloxacin hydrochloride (Avelox)
Mycophenolate mofetil (Cellcept)
Mycophenolic acid (Myfortic)
Olanzapine (Zyprexa)
Oprelvekin (Neumega)
Palivizumab (Synagis)
Pantoprazole sodium (Protonix)
Piperacillin sodium/Tazobactam sodium (Zosyn)
Pneumococcal vaccine, diphtheria conjugate (Prevnar)
Posaconazole (Noxafil)
Pramipexole dihydrochloride (Mirapex)
Salmeterol xinafoate (Serevent Diskus)
Sirolimus (Rapamune)
Tacrolimus (Prograf, Protopic)
Telithromycin (Ketek)
Thalidomide (Thalomid)
Tinidazole (Tindamax)
Tiotropium bromide (Spiriva)
Triamcinolone acetonide (Azmacort)
Venlafaxine hydrochloride (Effexor, Effexor XR)

Table 24. ORAL MANIFESTATIONS OF SYSTEMIC AGENTS *(Cont.)*

Candidiasis, pharynx

Beclomethasone dipropionate (Qvar)
Fluticasone propionate/Salmeterol xinafoate (Advair Diskus, Advair HFA)
Salmeterol xinafoate (Serevent Diskus)
Triamcinolone acetonide (Azmacort)

Carcinoma, laryngeal

Amoxicillin/Clarithromycin/Lansoprazole (PREVPAC)
Lansoprazole (Prevacid)

Cheek puffing

Amitriptyline hydrochloride
Chlorpromazine
Haloperidol (Haldol)
Molindone hydrochloride (Moban)
Pimozide (Orap)
Prochlorperazine (Compro)
Thiothixene hydrochloride (Navane)
Trifluoperazine hydrochloride

Cheilitis

Acitretin (Soriatane)
Amlodipine besylate/Atorvastatin calcium (Caduet)
Atorvastatin calcium (Lipitor)
Bexarotene (Targretin)
Candesartan cilexetil/Hydrochlorothiazide (Atacand)
Dactinomycin (Cosmegen)
Eprosartan mesylate/Hydrochlorothiazide (Teveten HCT)
Fentanyl citrate (Actiq)
Frovatriptan succinate (Frova)
Irbesartan (Avapro)
Irbesartan/Hydrochlorothiazide (Avalide)
Isotretinoin (Accutane)
Lisinopril (Prinivil, Zestril)
Lisinopril/Hydrochlorothiazide (Prinzide, Zestoretic)
Losartan potassium (Cozaar)
Losartan potassium/Hydrochlorothiazide (Hyzaar)
Penicillamine (Cuprimine)
Pramipexole dihydrochloride (Mirapex)
Riluzole (Rilutek)
Ritonavir (Norvir)
Saquinavir (Invirase)
Tacrolimus (Protopic)
Telmisartan/Hydrochlorothiazide (Micardis HCT)
Valsartan/Hydrochlorothiazide (Diovan HCT)
Venlafaxine hydrochloride (Effexor, Effexor XR)
Voriconazole (VFEND)
Zaleplon (Sonata)

Chewing movements

Chlorpromazine
Haloperidol (Haldol)
Molindone hydrochloride (Moban)
Perphenazine
Pimozide (Orap)
Prochlorperazine (Compro)
Thioridazine hydrochloride
Thiothixene hydrochloride (Navane)
Trifluoperazine hydrochloride (Stelazine)

Clotting time, prolongation

Cefditoren pivoxil (Spectracef)
Diclofenac sodium/Misoprostol (Arthrotec)
Oxymetholone (Anadrol)
Pegaspargase (Oncaspar)
Piperacillin sodium/Tazobactam sodium (Zosyn)
Sertraline hydrochloride (Zoloft)
Testosterone (Testim)

Coagulation dysfunction

Aldesleukin (Proleukin)
Alemtuzumab (Campath)
Aminocaproic acid (Amicar)
Amiodarone hydrochloride (Pacerone)
Amphotericin B (Abelcet, AmBisome)
Antihemophilic factor (recombinant) (NovoSeven)
Asparaginase (Elspar)
BCG, live (intravesical) (Tice BCG)
Capecitabine (Xeloda)
Cefdinir (Omnicef)
Citalopram hydrobromide (Celexa)
Clopidogrel bisulfate (Plavix)
Divalproex sodium (Depakote ER)
Estrogens, conjugated (Premarin)
Estrogens, esterified/Methyltestosterone (Estratest, Estratest H.S.)
Ethinyl estradiol/Norgestrel (Lo/Ovral-28)
Fluoxetine hydrochloride/Olanzapine (Symbyax)
Gabapentin (Neurontin)
Methyltestosterone (Android, Testred)
Muromonab-cd3 (Orthoclone OKT3)
Mycophenolate mofetil (CellCept)
Nimodipine (Nimotop)

Table 24. ORAL MANIFESTATIONS OF SYSTEMIC AGENTS *(Cont.)*

Coagulation dysfunction *(Cont.)*

Pegaspargase (Oncaspar)
Propofol (Diprivan)
Rituximab (Rituxan)
Sargramostim (Leukine)
Tacrolimus (Prograf)
Topotecan hydrochloride (Hycamtin)
Trastuzumab (Herceptin)
Valproate sodium (Depacon)
Valproic acid (Depakene)

Coagulopathy

Aldesleukin (Proleukin)
Aspirin (Bayer Aspirin, St. Joseph's Aspirin)
Aspirin/Dipyridamole (Aggrenox)
BCG, live (intravesical) (Tice BCG)
Caspofungin acetate (Cancidas)
Coagulation factor VIIa, recombinant (NovoSeven RT)
Etanercept (Enbrel)
Ixabepilone (Ixempra)
Micafungin sodium (Mycamine)
Pegaspargase (Oncaspar)
Sodium benzoate/Sodium phenylacetate (Ammonul)

Cold sore, non-herpetic

Interferon alfa-2b, recombinant (Intron A)
Naltrexone hydrochloride (Revia)
Varicella virus vaccine, live (Varivax)

Cough

Abacavir sulfate/Lamivudine (Epzicom)
Abacavir sulfate/Lamivudine/Zidovudine (Trizivir)
Adenosine (Adenoscan)
Agalsidase beta (Fabrazyme)
Albuterol sulfate (Ventolin HFA)
Albuterol sulfate/Ipratropium bromide (Combivent)
Aldesleukin (Proleukin)
Alefacept (Amevive)
Alemtuzumab (Campath)
Aliskiren (Tekturna)
Aliskiren hemifumarate/Hydrochlorothiazide (Tekturna HCT)
Alosetron hydrochloride (Lotronex)
Alpha1-Proteinase Inhibitor (human) (Aralast, Zemaira)
Alprostadil (Caverject)
Amiloride hydrochloride (Midamor)
Amiloride hydrochloride/Hydrochlorothiazide
Amiodarone hydrochloride (Pacerone, Cordarone)
Amlodipine besylate (Norvasc)
Amlodipine besylate/Atorvastatin calcium (Caduet)
Amlodipine besylate/Benazepril hydrochloride (Lotrel)
Amlodipine besylate/Valsartan (Exforge)
Amoxicillin/clarithromycin/lansoprazole (PREVPAC)
Amphotericin B, liposomal (AmBisome)
Anagrelide hydrochloride (Agrylin)
Anastrozole (Arimidex)
Antihemophilic factor (recombinant) (Advate, ReFacto)
Aprepitant (Emend)
Argatroban
Aripiprazole (Abilify)
Arsenic trioxide (Trisenox)
Aspirin/Dipyridamole (Aggrenox)
Atazanavir sulfate (Reyataz)
Atomoxetine hydrochloride (Strattera)
Atovaquone (Mepron)
Atovaquone/Proguanil hydrochloride (Malarone)
Azelastine hydrochloride (Astepro, Astelin)
Azithromycin (Zithromax)
Balsalazide disodium (Colazal)
Basiliximab (Simulect)
BCG, live (intravesical) (Tice BCG)
Beclomethasone dipropionate (QVAR)
Benazepril hydrochloride (Lotensin)
Bendamustine hydrochloride (Treanda)
Bendroflumethiazide/Nadolol (Corzide)
Betaxolol hydrochloride (Kerlone)
Bexarotene (Targretin)
Bicalutamide (Casodex)
Bortezomib (Velcade)
Botulinum toxin type A (Botox Purified Neurotoxin Complex)
Brimonidine tartrate (Alphagan P)
Brimonidine tartrate/Timolol maleate (Combigan)
Budesonide (Pulmicort, Rhinocort)
Buprenorphine hydrochloride (Subutex)
Buprenorphine HCl/Naloxone HCl (Suboxone)
Bupropion hydrochloride (Wellbutrin SR, Wellbutrin XL, Zyban SR)
Busulfan (Busulfex)
Calcitonin-salmon (Miacalcin)
Calcium carbonate/Risedronate sodium (Actonel with Calcium)
Candesartan cilexetil (Atacand)
Candesartan cilexetil/Hydrochlorothiazide (Atacand HCT)
Capecitabine (Xeloda)
Captopril
Carbidopa/Entacapone/Levodopa (Stalevo)
Carbidopa/Levodopa (Parcopa, Sinemet)
Carteolol hydrochloride
Carvedilol hydrochloride (Coreg)
Caspofungin acetate (Cancidas)
Cefaclor (Ceclor)
Cefpodoxime proxetil (Vantin)
Cefuroxime axetil (Ceftin)
Celecoxib (Celebrex)
Cetirizine hydrochloride (Zyrtec)
Cetirizine hydrochloride/Pseudoephedrine (Zyrtec-D)
Cetuximab (Erbitux)
Cevimeline hydrochloride (Evoxac)
Chlorambucil (Leukeran)

Table 24. ORAL MANIFESTATIONS OF SYSTEMIC AGENTS *(Cont.)*

Cough *(Cont.)*

Choriogonadotropin alfa (Ovidrel)
Ciclesonide (Alvesco)
Cilostazol (Pletal)
Citalopram hydrobromide (Celexa)
Cladribine (Leustatin)
Clindamycin phosphate/Tretinoin (Ziana)
Clofarabine (Clolar)
Clonazepam (Klonopin)
Clopidogrel bisulfate (Plavix)
Clozapine (Clozaril, Fazaclo)
Coagulation Factor IX (Recombinant) (BeneFIX)
Colesevelam hydrochloride (Welchol)
Cromolyn sodium (Intal)
Cyclosporine (Gengraf, Neoral)
Cytarabine liposome (DepoCyt)
Dapsone (Aczone)
Daptomycin (Cubicin)
Darbepoetin alfa (Aranesp)
Daxlizumab (Zenapax)
Decitabine (Dacogen)
Deferasirox (Exjade)
Delavirdine mesylate (Rescriptor)
Denileukin diftitox (Ontak)
Desflurane (Suprane)
Desloratadine (Clarinex)
Desmopressin acetate (DDAVP)
Desonide (Verdeso)
Dexlansoprazole (Kapidex)
Diazepam (Valium, Diastat)
Diclofenac sodium (Voltaren)
Diltiazem hydrochloride (Cardizem LA)
Diphtheria and tetanus toxoids and acellular pertussis adsorbed, inactivated poliovirus and haemophilus B conjugate (tetanus toxoid conjugate) vaccine (Pentacel)
Divalproex sodium (Depakote ER)
Docetaxel (Taxotere)
Dornase alfa (Pulmozyme)
Dorzolamide hydrochloride/Timolol maleate (Cosopt)
Doxapram hydrochloride (Dopram)
Doxercalciferol (Hectorol)
Doxorubicin hydrochloride liposome (Doxil)
Dronabinol (Marinol)
Drospirenone/Ethinyl estradiol (Yaz)
Duloxetine hydrochloride (Cymbalta)
Efavirenz (Sustiva)
Eletriptan hydrobromide (Relpax)
Emtricitabine (Emtriva)
Emtricitabine/Tenofovir disoproxil fumarate (Truvada)
Enalapril maleate (Vasotec)
Enalapril maleate/hydrochlorothiazide (Vaseretic)
Enfuvirtide (Fuzeon)
Epinastine hydrochloride (Elestat)
Eplerenone (Inspra)
Epoetin alfa (Epogen, Procrit)
Epoprostenol sodium (Flolan)
Eprosartan mesylate (Teveten)
Eprosartan mesylate/ Hydrochlorothiazide (Teveten HCT)
Erlotinib (Tarceva)
Ertapenem (Invanz)
Escitalopram oxalate (Lexapro)
Esomeprazole (Nexium)
Estradiol (Vivelle, Vivelle-dot)
Estradiol/Norgestimate (Prefest)
Estrogens, conjugated (Cenestin, Premarin)
Estrogens, conjugated/ Medroxyprogesterone acetate (Prempro, Premphase)
Etanercept (Enbrel)
Etonogestrel (Implanon)
Etoposide/etoposide phosphate (Vepesid, Etopophos)
Exemestane (Aromasin)
Ezetimibe (Zetia)
Febuxostat (Uloric)
Felodipine (Plendil)
Fenofibrate (Antara, Tricor)
Fentanyl (Duragesic, Actiq, Fentora)
Fexofenadine hydrochloride (Allegra)
Filgrastim (Neupogen)
Flunisolide hemihydrate (Aerobid, Aerobid M)
Fluoxetine hydrochloride (Prozac)
Fluticasone (Flonase, Flovent Diskus, Flovent HFA, Veramyst)
Fluticasone propionate/Salmeterol xinafoate (Advair Diskus, Advair HFA)
Fluvastatin sodium (Lescol, Lescol XL)
Fluvoxamine maleate (Luvox)
Follitropin alfa (Gonal-f)
Fondaparinux sodium (Arixtra)
Fosaprepitant dimeglumine (Emend)
Foscarnet sodium (Foscavir)
Fosinopril sodium (Monopril)
Fulvestrant (Faslodex)
Gabapentin (Neurontin)
Galantamine hydrobromide (Razadyne)
Ganciclovir
Gemcitabine hydrochloride (Gemzar)
Gemtuzumab ozogamicin (Mylotarg)
Glatiramer acetate (Copaxone)
Goserelin acetate (Zoladex)
Haemophilus B conjugate vaccine/ Hepatitis B vaccine, recombinant (Comvax)
Hepatitis A vaccine, inactivated (Vaqta)
Hepatitis B vaccine, recombinant (Recombivax HB)
Hydrochlorothiazide/Olmesartan medoxomil (Benicar HCT)
Hydrocodone bitartrate/Ibuprofen (Vicoprofen)
Ibritumomab tiuxetan (Zevalin)
Iloprost (Ventavis)
Imatinib mesylate (Gleevec)
Imiglucerase (Cerezyme)
Imiquimod (Aldara)
Immune globulin intravenous (human) (Flebogamma, Gammagard)
Indapamide
Indinavir sulfate (Crixivan)
Infliximab (Remicade)
Influenza virus vaccine (Fluarix, Flulaval)
Influenza virus vaccine live, intranasal (FluMist)
Interferon alfa-2b, recombinant (Intron A)
Interferon alfa-n3 (human leukocyte derived) (Alferon N)
Iodine I 131 Tositumomab (Bexxar)
Ipratropium bromide (Atrovent HFA)

Table 24. ORAL MANIFESTATIONS OF SYSTEMIC AGENTS *(Cont.)*

Cough *(Cont.)*

Irbesartan (Avapro)
Irbesartan/Hydrochlorothiazide (Avalide)
Irinotecan hydrochloride (Camptosar)
Isosorbide mononitrate (Ismo)
Isradipine (DynaCirc CR)
Itraconazole (Sporanox)
Ixabepilone (Ixempra)
Lamivudine (Epivir, Epivir-HBV)
Lamivudine/Zidovudine (Combivir)
Lamotrigine (Lamictal)
Lansoprazole (Prevacid)
Laronidase (Aldurazyme)
Lefluonimde (Arava)
Lepirudin (Refludan)
Letrozole (Femara)
Levalbuterol (Xopenex, Xopenex HFA)
Levetiracetam (Keppra)
Levocarnitine (Carnitor)
Levocetirizine dihydrochloride (Xyzal)
Levofloxacin (Levaquin)
Linezolid (Zyvox)
Lisinopril (Prinivil, Zestril)
Lisinopril/Hydrochlorothiazide (Prinzide, Zestoretic)
Loratadine (Claritin)
Loratadine/Pseudoephedrine sulfate (Claritin-D)
Losartan potassium (Cozaar)
Losartan potassium/ Hydrochlorothiazide (Hyzaar)
Lubiprostone (Amitiza)
Maraviroc (Selzentry)
Measles virus vaccine, live (Attenuvax)
Measles, mumps & rubella virus vaccine, live (M-M-R II, Proquad)
Measles, mumps, rubella and varicella virus vaccine live (ProQuad)
Megestrol acetate (Megace ES)
Meloxicam (Mobic)
Melphalan hydrochloride (Alkeran)
Memantine hydrochloride (Namenda)
Menotropins (Menopur)
Meropenem (Merrem)
Mesalamine (Asacol)
Methotrexate
Methylphenidate hydrochloride (Concerta, Concerta ER)
Metipranolol (OptiPranolol, Metipranolol)
Micafungin sodium (Mycamine)
Midazolam hydrochloride
Minocycline hydrochloride (Minocin, Dynacin)
Mirtazapine (Remeron)
Mitomycin (Mitomycin-C, Mutamycin)
Mitoxantrone hydrochloride (Novantrone)
Modafinil (Provigil)
Moexipril hydrochloride (Univasc)
Mometasone furoate monohydrate (Nasonex)
Montelukast sodium (Singulair)
Moxifloxacin hydrochloride (Vigamox)
Mumps virus vaccine, live (Mumpsvax)
Mupirocin calcium (Bactroban)
Mycophenolate mofetil (Cellcept)
Mycophenolic acid (Myfortic)
Nabumetone
Nadolol (Corgard)
Naltrexone hydrochloride (Revia)
Naratriptan hydrochloride (Amerge)
Nateglinide (Starlix)
Nedocromil (Alocril)
Nelarabine (Arranon)
Nesiritide (Natrecor)
Nicotine (Nicotrol)
Nifedipine (Procardia, Procardia XL)
Nilotinib (Tasigna)
Nisoldipine (Sular)
Nitrofurantoin (Furadantin)
Nizatidine (Axid)
Ofloxacin (Floxin)
Olanzapine (Zyprexa, Zyprexa ZYDIS)
Olopatadine hydrochloride (Patanase)
Omalizumab (Xolair)
Omega-3-acid ethyl esters (Lovaza)
Omeprazole (Prilosec)
Omeprazole/sodium bicarbonate/ magnesium (Zegerid w/Magnesium Hydroxide)
Oprelvekin (Neumega)
Oseltamivir phosphate (Tamiflu)
Oxaliplatin (Eloxatin)
Oxcarbazepine (Trileptal)
Oxybtuynin chloride (Ditropan)
Oxycodone hydrochloride (OxyContin)
Palivizumab (Synagis)
Pamidronate (Aredia)
Pancrelipase (Creon)
Panitumumab (Vectibix)
Pantoprazole sodium (Protonix)
Paroxetine hydrochloride (Paxil, Paxil CR)
Pegasparase (Oncaspar)
Peginterferon alfa-2b, alfa-2a (PegIntron, Pegasys)
Pemirolast potassium (Alamast)
Penbutolol sulfate (Levatol)
Pentostatin (Nipent)
Perindopril erbumine (Aceon)
Pimecrolimus (Elidel)
Piperacillin sodium/Tazobactam sodium (Zosyn)
Pirbuterol acetate (Maxair)
Porfimer sodium (Photofrin)
Posaconazole (Noxafil)
Pramipexole dihydrochloride (Mirapex)
Pravastatin sodium (Pravachol)
Procarbazine hydrochloride (Matulane)
Progesterone (Prometrium)
Propafenone hydrochloride (Rythmol, Rythmol SR)
Propofol (Diprivan)
Quadrivalent human papillomavirus (types 6, 11, 16, 18) recombinant vaccine (Gardasil)
Quetiapine fumarate (Seroquel, Seroquel XR)
Raloxifene hydrochloride (Evista)
Ramipril (Altace)
Ranibizumab (Lucentis)
Ribavirin (Rebetol)
Riluzole (Rilutek)
Rimantadine hydrochloride (Flumadine)
Risperidone (Risperdal Consta)
Ritonavir (Norvir)
Rituximab (Rituxan)
Rivastigmine tartrate (Exelon)

Table 24. ORAL MANIFESTATIONS OF SYSTEMIC AGENTS *(Cont.)*

Cough *(Cont.)*

Rizatriptan benzoate (Maxalt, Maxalt-MLT)
Ropinirole hydrochloride (Requip, Requip XL)
Ropivacaine hydrochloride (Naropin)
Rosuvastatin calcium (Crestor)
Rotavirus vaccine, live, oral (Rotarix)
Rotigotine (Neupro)
Rubella virus vaccine, live (Meruvax II)
Saquinavir mesylate (Invirase)
Selegiline (Emsam)
Sertraline hydrochloride (Zoloft)
Sevelamer hydrochloride (Renagel)
Sevoflurane (Ultane)
Sibutramine hydrochloride monohydrate (Meridia)
Sildenafil citrate (Viagra)
Sirolimus (Rapamune)
Sodium ferric gluconate (Ferrlecit)
Sodium oxybate (Xyrem)
Solifenacin succinate (VESIcare)
Somatropin (Humatrope)
Succimer (Chemet)
Sulfamethoxazole/trimethoprim (Bactrim, Septra)
Sumatriptan succinate (Imitrex)
Sumatriptan succinate/Naproxen sodium (Treximet)
Sunitinib malate (Sutent)
Tacrolimus (Prograf, Prototopic)
Tadalafil (Cialis)
Tamoxifen citrate
Tamsulosin hydrochloride (Flomax)
Telbivudine (Tyzeka)
Telmisartan (Micardis)
Telmisartan/Hydrochlorothiazide (Micardis HCT)
Temozolomide (Temodar)
Temsirolimus (Torisel)
Terbinafine hydrochloride (Lamisil)
Teriparatide (Forteo)
Tiagabine hydrochloride (Gabitril)
Timolol maleate (Timoptic, Timoptic-XE)
Tiotropium bromide (Spiriva)
Tipranavir (Aptivus)
Tolterodine tartrate (Detrol)
Topiramate (Topamax)
Topotecan hydrochloride (Hycamtin)
Torsemide (Demadex)
Tramadol hydrochloride (Ultram ER)
Trandolapril (Mavik)
Trandolapril/Verapamil hydrochloride (Tarka)
Trastuzumab (Herceptin)
Triamcinolone acetonide (Azmacort)
Triptorelin pamoate (Trelstar)
Valganciclovir hydrochloride (Valcyte)
Valproate sodium (Depacon)
Valproic acid (Depakene)
Valsartan (Diovan)
Valsartan/Hydrochlorothiazide (Diovan HCT)
Varicella virus vaccine, live (Varivax)
Venlafaxine hydrochloride (Effexor, Effexor XR)
Verteporfin (Visudyne)
Vinorelbine tartrate (Navelbine)
Voriconazole (VFEND)
Vorinostat (Zolinza)
Zanamivir (Relenza)
Zidovudine (Retrovir)
Ziprasidone hydrochloride (Geodon)
Zoledronic acid (Zometa)
Zolmitriptan (Zomig)
Zolpidem tartrate (Ambien, Ambien CR)

Cough reflex, depression

Acetaminophen/Hydrocodone bitartrate (Lortab, Vicodin)
Chlorpromazine
Fluoxetine hydrochloride (Prozac, Sarafem)
Morphine sulfate (Astramorph/PF, Avinza, Avinza ER, Depodur, Duramorph, Infumorph, Kadian ER, MS Contin, Oramorph ER)
Prochlorperazine (Compro)

Craniofacial deformities

Amlodipine besylate/Benazepril hydrochloride (Lotrel)
Candesartan cilexetil (Atacand)
Candesartan cilexetil/Hydrochlorothiazide (Atacand HCT)
Captopril (Capoten)
Enalapril maleate (Vasotec)
Enalapril maleate/Hydrochlorothiazide (Vaseretic)
Hydrochlorothiazide
Eprosartan mesylate (Teveten)
Eprosartan mesylate/Hydrochlorothiazide (Teveten HCT)
Hydrochlorothiazide/Irbesartan (Avalide)
Hydrochlorothiazide/Telmisartan (Micardis HCT)
Hydrochlorothiazide/Valsartan (Diovan HCT)
Lisinopril (Prinivil, Zestril)
Lisinopril/Hydrochlorothiazide (Prinzide, Zestoretic)
Losartan potassium (Cozaar)
Losartan potassium/Hydrochlorothiazide (Hyzaar)
Ramipril (Altace)

Table 24. ORAL MANIFESTATIONS OF SYSTEMIC AGENTS *(Cont.)*

Dental caries

Aripiprazole (Abilify)
Candesartan cilexetil/Hydrochlorothiazide (Atacand HCT)
Cetirizine hydrochloride/Pseudoephedrine hydrochloride (Zyrtec-D)
Eprosartan mesylate/Hydrochlorothiazide (Teveten HCT)
Fentanyl citrate (Actiq)
Fluoxetine hydrochloride/Olanzapine (Symbyax)
Fluvoxamine maleate (Luvox)
Glatiramer acetate (Copaxone)
Hydrochlorothiazide
Hydrochlorothiazide/Irbesartan (Avalide)
Hydrochlorothiazide/Lisinopril (Prinzide)
Hydrochlorothiazide/Losartan potassium (Hyzaar)
Hydrochlorothiazide/Telmisartan (Micardis HCT)
Hydrochlorothiazide/Valsartan (Diovan HCT)
Hyoscyamine
Lithium carbonate (Eskalith, Lithobid ER)
Loratadine (Claritin)
Paroxetine hydrochloride (Paxil)
Pramipexole dihydrochloride (Mirapex)
Quetiapine fumarate (Seroquel)
Selegiline (Eldepryl, Emsam)
Sertraline hydrochloride (Zoloft)
Sodium oxybate (Xyrem)
Tacrolimus (Protopic)
Tiagabine hydrochloride (Gabitril)
Zolpidem tartrate (Ambien, Ambien CR)

Dermatitis, perioral

Alclometasone dipropionate (Aclovate)
Bacitracin zinc/Hydrocortisone/Neomycin sulfate/Polymyxin B sulfate (Cortisporin)
Benzoyl peroxide/Hydrocortisone (Vanoxide-HC)
Betamethasone dipropionate (Diprolene AF, Luxiq)
Clobetasol propionate (Olux, Olux-E)
Clocortolone pivalate (Cloderm)
Betamethasone dipropionate/Clotrimazole (Lotrisone)
Desonide (Verdeso)
Desoximetasone (Topicort)
Diflorasone diacetate (Psorcon)
Fluocinolone acetonide (Synalar)
Fluocinolone acetonide/Hydroquinone/Tretinoin (Tri-Luma)
Fluocinonide (Vanos)
Fluticasone propionate (Cutivate)
Halobetasol propionate (Ultravate)
Hydrocortisone acetate/Pramoxine hydrochloride (Analpram HC, Pramosone)
Hydrocortisone butyrate (Lipocream, Locoid, Pandel)
Hydrocortisone/Neomycin sulfate/Polymyxin B sulfate (Pediotic)
Mometasone Furoate (Elocon)
Prednicarbate (Dermatop)

Drooling

Chlorpromazine
Dantrolene sodium (Dantrium)
Donepezil hydrochloride (Aricept)
Metyrosine (Demser)
Midazolam hydrochloride
Paliperidone (Invega)
Prochlorperazine (Compro)
Quetiapine fumarate (Seroquel, Seroquel XR)
Thioridazine hydrochloride
Thiothixene hydrochloride (Navane)

Dryness, mucous membrane

Busulfan (Myleran)
Candesartan cilexetil/Hydrochlorothiazide (Atacand HCT)
Carbetapentane tannate/Chlorpheniramine tannate (Tussi-12)
Carbetapentane tannate/Chlorpheniramine tannate/Ephedrine tannate/Phenyephrine tannate (Rynatuss)
Chlorpheniramine tannate/Phenylephrine tannate/Pyrilamine tannate (Rynatan-S)
Diflunisal
Eprosartan mesylate/Hydrochlorothiazide (Teveten HCT)
Ezetimibe/Simvastatin (Vytorin)
Hydrochlorothiazide/Timolol maleate (Timolide)
Hydrochlorothiazide/Irbesartan (Avalide)
Hydrochlorothiazide/Lisinopril (Prinzide)
Hydrochlorothiazide/Losartan potassium (Hyzaar)
Hydrochlorothiazide/Telmisartan (Micardis HCT)
Hydrochlorothiazide/Valsartan (Diovan HCT)
Lovastatin/Niacin (Advicor)
Pravastatin sodium (Pravachol)
Simvastatin (Zocor)
Tretinoin (Vesanoid)

Table 24. ORAL MANIFESTATIONS OF SYSTEMIC AGENTS *(Cont.)*

Dysphagia

Acamprosate calcium (Campral)
Acetaminophen/Tramadol hydrochloride (Ultracet, Ultram)
Alendronate sodium (Fosamax)
Alendronate sodium/Cholecalciferol (Fosamax Plus D)
Alprazolam (Xanax, Xanax XR)
Amantadine hydrochloride (Symmetrel)
Amlodipine besylate/Hydrochlorothiazide/Valsartan (Exforge HCT)
Amlodipine besylate/Valsartan (Exforge)
Amlodipine besylate/Atorvastatin calcium (Caduet)
Amoxicillin/Clarithromycin/Lansoprazole (PREVPAC)
Amphotericin B, Liposomal (AmBisome)
Aprepitant (Emend)
Aripiprazole (Abilify)
Atorvastatin calcium (Lipitor)
Betaxolol hydrochloride (Kerlone)
Bicalutamide (Casodex)
Bortezomib (Velcade)
Botulinum Toxin Type A (BOTOX)
Bupropion hydrochloride (Wellbutrin SR, Wellbutrin XL, Zyban SR)
Calcium carbonate/Risedronate sodium (Actonel with Calcium)
Candesartan cilexetil/Hydrochlorothiazide (Atacand HCT)
Capecitabine (Xeloda)
Carbidopa/Entacapone/Levodopa (Stalevo)
Carbidopa/Levodopa (Parcopa, Sinemet)
Celecoxib (Celebrex)
Cevimeline hydrochloride (Evoxac)
Ciprofloxacin (Cipro, Cipro XR)
Citalopram hydrobromide (Celexa)
Clozapine (Clozaril, Fazaclo)
Cyclosporine (Gengraf)
Cytarabine Liposome (DepoCyt)
Dactinomycin (Cosmegen)
Decitabine (Dacogen)
Delavirdine mesylate (Rescriptor)
Denileukin diftitox (Ontak)
Dexlansoprazole (Kapidex)
Dexrazoxane (Zinecard)
Diclofenac sodium/Misoprostol (Arthrotec)
Dihydroergotamine mesylate (Migranal)
Divalproex sodium (Depakote ER)
Docetaxel (Taxotere)
Donepezil hydrochloride (Aricept)
Doxorubicin hydrochloride liposome (Doxil)
Doxycycline monohydrate (Monodox)
Duloxetine hydrochloride (Cymbalta)
Eletriptan hydrobromide (Relpax)
Eprosartan mesylate/Hydrochlorothiazide (Teveten HCT)
Ertapenem (Invanz)
Esomeprazole (Nexium)
Eszopiclone (Lunesta)
Ethacrynate sodium (Edecrin)
Ethacrynic acid (Edecrin)
Etoposide (Etopophos, Vepesid)
Fentanyl citrate (Actiq, Fentora)
Fluoxetine hydrochloride (Prozac)
Fluoxetine hydrochloride/Olanzapine (Symbyax)
Fluvoxamine maleate (Luvox)
Fosaprepitant dimeglumine (Emend)
Foscarnet sodium (Foscavir)
Fosinopril sodium (Monopril)
Frovatriptan succinate (Frova)
Gabapentin (Neurontin)
Galantamine hydrobromide (Razadyne)
Glatiramer acetate (Copaxone)
Hydrochlorothiazide
Hydrochlorothiazide/Irbesartan (Avalide)
Hydrochlorothiazide/Lisinopril (Prinzide)
Hydrochlorothiazide/Losartan potassium (Hyzaar)
Hydrochlorothiazide/Telmisartan (Micardis HCT)
Hydrochlorothiazide/Valsartan (Diovan HCT)
Hydrocodone bitartrate/Ibuprofen (Vicoprofen)
Hydroxocobalamin (Cyanokit Antidote)
Infliximab (Remicade)
Influenza Virus Vaccine (Flulaval)
Interferon alfa-2B, Recombinant (Intron A)
Itraconazole (Sporanox)
Ixabepilone (Ixempra)
Lamotrigine (Lamictal, Lamictal CD, Lamictal XR)
Lansoprazole (Prevacid)
Leuprolide acetate (Lupron)
Levofloxacin (Levaquin)
Lopinavir/Ritonavir (Kaletra)
Memantine hydrochloride (Namenda)
Mesalamine (Pentasa)
Minocycline hydrochloride (Solodyn)
Modafinil (Provigil)
Morphine sulfate (Avinza)
Moxifloxacin hydrochloride (Avelox)
Mycophenolate mofetil (CellCept)
Nabumetone
Nifedipine (Procardia, Procardia XL)
Nisoldipine (Sular)
Norfloxacin (Noroxin)
Octreotide acetate (Sandostatin)
Olanzapine (Zyprexa, Zyprexa ZYDIS)
Omega-3-Acid Ethyl Esters (Lovaza)
Oxaliplatin (Eloxatin)
Oxcarbazepine (Trileptal)
Oxycodone hydrochloride (OxyContin)
Paliperidone (Invega)
Pantoprazole sodium (Protonix)
Paroxetine hydrochloride (Paxil, Paxil CR)
Pemetrexed (Alimta)
Pentostatin (Nipent)
Perphenazine
Pilocarpine hydrochloride (Salagen)
Pimozide (Orap)
Polifeprosan 20 with Carmustine (Gliadel)
Porfimer sodium (Photofrin)
Pramipexole dihydrochloride (Mirapex)
Pregabalin (Lyrica)
Procarbazine hydrochloride (Matulane)
Propafenone hydrochloride (Rythmol, Rythmol SR)
Quetiapine fumarate (Seroquel, Seroquel XR)

Table 24. ORAL MANIFESTATIONS OF SYSTEMIC AGENTS *(Cont.)*

Dysphagia *(Cont.)*

Rabeprazole sodium (Aciphex)
Ramipril (Altace)
Riluzole (Rilutek)
Rimantadine hydrochloride (Flumadine)
Risedronate sodium (Actonel)
Risperidone (Risperdal Consta)
Ritonavir (Norvir)
Rivastigmine tartrate (Exelon)
Rizatriptan benzoate (Maxalt, Maxalt MLT)
Ropinirole hydrochloride (Requip)
Saquinavir mesylate (Invirase)
Sargramostim (Leukine)
Selegiline (Emsam, Eldepryl)
Sertraline hydrochloride (Zoloft)
Sildenafil citrate (Viagra)
Sirolimus (Rapamune)
Sodium oxybate (Xyrem)
Sorafenib (Nexavar)
Sumatriptan succinate (Imitrex)
Sumatriptan succinate/Naproxen sodium (Treximet)
Tacrolimus (Prograf)
Tadalafil (Cialis)
Temozolomide (Temodar)
Thalidomide (Thalomid)
Tiagabine hydrochloride (Gabitril)
Tiotropium bromide (Spiriva)
Tolcapone (Tasmar)
Topiramate (Topamax)
Vardenafil hydrochloride (Levitra)
Varenicline tartrate (Chantix)
Venlafaxine hydrochloride (Effexor, Effexor XR)
Vinorelbine tartrate (Navelbine)
Voriconazole (VFEND)
Zaleplon (Sonata)
Zidovudine (Retrovir)
Ziprasidone hydrochloride (Geodon)
Zoledronic acid (Zometa)
Zolmitriptan (Zomig, Zomig-ZMT)
Zolpidem tartrate (Ambien, Ambien CR)
Zonisamide (Zonegran)

Edema, laryngeal

Acetaminophen/Oxycodone hydrochloride (Percocet)
Alteplase (Activase)
Amifostine (Ethyol)
Amlodipine besylate/Benazepril hydrochloride (Lotrel)
Antihemophilic factor (recombinant) (BeneFIX)
Aspirin (Bayer Aspirin, St. Joseph's Aspirin)
Aspirin/Dipyridamole (Aggrenox)
Aspirin/Oxycodone hydrochloride (Percodan)
Bortezomib (Velcade)
Candesartan cilexetil/Hydrochlorothiazide (Atacand HCT)
Cefdinir (Omnicef)
Ceftazidime (Fortaz)
Chloroprocaine hydrochloride (Nesacaine)
Chlorpromazine
Ciprofloxacin (Cipro, Cipro XR)
Cromolyn sodium (Intal)
Diclofenac sodium/Misoprostol (Arthrotec)
Dipyridamole (Persantine)
Enalapril maleate (Vasotec)
Enalapril maleate/Hydrochorothiazide (Vaseretic)
Eprosartan mesylate/Hydrochlorothiazide (Teveten HCT)
Esomeprazole (Nexium)
Fluoxetine hydrochloride (Prozac)
Gentamicin sulfate
Hydrochlorothiazide/Irbesartan (Avalide)
Hydrochlorothiazide/Losartan (Hyzaar)
Hydrochlorothiazide/Telmisartan (Micardis HCT)
Hydrochlorothiazide/Valsartan (Diovan HCT)
Infliximab (Remicade)
Lisinopril (Prinivil)
Hydrochlorothiazide/Lisinopril (Prinzide)
Menotropins (Menopur, Repronex)
Mepivacaine hydrochloride (Polocaine)
Metoclopramide (Reglan)
Moxifloxacin hydrochloride (Avelox)
Muromonab-cd3 (Orthoclone OKT3)
Nalbuphine hydrochloride
Nizatidine (Axid)
Ofloxacin (Floxin)
Ondansetron (Zofran, Zofran ODT)
Oprelvekin (Neumega)
Oxymorphone hydrochloride
Pegaspargase (Oncaspar)
Penicillin G benzathine (Bicillin C-R, Bicillin L-A)
Pentostatin (Nipent)
Prochlorperazine (Compro)
Ropivacaine hydrochloride (Naropin)
Tenecteplase (TNKase)
Thioridazine hydrochloride
Thiotepa
Thyrotropin alfa (Thyrogen)
Trandolapril/Verapamil hydrochloride (Tarka)
Tretinoin (Vesanoid)
Urofollitropin (Bravelle)
Vardenafil hydrochloride (Levitra)
Venlafaxine hydrochloride (Effexor, Effexor XR)
Zolmitriptan (Zomig, Zomig-ZMT)

Table 24. ORAL MANIFESTATIONS OF SYSTEMIC AGENTS *(Cont.)*

Edema, lips

- Agalsidase beta (Fabrazyme)
- Albuterol sulfate/Ipratropium bromide (Combivent)
- Ciprofloxacin (Cipro, Cipro XL)
- Delavirdine mesylate (Rescriptor)
- Finasteride (Propecia)
- Infliximab (Remicade)
- Losartan potassium (Cozaar)
- Muromonab-cd3 (Orthoclone OKT3)
- Pegaspargase (Oncaspar)
- Sumatriptan succinate (Imitrex)
- Trandolapril/Verapamil hydrochloride (Tarka)
- Zidovudine (Retrovir)

Edema, mouth

- Alemtuzumab (Campath)
- Bupropion hydrochloride (Wellbutrin)
- Cevimeline hydrochloride (Evoxac)
- Frovatriptan succinate (Frova)
- Paricalcitol (Zemplar)

Edema, oropharyngeal

- Albuterol sulfate (Proventil HFA, Ventolin HFA)
- Albuterol sulfate/Ipratropium bromide (Combivent)
- Ciprofloxacin (Cipro, Cipro XR)
- Diclofenac sodium/Misoprostol (Arthrotec)
- Fluticasone propionate/Salmeterol xinafoate (Advair Diskus, Advair HFA)
- Ipratropium bromide (Atrovent HFA)
- Penciclovir (Denavir)
- Sumatriptan succinate/Naproxen sodium (Treximet)
- Zanamivir (Relenza)

Edema, pharyngeal

- Candesartan cilexetil (Atacand)
- Ciprofloxacin (Cipro, Cipro XR)
- Febuxostat (Uloric)
- Infliximab (Remicade)
- Losartan potassium (Cozaar)
- Metyrosine (Demser)
- Moxifloxacin hydrochloride (Avelox)
- Nalidixic acid (NegGram)
- Norfloxacin (Noroxin)
- Omalizumab (Xolair)
- Rizatriptan benzoate (Maxalt, Maxalt MLT)
- Sodium phosphate (OsmoPrep)

Edema, tongue

- Acetaminophen/Tramadol (Ultracet)
- Albuterol sulfate/Ipratropium bromide (Combivent)
- Amitriptyline hydrochloride
- Aripiprazole (Abilify)
- Bisacodyl (Fleet)
- Budesonide (Entocort)
- Bupropion hydrochloride (Wellbutrin SR, Wellbutrin XL, Zyban SR)
- Candesartan cilexetil/Hydrochlorothiazide (Atacand HCT)
- Cetirizine hydrochloride (Zyrtec)
- Cetirizine hydrochloride/Pseudoephedrine hydrochloride (Zyrtec-D)
- Cilostazol (Pletal)
- Cyclobenzaprine hydrochloride (Amrix, Flexeril)
- Donepezil hydrochloride (Aricept)
- Eletriptan hydrobromide (Relpax)
- Eprosartan mesylate/Hydrochlorothiazide (Teveten HCT)
- Esomeprazole (Nexium)
- Eszopiclone (Lunesta)
- Etoposide (Vepesid, Etopophos)
- Fluoxetine hydrochloride (Prozac)
- Fluticasone propionate (Flonase)
- Fluticasone propionate/Salmeterol xinafoate (Advair Diskus, Advair HFA)
- Hydrochlorothiazide
- Hydrochlorothiazide/Irbesartan (Avalide)
- Hydrochlorothiazide/Lisinopril (Prinzide)
- Hydrochlorothiazide/Losartan potassium (Hyzaar)
- Hydrochlorothiazide/Telmisartan (Micardis HCT)
- Hydrochlorothiazide/Valsartan (Diovan HCT)
- Interferon Beta-1A (Avonex)
- Interferon Beta-1B (Betaseron)
- Lamotrigine (Lamictal)
- Levofloxacin (Levaquin)
- Losartan potassium (Cozaar)
- Metoclopramide (Reglan)
- Mirtazapine (Remeron, Remeron SolTab)
- Olanzapine (Zyprexa, Zyprexa ZYDIS)
- Omalizumab (Xolair)
- Oprelvekin (Neumega)
- Paroxetine hydrochloride (Paxil, Paxil CR)
- Polyethylene glycol/Potassium chloride/Sodium bicarbonate/Sodium chloride/Sodium sulfate (Colyte)
- Pramipexole dihydrochloride (Mirapex)
- Pregabalin (Lyrica)
- Quetiapine fumarate (Seroquel)
- Rasagiline mesylate (Azilect)
- Risperidone (Risperdal)
- Rizatriptan benzoate (Maxalt, Maxalt MLT)
- Ropinirole hydrochloride (Requip)
- Selegiline (Emsam)
- Sertraline hydrochloride (Zoloft)
- Sibutramine hydrochloride monohydrate (Meridia)
- Sodium phosphate (Fleet, EZ-Prep, Osmoprep)
- Topiramate (Topamax)
- Trandolapril/Verapamil hydrochloride (Tarka)

Table 24. ORAL MANIFESTATIONS OF SYSTEMIC AGENTS *(Cont.)*

Edema, tongue *(Cont.)*

Trimipramine maleate (Surmontil)
Venlafaxine hydrochloride (Effexor, Effexor XR)
Voriconazole (VFEND)
Zaleplon (Sonata)
Zidovudine (Retrovir)
Ziprasidone hydrochloride (Geodon)
Zolmitriptan (Zomig, Zomig-ZMT)

Gagging

Escitalopram oxalate (Lexapro)

Gingival disorder, unspecified

Daptomycin (Cubicin)
Nifedipine (Procardia, Procardia XL)
Orlistat (Xenical)
Rifaximin (Xifaxan)

Gingival hyperplasia

Acitretin (Soriatane)
Amlodipine besylate/Valsartan (Exforge)
Basiliximab (Simulect)
Cevimeline hydrochloride (Evoxac)
Cyclosporine (Gengraf, Neoral, Sandimmune)
Diltiazem hydrochloride (Cardizem LA)
Felodipine (Plendil ER)
Interferon alfa-2B, Recombinant (Intron A)
Lamotrigine (Lamictal)
Mycophenolate mofetil (CellCept)
Mycophenolic acid (Myfortic)
Nifedipine (Procardia, Procardia XL)
Nisoldipine (Sular)
Oxcarbazepine (Trileptal)
Paroxetine hydrochloride (Paxil, Paxil CR)
Phenytoin sodium (Phenytek)
Pimozide (Orap)
Sertraline hydrochloride (Zoloft)
Sirolimus (Rapamune)
Tiagabine hydrochloride (Gabitril)
Topiramate (Topamax)
Trandolapril/Verapamil hydrochloride (Tarka)
Voriconazole (VFEND)
Zonisamide (Zonegran)

Gingivitis

Acitretin (Soriatane)
Alemtuzumab (Campath)
Aripiprazole (Abilify)
Aurothioglucose (Solganal)
Bexarotene (Targretin)
Bupropion hydrochloride (Wellbutrin SR, Wellbutrin XL, Zyban SR)
Candesartan cilexetil/Hydrochlorothiazide (Atacand HCT)
Cevimeline hydrochloride (Evoxac)
Citalopram hydrobromide (Celexa)
Clonazepam (Klonopin)
Colchicine
Cyclosporine (Gengraf, Neoral)
Delavirdine mesylate (Rescriptor)
Donepezil hydrochloride (Aricept)
Doxorubicin hydrochloride liposome (Doxil)
Duloxetine hydrochloride (Cymbalta)
Eletriptan hydrobromide (Relpax)
Eprosartan mesylate (Teveten)
Eprosartan mesylate/Hydrochlorothiazide (Teveten HCT)
Fentanyl citrate (Actiq)
Fluoxetine hydrochloride/Olanzapine (Symbyax)
Fluvoxamine maleate (Luvox, Luvox CR)
Gabapentin (Neurontin)
Glatiramer acetate (Copaxone)
Interferon alfa-2B, Recombinant (Intron A)
Isotretinoin (Accutane)
Lamotrigine (Lamictal)
Leflunomide (Arava)
Leuprolide acetate (Lupron Depot)
Levetiracetam (Keppra)
Moexipril/Hydrochlorothiazide (Uniretic)
Methotrexate
Modafinil (Provigil)
Mycophenolate mofetil (CellCept)
Nabumetone
Octreotide (Sandostatin)
Oxaliplatin (Eloxatin)
Pantoprazole sodium (Protonix)
Paroxetine hydrochloride (Paxil, Paxil CR)
Pentostatin (Nipent)
Pilocarpine hydrochloride (Salagen)
Pramipexole dihydrochloride (Mirapex)
Probenecid
Quetiapine fumarate (Seroquel, Seroquel XL)
Rabeprazole sodium (Aciphex)
Rasagiline mesylate (Azilect)
Risperidone (Risperdal Consta)
Ritonavir (Norvir)
Rivastigmine tartrate (Exelon)
Ropinirole hydrochloride (Requip)
Saquinavir mesylate (Invirase)
Sildenafil citrate (Viagra)
Sirolimus (Rapamune)
Testosterone (Androgel, Androderm, Striant, Testim)
Tiagabine hydrochloride (Gabitril)
Topiramate (Topamax)
Varenicline tartrate (Chantix)
Venlafaxine hydrochloride (Effexor, Effexor XR)
Voriconazole (VFEND)
Zaleplon (Sonata)
Zolmitriptan (Zomig, Zomig-ZMT)
Zonisamide (Zonegran)

Table 24. ORAL MANIFESTATIONS OF SYSTEMIC AGENTS *(Cont.)*

Glossitis

Acetyl sulfisoxazole (Gantrisin)
Acitretin (Soriatane)
Albuterol sulfate (ProAir HFA)
Amlodipine besylate/Atorvastatin calcium (Caduet)
Amoxicillin/Clarithromycin/Lansoprazole (PREVPAC)
Amoxicillin/Clavulanate potassium (Augmentin, Augmentin XR)
Aripiprazole (Abilify)
Atorvastatin calcium (Lipitor)
Azelastine hydrochloride (Astelin, Astepro)
Balsalazide disodium (Colazal)
Betaxolol hydrochloride (Betoptic)
Bismuth subcitrate potassium/Metronidazole/Tetracyclinie hydrochloride (Pylera)
Budesonide (Entocort)
Bupropion hydrochloride (Wellbutrin SR, Wellbutrin XL, Zyban)
Captopril (Capoten)
Carbamazepine (Carbatrol, Equetro)
Ceftriaxone sodium (Rocephin)
Cevimeline hydrochloride (Evoxac)
Cilastatin sodium/Imipenem (Primaxin)
Citalopram hydrobromide (Celexa)
Clarithromycin (Biaxin, Biaxin XL)
Cyanocobalamin (Nascobal)
Cyclosporine (Gengraf, Neoral)
Diclofenac (Cataflam, Voltaren, Voltaren XR)
Diclofenac sodium/Misoprostol (Arthrotec)
Divalproex sodium (Depakote, Depakote ER)
Doxorubicin hydrochloride liposome (Doxil)
Doxycycline (Monodox, Oracea, Vibramycin)
Eletriptan hydrobromide (Relpax)
Enalapril maleate (Vasotec)
Enalapril maleate/Hydrochlorothiazide (Vaseretic)
Etidronate disodium (Didronel)
Fentanyl citrate (Actiq)
Flunisolide (Aerobid, Aerobid-M)
Fluoxetine hydrochloride (Prozac)
Fluvoxamine maleate (Luvox, Luvox CR)
Gabapentin (Neurontin)
Hydrocodone bitartrate/Ibuprofen (Vicoprofen)
Isosorbite mononitrate
Lamotrigine (Lamictal)
Lansoprazole (Prevacid)
Leuprolide acetate (Lupron)
Levofloxacin (Levaquin)
Mecamylamine hydrochloride (Inversine)
Mefenamic acid (Ponstel)
Meropenem (Merrem)
Minocycline hydrochloride (Solodyn)
Mirtazapine (Remeron)
Moxifloxacin hydrochloride (Avelox)
Nabumetone
Naproxen sodium (EC-Naprosyn, Naprosyn, Anaprox DS, Anaprox)
Nisoldipine (Sular)
Octreotide acetate (Sandostatin)
Olanzapine (Zyprexa, Zyprexa ZYDIS)
Pantoprazole sodium (Protonix)
Paroxetine hydrochloride (Paxil CR)
Penicillamine (Cuprimine)
Pentostatin (Nipent)
Pilocarpine hydrochloride (Salagen)
Pirbuterol acetate (Maxair)
Propafenone hydrochloride (Rythmol SR)
Pyrimethamine (Daraprim)
Quetiapine fumarate (Seroquel)
Rabeprazole sodium (Aciphex)
Riluzole (Rilutek)
Risedronate sodium/Calcium carbonate (Actonel With Calcium)
Rivastigmine tartrate (Exelon)
Ropinirole hydrochloride (Requip)
Saquinavir mesylate (Invirase)
Selegiline (Emsam)
Sertraline hydrochloride (Zoloft)
Sildenafil citrate (Viagra)
Sulfadoxine/Pyrimethamine (Fansidar)
Sulfamethoxazole/Trimethoprim (Bactrim, Septra)
Sulindac (Clinoril)
Telithromycin (Ketek)
Tiagabine hydrochloride (Gabitril)
Tiotropium bromide (Spiriva)
Tolmetin sodium (Tolectin DS, Tolectin 600)
Topiramate (Topamax)
Valproate sodium (Depacon)
Valproic acid (Depakene)
Venlafaxine hydrochloride (Effexor, Effexor XR)
Voriconazole (VFEND)
Zaleplon (Sonata)
Zonisamide (Zonegran)

Glossodynia

Adenosine (Adenoscan)
Clozapine (Clozaril, Fazaclo)
Decitabine (Dacogen)
Fentanyl citrate (Fentora)
Flecainide acetate (Tambocor)
Methyldopa/Hydrochlorothiazide
Propafenone hydrochloride (Rythmol SR)
Ramipril (Altace)
Sorafenib (Nexavar)
Sumatriptan succinate (Imitrex)
Sunitinib malate (Sutent)

Table 24. ORAL MANIFESTATIONS OF SYSTEMIC AGENTS *(Cont.)*

Glossoncus

Aripiprazole (Abilify)
Calcitonin-salmon (Miacalcin)
Cefuroxime axetil (Ceftin)
Flecainide acetate (Tambocor)
Flumazenil (Romazicon)
Influenza virus vaccine (Fluarix)
Hydrochlorothiazide/Irbesartan (Avalide)
Hydrochlorothiazide/Losartan potassium (Hyzaar)
Modafinil (Provigil)
Oseltamivir phosphate (Tamiflu)
Paliperidone (Invega)
Pregabalin (Lyrica)
Ramipril (Altace)
Rifaximin (Xifaxan)
Rizatriptan benzoate (Maxalt, Maxalt-MLT)
Sitagliptin phosphate (Januvia)
Sumatriptan succinate/Naproxen sodium (Treximet)
Ziprasidone hydrochloride (Geodon)

Glossoplegia

Risperidone

Glossotrichia

Amitriptyline hydrochloride (Elavil)
Amoxicillin (Amoxil)
Amoxicillin/Clarithromycin/Lansoprazole (PREVPAC)
Amoxicillin/Clavulanate potassium (Augmentin, Augmentin XR)
Clonazepam (Klonopin)
Protriptyline hydrochloride (Vivactil)
Trimipramine maleate (Surmontil)

Gums, sore

Bupropion hydrochloride (Wellbutrin)
Propafenone hydrochloride (Rythmol SR)
Testosterone (Androgel, Androderm, Striant, Testim)

Halitosis

Amoxicillin/Clarithromycin/Lansoprazole (PREVPAC)
Dexlansoprazole (Kapidex)
Duloxetine hydrochloride (Cymbalta)
Eletriptan hydrobromide (Relpax)
Eszopiclone (Lunesta)
Interferon alfa-2b, recombinant (Intron A)
Lansoprazole (Prevacid)
Ofloxacin (Floxin)
Pantoprazole sodium (Protonix)
Propafenone hydrochloride (Rythmol SR)
Rivastigmine tartrate (Exelon)
Selegiline (Emsam)
Tiagabine hydrochloride (Gabitril)

Herpes simplex

Abatacept (Orencia)
Acitretin (Soriatane)
Alefacept (Amevive)
Alemtuzumab (Campath)
Amphotericin B, liposomal (AmBisome)
Anti-thymocyte globulin (Thymoglobulin)
Aprepitant (Emend)
Arformoterol tartrate (Brovana)
Arsenic trioxide (Trisenox)
Azelastine hydrochloride (Astepro, Astelin)
Basiliximab (Simulect)
Bendamustine HCl (Treanda)
Bortezomib (Velcade)
Budesonide (Pulmicort, Rhinocort)
Celecoxib (Celebrex)
Cevimeline hydrochloride (Evoxac)
Clindamycin phosphate (Clindesse)
Clofarabine (Clolar)
Clonazepam (Klonopin)
Cyclosporine (Gengraf, Neoral)
Delavirdine mesylate (Rescriptor)
Dihydroergotamine mesylate (Migranal)
Donepezil hydrochloride (Aricept)
Doxorubicin hydrochloride liposome (Doxil)
Enfuvirtide (Fuzeon)
Eprosartan mesylate (Teveten)
Eprosartan mesylate/Hydrochlorothiazide (Teveten HCT)
Ertapenem (Invanz)
Estradiol (Vivelle, Vivelle-dot)
Fenofibrate (Tricor)
Fluorometholone (FML)
Fluorouracil
Fluticasone propionate (Cutivate)
Fosaprepitant dimeglumine (Emend for injection)
Gabapentin (Neurontin)
Gemtuzumab ozogamicin (Mylotarg)
Glatiramer acetate (Copaxone)
Goserelin acetate (Zoladex)
Hydrochlorothiazide/Lisinopril (Prinzid, Zestoretic)
Imatinib mesylate (Gleevec)
Imiquimod (Aldara)
Interferon alfa-2b, recombinant (Intron A)
Leflunomide (Arava)
Levofloxacin (Levaquin)
Loteprednol etabonate (Alrex, Lotemax)
Measles, mumps, varicella & rubella virus vaccine, live (ProQuad)

Table 24. ORAL MANIFESTATIONS OF SYSTEMIC AGENTS *(Cont.)*

Herpes simplex *(Cont.)*

Methotrexate (Trexall)
Mirtazapine (Remeron)
Modafinil (Provigil)
Mycophenolate mofetil (Cellcept)
Mycophenolic acid (Myfortic)
Nilotinib (Tasigna)
Nisoldipine (Sular)
Paclitaxel (Taxol)
Pantoprazole sodium (Protonix)
Paroxetine hydrochloride (Paxil)
Pegasparase (Oncaspar)
Pentostatin (Nipent)
Perindopril erbumine (Aceon)
Pilocarpine hydrochloride (Salagen)
Pimecrolimus (Elidel)
Prednisolone acetate (Flo-Pred)
Progesterone (Prometrium)
Raltegravir (Isentress)
Rivastigmine tartrate (Exelon)
Ropinirole hydrochloride (Requip)
Saquinavir mesylate (Invirase)
Selegiline (Emsam)
Sibutramine hydrochloride monohydrate (Meridia)
Sildenafil citrate (Viagra)
Sirolimus (Rapamune)
Sodium oxybate (Xyrem)
Somatropin recombinant (Serostim)
Tacrolimus (Prograf, Protopic)
Thalidomide (Thalomid)
Tiagabine hydrochloride (Gabitril)
Tipranavir (Aptivus)
Tolcapone (Tasmar)
Trastuzumab (Herceptin)
Voriconazole (VFEND)
Zolpidem tartrate (Ambien, Ambien CR)

Hoarseness

Albuterol sulfate (Ventolin HFA)
Albuterol sulfate/Ipatropium bromide (Combivent)
Beclomethsone dipropionate
Capecitabine (Xeloda)
Captopril (Capoten)
Carbidopa (Lodosyn)
Carbidopa/Levodopa (Parcopa, Sinemet)
Carbidopa/Entacapone/Levadopa (Stalevo)
Cetuximab (Erbitux)
Ciclesonide (Alvesco)
Clonazepam (Klonopin)
Cromolyn sodium (Intal)
Enalapril maleate (Vasotec)
Enalapril maleate/Hydrochlorothiazide (Vaseretic)
Estramustine phosphate sodium (Emcyt)
Flunisolide (Aerobid, Aerobid-M)
Fluticasone propionate (Flonase, Flovent Diskus, Flovent HFA)
Fluticasone propionate/Salmeterol xinafoate (Advair Diskus)
Fluvoxamine maleate (Luvox, Luvox CR)
Hydrocodone bitartrate/Ibuprofen (Vicoprofen)
Ipratropium bromide (Atrovent)
Levofloxacin (Levaquin)
Medroxyprogesterone acetate (Depo-SubQ Provera)
Methyltestosterone (Android)
Modafinil (Provigil)
Naltrexone hydrochloride (Revia)
Nicotine (Nicotrol)
Oxandrolone (Oxandrin)
Perindopril erbumine (Aceon)
Procarbazine hydrochloride (Matulane)
Rizatriptan benzoate (Maxalt, Maxalt-MLT)
Ropinirole hydrochloride (Requip)
Sorafenib (Nexavar)
Tiotropium bromide (Spiriva)
Triamcinolone acetonide (Azmacort)
Zidovudine (Retrovir)

Hyperesthesia, tongue

Interferon alfa-n3 (human leukocyte derived) (Alferon N)

Hypertrophy, gum

Ethotoin (Peganone)
Isotretinoin (Amnesteem)

Hypertrophy, tonsillar

Mecasermin [rDNA Origin] (Increlex)

Infection, pharyngeal

Budesonide
Flunisolide
Lamivudine (Epivir-HBV)

Table 24. ORAL MANIFESTATIONS OF SYSTEMIC AGENTS *(Cont.)*

Irritation, oral

Almotriptan malate (Axert)
Cyclosporine (Sandimmune)
Flunisolide (Aerobid, Aerobid-M)
Furosemide (Lasix)
Naratriptan hydrochloride (Amerge)
Nystatin (Mycostatin)
Pancrelipase (Creon)
Sumatriptan succinate (Imitrex)
Testosterone (Androgel, Androderm, Striant, Testim)

Irritation, oropharynx

Albuterol sulfate (Proventil HFA, Ventolin HFA)
Salmeterol xinafoate (Serevent Diskus)

Laryngismus

Acamprosate calcium (Campral)
Almotriptan malate (Axert)
Delavirdine mesylate (Rescriptor)
Fluoxetine hydrochloride/Olanzapine (Symbyax)
Fluvoxamine maleate (Luvox, Luvox CR)
Glatiramer acetate (Copaxone)
Iodine I 131/Tositumomab (Bexxar)
Oxcarbazepine (Trileptal)
Paroxetine hydrochloride (Paxil CR)
Pilocarpine hydrochloride (Salagen)
Pregabalin (Lyrica)
Selegiline (Emsam)
Sertraline hydrochloride (Zoloft)
Venlafaxine hydrochloride (Effexor, Effexor XR)

Laryngitis

Acitretin (Soriatane)
Agalsidase beta (Fabrazyme)
Albuterol sulfate (Ventolin HFA)
Almotriptan malate (Axert)
Alosetron hydrochloride (Lotronex)
Aripiprazole (Abilify)
Azelastine hydrochloride (Astelin, Astepro)
Botulinum Toxin Type A (Botox)
Capecitabine (Xeloda)
Celecoxib (Celebrex)
Cevimeline hydrochloride (Evoxac)
Citalopram hydrobromide (Celexa)
Clozapine (Clozaril, Fazaclo)
Dornase alfa (Pulmozyme)
Doxorubicin hydrochloride liposome (Doxil)
Duloxetine hydrochloride (Cymbalta)
Eletriptan hydrobromide (Relpax)
Escitalopram oxalate (Lexapro)
Eszopiclone (Lunesta)
Fenofibrate (Tricor)
Flunisolide (Aerobid, Aerobid-M)
Fluoxetine hydrochloride/Olanzapine (Symbyax)
Fluticasone propionate (Flovent Diskus, Flovent HFA)
Fluticasone propionate/Salmeterol xinafoate (Advair HFA)
Fluvoxamine maleate (Luvox, Luvox CR)
Fosinopril sodium (Monopril)
Frovatriptan succinate (Frova)
Gabapentin (Neurontin)
Glatiramer acetate (Copaxone)
Influenza virus vaccine (Flulaval)
Ixabepilone (Ixempra)
Leuprolide acetate (Lupron)
Lisinopril (Prinivil, Zestril)
Lisinopril/Hydrochlorothiazide (Prinzide, Zestoretic)
Loratadine (Claritin)
Loratadine/Pseudoephedrine sulfate (Claritin-D)
Mirtazapine (Remeron)
Montelukast sodium (Singulair)
Naltrexone (Vivitrol)
Nisoldipine (Sular)
Omega-3-acid ethyl esters (Lovaza)
Pantoprazole sodium (Protonix)
Paroxetine hydrochloride (Paxil CR)
Pilocarpine hydrochloride (Salagen)
Pramipexole dihydrochloride (Mirapex)
Rabeprazole sodium (Aciphex)
Raloxifene hydrochloride (Evista)
Riluzole (Rilutek)
Rivastigmine tartrate (Exelon)
Ropinirole hydrochloride (Requip)
Saquinavir mesylate (Invirase)
Selegiline (Emsam)
Sertraline hydrochloride (Zoloft)
Sibutramine hydrochloride monohydrate (Meridia)
Sodium oxybate (Xyrem)
Somatropin (rDNA origin) (Norditropin)
Tacrolimus (Protopic)
Tiagabine hydrochloride (Gabitril)
Tiotropium bromide (Spiriva)
Tolcapone (Tasmar)
Trastuzumab (Herceptin)
Venlafaxine hydrochloride (Effexor, Effexor XR)
Zaleplon (Sonata)
Zolmitriptan (Zomig, Zomig-ZMT)
Zolpidem tartrate (Ambien, Ambien CR)

Table 24. ORAL MANIFESTATIONS OF SYSTEMIC AGENTS *(Cont.)*

Laryngospasm

Albuterol sulfate/Ipratropium bromide (Combivent)
Aripiprazole (Abilify)
Atenolol (Tenormin)
Atenolol/Chlorthalidone (Tenoretic)
Bendroflumethiazide/Nadolol (Corzide)
Benzonatate (Tessalon)
Betaxolol hydrochloride (Kerlone)
Brimonidine tartrate/Timolol maleate (Combigan)
Desflurane (Suprane)
Diazepam (Valium)
Dorzolamide hydrochloride/Timolol maleate (Cosopt)
Doxapram hydrochloride (Dopram)
Etoposide (Etopophos, Vepesid)
Fluoxetine hydrochloride (Prozac)
Fluticasone propionate (Flovent Diskus, Flovent HFA)
Fluticasone propionate/Salmeterol xinafoate (Advair Diskus)
Haloperidol (Haldol)
Hydromorphone hydrochloride (Dilaudid)
Ipratropium bromide (Atrovent HFA)
Lidocaine (Lidoderm)
Metoclopramide (Reglan)
Metoprolol succinate (Toprol-XL)
Midazolam hydrochloride
Morphine sulfate (MS Contin)
Muromonab-cd3 (Orthoclone OKT3)
Nadolol
Ondansetron (Zofran ODT)
Oxymorphone hydrochloride (Opana)
Penbutolol sulfate (Levatol)
Pramipexole dihydrochloride (Mirapex)
Propofol (Diprivan)
Propranolol hydrochloride (InnoPran XL)
Salmeterol xinafoate (Serevent Diskus)
Sevoflurane (Ultane)
Sucralfate (Carafate)
Timolol maleate (Timoptic, Timoptic XE)

Laryngotracheobronchitis

Hepatitis A vaccine, inactivated (Vaqta)
Influenza virus vaccine (Flumist)
Palivizumab (Synagis)
Pneumococcal vaccine, diphtheria conjugate (Prevnar)

Lesions, oral

Arsenic trioxide (Trisenox)
Cefpodoxime proxetil (Vantin)
Fluticasone propionate/Salmeterol xinafoate (Advair Diskus)
Irbesartan (Avapro)
Nevirapine (Viramune)
Testosterone (Androgel, Androderm, Striant, Testim)

Leukoplakia, oral

Doxorubicin hydrochloride liposome (Doxil)
Interferon alfa-2b, recombinant (Intron A)
Ziprasidone hydrochloride (Geodon)

Lips, cracked

Acyclovir (Zovirax)

Lips, enlargement

Lithium carbonate (Eskalith)
Phenytoin sodium (Phenytek)

Lips, swelling

Ascorbic acid/Peg-3350/Potassium chloride/Sodium ascorbate/Sodium chloride/Sodium sulfate (MoviPrep)
Calcitriol (Rocaltrol)
Finasteride (Propecia, Proscar)
Flecainide acetate (Tambocor)
Influenza virus vaccine (Fluvirin)
Levofloxacin (Levaquin)
Lithium carbonate (Lithobid)
Modafinil (Provigil)
Ramipril (Altace)
Sitagliptin phosphate (Januvia)
Sodium phosphate dibasic anhydrous/Sodium phosphate monobasic monohydrate (OsmoPrep)

Table 24. ORAL MANIFESTATIONS OF SYSTEMIC AGENTS *(Cont.)*

Mouth, burning		
Acetaminophen/Butalbital/Caffeine/Codeine phosphate (Phrenilin)	Selegiline hydrochloride (Eldepryl)	
Mouth, discoloration		
Palifermin (Kepivance)		
Mouth, fissuring in corner of		
Tranylcypromine sulfate (Parnate)		
Mouth, puckering		
Molindone hydrochloride (Moban)	Pimozide (Orap)	Thiothixene hydrochloride (Navane)
Mouth, sore		
Atazanavir sulfate (Reyataz)	Haloperidol (Haldol)	Sumatriptan succinate (Imitrex)
Cyclosporine (Gengraf, Neoral)	Interferon alfa-n3 (human leukocyte derived) (Alferon N)	
Fluticasone propionate (Flovent Diskus)		
Mouth, thickening of		
Palifermin (Kepivance)		
Mouth ulceration		
Abacavir sulfate (Ziagen)	Fluoxetine hydrochloride (Prozac)	Tacrolimus (Prograf, Protopic)
Abacavir sulfate/Lamivudine (Epzicom)	Measles, mumps, varicella & rubella virus vaccine, live (ProQuad)	Tiotropium bromide (Spiriva)
Doxorubicin hydrochloride liposome (Doxil)	Mycophenolate mofetil (CellCept)	Varenicline tartrate (Chantix)
Febuxostat (Uloric)	Nilotinib (Tasigna)	Venlafaxine hydrochloride (Effexor, Effexor XR)
Fentanyl citrate (Actiq, Fentora)	Pregabalin (Lyrica)	Zidovudine (Retrovir)
	Rasagiline mesylate (Azilect)	
Mucosal pigmentation, changes		
Abacavir sulfate/Lamivudine/Zidovudine (Trizivir)	Interferon alfa-2b, recombinant (Intron A)	Minocycline hydrochloride (Dynacin, Minocin)
Mucositis		
Alemtuzumab (Campath)	Filgrastim (Neupogen)	Paclitaxel (Taxol)
Allopurinol sodium (Aloprim)	Gabapentin (Neurontin)	Panitumumab (Vectibix)
Amlexanox (Aphthasol)	Gemtuzumab ozogamicin (Mylotarg)	Pegaspargase (Oncaspar)
Amphotericin B, liposomal (AmBisome)	Hydroxyurea (Hydrea, Mylocel)	Pegfilgrastim (Neulasta)
Azithromycin (Zithromax)	Idarubicin hydrochloride (Idamycin)	Posaconazole (Noxafil)
Busulfan (Busulfex, Myleran)	Interferon alfa-2b, recombinant (Intron A)	Rasburicase (Elitek)
Cetuximab (Erbitux)	Interferon alfa-n3 (human leukocyte derived) (Alferon N)	Sorafenib (Nexavar)
Cevimeline hydrochloride (Evoxac)	Irinotecan hydrochloride (Camptosar)	Sunitinib malate (Sutent)
Daunorubicin hydrochloride (Cerubidine)	Ixabepilone (Ixempra)	Temsirolimus (Torisel)
Doxorubicin hydrochloride (Adriamycin)	Mitoxantrone hydrochloride (Novantrone)	Teniposide (Vumon)
Epirubicin hydrochloride (Ellence)	Oprelvekin (Neumega)	Tretinoin (Vesanoid)
Etoposide phosphate (Etopophos)	Oxaliplatin (Eloxatin)	Vinorelbine tartrate (Navelbine)
		Zoledronic acid (Zometa)

Table 24. ORAL MANIFESTATIONS OF SYSTEMIC AGENTS *(Cont.)*

Mucous membrane, abnormalities

- Abacavir sulfate/Lamivudine/Zidovudine (Trizivir)
- Aprepitant (Emend)
- Atropine sulfate/Chlorpheniramine maleate/Hyoscyamine sulfate/Phenylephrine hydrochloride/Phenylpropanolamine hydrochloride/Scopolamine hydrobromide (Atrohist)
- Captopril (Capoten)
- Fentanyl citrate (Actiq)
- Fluvastatin sodium (Lescol, Lescol XL)
- Fosaprepitant dimeglumine (Emend for injection)
- Gabapentin (Neurontin)
- Lovastatin (Mevacor)
- Minocycline hydrochloride (Dynacin, Minocin)
- Mirtazapine (Remeron)
- Perindopril erbumine (Aceon)
- Pilocarpine hydrochloride (Salagen)
- Sargramostim (Leukine)
- Simvastatin (Zocor)
- Sulindac (Clinoril)

Mucus, excess

- Naltrexone hydrochloride

Necrosis, buccal

- Ketoprofen

Neoplasm, laryngeal, malignant

- Ropinirole hydrochloride (Requip)

Numbness, buccal mucosa

- Clozapine (Clozaril, Fazaclo)
- Lidocaine hydrochloride (Xylocaine)
- Nicotine (Nicotrol)
- Sumatriptan succinate (Imitrex)

Numbness, lips

- Dipotassium phosphate/Disodium phosphate/Sodium phosphate (Uro-KP-Neutral)
- Methenamine mandelate/Sodium biphosphate (Uroqid-Acid No. 2)
- Pegaspargase (Oncaspar)
- Potassium acid phosphate (K-Phos Original [Sodium Free])
- Potassium phosphate/Sodium phosphate (K-Phos Neutral)

Osteonecrosis, jaw

- Alendronate sodium/Cholecalciferol (Fosamax Plus D)
- Calcium carbonate/Risedronate sodium (Actonel with Calcium)
- Etidronate disodium (Didronel)
- Ibandronate sodium (Boniva)
- Pamidronate disodium (Aredia)
- Tiludronate disodium (Skelid)
- Zoledronic acid (Reclast, Zometa)

Osteonecrosis, jaw

- Alendronate sodium/Cholecalciferol (Fosamax Plus D)
- Calcium carbonate/Risedronate sodium (Actonel with Calcium)
- Etidronate disodium (Didronel)
- Ibandronate sodium (Boniva)
- Pamidronate disodium (Aredia)
- Risedronate (Actonel)
- Tiludronate disodium (Skelid)
- Zoledronic acid (Reclast, Zometa)

Pain, dental

- Aripiprazole (Abilify)
- Atazanavir sulfate (Reyataz)
- Bupropion hydrochloride (Wellbutrin SR, Wellbutrin XL, Zyban SR)
- Cevimeline hydrochloride (Evoxac)
- Clonazepam (Klonopin)
- Eprosartan mesylate (Teveten)
- Eprosartan mesylate/Hydrochlorothiazide (Teveten HCT)
- Escitalopram oxalate (Lexapro)
- Estradiol (Vivelle, Vivelle-Dot)
- Fluticasone propionate (Flovent Diskus)
- Fluticasone propionate/Salmeterol xinafoate (Advair HFA)
- Frovatriptan succinate (Frova)
- Human papillomavirus quadrivalent (types 6, 11, 16, 18) vaccine, recombinant (Gardasil)
- Interferon alfacon-1 (Infergen)

Table 24. ORAL MANIFESTATIONS OF SYSTEMIC AGENTS *(Cont.)*

Pain, dental *(Cont.)*

- Losartan potassium (Cozaar)
- Losartan potassium/Hydrochlorothiazide (Hyzaar)
- Montelukast sodium (Singulair)
- Oxcarbazepine (Trileptal)
- Pimecrolimus (Elidel)
- Risperidone (Risperdal)
- Ropinirole hydrochloride (Requip)
- Salmeterol xinafoate (Serevent Diskus)
- Sumatriptan succinate (Imitrex)
- Telmisartan (Micardis)
- Telmisartan/Hydrochlorothiazide (Micardis HCT)
- Thalidomide (Thalidomid)
- Triamcinolone acetonide (Azmacort)

Pain, facial

- Botulinum toxin type A (Botox)
- Fluorouracil (Carac)
- Ritonavir (Norvir)
- Saquinavir mesylate (Invirase)
- Sumatriptan succinate (Imitrex)
- Tazarotene (Tazorac)

Pain, jaw

- Aripiprazole (Abilify)
- Ciprofloxacin (Cipro, Cipro XR)
- Clonazepam (Klonopin)
- Epoprostenol sodium (Flolan)
- Escitalopram oxalate (Lexapro)
- Nicotine (Nicotrol)
- Propafenone hydrochloride (Rythmol SR)
- Vinorelbine tatrate (Navelbine)
- Zolmitriptan (Zomig, Zomig-ZMT)

Pain, oral mucosa

- Ciprofloxacin (Cipro)
- Fluticasone propionate (Flovent Diskus, Flovent HFA)
- Fluticasone propionate/Salmeterol xinafoate (Advair Diskus)
- Ofloxacin (Floxin)
- Salmeterol xinafoate (Serevent Diskus)
- Sorafenib (Nexavar)
- Sunitinib malate (Sutent)

Pain, pharyngolaryngeal

- Agalsidase beta (Fabrazyme)
- Alprazolam (Xanax, Xanax XR)
- Amlodipine besylate/Valsartan (Exforge)
- Antihemophilic factor (recombinant) (Advate)
- Aprepitant (Emend)
- Aripiprazole (Abilify)
- Budesonide/Formoterol fumarate dihydrate (Symbicort)
- Bupropion hydrochloride (Wellbutrin SR, Wellbutrin XL, Zyban SR)
- Ciclesonide (Alvesco, Omnaris)
- Clindamycin phosphate/Tretinoin (Ziana)
- Daptomycin (Cubicin)
- Deferasirox (Exjade)
- Dexmethylphenidate hydrochloride (Focalin, Focalin XR)
- Duloxetine hydrochloride (Cymbalta)
- Fentanyl citrate (Fentora)
- Fluticasone furoate (Veramyst)
- Fosaprepitant dimeglumine (Emend for Injection)
- Imatinib mesylate (Gleevec)
- Influenza virus vaccine (Flulaval)
- Ixabepilone (Ixempra)
- Lubiprostone (Amitiza)
- Mesalamine (Lialda)
- Methylphenidate hydrochloride (Concerta)
- Mycophenolic acid (Myfortic)
- Naltrexone (Vivitrol)
- Nilotinib (Tasigna)
- Olopatadine hydrochloride (Patanase)
- Pramipexole dihydrochloride (Mirapex)
- Pregabalin (Lyrica)
- Rifaximin (Xifaxan)
- Ropinirole hydrochloride (Requip)
- Sodium oxybate (Xyrem)
- Telbivudine (Tyzeka)
- Terbinafine hydrochloride (Lamisil)
- Tiotropium bromide (Spiriva)
- Triamcinolone acetonide (Nasacort AQ)
- Valsartan/Hydrochlorothiazide (Diovan HCT)

Pain, pharynx

- Antihemophilic factor (recombinant) (Advate)
- Carbidopa/Entacapone/Levodopa (Stalevo)
- Carbidopa/Levodopa (Sinemet)
- Cilastatin/Imipenem (Primaxin)
- Estradiol (Vivelle, Vivelle-Dot)
- Lisinopril (Prinivil, Zestril)
- Lisinopril/Hydrochlorothiazide (Prinzide, Zestoretic)
- Omeprazole (Prilosec)
- Omeprazole/Sodium bicarbonate (Zegerid)

Table 24. ORAL MANIFESTATIONS OF SYSTEMIC AGENTS *(Cont.)*

Pain, salivary gland

Cevimeline hydrochloride (Evoxac)
Frovatriptan succinate (Frova)

Pain, throat

Alosetron hydrochloride (Lotronex)
Aripiprazole (Abilify)
Desmopressin acetate (DDAVP)
Naratriptan hydrochloride (Amerge)
Sumatriptan succinate (Imitrex)
Zanamivir (Relenza)
Zolmitriptan (Zomig, Zomig-ZMT)

Pain, tongue

Iloprost (Ventavis)

Paralysis, facial

Amlodipine besylate/Atorvastatin calcium (Caduet)
Atorvastatin calcium (Lipitor)
Bivalirudin (Angiomax)
Botulinum Toxin Type A (Botox)
Fentanyl citrate (Actiq)
Fluvastatin sodium (Lescol, Lescol XL)
Gabapentin (Neurontin)
Glatiramer acetate (Copaxone)
Influenza virus vaccine (Flulaval)
Lopinavir/Ritonavir (Kaletra)
Lovastatin (Altoprev, Altoprev ER)
Medroxyprogesterone acetate (Depo-provera)
Omega-3-acid ethyl esters (Lovaza)
Polifeprosan 20 with carmustine (Gliadel)
Rasagiline mesylate (Azilect)
Riluzole (Rilutek)
Sumatriptan succinate (Imitrex)
Tretinoin (Vesanoid)
Venlafaxine hydrochloride (Effexor, Effexor XR)
Zaleplon (Sonata)
Zonisamide (Zonegran)

Paralysis, tongue

Frovatriptan succinate (Frova)
Rizatriptan benzoate (Maxalt, Maxalt-MLT)
Topiramate (Topamax)

Paresthesia, oral

Amprenavir (Agenerase)
Dexlansoprazole (Kapidex)
Fosamprenavir calcium (Lexiva)
Indinavir sulfate (Crixivan)
Nicotine (Nicotrol)

Periodontitis

Carvedilol phosphate (Coreg, Coreg CR)
Donepezil hydrochloride (Aricept)
Eprosartan mesylate (Teveten)
Eprosartan mesylate/Hydrochlorothiazide (Teveten HCT)
Lopinavir/Ritonavir (Kaletra)
Pantoprazole sodium (Protonix)
Pramipexole dihydrochloride (Mirapex)
Ropinirole hydrochloride (Requip)
Thalidomide (Thalomid)
Venlafaxine hydrochloride (Effexor, Effexor XR)

Pharyngeal discomfort

Clozapine (Fazaclo)
Ertapenem sodium (Invanz)
Esomeprazole sodium (Nexium)
Lisinopril/Hydrochlorothiazide (Prinzide)
Losartan potassium (Cozaar)
Losartan/Hydrochlorothiazide (Hyzaar)

Pharyngitis

Abacavir sulfate (Ziagen)
Abacavir/Lamivudine (Epzicom)
Abacavir/Lamivudine/Zidovudine (Trizivir)
Acamprosate calcium (Campral)
Acebutolol hydrochloride (Sectral)
Acetylcysteine (Acetadote)
Acitretin (Soriatane)
Adefovir dipivoxil (Hepsera)
Agalsidase beta (Fabrazyme)
Albuterol/Ipatropium (Combivent, Duoneb)
Albuterol sulfate (ProAir HFA, Ventolin HFA)
Alefacept (Amevive)
Alemtuzumab (Campath)
Alfuzosin hydrochloride (Uroxatral)
Allopurinol sodium (Aloprim)

Table 24. ORAL MANIFESTATIONS OF SYSTEMIC AGENTS *(Cont.)*

Pharyngitis *(Cont.)*

Almotriptan malate (Axert)
Alpha1-proteinase inhibitor (human) (Aralast)
Amlodipine besylate (Exforge)
Amlodipine besylate/Atorvastatin calcium (Caduet)
Amlodipine besylate/Benazepril hydrochloride (Lotrel)
Amoxicillin/Clarithromycin/Lansoprazole (PREVPAC)
Amphotericin B, liposomal (AmBisome)
Anagrelide hydrochloride (Agrylin)
Anastrozole (Arimidex)
Antihemophilic factor (human) (Alphanate)
Antihemophilic factor (recombinant) (ReFacto)
Aprepitant (Emend)
Atorvastatin calcium (Lipitor)
Azelastine hydrochloride (Astelin, Astepro)
Azithromycin dihydrate (Zithromax)
Balsalazide disodium (Colazal)
Basiliximab (Simulect)
Beclomethasone dipropionate (Qvar)
Bepridil hydrochloride (Vascor)
Betaxolol hydrochloride (Kerlone)
Bexarotene (Targretin)
Bicalutamide (Casodex)
Botulinum toxin type A (Botox)
Brimonidine tartrate (Alphagan P)
Brimonidine tartrate/Timolol maleate (Combigan)
Brinzolamide (Azopt)
Budesonide (Pulmicort)
Buprenorphine hydrochloride (Subutex)
Buprenorphine hydrochloride/Naloxone hydrochloride (Suboxone)
Bupropion hydrochloride (Wellbutrin, Wellbutrin SR, Wellbutrin XL, Zyban SR)
Busulfan (Busulfex)
Calcitonin-salmon (Miacalcin)
Candesartan cilexetil (Atacand)
Candesartan cilexetil/Hydrochlorothiazide (Atacand HCT)
Carbamazepine (Carbatrol, Equetro, Tegretol)
Cefaclor (Ceclor)
Cefditoren pivoxil (Spectracef)
Celecoxib (Celebrex)
Cetirizine hydrochloride (Zyrtec)
Cetirizine hydrochloride/Pseudoephedrine hydrochloride (Zyrtec-D)
Cetuximab (Erbitux)
Cevimeline hydrochloride (Evoxac)
Cilostazol (Pletal)
Citalopram hydrobromide (Celexa)
Clindamycin phosphate (Clindesse)
Clonazepam (Klonopin)
Colesevelam hydrochloride (WelChol)
Cyclosporine (Gengraf, Neoral)
Daclizumab (Zenapax)
Dactinomycin (Cosmegen)
Dapsone (Aczone)
Darifenacin (Enablex)
Decitabine (Dacogen)
Deferasirox (Exjade)
Delavirdine mesylate (Rescriptor)
Denileukin diftitox (Ontak)
Desflurane (Suprane)
Desloratadine (Clarinex)
Desloratadine/Pseudoephedrine hydrochloride (Clarinex-D)
Desonide (Verdeso)
Dexlansoprazole (Kapidex)
Dihydroergotamine mesylate (Migranal)
Diltiazem hydrochloride (Dilacor XR, Tiazac)
Divalproex sodium (Depakote ER)
Docetaxel (Taxotere)
Donepezil hydrochloride (Aricept)
Dornase alfa (Pulmozyme)
Dorzolamide hydrochloride (Trusopt)
Dorzolamide hydrochloride/Timolol maleate (Cosopt)
Doxorubicin hydrochloride liposome (Doxil)
Drospirenone/Ethinyl estradiol (Yasmin, Yaz)
Eletriptan hydrobromide (Relpax)
Epinastine hydrochloride (Elestat)
Epoetin alfa (Epogen)
Epoprostenol sodium (Flolan)
Eprosartan mesylate (Teveten)
Eprosartan mesylate/Hydrochlorothiazide (Teveten HCT)
Ertapenem sodium (Invanz)
Escitalopram oxalate (Lexapro)
Esomeprazole sodium (Nexium I.V.)
Esomeprazole magnesium/Esomeprazole sodium (Nexium)
Estradiol (Climara)
Estradiol/Norethindrone acetate (Combipatch)
Estrogens, conjugated (Premarin)
Estrogens, conjugated, synthetic A (Cenestin)
Estrogens/Medroxyprogesterone (Premphase, Prempro)
Eszopiclone (Lunesta)
Etanercept (Enbrel)
Etonogestrel (Implanon)
Exemestane (Aromasin)
Ezetimibe/Simvastatin (Vytorin)
Famciclovir (Famvir)
Felodipine (Plendil, Felodipine, Felodipine ER)
Fenofibrate (Tricor)
Fentanyl (Duragesic, Ionsys)
Fentanyl citrate (Actiq)
Flunisolide hemihydrate (Aerobid, Aerobid-M)
Fluoxetine hydrochloride (Prozac)
Fluoxetine hydrochloride/Olanzapine (Symbyax)
Fluticasone propionate (Flonase, Flovent Diskus, Flovent HFA)
Fluvastatin sodium (Lescol, Lescol XL)
Fluvoxamine maleate (Luvox, Luvox CR)
Follitropin alfa (Gonal-F)
Formoterol fumarate (Foradil)
Fosaprepitant dimeglumine (Emend for Injection)
Foscarnet sodium (Foscavir)
Fosinopril sodium (Monopril)
Frovatriptan succinate (Frova)
Fulvestrant (Faslodex)
Gabapentin (Neurontin)
Gemcitabine hydrochloride (Gemzar)

Table 24. ORAL MANIFESTATIONS OF SYSTEMIC AGENTS *(Cont.)*

Pharyngitis *(Cont.)*

Gemifloxacin mesylate (Factive)
Gemtuzumab ozogamicin (Mylotarg)
Glatiramer acetate (Copaxone)
Glimepiride/Pioglitazone hydrochloride (Duetact)
Goserelin acetate (Zoladex)
Hepatitis A vaccine, inactivated (Havrix, Vaqta)
Hepatitis B vaccine, recombinant (Recombivax HB)
Hydrocodone bitartrate (Vicoprofen)
Ibandronate sodium (Boniva)
Ibuprofen/Oxydone hydrochloride (Combunox)
Imatinib mesylate (Gleevec)
Imiquimod (Aldara)
Immune globulin intravenous (human) (Flebogamma, Gamunex)
Indapamide (Indapamide)
Indinavir sulfate (Crixivan)
Infliximab (Remicade)
Influenza virus vaccine (Fluarix, Flulaval)
Interferon alacon-1 (Infergen)
Interferon alfa-2b, recombinant (Intron A)
Interferon alfa-n3 (human leukocyte derived) (Alferon N)
Iodine I 131 tositumomab (Bexxar)
Ipratropium bromide (Atrovent)
Irbesartan (Avapro)
Irbesartan/Hydrochlorothiazide (Avalide)
Isosorbite mononitrate (Imdur, Ismo, Monoket)
Itraconazole (Sporanox)
Ketotifen fumarate (Zaditor)
Lamotrigine (Lamictal, Lamictal CD)
Lansoprazole (Prevacid)
Lefluomide (Arava)
Levalbuterol hydrochloride (Xopenex, Xopenex HFA)
Levetiracetam (Keppra, Keppra XR)
Levocarnitine (Carnitor)
Levocetirizine dihydrochloride (Xyzal)
Levofloxacin (Quixin, Levaquin)
Linezolid (Zyvox)
Lisinopril (Prinivil, Zestril)
Lisinopril/Hydrochlorothiazide (Prinzide, Zestoretic)
Lopinavir/Ritonavir (Kaletra)
Loratadine/Pseudoephedrine sulfate (Claritin-D)
Losartan potassium (Cozaar)
Losartan/Hydrochlorothiazide (Hyzaar)
Loteprednol etabonate (Lotemax)
Measles, mumps, varicella & rubella virus vaccine, live (ProQuad)
Megestrol acetate (Megace ES)
Meloxicam (Mobic)
Meropenem (Merrem)
Mesalamine (Asacol)
Methotrexate
Methylphenidate hydrochloride (Concerta)
Mitoxantrone hydrochloride (Novantrone)
Modafinil (Provigil)
Moexipril hydrochloride (Univasc)
Mometasone furoate (Asmanex)
Mometasone furoate monohydrate (Nasonex)
Montelukast sodium (Singulair)
Moxifloxacin hydrochloride (Vigamox)
Mupirocin calcium (Bactroban)
Mycophenolate mofetil hydrochloride (CellCept)
Naltrexone (Vivitrol)
Nedocromil sodium (Alocril)
Nelfinavir mesylate (Viracept)
Nicotine (Nicotrol)
Nifedipine (Procardia, Procardia XL)
Nilotinib (Tasigna)
Nisoldipine (Sular)
Nitazoxanide (Alinia)
Nizatidine (Axid)
Octreotide acetate (Sandostatin)
Ofloxacin (Floxin)
Olanzapine (Zyprexa, Zyprexa ZYDIS)
Olopatadine hydrochloride (Pataday, Patanol)
Omalizumab (Xolair)
Omega-3-acid ethyl esters (Lovaza)
Omeprazole (Prilosec, Zegerid)
Oprelvekin (Neumega)
Oxaliplatin (Eloxatin)
Oxcarbazepine (Trileptal)
Oxybutynin chloride (Ditropan XL)
Oxycodone hydrochloride (OxyContin)
Palivizumab (Synagis)
Pancrelipase (Creon)
Pantoprazole sodium (Protonix)
Paroxetine hydrochloride (Paxil CR, Paxil)
Peginterferon alfa-2b (PegIntron)
Pemetrexed (Alimta)
Pentosan polysulfate sodium (Elmiron)
Pentostatin (Nipent)
Perindopril erbumine (Aceon)
Pilocarpine hydrochloride (Salagen)
Pimecrolimus (Elidel)
Pioglitazone hydrochloride (Actos)
Pioglitazone hydrochloride/Metformin hydrochloride (ActoPlus Met)
Piperacillin sodium/Tazobactam sodium (Zosyn)
Pneumococcal vaccine, diphtheria conjugate (Prevnar)
Porfimer sodium (Photofrin)
Posaconazole (Noxafil)
Pramipexole dihydrochloride (Mirapex)
Progesterone (Crinone, Prometrium)
Propofol (Diprivan)
Propranolol hydrochloride (Inderal, InnoPran XL)
Quetiapine fumarate (Seroquel, Seroquel XR)
Rabeprazole sodium (Aciphex T)
Raloxifene hydrochloride (Evista)
Ribavirin (Rebetol)
Rifaximin (Xifaxan)
Risedronate sodium (Actonel)
Risedronate sodium/Calcium carbonate (Actonel With Calcium)
Risperidone (Risperdal)
Ritonavir (Norvir)
Rivastigmine tartrate (Exelon)
Rizatriptan benzoate (Maxalt, Maxalt-MLT)
Ropinirole hydrochloride (Requip)

Table 24. ORAL MANIFESTATIONS OF SYSTEMIC AGENTS *(Cont.)*

Pharyngitis *(Cont.)*

Rosuvastatin calcium (Crestor)
Rotavirus vaccine, live, oral, tetravalent (Rotashield)
Salmeterol xinafoate (Serevent Diskus)
Saquinavir mesylate (Invirase)
Sargramostim (Leukine)
Selegiline (Emsam)
Sertraline hydrochloride (Zoloft)
Sevoflurane (Ultane)
Sibutramine hydrochloride monohydrate (Meridia)
Sildenafil citrate (Viagra)
Sirolimus (Rapamune)
Sodium ferric gluconate (Ferrlecit)
Sodium oxybate (Xyrem)
Solifenacin succinate (VESIcare)
Somatropin (Humatrope)
Tacrolimus (Prograf, Protopic)
Tadalafil (Cialis)
Tamsulosin hydrochloride (Flomax)
Telmisartan (Micardis)
Telmisartan/Hydrochlorothiazide (Micardis HCT)
Temozolomide (Temodar)
Temsirolimus (Torisel)
Terazson hydrochloride (Hytrin)
Teriparatide (Forteo)
Thalidomide (Thalomid)
Tiagabine hydrochloride (Gabitril)
Tinidazole (Tindamax)
Tiotropium bromide (Spiriva)
Tobramycin (TOBI)
Tolcapone (Tasmar)
Tolterodine tartrate (Detrol, Detrol LA)
Topiramate (Topamax)
Topotecan hydrochloride (Hycamtin)
Tositumomab (Bexxar)
Trastuzumab (Herceptin)
Triamcinolone acetonide (Azmacort, Nasacort AQ)
Triptorelin pamoate (Trelstar)
Valganciclovir hydrochloride (Valcyte)
Valproate (Depacon)
Valproic acid (Depakene)
Valsartan (Diovan)
Valsartan/Hydrochlorothiazide (Diovan HCT)
Vardenafil hydrochloride (Levitra)
Varicella virus vaccine, live (Varivax)
Venlafaxine hydrochloride (Effexor, Effexor XR)
Verapamil hydrochloride (Verelan, Verapamil)
Verteporfin (Visudyne)
Voriconazole (VFEND)
Zidovudine (Retrovir)
Ziprasidone hydrochloride (Geodon)
Zolmitriptan (Zomig, Zomig-ZMT)
Zolpidem tartrate (Ambien)
Zonisamide (Zonegran)

Pharyngolaryngeal pain

Duloxetine hydrochloride (Cymbalta)
Imatinib mesylate (Gleevec)

Pharyngoxerosis

Carbamazepine (Carbatrol)

Prothrombin time, decrease

Ciprofloxacin (Cipro, Cipro XR)
Estrogens, conjugated (Premarin)
Flavocoxid (Limbrel)
Estrogen, conjugated/Medroxyprogesterone acetate (Premphase, Prempro)
Moxifloxacin hydrochloride (Avelox)

Prothrombin time, deviation

Cefepime hydrochloride (Maxipime)
Moxifloxacin hydrochloride (Avelox)
Thrombin (Thrombin-JMI)

Prothrombin time, elevation

Aspirin (St. Joseph's Aspirin)
Caspofungin acetate (Cancidas)
Lovastatin/Niacin (Advicor)

Prothrombin time, prolongation

Amoxicillin/Clarithromycin/Lansoprazole (PREVPAC)
Asparaginase (Elspar)
Aspirin (Bayer Aspirin)
Aspirin/Dipyridamole (Aggrenox)
Aspirin/Oxycodone hydrochloride (Percodan)
Balsalazide disodium (Colazal)
Busulfan (Busulfex)
Cefadroxil (Duricef)
Cefixime (Suprax)
Cefoxitin sodium (Mefoxin)
Cefpodoxime proxetil (Vantin)
Cefprozil (Cefzil)
Ceftazidime (Fortaz)
Ceftriaxone sodium (Rocephin)
Cefuroxime (Zinacef)
Cefuroxime axetil (Ceftin)
Cephalexin hydrochloride (Keflex)
Ciprofloxacin (Cipro, Cipro XR)
Clarithromycin (Biaxin, Biaxin XL)
Daptomycin (Cubicin)
Delavirdine mesylate (Rescriptor)
Ertapenem sodium (Invanz)

Table 24. ORAL MANIFESTATIONS OF SYSTEMIC AGENTS *(Cont.)*

Prothrombin time, prolongation *(Cont.)*

Ethinyl estradiol/Norgestimate (Ortho Tri-Cyclen Lo, Ortho Tri-Cyclen, Ortho-Cyclen)
Febuxostat (Uloric)
Flavocoxid (Limbrel)
Hemin (Panhematin)
Imipenem/Cilastatin (Primaxin)
Interferon alfacon-1 (Infergen)
Levofloxacin (Levaquin)
Meropenem (Merrem)
Moxifloxacin hydrochloride (Avelox)
Mycophenolate mofetil hydrochloride (CellCept)
Niacin (Niaspan)
Norfloxacin (Noroxin)
Ofloxacin (Floxin)
Oxaliplatin (Eloxatin)
Oxandrolone (Oxandrin)
Oxymetholone (Anadrol)
Pegaspargase (Oncaspar)
Pentosan polysulfate sodium (Elmiron)
Piperacillin sodium/Tazobactam sodium (Zosyn)
Sertraline hydrochloride (Zoloft)
Sulindac (Clinoril)
Testosterone (Testim)
Ticarcillin disodium/Clavulanate potassium (Timentin)
Tigecycline (Tygacil)

Saliva, discoloration

Carbidopa (Lodosyn)
Carbidopa/Levadopa/Entacapone (Stalevo)
Carbidopa/Levodopa (Parcopa, Sinemet)

Salivary gland enlargement

Acetyl sulfisoxazole (Gantrisin)
Cevimeline hydrochloride (Evoxac)
Clozapine (Clozaril, Fazaclo)
Cyclosporine (Gengraf, Neoral)
Fluoxetine hydrochloride (Prozac)
Gabapentin (Neurontin)
Glatiramer acetate (Copaxone)
Leflunomide (Arava)
Lithium carbonate (Lithobid)
Mirtazapine (Remeron)
Nitazoxanide (Alinia)
Paroxetine hydrochloride (Paxil, Paxil CR)
Pilocarpine hydrochloride (Salagen)
Rabeprazole sodium (Aciphex)
Riluzole (Rilutek)
Sumatriptan succinate (Imitrex)

Sialadenitis

Aliskiren/Hydrochlorothiazide (Tekturna HCT)
Benazepril (Lotensin)
Bendroflumethiazide/Nadolol (Corzide)
Candesartan cilexetil/Hydrochlorothiazide (Atacand HCT)
Cevimeline hydrochloride (Evoxac)
Chlorothiazide sodium (Diuril)
Delavirdine mesylate (Rescriptor)
Enalapril maleate/Hydrochlorothiazide (Vaseretic)
Eprosartan mesylate/Hydrochlorothiazide (Teveten HCT)
Fosinopril sodium (Monopril)
Indapamide
Irbesartan/Hydrochlorothiazide (Avalide)
Lisinopril/Hydrochlorothiazide (Prinzide)
Lopinavir/Ritonavir (Kaletra)
Losartan potassium/Hydrochlorothiazide (Hyzaar)
Methyclothiazide (Enduron)
Methyldopate hydrochloride (Aldomet)
Naratriptan hydrochloride (Amerge)
Nitrofurantoin (Furadantin, Nitrofurantoin)
Oxcarbazepine (Trileptal)
Paroxetine hydrochloride (Paxil CR, Paxil)
Telmisartan/Hydrochlorothiazide (Micardis HCT)
Triamterene/Hydrochlorothiazide (Dyazide)
Valsartan/Hydrochlorothiazide (Diovan HCT)
Zolmitriptan (Zomig, Zomig-ZMT)

Stomatitis

Abacavir sulfate/Lamivudine (Epzicom)
Abacavir/Lamivudine/Zidovudine (Trizivir)
Acetyl sulfisoxazole (Gantrisin)
Acitretin (Soriatane)
Aldesleukin (Proleukin)
Alemtuzumab (Campath)
Amitriptyline hydrochloride (Elavil)
Amlodipine besylate/Atorvastatin calcium (Caduet)
Amoxicillin/Clavulanate potassium (Augmentin, Augmentin XR)
Amoxicillin/Clarithromycin/Lansoprazole (PREVPAC)
Amphotericin B, liposomal (AmBisome)
Aprepitant (Emend)
Aripiprazole (Abilify)
Atorvastatin calcium (Lipitor)

Table 24. ORAL MANIFESTATIONS OF SYSTEMIC AGENTS *(Cont.)*

Stomatitis *(Cont.)*

Atovaquone/Proguanil (Malarone)
Azithromycin dihydrate (Zithromax)
Bendamustine hydrochloride (Treanda)
Bevacizumab (Avastin)
Bismuth subcitrate potassium/Metronidazole/Tetracycline (Pylera)
Bleomycin sulfate (Blenoxane)
Bortezomib (Velcade)
Bupropion hydrochloride (Wellbutrin SR, Wellbutrin XL, Zyban SR)
Busulfan (Busulfex)
Capecitabine (Xeloda)
Carbamazepine (Carbatrol, Equetro, Tegretol)
Cefdinir (Omnicef)
Cefditoren pivoxil (Spectracef)
Ceftriaxone sodium (Rocephin)
Celecoxib (Celebrex)
Cetirizine hydrochloride (Zyrtec)
Cetirizine hydrochloride/Pseudoephedrine hydrochloride (Zyrtec-D)
Cetuximab (Erbitux)
Cevimeline hydrochloride (Evoxac)
Citalopram hydrobromide (Celexa)
Clarithromycin potassium (Biaxin, Biaxin XL)
Clofibrate
Clopidogrel bisulfate (Plavix)
Cyclobenzaprine hydrochloride (Flexeril)
Cyclosporine (Gengraf, Neoral)
Cytarabine (Cytosar-U)
Dalfopristin/Quinupristin (Synercid)
Daptomycin (Cubicin)
Decitabine (Dacogen)
Delavirdine mesylate (Rescriptor)
Dexrazoxane (Zinecard)
Diclofenac sodium (Voltaren, Voltaren-XR)
Diclofenac sodium/Misoprostol (Arthrotec)
Diflunisal
Divalproex sodium (Depakote, Depakote ER)
Docetaxel (Taxotere)
Doxorubicin hydrochloride (Adriamycin)
Doxorubicin hydrochloride liposome (Doxil)
Duloxetine hydrochloride (Cymbalta)
Eletriptan hydrobromide (Relpax)
Enalapril maleate (Vasotec)
Enalapril maleate/Hydrochlorothiazide (Vaseretic)
Epirubicin hydrochloride (Ellence)
Erlotinib (Tarceva)
Ertapenem sodium (Invanz)
Esomeprazole magnesium/Esomeprazole sodium (Nexium)
Estrogens, esterified/Methyltestosterone (Estratest H.S.)
Eszopiclone (Lunesta)
Ethionamide (Trecator)
Etoposide (Vepesid)
Etoposide phosphate (Etopophos)
Etravirine (Intelence)
Fentanyl citrate (Actiq, Fentora)
Filgrastim (Neupogen)
Fluorouracil
Fluoxetine hydrochloride (Prozac)
Fluoxetine hydrochloride/Olanzapine (Symbyax)
Fluvoxamine maleate (Luvox, Luvox CR)
Fosaprepitant dimeglumine (Emend)
Frovatriptan succinate (Frova)
Gabapentin (Neurontin)
Gemcitabine hydrochloride (Gemzar)
Gemtuzumab ozogamicin (Mylotarg)
Glatiramer acetate (Copaxone)
Hydroxyurea (Droxia, Hydrea)
Interferon alfa-2b, recombinant (Intron A)
Interferon alfa-n3 (human leukocyte derived) (Alferon N)
Irinotecan hydrochloride (Camptosar)
Ixabepilone (Ixempra)
Lamivudine (Epivir, Epivir-HBV)
Lamivudine/Zidovudine (Combivir)
Lamotrigine (Lamictal)
Lansoprazole (Prevacid)
Lapatinib (Tykerb)
Leflunomide (Arava)
Leucovorin calcium (Leucovorin)
Levofloxacin (Levaquin)
Lomustine (CCNU) (CeeNu)
Lopinavir/Ritonavir (Kaletra)
Loratadine (Claritin)
Loratadine/Pseudoephedrine sulfate (Claritin-D)
Mefenamic acid (Ponstel)
Mesalamine (Asacol)
Methotrexate
Minocycline hydrochloride (Minocin, Dynacin)
Mirtazapine (Remeron, Remeron SolTab)
Mitomycin (Mitomycin-C, Mutamycin)
Mitoxantrone hydrochloride (Novantrone)
Moxifloxacin hydrochloride (Avelox)
Mycophenolate mofetil (CellCept)
Nabumetone
Naproxen (EC-Naprosyn, Naprosyn)
Naproxen sodium (Anaprox DS)
Nelarabine (Arranon)
Nicotine (Nicotrol)
Nilotinib (Tasigna)
Norfloxacin (Noroxin)
Octreotide (Sandostatin)
Oxaliplatin (Eloxatin)
Oxcarbazepine (Trileptal)
Oxycodone hydrochloride (OxyContin)
Pamidronate disodium (Aredia)
Panitumumab (Vectibix)
Pantoprazole sodium (Protonix)
Paroxetine hydrochloride (Paxil, Paxil CR)
Pegfilgrastim (Neulasta)
Peginterferon alfa-2b (PegIntron)
Pemetrexed (Alimta)
Pentostatin (Nipent)
Pilocarpine hydrochloride (Salagen)
Pirbuterol acetate (Maxair)

Table 24. ORAL MANIFESTATIONS OF SYSTEMIC AGENTS *(Cont.)*

Stomatitis *(Cont.)*

Procarbazine hydrochloride (Matulane)
Protriptyline hydrochloride (Vivactil)
Pyrimethamine/Sulfadoxine (Fansidar)
Quetiapine fumarate (Seroquel)
Rabeprazole sodium (Aciphex)
Rasagiline mesylate (Azilect)
Riluzole (Rilutek)
Rimantadine hydrochloride (Flumadine)
Risperidone (Risperdal Consta)
Ropinirole hydrochloride (Requip)
Saquinavir mesylate (Invirase)
Sargramostim (Leukine)
Sertraline hydrochloride (Zoloft)
Sildenafil citrate (Viagra)
Sirolimus (Rapamune)
Sodium oxybate (Xyrem)
Sorafenib (Nexavar)
Sulfamethoxazole/Trimethoprim (Bactrim, Septra)
Sulindac (Clinoril)
Sunitinib maleate (Sutent)
Tacrolimus (Prograf, Protopic)
Telithromycin (Ketek)
Temozolomide (Temodar)
Testosterone (Androgel, Androderm, Striant, Testim)
Thalidomide (Thalomid)
Thioguanine (Tabloid)
Tiagabine hydrochloride (Gabitril)
Ticarcillin disodium/Clavulanate potassium (Timentin)
Tinidazole (Tindamax)
Tiotropium bromide (Spiriva)
Tolmetin sodium (Tolectin DS)
Topiramate (Topamax)
Topotecan hydrochloride (Hycamtin)
Trastuzumab (Herceptin)
Trimipramine maleate (Surmontil)
Valproate sodium (Depacon)
Valproic acid (Depakene)
Venlafaxine hydrochloride (Effexor, Effexor XR)
Vinorelbine tartrate (Navelbine)
Voriconazole (VFEND)
Zaleplon (Sonata)
Zoledronic acid (Zometa)
Zolmitriptan (Zomig, Zomig-ZMT)
Zonisamide (Zonegran)

Stomatitis, ulcerative

Acitretin (Soriatane)
Alemtuzumab (Campath)
Amlodipine besylate/Atorvastatin (Caduet)
Amoxicillin/Clarithromycin/Lansoprazole (Prevpac)
Amphotericin B, liposomal (AmBisome)
Anagrelide hydrochloride (Agrylin)
Atazanavir sulfate (Reyataz)
Atorvastatin calcium (Lipitor)
Azelastine hydrochloride (Astelin)
Balsalazide disodium (Colazol)
Basiliximab (Simulect)
Cetirizine hydrochloride (Zyrtec)
Cetirizine hydrochloride/Pseudoephedrine hydrochloride (Zyrtec-D)
Cevimeline hydrochloride (Evoxac)
Dactinomycin (Cosmegen)
Diclofenac sodium/Misoprostol (Arthrotec)
Doxorubicin hydrochloride liposome (Doxil)
Duloxetine hydrochloride (Cymbalta)
Esomeprazole magnesium (Nexium)
Eszopiclone (Lunesta)
Fluoxetine hydrochloride (Prozac)
Follitropin alfa (Gonal-F SQ)
Foscarnet sodium (Foscavir)
Gabapentin (Neurontin)
Ganciclovir sodium (Cytovene)
Glatiramer acetate (Copaxone)
Indomethacin (Indocin)
Interferon alfa-2b, recombinant (Intron A)
Itraconazole (Sporanox)
Lansoprazole (Prevacid)
Lopinavir/Ritonavir (Kaletra)
Meloxicam (Mobic)
Methotrexate
Mirtazapine (Remeron)
Mitoxantrone hydrochloride (Novantrone)
Mupirocin calcium (Bactroban)
Naproxen (EC-Naprosyn, Naprosyn)
Naproxen sodium (Anaprox)
Nevirapine (Viramune)
Olanzapine/Fluoxetine hydrochloride (Symbyax)
Oxcarbazepine (Trileptal)
Pantoprazole sodium (Protonix)
Paroxetine hydrochloride (Paxil, Paxil Cr)
Peginterferon alfa-2b (PegIntron)
Piperacillin sodium/Tazobactam sodium (Zosyn)
Pramipexole dihydrochloride (Mirapex)
Pregabalin (Lyrica)
Risperidone (Risperdal Consta)
Rivastigmine tartrate (Exelon)
Ropinirole hydrochloride (Requip)
Sertaline hydrochloride (Zoloft)
Tiagabine hydrochloride (Gabitril)
Tiotropium bromide (Spiriva)
Zaleplon (Sonata)
Zonisamide (Zonegran)

Swallowing, impairment

Aprepitant (Emend)
Captopril
Cyclosporine (Gengraf, Neoral, Sandimmune)
Dantrolene sodium (Dantrium)
Daptomycin (Cubicin)
Enalapril maleate (Vasotec)
Enalapril maleate/Hydrochlorothiazide (Vaseretic)
Escitalopram oxalate (Lexapro)
Fosinopril sodium (Monopril)
Levofloxacin (Levaquin)
Lidocaine hydrochloride (Xylocaine)
Lisinopril (Prinivil, Zestril)

Table 24. ORAL MANIFESTATIONS OF SYSTEMIC AGENTS *(Cont.)*

Swallowing, impairment *(Cont.)*

Lisinopril/Hydrochlorothiazide (Prinzide, Zestoretic)	Prochloroperazine (Compro)	Thioridazine hydrochloride
Muromonab-cd3 (Orthoclone OKT3)	Sitagliptin phosphate (Januvia)	Trandolapril (Mavik)
	Sumatriptan succinate (Imitrex)	Warfarin (Coumadin)

Swelling, mouth

Diphtheria & tetanus toxoids and acellular pertussis vaccine adsorbed (Infanrix, Pediarix, Adacel, Boostrix)	Flecainide acetate (Tambocor)	Influenza virus vaccine (Fluarix)
	Hepatitis B vaccine, recombinant (Pediarix)	Poliovirus vaccine inactivated (Pediarix)

Swelling, oropharyngeal

Duloxetine hydrochloride (Cymbalta)	Sodium oxybate (Xyrem)	

Swelling, salivary gland

Cyclobenzaprine hydrochloride (Flexeril)	Lithium carbonate (Eskalith)	

Tardive dyskinesia

Aripiprazole (Abilify)	Haloperdiol (Haldol)	Selegiline hydrochloride (Eldepryl)
Amitriptyline hydrochloride (Elavil)	Memantine hydrochloride (Namenda)	Thioridazine hydrochloride
Bupropion hydrochloride (Zyban SR)	Metoclopramide (Reglan)	Thiothixene hydrochloride (Navane)
Buspirone hydrochloride (Buspar)	Molindone hydrochloride (Moban)	Valproate sodium (Depacon)
Clozapine (Clozaril, Fazaclo ODT)	Olanzapine (Zyprexa, Zyprexa ZYDIS)	Valproic acid (Depakene)
Divalproex sodium (Depakote, Depakote ER)	Paliperidone (Invega)	Venlafaxine hydrochloride (Effexor, Effexor XR)
Escitalopram oxalate (Lexapro)	Pimozide (Orap)	Ziprasidone hydrochloride (Geodon)
Fluoxetine hydrochloride/Olanzapine (Symbyax)	Prochlorperazine (Compro)	Zolmitriptan (Zomig, Zomig ZMT)
Fluvoxamine maleate (Luvox, Luvox CR)	Quetiapine fumarate (Seroquel, Seroquel XR)	
	Risperidone (Risperdal Consta)	

Taste, altered

Acamprosate calcium (Campral)	Antihemophilic factor (recombinant) (BeneFIX, Kogenate FS, ReFacto)	Carbidopa/Levodopa/Entacapone (Stalevo)
Acitretin (Soriatane)	Aprepitant (Emend)	Cefditoren pivoxil (Spectracef)
Albuterol sulfate (ProAir HFA, Proventil HFA)	Atorvastatin calcium (Lipitor)	Cefpodoxime proxetil (Vantin)
Albuterol sulfate/Ipratropium bromide (Combivent)	Atovaquone (Mepron)	Celecoxib (Celebrex)
Aldesleukin (Proleukin)	Azithromycin (Zithromax, Zmax)	Cetirizine hydrochloride (Zyrtec)
Alendronate sodium (Fosamax)	Balsalazide disodium (Colazal)	Cetirizine hydrochloride/Pseudoephedrine (Zyrtec-D)
Alendronate sodium/Cholecalciferol (Fosamax Plus D)	Betaxolol hydrochloride (Kerlone)	Cevimeline hydrochloride (Evoxac)
Almotriptan malate (Axert)	Bevacizumab (Avastin)	Cilastatin sodium/Imipenem (Primaxin)
Alprazolam (Niravam, Xanax)	Brimonidine tartrate (Alphagan P)	Ciprofloxacin (Ciprodex)
Alsetron hydrochloride (Lotronex)	Budesonide (Pulmicort)	Citalopram hydrobromide (Celexa)
Amiodarone hydrochloride (Pacerone)	Bupropion hydrochloride (Wellbutrin SR, Wellbutrin XL, Zyban SR)	Clarithromycin (Biaxin, Biaxin XL)
Amlodipine besylate (Norvasc)	Buspirone hydrochloride (Buspar)	Clavulanate potassium (Timentin)
Amoxicillin/Clarithromycin/Lansoprazole (Prevpac)	Calcitonin-salmon (Miacalcin)	Clonidine (Catapres-TTS)
Atazanavir sulfate (Reyataz)	Captopril	Clopidogrel bisulfate (Plavix)
	Carbidopa (Lodosyn)	Cyclosporine (Gengraf, Neoral)
	Carbidopa/Levodopa (Parcopa, Sinemet)	Dantrolene sodium (Dantrium)
		Daptomycin (Cubicin)

Table 24. ORAL MANIFESTATIONS OF SYSTEMIC AGENTS *(Cont.)*

Taste, altered *(Cont.)*

Delavirdine mesylate (Rescriptor)
Dexamethasone (Ciprodex)
Dexlansoprazole (Kapidex)
Diclofenac sodium/Misoprostol (Arthrotec)
Dihydroergotamine mesylate (Migranal)
Diltazem hydrochloride (Dilacor XR)
Disulfiram (Antabuse)
Divalproex sodium (Depakote, Depakote ER)
Docetaxel (Taxotere)
Dolasetron mesylate (Anzemet)
Dorzolamide hydrochloride/Timolol maleate (Cosopt)
Doxorubicin hydrochloride liposome (Doxil)
Efavirenz (Sustiva)
Eletriptan hydrobromide (Relpax)
Enalapril maleate (Vasotec)
Enalapril maleate/Hydrochlorothiazide (Vaseretic)
Enfuvirtide (Fuzeon)
Entacapone (Comtan)
Ertapenem sodium (Invanz)
Escitalopram oxalate (Lexapro)
Esmolol hydrochloride (Brevibloc)
Esomeprazole magnesium (Nexium)
Esomeprazole sodium (Nexium I.V.)
Etanercept (Enbrel)
Etidronate disodium (Didronel)
Etoposide phosphate (Etopophos)
Ezetimibe/Simvastatin (Vytorin)
Famotidine (Pepcid)
Febuxostat (Uloric)
Fentanyl citrate (Actiq)
Flecainide acetate (Tambocor)
Fluconazole (Diflucan)
Fluorometholone (FML, FML Forte)
Fluoxetine hydrochloride (Prozac, Symbyax)
Fluticasone propionate (Flonase)
Fluticasone propionate/Salmeterol xinafoate (Advair Diskus)
Fluvastatin sodium (Lescol, Lescol XL)
Fluvoxamine maleate (Luvox, Luvox CR)
Foscarnet sodium (Foscavir)
Fosinopril sodium (Monopril)
Frovatriptan succinate (Frova)
Gabapentin (Neurontin)
Ganciclovir sodium (Cytovene)
Gatifloxacin (Zymar)
Gemifloxacin mesylate (Factive)
Glatiramer acetate (Copaxone)
Granisetron hydrochloride (Kytril)
Hydrochlorothiazide/Lisinopril (Prinzide)
Hydromorphone hydrochloride (Dilaudid, Dilaudid HP)
Ibuprofen/Oxycodone hydrochloride (Combunox)
Imatinib mesylate (Gleevec)
Indinavir sulfate (Crixivan)
Interferon alfa-2b, recombinant (Intron A)
Interferon alfacon-1 (Infergen)
Interferon alfa-n3 (human leukocyte derived) (Alferon N)
Ipratropium bromide (Atrovent HFA)
Iron dextran (Infed)
Itraconazole (Sporanox)
Lamotrigine (Lamictal)
Lansoprazole (Prevacid)
Leflunomide (Arava)
Leuprolide acetate (Lupron Depot)
Levocarnitine (Carnitor)
Levofloxacin (Levaquin)
Lidocaine (Lidoderm)
Linezolid (Zyvox)
Lisinopril (Prinivil)
Lithium carbonate (Lithobid)
Lopinavir/Ritonavir (Kaletra)
Loratadine (Claritin)
Loratadine/Pseudoephedrine sulfate (Claritin-D)
Losartan potassium (Cozaar)
Losartan potassium/Hydrochlorothiazide (Hyzaar)
Lovastatin (Mevacor)
Meloxicam (Mobic)
Mesalamine (Asacol)
Metformin hydrochloride (Glucophage)
Metoprolol succinate (Toprol-XL)
Metronidazole (Metrogel)
Modafinil (Provigil)
Moexipril hydrochloride (Univasc)
Mometasone furoate monohydrate (Nasonex)
Morphine sulfate (Avinza, MS Contin)
Moxifloxacin hydrochloride (Avelox)
Mupirocin calcium (Bactroban)
Nabumetone
Naratriptan hydrochloride (Amerge)
Nicotine (Nicotrol)
Nisoldipine (Sular)
Octreotide acetate (Sandostatin)
Ofloxacin (Floxin)
Olopatadine hydrochloride (Patanol)
Omega-3-acid ethyl esters (Lovaza)
Omeprazole (Prilosec)
Omeprazole/Sodium bicarbonate (Zegerid)
Oxaliplatin (Eloxatin)
Oxcarbazepine (Trileptal)
Oxycodone hydrochloride (OxyContin)
Palifermin (Kepivance)
Pantoprazole sodium (Protonix)
Paricalcitol (Zemplar)
Paroxetine hydrochloride (Paxil, Paxil CR)
Pegfilgrastim (Neulasta)
Peginterferon alfa-2b (PegIntron)
Penciclovir (Denavir)
Penicillamine (Cuprimine)
Penicillin g benzathine/Penicillin g procaine (Bicillin C-R)
Pentostatin (Nipent)
Pimozide (Orap)
Piperacillin sodium (Zosyn)
Pirbuterol acetate (Maxair)
Pramipexole dihydrochloride (Mirapex)
Pravastatin sodium (Pravachol)
Pregabalin (Lyrica)
Propafenone hydrochloride (Rythmol SR)
Propofol (Diprivan)
Quetiapine fumarate (Seroquel)
Ramipril (Altace)
Ribavirin (Rebetol)
Rimantadine hydrochloride (Flumadine)
Ritonavir (Kaletra, Norvir)

Table 24. ORAL MANIFESTATIONS OF SYSTEMIC AGENTS *(Cont.)*

Taste, altered *(Cont.)*

Rituximab (Rituxan)
Rivastigmine tartrate (Exelon)
Saquinavir mesylate (Invirase)
Selegiline hydrochloride (Eldepryl)
Sevoflurane (Ultane)
Sibutramine hydrochloride monohydrate (Meridia)
Simvastatin (Zocor)
Sodium phenylbutyrate (Buphenyl)
Sumatriptan succinate (Imitrex)
Sunitinib malate (Sutent)
Tacrolimus (Protopic)
Tazobactam sodium (Zosyn)
Temozolomide (Temodar)
Terbinafine hydrochloride (Lamisil)
Testosterone (Testim)
Tiagabine hydrochloride (Gabitril)
Tigecycline (Tygacil)
Tinidazole (Tindamax)
Tobramycin (TOBI)
Tolcapone (Tasmar)
Tolterodine tartrate (Detrol, Detrol LA)
Topiramate (Topamax)
Triamcinolone acetonide (Nasacort AQ)
Trimipramine maleate (Surmontil)
Valproate sodium (Depacon)
Valproic acid (Depakene)
Valrubicin (Valstar)
Venlafaxine hydrochloride (Effexor, Effexor XR)
Vinorelbine tartrate (Navelbine)
Voriconazole (VFEND)
Warfarin sodium (Coumadin)
Zaleplon sodium (Sonata)
Zidovudine (Retrovir)
Zolmitriptan (Zomig, Zomig-ZMT)
Zolpidem tartrate (Ambien, Ambien CR)
Zonisamide (Zonegran)

Taste, bad

Albuterol sulfate (Ventolin HFA)
Antithrombin III (Thrombate)
Budesonide (Rhinocort)
Ciprofloxacin hydrochloride (Cipro)
Cromolyn sodium (Intal)
Donepezil hydrochloride (Aricept)
Fluorescein sodium (Fluorescite)
Hydrocodone bitartrate/Ibuprofen (Vicoprofen)
Mesna (Mesnex)
Sodium phenylbutyrate (Buphenyl)
Sumatriptan succinate (Imitrex)

Taste, bitter

Azelastine hydrochloride (Astelin, Optivar)
Brinzolamide (Azopt)
Cefuroxime axetil (Ceftin)
Clozapine (Clozaril, Fazaclo ODT)
Dorzolamide hydrochloride (Trusopt)
Flurazepam hydrochloride (Dalmane)
Isosorbide mononitrate (Monoket)
Norfloxacin (Noroxin)
Olopatadine hydrochloride (Patanase)
Risperidone (Risperdal, Risperdal ODT)
Sulindac (Clinoril)
Tinidazole (Tindamax)

Taste, metallic

Adenosine (Adenocard, Adenoscan)
Bismuth/Metronidazole/Tetracycline (Pylera)
Calcitriol (Calcijex, Rocaltrol)
Disulfiram (Antabuse)
Doxercalciderol (Hectorol)
Escitalopram oxalate (Lexapro)
Ethionamide (Trecator)
Etidronate disodium (Didronel)
Fenoprofen calcium (Nalfon)
Lidocaine (Lidoderm)
Lithium carbonate (Lithobid)
Methocarbamol (Robaxin)
Succimer (Chemet)
Sulindac (Clinoril)
Tetracycline hydrochloride
Tinidazole (Tindamax)

Taste, salty

Calcitonin-salmon (Miacalcin)

Taste, unpleasant

Amphetamine aspartate/Amphetamine sulfate/Dextroamphetamine saccharate/Dextroamphetamine sulfate (Adderall XR)
Amitriptyline hydrochloride
Antihemophilic factor (recombinant) (Kogenate FS with Bio-Set)
Beclomethasone dipropionate monohydrate (Beconase AQ)
Brinzolamide (Azopt)
Cefuroxime axetil (Ceftin)
Ciprofloxacin (Cipro)
Clotrimazole (Mycelex)
Cyclobenazprine hydrochloride (Flexeril)
Dextroamphetamine sulfate (Dexedrine, Dexedrine SR)
Eszopiclone (Lunesta)
Flunisolide (Aerobid, Aerobid-M)
Fluorouracil
Fluticasone propionate (Flonase)
Lisdexamfetamine dimesylate (Vyvanse)
Methamphetamine hydrochloride (Desoxyn)
Moxifloxacin hydrochloride (Avelox)
Phentermine hydrochloride (Adipex-P)
Vitamin K1 (Mephyton)

Table 24. ORAL MANIFESTATIONS OF SYSTEMIC AGENTS *(Cont.)*

Teeth grinding

- Citalopram hydrobromide (Celexa)
- Setraline hydrochloride (Zoloft)

Throat burning

- Selegiline hydrochloride (Eldepryl)
- Azelastine hydrochloride (Astelin)
- Budesonide (Rhinocort)
- Estramustine phosphate sodium (Emcyt)
- Propofol (Diprivan)

Throat dryness

- Beclomethasone dipropionate monohydrate (Beconase AQ)
- Brompheniramine maleate (Veltane)
- Cefpodoxime proxetil (Vantin)
- Chlorpheniramine maleate
- Ciclesonide (Alvesco)
- Clonidine (Catapres-TTS)
- Clozapine (Clozaril, Fazaclo ODT)
- Cromolyn sodium (Intal)
- Cyclobenzaprine hydrochloride (Amrix)
- Flunisolide hemihydrate (Aerobid, Aerobid-M)
- Fluticasone propionate (Flonase)
- Gabapentin (Neurontin)
- Glycopyrrolate (Robinul)
- Hydroxocobalamin (Cyanokit Antidote)
- Ipratropium bromide (Atrovent)
- Levalbuterol hydrochloride (Xopenex)
- Levalbuterol tartrate (Xopenex HFA)
- Mometasone furoate (Asmanex)
- Pramipexole dihydrochloride (Mirapex)
- Propafenone hydrochloride (Rythmol SR)
- Rifaximin (Xifaxan)
- Rizatriptan benzoate (Maxalt, Maxalt-MLT)
- Ropinirole hydrochloride (Requip)
- Sodium oxybate (Xyrem)
- Triamcinolone acetonide (Azmacort)
- Trospium chloride (Sanctura)
- Zolpidem tartrate (Ambien, Ambien CR)

Throat irritation

- Albuterol sulfate (Proair HFA, Ventolin HFA)
- Budesonide (Rhinocort)
- Clozapine (Clozaril)
- Cromolyn sodium (Intal)
- Dorzolamide hydrochloride (Trusopt)
- Dorzolamide hydrochloride/Timolol maleate (Cosopt)
- Febuxostat (Uloric)
- Fexofenadine hydrochloride (Allegra)
- Fexofenadine hydrochloride/Pseudoephedrine hydrochloride (Allegra-D)
- Flunisolide hemihydrate (Aerobid, Aerobid-M)
- Fluticasone propionate (Flonase, Flovent Diskus, Flovent HFA)
- Fluticasone propionate/Salmeterol xinafoate (Advair HFA, Advair Diskus)
- Ibritumomab tiuxetan (Zevalin)
- Lamivudine (Epivir-HBV)
- Levofloxacin (Iquix)
- Nicotine (Nicotrol)
- Nilotinib (Tasigna)
- Olopatadine hydrochloride (Patanase)
- Pamidronate disodium (Aredia)
- Paroxetine hydrochloride (Paxil)
- Ritonavir (Norvir)
- Rituximab (Rituxan)
- Tiotropium bromide (Spiriva)
- Triamcinolone acetonide (Azmacort)
- Zolpidem tartrate (Ambien CR)

Throat soreness

- Acebutolol (Sectral)
- Adenosine (Adenoscan)
- Albuterol sulfate/Ipatropium bromide (Duoneb)
- Alpha1-proteinase inhibitor (human) (Zemaira)
- Antihemophilic factor (recombinant) (Kogenate)
- Arsenic trioxide (Trisenox)
- Atenolol (Tenormin)
- Atenolol/Chlorthalidone (Tenoretic)
- Atomoxetine hydrochloride (Strattera)
- Bendroflumethiazide/Nadolol (Corzide)
- Betaxolol hydrochloride (Kerlone)
- Brimonidine tartrate/Timolol maleate (Combigan)
- Bupropion hydrochloride (Wellbutrin SR, Wellbutrin XL)
- Buspirone hydrochloride (Buspar)
- Capecitabine (Xeloda)
- Captopril (Capoten)
- Carbamazepine (Carbatrol)
- Clofarabine (Clolar)
- Clozapine (Clozaril, Fazaclo ODT)
- Cytarabine (Cytosar-U)
- Dapsone
- Daptomycin (Cubicin)
- Desmopressin acetate (DDAVP)
- Dexlansoprazole (Kapidex)
- Diazepam (Valium)
- Donepezil hydrochloride (Aricept)
- Dorzolamide hydrochloride/Timolol maleate (Cosopt)
- Drospirenone/Ethinyl estradiol (Yaz)
- Enalapril maleate (Vasotec)

Table 24. ORAL MANIFESTATIONS OF SYSTEMIC AGENTS *(Cont.)*

Throat soreness *(cont.)*

Enalapril maleate/Hydrochlorothiazide (Vaseretic)
Filgrastim (Neupogen)
Flunisolide hemihydrate (Aerobid, Aerobid-M)
Fluticasone propionate/Salmeterol xinafoate (Advair HFA)
Globulin, immune (human) (Flebogamma 5%)
Guanidine
Imatinib mesylate (Gleevec)
Infliximab (Remicade)
Influenza virus vaccine (Flulaval)
Influenza virus vaccine live, intranasal (FluMist)
Lisinopril (Prinivil)
Lisinopril/Hydrochlorothiazide (Prinzide)
Measles, mumps & rubella virus vaccine, live (M-M-R II)
Measles, mumps, rubella and varicella virus vaccine live (ProQuad)
Metoprolol succinate (Toprol-XL)
Mirtazapine (Remeron, Remeron SolTab)
Mycophenolic acid (Myfortic)
Nadolol (Corgard)
Naltrexone hydrochloride (Revia)
Paclitaxel (Taxol)
Penbutolol sulfate (Levatol)
Perindopril erbumine (Aceon)
Pimecrolimus (Elidel)
Pirbuterol acetate (Maxair)
Prochlorperazine (Compro)
Propafenone hydrochloride (Rythmol SR)
Propranolol hydrochloride (InnoPran XL)
Ramipril (Altace)
Rubella virus vaccine, live (Meruvax II)
Succimer (Chemet)
Sulfamethoxazole/Trimethoprim (Septra)
Sumatriptan succinate (Imitrex)
Ticlopidine hydrochloride (Ticlid)
Torsemide (Demadex)
Tramadol hydrochloride (Ultram ER)
Trandolapril (Mavik)
Vitamin B12 (Nascobal)
Zoledronic acid (Zometa)

Throat swelling

Budesonide (Rhinocort)
Calcitonin-salmon (Fortical, Miacalcin)
Fluticasone propionate (Cutivate)

Throat tightness

Acetylcysteine (Acetadote)
Adenosine (Adenocard)
Agalsidase beta (Fabrazyme)
Amitripyline hydrochloride
Aripiprazole (Abilify)
Atemtuzumab (Campath)
Atovaquone (Mepron)
Doxorubicin hydrochloride liposome (Doxil)
Duloxetine hydrochloride (Cymbalta)
Etoposide (Vepesid)
Etoposide phosphate (Etopophos)
Fluoxetine hydrochloride/Olanzapine (Symbyax)
Hydroxocobalamin (Cyanokit Antidote)
Influenza (Flulaval)
Interferon alfa-n3 (human leukocyte derived) (Alferon N)
Levofloxacin (Levaquin)
Lubiprostone (Amitiza)
Molindone hydrochloride (Moban)
Olanzapine (Zyprexa, Zyprexa ZYDIS)
Oprelvekin (Neumega)
Paliperidone (Invega)
Paroxetine hydrochloride (Paxil, Paxil CR)
Peg-3350/Potassium chloride/Sodium ascorbate/Sodium chloride/Sodium sulfate/Ascorbic acid (MoviPrep)
Propafenone hydrochloride (Rythmol, Rythmol SR)
Quetiapine fumarate (Seroquel, Seroquel XR)
Risperidone (Risperdal Consta)
Rizatriptan benzoate (Maxalt, Maxalt-MLT)
Sodium phosphate (OsmoPrep)
Sodium phosphate/Bisacodyl (Fleet Phospho-soda, Phospho-soda EZ-PREP, Prep Kits)
Sumatriptan succinate (Imitrex)
Sumatriptan succinate/Naproxen sodium (Treximet)
Thiothixene hydrochloride (Navane)
Tipranavir (Aptivus)
Ziprasidone (Geodon)
Zolmitriptan (Zomig, Zomig-ZMT)
Zolpidem tartrate (Ambien, Ambien CR)

Tightness, tongue

Aripiprazole (Abilify)

Table 24. ORAL MANIFESTATIONS OF SYSTEMIC AGENTS *(Cont.)*

Tongue, burning

- Buspirone hydrochloride (Buspar)
- Carbidopa (Lodosyn)
- Carbidopa/Entacapone/Levodopa (Stalevo)
- Carbidopa/Levodopa (Parcopa, Sinemet)
- Fenoprofen calcium (Nalfon)
- Sumatriptan succinate (Imitrex)

Tongue discoloration

- Amitriptyline hydrochloride
- Amoxicillin/Clarithromycin/Lansoprazole (Prevpac)
- Balsalazide disodium (Colazal)
- Bismuth subsalicylate (Pepto-Bismol)
- Cetirizine hydrochloride (Zytrec)
- Cetirizine hydrochloride/Pseudoephedrine (Zytrec-D)
- Cilastatin/Imipenem (Primaxin)
- Clarithromycin (Biaxin)
- Glatiramer acetate (Copaxone)
- Hydrochlorothiazide/Moexipril (Uniretic)
- Linezolid (Zyvox)
- Mirtazapine (Remeron)
- Moxifloxacin hydrochoride (Avelox)
- Olanzapine (Zyprexa)
- Omeprazole (Prilosec)
- Omeprazole/Sodium bicarbonate (Zegerid)
- Palifermin (Kepivance)
- Pantoprazole sodium (Protonix)
- Paroxetine hydrochloride (Paxil)
- Riluzole (Rilutek)
- Risperidone (Risperdal)
- Thalidomide (Thalomid)
- Tinidazole (Tindamax)
- Venlafaxine hydrochloride (Effexor)
- Zalpelon (Sonata)

Tongue disorder, unspecified

- Acitretin (Soriatane)
- Amoxicillin/Clarithromycin/Lansoprazole (Prevpac)
- Cevimeline hydrochloride (Evoxac)
- Cyclosporine (Gengraf, Neoral)
- Eletriptan hydrobromide (Relpax)
- Esomeprazole magnesium (Nexium)
- Fluticasone propionate (Flovent)
- Gabapentin (Neurontin)
- Lansoprazole (Prevacid)
- Tolcapone (Tasmar)

Tongue, fine vermicular movements

- Amitriptyline hydrochloride
- Lithium carbonate (Lithobid)
- Metoclopramide (Reglan)
- Molindone hydrochloride (Moban)
- Pimozide (Orap)
- Prochlorperazine (Compro)
- Thioridazine hydrochloride
- Thiothixene hydrochloride (Navane)

Tongue, furry

- Bismuth subcitrate potassium/Metronidazole/Tetracycline hydrochloride (Pylera)
- Tinidazole (Tindamax)

Tongue, geographic

- Cevimeline hydrochloride (Evoxac)

Tongue, mucosal atrophy

- Omeprazole (Prilosec)
- Omeprazole/Sodium bicarbonate (Zegerid)

Tongue, protrusion

- Amitriptyline hydrochloride
- Fluoxetine hydrochloride (Sarafem)
- Fluoxetine hydrochloride/Olanzapine (Symbyax)
- Haloperidol (Haldol)
- Metoclopramide (Reglan)
- Molindone hydrochloride (Moban)
- Paliperidone (Invega)
- Pimozide (Orap)
- Prochlorperazine (Compro)
- Promethazine hydrochloride
- Quetiapine fumarate (Seroquel, Seroquel XR)
- Risperidone (Risperdal Consta)
- Thioridazine hydrochloride
- Thiothixene hydrochloride (Navane)
- Ziprasidone (Geodon)

Table 24. ORAL MANIFESTATIONS OF SYSTEMIC AGENTS *(Cont.)*

Tongue, thickening of

Palifermin (Kepivance)

Tonsillitis

Amlodipine besylate/Valsartan (Exforge)
Cyclosporine (Gengraf, Neoral)
Dexlansoprazole (Kapidex)
Fluticasone propionate (Flovent Diskus)
Fluticasone propionate/Salmeterol xinafoate (Advair HFA)
Formoterol fumarate (Foradil)
Influenza virus vaccine (Fluarix)
Montelukast sodium (Singulair)
Pimecrolimus (Elidel)
Ropinirole hydrochloride (Requip)
Somatropin (Genotropin)

Tooth discoloration

Amoxicillin (Amoxil, Moxatag)
Amoxicillin/Clavulanate potassium (Augmentin, Augmentin XR)
Amoxicillin/Clarithromycin/Lansoprazole (Prevpac)
Cilastatin sodium/Imipenem (Primaxin)
Clarithromycin (Biaxin, Biaxin XL)
Doxycycline monohydrate (Monodox)
Gabapentin (Neurontin)
Linezolid (Zyvox)
Minocycline hydrochloride (Solodyn ER)
Tetracycline hydrochloride (Pylera)

Tooth disorder

Amphetamine aspartate monohydrate/Amphetamine sulfate/Dextroamphetamine saccharate/Dextroamphetamine sulfate (Adderall XR)
Benazepril hydrochloride (Lotensin)
Botulinum toxin type A (Botox)
Budesonide (Entocort)
Bupropion hydrochloride (Wellbutrin, Wellbutrin SR, Wellbutrin XL)
Calcium carbonate (Actonel with Calcium)
Cefpodoxime proxetil (Vantin)
Celecoxib (Celebrex)
Cetirizine hydrochloride (Zytrec)
Cetirizine hydrochloride/Pseudoephedrine (Zytrec-D)
Cevimeline hydrochloride (Evoxac)
Cyclosporine (Gengraf, Neoral)
Delavirdine mesylate (Rescriptor)
Diltazem hydrochloride (Dilacor XR)
Divalproex sodium (Depakote ER)
Drospirenone/Ethinyl estradiol (Yaz)
Eletriptan hydrobromide (Relpax)
Estadiol (Vivelle, Vivelle-Dot)
Estradiol/Norgestimate (Prefest)
Estradiol/Norethindrone acetate (Combipatch)
Fenofibrate (Tricor)
Fentanyl citrate (Actiq)
Fluoxetine hydrochloride (Prozac)
Fluoxetine hydrochloride/Olanzapine (Symbyax)
Fluticasone propionate (Flovent Diskus)
Fluticasone propionate/Salmeterol xinafoate (Advair HFA)
Fluvastatin sodium (Lescol XL, Lescol)
Fluvoxamine maleate (Luvox, Luvox CR)
Gabapentin (Neurontin)
Glimepiride/Pioglitazone hydrochloride (Duetact)
Ibandronate sodium (Boniva)
Isosorbide mononitrate (Ismo)
Lamotrigine (Lamictal)
Leflunomide (Arava)
Loratadine (Claritin)
Loratadine/Pseudoephedrine sulfate(Claritin-D)
Metformin hydrochloride (Glucophage)
Modafinil (Provigil)
Nizatidine (Axid)
Orlistat (Xenical)
Paroxetine hydrochloride (Paxil, Paxil CR)
Pentostatin (Nipent)
Pilocarpine hydrochloride (Salagen)
Pioglitazone hydrochloride (Actos)
Pioglitazone hydrochloride/Metformin hydrochloride (ActoPlus Met)
Pramipexole dihydrochloride (Mirapex)
Progesterone (Prometrium)
Repaglinide (Prandin)
Riluzole (Rilutek)
Risedronate sodium (Actonel)
Risedronate sodium/Calcium carbonate (Actonel with Calcium)
Risperidone (Risperdal Consta)
Saquinavir mesylate (Invirase)
Sibutramine hydrochloride monohydrate (Meridia)
Tacrolimus (Protopic)
Tamsulosin hydrochloride (Flomax)
Teriparatide (Forteo)
Thalidomide (Thalomid)
Tolcapone (Tasmar)
Topiramate (Topamax)
Triamcinolone acetonide (Nasacort AQ)
Ziprasidone mesylate (Geodon)

Table 24. ORAL MANIFESTATIONS OF SYSTEMIC AGENTS *(Cont.)*

Toothache

Agalsidase beta (Fabrazyme)
Aripiprazole (Abilify)
Bupropion hydrochloride (Wellbutrin)
Cefpodoxime proxetil (Vantin)
Cevimeline hydrochloride (Evoxac)
Clonazepam (Klonopin)
Delavirdine mesylate (Rescriptor)
Donepezil hydrochloride (Aricept)
Eprosartan mesylate (Teveten)
Eprosartan mesylate/Hydrochlorothiazide (Teveten HCT)
Escitalopram oxalate (Lexapro)
Estadiol (Vivelle, Vivelle-Dot)
Estradiol/Norgestimate (Prefest)
Follitropin alfa (Gonal-F SQ)
Frovatriptan succinate (Frova)
Interferon beta-1a (Avonex)
Naltrexone (Vivitrol)
Oxcarbazepine (Trileptal)
Paroxetine hydrochloride (Paxil, Paxil CR)
Pimecrolimus (Elidel)
Pramipexole dihydrochloride (Mirapex)
Progesterone (Crinone)
Quadrivalent human papillomavirus (types 6, 11, 16, 18) recombinant vaccine (Gardasil)
Risperidone (Risperdal Consta)
Ropinirole hydrochloride (Requip)
Sodium oxybate (Xyrem)
Telmisartan (Micardis)
Telmisartan/Hydrochlorothiazide (Micardis HCT)
Terbinafine hydrochloride (Lamisil)
Testosterone (Testim)
Tramadol hydrochloride (Ultram ER)
Triamcinolone acetonide (Azmacort)

Trismus

Carbidopa/Levodopa (Sinemet, Parcopa)
Carbidopa/Levodopa/Entacapone (Stalevo)
Cefuroxime axetil (Ceftin)
Duloxetine hydrochloride (Cymbalta)
Fluvoxamine maleate (Luvox, Luvox CR)
Ixabepilone (Ixempra)
Iloprost (Ventavis)
Metoclopramide (Reglan)
Metyrosine (Demser)
Paliperidone (Invega)
Paroxetine hydrochloride (Paxil, Paxil CR)
Pregabalin (Lyrica)
Prochlorperazine (Compro)
Riluzole (Rilutek)
Thioridazine hydrochloride
Venlafaxine hydrochloride (Effexor, Effexor XR)
Zaleplon (Sonata)
Ziprasidone hydrochloride (Geodon)

Ulceration, tongue

Acitretin (Soriatane)
Cevimeline hydrochloride (Evoxac)
Decitabine (Dacogen)
Delaviridine mesylate (Rescriptor)
Loratadine (Claritin)
Loratadine/Pseudoephedrine sulfate (Claritin-D)
Saquinavir mesylate (Invirase)
Sertaline hydrochloride (Zoloft)

Ulcers, oral mucosal

Abacavir sulfate (Ziagen)
Abacavir sulfate/Lamivudine/Zidovudine (Trizivir)
Acamprosate calcium (Campral)
Albuterol sulfate (Combivent)
Amlodipine besylate/Atorvastatin (Caduet)
Amoxicillin/Clarithromycin/Lansoprazole (Prevpac)
Aripiprazole (Abilify)
Atazanavir sulfate (Reyataz)
Atorvastatin calcium (Lipitor)
Atovaquone/Proguanil hydrochloride (Malarone, Malarone Pediatric)
Betaxolol hydrochloride (Kerlone)
Bupropion hydrochloride (Wellbutrin SR, Wellbutrin XL, Zyban SR)
Carbamazepine (Carbatrol, Equetro, Tegretol)
Cefpodoxime proxetil (Vantin)
Cefuroxime axetil (Ceftin)
Chlorambucil (Leukeran)
Ciprofloxacin (Cipro)
Clozapine (Cloazaril)
Cytarabine (Cytosar-U)
Delavirdine mesylate (Rescriptor)
Denileukin diftitox (Ontak)
Divalproex sodium (Depakote ER)
Doxorubicin hydrochloride liposome (Doxil)
Ertapenem sodium (Invanz)
Eszopiclone (Lunesta)
Etanercept (Enbrel)
Fentanyl citrate (Actiq)
Fluoxetine hydrochloride (Prozac)
Fluoxetine hydrochloride/Olanzapine (Symbyax)
Fluticasone propionate (Flovent)
Gabapentin (Neurontin)
Gefitinib (Iressa)
Glatiramer acetate (Copaxone)
Hydrocodone bitartrate/Ibuprofen (Vicoprofen)
Imatinib mesylate (Gleevec)
Interferon alfa-2b, recombinant (Intron A)
Lamotrigine (Lamictal)
Lansoprazole (Prevacid)
Leflunomide (Arava)
Lopinavir/Ritonavir (Kaletra)
Melphalan hydrochloride (Alkeran)

Table 24. ORAL MANIFESTATIONS OF SYSTEMIC AGENTS *(Cont.)*

Ulcers, oral mucosal *(Cont.)*

Mesalamine (Asacol, Pentasa)
Midodrine hydrochloride (ProAmatine)
Modafinil (Provigil)
Mycophenolate mofetil (Cellept)
Nelfinavir mesylate (Viracept)
Nisoldipine (Sular)
Norfloxacin (Noroxin)
Olanzapine (Zyprexa)
Pantoprazole sodium (Protonix)
Paroxetine hydrochloride (Paxil CR)
Penicillamine (Cuprimine)
Pentosan polysulfate sodium (Elmiron)
Propafenone hydrochloride (Rythmol SR)
Quetiapine fumarate (Seroquel)
Rabeprazole sodium (Aciphex)
Ritonavir (Norvir)
Ropinirole hydrochloride (Requip)
Sibutramine hydrochloride monohydrate (Meridia)
Sirolimus (Rapamune)
Sodium oxybate (Xyrem)
Tiagabine hydrochloride (Gabitril)
Tolcapone (Tasmar)
Venlafaxine hydrochloride (Effexor XR)
Voriconazole (VFEND)
Zaleplon (Sonata)
Zidovudine (Retrovir)
Zonisamide (Zonegran)

Ulcers, oropharyngeal

Alendronate sodium (Fosamax)
Alendronate sodium/Cholecalciferol (Fosamax Plus D)

Xerochilia

Acyclovir (Zovirax)
Escitalopram oxalate (Lexapro)
Rifaximin (Xifaxan)
Saquinavir mesylate (Inivirase)

Xerostomia

Abciximab (ReoPro)
Acamprosate calcium (Campral)
Acetaminophen/Butalbital/Caffeine/Codeine phosphate (Phrenilin)
Acetaminophen/Tramadol (Ultracet)
Adenosine (Adenoscan)
Albuterol sulfate (Proventil HFA)
Albuterol sulfate/Ipratropium bromide (Combivent)
Almotriptan malate (Axert)
Alprazolam (Niravam, Xanax)
Alprostadil (Caverject)
Amantadine hydrochloride (Symmetrel)
Amiloride hydrochloride (Midamor)
Amitriptyline hydrochloride (Elavil)
Amlodipine besylate/Atorvastatin (Caduet)
Amlodipine besylate/Benazepril (Lotrel)
Amoxicillin/Clarithromycin/Lansoprazole (Prevpac)
Amphetamine aspartate/Amphetamine sulfate/Dextroamphetamine saccharate/Dextroamphetamine sulfate (Adderall XR)
Amphotericin B, liposomal (AmBisome)
Anastrozole (Arimidex)
Aprepitant (Emend)
Arformoterol tartrate (Brovana)
Aripiprazole (Abilify)
Arsenic trioxide (Trisenox)
Aspirin/Caffeine/Orphenadrine (Norgesic)
Atenolol (Tenormin)
Atenolol/Chlorthalidone (Tenoretic)
Atomoxetine hydrochloride (Strattera)
Atorvastatin calcium (Lipitor)
Azelastine hydrochloride (Astelin)
Balsalazide disodium (Colazal)
Benazepril hydrochloride (Lotensin)
Bendamustine hydrochloride (Treanda)
Bendroflumethiazid/Nadolol (Corzide)
Benztropine mesylate (Cogentin)
Betaxolol hydrochloride (Kerlone)
Bevacizumab (Avastin)
Bexarotene (Targretin)
Bicalutamide (Casodex)
Biperiden hydrochloride (Akineton)
Bismuth subcitrate potassium/Metronidazole/Tetracycline (Pylera)
Brimonidine tartrate (Alphagan P)
Brimonidine tartrate/Timolol maleate (Combigan)
Brinzolamide (Azopt)
Brompheniramine maleate/Dextromethorrphan hydrobromide/Pseudoephedrine hydrochloride (Bromfed)
Budesonide (Pulmicort)

Table 24. ORAL MANIFESTATIONS OF SYSTEMIC AGENTS *(Cont.)*

Xerostomia *(Cont.)*

Bupropion hydrochloride (Buspar, Wellbutrin SR, Wellbutrin XL, Zyban SR)
Busulfan (Busulfex)
Calcitonin-salmon (Miacalcin)
Calcitriol (Calcijex, Rocaltrol)
Capecitabine (Xeloda)
Captopril
Carbamazepine (Carbatrol, Equetro)
Carbidopa/Levodopa (Parcopa, Sinemet)
Carvedilol (Coreg, Coreg CR)
Cefdinir (Omnicef)
Cefditoren pivoxil (Spectracef)
Cefpodoxime proxetil (Vantin)
Celecoxib (Celebrex)
Cetirizine hydrochloride (Zyrtec)
Cetirizine hydrochloride/Pseudoephedrine (Zyrtec-D)
Cetuximab (Erbitux)
Cevimeline hydrochloride (Evoxac)
Chlorothiazide sodium (Diuril)
Chlorpheniramine maleate
Chlorthalidone (Clorpres)
Ciclesonide (Alvesco)
Ciprofloxacin (Cipro, Cipro XR)
Citalopram hydrobromide (Celexa)
Clonazepam (Klonopin)
Clonidine (Catapres, Catapres-TTS)
Clonidine hydrochloride/Chlorthalidone (Clorpres)
Clozapine (Clozaril)
Conivaptan hydrochloride (Vaprisol)
Cyclobenzaprine hydrochloride (Amrix)
Cyclosporine (Gengraf, Neoral)
Daptomycin (Cubicin)
Darifenacin hydrobromide (Enablex)
Delavirdine mesylate(Rescriptor)
Desloratadine (Clarinex)
Desloratadine/Pseudophedrine hydrochloride (Clarinex-D)
Desvenlafaxine succinate (Pristiq)
Dexlansoprazole (Kapidex)
Dexmethylphenidate hydrochloride (Focalin, Focalin XR)
Dextroamphetamine sulfate (Dexedrine SR)
Diazepam (Valium)
Diclofenac epolamine (Flector)
Diclofenac sodium (Voltaren, Voltaren XR)
Diclofenac sodium/Misoprostol (Arthrotec)
Dicyclomine hydrochloride (Bentyl)
Dihydroergotamine mesylate (Migranal)
Diltiazem hydrochloride (Cardizem LA)
Divalproex sodium (Depakote ER)
Donepezil hydrochloride (Aricept)
Dorzolamide hydrochloride (Trusopt)
Dorzolamide hydrochloride/Timolol maleate (Cosopt)
Doxercalciferol (Hectorol)
Doxorubicin hydrochloride liposome (Doxil)
Duloxetine hydrochloride (Cymbalta)
Eletriptan hydrobromide (Relpax)
Enalapril maleate (Vasotec)
Enalapril maleate/Hydrochlorothiazide (Vaseretic)
Enfuvirtide (Fuzeon)
Entacapone (Comtan)
Entacapone/Carbidopa/Levodopa (Stalevo)
Eprosartan mesylate/Hydrochlorothiazide (Teveten HCT)
Escitalopram oxalate (Lexapro)
Esmolol hydrochloride (Brevibloc)
Esomeprazole (Nexium)
Estazolam (Prosom)
Eszopiclone (Lunesta)
Etanercept (Enbrel)
Etravirine (Intelence)
Famotidine (Pepcid)
Febuxostat (Uloric)
Felodipine (Plendil ER)
Fenofibrate (Tricor)
Fenoprofen calcium (Nalfon)
Fentanyl (Duragesic, Ionsys)
Fentanyl citrate (Actiq, Fentora)
Fexofenadine hydrochloride/Pseudoephedrine (Allegra-D)
Fexofenadine hydrochloride (Allegra)
Flecainide acetate (Tambocor)
Flumazenil (Romazicon)
Fluocinolone acetonide/Hydroquinone/Tretinoin (Tri-Luma)
Fluoxetine hydrochloride (Prozac)
Fluoxetine hydrochloride/Olanzapine (Symbyax)
Flurazepam hydrochloride (Dalamane)
Fluticasone propionate/Salmeterol xinafoate (Advair Diskus, Advair HFA)
Fluvoxamine maleate (Luvox CR)
Formoterol fumarate (Foradil, Perforomist)
Fosaprepitant dimeglumine (Emend for Injection)
Foscarnet sodium (Foscavir)
Fosinopril sodium (Monopril)
Frovatriptan succinate (Frova)
Furosemide
Gabapentin (Neurontin)
Galantamine hydrobromide (Razadyne)
Gemifloxacin mesylate (Factive)
Glatiramer acetate (Copaxone)
Glycopyrrolate (Robinul)
Goserelin acetate (Zoladex)
Guanidine hydrochloride (Guanidine)
Haloperidol (Haldol)
Hydrochlorothiazide/Eprosartan mesylate (Teveten HCT)
Hydrochlorothiazide/Lisinopril (Prinzide)
Hydrochlorothiazide/Losartan (Hyzaar)
Hydrochlorothiazide/Telmisartan (Micardis HCT)
Hydrochlorothiazide/Triamterene (Dyazide)
Hydrochlorothiazide/Valsartan (Diovan HCT)
Hydrocodone bitartrate/Ibuprofen (Vicoprofen)
Hydromorphone hydrochloride (Dilaudid, Dilaudid-HP)
Interferon alfa-2b, recombinant (Intron A)
Interferon alfacon-1 (Infergen)

Table 24. ORAL MANIFESTATIONS OF SYSTEMIC AGENTS *(Cont.)*

Xerostomia *(Cont.)*

Interferon alfa-n3 (human leukocyte derived) (Alferon N)
Interferon beta-1a (Rebif)
Ipratropium bromide (Atrovent, Atrovent HFA)
Irbesartan/Hydrochlorothiazide (Avalide)
Isocarboxazid (Marplan)
Isosorbide mononitrate (Imdur LA, Monoket)
Isotretinoin (Accutane)
Isradipine (DynaCirc CR)
Lamotrigine (Lamictal)
Leuprolide acetate (Eligard, Lupron Depot)
Levalbuterol hydrochloride (Xopenex)
Levalbuterol tartrate (Xopenex HFA)
Levocetirizine dihydrochloride (Xyzal)
Lisdexamfetamine dimesylate (Vyvanse)
Lisinopril (Prinivil, Zestril)
Lopinavir/Ritonavir (Kaletra)
Losartan potassium (Cozaar)
Lovastatin (Mevacor)
Lovastatin (Advicor)
Lubiprostone (Amitiza)
Megestrol acetate (Megace ES)
Meloxicam (Mobic)
Mesalamine (Asacol)
Methylphenidate hydrochloride (Concerta, Concerta XL)
Metoprolol succinate (Toprol-XL)
Metyrosine (Demser)
Midodrine hydrochloride (ProAmatine)
Minocycline hydrochloride (Solodyn)
Mirtazapine (Remeron, Remeron SolTab)
Modafinil (Provigil)
Moexipril hydrochloride (Univasc)
Molindone hydrochloride (Moban)
Mometasone furoate (Elocon)
Morphine sulfate (Avinza, MS Contin)
Moxifloxacin hydrochloride (Avelox)
Mupirocin calcium (Bactroban)
Mycophenolate mofetil (CellCept)
Nabumetone
Nadolol (Corgard)
Naltrexone (Vivitrol)
Naproxen (EC-Naprosyn, Naprosyn)
Naproxen sodium (Anaprox, Anaprox DS T)
Niacin (Advicor, Niaspan ER)
Nicotine (Nicotrol)
Nilotinib (Tasigna)
Nisoldipine (Sular ER)
Nizatidine (Axid)
Norfloxacin (Noroxin)
Octreotide acetate (Sandostatin)
Ofloxacin (Floxin)
Olanzapine (Zyprexa, Zyprexa ZYDIS)
Olopatadine hydrochloride (Patanase)
Omega-3-acid ethyl esters (Lovaza)
Omeprazole (Prilosec)
Omeprazole/Sodium bicarbonate (Zegerid)
Ondansetron hydrochloride (Zofran ODT)
Oxaliplatin (Eloxatin)
Oxcarbazepine (Trileptal)
Oxybutynin (Oxytrol ER)
Oxybutynin chloride (Ditropan)
Oxycodone hydrochloride (OxyContin)
Oxycodone hydrochloride/Acetaminophen (Percocet)
Oxycodone hydrochloride/Aspirin (Percodan)
Oxycodone hydrochloride/Ibuprofen (Combunox)
Oxymorphone hydrochloride (Opana, Opana ER)
Paliperidone (Invega)
Palonosetron hydrochloride (Aloxi)
Pantoprazole sodium (Protonix)
Paricalcitol (Zemplar)
Paroxetine hydrochloride (Paxil, Paxil CR)
Peginterferon alfa-2a (Pegasys)
Peginterferon alfa-2b (PEG-Intron, PegIntron)
Pemetrexed (Alimta)
Perindopril erbumine (Aceon)
Phendimetrazine tartrate (Bontril ER)
Phenobarbital/Hyoscyamine/Atropine/Scopolamine (Donnatal)
Phentermine hydrochloride (Adipex-P)
Pilocarpine hydrochloride (Salagen)
Pimozide (Orap)
Pirbuterol acetate (Maxair)
Posaconazole (Noxafil)
Pramipexole dihydrochloride (Mirapex)
Pregabalin (Lyrica)
Procarbazine hydrochloride (Matulane)
Prochlorperazine (Compro)
Progesterone (Crinone, Prometrium)
Promethazine hydrochloride
Propafenone hydrochloride (Rythmol SR)
Propofol (Diprivan)
Protriptyline hydrochloride (Vivactil)
Quetiapine fumarate (Seroquel, Seroquel XR)
Rabeprazole sodium (Aciphex)
Ramipril (Altace)
Rasagiline mesylate (Azilect)
Ribavirin (Rebetol)
Riluzole (Rilutek)
Rimantadine hydrochloride (Flumadine)
Risedronate sodium/Calcium carbonate (Actonel with Calcium)
Risperidone (Risperdal Consta)
Ritonavir (Norvir)
Rivastigmine tartrate (Exelon)
Rizatriptan benzoate (Maxalt, Maxalt MLT)
Ropinirole hydrochloride (Requip, Requip XL)
Rotigotine (Neupro)
Saquinavir mesylate (Invirase)
Scopolamine (Transderm-Scop)
Selegiline (Emsam)
Selegiline hydrochloride (Eldepryl)
Sertaline hydrochloride (Zoloft)
Sevoflurane (Ultane)
Sibutramine hydrochloride monohydrate (Meridia)
Sidenafil citrate (Viagra)
Sodium ferric gluconate (Ferrlecit)
Solifenacin succinate (VESIcare)
Sorafenib (Nexavar)

Table 24. ORAL MANIFESTATIONS OF SYSTEMIC AGENTS *(Cont.)*

Xerostomia *(Cont.)*

Sucralfate (Carafate)
Sulindac (Clinoril)
Sumatriptan succinate (Imitrex)
Sumatriptan succinate/Naproxen sodium (Treximet)
Sunitinib maleate (Sutent)
Tacrolimus (Protopic)
Tadalafil (Cialis)
Telithromycin (Ketek)
Telmisartan (Micardis)
Terazosin hydrochloride (Hytrin)
Testosterone (Testim)
Thalidomide (Thalomid)
Thiabendazole (Mintezol)
Thioridazine hydrochloride
Thiothixene hydrochloride (Navane)
Tiagabine hydrochloride (Gabitril)
Tigecycline (Tygacil)
Timolol hemihydrate (Betimol)
Timolol maleate (Timoptic, Timoptic XE)
Tinidazole (Tindamax)
Tiotropium bromide (Spiriva)
Tolacapone (Tasmar)
Tolterodine tartrate (Detrol)
Topiramate (Topamax)
Torsemide (Demadex)
Tramadol hydrochloride (Ultram ER)
Trandolapril/Verapamil (Tarka)
Tranylcypromine sulfate (Parnate)
Triamcinolone acetonide (Azmacort)
Triamterene (Dyrenium)
Trimipramine maleate (Surmontil)
Trospium chloride (Sanctura)
Valproate sodium (Depacon)
Valproic acid (Depakene)
Valsartan (Diovan)
Valsartan/Hydrochlorothiazide (Diovan HCT)
Vardenafil hydrochloride (Levitra)
Varenicline tartrate (Chantix)
Venlafaxine hydrochloride (Effexor, Effexor XR)
Verapamil hydrochloride (Verelan)
Voriconazole (VFEND T)
Vorinostat (Zolinza)
Zaleplon (Sonata)
Ziprasidone (Geodon)
Zoledronic acid (Zometa)
Zolmitriptan (Zomig, Zomig-ZMT)
Zolpidem tartrate (Ambien, Ambien CR)
Zonisamide (Zonegran)

Chapter 25

Herbs and Dietary Supplements

Adriane Fugh-Berman, M.D.; Maria Salnik, M.S., D.D.S. candidate

HERBS AND DENTAL HEALTH

Many drugs used in dentistry have their origins in the plant world, including lidocaine and novocaine, derived from the coca plant (*Erythroxylum coca*); opioids, derived from the poppy (*Papaver somniferum*); and several antibiotics derived from fungi, including penicillin from *Penicillium notatum* and cephalosporins from a marine fungus (*Cephalosporium acremonium*). Clove oil, which contains eugenol, is the essential oil of *Eugenia caryophyllus*.[1] In fact, the best-selling herbal products in the United States may well be oral hygiene products, which rely heavily on essential oils (or their components), including eucalyptol, derived from eucalyptus (*E. globulus*); thymol, derived from thyme (*Thymus vulgaris*), and menthol, derived from peppermint (*Mentha piperita*).

Chewing sticks, used in African and Southern Asian communities, are oral hygiene products made from a variety of plants, including neem (*Azadirachta indica*), salvadora (*S. persica*) and species of *Garcinia and Diospyros*.[1] Chewing sponges made from *Hibiscus* species and other plants are popular in Ghana. A study comparing the periodontal status of Sudanese miswak and toothbrush users found the two comparable for oral hygiene.[2] A group of 109 men who used miswak sticks prepared from the roots or twigs of *S. persica* were compared with 104 toothbrush users (all had ≥18 teeth). Attachment level was measured, and gingival bleeding, supragingival dental calculus, and probing pocket depth of teeth were scored by the Community Periodontal Index.

Gingival bleeding and dental calculus were common in the study population, especially among those >40 years. Compared to toothbrush users, miswak users had significantly lower numbers of posterior sextants with dental calculus and ≥4 mm probing depth. However, miswak use demonstrated no advantage over toothbrush use in the anterior teeth, and probing depth ≥4 mm was more common in the anterior teeth of miswak users. The results did not show a significant benefit of miswak use versus toothbrush use in gingival bleeding. *Camellia* and other plants are rich in fluoride; the chewing stick with the highest fluoride content is from a plant related to persimmon (*Diospyros tricolor*). *Fagara zanthoxyloides* and *Massularia acuminata* reduce both acid production and bacterial growth. Extracts from *Rhus natalensis* and *Euclea divinorum*, used in Kenya as chewing sticks, inhibited the proteolytic activity of *Bacteroides gingivalis, B. intermedius*, and *Treponema denticola*.[3]

A recent study compared the antibacterial properties of aqueous extracts from 17 plants used as chewing sticks in Nigeria and the fruit of *Cnestis ferruginea*, which is used in oral hygiene.[4] *C. ferruginea* fruit and *Terminalia glaucescens* were active against cultures of *Staphylococcus aureus, Bacillus subtilis, Escherichia coli,* and *Pseudomonas aeruginosa*; nine other extracts showed some activity. When tested against clinical isolates from orofacial infections, three extracts (*Bridellia ferruginea, Terminalia glaucescens,* and *Anogeissus leiocarpus*) were active against facultative gram-negative rods (*Escherichia, citrobacter,* and *Enterobacter* species). Ten of 11 extracts tested were active against obligate anaerobes; the most active were *Phyllanthus, muellerianus, Anogeissus leiocarpus,* and *C. ferruginea* fruit.

Commercial toothpastes have been made from neem (*Azadirachta indica*) and arak (*Salvadora persica,* one of several plants called "toothbrush tree"). Powdered plants used in abrasive dentrifices include sweet flag root (*Acorus calamus*), gum-resin of myrrh (*Commiphora myrrha*), yellow dock root (*Rumex crispus*), toothbrush tree (*Gouania lupuloides,*) and ashes from the branches of the European grape (*Vitis vinifera*). Commercial mouthwashes commonly contain essential oils; Listerine, for example, contains thymol, menthol, eucalyptol, and methyl salicylate--all derived from botanicals.[1]

Several herbs have been tested against pathogenic oral bacteria. Licorice (*Glycyrrhiza glabra*) and glycyrrhizin (a component of licorice) both inhibit bacterial adherence. In the presence of sucrose, glycyrrhizin did not affect growth of *S. mutans* but did reduce plaque formation; inhibition was almost complete at concentrations of 0.5% to 1% glycyrrhizin or 5% to 10% licorice.[5]

A high–molecular-weight constituent of cranberry (*Vaccinium macrocarpon*) juice reversed the coaggregation of 58% of 84 coaggregating bacterial pairs tested.[6] This effect was strongest when at least one species was a gram-negative anaerobe; thus, it may alter subgingival microflora. Most cranberry juice, however, contains large amounts of sugar.

An *in vitro* study found no effect against microorganisms in biofilms from saliva or dental plaque with the use of an infant dentifrice containing calendula (*Calendula officinalis*) or a dentifrice containing lactoperoxidase, glucose oxidase, and lactoferrin; the calendula preparation also had no significant effect on any microorganism evaluated. Compared to controls, only a dentifrice containing sodium fluoride and sodium lauryl sulfate significantly reduced viable microorganisms.[7]

Herbal Teas

Although herbal teas are perceived to be healthful, many are as acidic as orange juice (pH 3.73). An *in vitro* study of 10 herbal teas found that the pH of nine mixed herbal teas ranged from 3.15 to 3.78; by comparison, traditional black tea (*Camellia sinensis*) has a pH of 5.67.[8] The pH of one chamomile, apple, and cinnamon herbal tea was 7.08, but in a molar immersion test, all the herbal teas tested except for the chamomile/cinnamon tea caused significantly higher enamel loss than black tea. It bears noting that all herbal teas in this experiment were mixed herbals, so effects cannot be attributed to specific herbs. Further research should be done on single-herb teas.

Adverse Dental Effects of Herbs and Dietary Supplements

Betel. Betel nut (*Areca catechu*), a masticant with mild stimulatory effects, is traditionally viewed as beneficial to the teeth and gums. Betel stains the saliva a reddish color and can stain the teeth, gingival, and oral mucosa red or black. Some evidence suggests that chewing betel helps to prevent dental caries, possibly via mechanical cleansing, altering salivary pH, or formation of a protective barrier to cariogenic agents.[9] Other evidence shows that populations that chew betel have a high rate of caries and periodontal disease. Any protective effects of betel that exist are minor and are overwhelmed by its carcinogenic effects. Betel chewing causes oral and esophageal cancers.[10] Oral squamous cell carcinoma usually occurs in the midbuccal mucosa and the lateral borders of the tongue--parts of the mouth directly contacted by betel quid. Betel use also causes oral submucous fibrositis, a precancerous condition.[11]

The addition of tobacco clearly increases the carcinogenic risk of betel.[10] Lime, another addition to betel quids, may increase the generation of reactive oxygen species; oral squamous cell cancers were noted to correspond to the site of lime application in 77% of 169 cases in Papua New Guinea.[9]

Khat. Another stimulatory masticant, khat (*Catha edulis*), is cariogenic, can stain teeth, and causes thickened oropharyngeal mucosa. Khat contains an amphetamine-like substance and can cause dependence.[12]

Colloidal silver. With a long history as an antibacterial agent, colloidal silver is marketed as a "natural" antibiotic. Argyria (discoloration caused by silver deposition) often manifests first in the mouth, causing a slate-blue or silver line in the gingiva. Deposits in the skin or mucosa cause a permanent gray-blue discoloration. Contrary to proponents' claims that colloidal silver is different from noncolloidal, colloidal silver protein does in fact cause argyria.[13, 14]

VITAMIN AND MINERAL DEFICIENCY

Nutrition is important in craniofacial and oral tissue development. Prolonged vitamin A deficiency during tooth development can result in enamel hypoplasia. Deficiencies of vitamin D or phosphorus can cause incomplete calcification of teeth. Deficiency of calcium, vitamin D, magnesium, or copper can cause defects in alveolar bone. Iodine deficiency can delay the eruption of both primary and secondary teeth and can cause malocclusion.[15]

Many nutritional deficiencies manifest first in the oral cavity. Glossitis can occur from multiple nutritional deficiencies; vitamin E appears to be particularly important in papillary health. Angular cheilosis can be caused by too little vitamin B_2 (riboflavin), B_3 (niacin), B_6 (pyridoxine), B_{12} (cobalamin), folic acid, or iron. Burning mouth syndrome may be the result of deficiency of vitamin B complex, protein, or iron.[15] Zinc deficiency can cause distortions of taste and smell, delayed wound healing, atrophic oral mucosa, xerostomia, and increased susceptibility to periodontal disease.[15] Vitamin A deficiency also can cause desquamation of oral mucosa, leukoplakia, xerostomia, or gingival hypertrophy; it also increases the risk of candidiasis. Either inadequate or excessive vitamin A intake can impair healing.

Vitamin C deficiency causes impaired wound healing, gingival inflammation and bleeding, and swollen interdental papillae. In a case report, an epileptic child on a ketogenic diet developed vitamin C deficiency, which resulted in gingival erythema, edema, and bleeding, as well as aspiration of a primary molar following a routine dental cleaning.[16]

Inadequate intake of magnesium can cause gingival hypertrophy. Magnesium deficiency may also cause tooth loss, decreased alveolar crestal bone height, and other manifestations of low bone mass. An epidemiologic study of 4,290 subjects aged 20 to 80 years in northeastern Germany found that about a third had low serum (<0.75 mmol/L) magnesium levels. Magnesium regulates cell functions; physiologically, it antagonizes calcium so the ratio between the two minerals was assessed. In a subset study, no influence of the Mg/Ca ratio on periodontal status was found in subjects <40 years old. However, in subjects >40 years, a statistically significant inverse association was noted between Mg/Ca ratio and level of periodontitis. Additionally, subjects who used magnesium-containing drugs had fewer signs of periodontal disease than matched controls.[17]

Inadequate calcium can cause increased tooth mobility and premature loss. A case-control study of 54 female adolescents (aged 17 to 19 years) found that low intakes of riboflavin, calcium, and fiber were correlated with gingivitis risk.[18] Calcium (500 mg daily calcium citrate malate) and vitamin D (700 IU/day cholecalciferol) supplementation was found to significantly reduce tooth loss in a 3-year, randomized, placebo-controlled, double-blind trial of 145 subjects aged ≥65 years. In a 2-year follow-up study, higher self-reported intake of supplemental calcium (1,166 ± 294 mg daily) was found to significantly reduce tooth loss when compared to lower intake (705 ± 261 mg daily). Vitamin D supplementation was not significantly related to tooth loss.[19]

CLINICAL TRIALS OF HERBS AND SUPPLEMENTS FOR TREATING DENTAL CONDITIONS

Oral Lesions

Labial Herpes

A study in 16 adults with recurrent herpes (eight genital, eight labial; viral type unspecified) compared the effects of topical honey with 5% acyclovir on duration of outbreaks, pain, and healing time.[20] For labial herpes outbreaks, topical honey was more effective than acyclovir for all parameters measured, including mean duration of attacks (35%), mean duration of pain (39%), occurrence of crusting (28%), and mean healing time (43%). Results were similar for genital herpes. No side effects associated with the application of honey were reported; three patients reported itching with acyclovir.

Aphthous Ulcers

Acemannan, a component of *Aloe vera* gel, may be effective for aphthous stomatitis.[21] A double-blind randomized trial of 60 patients with recurrent aphthae compared acemannan hydrogel to an over-the-counter product as an active control. Lesions treated with acemannan hydrogel healed in 5.89 days, while those treated with control healed in 7.8 days.

Chemotherapy-Induced Mucositis

Honey

A randomized, controlled trial tested honey to treat mucositis in 40 patients undergoing radiation for head and neck cancer. Twenty patients were instructed to swish and swallow 20 mL of raw honey from tea flowers (*Camellia sinensis*) before, after, and 6 hours following radiotherapy, while the remaining patients received no such instructions. There was no difference between groups in overall incidence of mucositis, but the incidence of grade 3 or 4 mucositis was significantly lower in the experimental group. While treatment was interrupted because of mucositis in four controls, no interruptions occurred in the honey-treated group.[22] Honey may contain pharmacologically active compounds from the plants' nectar that it is collected from, so it is unclear whether all honey would have a similar effect.

Chamomile

A randomized, double-blind, placebo-controlled trial of chamomile mouthwash in 164 patients entering their first cycle of 5-fluorouracil (5FU)-based chemotherapy tested chamomile mouthwash three times daily for 2 weeks against placebo. All patients also received oral cryotherapy.[23] Physicians and patients each scored stomatitis severity on a scale from 1 to 4. Daily mean mucositis scores were similar between the chamomile group and the placebo group. No toxicity was noted.

Vitamin E

A randomized, double-blind, controlled trial compared topical vitamin E against placebo oil for treatment of oral mucositis in 18 patients receiving chemotherapy. After 5 days of topical application (1 mL of 400 mg/mL vitamin E oil twice daily), six of nine patients had complete resolution of lesions; only one of nine subjects in the placebo group had complete resolution.[24]

Vitamin E was previously thought to increase bleeding risk, but a study specifically designed to examine bleeding risk found no effect. A substudy of 409 male cigarette smokers in a study of vitamin E and β-carotene found gingival bleeding on probing to be more common in those with a high prevalence of dental plaque assigned to α-tocopherol (50 mg daily), especially when combined with aspirin.[25] In this study, aspirin alone did not increase bleeding significantly, an unusual finding that should have called other findings into question.

A study specifically designed to address the risk of bleeding with vitamin E supplementation found no effect of the most popular form of vitamin E, all-rac-α-tocopherol (60, 200, or 800 IU for 4 months), on bleeding time in 88 healthy elders.[26]

Burning Mouth Syndrome

A randomized, double-blind, placebo-controlled trial found that St. John's wort (*Hypericum perforatum*) extract (300-mg capsules three times per day for 12 weeks) did not significantly reduce pain, compared to placebo. St. John's wort treatment significantly reduced the number of oral sites affected by symptoms (a secondary outcome of the study).[27]

Oral Leukoplakia

A placebo-controlled trial of 87 tobacco chewers with oral leukoplakia tested 1 gram daily of a blue-green algae, *Spirulina fusiformis*, against placebo for 12 months.[28] Complete regression of lesions was noted in 20 of 44 (45%) subjects in the *Spirulina*-treated group, vs three of 43 (7%) subjects in the placebo group. No effect was seen in those with ulcerated or nodular lesions. Within 1 year of discontinuing use of *Spirulina fusiformis*, nine of 20 subjects experienced complete regression of lesions. No toxicity was noted.

Oral Lichen Planus

A randomized, double-blind, placebo-controlled trial tested turmeric abstract (2,000 mg of at least 95% curcuminoids daily for 7 weeks) as an adjunct to short-course corticosteroid therapy (60 mg prednisone daily for 1 week) in 33 patients with oral lichen planus. No significant changes in symptoms (pain, erythema, ulceration, and total clinical scores of erythema plus ulceration) were observed in the treated group, compared with placebo.[29]

Topical *Aloe vera* gel application (twice daily for 8 weeks) was tested in a randomized, double-blind, placebo-controlled trial in 54 subjects with oral lichen planus lesions; aloe significantly improved clinical signs and significantly reduced pain scores. The treatment also resulted in a significantly higher rate of complete remissions, compared to placebo.[30]

Caries and Oral Microbial Growth

Lactic bacteria

A clinical trial in 245 7-year-olds compared chewable tablets containing vitamin B_6 and heat-killed lactic bacteria (streptococci and lactobacilli) against placebo (vitamin B_6 only) to prevent caries.[31] Treatments were given once weekly for 16 weeks. Permanent teeth were evaluated four times during 24 months of follow-up using the Decayed, Missing, and Filled Surfaces (DMFS) Index. The incidence of dental caries in the lactic bacteria group was reduced at all time points; compared to controls, the experimental group had a 42% reduction in incidence of caries at the end of the study.

A randomized, double-blind, crossover study found that subjects who consumed yogurt (200 mg once daily for 2 weeks) containing *Bifidobacterium animalis* subspecies *animalis*, strain DN-173 010 (7x107 cfu/g) reported significantly reduced salivary *S. mutans* and reduced salivary lactobacilli levels.[32] Another randomized, double-blind, crossover study found that following the active treatment periods, consumption of ice cream (153 g daily for 10 days) containing *Bifidobacterium animalis* subspecies *lactis* strain Bb-12 (1x107 cfu/g) significantly reduced salivary *S. mutans* levels and did not significantly affect salivary lactobacilli levels.[33]

Polyols: xylitol and sorbitol

Chewing sugarless gum after meals stimulates saliva production and may reduce caries. Some sugar substitutes may be superior to others. Xylitol (birch sugar) is as sweet as sucrose; sorbitol, another sugar alcohol used as a sugar substitute, is less sweet but more popular commercially than xylitol, because sorbitol is less expensive and easier to formulate into products. Although both stimulate saliva production, xylitol is not fermented by oral microbes, while sorbitol, when consumed in doses exceeding two sticks of chewing gum daily, is very slowly fermented and can increase plaque acid production.[34] Furthermore, in an animal study, cariogenic microorganisms were found to adaptively metabolize sorbitol under restricted sucrose conditions.[35]

A controlled trial of 583 mixed dentition subjects found that a group that chewed sorbitol-flavored gum (one stick of gum for 20 minutes after meals for 2 years), experienced 33.1% fewer carious lesions and 38.7% fewer cavitated lesions compared to an untreated control group.[36] Another controlled trial of 2,601 mixed dentition subjects living in an area without fluoridated water found that the group that chewed sorbitol gum (one pellet for 20 minutes after every meal) experienced significantly fewer caries at 2 and 3 years, compared with a non-gum-chewing group. An intention-to-treat analysis at 3 years found that, compared with controls, a high-risk subgroup had about one less decayed, missing, or filled surface.[37]

In four clinical trials, xylitol gum (one stick of gum at least two times per day for 2 years, starting 3 months post-delivery) significantly reduced maternal transmission of *S. mutans* to infants, compared to chlorhexidine and fluoride varnish treatments administered at 6, 12, and 18 months post-delivery.[38,39,40,41] A more recent randomized controlled trial (n=173) compared three gums. At 4 years of age, the children of mothers who chewed xylitol gum (one piece containing 650 mg xylitol chewed for 5 minutes three times daily for 1 year) had significantly fewer decayed, extracted, and filled surfaces compared to a group that chewed a gum containing sodium fluoride 0.55 mg, xylitol 289 mg, and sorbitol 189 mg.[42] A gum containing 142 mg sorbitol, 5 mg chlorhexidine, and 533 mg xylitol was not significantly better than control.

An analysis of four published double-blind trials (all performed by the same investigator) of sorbitol and xylitol chewing gums administered three to five times daily found that xylitol gums were superior to sorbitol gums in two secondary dentition trials but not in two primary dentition trials.[43] All gums reduced caries compared to non-gum-chewing groups. A more recent nonrandomized, multicenter study by the same investigator compared xylitol or xylitol/sorbitol gum use (one stick of gum for 5 minutes five times per day for 454 days) in 892 school children to a non-gum-chewing group over 2 years. Neither gum reduced Plaque Index scores significantly. Salivary *S. mutans* counts were significantly reduced in both groups after 2 years, with no significant differences between the treated groups; reductions in *S. mutans* persisted for 15 months after gum administration was terminated.[44]

Another double-blind, randomized, controlled trial in 160 10- to 12-year-olds with high caries risk found that lozenges containing xylitol (2.5 g) or xylitol 2.5 g/fluoride 1.5 mg (two lozenges three times daily) did not significantly reduce caries over 2 years.[45] Most, but not all, studies have shown that xylitol reduces salivary *Streptococcus mutans* levels;[46] one comparison trial found that xylitol was superior to sorbitol in reducing *S. mutans* levels.[47] In rats, xylitol-resistant strains of *S. mutans* developed following regular exposure to xylitol,[48] although these strains were less cariogenic.[49]

Calcium

A calcium-fortified chewing gum ameliorated the cariogenic effects of sucrose more than a conventional gum, as measured by increased pH, calcium, and phosphate concentrations in plaque fluid and saliva.[50]

Propolis

Propolis, or "bee glue," is an adhesive, resinous substance used by honeybees in building and sealing a hive. A double-blind study comparing a propolis-containing mouthwash with a positive control (chlorhexidine) and a negative control found that the chlorhexidine mouthrinse was best; there was no significant difference between the propolis-containing mouthrinse and the negative control.[51] Another study in 10 volunteers tested propolis and honey against oral bacteria; propolis reduced streptococci counts both in vitro and clinically.[52]

Periodontal Disease

Herbal Mixtures

An herbal extract containing a mixture of equal parts juniper (*Juniperus communis*), nettle (*Urtica dioca*), and yarrow (*Achillea millefolium*) was tested in 45 subjects with moderate gingival inflammation, randomized to treatment or control in a 2:1 ratio.[53] All were asked to rinse with 10 mL of mouthwash twice a day for 3 months. Plaque index, modified gingival index, and angulated bleeding index were assessed at baseline, at 6 weeks, and at 3 months. There was no difference between the treated group and the control group. Another recent study found no benefit of an herbal rinse over a placebo rinse on the gingival health in 63 participants over 3 months.[54]

A randomized, double-blind, placebo-controlled clinical trial compared a toothpaste containing *P. vulgaris* (0.5%) and *M. conrata* (0.005%) extracts to a placebo toothpaste for gingivitis in 40 subjects. Compared to placebo, the treated group showed a statistically significant improvement in inflammation, assessed by the papillary bleeding index and the community periodontal index of treatment needs. There was no difference between groups in plaque reduction, measured by the plaque index.[55]

Folate

A randomized, double-blind, placebo-controlled study tested folate mouthwash against established gingivitis in 60 subjects who had >20 teeth and visible gingival inflammation around >6 teeth.[56] Subjects rinsed with 5 mL of placebo or folate-containing mouthwash (5 mg folate/5 mL) for 1 minute twice daily for 4 weeks. Oral examination was done at baseline and at 4 weeks. Compared with the control group, the treated group showed a significant decrease in mean number of color change sites (from 70.17 ± 12.89 to 56.62 ± 17.42) and in bleeding sites (from 48.59 ± 24.28 to 29.28 ± 19.64).

Vitamin E

A double-blind trial compared the effect of a topical vitamin E gel (5%), a placebo gel, and a chlorhexidine rinse on established and developing plaque and periodontal disease in 48 adults.[57] The first two groups applied either 12 mL of placebo or vitamin E gel (containing 800 mg α-tocopherol) daily; the chlorhexidine group rinsed with 0.5 oz of 0.12% chlorhexidine gluconate. Plaque index, gingival index, and periodontal probing depth were assessed at baseline and at 2 weeks; root planing and scaling were done at 2 weeks, with additional data collection at 4 and 6 weeks. Only chlorhexidine significantly reduced plaque; vitamin E had no significant effects on plaque or gingivitis, compared with placebo.

Coenzyme Q10

A review of coenzyme Q10 (involved in electron transport in mitochondria) to treat periodontal disease identified two controlled trials, neither of which was published in the periodontal literature, and found that both trials were methodologically deficient.[58]

Polyunsaturated Fatty Acids

Fish oil contains the omega-3 fatty acids eicosapentaenoic acid (EPA) and doxahexanoic acid (DHA). Evening primrose oil and borage seed oil are rich in gamma-linolenic acid. A double blind, randomized, placebo-controlled study of 30 periodontitis patients compared EPA supplements (3,000 mg daily), borage oil supplements (3,000 mg daily), and a combination (1,500 mg each daily) for 12 weeks. A significant improvement in the modified gingival index score and periodontal probing depths was reported for the borage oil group.[59]

Lactic Bacteria

A double-blind, randomized, placebo-controlled trial of 59 patients with moderate to severe gingivitis found that gum containing live cultures of *Lactobacillus reuteri* ($2x10^8$ cfu daily for 2 weeks) showed that *L. reuteri*-1 strains significantly improved gingival index scores at day 14, while *L. reuteri*-1 and *L.reuteri*-2 strains significantly reduced plaque index scores. *L. reuteri*-2 strains were also found to more readily colonize the oral cavity.[60]

Other Conditions

Phenytoin-induced Gingival Enlargement

Two controlled trials assessed the effect of folic acid (3 mg for 4 months and 5 mg for 1 year) on phenytoin-induced gingival enlargement.[61,62] Neither found an effect. A third small study of eight institutionalized disabled residents tested 5 mg folic acid for 6 months in an effort to reduce recurrence of phenytoin-induced gingival enlargement after gingivectomy. The treatment group had significantly less recurrence of gingival enlargement, but the mean difference was only 7% at 6 months.[63]

Xerostomia

Yohimbine, an α_2-antagonist used to treat impotence, has been tested for its effect on salivary secretion in 11 healthy volunteers and in volunteers treated with tricyclic antidepressants.[64] A regimen of yohimbine (4 mg three times daily for 3 weeks) did not affect resting salivary secretion levels (tested at baseline and weekly thereafter) in either group; acute administration, however, significantly increased salivary volume within 1 hour in both groups.

Bleeding Risks

Several herbs can increase the risk of bleeding, especially when combined with anticoagulants. Garlic (*Allium sativum*) inhibits platelet-activating factor, and large amounts of dietary garlic prior to surgery has been associated with bleeding episodes. The Chinese herbs dong quai (*Angelica sinensis*) and danshen (*Salvia miltiorrhiza*) are associated with increased anticoagulant effect when combined with warfarin.

Other herbs and supplements previously thought to increase bleeding risk have been exonerated. Studies designed to assess bleeding risk have found no effect of ginkgo (*G. biloba*)[64] extract or vitamin E (up to 800 IUs/day for 4 months) in normal subjects.[66] A 6-month study found no effect of EPA+DHA (0.8 or 1.7 g/day) on clotting factors compared with the control.[67] Fish oil did not increase bleeding risk when combined with aspirin[6,69] or warfarin.[69] In a controlled trial, vitamin E did not affect INR in those taking warfarin.[70] Ginkgo does not increase bleeding risk over aspirin alone[71,72] or warfarin.[73,74] Little is known about bleeding effects of many other herbs and dietary supplements; it is advisable to discontinue the use of herbs and dietary supplements a week before surgery.[75]

CONCLUSION

Herbs and dietary supplements are used commonly by the general public and may have both beneficial and adverse effects relevant to dentistry. (**Table 25** shows adverse effects—those described previously as well as others[75,15,76-78]—of herbs and dietary supplements.) Nutritional deficiencies can manifest first in the mouth; stained gingiva can indicate the use of betel, khat, or silver; garlic, danshen, and other herbs can increase the risk of bleeding after an invasive procedure. Therefore, it is worthwhile to include questions about the use of herbs and dietary supplements in the patient's health history, and to be aware of possible adverse effects or interactions. Several herbs may hold promise in dental treatment and should be researched further.

Editor's note: Because herbs and dietary supplements are not regulated as drugs by the U.S. Food and Drug Administration, claims regarding their therapeutic benefit should not be accepted without support from well-controlled studies published in peer-reviewed journals. Only a limited number of controlled clinical trials have been conducted with these agents; more are needed. This chapter reviews both positive and negative controlled trials published in peer-reviewed journals and methodological flaws are noted.

References

1. Lewis WH, Elvin-Lewis PF. *Medical botany: Plants Affecting Man's Health*. New York: John Wiley and Sons; 2003:379-459.
2. Darout IA, Albandar JM, Skaug N. Periodontal status of adult Sudanese habitual users of miswak chewing sticks or toothbrushes. *Acta Odontol Scand*. 2000;58(1):25-30.
3. Homer KA, Manji F, Beighton D. Inhibition of protease activities of periodontopathic bacteria by extracts of plants used in Kenya as chewing sticks (mswaki). *Arch Oral Biol*. 1990;35:421-424.
4. Biswal BM, Zakaria A, Ahmad NM. Topical application of honey in the management of radiation mucositis: a preliminary study. *Support Care Cancer*. 2003;11(4):242-248.
5. Segal R, Pisanti S, Wormser R, et al. Anticariogenic activity of licorice and glycyrrhizin inhibition of in vitro plaque formation by *Streptococcus mutans*. *J Pharm Sci*. 1985;74(1):79-81.
6. Weiss EI, Lev-Dor R, Kashamn Y, et al. Inhibiting interspecies coaggregation of plaque bacteria with a cranberry juice constituent. *JADA*. 1998;129:1719-1723.
7. Modesto A, Lima KC, de Uzeda M. Effects of three different infant dentifrices on biofilms and oral microorganisms. *J Clin Pediatr Dent*. 2000;24(3):237-243.
8. Phelan J, Rees J. The erosive potential of some herbal teas. *J Dent*. 2003;31(4):241-246.
9. Thomas SJ, MacLenna R. Slaked lime and betel nut cancer in Papua New Guinea. *Lancet*. 1992;340:577-578.
10. Morton JF. Widespread tannin intake via stimulants and masticatories, especially guarana, kola nut, betel vine, and accessories. In: Hemingway RW, Laks PE, eds. *Plant Polyphenols*. New York: Plenum Press; 1992:739-765.
11. Norton SA. Betel: consumption and consequences. *J Am Acad Dermatol*. 1998;38(1):81-88.
12. D'Arcy PF. Adverse reactions and interactions with herbal medicines. *Adverse Drug React Toxicol Rev*. 1991;10:189-208.
13. Kim CS. Argyria secondary to chronic ingestion of colloidal silver (abstract 121). *Clin Tox*. 2000;38(5):552.
14. Gulbranson SH, Hud JA, Hansen RC. Argyria following the use of dietary supplements containing colloidal silver protein. *Cutis*. 2000;66:373-374.
15. Depaola DP, Faine MP, Palmer CA. Nutrition in relation to dental medicine. In: Shils ME, Olson JA, Shike M, Ross AC, eds. *Modern Nutrition in Health and Disease*. 9th ed. Baltimore: Williams & Wilkins; 1999:1099-1124.
16. Willmott NS, Bryan RA. Case report: scurvy in an epileptic child on a ketogenic diet with oral complications. *Eur Arch Paediatr Dent*. 2008;9(3):148-152.
17. Meisel P, Schwahn C, Luedemann J, et al. Magnesium deficiency is associated with periodontal disease. *J Dent Res*. 2005; 84(10):937-941.
18. Petti S, Cairella G, Tarsitani G. Nutritional variables related to gingival health in adolescent girls. *Community Dent Oral Epidemiol*. 2000;28(6):407-413.
19. Krall EA, Wehler C, Garcia RI, et al. Calcium and vitamin D supplements reduce tooth loss in the elderly. *Am J Med*. 2001;111(6):452-456.
20. Al-Waili NS. Topical honey application vs. acyclovir for the treatment of recurrent herpes simplex lesions. *Med Sci Monit*. 2004;10(8):MT94-98.
21. Plemons JM, Rees TD, Binnie WH, et al. Evaluation of acemannan in the treatment of recurrent aphthous stomatitis. *Wounds*. 1994;6(2):40-45.
22. Biswal BM, Zakaria A, Ahmad NM. Topical application of honey in the management of radiation mucositis: a preliminary study. *Support Care Cancer*. 2003;11(4):242-248.
23. Fidler P, Loprinzi CL, O'Fallon JR, et al. Prospective evaluation of a chamomile mouthwash for prevention of 5-FU-induced oral mucositis. *Cancer*. 1996;77:522-525.
24. Wadleigh RG, Redman RS, Graham ML, et al. Vitamin E in the treatment of chemotherapy-induced mucositis. *Am J Med*. 1992;92:481-484.
25. Liede KE, Haukka JK, Saxen LM, et al. Increased tendency towards gingival bleeding caused by joint effect of α-tocopherol supplementation and acetylsalicylic acid. *Ann Med*. 1998;30:542-546.
26. Meydani SN, Meydani M, Blumberg JB, et al. Assessment of the safety of supplementation with different amounts of vitamin E in healthy older adults. *Am J Clin Nutr*. 1998;68:311-318.
27. Sardella A, Lodi G, Demarosi F, et al. *Hypericum perforatum* extract in burning mouth syndrome: a randomized placebo-controlled study. *J Oral Pathol Med*. 2008;37(7):395-401.
28. Mathew B, Sankaranarayanan R, Nair PP, et al. Evaluation of chemoprevention of oral cancer with *Spirulina fusiformis*. *Nutr Cancer*. 1995;24(2):197-202.
29. Chainani-Wu N, Silverman S Jr, Reingold A, et al. A randomized, placebo-controlled, double-blind clinical trial of curcuminoids in oral lichen planus. *Phytomedicine*. 2007;14(7-8):437-446.
30. Choonhakarn C, Busaracome P, Sripanidkulchai B, et al. The efficacy of aloe vera gel in the treatment of oral lichen planus: a randomized controlled trial. *Br J Dermatol*. 2008;158(3):573-577.
31. Bayona-Gonzalez A, Lopez-Camara V, Gomez-Castellanos A. Final results of a dental caries clinical trial using heat killed lactic bacteria (streptococci and lactobacilli) orally. *Pract Odontol*. 1990;11(6):41-47.
32. Caglar E, Sandalli N, Twetman S, et al. Effect of yogurt with *Bifidobacterium* DN-173 010 on salivary mutans streptococci and lactobacilli in young adults. *Acta Odontol Scand*. 2005;63(6):317-20.

33. Caglar E, Kuscu OO, Selvi Kuvvetli S, et al. Short-term effect of ice cream containing *Bifidobacterium lactis* Bb-12 on the number of salivary mutans streptococci and lactobacilli. *Acta Odontol Scand.* 2008;66(3):154-8.
34. Birkhed D, Svensäter G, Edwardsson S. Cariological studies of individuals with long-term sorbitol consumption. *Caries Res.* 1990;24:220-3.
35. Firestone AR, Navia JM. In vivo measurements of sulcal plaque pH after topical applications of sorbitol and sucrose in rats fed sorbitol or sucrose. *J Dent Res.* 1986;65:1020-3.
36. Szoke J, Banoczy J, Proskin HM. Effect of after-meal sucrose-free gum-chewing on clinical caries. *J Dent Res.* 2001;80:1725-9.
37. Bradley B, Beiswanger, Boneta AE, et al. The effect of chewing sugar-free gum after meals on clinical caries incidence. *JADA.* 1998;129:1623-6.
38. Isokangas P, Söderling E, Pienihakkinen K, et al. Occurrence of dental decay in children after maternal consumption of xylitol chewing gum, a follow-up from 0 to 5 years of age. *J Dent Res.* 2000;79:1885-9.
39. Söderling E, Isokangas P, Pienihakkinen K, et al. Influence of maternal xylitol consumption on acquisition of mutans streptococci by infants. *J Dent Res.* 2000;79:882-7.
40. Söderling E, Isokangas P, Pienihakkinen K, et al. Influence of maternal xylitol consumption on mother-child transmission of mutans streptococci: 6-year follow-up. *Caries Res.* 2001;35(3): 173-7.
41. Thorild I, Lindau B, Twetman S. Effect of maternal use of chewing gums containing xylitol, chlorhexidine or fluoride on mutans streptococci colonization in the mothers' infant children. *Oral Health Prev Dent.* 2003;1(1):53-7.
42. Thorild I, Lindau B, Twetman S. Caries in 4-year-old children after maternal chewing of gums containing combinations of xylitol, sorbitol, chlorhexidine and fluoride. *Eur Arch Paediatr Dent.* 2006;7(4):241-5.
43. Gales MA, Nguyen T-M. Sorbitol compared with xylitol in prevention of dental caries. *Ann Pharmacother.* 2000;34:98-100.
44. Mäkinen KK, Alanen P, Isokangas P, et al. Thirty-nine-month xylitol chewing-gum programme in initially 8-year-old school children: a feasibility study focusing on mutans streptococci and lactobacilli. *Int Dent J.* 2008;58(1):41-50.
45. Stecksen-Blicks C, Holgerson PL, Twetman S. Effect of xylitol and xylitol-fluoride lozenges on approximal caries development in high-caries-risk children. *Int J Paediatr Dent.* 2008;18(3):170-7.
46. Burt BA. The use of sorbitol- and xylitol-sweetened chewing gum in caries control. *JADA.* 2006 Feb;137(2):190-6. Erratum in: *J Am Dent Assoc.* 2006 Apr;137(4):447.
47. Hildebrandt GH, Sparks BS. Maintaining mutans streptococci suppression with xylitol chewing gum. *JADA.* 2000;131: 909-16.
48. Beckers HJ. Influence of xylitol on growth, establishment and cariogenicity of Streptococcus mutans in dental plaque of rats. Caries Res. 1988;22:166–73.
49. Trahan L. Xylitol: a review of its action on mutans streptococci and dental plaque—its clinical significance. *Int Dent J.* 1995;45:77–92.
50. Vogel GL, Zhang Z, Carey CM, et al. Composition of plaque and saliva following a sucrose challenge and use of an α-tricalcium-phosphate-containing chewing gum. *J Dent Res.* 1998;77(3):518-524.
51. Murray MC, Worthington HV, Blinkhorn AS. A study to investigate the effect of a propolis-containing mouthrinse on the inhibition of de novo plaque formation. *J Clin Periodontol.* 1997;24:796-798.
52. Steinberg D, Kaine G, Gedalia J. Antibacterial effect of propolis and honey on oral bacteria. *Am J Dent.* 1996;9(6):236-239.
53. Van der Weijden GA, Timmer CJ, Timmerman MF, et al. The effect of herbal extracts in an experimental mouthrinse on established plaque and gingivitis. *J Clin Periodontol.* 1998;25: 399-403.
54. Southern EN, McCombs GB, Tolle SL, et al. The comparative effects of 0.12% chlorhexidine and herbal oral rinse on dental plaque-induced gingivitis. *J Dent Hyg.* 2006;80(1):12.
55. Adámková H, Vicar J, Palasová J, et al. Macleya cordata and Prunella vulgaris in oral hygiene products—their efficacy in the control of gingivitis. *Biomed Pap Med Fac Univ Palacky Olomouc Czech Repub.* 2004;148(1):103-105.
56. Pack AR. Folate mouthwash: effects on established gingivitis in periodontal patients. *J Clin Periodontol.* 1984;11:619-628.
57. Cohen RE, Ciancio SG, Mather ML, et al. Effect of vitamin E gel, placebo gel and chlorhexidine on periodontal disease. *Clin Prev Dent.* 1991;13(5):20-24.
58. Watts TLP. Coenzyme Q10 and periodontal treatment: is there any beneficial effect? *Br Dent J.* 1995;178:209-213.
59. Rosenstein ED, Kushner LJ, Kramer N, et al. Pilot study of dietary fatty acid supplementation in the treatment of adult periodontitis. *Prostaglandins Leukot Essent Fatty Acids.* 2003;68:213-18.
60. Krasse P, Carlsson B, Dahl C, et al. Decreased gum bleeding and reduced gingivitis by the probiotic *Lactobacillus reuteri. Swed Dent J.* 2005;30: 55-60.
61. Brown RS, Di Stanislao PT, Beaver WT, et al. The administration of folic acid to institutionalized epileptic adults with phenytoin-induced gingival hyperplasia. A double-blind, randomized, placebo-controlled, parallel study. *Oral Surg Oral Med Oral Pathol.* 1991;71:565-568.
62. Backman N, Holm AK, Hanstrom L, et al. Folate treatment of diphenylhydantoin-induced gingival hyperplasia. *Scand J Dent Res.* 1989;97:222-232.
63. Poppell TD, Keeling SD, Collins JF, et al. Effect of folic acid on recurrence of phenytoin-induced gingival overgrowth following gingivectomy. *J Clin Periodontol.* 1991;18(2):134-139.
64. Bagheri H, Schmitt L, Berlan M, et al. Effect of 3 weeks' treatment with yohimbine on salivary secretion in healthy volunteers and in depressed patients treated with tricyclic antidepressants. *Br J Clin Pharmacol.* 1992;34:555-558.
65. Bal Dit Sollier C, Caplain H, Drouet L.No alteration in platelet function or coagulation induced by EGb761 in a controlled study. *Clin Lab Haematol.* 2003;25(4):251-3.
66. Meydani SN, Meydani M, Blumberg JB, Leka LS, Pedrosa M, Diamond R, Schaefer EJ. Assessment of the safety of supplementation with different amounts of vitamin E in healthy older adults. *Am J Clin Nutr.* 1998;68(2):311-8.
67. Finnegan YE, Howarth D, Minihane AM, Kew S, Miller GJ, Calder PC, Williams CM. Plant and marine derived (n-3) polyunsaturated fatty acids do not affect blood coagulation and fibrinolytic factors in moderately hyperlipidemic humans. *J Nutr.* 2003;133(7):2210-3.
68. Bender NK, Kraynak MA, Chiquette E, Linn WD, Clark GM, Bussey HI. Effects of Marine Fish Oils on the Anticoagulation Status of Patients Receiving Chronic Warfarin Therapy. *J Thromb Thrombolysis.* 1998;5:257.
69. Eritsland J, Arnesen H, Gronseth K, Fjeld NB, Abdelnoor M. Effect of dietary supplementation with n-3 fatty acids on coronary artery bypass graft patency. *Am J Cardiol.* 1996;77(1):31-6.
70. Kim JM, White RH. Effect of vitamin E on the anticoagulant response to warfarin. *Am J Cardiol.* 1996;77:545.
71. Gardner CD, Zehnder JL, Rigby AJ, Nicholus JR, Farquhar JW. Effect of Ginkgo biloba (EGb 761) and aspirin on platelet aggregation and platelet function analysis among older adults at risk of cardiovascular disease: a randomized clinical trial. *Blood Coagul Fibrinolysis.* 2007;18(8):787-93.
72. Wolf HR. Does *Ginkgo biloba* special extract EGb 761 provide additional effects on coagulation and bleeding when added to acetylsalicylic acid 500 mg daily? *Drugs R D.* 2006;7(3): 163-72.
73. Jiang X, Williams KM, Liauw WS, et al. Effect of ginkgo and ginger on the pharmacokinetics and pharmacodynamics of warfarin in healthy subjects. *Br J Clin Pharmacol.* 2005;59:425.
74. Engelsen J, Nielsen JD, Winther K. Effect of coenzyme Q10 and *Ginkgo biloba* on warfarin dosage in stable, long-term warfarin treated outpatients. A randomised, double blind, placebo-crossover trial. *Thromb Haemost.* 2002;87:1075.
75. Fugh-Berman A, Ernst E. Herb-drug interactions: review and assessment of report reliability. *Br J Clin Pharmacol.* 2001;52: 587-595.
76. Ernst E. Harmless herbs? A review of the recent literature. *Am J Med.* 1998;104:170-178.
77. Garty BZ. Garlic burns. *Pediatrics.* 1993;91(3):658-659.
78. D'Arcy PF. Adverse reactions and interactions with herbal medicines. *Adverse Drug React Toxicol Rev.* 1991;10:189-208.

Table 25. USAGE INFORMATION FOR HERBS AND DIETARY SUPPLEMENTS

COMMON USE(S)	ADVERSE EFFECTS/INTERACTIONS
Aloe *(A. vera)*	
Burns, skin/mucosal irritation	Diarrhea from anthraquinones in leaf (not gel)[76]
Betel nut *(Areca catechu)*	
Masticatory stimulant	Oral leukoplakia; oral cancer; stained teeth and gingiva; bronchoconstriction; can interact with the antipsychotics flupenthixol and fluphenazine, causing bradykinesia, jaw tremor, rigidity[45]
Chaparral *(Larrea tridentata)*	
Cancer	Hepatotoxicity[45]
Coltsfoot *(Tussilago farfara)*	
Cough	Hepatotoxicity[75]
Comfrey *(Symphytum officinale)*	
Ulcers, wound healing	Hepatotoxicity[75]
Danshen *(Salvia miltiorrhiza)*	
Cardiovascular disease	Potentiates warfarin[75]
Dong quai *(Angelica sinensis)*	
Gynecologic conditions	Potentiates warfarin[40]
Ephedra *(E. sinica)*	
Respiratory conditions, weight loss	Hypertension, cardiac dysrhythmias, anxiety; can potentiate sympathomimetic drugs[75]
Feverfew *(Tanacetum parthenium)*	
Migraine	Aphthous ulcers[75]
Garlic *(Allium sativum)*	
Cardiovascular health	Anticoagulant effects[78]; topical garlic may cause a chemical burn[77]
Germander *(Teucrium chamaedrys)*	
Weight control	Hepatotoxicity[45]
Khat *(Catha edulis)*	
Masticatory stimulant	Caries, stained teeth, thickened oropharyngeal mucosa, psychosis, dependence[78]
Licorice *(Glycyrrhiza glabra)*	
Oral or gastrointestinal ulcers, inflammation	Hypokalemia, hypertension, edema; may potentiate glucocorticoids[75] *Note:* Deglycyrrhizinated licorice (DGL) preparations will not cause these effects.

Table 25. USAGE INFORMATION FOR HERBS AND DIETARY SUPPLEMENTS *(Cont.)*

COMMON USE(S)	ADVERSE EFFECTS/INTERACTIONS
St. John's wort *(Hypericum perforatum)*	
Depression	Phototoxic reactions; decreases levels of many drugs; increases serotonergic effects when combined with sertraline, trazodone, or nefazodone[76]
Silver	
Antibiotic	Argyria (slate-blue or silver line in the gingiva)[14]
Vitamin A	
Acne	Excessive vitamin A can cause hepatotoxicity and delay wound healing; in early pregnancy, excess can cause severe craniofacial and oral clefts and other birth defects[15]
Vitamin D	
Osteoporosis	Excessive vitamin D can cause pulp calcification and enamel hypoplasia[15]

Chapter 26

Legal Implications of Using Drugs in Dental Practice

ADA Division of Legal Affairs

Editor's Note: See page ii of this book for a disclaimer regarding the information provided in this section.

Dentists often fear that they need a law license to practice their profession successfully in today's climate of excessive federal regulation and burgeoning litigation. This fear is sometimes manifested when doctors face difficult choices about the types of drugs they prescribe in their practices.

Two types of approval processes can assist dentists in making difficult choices: the federal Food, Drug, and Cosmetic Act approval process, and the American Dental Association's Seal of Acceptance Program. Generally, a dentist who prescribes a drug approved by the U.S. Food and Drug Administration in a manner that is consistent with the label approved by the FDA—according to the approved directions for dosage, indications for usage and so forth—can feel relatively confident that the drug is safe and effective for its approved uses. Similarly, products that bear the ADA's Seal have been found by the ADA Council on Scientific Affairs to meet ADA guidelines for safety and effectiveness. An FDA-approved, ADA-accepted drug is a wise choice.

However, the wise choice may not always be the reasonable choice. In court, a doctor will be judged according to the applicable standard of care. Generally, doctors are judged according to a reasonableness standard; in a malpractice action, courts look to see how a reasonably prudent doctor would have acted in the same or similar circumstances. This means the doctor must be able to show at all times that his or her decision about which drug to prescribe was reasonable.

For example, it may be unreasonable to prescribe a drug approved for pain relief to a patient who has no pain. Although the safety and efficacy of the drug may be well established by the FDA, prescribing the drug for a pain-free patient could be inappropriate and might well constitute a breach of the standard of care.

Conversely, there may be instances in which it is reasonable for a doctor to prescribe an approved drug for a nonapproved use or even to prescribe a non–FDA-approved drug. In this situation, in the absence of state regulations that might prohibit the use of a non–FDA-approved drug, the doctor's actions will be judged primarily by the same standard of reasonableness that would be used in a typical dental or medical malpractice action. However, the analysis is trickier, because some jurisdictions have found that use of nonapproved drugs or use of approved drugs in nonapproved ways is prima facie negligence—in other words, negligence on the face of it. Such a finding does not end the inquiry, but it does place the burden on the doctor to justify the scientific basis for his or her decision, to show that a reasonably prudent doctor acting in the same or similar circumstances would have made the same decision. In some situations, it may be appropriate to obtain specific informed consent for the use prescribed.

Overall, the law defers to the doctor's need and ability to exercise independent professional judgment in the prescription of all drugs but holds doctors accountable for the results of negligent decisions. This chapter will discuss the legal ramifications of various decisions that are made in the context of making difficult prescription choices.

Use of FDA-Approved Drugs for Unapproved Uses

Generally, the FDA does not regulate dentists and physicians.[1] Thus, if an approved drug is shipped in interstate commerce with an approved package insert, and neither the shipper nor the recipient intends that it be used for an unapproved purpose; all requirements of the Food, Drug, and Cosmetic Act (the Act) are satisfied. Once the drug is in a local pharmacy, a dentist or physician may lawfully prescribe a different dosage for his or her patient, or may otherwise vary the conditions of use from those approved in the package insert, without informing or obtaining the approval of the FDA.[1,2]

The FDA has itself explained that Congress did not intend the FDA to interfere with medical practice or to regulate the practice of medicine between the doctor and the patient. Congress recognized that patients have the right to seek civil damages in the courts if there should be evidence of malpractice and declined to place any legislative restrictions on the medical profession.[3,4] (The FDA stated in an issue of FDA Drug Bulletin, "Accepted medical practice often includes drug use that is not reflected in approved drug labeling."[3] And in Chaney vs. Heckler, the court stated, "Congress would have created havoc in the medical profession had it required physicians to follow the expensive and time-consuming procedure of obtaining FDA approval before putting drugs to new uses."[4]) These pronouncements also should apply to the practice of dentistry, although the FDA has not made any specific statements to that effect.

In 1997, Congress adopted sweeping reforms of the Food Drug and Cosmetic Act via the Food and Drug Administration Modernization Act (FDAMA).[5] The FDAMA was approved in part because Congress recognized that the "prompt approval of safe and effective new drugs and other therapies is critical to the improvement of the public health so that patients may enjoy the benefits provided by these therapies to treat and prevent illness and disease."[6]

Nothing in the FDAMA changes the FDA's fundamental position on noninterference in the doctor-patient relationship. However, the Act does make it easier for drug manufacturers to at least discuss, if not promote, off-label or unapproved uses for their drug products by abolishing the previous prohibition on dissemination of information about unapproved uses of drugs and medical devices. It allows, among other things, a manufacturer to disseminate certain written information (primarily a reprint or copy of a peer-reviewed article) concerning the safety, effectiveness, or benefit of a use not described in the approved labeling of a drug or device if the manufacturer meets the specific requirements set forth in the Act.[7] The manufacturer must include with the information to be disseminated a prominently displayed statement disclosing that the information concerns a use of a drug or device that has not been approved or cleared by the Food and Drug Administration.

The FDA's policy on dissemination of information on off-label uses was the subject of long-standing litigation initiated by the Washington Legal Foundation. In July 1999, the U.S. District Court of the District of Columbia ruled that the FDAMA was unconstitutional to the extent that it impermissibly restrained a manufacturer's First Amendment right to disseminate truthful and non-misleading information about its product.[8] The FDA appealed to the U.S. Court of Appeals for the District of Columbia. In February 2000, the appeals court dismissed the FDA's appeal after FDA attorneys assured the court during oral argument that the agency did not interpret the FDAMA to give the agency new powers to prohibit or sanction constitutionally protected speech. In dismissing the appeal, the court vacated a district court injunction against FDA enforcement of the act. However, the appellate court did not disturb the district court's opinion about the limits the First Amendment places on the FDA's ability to regulate manufacturers' communications about off-label uses of drugs and devices.[9]

Determining Liability in Malpractice Cases

Although the FDA does not regulate the prescription by doctors of FDA-approved drugs, doctors are subject to civil liability for their actions. Thus, while it is not uncommon for doctors to prescribe approved drugs for unapproved purposes, in doing so they take upon themselves the burden of justifying their actions and assume potential liability if a mistake is made. In a typical dental or medical malpractice case, the plaintiff must prove these elements[10]:

- the existence of a duty, created by a doctor-patient relationship between the plaintiff and defendant;
- evidence of the standard of care owed by the defendant doctor to the plaintiff;
- evidence that the standard of care was violated or breached;
- proof that the breach of the standard of care was the proximate cause of the plaintiff's injury.

Generally, the standard of care in a malpractice case is determined under state law and must be established through the use of expert testimony. The rationale for the rule requiring expert testimony is that laypeople (in other words, jurors) cannot comprehend technical information without expert assistance.[11-13]

Courts have relied heavily on FDA-approved uses for approved drugs as evidence of the standard of care. In a malpractice action involving administration of a drug, some courts have gone so far as to hold that a drug manufacturer's clear and explicit instructions regarding the proper manner of administering a drug, accompanied by specific warnings of the hazards encountered in its improper administrations, are prima facie evidence of the standard of care. Under these decisions, no expert testimony is needed for the plaintiff to show the standard of care.

For example, in Haught vs. Maceluch,[14] the *Physicians' Desk Reference®* (*PDR*), which publishes drug manufacturers' instructions and package inserts, was cited as independent evidence of the medical standard for the administration of the drug oxytocin (Pitocin). This drug induces or augments labor. In the Haught case, the plaintiff claimed the defendant physician was negligent for failing to recognize well-established signs of fetal distress and to take appropriate action, and that the defendant negligently administered Pitocin. At trial, the court accepted evidence directly from the *PDR* that specifically contraindicated the use of Pitocin when fetal distress is suspected. The court held that the *PDR* established the standard because the physician ignored two important indicators of fetal distress.

In another case, a physician was found to have ignored the manufacturer's instructions for the intravenous injection of promazine hydrochloride (Sparine), as well as the warnings about complications that would arise from its improper administration.[15] The court relied directly on the FDA-approved manufacturer's instructions as evidence of the standard of care. The court held that where a drug manufacturer recommends to the medical profession the conditions under which its drug should be prescribed, the disorders it is designed to relieve, and the precautionary measures that should be observed and warns of the dangers inherent in its use, a doctor's deviation from such recommendations is prima facie evidence of negligence.[15,16] This evidence creates a rebuttable presumption that the doctor acted negligently and requires the doctor to come forward at trial with evidence as to why he or she was not negligent in deviating from the instructions.

Is it sufficient to follow manufacturer's instructions?

The cases mentioned above represent an extreme view.[17] Other cases, even from the same jurisdictions as the cases discussed above, have been careful to require that the manufacturer's instructions be absolutely clear and explicit before the courts will presume negligence. In Young vs. Cerniak,[18] for example, the defendant physicians were accused of deviating from the standard of care in failing to administer a proper dosage of the anticoagulant heparin. The plaintiff had an expert witness who relied at trial not on the manufacturer's instructions about the appropriate dosage, but on texts and treatises of experts in the field. The manufacturer's instructions were not, in the appellate court's opinion, explicit about the proper dosage and method of administration of the drug, and did not contain warnings about undesirable results if the physician deviated from the precise instructions. Moreover, the defendant physicians' experts testified that the manufacturer's recommendations contained one acceptable procedure for determining dosage, but the defendants followed an equally acceptable alternative method. The appellate court held that the manufacturer's instructions were not evidence of the standard of care, and the trial court had erred by telling the jury that the drug company's recommendations were a standard against which defendant's conduct was to be measured.

Similarly, in Nicolla vs. Fasulo,[19] an oral surgeon was sued for injuries allegedly resulting from his prescribing the drug oxycodone and acetaminophen (Percodan). The plaintiff asked the court to instruct the jury that the defendant would be prima facie negligent if the defendant deviated from the manufacturer's recommendations contained in the *PDR*. The appellate court held that the trial judge acted appropriately by refusing the request, because there was no clear and explicit contraindication or warning about Percodan in the *PDR* from which the defendant deviated.[20]

In any case, even in those jurisdictions that do not treat departure from *PDR* recommendations as prima facie evidence of malpractice, manufacturer recommendations will undoubtedly still be cited as some evidence of the standard of care.

Product inserts and expert testimony

An even more common approach is to allow product inserts and their parallel *PDR* references into evidence to show the standard of care, but only if expert testimony is also presented to explain the standard to the jury. This rule was followed in the case of Morlino vs. Medical Center of Ocean County.[21,22] In Morlino, a physician prescribed the antibiotic ciprofloxacin hydrochloride to the plaintiff, who was 8 months pregnant and suffering from acute pharyngitis. Earlier treatment with another antibiotic had been ineffective. The plaintiff's fetus died 1 day after she ingested the drug. Experts for the plaintiff testified that a reasonable and prudent physician would not have used ciprofloxacin in a pregnant patient and pointed to the explicit warning in the *PDR* against such use. The defendant physician acknowledged that he was familiar with the *PDR* warning but produced an expert who testified that the suspected infectious agent (*Haemophilus influenzae*) was much more risky to the mother and the developing fetus than ciprofloxacin. The defendant argued that it was reasonable for him to prescribe ciprofloxacin in these circumstances.

The jury rendered a verdict for the defendant, and the plaintiff appealed. On appeal, the plaintiff argued that the jury should have been allowed to find that the physician was prima facie negligent for deviating from the *PDR* warning, without reference to conflicting expert testimony. The appellate court disagreed. It reasoned that to have allowed the jury to find that failure to follow the *PDR* warning alone was negligence would force a physician to follow the *PDR* directives or automatically suffer the consequences of a malpractice action. The court pointed out the differences between a package insert and accepted medical practice. The former is based on the rigorous proof a regulatory agency demands, the latter on the clinical judgment of a doctor based on the doctor's training, experience, and skill and the specific needs of the individual patient. The court (quoting Peter H. Rheinstein, Drug Labeling as Standard for Medical Care,[4] *J. Legal Med.*[22, 24] [1976]) held that one cannot be taken as a standard for the other.[21]

The cases discussed above deal with the use of FDA-approved drugs for unapproved purposes, or the simple use of drugs in a manner inconsistent with the manufacturer's instructions. There appear to be no reported cases discussing the legal effect of a dentist's use of an ADA-accepted drug. It is logical to assume, however, that if the dentist used the drug in the manner recommended by the manufacturer, the dentist would certainly try to introduce testimony about the product's acceptance by the ADA as evidence of the reasonableness of the dentist's action. When the ADA accepts a dental product, all of the packaging claims made by the manufacturer about the product are also reviewed and approved. In fact, attorneys representing dentists frequently contact the ADA to find out whether a product used by a dentist bears the ADA Seal.

In summary, dentists and physicians may prescribe and use FDA-approved drugs in ways that differ from the uses approved by the FDA. Doctors should always base these decisions on sound professional judgment and should recognize that the decisions may need to be justified if the doctor is accused of malpractice.

Failure to Obtain Adequate Informed Consent

A related issue that needs to be considered is whether a doctor must obtain a special informed consent from a patient if the doctor prescribes an FDA-approved drug for a nonapproved purpose. A doctor's failure to obtain adequate informed consent can form a basis of liability to a patient that is separate and distinct from a negligence claim.

Traditionally, the standard of disclosure has been based on the customary practice of the community. Thus, courts look at what risks of treatment a reasonably prudent doctor would disclose in similar circumstances.[23,24] A more contemporary approach focuses on a lay standard of disclosure. While the details of this patient-centered approach vary by jurisdiction, courts generally look at what information a reasonable patient would consider material to the decision about whether or not to undergo treatment or diagnosis.[25-29]

The case of Reinhardt vs. Colton[30] is informative on the issue of informed consent in the context of using FDA-approved drugs for unapproved uses. In this case, the plaintiff's physician prescribed the drug penicillamine for the treatment of rheumatoid arthritis. At the time the drug was prescribed for her, it was used by other doctors to treat rheumatoid arthritis, but it was not approved by the FDA for this purpose. Penicillamine has the potential to cause many side effects, including destruction of the capacity to make red blood cells, which causes aplastic anemia. The plaintiff developed aplastic anemia after using penicillamine and brought suit against her physician.

One of the theories on which she based her lawsuit was a theory of "negligent nondisclosure of risk." Under this theory (a contemporary version of lack of informed consent), the plaintiff was required to prove that the physician had a duty to know of a risk or alternative treatment plan, that the physician had a duty to disclose the risk or alternative, that the duty was breached and that the plaintiff was harmed because of the nondisclosure of the risk. The standard used to judge the duty to disclose was based on the significance that a reasonable person in the plaintiff's position would have attached to the risk or the alternative in deciding whether to consent to treatment.

At trial, there was conflicting testimony about whether the plaintiff was informed that the use of penicillamine for rheumatoid arthritis was not approved by the FDA. However, the important testimony was the doctor's own statement about the risks of aplastic anemia associated with using the drug, the wide recognition of this risk in the medical community, and other testimony about whether the patient had been sufficiently warned about this risk. The court held that this testimony was sufficient to create an issue that had to be decided by the jury.

In addition to informed consent for using drugs for unapproved purposes, there has recently been a flurry of litigation involving the use of unapproved medical devices. In the case of Blazoski vs. Cook, 787 A.2d 910 (N.J. Super. A.D., 2002), the appeals court of New Jersey held that an orthopedic surgeon who performed spinal-fusion surgery on a patient need not disclose to the patient prior to surgery that the pedicle screws were not approved by the Food and Drug Administration (FDA) for use on lumbar spine. The Blazoski case was representative of a majority view that the FDA status of a medical device is not a material fact that must be disclosed to a patient to get informed consent. See Southard vs. Temple University Hospital, 781 A.2d 101, 107 (Pa. 2001). However, this case is not binding precedent throughout the United States.

These cases show that standard principles of informed consent, just like standard principles of negligence, govern the doctor's treatment decisions. It may not be necessary always to disclose whether a particular drug or device has been approved by the FDA. The overall analysis will focus on the total circumstances, as well as on whether the doctor acted within the applicable standard of care and informed the patient of risks and alternatives in a manner consistent with the standard applicable in the doctor's jurisdiction.

Use of Drugs Not Approved by the FDA

As discussed in the previous section, the FDA does not generally have jurisdiction over the practice of dentistry or medicine. Therefore, the FDA cannot, as a general rule, take action against a dentist or physician who prescribes drugs that do not have FDA approval.

Pharmacy as Manufacturer

An exception to this general principle arises if a dentist or physician places bulk orders from a pharmacy for unapproved prescription drugs. In this situation, the doctor may not be exempt from regulation by the FDA. For example, the FDA has stated that the dental drug called Sargenti Paste, Sargenti Compound, or N2 is an unapproved new drug (letter from Carl C. Peck, M.D., director, Center for Drug Evaluation and Research, Food and Drug Administration, to Newell Yaple, D.D.S., secretary, Ohio State Dental Board, Aug. 12, 1991).[31] Single prescriptions for individual patients may be lawfully prepared by pharmacies according to the Food, Drug, and Cosmetic Act, but bulk shipments by pharmacists to dentists are not permitted. The maximum amount of the formulation that the FDA permits to be dispensed is five grams (letter from Carl C. Peck, M.D., to Newell Yaple, D.D.S., Aug. 12, 1991). Conceivably, the FDA could take enforcement action against a dentist who ordered Sargenti Paste in bulk from a pharmacy.

A note about the above situation: Under the "pharmacy" exception to the Act, pharmacies are exempt from regulation under the Act if they are regularly engaged in dispensing prescription drugs or devices for prescriptions of practitioners licensed to administer such drugs or devices to patients under the care of such practitioners in the course of their professional practice; and if they do not manufacture, prepare, propagate, compound, or process drugs or devices for sale other than in the regular course of their business of dispensing or selling drugs or devices at retail. On the other hand, where a pharmacy compounds drugs in bulk, and sells them at wholesale prices with nationwide distribution, the pharmacy becomes a "manufacturer" under the act and is subject to FDA regulation. Relevant factors used to determine whether a pharmacy qualifies for the "pharmacy" exception to the Act are:

- whether particular drugs are being compounded on a regular basis, as opposed to periodic compounding of different drugs;
- whether drugs are being compounded primarily for individual patient prescriptions as opposed to orders contemplating larger amounts for office use;
- the geographic area of distribution;
- whether any form of advertising or promotion is being used;
- the percentage of gross income received from sales of particular compounded drugs;
- whether particular compounded drugs are being offered at wholesale prices.[32]

A dentist's use of non–FDA-approved drugs could conceivably also be limited by state law or by rules issued by a state licensing board. Some years ago, the Ohio State Dental Board considered a rule that would have prohibited dentists in that state from using any drug or medication not approved by the FDA in the treatment of patients. The rule was not adopted.

Use of Drugs Not Accepted by the ADA

The American Dental Association does not require its members to use only products that bear the ADA Seal of Acceptance. This policy reflects the voluntary nature of the ADA's Seal Program. While the Seal is an important indicator that a product meets ADA guidelines, the fact that a product has not been evaluated by the ADA Council on Scientific Affairs does not necessarily mean the product is unsafe or ineffective. Manufacturers of many safe and effective products may simply not have submitted those products to the ADA Seal Program.

Therefore, lack of the Seal should not be used to create any presumptions about the safety or efficacy of the unaccepted product.

Unproven Reliability and Effectiveness

Potential civil liability in a malpractice suit remains the most significant legal consequence of using a non–FDA-approved drug. In this area of inquiry, the existence of informed consent can be crucial, but will not always be enough to protect a doctor from later claims of negligence. Another crucial fact is whether alternative drugs of known effectiveness and proven reliability were available. In some cases, the outcome seems to depend upon the apparent egregiousness of the doctor's conduct.

The case of Sullivan vs. Henry illustrates the problems that can arise when a doctor prescribes a non–FDA-approved drug.[33] Sullivan involved a general physician who diagnosed his patient with cancer, determined it could not be treated with conventional cancer therapies, and suggested that the patient try amygdalin (Laetrile). Use of Laetrile was not approved by the FDA except for investigational use by experts qualified by scientific training and experience to investigate the safety and efficacy of the drug. The doctor in this case was not participating in such an investigation.

The patient was informed about the experimental nature of her treatment with Laetrile and knew that the drug was not approved by the FDA. The key issue was whether the physician acted negligently in choosing this course of treatment. The defendant asserted that he should win as a matter of law because he acted reasonably and within the standard of care. In opposition to that claim, the plaintiffs (the patient's family) produced affidavits from expert witnesses stating that Laetrile was not listed in the *PDR*, was a known poison with no known benefits, and was unsafe at any dosage. Another expert for the plaintiffs expressed the opinion that the defendant doctor did not fully explore the nature of the patient's malignancy. This raised questions about the doctor's conclusion that conventional cancer therapies, such as chemotherapy and radiotherapy, were not suitable for this patient's cancer. These facts created a jury question as to whether the defendant was negligent.

It is interesting to note that the plaintiffs' expert in Sullivan focused on the potential that experimental treatment was unnecessary. Failure to prescribe a drug of known effectiveness and proven reliability, which could have been used instead of a non–FDA-approved drug, may constitute a breach of the standard of care. This occurred in Blanton vs. U.S.,[34] in which the plaintiff was asked to participate in an experiment to test whether the drug Rho(D) immune globulin (HypRho-D) had effectiveness beyond its FDA-approved shelf life. The plaintiff, a hospital patient, refused to participate in the experiment, but she received the drug anyway by mistake.

The court noted that this was not a simple case of the plaintiff receiving one drug that was inaccurately represented as another. Rather, the drug was in effect a "new drug" that was not FDA-approved, and "it was administered despite the availability of a drug of known effectiveness and proven reliability." The court held that the hospital, by administering the drug to plaintiff without her consent, violated "accepted medical standards."[34 (at 362)] While this case involved a hospital's conduct, not that of a physician or dentist, the rationale could be extended to a health professional as well.

Duty of Disclosure

In truly egregious cases, courts may look beyond a negligence theory to impose liability on doctors who act improperly in prescribing non–FDA-approved therapies. For example, in Nelson vs. Gaunt, the plaintiff received from the defendant a series of silicone injections for breast augmentation.[35] The uncontested evidence showed that at the time the plaintiff received the injections, the FDA considered silicone injections dangerous for use in human body tissues, and only persons who obtained a special permit to administer the injections under scientific circumstances could use silicone for this purpose. The defendant physician not only had no such permit, but he told the plaintiff that the substance was safe, inert, and had absolutely no side effects. He did not tell her the name of the substance, the fact that it could be used only for the purposes of scientific research, that even under those conditions its use required state or federal approval, and that he did not have a permit to perform the injections.

These facts, the court found, went beyond an ordinary negligence theory and even beyond a claim of battery, which would exist if, for example, a doctor performed an operation without the patient's consent. The theory applicable on these facts was fraud, based on the physician's fiduciary duty to disclose information to the patient that may be relevant to a meaningful decision-making process and necessary to form the basis of an intelligent consent by the patient to the proposed treatment. In this case, the court found, the doctor provided the patient with false and misleading information and knowingly concealed information that was material to the cause of the plaintiff's injuries.[35]

The fact that a doctor is participating in an FDA-approved clinical investigation is not in itself sufficient to protect the doctor from claims of negligence. In a case involving use of a medical device, Daum vs. Spinecare Medical Group, Inc.,[36] a physician was required to defend himself against the charge that he failed to obtain the patient's informed consent to use the investigational device—a metal screw—in spinal fusion surgery. Applicable federal and state laws incorporated in the manufacturer's protocol for clinical trials required that patients be informed of the device's investigational status, give written consent to participate in the trial, and be provided with a copy of their consent form.

The patient claimed that he was not told that the device was investigational or provided with the consent form until he was sedated and on a gurney being wheeled to the operating room; this raised an issue of whether the patient's consent was truly informed. However, the immediate question for the appellate court was whether the jury could find that simple failure to comply with the rules for conduct of the clinical trial, including the rule on informed consent, was negligence per se. The court held that it could, reasoning that the physician was not required to participate in the clinical trials but that once he did, he was required to abide by its rules. The jury was entitled to consider the physician's failure to comply with the rules on informed consent as evidence of negligence per se, shifting to the physician the burden of proving that he did what might reasonably be expected of a person of ordinary prudence, acting under similar circumstances who desired to comply with the law. There is no reason to believe that the court would not apply the same rule to a new drug.

Conclusion

Dentists, in using drugs in their practices, need to be cognizant of the status of those agents within the FDA and the ADA. However, the more important concern is to exercise sound professional judgment in making choices and to be sure that patients are fully cognizant of material information concerning their treatments and the alternatives available to them.

Editor's note: This chapter was originally based on a 1992 article by Linda M. Wakeen, J.D., that appeared in the *Journal of Public Health Dentistry*[37] and was edited by Kathleen M. Todd, J.D., and Jill Wolowitz, J.D., LL.M. The chapter has since been further edited for this publication.

References

1. *See Generally* 21 C.F.R. § 1.1, et. al.
2. Beck JM, Azari ED. FDA, off-label use, and informed consent: debunking myths and misconceptions. *Food and Drug Law J.* 1998;53:71-104.
3. See also "Use of Approved Drugs for Unlabeled Indications," 12 FDA Drug Bulletin 4 (April 1982).
4. See also Chaney vs. Heckler, 718 F.2d 1174, 1180 (D.C. App. 1983), rev'd on other grounds, 470 U.S. 821 (1985).
5. Pub L No. 105-115 §101 (1997).
6. Pub. L. 105-115 § 101(1997); *See generally*21 U.S.C.A § 301 et. seq.
7. 21 U.S.C.A. § 360aaa, et seq., Requirements for dissemination of treatment information on drugs or devices.
8. Washington Legal Foundation vs. Henney, 56 F.Supp.2d 81 (D.D.C. 1999).
9. Washington Legal Foundation v. Henney, 202 F.3d 331 (D.C. Cir., 2000).
10. See, e.g., Nold v. Binyon, 272 Kan. 87 (Kan. 2001); and Winkjer vs. Herr, 277 N.W.2d 579, 583 (N.D. 1979).
11. See, e.g., Olivier v. Robert L. Yeager Mental Health Center, 398 F.3d 183, 190 (2d Cir. 2005) ("we note that a jury composed of non-experts typically cannot discern generally accepted medical standards for itself. In order to demonstrate an objective violation of those standards, therefore, a plaintiff ordinarily must introduce expert testimony to establish the relevant medical standards that were allegedly violated."); and, Blackwell vs. Hurst, 46 Cal. App. 4th 939, 942 (Cal. App. 1996).
12. See, e.g., Rallings vs. Evans, 930 S.W.2d 259, 262 (Texas Ct. App. 1996).
13. See, e.g., Ellis vs. Oliver, 323 S.C. 121, 125 (1996).
14. Haught vs. Maceluch, 681 F.2d 291 (5th Cir. 1982).
15. Ohligschlager vs. Proctor Community Hospital, 303 N.E.2d 392 (Ill. 1973).
16. See also Mulder vs. Parke Davis & Company, 181 N.W.2d 882 (Minn. 1970).
17. See, e.g., Spensieri v. Lasky, 94 N.Y. 2d 231 (N.Y. 1999) (holding that a PDR by itself cannot be used to establish a standard of care for prescribing of drugs) (declining to follow Ohligschlager vs. Proctor Community Hospital, 303 N.E.2d 392 [Ill. 1973]).
18. See Young vs. Cerniak, 467 N.E.2d 1045 (Ill. App. 1984).
19. See Nicolla vs. Fasulo, 557 N.Y.S.2d 539 (App. Div. 1990).

20. See, e.g., Ramon By and Through Ramon v. Farr, 770 P.2d 131 (Utah. 1991), for a case distinguishing Mulder.
21. Morlino vs. Medical Center of Ocean County, 295 N.J.Super. 113, 122 (1996).
22. See also Ramon vs. Farr, 770 P.2d 131 (Utah 1989).
23. See, e.g., Ross vs. Hodges, 234 So.2d 905 (Miss. 1970).
24. See, e.g., Aiken vs. Clary, 396 S.W.2d 668 (Mo. 1965).
25. See, e.g., Howard v. University of Medicine and Dentistry of New Jersey, 172 N.J. 537, 547 (N.J.. 2002); and Cobbs vs. Grant, 502 P.2d 1 (Cal. 1972).
26. See, e.g., Wilkinson vs. Vesey, 295 A.2d 676 (R.I. 1972).
27. See also R.I. Gen. Laws § 9–19–32 (2009).
28. See also Wash. Rev. Code Ann. § 7.70.050(1)(c) (2009).
29. Reinhardt vs. Colton, 337 N.W.2d 88 (Minn. 1983).
30. See 21 U.S.C. § 360(g)(1).
31. *See* Cedars North Towers Pharmacy, Inc. v. U.S. (DC Fla. 1978); 1978-79 FDC L. Rept. Dev. Trans. Bind ¶ 38, 200.
32. Sullivan vs. Henry, 287 S.E.2d 652 (Ga. App. 1982).
33. Blanton vs. United States, 428 F. Supp. 360 (D.D.C. 1977).
34. Nelson vs. Gaunt, 125 Cal.App.3d 623 (1981).
35. Daum vs. Spinecare Medical Group, Inc., 52 Cal. App.4th 1285 (Cal. App. 1997).
36. Wakeen LM. Legal implications of using drugs and devices in the dental office. *J Public Health Dent*. 1992;52(6):403-408.

Appendices

U.S. Schedules for Controlled Substances

U.S. CLASSIFICATIONS	
Schedule I	No recognized legal medical use; used in research with appropriate registration.
Schedule II	High potential for abuse. Use may lead to severe physical or psychological dependence. Prescriptions must be written in ink, or typewritten and signed by the practitioner. Verbal prescriptions must be confirmed in writing within 72 hours, and may be given only in a genuine emergency. No renewals are permitted.
Schedule III	Some potential for abuse. Use may lead to low-to-moderate physical dependence or high psychological dependence. Prescriptions may be oral or written. Up to 5 renewals are permitted within 6 months.
Schedule IV	Low potential for abuse. Use may lead to limited physical or psychological dependence. Prescriptions may be oral or written. Up to 5 renewals are permitted within 6 months.
Schedule V	Subject to state and local regulation. Abuse potential is low; a prescription may not be required.

SCHEDULES FOR CONTROLLED SUBSTANCES	
Heroin, LSD, peyote, marijuana, mescaline	Schedule I (CI)
Opium, fentanyl, morphine, meperidine, methadone, oxycodone (and combinations), hydromorphone, codeine (single-drug entity), cocaine, phencyclidine	Schedule II (CII)
Short-acting barbiturates	Schedule II (CII)
Amphetamine, methylphenidate	Schedule II (CII)
Codeine combinations, hydrocodone combinations, paregoric, phendimetrazine, testosterone, other androgens	Schedule III (CIII)
Benzodiazepines (e.g., diazepam, midazolam), chloral hydrate, meprobamate, phenobarbital, propoxyphene (and combinations), pentazocine (and combinations), methohexital	Schedule IV (CIV)
Antidiarrheals and antitussives with opioid derivatives	Schedule V (CV)

Key to FDA Use-in-Pregnancy Ratings

FDA USE-IN-PREGNANCY CLASSIFICATIONS	
CATEGORY	**INTERPRETATION**
A	CONTROLLED STUDIES SHOW NO RISK. Adequate, well-controlled studies in pregnant women have failed to demonstrate a risk to the fetus in any trimester of pregnancy.
B	NO EVIDENCE OF RISK IN HUMANS. Adequate, well-controlled studies in pregnant women have not shown increased risk of fetal abnormalities despite adverse findings in animals, or, in the absence of adequate human studies, animal studies show no fetal risk. The chance of fetal harm is remote, but remains a possibility.
C	RISK CANNOT BE RULED OUT. Adequate, well-controlled human studies are lacking, and animal studies have shown a risk to the fetus or are lacking as well. There is a chance of fetal harm if the drug is administered during pregnancy; but the potential benefits may outweigh the potential risk.
D	POSITIVE EVIDENCE OF RISK. Studies in humans, or investigational or post-marketing data, have demonstrated fetal risk. Nevertheless, potential benefits from the use of the drug may outweigh the potential risk. For example, the drug may be acceptable if needed in a life-threatening situation or serious disease for which safer drugs cannot be used or are ineffective.
X	CONTRAINDICATED IN PREGNANCY. Studies in animals or humans, or investigational or post-marketing reports, have demonstrated positive evidence of fetal abnormalities or risk which clearly outweighs any possible benefit to the patient.

Agents That Affect the Fetus and Nursing Infant

Angelo J. Mariotti, D.D.S., Ph.D.

A teratogen is a drug or chemical that induces alterations in the formation of cells, tissues, and organs and thus creates physical defects in a developing embryo or fetus. Teratogens act via a number of diverse mechanisms to ultimately damage the developing fetus. Drug-induced teratogenic changes can occur only during organogenesis; however, drug-induced toxicological changes affect the fetus after completion of tissue or organ formation because these drugs induce degenerative changes in formed tissue or organs. Unfortunately, the teratogenic or toxicological potential of many drugs has not been evaluated in utero.

To be safe, drugs that are known to be innocuous to the embryo or fetus should be the drugs of choice in the dental management of pregnant women. Drugs with unknown teratogenic or toxicological potential should be prescribed in consultation with the patient's obstetrician and used sparingly. Drugs with known teratogenic or toxicological effects should not be considered for use during dental procedures.

To aid health care providers, the U.S. Food and Drug Administration has developed a rating system for drugs that affect the fetus. The five categories the FDA uses to evaluate drug effects during pregnancy are shown in **Appendix B**.

The first list on the following page contains examples of drugs that require special precautions when used during pregnancy. Many of these drugs are not teratogenic, but the potential side effect of each agent may affect the embryo or fetus; therefore, each drug should be carefully investigated. If you have questions about any drug that might cause problems during pregnancy, contact an obstetrician or the Organization of Teratology Information Services (866-626-6847 or *www.otispregnancy.org*) for agencies in your region that deal with potential harmful drugs to pregnant women.

The second list contains examples of drugs that are excreted in breast milk. Please keep in mind that neither list is meant to be comprehensive. For further pregnancy and nursing precautions, consult the prescribing information tables within each chapter or the manufacturer's labeling.

PREGNANCY CAUTION INFORMATION LIST

Alprazolam (systemic)
Amitriptyline (systemic)
Amobarbital (systemic)
Aprobarbital (systemic)
Ascorbic acid (systemic)
Aspirin, alone and in combination (systemic)
Atropine (systemic)
Bupivacaine (parenteral-local)
Butabarbital, alone and in combinations (systemic)
Butorphanol (systemic)
Caffeine (systemic)
Calcium carbonate (oral-local)
Carbamazepine (systemic)
Cefoxitin (systemic)
Chloral hydrate (systemic)
Chloramphenicol (systemic)
Chlordiazepoxide, alone and in combination (systemic)
Ciprofloxacin (ophthalmic)
Clarithromycin (systemic)
Clonazepam (systemic)
Clonidine (systemic)
Clorazepate (systemic)
Clotrimazole
Codeine
Cortisone (systemic)
Cyanocobalamin Co 57 (systemic)
Demeclocycline (systemic)
Desoximetasone
Dexamethasone
Diclofenac (systemic)
Diflunisal
Epinephrine
Erythromycin estolate
Ethchlorvynol (systemic)
Etidocaine (parenteral-local)
Etodolac (systemic)
Fenoprofen (systemic)
Fentanyl (systemic)
Fluconazole (systemic)
Flurazepam (systemic)
Flurbiprofen (systemic)
Griseofulvin (systemic)
Halazepam (systemic)
Haloperidol (systemic)
Halothane (systemic)
Hydralazine (systemic)
Hydrocodone (systemic)
Hydrocortisone (systemic)
Hydromorphone (systemic)
Hyoscyamine (systemic)
Ibuprofen (systemic)
Indomethacin (systemic)
Iodine (topical)
Ketazolam (systemic)
Ketoprofen (systemic)
Ketorolac (systemic)
Labetalol (systemic)
Lidocaine (parenteral-local)
Lorazepam (systemic)
Meclizine (systemic)
Meclofenamate (systemic)
Mefenamic acid (systemic)
Meperidine (systemic)
Methadone (systemic)
Metronidazole (systemic)
Miconazole (vaginal)
Minocycline (systemic)
Morphine (systemic)
Naproxen (systemic)
Neomycin (oral-local)
Nicotine (systemic)
Nitrous oxide (systemic)
Norfloxacin (systemic)
Ofloxacin (ophthalmic)
Orphenadrine, aspirin and caffeine (systemic)
Oxazepam (systemic)
Oxycodone (systemic)
Oxytetracycline (systemic)
Paregoric (systemic)
Penbutolol (systemic)
Pentazocine (systemic)
Phenobarbital (systemic)
Phenylbutazone (systemic)
Prednisone (systemic)
Procaine (parenteral-local)
Promazine (systemic)
Promethazine (systemic)
Propoxyphene (systemic)
Pseudoephedrine (systemic)
Rifampin (systemic)
Salicylic acid (topical)
Salsalate (systemic)
Secobarbital (systemic)
Sufentanil (systemic)
Sulindac (systemic)
Tetracaine (parenteral-local)
Tetracycline (systemic)
Triamcinolone (systemic)
Triazolam (systemic)
Vitamin A (systemic)

DRUGS EXCRETED IN BREAST MILK

Ampicillin
Antihistamines*
Aspirin
Atropine
Barbiturates
Cephalexin*
Cephalothin*
Chloral hydrate
Chloramphenicol
Codeine
Corticosteroids
Demeclocycline*
Diazepam
Diphenhydramine*
Erythromycin*
Fluorides*
Lincomycin*
Meperidine
Meprobamate
Methacycline
Methadone
Morphine
Narcotics
Oxacillin*
Penicillins*
Pentazocine*
Phenobarbital
Propantheline bromide*
Propoxyphene
Salicylates
Scopolamine*
Streptomycin
Tetracyclines*
Thiopental sodium*

*No adverse effects reported.

Prevention of Infective Endocarditis:

Guidelines from the American Heart Association

A guideline from the American Heart Association Rheumatic Fever, Endocarditis and Kawasaki Disease Committee, Council on Cardiovascular Disease in the Young, and the Council on Clinical Cardiology, Council on Cardiovascular Surgery and Anesthesia, and the Quality of Care and Outcomes Research Interdisciplinary Working Group

Walter Wilson, MD; Kathryn A. Taubert, PhD, FAHA; Michael Gewitz, MD, FAHA; Peter B. Lockhart, DDS; Larry M. Baddour, MD; Matthew Levison, MD; Ann Bolger, MD, FAHA; Christopher H. Cabell, MD, MHS; Masato Takahashi, MD, FAHA; Robert S. Baltimore, MD; Jane W. Newburger, MD, MPH, FAHA; Brian L. Strom, MD; Lloyd Y. Tani, MD; Michael Gerber, MD; Robert O. Bonow, MD, FAHA; Thomas Pallasch, DDS, MS; Stanford T. Shulman, MD, FAHA; Anne H. Rowley, MD; Jane C. Burns, MD; Patricia Ferrieri, MD; Timothy Gardner, MD, FAHA; David Goff, MD, PhD, FAHA; David T. Durack, MD, PhD

The Council on Scientific Affairs of the American Dental Association has approved these guidelines as they relate to dentistry.

ABSTRACT

Background. The purpose of this statement is to update the recommendations by the American Heart Association (AHA) for the prevention of infective endocarditis, which were last published in 1997.

Methods and Results. A writing group appointed by the AHA for their expertise in prevention and treatment of infective endocarditis (IE) with liaison members representing the American Dental Association, the Infectious Diseases Society of America and the American Academy of Pediatrics. The writing group reviewed input from national and international experts on IE. The recommendations in this document reflect analyses of relevant literature regarding procedure-related bacteremia and IE; in vitro susceptibility data of the most common microorganisms, which cause IE; results of prophylactic studies in animal models of experimental endocarditis; and retrospective and prospective studies of prevention of IE. MEDLINE database searches from 1950 through 2006 were done for English language articles using the following search terms: endocarditis, infective endocarditis, prophylaxis, prevention, antibiotic, antimicrobial, pathogens, organisms, dental, gastrointestinal, genitourinary, streptococcus, enterococcus, staphylococcus, respiratory, dental surgery, pathogenesis, vaccine, immunization and bacteremia. The reference lists of the identified articles were also searched. The writing group also searched

ABBREVIATION KEY. ACC: American College of Cardiology. **ADA:** American Dental Association. **AHA:** American Heart Association. **CFU:** Colony-forming unit. **CHD:** Congenital heart disease. **FimA:** Fimbrial adhesion protein. **GI:** Gastrointestinal. **GU:** Genitourinary. **IE:** Infective endocarditis. **LOE:** Level of evidence. **MVP:** Mitral valve prolapse. **NBTE:** Nonbacterial thrombotic endocarditis. **PVE:** Prosthetic valve endocarditis. **RHD:** Rheumatic heart disease.

Wilson W, Taubert KA, Gewitz M, et al. Prevention of infective endocarditis: Guidelines from the American Heart Association. *JADA*. 2008;139(1):3S-24S. Copyright © 2008 American Dental Association. All rights reserved. Reprinted by permission.

the AHA online library. The American College of Cardiology/AHA classification of recommendations and levels of evidence for practice guidelines were used. The article subsequently was reviewed by outside experts not affiliated with the writing group and by the AHA Science Advisory and Coordinating Committee.

Conclusions. The major changes in the updated recommendations include the following. (1) The committee concluded that only an extremely small number of cases of IE might be prevented by antibiotic prophylaxis for dental procedures even if such prophylactic therapy were 100 percent effective. (2) IE prophylaxis for dental procedures should be recommended only for patients with underlying cardiac conditions associated with the highest risk of adverse outcome from IE. (3) For patients with these underlying cardiac conditions, prophylaxis is recommended for all dental procedures that involve manipulation of gingival tissue or the periapical region of teeth or perforation of the oral mucosa. (4) Prophylaxis is not recommended based solely on an increased lifetime risk of acquisition of IE. (5) Administration of antibiotics solely to prevent endocarditis is not recommended for patients who undergo a genitourinary or gastrointestinal tract procedure. These changes are intended to define more clearly when IE prophylaxis is or is not recommended and to provide more uniform and consistent global recommendations.

Key Words. AHA Scientific Statements; cardiovascular disease; endocarditis; prevention; antibiotic prophylaxis. *JADA*. 2008;139(1):3S-24S.

Editor's note: Of the complete text of Prevention of Infective Endocarditis: Guidelines From the American Heart Association—A Guideline From the American Heart Association Rheumatic Fever, Endocarditis and Kawasaki Disease Committee, Council on Cardiovascular Disease in the Young, and the Council on Clinical Cardiology, Council on Cardiovascular Surgery and Anesthesia, and the Quality of Care and Outcomes Research Interdisciplinary Working Group, the following text represents the portions that are pertinent to dentistry. The American Dental Association Council on Scientific Affairs has approved these guidelines as they relate to dentistry. These guidelines have been endorsed by the Infectious Diseases Society of America and by the Pediatric Infectious Diseases Society.

Throughout this article, readers will see references to gastrointestinal, genitourinary and respiratory tract procedures; surgical procedures that involve infected skin, skin structures or musculoskeletal tissue; and some types of cardiac surgery. Reference to these conditions has been retained in this version of the American Heart Association (AHA) antibiotic prophylaxis recommendations directed toward dentistry because of the historical context of their inclusion by the AHA. However, the sections of the original AHA Prevention of Infective Endocarditis Guidelines that go into detail on these conditions have been removed from this article. Interested readers should consult the complete AHA Guidelines available at *http://circ.ahajournals.org/cgi/content/full/116/15/1736*. To check for ADA statement updates, visit *www.ada.org/prof/resources/positions/statements/index.asp*.

Infective endocarditis (IE) is an uncommon but life-threatening infection. Despite advances in diagnosis, antimicrobial therapy, surgical techniques and management of complications, patients with IE still have substantial morbidity and mortality related to this condition. Since the last American Heart Association (AHA) publication on prevention of IE in 1997,[1] many authorities, societies and the conclusions of published studies have questioned the efficacy of antimicrobial prophylaxis to prevent IE in patients who undergo a dental, gastrointestinal (GI) or genitourinary (GU) tract procedure and have suggested that the AHA guidelines should be revised.[2-5] Members of the Rheumatic Fever, Endocarditis and Kawasaki Disease Committee of the AHA Council on Cardiovascular Disease in the Young (the Committee), and a national and international group of experts on IE extensively reviewed data published on the prevention of IE. The revised guidelines for IE prophylaxis are the subject of this report. The writing group was charged with the task of performing an assessment of the evidence and giving a classification of recommendations and a level of evidence (LOE) to each recommendation. The American College of Cardiology (ACC)/AHA classification system was used (**Box 1**).[6]

HISTORY OF AMERICAN HEART ASSOCIATION STATEMENTS ON PREVENTION OF INFECTIVE ENDOCARDITIS

The AHA has made recommendations for the prevention of IE for more than 50 years. In 1955, the first AHA document was published in Circulation.[7] **Table 1** shows a summary of the documents published from 1955 through 1997.[1,7-14] The 1960 document called attention to the possible emergence of penicillin-resistant oral microflora as a result of prolonged therapy for prevention of IE, and pediatric patients were included for the first time.[9] Chloramphenicol was recommended for patients allergic to penicillin. In 1965, the Committee published for the first time a document devoted solely to the prophylaxis of IE and recognized the importance of enterococci after GI or GU tract procedures.[10] The revised recommendations published in 1972 were endorsed for the first time by the American Dental Association (ADA) and emphasized the importance of maintenance of good oral hygiene.[11] This version introduced a recommendation for ampicillin in patients undergoing a GI or GU tract procedure. The 1977 revisions categorized both patients and procedures into high- and low-risk groups.[12] This resulted in complex tables with many footnotes. The duration of post-procedure therapy was reduced from two days to two doses. The 1984 recommendations attempted to simplify prophylactic regimens by providing clear lists of procedures for which prophylaxis was and was not recommended and reduced post-procedure prophylaxis for dental, GI and GU tract procedures to only one oral or parenteral dose.[13] In 1990, a more complete list of cardiac conditions and dental or surgical procedures for which prophylaxis was and was not recommended was provided.[14] These previous recommendations recognized the potential medicolegal risks associated with IE prophylaxis and suggested that the recommendations were intended to serve as a guideline, not as established standard of care. The most recent AHA document on IE prophylaxis was published in 1997.[1] The 1997 document stratified cardiac conditions into high-, moderate- and low-risk (negligible risk) categories with prophylaxis not recommended for the low-risk group.[1] An even more detailed list of dental, respiratory, GI and GU tract procedures for which prophylaxis was and was not recommended was provided. The 1997 document was notable for its acknowledgment that most cases of IE are not attributable to an invasive procedure but rather are the result of randomly occurring bacteremias from routine daily activities and for acknowledging possible IE prophylaxis failures.

RATIONALE FOR REVISING THE 1997 DOCUMENT

It is clear from the above chronology that the AHA guidelines for IE prophylaxis have been in a process of evolution for more than 50 years. The rationale for prophylaxis was based largely on expert opinion and what seemed to be a rational and prudent attempt to prevent a life-threatening infection. On

Box 1

CLASSIFICATION OF RECOMMENDATIONS AND LEVELS OF EVIDENCE.*

CLASSIFICATION OF RECOMMENDATIONS

Class I	Conditions for which there is evidence and/or general agreement that a given procedure or treatment is useful and effective
Class II	Conditions for which there is conflicting evidence and/or a divergence of opinion about the usefulness or efficacy of a procedure or treatment
	IIa Weight of evidence/opinion is in favor of usefulness/efficacy
	IIb Usefulness/efficacy is less well-established by evidence/opinion
Class III	Conditions for which there is evidence and/or general agreement that the procedure or treatment is not useful or effective and, in some cases, may be harmful

LEVEL OF EVIDENCE

A	Data derived from multiple randomized clinical trials or meta-analysis
B	Data derived from a single randomized trial or from nonrandomized studies
C	Only consensus opinion of experts, case studies or standard of care

* Adapted from the American College of Cardiology Foundation and American Heart Association Task Force on Practice Guidelines.[6]

the basis of the ACC and AHA Task Force on Practice Guidelines' evidence-based grading system for ranking recommendations, the recommendations in the AHA documents published during the last 50 years would be Class IIb, LOE C. Accordingly, the basis for recommendations for IE prophylaxis was not well-established, and the quality of evidence was limited to a few case-control studies or was based on expert opinion, clinical experience and descriptive studies, which used surrogate measures of risk.

Over the years, other international societies have published recommendations and guidelines for the prevention of IE.[15,16] Recently, the British Society for Antimicrobial Chemotherapy issued new IE prophylaxis recommendations.[16] This group now recommends prophylaxis before dental procedures only for patients who have a history of previous IE or who have had cardiac valve replacement or surgically constructed pulmonary shunts or conduits.

Fundamental underlying principles that drove the formulation of the AHA guidelines and the nine previous AHA documents were that (1) IE is an uncommon but life-threatening disease and prevention is preferable to treatment of established infection; (2) certain underlying cardiac conditions predispose to IE; (3) bacteremia with organisms known to cause IE occurs commonly in association with invasive dental, GI or GU tract procedures; (4) antimicrobial prophylaxis was proven to be effective for prevention of experimental IE in animals; and (5) antimicrobial prophylaxis was thought to be effective in humans for prevention of IE associated with dental, GI or GU tract procedures. The Committee believes that of these five underlying principles, the first four are valid and have not changed during the past 30 years. Numerous publications questioned the validity of the fifth principle and suggested revision of the guidelines, primarily for reasons shown in **Box 2**.

Another reason that led the Committee to revise the 1997 document was that over the past 50 years, the AHA guidelines on prevention of IE became overly complicated, making it difficult for patients and health care providers to interpret or remember specific details, and they contained ambiguities and some inconsistencies in the recommenda-

TABLE 1. SUMMARY OF NINE ITERATIONS OF AMERICAN HEART ASSOCIATION–RECOMMENDED ANTIBIOTIC REGIMENS* FROM 1955 TO 1997 FOR DENTAL/RESPIRATORY TRACT PROCEDURES.

YEAR	PRIMARY REGIMENS FOR DENTAL PROCEDURES
1955[7]	Aqueous penicillin 600,000 units IM† and procaine penicillin in oil containing 2 percent aluminum monostearate 600,000 U IM administered 30 minutes before the operative procedure.
1957[8]	For two days before surgery, penicillin 200,000 to 250,000 U by mouth four times per day. On day of surgery, penicillin 200,000 to 250,000 U by mouth four times per day and aqueous penicillin 600,000 U with procaine penicillin 600,000 U IM 30 to 60 minutes before surgery. For two days after, 200,000 to 250,000 U by mouth four times per day.
1960[9]	Step I: prophylaxis two days before surgery with procaine penicillin 600,000 U IM on each day. Step II: day of surgery: procaine penicillin 600,000 U IM supplemented by crystalline penicillin 600,000 U IM one hour before surgical procedure. Step III: for two days after surgery: procaine penicillin 600,000 U IM each day.
1965[10]	Day of procedure: Procaine penicillin 600,000 U, supplemented by crystalline penicillin 600,000 U IM one to two hours before the procedure. For two days after procedure: procaine penicillin 600,000 U IM each day.
1972[11]	Procaine penicillin G 600,000 U mixed with crystalline penicillin G 200,000 U IM one hour before procedure and once daily for the two days after the procedure.
1977[12]	Aqueous crystalline penicillin G 1,000,000 U IM mixed with procaine penicillin G 600,000 U IM. Give 30 minutes to one hour before procedure and then give penicillin V 500 milligrams orally every two hours for eight doses.
1984[13]	Penicillin V 2 grams orally one hour before; then 1 g six hours after initial dose.
1990[14]	Amoxicillin 3 g orally one hour before procedure; then 1.5 g six hours after initial dose.
1997[1]	Amoxicillin 2 g orally one hour before procedure.

* These regimens were for adults and represented the initial regimen listed in each version of the recommendations. In some versions, more than one regimen was included.

† IM: Intramuscularly.

tions. The decision to substantially revise the 1997 document was not taken lightly. The present revised document was not based on the results of a single study but rather on the collective body of evidence published in numerous studies over the past two decades. The Committee sought to construct the present recommendations such that they would be in the best interest of patients and providers, would be reasonable and prudent, and would represent the conclusions of published studies and the collective wisdom of many experts on IE and relevant national and international societies.

POTENTIAL CONSEQUENCES OF SUBSTANTIVE CHANGES IN RECOMMENDATIONS

Substantive changes in recommendations could (1) violate long-standing expectations and practice patterns, (2) make fewer patients eligible for IE prophylaxis, (3) reduce malpractice claims related to IE prophylaxis and (4) stimulate prospective studies on IE prophylaxis. The Committee and Ashrafian and Bogle[17] recognize that substantive changes in IE prophylaxis guidelines may violate long-standing expectations of and practice patterns by patients and health care providers. The Committee recognizes that these new recommendations may cause concern among patients who have previously taken antibiotic prophylaxis to prevent IE before dental or other procedures and are now advised that such prophylaxis is unnecessary. **Box 2** includes the main talking points that may be helpful for clinicians in re-educating their patients regarding these changes. To recommend such changes demands due diligence and critical analysis. For 50 years, since the publication of the first AHA guidelines on the prevention of IE,[7] patients and health care providers assumed that antibiotics administered in association with a bacteremia-producing procedure effectively prevented IE in patients with underlying cardiac risk factors. Patients were educated about bacteremia-producing procedures and risk factors for IE, and they expected to receive antibiotic prophylaxis; health care providers, especially dentists, were expected to administer them. Patients with underlying cardiac conditions that have a lifetime risk of acquisition of IE, such as mitral valve prolapse (MVP), had a sense of reassurance and comfort that antibiotics administered in association with a dental procedure was effective and usually safe to prevent IE. Health care providers, especially dentists, felt a sense of obligation and professional and legal responsibility to protect their patients from IE that might result from a procedure. On the basis of recommendations in this revised document, substantially fewer patients will be recommended for IE prophylaxis.

Cases of IE either temporally or remotely associated with an invasive procedure, especially a dental procedure, have frequently been the basis for malpractice claims against health care providers. Unlike many other infections for which there is conclusive evidence for the efficacy of preventive therapy, the prevention of IE is not a precise science. Because previously published AHA guidelines for the prevention of IE contained ambiguities and inconsistencies and often were based on minimal published data or expert opinion, they were subject to conflicting interpretations among patients, health care providers and the legal system about patient eligibility for prophylaxis and whether there was strict adherence by health care providers to AHA recommendations for prophylaxis. This document is intended to identify which, if any, patients may possibly benefit from IE prophylaxis and to define, to the extent possible, which dental procedures should have prophylaxis in this select group of patients. Accordingly, the Committee hopes that this document will result in greater clarity for patients, health care providers and consulting professionals.

The Committee believes that recommendations for IE prophylaxis must be evidence-based. A placebo-controlled, multicenter, randomized, double-blinded study to evaluate the efficacy of IE prophylaxis in patients who undergo a dental, GI or GU tract procedure has not been done. Such a study would require a large number of patients per treatment group and standardization of the specific invasive procedures and the patient populations.

This type of study would be necessary to answer definitively long-standing unresolved questions regarding the efficacy of IE prophylaxis. The Committee hopes that this revised document will stimulate additional studies on the prevention of IE. Future published data will be reviewed carefully by the AHA Rheumatic Fever, Endocarditis and Kawasaki Disease Committee, and other societies, and further revisions to the current document will be based on relevant studies.

PATHOGENESIS OF INFECTIVE ENDOCARDITIS

The development of IE is the net result of the complex interaction between the bloodstream pathogen with matrix molecules and platelets at sites of endocardial cell damage. In addition, many of the clinical manifesta-

Box 2

PRIMARY REASONS FOR REVISION OF THE INFECTIVE ENDOCARDITIS PROPHYLAXIS GUIDELINES.

- Infective endocarditis (IE) is much more likely to result from frequent exposure to random bacteremias associated with daily activities than from bacteremia caused by a dental, gastrointestinal (GI) tract or genitourinary (GU) tract procedure
- Prophylaxis may prevent an exceedingly small number of cases of IE, if any, in people who undergo a dental, GI tract or GU tract procedure
- The risk of antibiotic-associated adverse events exceeds the benefit, if any, from prophylactic antibiotic therapy
- Maintenance of optimal oral health and hygiene may reduce the incidence of bacteremia from daily activities and is more important than prophylactic antibiotics for a dental procedure to reduce the risk of IE

tions of IE emanate from the host's immune response to the infecting microorganism. The following sequence of events is thought to result in IE: formation of nonbacterial thrombotic endocarditis (NBTE) on the surface of a cardiac valve or elsewhere that endothelial damage occurs, bacteremia, adherence of the bacteria in the bloodstream to NBTE and proliferation of bacteria within a vegetation.

Formation of NBTE. Turbulent blood flow produced by certain types of congenital or acquired heart disease, such as flow from a high to a low-pressure chamber or across a narrowed orifice, traumatizes the endothelium. This creates a predisposition for deposition of platelets and fibrin on the surface of the endothelium, which results in NBTE. Invasion of the bloodstream with a microbial species that has the pathogenic potential to colonize this site can then result in IE.

Transient bacteremia. Mucosal surfaces are populated by a dense endogenous microflora. Trauma to a mucosal surface, particularly the gingival crevice around teeth, oropharynx, GI tract, urethra or vagina, releases many different microbial species transiently into the bloodstream. Transient bacteremia caused by viridans group streptococci and other oral microflora occurs commonly in association with dental extractions or other dental procedures or with routine daily activities. Although controversial, the frequency and intensity of the resulting bacteremias are believed to be related to the nature and magnitude of the tissue trauma, the density of the microbial flora and the degree of inflammation or infection at the site of trauma. The microbial species entering the circulation depends on the unique endogenous microflora that colonizes the particular traumatized site.

Bacterial adherence. The ability of various microbial species to adhere to specific sites determines the anatomical localization of infection caused by these microorganisms. Mediators of bacterial adherence serve as virulence factors in the pathogenesis of IE. Numerous bacterial surface components present in streptococci, staphylococci and enterococci have been shown in animal models of experimental endocarditis to function as critical adhesins. Some viridans group streptococci contain a fimbrial adhesion protein (FimA), which is a lipoprotein receptor antigen I that serves as a major adhesin to the fibrin platelet matrix of NBTE.[18] Staphylococcal adhesins function in at least two ways. In one, microbial surface components recognizing adhesive matrix molecules facilitate the attachment of staphylococci to human extracellular matrix proteins and to medical devices, which become coated with matrix proteins after implantation. In the other, bacterial extracellular structures contribute to the formation of biofilm, which forms on the surface of implanted medical devices. In both cases, staphylococcal adhesins are important virulence factors.

Both FimA and staphylococcal adhesins are immunogenic in experimental infections.

Vaccines prepared against FimA and staphylococcal adhesins provide some protective effect in experimental endocarditis caused by viridans group streptococci and staphylococci.[19,20] The results of these experimental studies are highly intriguing, because the development of an effective vaccine for use in humans to prevent viridans group streptococcal or staphylococcal IE would be of major importance.

Proliferation of bacteria within a vegetation. Microorganisms adherent to the vegetation stimulate further deposition of fibrin and platelets on their surface. Within this secluded focus, the buried microorganisms multiply as rapidly as do bacteria in broth cultures to reach maximal microbial densities of 10^8 to 10^{11} colony forming units (CFUs) per gram of vegetation within a short time on the left side of the heart, apparently uninhibited by host defenses in left-sided lesions. Right-sided vegetations have lower bacterial densities, which may be the consequence of host defense mechanisms active at this site, such as polymorphonuclear activity or platelet-derived antibacterial proteins. More than 90 percent of the microorganisms in mature left- or right-sided valvular vegetations are metabolically inactive, rather than in an active growth phase, and are, therefore, less responsive to the bactericidal effects of antibiotics.[21]

RATIONALE FOR OR AGAINST PROPHYLAXIS OF INFECTIVE ENDOCARDITIS

Historical background. Viridans group streptococci are part of the normal skin, oral, respiratory and GI tract flora, and they cause at least 50 percent of cases of community-acquired native valve IE not associated with intravenous drug use.[22] More than a century ago, the oral cavity was recognized as a potential source of the bacteremia that caused viridans group streptococcal IE. In 1885, Osler[23] noted an association between bacteremia from surgery and IE. Okell and Elliott[24] in 1935 reported that 11 percent of patients with poor oral hygiene had positive blood cultures with viridans group streptococci, and that 61 percent of patients had viridans group streptococcal bacteremia with dental extraction.

As a result of these early and subsequent studies, during the past 50 years the AHA guidelines recommended antimicrobial prophylaxis to prevent IE in patients with underlying cardiac conditions who underwent bacteremia-producing procedures based on the following factors: (1) bacteremia causes endocarditis; (2) viridans group streptococci are part of the normal oral flora and enterococci are part of the normal GI and GU tract flora; (3) these microorganisms were usually susceptible to antibiotics recommended for prophylaxis; (4) antibiotic prophylaxis prevents viridans group streptococcal or enterococcal experimental endocarditis in animals; (5) a large number of poorly documented case reports implicated a dental procedure as a cause of IE; (6) in some cases, there was a temporal relationship between a dental procedure and the onset of symptoms of IE; (7) an awareness of bacteremia caused by viridans group streptococci associated with a dental procedure exists; (8) the risk of significant adverse reactions to an antibiotic is low in an individual patient; and (9) morbidity and mortality of IE are high. Most of these factors remain valid, but collectively they do not compensate for the lack of published data that demonstrate a benefit from prophylaxis.

Bacteremia-producing dental procedures. The large majority of published studies have focused on dental procedures as a cause of IE and the use of prophylactic antibiotics to prevent IE in patients at risk. Few data exist on the risk of or prevention of IE associated with a GI or GU tract procedure. Accordingly, the Committee undertook a critical analysis of published data in the context of the historical rationale for recommending antibiotic prophylaxis for IE before a dental procedure. The following factors were considered: (1) frequency, nature, magnitude and duration of bacteremia associated with dental procedures; (2) impact of dental disease, oral hygiene and type of dental procedure on bacteremia; (3) impact of antibiotic prophylaxis on bacteremia from a dental procedure; and (4) the exposure over time of frequently occurring bacteremia from routine daily activities compared with bacteremia from various dental procedures.

Frequency, nature, magnitude and duration of bacteremia associated with a dental procedure. Transient bacteremia is common with manipulation of the teeth and periodontal tissues, and there is a wide variation in reported frequencies of bacteremia in patients resulting from dental procedures: tooth extraction (10-100 percent), periodontal surgery (36-88 percent), scaling and root planing (8-80 percent), teeth cleaning (up to 40 percent), rubber dam matrix/wedge placement (9-32 percent) and endodontic procedures (up to 20 percent).[25-31] Transient bacteremia also occurs frequently during routine daily activities unrelated to a dental procedure: tooth brushing and flossing (20-68 percent), use of wooden toothpicks (20-40 percent), use of water irrigation devices (7-50 percent) and chewing food (7-51 percent).[27-30,32-27] Considering that the average person living in the United States has fewer than two dental visits per year, the frequency of bacteremia from routine daily activities is far greater.

There has been a disproportionate focus on the frequency of bacteremia associated with dental procedures rather than the species of bacteria recovered from blood cultures. Studies suggest that more than 700 species of bacteria, including aerobic and anaerobic gram-positive and gram-negative microorganisms, may be identified in the human mouth, particularly on the teeth and in the gingival crevices.[25,38-41] Approximately 30 percent of the flora of the gingival crevice is streptococci, predominantly of the viridans group. Of the more than 100 oral bacterial species recovered from blood cultures after dental procedures, the most prevalent of these are viridans group streptococci, the most common microbiological cause of community-acquired native valve IE in nonintravenous drug users.[22] In healthy mouths, a thin surface of mucosal epithelium separates potentially pathogenic bacteria from entering the bloodstream and lymphatic system. Anaerobic microorganisms commonly are responsible for periodontal disease and frequently enter the bloodstream but rarely cause IE, with fewer than 120 cases reported.[42] Viridans group streptococci are antagonistic to periodontal pathogens and predominate in a clean, healthy mouth.[43]

Few published studies exist on the magnitude of bacteremia after a dental procedure or from routine daily activities, and most of the published data used older, often unreliable microbiological methodology. There are no published data that demonstrate that a greater magnitude of bacteremia, compared with a lower magnitude, is more likely to cause IE in humans. The magnitude of bacteremia resulting from a dental procedure is relatively low <104 CFUs of bacteria per milliliter), similar to that resulting from routine daily activities, and is less than that used to cause experimental IE in animals (106-108 CFUs of bacteria/mL).[21,44,45] Although the infective dose required to cause IE in humans is unknown, the number of microorganisms in blood after a dental procedure or associated with daily activities is low. Cases of IE caused by oral bacteria probably result from the exposures to low inocula of bacteria in the bloodstream that result from routine daily activities and not from a dental procedure. Additionally, the vast majority of patients with IE have not had a dental procedure within two weeks before the onset of symptoms of IE.[2-4]

The role of duration of bacteremia on the risk of acquisition of IE is uncertain.[46-47] Early studies reported that sequential blood cultures were positive for up to 10 minutes after tooth extraction and that the number of positive blood cultures dropped sharply after 10 to 30 minutes.[25,46-52] More recent studies support these data but report a small percentage of positive blood cultures from 30 to 60 minutes after tooth extraction.[44,53,54] Intuitively, it seems logical to assume that the longer the duration of bacteremia, the greater the risk of IE, but no published studies support this assumption. Given the preponderance of published data, there may not be a clinically significant difference in the frequency, nature, magnitude and duration of bacteremia associated with a dental procedure compared with that resulting from routine daily activities. Accordingly, it is inconsistent to recommend prophylaxis of IE for dental procedures but not for these same patients during routine daily activities. Such a recommendation for prophylaxis for routine daily activities would be impractical and unwarranted.

Impact of dental disease, oral hygiene and type of dental procedure on bacteremia. It is assumed that a relationship exists between poor oral hygiene; the extent of dental and periodontal disease; the type of dental procedure; and the frequency, nature, magnitude and duration of bacteremia, but the presumed relationship is controversial.[24,30,31,39,46,55-62] Nevertheless, available evidence supports an emphasis on maintaining good oral hygiene and eradicating dental disease to decrease the frequency of bacteremia from routine daily activities.[46,57-59,63,64] In patients with poor oral hygiene, the frequency of positive blood cultures just before dental extraction may be similar to that after extraction.[63,64]

More than 80 years ago, it was suggested that poor oral hygiene and dental disease were more important as a cause of IE than were dental procedures.[65] Most studies since that time have focused instead on the risks of bacteremia associated with dental procedures. For example, tooth extraction is thought to be the dental procedure most likely to cause bacteremia, with an incidence ranging from 10 to 100 percent.[24,25,28,30,46,49,53,55,58,66-68] However, numerous other dental procedures have been reported to be associated with risks of bacteremia that are similar to that resulting from tooth extraction.[28,29,48,52,55,57,59,69-72] A precise determination of the relative risk of bacteremia resulting from a specific dental procedure in patients with or without dental disease probably is not possible.[28,73,74]

Bleeding often occurs during a dental procedure in patients with or without periodontal disease. Previous AHA guidelines recommended antibiotic prophylaxis for dental procedures for which bleeding was anticipated but not for procedures or which bleeding was not anticipated.[1] However, no data show that visible bleeding during a dental procedure is a reliable predictor for bacteremia.[63] These ambiguities in the previous AHA guidelines led to further uncertainties among health care providers about which dental procedures should be covered by prophylaxis.

These factors complicated recommendations in previous AHA guidelines on prevention of IE, which suggested antibiotic prophylaxis for some dental procedures but not for others. The collective published data suggest that the vast majority of dental office visits result in some degree of bacteremia; however, there is no evidence-based method to decide which procedures should require prophylaxis because no data show that the incidence, magnitude or duration of bacteremia from any dental procedure increases the risk of IE. Accordingly, it is not clear which dental procedures are more or less likely to cause a transient bacteremia or result in a greater magnitude of bacteremia than that which results from routine daily activities such as chewing food, tooth brushing or flossing.

In patients with underlying cardiac conditions, lifelong antibiotic therapy is not recommended to prevent IE that might result from bacteremias associated with routine daily activities.[5] In patients with dental disease, the focus on the frequency of bacteremia associated with a specific dental procedure and the AHA guidelines for prevention of IE have resulted in an overemphasis on antibiotic prophylaxis and an underemphasis on maintenance of good oral hygiene and access to routine dental care, which are likely more important in reducing the lifetime risk of IE than is the administration of antibiotic prophylaxis for a dental procedure. However, there are no observational or controlled studies to support this contention.

Impact of antibiotic therapy on bacteremia from a dental procedure. The ability of antibiotic therapy to prevent or reduce the frequency, magnitude or duration of bacteremia associated with a dental procedure is controversial.[25,75] Some studies reported that antibiotics administered before a dental procedure reduced the frequency, nature or duration of bacteremia,[54,76,77] while others did not.[25,67,78,79] Recent studies suggest that amoxicillin therapy has a statistically significant impact on reducing the incidence, nature and duration of bacteremia from dental procedures, but it does not eliminate bacteremia.[53,54,77] However, no data show that such a reduction as a result of amoxicillin therapy reduces the risk of or prevents IE. Hall and colleagues[79] reported that neither penicillin V nor amoxicillin therapy was effective in reducing the frequency of bacteremia compared with untreated control subjects. In patients who underwent a dental extraction, penicillin or ampicillin therapy compared with placebo diminished the percentage of viridans group streptococci and anaerobes in culture, but there was no significant difference in the percentage of patients with positive cultures 10 minutes after tooth extraction.[25,67] In a separate study, Hall and colleagues[78] reported that patients treated with cefaclor did not have a reduction of post-procedure bacteremia compared with untreated control subjects. Contradictory published results from two studies showed reduction of post-procedure bacteremia by erythromycin in one[76] but lack of efficacy for erythromycin or clindamycin in another,[79] Finally, results are contradictory regarding the efficacy of the use of topical antiseptics in reducing the frequency of bacteremia associated with dental procedures, but the preponderance of evidence suggests that there is no clear benefit. One study reported that chlorhexidine and povidone-iodine mouthrinse were effective,[80] while others showed no statistically significant benefit.[53,81] Topical antiseptic rinses do not penetrate beyond 3 mm into the periodontal pocket and, therefore, do not reach areas of ulcerated tissue where bacteria most often gain entrance to the circulation. On the basis of these data, it is unlikely that topical antiseptics are effective to significantly reduce the frequency, magnitude and duration of bacteremia associated with a dental procedure.

Cumulative risk over time of physiological bacteremias from routine daily activities compared with the bacteremia from a dental procedure. Guntheroth[82] estimated a cumulative exposure of 5,370 minutes of bacteremia over a one-month period in dentulous patients resulting from random bacteremia from chewing food and from oral hygiene measures, such as tooth brushing and flossing, and compared that to a duration of bacteremia lasting six to 30 minutes associated with a single tooth extraction. Roberts[63] estimated that tooth brushing two times daily for one year had a 154,000 times greater risk of exposure to bacteremia than that resulting from a single tooth extraction. The cumulative exposure during one year to bacteremia from routine, daily activities may be as high as 5.6 million times greater than that resulting from a single tooth extraction, the dental procedure reported to be most likely to cause a bacteremia.[63]

Data exist for the duration of bacteremia from a single tooth extraction, and it is possible to estimate the annual cumulative exposure from dental procedures for the average patient. However, calculations for the incidence, nature and duration of bacteremia from routine daily activities are at best rough estimates, and it is, therefore, not possible to compare precisely the cumulative monthly or annual duration of exposure for bacteremia from dental procedures compared with routine daily activities. Nevertheless, even if the estimates of bacteremia from routine daily activities are off by a factor of 1,000, it is likely that the frequency and cumulative duration of exposure to bacteremia from routine daily events over one year are much higher than those resulting from dental procedures.

Results of clinical studies of IE prophylaxis for dental procedures. There are no prospective randomized placebo-controlled studies on the efficacy of antibiotic prophylaxis to prevent IE in patients who undergo a dental procedure. Data from published retrospective or prospective case-control studies are limited by the following factors: (1) the low incidence of IE, which requires a large number of patients per cohort for statistical significance; (2) the wide variation in the types and severity of underlying cardiac conditions, which would require a large number of patients with specific matched control subjects for each cardiac condition; and (3) the large variety of invasive dental procedures and dental disease states, which would be difficult to standardize for control groups. These and other limitations complicate the interpretation of the results of published studies of the efficacy of IE prophylaxis in patients who undergo dental procedures.

Although some retrospective studies suggested that there was a benefit from prophylaxis, these studies were small and reported insufficient clinical data. Furthermore, in a number of cases, the incubation period between the dental procedure and the onset of symptoms of IE was prolonged.[81,83-85] van der Meer and colleagues[86] published a study of dental procedures in the Netherlands and the efficacy of antibiotic prophylaxis to prevent IE in patients with native or prosthetic cardiac valves. They concluded that dental or other procedures probably caused only a small fraction of cases of IE and that prophylaxis would prevent only a small number of cases even if it were 100 percent effective. van der Meer and colleagues[87] performed a two-year case-control study. Among patients for whom prophylaxis was recommended, five of 20 cases of IE occurred despite receiving antibiotic prophylaxis. They concluded that prophylaxis was not effective. In a separate study, van der Meer and colleagues[88] reported that there was poor awareness of recommendations for prophylaxis among both patients and health care providers.

Strom and colleagues[2] evaluated dental prophylaxis and cardiac risk factors in a multicenter case-control study. These authors reported that MVP, congenital heart disease (CHD), rheumatic heart disease (RHD) and previous cardiac valve surgery were risk factors for the development of IE. In this study, control subjects without IE were more likely to have undergone a dental procedure than patients with IE (P= .03). The authors concluded that dental treatment was not a risk factor for IE even in patients with valvular heart disease and that few cases of IE could be prevented with prophylaxis even if it were 100 percent effective.

The studies are in agreement with a recently published French study of the estimated risk of IE in adults with predisposing cardiac conditions who underwent dental procedures with or without antibiotic prophylaxis.[89] These authors concluded that a "huge number of prophylaxis doses would be necessary to prevent a very low number of IE cases."

Absolute risk of IE resulting from a dental procedure. No published data accurately determine the absolute risk of IE resulting from a dental procedure. One study reported that 10 to 20 percent of patients with IE caused by oral flora underwent a preceding dental procedure (within 30 or 180 days of onset).[86] The evidence linking bacteremia associated with a dental procedure with IE is largely circumstantial, and the number of cases related to a dental procedure is overestimated for a number of reasons. For 60 years, noted opinion leaders in medicine suggested a link between bacteremia-causing dental procedures and IE,[24] and for 50 years the AHA published regularly updated guidelines that emphasized the association between dental procedures and IE and recommended antibiotic prophylaxis.[1] Additionally, bacteremia-producing dental procedures are common; it is estimated that at least 50 percent of the population in the United States visits a dentist at least once a year. Furthermore, there are numerous poorly documented case reports that implicate dental procedures associated with the development of IE, but these reports did not prove a direct causal relationship. Even in the event of a close temporal relationship between a dental procedure and IE, it is not possible to determine with certainty whether the bacteremia that caused IE originated from a dental procedure or from a randomly occurring bacteremia as a result of routine daily activities during the same period. Many case reports and reviews have included cases with a remote preceding dental procedure, often three to six months before the diagnosis of IE. Studies suggest that the time frame between bacteremia and the onset of symptoms of IE is usually seven to 14 days for viridans group streptococci or enterococci. Reportedly, 78 percent of such cases of IE occur within seven days of bacteremia and 85 percent within 14 days.[90] Although the upper time limit is not known, it is likely that many cases of IE with incubation periods longer than two weeks after a dental procedure were attributed incorrectly to the procedure. These and other factors have led to a heightened awareness among patients and health care providers of the possible association with dental procedures and IE, which likely has led to substantial over-reporting of cases attributable to dental procedures.

Although the absolute risk for IE from a dental procedure is impossible to measure precisely, the best available estimates are as follows: if dental treatment causes 1 percent of all cases of viridans group streptococcal IE annually in the United States, the overall risk in the general population is estimated to be as low as one case of IE per 14 million dental procedures.[42,91,92] The estimated absolute risk rates for IE from a dental procedure in patients with underlying cardiac conditions are MVP, one per 1.1 million procedures; CHD, one per 475,000; RHD, one per 142,000; presence of a prosthetic cardiac valve, one per 114,000; and previous IE, one per 95,000 dental procedures.[42,92] Although these calculations of risk are estimates, it is likely that the number of cases of IE that results from a dental procedure is exceedingly small. Therefore, the number of cases that could be prevented by antibiotic prophylaxis, even if 100 percent effective, is similarly small. One would not expect antibiotic prophylaxis to be near 100 percent effective, however, because of the nature of the organisms and choice of antibiotics.

Risk of adverse reactions and cost-effectiveness of prophylactic therapy. Nonfatal adverse reactions, such as rash, diarrhea and GI upset, occur commonly with use of the antimicrobials; however, only single-dose therapy is recommended for dental prophylaxis, and these common adverse reactions are usually not severe and are self-limited. Fatal anaphylactic reactions were estimated to occur in 15 to 25 patients per 1 million patients who receive a dose of penicillin.[93,94] Among patients with a prior penicillin use, 36 percent of fatalities from anaphylaxis occurred in those with a known allergy to penicillin, compared with 64 percent of fatalities among those with no history of penicillin allergy.[95] These calculations are at best rough estimates of, and may overestimate, the true risk of death caused by fatal anaphylaxis from administration of a penicillin. They are based on retrospective reviews or surveys of patients or on health care providers' recall of events. A prospective study is necessary to accurately determine the risk of fatal anaphylaxis resulting from administration of a penicillin.

For 50 years, the AHA has recommended a penicillin as the preferred choice for dental prophylaxis for IE. During these 50 years, the Committee is unaware of any cases reported to the AHA of fatal anaphylaxis resulting from the administration of a penicillin recommended in the AHA guidelines for IE prophylaxis. The Committee believes that a single dose of amoxicillin or ampicillin is safe and is the preferred prophylactic agent for patients who do not have a history of type I hypersensitivity reaction to a penicillin, such as anaphylaxis, urticaria or angioedema. Fatal anaphylaxis from a cephalosporin is estimated to be less common than from penicillin and is estimated to be approximately one case per 1 million patients.96 Fatal reactions to a single dose of a macrolide or clindamycin are extremely rare.[97,98] There has been only one case report of documented *Clostridium difficile* colitis after a single dose of prophylactic clindamycin.[99]

Summary. Although it has long been assumed that dental procedures may cause IE in patients with underlying cardiac risk factors and that antibiotic prophylaxis is effective, scientific proof is lacking to support these assumptions. The collective published evidence suggests that of the total number of cases of IE that occur annually, it is likely that an exceedingly small number of these cases is caused by bacteremia-producing dental procedures. Accordingly, only an extremely small number of cases of IE might be prevented by antibiotic prophylaxis even if it were 100 percent effective. The vast majority of cases of IE caused by oral microflora most likely result from random bacteremias caused by routine daily activities, such as chewing food, tooth brushing, flossing, use of toothpicks, use of water irrigation devices and other activities. The presence of dental disease may increase the risk of bacteremia associated with these routine activities. There should be a shift in emphasis away from a focus on a dental procedure and antibiotic prophylaxis toward a greater emphasis on improved access to dental care and oral health in patients with underlying cardiac conditions associated with the highest risk of adverse outcome from IE and those conditions that predispose to the acquisition of IE.

CARDIAC CONDITIONS AND ENDOCARDITIS

Previous AHA guidelines categorized underlying cardiac conditions associated with the risk of IE as those with high risk, moderate risk and negligible risk and recommended prophylaxis for patients in the high- and moderate-risk categories.[1] For the present guidelines on prevention of IE, the Committee considered three distinct issues: (1) What underlying cardiac conditions over a lifetime have the highest predisposition to the acquisition of endocarditis? (2) What underlying cardiac conditions are associated with the highest risk of adverse outcome from endocarditis? (3) Should recommendations for IE prophylaxis be based on either or both of these two conditions?

Underlying conditions over a lifetime that have the highest predisposition to the acquisition of endocarditis. In Olmsted County, Minn., the incidence of IE in adults ranged from five to seven cases per 100,000 person-years.[100] This incidence has remained stable during the past four decades and is similar to that reported in other studies.[101-104] Previously, RHD was the most common

AN UPDATED LEGAL PERSPECTIVE ON ANTIBIOTIC PROPHYLAXIS

American Dental Association Division of Legal Affairs

Editor's note: The following statement is intended as a companion to the 2007 American Heart Association (AHA) guidelines for prevention of infective endocarditis reprinted in this supplement. When referring to the AHA guidelines, readers also should consult this statement.

The American Heart Association (AHA)[1] states that its document "Prevention of Infective Endocarditis: Guidelines From the American Heart Association" was developed through an evidence-based approach and attempts to reduce ambiguities about the patients for whom antibiotic prophylaxis may be indicated and under what conditions, as well as what antibiotics to use. Dentists should be aware that, while the precise standard of care may vary based on locale, the guidelines likely will be cited as some evidence of the standard of care in any malpractice litigation. Nonetheless, it is the American Dental Association's recommendation that a dentist exercise independent professional judgment in applying these or any other guidelines as necessary in any clinical situation.

Should the patient present a recommendation from a treating physician with which the dentist disagrees, the dentist may wish to consult with the physician, as the goal in treatment should be to reach consensus among professionals. Communication between professionals should provide information about the bases for the physician's recommendations and why the dentist disagrees.

If consensus on treatment cannot be reached, the answer may lie in informed consent, which usually can be relied on to protect the practitioner who respects the patient's treatment decisions from legal liability as long as the treatment is within the standard of care. To be effective, the patient's consent must be given after all reasonable treatment options and each option's benefits and risks are fully disclosed. When treatment consensus among treating professionals is absent, it is prudent also to disclose that the treatment recommendations differ and to encourage the patient to discuss treatment options with the physician before making a decision regarding treatment. The dentist should note or copy all communications regarding treatment options.

It should be remembered that the dentist and not the patient ultimately is responsible for patient treatment. The dentist, therefore, is not obligated to perform a treatment he or she does not believe to be in the best interests of the patient.

The above information should not be construed as legal advice or a standard of care. A practitioner always should consult his or her own attorney for answers to specific legal questions.

1. Wilson W, Taubert KA, Gewitz M, et al. Prevention of infective endocarditis: guidelines from the American Heart Association—a guideline from the American Heart Association Rheumatic Fever, Endocarditis and Kawasaki Disease Committee, Council on Cardiovascular Disease in the Young, and the Council on Clinical Cardiology, Council on Cardiovascular Surgery and Anesthesia, and the Quality of Care and Outcomes Research Interdisciplinary Working Group. *Circulation*. 2007;116:1736-54.

American Dental Association Division of Legal Affairs. An updated legal perspective on antibiotic prophylaxis. *JADA*. 2008;139(1):10S.
Copyright © 2008 American Dental Association. All rights reserved. Reprinted by permission.

underlying condition predisposing to endocarditis, and RHD is still common in developing countries.[100] In developed countries, the frequency of RHD has declined, and MVP is the most common underlying condition in patients with endocarditis.[105]

Few published data quantitate the lifetime risk of acquisition of IE associated with a specific underlying cardiac condition. Steckelberg and Wilson[91] reported the lifetime risk of acquisition of IE, which ranged from five per 100,000 patient-years in the general population with no known cardiac conditions to 2,160 per 100,000 patient-years in patients who underwent replacement of an infected prosthetic cardiac valve. In that study, the risk of IE per 100,000 patient-years was 4.6 in patients with MVP without an audible cardiac murmur and was 52 in patients with MVP with an audible murmur of mitral regurgitation. Per 100,000 patient-years, the lifetime risk (380-440) for RHD was similar to that (308-383) for patients with a mechanical or bioprosthetic cardiac valve. The highest lifetime risks per 100,000 patient-years were as follows: cardiac valve replacement surgery for native valve IE, 630; previous IE, 740; and prosthetic valve replacement done in patients with prosthetic valve endocarditis (PVE), 2,160. In a separate study, the risk of IE per 100,000 patient-years was 271 in patients with congenital aortic stenosis and was 145 in patients with ventricular septal defect.[106] In that study, the risk of IE before closure of ventricular septal defect was more than twice that after closure. Although these data provide useful ranges of risk in large populations, it is difficult to use them to define accurately the lifetime risk of acquisition of IE in an individual patient with a specific underlying cardiac risk factor. This difficulty is based in part on the fact that each cardiac condition, such as RHD or MVP, represents a broad spectrum of pathology from minimal to severe, and the risk of IE would likely be influenced by the severity of valvular disease.

CHD is another underlying condition with multiple different cardiac abnormalities that range from relatively minor to severe complex cyanotic heart disease. During the past 25 years, there has been an increasing use of various different intracardiac valvular prostheses and intravascular shunts, grafts and other devices for repair of valvular heart disease and CHD. The diversity and nature of these prostheses and procedures likely present different levels of risk for acquisition of IE. These factors complicate an accurate assessment of the true lifetime risk of acquisition of IE in patients with a specific underlying cardiac condition.

On the basis of data from Steckelberg and Wilson[91] and Strom and colleagues,[2] it is clear that the underlying conditions discussed above represent a lifetime increased risk of acquisition of IE compared with patients with no known underlying cardiac condition. Accordingly, when using previous AHA guidelines in the decision to recommend IE prophylaxis for a patient scheduled to undergo a dental, GI or GU tract procedure, health care providers were required to base their decision on population-based studies of risk of acquisition of IE that may or may not be relevant to their specific patient. Furthermore, practitioners had to weigh the potential efficacy of IE prophylaxis in a patient who may neither need nor benefit from such therapy against the risk of adverse reaction to the antibiotic prescribed. Finally, health care providers had to consider the potential medicolegal risk of not prescribing IE prophylaxis. For dental procedures, there is a growing body of evidence that suggests that IE prophylaxis may prevent only an exceedingly small number of cases of IE, as discussed in detail above.

Cardiac conditions associated with the highest risk of adverse outcome from endocarditis. Endocarditis, irrespective of the underlying cardiac condition, is a serious, life-threatening disease that was always fatal in the preantibiotic era. Advances in antimicrobial therapy, early recognition and management of complications of IE, and improved surgical technology have reduced the morbidity and mortality of IE. Numerous comorbid factors, such as older age, diabetes mellitus, immunosuppressive conditions or therapy, and dialysis, may complicate IE. Each of these comorbid conditions independently increases the risk of adverse outcome from IE, and they often occur in combination, which further increases morbidity and mortality. Additionally, there may be long-term consequences of IE. Over time, the cardiac valve damaged by IE may undergo progressive functional deterioration that may result in the need for cardiac valve replacement.

In native valve viridans group streptococcal or enterococcal IE, the spectrum of disease may range from a relatively benign infection to severe valvular dysfunction, dehiscence, congestive heart failure, multiple embolic events and death; however, the underlying conditions shown in **Box 3** virtually always have an increased risk of adverse outcome. For example, patients with viridans group streptococcal PVE have a mortality of approximately 20 percent or greater,[107-110] whereas the mortality for patients with viridans group streptococcal native valve IE is 5 percent or less.[109,111-117] Similarly, the mortality of enterococcal PVE is higher than that of native valve enterococcal IE.[108,109,115,118] Moreover, patients with PVE are more likely than those with native valve endocarditis to develop heart failure, the need for cardiac valve replacement surgery, perivalvular extension of infection and other complications.

Patients with relapsing or recurrent IE are at greater risk of congestive heart failure and increased need for cardiac valve replacement surgery, and they have a higher mortality than do patients with a first episode of native valve IE.[119-125] Additionally, patients with multiple episodes of native or prosthetic valve IE are at greater risk of additional episodes of endocarditis, each of which is associated with the risk of more serious complications.[91]

Published series regarding endocarditis in patients with CHD are underpowered to determine the extent to which a specific form of CHD is an independent risk factor for morbidity and mortality. Nevertheless, most retrospective case series suggest that patients with complex cyanotic heart disease and those who have postoperative palliative shunts, conduits or other prostheses have a high lifetime risk of acquiring IE, and these same groups appear at highest risk for morbidity and mortality among all patients with CHD.[126-130] In addition, multiple series and reviews reported that the presence of prosthetic material[131,132] and complex cyanotic heart disease in patients of very young age (newborns and infants younger than 2 years)[133,134] are two factors associated with the worst prognoses from IE. Some types of CHD may be repaired completely without residual cardiac defects. In **Box 3**, the Committee concludes that prophylaxis is reasonable for dental procedures for these patients during the first six months after the procedure. In these patients, endothelialization of prosthetic material or devices occurs within six months after the procedure.[135] The Committee does not recommend prophylaxis for dental procedures more than six months after the procedure provided that there is no residual defect from the repair. In most instances, treatment of patients who have infected prosthetic materials requires surgical removal in addition to medical therapy with associated high morbidity and mortality rates.

Should IE prophylaxis be recommended for patients with the highest risk of acquisition of IE or for patients with the highest risk of adverse outcome from IE? In a major departure from previous AHA guidelines, the Committee no longer recommends IE prophylaxis based solely on an increased lifetime risk of acquisition of IE. It is noteworthy that patients with the conditions listed in **Box 3** with a prosthetic cardiac valve, those with a previous episode of IE and some patients with CHD are also among

Box 3

CARDIAC CONDITIONS ASSOCIATED WITH THE HIGHEST RISK OF ADVERSE OUTCOME FROM ENDOCARDITIS FOR WHICH PROPHYLAXIS WITH DENTAL PROCEDURES IS REASONABLE.

- Prosthetic cardiac valve or prosthetic material used for cardiac valve repair
- Previous infective endocarditis
- Congenital heart disease (CHD)*
- Unrepaired cyanotic CHD, including palliative shunts and conduits
- Completely repaired congenital heart defect with prosthetic material or device, whether placed by surgery or by catheter intervention, during the first six months after the procedure†
- Repaired CHD with residual defects at the site or adjacent to the site of a prosthetic patch or prosthetic device (which inhibit endothelialization)
- Cardiac transplantation recipients who develop cardiac valvulopathy

* Except for the conditions listed above, antibiotic prophylaxis is no longer recommended for any other form of CHD.
† Prophylaxis is reasonable because endothelialization of prosthetic material occurs within six months after the procedure.

those patients with the highest lifetime risk of acquisition of endocarditis. No published data demonstrate convincingly that the administration of prophylactic antibiotics prevents IE associated with bacteremia from an invasive procedure. We cannot exclude the possibility that there may be an exceedingly small number of cases of IE that could be prevented by prophylactic antibiotics in patients who undergo an invasive procedure. However, if prophylaxis is effective, such therapy should be restricted to those patients with the highest risk of adverse outcome from IE who would derive the greatest benefit from prevention of IE. In patients with underlying cardiac conditions associated with the highest risk of adverse outcome from IE (**Box 3**), IE prophylaxis for dental procedures is reasonable, even though we acknowledge that its effectiveness is unknown (Class IIb, LOE B).

Compared with previous AHA guidelines, under these revised guidelines, many fewer patients would be candidates to receive IE prophylaxis. We believe these revised guidelines are in the best interest of the patients and health care providers and are based on the best available published data and expert opinion. Additionally, the change in emphasis to restrict prophylaxis to only those patients with the highest risk of adverse outcome should reduce the uncertainties among patients and providers about who should receive prophylaxis. MVP is the most common underlying condition that predisposes to acquisition of IE in the Western world; however, the absolute incidence of endocarditis is extremely low for the entire population with MVP, and it is not usually associated with the grave outcome associated with the conditions identified in **Box 3**. Thus, IE prophylaxis is no longer recommended in this group of patients.

Finally, the administration of prophylactic antibiotics is not risk-free as discussed above. Additionally, the widespread use of antibiotic therapy promotes the emergence of resistant microorganisms most likely to cause endocarditis, such as viridans group streptococci and enterococci. The frequency of multidrug-resistant viridans group streptococci and enterococci has increased dramatically during the past two decades. This increased resistance has reduced the efficacy and number of antibiotics available for the treatment of IE.

ANTIBIOTIC REGIMENS

General principles. An antibiotic for prophylaxis should be administered in a single

Box 4

DENTAL PROCEDURES FOR WHICH ENDOCARDITIS PROPHYLAXIS IS REASONABLE FOR PATIENTS IN BOX 3.

All dental procedures that involve manipulation of gingival tissue or the periapical region of teeth or perforation of the oral mucosa.*

* The following procedures and events do not need prophylaxis: routine anesthetic injections through noninfected tissue, taking dental radiographs, placement of removable prosthodontic or orthodontic appliances, adjustment of orthodontic appliances, placement of orthodontic brackets, shedding of primary teeth, and bleeding from trauma to the lips or oral mucosa.

dose before the procedure. If the dosage of antibiotic is inadvertently not administered before the procedure, the dosage may be administered up to two hours after the procedure. However, administration of the dosage after the procedure should be considered only when the patient did not receive the preprocedural dose. Some patients who are scheduled for an invasive procedure may have a coincidental endocarditis. The presence of fever or other manifestations of systemic infection should alert the provider to the possibility of IE. In these circumstances, it is important to obtain blood cultures and other relevant tests before administration of antibiotics intended to prevent IE. Failure to do so may result in delay in diagnosis or treatment of a concomitant case of IE.

Regimens for dental procedures. Previous AHA guidelines on prophylaxis listed a substantial number of dental procedures and events for which antibiotic prophylaxis was recommended and those procedures for which prophylaxis was not recommended. On the basis of a critical review of the published data, it is clear that transient viridans group streptococcal bacteremia may result from any dental procedure that involves manipulation of the gingival or periapical region of teeth or perforation of the oral mucosa. It cannot be assumed that manipulation of a healthy-appearing mouth or a minimally invasive dental procedure reduces the likelihood of a bacteremia. Therefore, antibiotic prophylaxis is reasonable for patients with the conditions listed in **Box 3** who undergo any dental procedure that involves the gingival tissues or periapical region of a tooth and for those procedures that perforate the oral mucosa (**Box 4**). Although IE prophylaxis is reasonable for these patients, its effectiveness is unknown (Class IIa, LOE C). This includes procedures such as biopsies, suture removal and placement of orthodontic bands, but does not include routine anesthetic injections through noninfected tissue, taking dental radiographs, placement of removable prosthodontic or orthodontic appliances, placement of orthodontic brackets or adjustment of orthodontic appliances. Finally, there are other events that are not dental procedures and for which prophylaxis is not recommended, such as shedding of primary teeth and trauma to the lips and oral mucosa.

In this limited patient population, prophylactic antimicrobial therapy should be directed against viridans group streptococci. During the past two decades, there has been a significant increase in the percentage of strains of viridans group streptococci resistant to antibiotics recommended in previous AHA guidelines for the prevention of IE. Prabhu and colleagues[136] studied susceptibility patterns of viridans group streptococci recovered from patients with IE diagnosed during a period from 1971 to 1986 and compared these susceptibilities with those of viridans group streptococci from patients with IE diagnosed from 1994 to 2002. In this study, none of the strains of viridans group streptococci were penicillin-resistant in the early period, compared with 13 percent of strains that were intermediate or fully penicillin-resistant during the later period. In this study, macrolide resistance increased from 11 to 26 percent and clindamycin resistance from 0 to 4 percent.

Among 352 blood culture isolates of viridans group streptococci, resistance rates were 13 percent for penicillin, 15 percent for amoxicillin, 17 percent for ceftriaxone,

38 percent for erythromycin and 96 percent for cephalexin.[137] The rank order of decreasing level of activity of cephalosporins in that study was cefpodoxime equal to ceftriaxone, greater than cefprozil, equal to cefuroxime, and cephalexin was the least active. In other studies, resistance of viridans group streptococci to penicillin ranged from 17 to 50 percent[138-143] and resistance to ceftriaxone from 22 to 42 percent.[132,141] Ceftriaxone was two to four times more active in vitro than was cefazolin.[132,141] Similarly high rates of resistance were reported for macrolides, ranging from 22 to 58 percent;[138,142,144,145] resistance to clindamycin ranged from 13 to 27 percent.[129,130,132,138,139,141]

Most of the strains of viridans group streptococci in the above-cited studies were recovered from patients with serious underlying illnesses, including malignancies and febrile neutropenia. These patients are at increased risk of infection and colonization by multiple drug-resistant microorganisms, including viridans group streptococci. Accordingly, these strains may not be representative of susceptibility patterns of viridans group streptococci recovered from presumably normal patients who undergo a dental procedure. Diekema and colleagues[138] reported that 32 percent of strains of viridans group streptococci were resistant to penicillin in patients without cancer. King and colleagues[145] reported erythromycin resistance in 41 percent of streptococci recovered from throat cultures in otherwise healthy patients who presented with mild respiratory tract infections. In that study, after treatment with either azithromycin or clindamycin, the percentage of resistant streptococci increased to 82 percent and 71 percent, respectively. Accordingly, the resistance rates of viridans group streptococci are similarly high in otherwise healthy patients or in patients with serious underlying diseases.

The impact of viridans group streptococcal resistance on antibiotic prevention of IE is unknown. If resistance in vitro is predictive of lack of clinical efficacy, the high resistance rates of viridans group streptococci provide additional support for the assertion that prophylactic therapy for a dental procedure is of little, if any, value. It is impractical to recommend prophylaxis with only those antibiotics, such as vancomycin or a fluoroquinolone, that are highly active in vitro against viridans group streptococci. There is no evidence that such therapy is effective for prophylaxis of IE, and their use might result in the development of resistance of viridans group streptococci and other microorganisms to these and other antibiotics.

In **Table 2**, amoxicillin is the preferred choice for oral therapy because it is well-absorbed in the GI tract and provides high and sustained serum concentrations. For patients who are allergic to penicillins or amoxicillin, the use of cephalexin or another first-generation oral cephalosporin, clindamycin, azithromycin or clarithromycin is recommended. Even though cephalexin was less active against viridans group streptococci than other first-generation oral cephalosporins in one study,[137] cephalexin is included in **Table 2**. No data show superiority of one oral cephalosporin over another for prevention of IE, and generic cephalexin is widely available and is relatively inexpensive. Because of possible cross-reactions, a cephalosporin should not be administered to patients with a history of anaphylaxis, angioedema or urticaria after treatment with any form of penicillin, including ampicillin or amoxicillin. Patients who are unable to tolerate an oral antibiotic may be treated with ampicillin, ceftriaxone or cefazolin administered intramuscularly or intravenously. For patients who are allergic to ampicillin and are unable to tolerate an oral agent, therapy is recommended with parenteral cefazolin, ceftriaxone or clindamycin.

A summary of the major changes in these updated recommendations for prevention of IE compared with previous AHA recommendations is shown in **Box 5**.

TABLE 2. REGIMENS FOR A DENTAL PROCEDURE

Situation	Agent	Regimen: Single dose 30-50 minutes before procedure	
		Adults	**Children**
Oral	Amoxicillin	2 grams	50 milligrams per kilogram
Unable to take oral medication	Ampicillin OR Cefazolin or ceftriaxone	2 g IM* or IV† 1 g IM or IV	50 mg/kg IM or IV 50 mg/kg IM or IV
Allergic to Penicillins or Ampicillin Oral	Cephalexin‡§ OR Clindamycin OR Azithromycin or clarithromycin	2 g 600 mg 500 mg	50 mg/kg 20 mg/kg 15 mg/kg
Allergic to Penicillins or Ampicillin and Unable to Take Oral Medication	Cefazolin or ceftriaxone§ OR Clindamycin	1 g IM or IV 600 mg IM or IV	50 mg/kg IM or IV 20 mg/kg IM or IV

* IM: Intramuscular.

† IV: Intravenous.

‡ Or other first- or second-generation oral cephalosporin in equivalent adult or pediatric dosage.

§ Cephalosporins should not be used in a person with a history of anaphylaxis, angioedema or urticaria with penicillins or ampicillin.

SPECIFIC SITUATIONS AND CIRCUMSTANCES

Patients already receiving antibiotics. If a patient is already receiving chronic antibiotic therapy with an antibiotic that is also recommended for IE prophylaxis for a dental procedure, it is prudent to select an antibiotic from a different class rather than to increase the dosage of the current antibiotic. For example, antibiotic regimens used to prevent the recurrence of acute rheumatic fever are administered in dosages lower than those recommended for the prevention of IE. Patients who take an oral penicillin for secondary prevention of rheumatic fever or for other purposes are likely to have viridans group streptococci in their oral cavity that are relatively resistant to penicillin or amoxicillin. In such cases, the provider should select either clindamycin, azithromycin or clarithromycin for IE prophylaxis for a dental procedure, but only for patients shown in **Box 3**. Because of possible cross-resistance of viridans group streptococci with cephalosporins, this class of antibiotics should be avoided. If possible, it would be preferable to delay a dental procedure until at least 10 days after completion of the antibiotic therapy. This may allow time for the usual oral flora to be re-established. Patients receiving parenteral antibiotic therapy for IE may require dental procedures during antimicrobial therapy, particularly if subsequent cardiac valve replacement surgery is anticipated. In these cases, the parenteral antibiotic therapy for IE should be continued and the timing of the dosage adjusted to be administered 30 to 60 minutes before the dental procedure. This parenteral antimicrobial therapy is administered in such high doses that the high concentration would overcome any possible low-level resistance developed among mouth flora (unlike the concentration that would occur after oral administration).

Box 5

SUMMARY OF MAJOR CHANGES IN UPDATED DOCUMENT.

- We concluded that bacteremia resulting from daily activities is much more likely to cause infective endocarditis (IE) than bacteremia associated with a dental procedure.
- We concluded that only an extremely small number of cases of IE might be prevented by antibiotic prophylaxis even if prophylaxis is 100 percent effective.
- Antibiotic prophylaxis is not recommended based solely on an increased lifetime risk of acquisition of IE.
- Limit recommendations for IE prophylaxis only to those conditions listed in Box 3.
- Antibiotic prophylaxis is no longer recommended for any other form of congenital heart disease, except for the conditions listed in Box 3.
- Antibiotic prophylaxis is reasonable for all dental procedures that involve manipulation of gingival tissues or periapical region of teeth or perforation of oral mucosa only for patients with underlying cardiac conditions associated with the highest risk of adverse outcome from IE (Box 3).
- Antibiotic prophylaxis is reasonable for procedures on respiratory tract or infected skin, skin structures or musculoskeletal tissue only for patients with underlying cardiac conditions associated with the highest risk of adverse outcome from IE (Box 3).
- Antibiotic prophylaxis solely to prevent IE is not recommended for gastrointestinal or genitourinary tract procedures.
- Although these guidelines recommend changes in indications for IE prophylaxis with regard to selected dental procedures (see text), the writing group reaffirms that those medical procedures listed as not requiring IE prophylaxis in the 1997 statement remain unchanged and extends this view to vaginal delivery, hysterectomy, and tattooing. Additionally, the writing group advises against body piercing for patients with conditions listed in Box 3 because of the possibility of bacteremia, while recognizing that there are minimal published data regarding the risk of bacteremia or endocarditis associated with body piercing.

Patients who receive anticoagulants. Intramuscular injections for IE prophylaxis should be avoided in patients who are receiving anticoagulant therapy (Class I, LOE A). In these circumstances, orally administered regimens should be given whenever possible. Intravenously administered antibiotics should be used for patients who are unable to tolerate or absorb oral medications.

Patients who undergo cardiac surgery. A careful dental evaluation is recommended so that required dental treatment may be completed whenever possible before cardiac valve surgery or replacement or repair of CHD. Such measures may decrease the incidence of late PVE caused by viridans group streptococci.

OTHER CONSIDERATIONS

There is no evidence that coronary artery bypass graft surgery is associated with a long-term risk for infection. Therefore, antibiotic prophylaxis for dental procedures is not needed for patients who have undergone this surgery. Antibiotic prophylaxis for dental procedures is not recommended for patients with coronary artery stents (Class III, LOE C). The treatment and prevention of infection for these and other endovascular grafts and prosthetic devices are addressed in a separate AHA article.[146] There are insufficient data to support specific recommendations for patients who have undergone heart transplantation. Such patients are at risk of acquired valvular dysfunction, especially during episodes of rejection. Endocarditis that occurs in a heart transplant patient is associated with a high risk of adverse outcome (**Box 3**).[147] Accordingly, the use of IE prophylaxis for dental procedures in cardiac transplant recipients who develop cardiac valvulopathy is reasonable, but the usefulness is not well-established (Class IIa, LOE C) (**Box 4**). The use of prophylactic antibiotics to prevent infection of joint prostheses during potentially bacteremia-inducing procedures is not within the scope of this document.

FUTURE CONSIDERATIONS

Prospective placebo-controlled double-blinded studies of antibiotic prophylaxis of IE in patients who undergo a bacteremia-producing procedure would be necessary to evaluate accurately the efficacy of IE prophylaxis. Additional prospective case-control studies are needed. The AHA has made substantial revisions to previously published guidelines on IE prophylaxis. Based on our current recommendations, we anticipate that significantly fewer patients will receive IE prophylaxis for a dental procedure. Studies are necessary to monitor the effects, if any, of these recommended changes in IE prophylaxis. The incidence of IE could change or stay the same. Because the incidence of IE is low, small changes in incidence may take years to detect. Accordingly, we urge that such studies be designed and instituted promptly so that any change in incidence may be detected sooner rather than later. Subsequent revisions of the AHA guidelines on the prevention of IE will be based on the results of these studies and other published data.

The writing group thanks the following international experts on infective endocarditis for their valuable comments: Drs. Christa Gohlke-Bärwolf, Roger Hall, Jae-Hoon Song, Catherine Kilmartin, Catherine Leport, José M. Miró, Christopher Naber, Graham Roberts and Jan T.M. van der Meer. The writing group also thanks Dr. George Meyer for his helpful comments regarding gastroenterology. Finally, the writing group would like to thank Lori Hinrichs for her superb assistance with the preparation of this manuscript.

This article was adapted from Wilson W, Taubert KA, Gewitz M, et al. Prevention of Infective Endocarditis: Guidelines From the American Heart Association—A Guideline From the American Heart Association Rheumatic Fever, Endocarditis and Kawasaki Disease Committee, Council on Cardiovascular Disease in the Young, and the Council on Clinical Cardiology, Council on Cardiovascular Surgery and Anes- thesia, and the Quality of Care and Outcomes Research Interdisciplinary Working Group. Circulation 2007;116:1736-54. Copyright 2007 American Heart Association. All rights reserved. Any reproduction or use is prohibited without the express permission of the AHA.

Dr. Wilson is a professor of medicine, Mayo Clinic, Rochester, Minn. Dr. Taubert is a senior scientist, American Heart Association, Dallas, and a professor, University of Texas Southwest Medical School, Dallas. Dr. Gewitz is a professor and the vice chair, Department of Pediatrics, Children's Hospital of Westchester, New York Medical College, Valhalla.

Dr. Lockhart is the chairman, Department of Oral Medicine, Carolinas Medical Center, Charlotte, N.C.

Dr. Baddour is a professor of medicine, Mayo Clinic, Rochester, Minn. Dr. Levison is a professor medicine and public health, Drexel University College of Medicine, Philadelphia.

Dr. Bolger is a William Watt Kerr professor of clinical medicine, University of California, San Francisco.

Dr. Cabell is a professor of medicine, Duke University, Durham, N.C. Dr. Takahashi is a professor of pediatrics, Childrens Hospital Los Angeles, University of Southern California.

Dr. Baltimore is a professor, pediatrics infectious diseases and epidemiology/public health, Yale University School of Medicine, New Haven, Conn.

Dr. Newburger is a professor of pediatrics, Harvard Medical School, Boston, and associate chief for academic affairs, Department of Cardiology, Children's Hospital, Boston.

Dr. Strom is the chair and a professor of biostatistics and epi-demi- ology, University of Pennsylvania School of Medicine, Philadelphia.

Dr. Tani is a professor of pediatrics, University of Utah School of Medicine, Salt Lake City.

Dr. Gerber is a professor of pediatrics, Cincinnati Children's Hospital Medical Center.

Dr. Bonow is the chief, Division of Cardiology, and a professor of medicine, Northwestern Memorial Hospital, Chicago.

Dr. Pallasch is a professor emeritus of dentistry, University of Southern California, Los Angeles.

Dr. Shulman is a professor of pediatrics and the chief, infectious diseases, Children's Memorial Hospital, Chicago.

Dr. Rowley is a professor of pediatrics, Children's Memorial Hospital, Chicago.

Dr. Burns is a professor and the chief, Division of Allergy, Immunology, Department of Pediatrics, University of California, San Diego.

Dr. Ferrieri is a professor, Department of Laboratory Medicine and Pathology, and a professor of pediatrics, University of Minnesota Med- ical School, Minneapolis.

Dr. Gardner is the medical director, Christiana Care Health Systems, Newark, Del.

Dr. Goff is a professor, Public Health Sciences and Internal Medicine, Wake Forest University School of Medicine, Winston-Salem, N.C.

Dr. Durack is senior vice president, Corporate Medical Affairs, Becton, Dickinson and Company, Franklin Lakes, N.J. and the director of pre-clinical and clinical development, Becton, Dickinson and Company, and a consulting professor of medicine, Duke University, Durham, N.C.

Address reprint requests to Division of Science, American Dental Association Council on Scientific Affairs, 211 E. Chicago Ave., Chicago, Ill. 60611, e-mail "science@ada.org".

Readers interested in additional information regarding the authors' conflicts of interest may access it via the Supplemental Data link in the online version of the article on the JADA Web site (*"http://jada.ada.org"*).

References

1. Dajani AS, Taubert KA, Wilson W, et al. Prevention of bacterial endocarditis: recommendations by the American Heart Association. *JAMA*. 1997;277(22):1794-801.
2. Strom BL, Abrutyn E, Berlin JA, et al. Dental and cardiac risk factors for infective endocarditis: a population-based, case-control study. *Ann Intern Med*. 1998;129(10):761-9.
3. Durack DT. Prevention of infective endocarditis. *N Engl J Med*. 1994(1);332:38-44.
4. Durack DT. Antibiotics for prevention of endocarditis during dentistry: time to scale back? *Ann Intern Med*. 1998;129(10):829-31.
5. Lockhart PB, Brennan MT, Fox PC, Norton HJ, Jernigan DB, Strausbaugh LJ. Decision-making on the use of antimicrobial prophylaxis for dental procedures: a survey of infectious disease consultants and review. *Clin Infect Dis*. 2002;34(12):1621-6.
6. American College of Cardiology and American Heart Association Task Force on Practice Guidelines. Manual for ACC/AHA guideline writing committees: Methodologies and policies from the ACC/AHA Task Force on Practice Guidelines. Available at: "*http://circ.ahajournals.org/manual/*". Accessed May 2, 2007.
7. Jones TD, Baumgartner L, Bellows MT, et al. Prevention of rheumatic fever and bacterial endocarditis through control of streptococcal infections. *Circulation*. 1955;11:317-20.
8. Rammelkamp CH, Breese BB, Griffeath HI, et al. (Committee on Prevention of Rheumatic Fever and Bacterial Endocarditis, American Heart Association). Treatment of streptococcal infections in the general population. *Circulation*. 1957;15:154-8.
9. Committee on Prevention of Rheumatic Fever and Bacterial Endocarditis, American Heart Association. Prevention of rheumatic fever and bacterial endocarditis through control of streptococcal infections. *Circulation*. 1960;21:151-5.
10. Wannamaker LW, Denny FW, Diehl, et al. (Committee on Prevention of Rheumatic Fever and Bacterial Endocarditis, American Heart Association). Prevention of bacterial endocarditis. *Circulation*. 1965;31:953-4.
11. Rheumatic Fever Committee and the Committee on Congenital Cardiac Defects, American Heart Association. Prevention of bacterial endocarditis. *Circulation*. 1972;46:S3-S6.
12. Kaplan EL, Anthony BF, Bisno A, et al. (Committee on Prevention of Rheumatic Fever and Bacterial Endocarditis, American Heart Association). Prevention of bacterial endocarditis. *Circulation*. 1977;56(1):139A-143A.
13. Shulman ST, Amren DP, Bisno AL, et al. (Committee on Prevention of Rheumatic Fever and Bacterial Endocarditis, American Heart Association). Prevention of bacterial endocarditis: a statement for health professionals by the Committee on Rheumatic Fever and Infective Endocarditis of the Council on Cardiovascular Disease in the Young. *Circulation*. 1984;70(6):1123A-1127A.
14. Dajani AS, Bisno AL, Chung KJ, et al. Prevention of bacterial endocarditis: recommendations by the American Heart Association. *JAMA*. 1990;264(22):2919-22.
15. Selton-Suty C, Duval X, Brochet E, et al. New French recomme dations for the prophylaxis of infectious endocarditis [in French]. *Arch Mal Coeur Vaiss*. 2004;97(6):626-31.
16. Gould FK, Elliott TS, Foweraker J, et al. Guidelines for the prevention of endocarditis: report of the Working Party of the British Society for Antimicrobial Chemotherapy—authors' response. *J Antimicrob Chemother*. 2006;57(4):1035-42.
17. Ashrafian H, Bogle RG. Antimicrobial prophylaxis for endocarditis: emotion or science. *Heart*. 2007;93(1):5-6.
18 Burnette-Curley D, Wells V, Viscount H, et al. FimA, a major virulence factor associated with Streptococcus parasanguis endocarditis. *Infect Immun*. 1995;63(12):4669-74.
19. Viscount HB, Munro CL, Burnette-Curley D, Peterson DL, Macrina FL. Immunization with FimA protects against Streptococcus parasanguis endocarditis in rats. *Infect Immun*. 1997;65(3):994-1002.
20. Kitten T, Munro CL, Wang A, Macrina FL. Vaccination with FimA from Streptococcus parasanguis protects rats from endocarditis caused by other viridans streptococci. *Infect Immun*. 2002;70(1):422-5.
21. Durack DT, Beeson PB. Experimental bacterial endocarditis, part II: survival of a bacteria in endocardial vegetations. *Br J Exp Pathol*. 1972;53(1):50-3.
22. Fowler VG, Scheld WM, Bayer AS. Endocarditis and intravascular infections. In: Mandell GL, Douglas RG, Bennett JE, Dolin R, eds. Principles and practices of infectious diseases. 6th ed. New York: Elsevier/Churchill Livingstone; 2005:975-1021.
23. Osler W. Gulstonian lectures on malignant endocarditis: lecture I and lecture II. *Lancet*. 1885;1:415-8, 459-64.
24. Okell CC, Elliott SD. Bacteraemia and oral sepsis: with special reference to the aetiology of subacute endocarditis. *Lancet*. 1935;2:869-72.
25. Lockhart PB, Durack DT. Oral microflora as a cause of endocarditis and other distant site infections. *Infect Dis Clin North Am*. 1999;13(4):833-50, vi.
26. Roberts GJ, Holzel HS, Sury MR, Simmons NA, Gardner P, Longhurst P. Dental bacteremia in children. *Pediatr Cardiol*. 1997;18(1):24-7.
27. Pallasch TJ, Slots J. Antibiotic prophylaxis and the medically compromised patient. *Periodontol*. 2000 1996;10:107-38.
28. Lockhart PB. The risk for endocarditis in dental practice. Periodontol. 2000 2000;23:127-35.
29. Cobe HM. Transitory bacteremia. *Oral Surg Oral Med Oral Pathol*.1954;7(6):609-15.
30. Sconyers JR, Crawford JJ, Moriarty JD. Relationship of bacteremia to toothbrushing in patients with periodontitis. *JADA*. 1973;87(3):616-22.
31. Forner L, Larsen T, Kilian M, Holmstrup P. Incidence of bacteremia after chewing, tooth brushing and scaling in individuals with periodontal inflammation. *J Clin Periodontol*. 2006;33(6):401-7.
32. Rise E, Smith JF, Bell J. Reduction of bacteremia after oral manipulations. *Arch Otolaryngol*. 1969;90(2):198-201.
33. Schlein RA, Kudlick EM, Reindorf CA, Gregory J, Royal GC. Toothbrushing and transient bacteremia in patients undergoing orthodontic treatment. *Am J Orthod Dentofacial*. Orthop 1991;99(5):466-72.
34. Faden HS. Dental procedures andbacteremia (letter). *Ann Intern Med*. 1974;81(2):274.
35. Round H, Kirkpatrick HJR, Hails CG. Further investigations on bacteriological infections of the mouth. *Proc R Soc Med*. 1936;29:1552-6.
36. Felix JE, Rosen S, App GR. Detection of bacteremia after the use of an oral irrigation device in subjects with periodontitis. *J Periodontol*. 1971;42(12):785-7.
37. O'Leary TJ, Shafer WG, Swenson HM, Nesler DC, Van Dorn PR. Possible penetration of crevicular tissue from oral hygiene procedures, part I: use of oral irrigating devices. *J Periodontol*. 1970;41(3):158-62.
38. Socransky SS, Haffajee AD, Smith GL, Dzink JL. Difficulties encountered in the search for the etiologic agents of destructive periodontal diseases. *J Clin Periodontol*. 1987;14(10):588-93.
39. Tanner A, Maiden MF, Paster BJ, Dewhirst FE. The impact of 16S ribosomal RNA-based phylogeny on the taxonomy of oral bacteria. *Periodontol*. 2000 1994;5:26-51.
40. Paster BJ, Boches SK, Galvin JL, et al. Bacterial diversity in human subgingival plaque. *J Bacteriol*. 2001;183(12):3770-83.
41. Aas JA, Paster BJ, Stokes LN, Olsen I, Dewhirst FE. Defining the normal bacterial flora of the oral cavity. *J Clin Microbiol*. 2005;43(11):5721-32.
42. Pallasch TJ. Antibiotic prophylaxis: problems in paradise. *Dent Clin North Am*. 2003;47(4):665-79.
43. Hillman JD, Socransky SS, Shivers M. The relationships between streptococcal species and periodontopathic bacteria in human dental plaque. *Arch Oral Biol*. 1985;30(11-12):791-5.
44. Roberts GJ, Jaffray EC, Spratt DA, et al. Duration, prevalence and intensity of bacteraemia after dental extractions in children. *Heart*. 006;92(9):1274-7.
45. Lucas VS, Lytra V, Hassan T, Tatham H, Wilson M, Roberts GJ. Comparison of lysis filtration and an automated blood culture system (BACTEC) for detection, quantification, and identification of odontogenic bacteremia in children. *J Clin Microbiol*. 2002;40(9):3416-20.
46. Lockhart PB, Schmidtke MA. Antibiotic considerations in medically compromised patients. *Dent Clin North Am*. 1994;38(3):381-402.
47. Overholser CD, Moreillon P, Glauser MP. Experimental endocarditis following dental extractions in rats with periodontitis (published correction appears in J Oral Maxillofac Surg. 1989;47[2]:215). *J Oral Maxillofac Surg*. 1988;46(10):857-61.
48. Baltch AL, Schaffer C, Hammer MC, et al. Bacteremia following dental cleaning in patients with and without penicillin prophylaxis. *Am Heart J*. 1982;104(6):1335-9.

49. Baltch AL, Pressman HL, Schaffer C, et al. Bacteremia in patients undergoing oral procedures. Study following parenteral antimicrobial prophylaxis as recommended by the American Heart Association, 1977. *Arch Intern Med.* 1988;148(5):1084-8.
50. Coffin F, Thompson RE. Factors influencing bacteraemia following dental extraction. *Lancet.* 1956;271(6944):654-6.
51. Heimdahl A, Hall G, Hedberg M, et al. Detection and quantitation by lysis-filtration of bacteremia after different oral surgical procedures. *J Clin Microbiol.* 1990;28(10):2205-9.
52. Lucartorto FM, Franker CK, Maza J. Postscaling bacteremia in HIV-associated gingivitis and periodontitis. *Oral Surg Oral Med Oral Pathol.* 1992;73(5):550-4.
53. Lockhart PB. An analysis of bacteremias during dental extractions: a double-blind, placebo-controlled study of chlorhexidine. *Arch Intern Med.* 1996;156(5):513-20.
54. Lockhart PB, Brennan MT, Kent ML, Norton HJ, Weinrib DA. Impact of amoxicillin prophylaxis on the incidence, nature, and duration f bacteremia in children after intubation and dental procedures. *Circulation.* 2004;109(23):2878-84.
55. Lazansky JP, Robinson L, Rodofsky L. Factors influencing the incidence of bacteremias ollowing surgical procedures in the ral cavity. *J Dent Res.* 1949;28(6):533-43.
56. Bender IB, Montgomery S. Nonsurgical endodontic procedures for the patient at risk for infective endocarditis and other systemic disorders. *J Endod.* 1986;12(9):400-7.
57. Conner HD, Haberman S, Collings CK, Winford TE. Bacteremias following periodontal scaling in patients with healthy appearing gingival. *J Periodontol.* 1967;38(6):466-72.
58. McEntegart MD, Porterfield JS. Bacteraemia following dental extractions. *Lancet.* 1949;2:596-8.
59. Robinson L, Kraus FW, Lazansky JP, Wheeler RE, Gordon S, Johnson V. Bacteremias of dental origin, II: a study of the factors influencing occurrence and detection. *Oral Surg Oral Med Oral Pathol.* 1950;3:923-36.
60. Eldirini AH. Effectiveness of epinephrine in local anesthetic solutions on the bacteremia following dental extraction. *J Oral Ther Pharmacol.* 1968;4(4):317-26.
61. Elliott RH, Dunbar JM. Streptococcal bacteraemia in children following dental extractions. *Arch Dis Child.* 1968;43(230):451-4.
62. Vargas B, Collings CK, Polter L, Haberman S. Effects of certain factors on bacteremias resulting from gingival resection. *J Periodontol.* 1959;30:196-207.
63. Roberts GJ. Dentists are innocent! "Everyday" bacteremia is the real culprit: a review and assessment of the evidence that dental surgical procedures are a principal cause of bacterial endocarditis in children. *Pediatr Cardiol.* 1999;20(5):317-25.
64. Hockett RN, Loesche WJ, Sodeman TM. Bacteraemia in asymptomatic human subjects. *Arch Oral Biol.* 1977;22(2):91-8.
65. Thayer W. Studies on bacterial (infective) endocarditis. *Hopkins Hospital Report.* 1926;22:1-185.
66. Okabe K, Nakagawa K, Yamamoto E. Factors affecting the occurrence of bacteremia associated with tooth extraction. *Int J Oral Maxillofac Surg.*1995;24(3):239-42.
67. Hall G, Hedstrom SA, Heimdahl A, Nord CE. Prophylactic administration of penicillins for endocarditis does not reduce the incidence of postextraction bacteremia. *Clin Infect Dis.* 1993;17(2):188-94.
68. Lineberger LT, De Marco TJ. Evaluation of transient bacteremia following routine periodontal procedures. *J Periodontol.* 1973;44(12):757-62.
69. Witzenberger T, O'Leary TJ, Gillette WB. Effect of a local germi- cide on the occurrence of bacteremia during subgingival scaling. *J Periodontol.* 1982;53(3):172-9.
70. Rogosa M, Hampp EG, Nevin TA, Wagner HN Jr, Driscoll EJ, Baer PN. Blood sampling and cultural studies in the detection of post-operative bacteremias. *JADA.* 1960;60:171-80.
71. Bandt CL, Korn NA, Schaffer EM. Bacteremias from ultrasonic and hand instrumentation. *J Periodontol.* 1964;35:214-5.
72. De Leo AA, Schoenknecht FD, Anderson MW, Peterson JC. The incidence of bacteremia following oral prophylaxis on pediatric patients. *Oral Surg Oral Med Oral Pathol.* 1974;37(1):36-45.
73. Barco CT. Prevention of infective endocarditis: a review of the medical and dental literature. *J Periodontol.* 1991;62(8):510-23.
74. Bayliss R, Clarke C, Oakley C, Somerville W, Whitfield AG. The teeth and infective endocarditis. *Br Heart J.* 1983;50(6):506-12.
75. Hirsh HL, Vivino JJ, Merril A, Dowling HF. Effect of prophylactically administered penicillin on incidence of bacteremia following extraction of teeth. *Arch Intern Med.* 1948;81:868-78.
76. Shanson DC, Akash S, Harris M, Tadayon M. Erythromycin stearate, 1.5 g, for the oral prophylaxis of streptococcal bacteraemia in patients undergoing dental extraction: efficacy and tolerance. *J Antimicrob Chemother.* 1985;15(1):83-90.
77. Roberts GJ, Radford P, Holt R. Prophylaxis of dental bacteraemia with oral amoxycillin in children. *Br Dent J.* 1987;162(5):179-82.
78. Hall G, Heimdahl A, Nord CE. Effects of prophylactic administration of cefaclor on transient bacteremia after dental extraction. *Eur J Clin Microbiol Infect Dis.* 1995;15:646-9.
79. Hall G, Heimdahl A, Nord CE. Bacteremia after oral surgery and antibiotic prophylaxis for endocarditis. *Clin Infect Dis.* 1999;29(1):1-8.
80. Macfarlane TW, Ferguson MM, Mulgrew CJ. Post-extraction bacteraemia: role of antiseptics and antibiotics. *Br Dent J.* 1984;156(5):179-81
81. Oliver R, Roberts GJ, Hooper L. Penicillins for the prophylaxis of bacterial endocarditis in dentistry. *Cochrane Database Syst Rev.* 2004(2):CD003813.
82. Guntheroth WG. How important are dental procedures as a cause of infective endocarditis? *Am J Cardiol.* 1984;54(7):797-801.
83. Everett ED, Hirschmann JV. Transient bacteremia and endocarditis prophylaxis: a review. *Medicine* (Baltimore). 1977;56(1):61-77.
84. Horstkotte D, Rosin H, Friedrichs W, Loogen F. Contribution for choosing the optimal prophylaxis of bacterial endocarditis. *Eur Heart J.* 1987;8(supplement J):379-81.
85. Imperiale TF, Horwitz RI. Does prophylaxis prevent post-dental infective endocarditis? A controlled evaluation of protective efficacy. *Am J Med.* 1990;88(2):131-6.
86. van der Meer JT, Thompson J, Valkenburg HA, Michel MF. Epidemiology of bacterial endocarditis in The Netherlands, part II: antecedent procedures and use of prophylaxis. *Arch Intern Med.* 1992;152(9):1869-73.
87. van der Meer JT, van Wijk W, Thompson J, Vandenbroucke JP, Valkenburg HA, Michel MF. Efficacy of antibiotic prophylaxis for prevention of native-valve endocarditis. *Lancet.* 1992;339(8786):135-9.
88. van der Meer JT, van Wijk W, Thompson J, Valkenburg HA, Michel MF. Awareness of need and actual use of prophylaxis: lack of patient compliance in the prevention of bacterial endocarditis. *J Antimicrob Chemother.* 1992;29(2):187-94.
89. Duval X, Alla F, Hoen B, et al. Estimated risk of endocarditis in adults with predisposing cardiac conditions undergoing dental procedures with or without antibiotic prophylaxis. *Clin Infect Dis.* 2006;42(12):e102-7.
90. Starkebaum M, Durack D, Beeson P. The "incubation period" of subacute bacterial endocarditis. *Yale J Biol Med.* 1977;50(1):49-58.
91. Steckelberg JM, Wilson WR. Risk factors for infective endocarditis. *Infect Dis Clin North Am.* 1993;7(1):9-19.
92. Pallasch TJ, Wahl MJ. Focal infection: new age or ancient history? *Endodontic Topics.* 2003;4:32-45.
93. Idsoe O, Guthe T, Willcox RR, de Weck AL. Nature and extent of penicillin side-reactions, with particular reference to fatalities from anaphylactic shock. *Bull World Health Organ.* 1968;38(2):159-88.
94. Ahlstedt S. Penicillin allergy: can the incidence be reduced? *Allergy.* 1984;39(3):151-64.
95. Agha Z, Lofgren RP, Van Ruiswyk JV. Is antibiotic prophylaxis for bacterial endocarditis cost-effective? *Med Decis Making.* 2005;25(3):308-20.
96. Kelkar PS, Li JT. Cephalosporin allergy. *N Engl J Med.* 2001;345(11):804-9.
97. Guay DR, Patterson DR, Seipman N, Craft JC. Overview of the tolerability profile of clarithromycin in preclinical and clinical trials. *Drug Saf.* 1993;8(5):350-64.
98. Mazur N, Greenberger PA, Regalado J. Clindamycin hypersensitivity appears to be rare. *Ann Allergy Asthma Immunol.* 1999;82(5): 443-5.
99. Bombassaro AM, Wetmore SJ, John MA. Clostridium difficile colitis following antibiotic prophylaxis for dental procedures. *J Can Dent Assoc.* 2001;67(1):20-2.
100. Tleyjeh IM, Steckelberg JM, Murad HS, et al. Temporal trends in infective endocarditis: a population-based study in Olmsted County, Minnesota. *JAMA.* 2005;293(24):3022-8.

101. Griffin MR, Wilson WR, Edwards WD, O'Fallon WM, Kurland LT. Infective endocarditis. Olmsted County, Minnesota, 1950 through 1981. *JAMA*. 1985;254(9):1199-202.
102. Durack DT, Petersdorf RG. Changes in the epidemiology of endocarditis. Dallas: American Heart Association; 1977. AHA Monograph No. 52.
103. Delahaye F, Goulet V, Lacassin F, et al. Characteristics of infective endocarditis in France in 1991: a 1-year survey. *Eur Heart J*. 1995;16(3):394-401.
104. Hoen B, Alla F, Selton-Suty C, et al. Changing profile of infective endocarditis: results of a 1-year survey in France. *JAMA*. 2002;288(1):75-81.
105. Mylonakis E, Calderwood SB. Infective endocarditis in adults. *N Engl J Med*. 2001;345(18):1318-30.
106. Gersony WM, Hayes CJ, Driscoll DJ, et al. Bacterial endocarditis in patients with aortic stenosis, pulmonary stenosis, or ventricular septal defect. *Circulation*. 1993;87(2 supplement):1121-6.
107. Wilson WR, Jaumin PM, Danielson GK, Giuliani ER, Washington JA II, Geraci JE. Prosthetic valve endocarditis. *Ann Intern Med*. 1975;82(6):751-6.
108. Baddour LM, Wilson WR. Infections of prosthetic valves and other cardiovascular devices. In: Mandell GL, Douglas RG, Bennett JE, Dolin R, eds. Mandell, Douglas, and Bennett's principles and practice of infectious diseases. 6th ed. New York: Elsevier/Churchill Livingstone; 2005:1022-44.
109. Baddour LM, Wilson WR, Bayer AS, et al. Infective endocarditis: diagnosis, antimicrobial therapy, and management of complications: a statement for healthcare professionals from the Committee on Rheumatic Fever, Endocarditis, and Kawasaki Disease, Council on Cardiovascular Disease in the Young, and the Councils on Clinical Cardiology, Stroke, and Cardiovascular Surgery and Anesthesia, American Heart Association: endorsed by th Infectious Diseases Society of America (published corrections appear in *Circulation* 2005;112[15]:2373 and *Circulation* 2007;115[15]:e408). *Circulation* 2005;111(23):e394-434.
110. Wilson WR, Danielson GK, Giuliani ER, Geraci JE. Prosthetic valve endocarditis. *Mayo Clin Proc*. 1982;57(3):155-61.
111. Wilson WR, Geraci JE, Wilkowske CJ, Washington JA 2nd. Short-term intramuscular therapy with procaine penicillin plus streptomycin for infective endocarditis due to viridans streptococci. *Circulation*. 1978;57(6):1158-61.
112. Anderson DJ, Olaison L, McDonald JR, et al. Enterococcal prosthetic valve infective endocarditis: report of 45 episodes from the International Collaboration on Endocarditis-merged database. *Eur J Clin Microbiol Infect Dis*. 2005;24(10):665-70.
113. Chu VH, Cabell CH, Abrutyn E, et al. Native valve endocarditis due to coagulase-negative staphylococci: report of 99 episodes from the International Collaboration on Endocarditis Merged Database. *Clin Infect Dis*. 2004;39(10):1527-30.
114. Lalani T, Kanafani ZA, Chu VH, et al. Prosthetic valve endocarditis due to coagulase-negative staphylococci: findings from the International Collaboration on Endocarditis Merged Database. *Eur J Clin Microbiol Infect Dis*. 2006;25(6):365-8.
115. McDonald JR, Olaison L, Anderson DJ, et al. Enterococcal endocarditis: 107 cases from the international collaboration on endocarditis merged database. *Am J Med*. 2005;118(7):759-66.
116. Sexton DJ, Tenenbaum MJ, Wilson WR, et al. Ceftriaxone once daily for four weeks compared with ceftriaxone plus gentamicin once daily for two weeks for treatment of endocarditis due to penicillin-susceptible streptococci. Endocarditis Treatment Consortium Group. *Clin Infect Dis*. 1998;27(6):1470-4.
117. Francioli P, Etienne J, Hoigne R, Thys JP, Gerber A. Treatment of streptococcal endocarditis with a single daily dose of ceftriaxone sodium for 4 weeks: efficacy and outpatient treatment feasibility. *JAMA*. 1992;267(2):264-7.
118. Wilson WR, Wilkowske CJ, Wright AJ, Sande MA, Geraci JE. Treatment of streptomycin-susceptible and streptomycin-resistant enterococcal endocarditis. *Ann Intern Med*. 1984;100(6):816-23.
119. Mansur AJ, Dal Bo CM, Fukushima JT, Issa VS, Grinberg M, Pomerantzeff PM. Relapses, recurrences, valve replacements, and mortality during the long-term follow-up after infective endocarditis. *Am Heart J*. 2001;141(1):78-86.
120. Baddour LM. Twelve-year review of recurrent native-valve infective endocarditis: a disease of the modern antibiotic era. *Rev Infect Dis*. 1988;10(6):1163-70.
121. Chu VH, Sexton DJ, Cabell CH, et al. Repeat infective endocarditis: differentiating relapse from reinfection. *Clin Infect Dis*. 2005;41(3):406-9.
122. Welton DE, Young JB, Gentry WO, et al. Recurrent infective endocarditis: analysis of predisposing factors and clinical features. *Am J Med*. 1979;66(6):932-8.
123. Levison ME, Kaye D, Mandell GL, Hook EW. Characteristics of patients with multiple episodes of bacterial endocarditis. *JAMA*. 1970;211(8):1355-7.
124. Renzulli A, Carozza A, Romano G, et al. Recurrent infective endocarditis: a multivariate analysis of 21 years of experience. *Ann Thorac Surg*. 2001;72(1):39-43.
125. Erbel R, Liu F, Ge J, Kupferwasser I. Identification of high-risk subgroups in infective endocarditis and the role of echocardiography. *Eur Heart J*. 1995;16(5):588-602.
126. Kaplan EL, Rich H, Gersony W, Manning J. A collaborative study of infective endocarditis in the 1970s: emphasis on infections in patients who have undergone cardiovascular surgery. *Circulation*. 1979;59(2):327-35.
127. Coward K, Tucker N, Darville T. Infective endocarditis in Arkansan children from 1990 through 2002. *Pediatr Infect Dis J*. 2003;22(12):1048-52.
128. Saiman L, Prince A, Gersony WM. Pediatric infective endocarditis in the modern era. *J Pediatr*. 1993;122(6):847-53.
129. Dodo H, Child JS. Infective endocarditis in congenital heart disease. *Cardiol Clin*. 1996;14(3):383-92.
130. Martin JM, Neches WH, Wald ER. Infective endocarditis: 35 years of experience at a children's hospital. *Clin Infect Dis*. 1997;24(4):669-75.
131. Parras F, Bouza E, Romero J, et al. Infectious endocarditis in children. *Pediatr Cardiol*. 1990;11(2):77-81.
132. Takeda S, Nakanishi T, Nakazawa M. A 28-year trend of infective endocarditis associated with congenital heart diseases: a single institute experience. *Pediatr Int*. 2005;47(4):392-6.
133. Ferrieri P, Gewitz MH, Gerber MA, et al. Unique features of infective endocarditis in childhood. *Circulation*. 2002;105(17):2115-26.
134. Ishiwada N, Niwa K, Tateno S, et al. Causative organism influences clinical profile and outcome of infective endocarditis in pediatric patients and adults with congenital heart disease. *Circ J*. 2005;69(10):1266-70.
135. Han YM, Gu X, Titus JL, et al. New self-expanding patent foramen ovale occlusion device. *Catheter Cardiovasc Interv*. 1999;47(3):370-6.
136. Prabhu RM, Piper KE, Baddour LM, Steckelberg JM, Wilson WR, Patel R. Antimicrobial susceptibility patterns among viridans group streptococcal isolates from infective endocarditis patients from 1971 to 1986 and 1994 to 2002. *Antimicrob Agents Chemother*. 2004;48(11):4463-5.
137. Doern GV, Ferraro MJ, Brueggemann AB, Ruoff KL. Emergence of high rates of antimicrobial resistance among viridans group streptococci in the United States. *Antimicrob Agents Chemother*. 1996;40(4):891-4.
138. Diekema DJ, Beach ML, Pfaller MA, Jones RN; SENTRY Participants Group. Antimicrobial resistance in viridans group streptococci among patients with and without the diagnosis of cancer in the USA, Canada and Latin America. *Clin Microbiol Infect*. 2001;7(3):152-7.
139. Groppo FC, Castro FM, Pacheco AB, et al. Antimicrobial resistance of Staphylococcus aureus and oral streptococci strains from high-risk endocarditis patients. *Gen Dent*. 2005;53(6):410-3.
140. Teng LJ, Hsueh PR, Chen YC, Ho SW, Luh KT. Antimicrobial susceptibility of viridans group streptococci in Taiwan with an emphasis on the high rates of resistance to penicillin and macrolides in Streptococcus oralis. *J Antimicrob Chemother*. 1998;41(6):621-7.
141. Tuohy M, Washington JA. Antimicrobial susceptibility of viridans group streptococci. *Diagn Microbiol Infect Dis*. 1997;29(4):277-80.
142. Seppala H, Haanpera M, Al-Juhaish M, Jarvinen H, Jalava J, Huovinen P. Antimicrobial susceptibility patterns and macrolide resistance genes of viridans group streptococci from normal flora. *J Antimicrob Chemother*. 2003;52(4):636-44.
143. Marron A, Carratala J, Alcaide F, Fernandez-Sevilla A, Gudiol F. High rates of resistance to cephalosporins among viridans-group streptococci causing bacteraemia in neutropenic cancer patients. *J Antimicrob Chemother*. 2001;47(1):87-91.
144. Wu JJ, Lin KY, Hsueh PR, Liu JW, Pan HI, Sheu SM. High incidence of erythromycin-resistant streptococci in Taiwan. *Antimicrob Agents Chemother*. 1997;41(4):844-6.

145. King A, Bathgate T, Phillips I. Erythromycin susceptibility of viridans streptococci from the normal throat flora of patients treated with azithromycin or clarithromycin. *Clin Microbiol Infect.* 2002;8(2):85-92.
146. Baddour LM, Bettmann MA, Bolger AF, et al. Nonvalvular cardiovascular device-related infections. *Circulation.* 2003;108(16):2015-31.
147. Sherman-Weber S, Axelrod P, Suh B, et al. Infective endocarditis following orthotopic heart transplantation: 10 cases and a review of the literature. *Transpl Infect Dis.* 2004;6(4):165-70.

Antibiotic Prophylaxis for Dental Patients With Total Joint Replacements

American Dental Association

Guidelines for patients who have a **total joint replacement** were updated by the American Academy of Orthopedic Surgeons (AAOS) in 2009. In 1997, the ADA and the AAOS developed an Advisory Statement on Antibiotic Prophylaxis for Dental Patients with Total Joint Replacements. The Advisory Statement was reviewed and revised in 2003, consistent with the ADA's practice of periodically reviewing all its guidelines to make sure they take into consideration any new information. The 2003 Total Joint Advisory Statement issued by the ADA and AAOS was retired by AAOS consistent with their process requiring review of statements every five years. AAOS issued a new statement in 2009 that consolidates their prophylaxis recommendations for dental and medical procedures. The AAOS 2009 Information Statement differs from the 2003 AAOS/ADA Advisory Statement on the following topics:

- AAOS now states that, *"Given the potential adverse outcomes and cost of treating an infected joint replacement, the AAOS recommends that clinicians consider antibiotic prophylaxis for all total joint replacement patients prior to any invasive procedure that may cause bacteremia."*

By contrast, the 2003 advisory statement recommended antibiotic prophylaxis for all patients within the first two years after replacement surgery only; after two years, the recommendation for prophylaxis was limited to patients who had comorbidities that might place them at increased risk for hematogenous total joint infection (ie, immunocompromised patients).

- Specific dental procedures that may potentially cause a bacteremia are not identified in the new statement. In the 2003 statement, the following procedures were identified as having a higher incidence of bacteremia: dental extractions; periodontal procedures, including surgery, subgingival placement of antiobiotic fibers/strips, scaling and root planing, probing, recall maintenance; dental implant placement and replantation of avulsed teeth; endodontic (root canal) instrumentation or surgery only beyond the apex; initial placement of orthodontic bands but not brackets; intraligamentary and intraosseous local anesthetic injections; and prophylactic cleaning of teeth or implants where bleeding is anticipated.

- AAOS does not include a recommendation for an antibiotic regimen for patients who are allergic to penicillin. In the 2003 statement, clindamycin (600 milligrams 1 hour before the procedure) was the recommended antibiotic.

(continued on next page)

The updated AAOS Information Statement is available at *http://www.aaos.org/about/papers/advistmt/1033.asp*.

Editor's note: For dental procedures, the AAOS currently recommends amoxicillin, cephalexin or cephadrine, 2 grams, given 1 hour before the procedure. To check for ADA statement updates, visit *www.ada.org/prof/resources/positions/statements/index.asp*.

Nitrous Oxide in the Dental Office

ADA Council on Scientific Affairs; ADA Council on Dental Practice

The safe use of nitrous oxide in the dental office has been an issue the ADA has monitored for many years. In 1977, an ad hoc committee convened by the Association published a report on the potential health hazards of trace anesthetics in dentistry.[1] Also in 1977, the National Institute of Occupational Safety and Health (NIOSH) reported that, by using several control measures, nitrous oxide levels of approximately 50 parts per million (ppm) were achievable in dental operatories during routine dental anesthesia/analgesia.[2] A few years later, in 1980, the ADA Council on Dental Materials, Instruments and Equipment recommended that effective scavenging devices be installed and monitoring programs be instituted in dental offices in which nitrous oxide is used, and the council indicated that using these methods or devices would assist in keeping the levels of nitrous oxide at the lowest possible level[3]

NIOSH continued its activities relating to nitrous oxide concentrations in the dental office and, in 1994, published an alert called "Request for Assistance in Controlling Exposures to Nitrous Oxide During Anesthetic Administration."[4] In the same year, NIOSH also reported on field evaluations and laboratory studies evaluating nitrous oxide scavenging systems and modifications in attempts to achieve the current NIOSH recommended exposure limit of 25 ppm during administration. NIOSH concluded that nitrous oxide levels may be controlled to about 25 ppm by maintaining leak-free delivery systems and using proper exhaust rates, better-fitting masks, and auxiliary exhaust ventilation.[5]

In 1995 the ADA Council on Scientific Affairs convened an expert panel to review scientific literature on nitrous oxide and to revise recommendations on controlling nitrous oxide concentrations in the dental office. What follows is an overview of the conclusions reached by that panel.

Conclusions and Recommendations of the Expert Panel

Nitrous oxide continues to be a valuable agent for the control of pain and anxiety. However, chronic occupational exposure to nitrous oxide in offices not using scavenging systems may be associated with possible deleterious neurological and reproductive effects on dental personnel. Limited studies show that as little as three to five hours per week of unscavenged nitrous oxide exposure could result in adverse reproductive effects. In contrast, in dental offices using nitrous oxide scavenging systems, there has been no evidence of adverse health effects.[6] It is strongly recommended, therefore, that while there is no consensus on a recommended exposure limit to nitrous oxide, appropriate scavenging systems and methods of administration should be adopted. A protocol for controlling nitrous oxide is outlined below.

Recommendations for Controlling Nitrous Oxide Exposure

The expert panel identified a number of recommendations that are important to consider in the safe and effective use of nitrous oxide:

- The dental office should have a properly installed nitrous oxide delivery system. This includes appropriate scavenging equipment with a readily visible and accurate flow meter (or equivalent measuring device), a vacuum pump with the capacity for up to 45 L of air per min per workstation, and a variety of sizes of masks to ensure proper fit for individual patients.
- The vacuum exhaust and ventilation exhaust should be vented to the outside (for example, through the vacuum system) and not in close proximity to fresh air intake vents.
- The general ventilation should provide good room air mixing.
- Each time the nitrous oxide machine is first turned on and every time a gas cylinder is changed, the pressure connections should be tested for leaks. High-pressure–line connections should be tested for leaks on a quarterly basis. A soap solution may be used to test for leaks. Alternatively, a portable infrared spectrophotometer can be used to diagnose an insidious leak.
- Prior to first daily use, all nitrous oxide equipment (reservoir bag, tubings, mask, connectors) should be inspected for worn parts, cracks, holes or tears. Replace as necessary.
- The mask may then be connected to the tubing and the vacuum pump turned on. All appropriate flow rates (that is, up to 45 L/min or per manufacturer's recommendations) should be verified.
- A properly sized mask should be selected and placed on the patient. A good, comfortable fit should be ensured. The reservoir (breathing) bag should not be over- or underinflated while the patient is breathing oxygen (before administering nitrous oxide).
- The patient should be encouraged to minimize talking and mouth breathing while the mask is in place.
- During administration, the reservoir bag should be periodically inspected for changes in tidal volume and the vacuum flow rate should be verified.
- On completing administration, 100% oxygen should be delivered to the patient for 5 minutes before removing the mask. In this way, both the patient and the system will be purged of residual nitrous oxide. Do not use an oxygen flush.
- Periodic (semiannual interval is suggested) personal sampling of dental personnel, with emphasis to chairside personnel exposed to nitrous oxide, should be conducted (for example, use of diffusive sampler [dosimeters] or infrared spectrophotometer).

Research Priorities

The expert panel identified a number of areas that require high-priority research:

- The elucidation of biological mechanisms that result in the adverse health effects associated with exposure to nitrous oxide.
- Studies to gain a full understanding of the potential health effects of chronic low-level exposure to nitrous oxide, with emphasis on prospective studies that use direct nitrous oxide exposure measurement.
- The investigation of possible cognitive effects related to exposure to low levels of nitrous oxide.
- The development of equipment to evaluate and control exposure to nitrous oxide.
- The study of ventilation systems and air exchange mechanisms for dental office designs.

- The evaluation of advantages associated with the use of nitrous oxide in combination with other sedative drugs.

The councils will continue to work with industry and the research community to address research and development needs that will further reduce occupational exposure to nitrous oxide.

Editor's note: To check for ADA statement updates, visit *www.ada.org/prof/resources/positions/statements/index.asp.*

References

1. ADA Ad Hoc Committee on Trace Anesthetics as Potential Health Hazard in Dentistry. Reports of subcommittees of the ADA Ad Hoc Committee on Trace Anesthetics as Potential Health Hazard in Dentistry: review and current status of survey. *JADA*. 1977;95(10):787-90.
2. Whitcher CE, Zimmerman DC, Piziali RL. Control of occupational exposure to N_2O in the dental operatory. Cincinnati: National Institute of Occupational Safety and Health, 1977; DHEW publication no. (NIOSH) 77-171.
3. Council on Dental Materials, Instruments and Equipment. Council position on nitrous oxide scavenging and monitoring devices. *JADA*. 1980;101(1):62.
4. Alert: request for assistance in controlling exposures to nitrous oxide during anesthetic administration. Cincinnati: U.S. Department of Health and Human Services, Public Health Service, Centers for Disease Control, National Institute of Occupational Safety and Health, 1994; DHHS publication no. (NIOSH) 94100.
5. Technical report: control of nitrous oxide in dental operatories. Cincinnati: U.S. Department of Health and Human Services, Public Health Service, Centers for Disease Control and Prevention, National Institute of Occupational Safety and Health, Division of Physical Sciences and Engineering, Engineering Control Technology Branch, 1994; DHHS publication no. (NIOSH) 94-129.
6. Rowland AS, Baird DD, Weinberg CR, Shore DL, Shy CM, Wilcox AJ. Reduced fertility among women employed as dental assistants exposed to high levels of nitrous oxide. *N Engl J Med*. 1992;327:993-7.

This material first appeared in ADA Council on Scientific Affairs and ADA Council on Dental Practice. Nitrous oxide in the dental office. *JADA*. 1997; 128:864-5.

Weights and Measures

COMMON METRIC MEASUREMENTS AND THEIR ABBREVIATIONS	
METRIC MEASUREMENTS	**ABBREVIATIONS**
WEIGHT	
gram	g
kilogram	kg
milligram	mg
microgram	µg
VOLUME	
Liter	L
Milliliter	mL
Microliter	µL

COMMON METRIC EQUIVALENTS	
METRIC MEASUREMENTS	**EQUIVALENTS**
WEIGHT	
0.000001 gram (g)	1 microgram (µg)
0.001 g	1 milligram (mg)
1 g	1,000 milligrams (mg) 1,000,000 µg
1 kg	1,000 g
VOLUME	
0.001 milliliter (mL)	1 microliter (µL)
1 mL	0.001 liter (L)
1,000 mL	1 L

MEASURES OF VOLUME	
METRIC MEASUREMENTS	**APOTHECARY**
3.697 mL	1 fluid dram
5 milliliters (mL)	1 teaspoonful
30 mL	1 fluid ounce
480 mL	1 pint
960 mL	1 quart

MEASURES OF WEIGHT	
METRIC MEASUREMENTS	**APOTHECARY**
1 gram (g)	15 grains (gr)
4 g	60 gr = 1 dram
30 g	1 ounce (oz)
1 kilogram (kg)	2.2 pounds (lb)
60 milligram (mg)	1 gr

Calculation of Local Anesthetic and Vasoconstrictor Dosages

LOCAL ANESTHETIC DOSAGES

PERCENTAGE CONCENTRATION	= mg/mL	X 1.8 = mg/CARTRIDGE
0.5	5	9
1.5	15	27
3	30	54
1	10	18
2	20	36
4	40	72

VASOCONSTRICTOR CONCENTRATIONS (EQUIVALENCY FORMULA AND USE)

DILUTION OR	mg/mL X 1.8	= mg/CARTRIDGE	RECOMMENDED USE
1:1,000	1	—	Anaphylaxis (IM, SC)
1:10,000	0.1	—	Cardiac arrest (IV)
1:20,000	0.05	0.09	Local anesthesia; levonordefrin
1:50,000	0.02	0.036	Local anesthesia; epinephrine
1:80,000	0.0125	0.0225	Local anesthesia; epinephrine (UK)
1:100,000	0.01	0.018	Local anesthesia; epinephrine
1:200,000	0.005	0.009	Local anesthesia; epinephrine

HIV and Common Antiretroviral Medications

Lida Radfar, D.D.S., M.S.

Treatment regimens for human immunodeficiency virus (HIV) disease include prophylactic and maintenance medications. Prophylactic medications usually are indicated when the patient's immune system has deteriorated to a point at which opportunistic infections can be expected. The more common medications include anti–*Pneumocystis-carinii*-pneumonia (PCP) agents such as trimethoprim-sulfamethoxazole; antifungal medications such as fluconazole; and antimycobacterial agents such as rifampin and isoniazid. Many of these medications interact with other medications commonly used in dentistry.

More than 20 antiretroviral medications, representing five drug classes, have been approved by the FDA for treatment of HIV disease, with many more in development. These medications directly or indirectly inhibit HIV replication through different mechanisms. Nucleoside reverse transcriptase inhibitors (NRTIs) and non-nucleoside reverse transcriptase inhibitors (NNRTIs) act as competitive inhibitors to an enzyme, reverse transcriptase, which the virus carries for the purpose of transcribing the viral RNA into viral DNA. Protease inhibitors (PI) prevent the breakdown of proteins produced by the HIV-infected cell into appropriate sizes for viral production. One of the newer antiretroviral classes–entry inhibitors–act at a specific site to prevent viral replication in the CD4 cell. These drugs can target the gp 120 or gp 41 proteins on the HIV cell surface (enfurvirtide) or the chemokine receptors (CCR5) of the CD4 cell to prevent HIV entering the host cells (maraviroc). Integrase inhibitors, the latest class of antiretroviral medications, received FDA approval in October 2007. This group of drugs acts by blocking the integrase enzyme and hence interrupts facilitating incorporation of the viral genetic material into the DNA of the host cells.

To maximize the treatment effect, a combination of several antiretroviral medications is recommended. This approach has been named highly active antiretroviral therapy, or HAART. This combination regimen has been shown to suppress the plasma viral load titer and raise CD4 cell counts. Although combination antiretroviral therapy has dramatically improved the lives of patients with HIV infection, viral strains resistant to multiple medications are a serious problem. Continuous development of antiretroviral medications will challenge all healthcare workers treating HIV-infected patients to keep apprised of new agents that are often associated with a high degree of toxicity, including liver toxicity, hyperglycemia, and lipid dystrophy.

The table on the following page presents antiretroviral medications used for HIV disease, which may interact with a number of drugs prescribed by dentists.

COMMON ANTIRETROVIRAL MEDICATIONS: DENTAL CONSIDERATIONS

GENERIC NAME	BRAND NAME(S)	INTERACTIONS WITH DRUGS IN DENTISTRY	ADVERSE EFFECTS RELEVANT TO DENTISTRY
ENTRY INHIBITORS			
Enfuvirtide (T-20)	Fuzeon	None noted.	Nerve pain.
Maraviroc (MVC)	Selzentry	Substrate of CYP3A and P-gp.	Cough, esophageal candidiasis, peripheral neuropathies, breathing abnormalities.
INTEGRASE INHIBITOR			
Raltegravir (RAL)	Isentress	Metabolized by UGT1A1-mediated glucuronidation pathway. Levels are decreased by rifampin. Increase dose of RAL to 800mg bid during concomitant administration with rifampin.	None noted.
NUCLEOSIDE REVERSE TRANSCRIPTASE INHIBITORS (NRTIs)			
Abacavir (ABC)	Ziagen	None noted.	Xerostomia.
Didanosine (ddI)	Videx	Reduces efficacy of itraconazole and ketoconazole; administer >2 hrs from ddI. Reduces efficacy of quinolones and tetracyclines; administer 2 hrs before or 6 hrs after ddI. Levels are increased by ganciclovir.	Peripheral neuropathy, xerostomia, thrombocytopenia.
Emtricitabine (FTC)	Emtriva	None noted.	Increased cough.
Lamivudine (3TC)	Epivir	Eliminated in urine by active organic cationic secretion. May compete with other similarly eliminated drugs.	Neuropathy, stomatitis, parasthesia, anemia.
Stavudine (d4T)	Zerit	None noted.	Peripheral neuropathy, anemia, neutropenia, thrombocytopenia.
Zalcitabine (ddC)	Hivid	Avoid use with amphotericin B and aminoglycosides due to increased risk of peripheral neuropathy.	Peripheral neuropathy, oral ulcerations.
Zidovudine (AZT, ZDV)	Retrovir	None noted.	Anemia, neutropenia, mouth ulcers, oral mucosa pigmentation, leukopenia.
Zidovudine/lamivudine	Combivir	None noted.	Anemia, neutropenia, thrombocytopenia (rare), neuropathy, oral mucosa pigmentation stomatitis.

COMMON ANTIRETROVIRAL MEDICATIONS: DENTAL CONSIDERATIONS

GENERIC NAME	BRAND NAME(S)	INTERACTIONS WITH DRUGS IN DENTISTRY	ADVERSE EFFECTS RELEVANT TO DENTISTRY
Zidovudine/lamivudine/abacvir	Trizivir	Lamivudine levels are increased by trimethoprim-sulfamethoxazole 160mg/800mg qd.	Anemia, neutropenia, oral mucosal pigmentation, peripheral neuropathy.
NON-NUCLEOSIDE REVERSE TRANSCRIPTASE INHIBITORS (NNRTIs)			
Delavirdine (DLV)	Rescriptor	Inhibits CYP450 enzymes. Levels decreased by phenobarbitol and dexamethasone. Increases levels of clarithromycin and dapsone. Administer buffered medications >2 hrs apart from DLV. Contraindicated for concomitant administration with midazolam, triazolam, alprazolam.	None noted.
Efavirenz (EFV)	Sustiva	Induces CYP450 enzymes. Decreases levels of clarithromycin but increases plasma concentrations of active metabolite. Decreases levels of voriconazole, ketoconazole, and itraconazole. Avoid concurrent use with midazolam, triazolam and clarithromycin.	Xerostomia.
Etravirine (ETR)	Intelence	Induces, inhibits, and is metabolized by CYP450 enzymes. Decreases levels of itraconazole, ketoconazole, clarithromycin. Increases levels of voriconazole, active metabolite of clarithromycin, and diazepam. Levels decreased by dexamethasone.	Peripheral neuropathy.
Nevirapine (NVP)	Viramune	Induces CYP450 enzymes. Decreases levels of clarithromycin but increases levels of active metabolite. Decreases levels of ketoconazole.	None noted.
NUCLEOTIDE REVERSE TRANSCRIPTASE INHIBITORS			
Tenofovir (TDF)	Viread	Renally eliminated; coadministration with drugs that reduce renal function or compete for active tubular secretion may increase levels (eg, acyclovir, valacyclovir, ganciclovir, and valganciclovir).	Decreases bone mineral density.

COMMON ANTIRETROVIRAL MEDICATIONS: DENTAL CONSIDERATIONS

GENERIC NAME	BRAND NAME(S)	INTERACTIONS WITH DRUGS IN DENTISTRY	ADVERSE EFFECTS RELEVANT TO DENTISTRY
PROTEASE INHIBITORS*			
Atazanavir (ATV)	Reyataz	Inhibits CYP450 and UGT1A1 enzymes. Also metabolized by CYP450 enzymes. Increases levels of ketoconazole, itraconazole, rifabutin, and clarithromycin. Contraindicated for concomitant administration with triazolam, midazolam, and rifampin.	Hemophilia.
Darunavir (DRV)	Prezista	Inhibits and is metabolized by CYP450 enzymes. Increases levels of clarithromycin, ketoconazole, itraconazole, rifabutin. Decreases levels of voriconazole. Levels are decreased by dexamethasone. Contraindicated for concomitant administration with midazolam, triazolam, and rifampin.	Hemophilia.
Fosamprenavir (FPV)	Lexiva	Contraindicated for concomitant administration with rifampin, midazolam, and triazolam. Amprenavir, the active metabolite of fosamprenavir, is an inhibitor of CYP450 and is also metabolized by CYP450. Increases levels of ketoconazole, itraconazole, rifabutin, benzodiazepines (eg, alprazolam, clorazepate, diazepam, flurazepam). Levels are decreased by dexamethasone.	Acute hemolytic anemia, spontaneous bleeding.
Indinavir (IDV)	Crixivan	Inhibits and is metabolized by CYP450 enzymes. Avoid concurrent use with midazolam, alprazolam, and triazolam. Levels increased by ketoconazole. Adequate hydration is recommended in all patients treated with IDV.	Thrombocytopenia, chapped lips, metallic taste, dry mouth, acute hemolytic anemia, spontaneous bleeding in patients with hemophilia, taste perversion, oral parasthesia.
Lopinavir/ritonavir (LPV/r)	Kaletra	Induces, inhibits, and is metabolized by CYP450 enzymes. Increases levels of clarithromycin, ketoconazole, itraconazole, and rifabutin. Decreases levels of voriconazole. Lopinavir levels decreased by rifampin and dexamethasone. Contraindicated for concomitant administration with triazolam and midazolam.	Spontaneous bleeding, dysgeusia.

*Protease inhibitors have been associated with reactivation of hepatitis, diabetes mellitus, and diminished response to narcotics.

COMMON ANTIRETROVIRAL MEDICATIONS: DENTAL CONSIDERATIONS

GENERIC NAME	BRAND NAME(S)	INTERACTIONS WITH DRUGS IN DENTISTRY	ADVERSE EFFECTS RELEVANT TO DENTISTRY
Nelfinavir (NFV)	Viracept	Inhibits CYP450 enzymes. Avoid concurrent use with midazolam and triazolam. Increases levels of rifabutin and azithromycin. Levels increased by ketoconazole.	None noted.
Ritonavir (RTV)	Norvir	Inhibits CYP450 enzymes (potent). Increases levels of clarithromycin, propoxyphene, tramadol, ketoconazole, itrazonazole, dexamethasone. Decreases levels of meperidine but increases levels of its active metabolite. Decreases levels of trimethoprim-sulfamethoxazole. Contraindicated for concomitant administration with diazepam, meperidine, voriconazole, triazolam, midazolam, piroxicam, propoxyphene.	Dysgeusia, perioral parasthesia.
Saquinavir (SQV)	Fortovase, Invirase	Inhibits CYP450 enzymes. Metabolized by CYP450 and P-gp. Increases levels of clarithromycin and benzodiazepines. Levels decreased by dexamethasone. Contraindicated for concomitant administration with triazolam, midazolam, rifampin.	None noted.
Tipranavir (TPV)	Aptivus	Inhibits CYP450 enzymes and is metabolized by CYP450 and P-gp. Levels are increased by fluconazole. Increases levels of itraconazole, ketoconazole, rifabutin. Decreases levels of meperidine. Contraindicated for concomitant administration with rifampin, midazolam, and triazolam.	Fatal intracranial hemorrhage, rash, increased bleeding, neutropenia, anemia, peripheral neuropathy.
COMBINATIONS			
Emtricitabine/tenofovir	Truvada	See individual drugs. Caution with renally eliminated drugs (eg, acyclovir, valacyclovir, ganciclovir, valganciclovir); may increase levels.	Decreases bone density.
Emtricitabine/tenofovir/efavirenz	Atripla	See individual drugs. Contraindicated for concomitant administration with midazolam and triazolam.	Decreases in bone mineral density, convulsions (efavirenz).

COMMON ANTIRETROVIRAL MEDICATIONS: DENTAL CONSIDERATIONS

GENERIC NAME	BRAND NAME(S)	INTERACTIONS WITH DRUGS IN DENTISTRY	ADVERSE EFFECTS RELEVANT TO DENTISTRY
Lamivudine/zidovudine	Combivir	See NRTIs section.	See NRTIs section.
Lamivudine/zidovudine/abacavir	Trizivir	See NRTIs section.	See NRTIs section.

Sample Prescriptions and Prescription Abbreviations

SAMPLE PRESCRIPTIONS

The following prescriptions are not all-inclusive; they are provided only as examples of prescriptions commonly written by dentists. Consult the product labeling before prescribing any dosage listed in this appendix.

For these examples, it's important to note the following: 1) suggested dosages are for adults; 2) route of administration is oral unless otherwise noted; 3) drugs are listed by generic name; those listed as drug combinations are available under a variety of brand names; and 4) selection of any particular drug for inclusion in these examples in no way indicates a recommendation of that agent over another.

The last table in this appendix shows abbreviations for prescription directions. However, if in doubt, write out the full directions.

ANTIBIOTICS FOR PATIENTS REQUIRING ANTIBIOTIC PREMEDICATION

DRUG	NUMBER	DIRECTIONS	ABBREVIATED DIRECTIONS
Penicillin			
Amoxicillin 500 mg	4	Sig: 4 capsules 1 hour before procedure	Sig: 4 caps po 1 h ā procedure
For patients allergic to penicillins			
Clindamycin HCl 150 mg	4	Sig: 4 capsules 1 hour before procedure	Sig: 4 caps po 1 h ā procedure
Cephalexin 500 mg†	4	Sig: 4 capsules 1 hour before procedure	Sig: 4 caps po 1 h ā procedure
Azithromycin 250 mg	2	Sig: 2 tablets 1 hour before procedure	Sig: 2 tabs po 1 h ā procedure
Clarithromycin 500 mg	1	Sig: 1 tablet 1 hour before procedure	Sig: 1 tab po 1 h ā procedure

†Do not use cephalosporins in patients with a history of recent, severe, or immediate-type hypersensitivity reaction (urticaria, angioedema, or anaphylaxis) to penicillins.

TO REDUCE EXCESS SALIVATION

DRUG	NUMBER	DIRECTIONS	ABBREVIATED DIRECTIONS
Atropine sulfate 0.4 mg	2	Sig: 1-2 tablets 1 hour before procedure	Sig: 1-2 tab po 1 h ā procedure
Propantheline bromide 15 mg	2	Sig: 1-2 tablets 1 hour before procedure	Sig: 1-2 tab po 1 h ā procedure

TO INCREASE SALIVATION

DRUG	NUMBER	DIRECTIONS	ABBREVIATED DIRECTIONS
Cevimeline HCl 30 mg	90	Sig: 1 capsule three times daily	Sig: 1 cap po tid
Pilocarpine 5 mg‡	30	Sig: 1-2 tablets three times daily	Sig: 1-2 tab po tid

‡Dosage shown is for dry mouth due to radiation. Dosage for dry mouth due to Sjögren's syndrome is 1 tab qid.

TO REDUCE PATIENT ANXIETY BEFORE A DENTAL PROCEDURE

DRUG	NUMBER	DIRECTIONS	ABBREVIATED DIRECTIONS
Diazepam 5 mg	V	Sig: 1-2 tablets 1 hour before sleep; 1-2 tablets 1 hour before procedure	Sig: 1-2 tab po 1 h ā hs; 1-2 tab po 1 h ā procedure
Lorazepam 1 mg	V	Sig: 1-2 tablets 1 hour before sleep; 1-2 tablets 1-2 hours before procedure	Sig: 1-2 tab po 1 h ā hs; 1-2 tab po 1-2 h ā procedure
Triazolam 0.25 mg	V	Sig: 1 tablet ½ hour before sleep; 1 tablet ½-1 hour before procedure	Sig: 1 tab po ½ h ā hs; 1 tab po ½-1 h ā procedure
Hydroxyzine pamoate 50 mg	V	Sig: 2 capsules 1 hour before sleep; 1-2 tablets 1 hour before procedure	Sig: 2 caps po 1 h ā hs; 1-2 tab po 1 h ā procedure

V: Varies with number of appointments.

FOR ANALGESIA

DRUG	NUMBER	DIRECTIONS	ABBREVIATED DIRECTIONS
For mild-to-moderate pain			
Ibuprofen 400 mg	18	Sig: 1 tablet every 4-6 hours as needed for pain; maximum daily dose 8 tablets	Sig: 1 tab po q 4-6 h prn pain; MDD 8 tab
Acetaminophen with codeine #3 (30 mg)	24	Sig: 1-2 tablets every 4 hours as needed for pain; maximum daily dose 12 tablets, acetaminophen 4,000 mg	Sig: 1-2 tab po q 4 h prn pain; MDD 12 tab, acetaminophen 4,000 mg
Ketoprofen 25 mg or 50 mg	12	Sig: 1 tablet every 6-8 hours as needed for pain; maximum daily dose 300 mg	Sig: 1 tab po q 6-8 h prn pain; MDD 300 mg
For moderate-to-severe pain (unresponsive to NSAIDs)			
Hydrocodone bitartrate 5 mg and acetaminophen 500 mg, 650 mg, or 750 mg	18	Sig: 1-2 tablets every 4-6 hours; maximum daily dose 5 tablets, acetaminophen 4,000 mg	Sig: 1-2 tab po q 4-6 h; MDD 5 tab, acetaminophen 4,000 mg
Oxycodone HCl 5 mg and acetaminophen 325 mg or 500 mg	18	Sig: 1-2 tablets every 6 hours; maximum daily dose 8 tablets, acetaminophen 4,000 mg	Sig: 1-2 tab po q 6 h; MDD 8 tab, acetaminophen 4,000 mg
For severe pain (unresponsive to opioid combinations)			
Hydromorphone HCl 2 mg	30	Sig: 1-2 tablets every 4-6 hours as needed for pain; maximum daily dose 8 tablets	Sig: 1-2 tab po q 4-6 h prn pain; MDD 8 tab

FOR INFECTIONS IN THE MOUTH AND ADJACENT TISSUES

DRUG	NUMBER	DIRECTIONS	ABBREVIATED DIRECTIONS
Penicillin V potassium 500 mg	30	Sig: 2 tablets at once, then 1 tablet every 6 hours until gone	Sig: 2 tabs po stat, then 1 tab po q 6 h until gone
Amoxicillin 500 mg	30	Sig: 1 capsule every 8 hours until gone	Sig: 1 cap po q 8 h until gone
Metronidazole 250 mg	28	Sig: 1 tablet every 6 hours until gone	Sig: 1 tab po q 6 h until gone
Clindamycin HCl 150 mg	28	Sig: 1 capsule every 6 hours until gone	Sig: 1 cap po q 6 h until gone
Erythromycin stearate 250 mg	30	Sig: 1 tablet every 6 hours until gone	Sig: 1 tab po q 6 h until gone
Doxycycline HCl 100 mg	15	Sig: 1 capsule twice on day one; 1 capsule once daily until gone	Sig: 1 cap po bid day one; 1 cap po d until gone
Tetracycline HCl 250 mg	40	Sig: 1 capsule every 6 hours until gone	Sig: 1 cap po q 6 h until gone
Cephalexin 250 mg	30	Sig: 1 capsule every 6 hours until gone	Sig: 1 cap po q 6 h until gone

FOR ORAL CANDIDIASIS

DRUG	NUMBER	DIRECTIONS	ABBREVIATED DIRECTIONS
Nystatin oral suspension 100,000 units/mL	480 mL	Sig: Rinse for 2 minutes and swallow one teaspoonful four times daily until symptoms disappear	Sig: 1 teaspoonful qid, rinse 2 min and swallow
Chlorhexidine 0.12%	16 oz	Sig: Rinse for 30 seconds and spit 0.5 oz twice a day until symptoms disappear	Sig: 0.5 oz bid, rinse 30 sec and spit
Clotrimazole troche 10 mg	70	Sig: Dissolve completely 1 troche by mouth five times daily until symptoms disappear	Sig: Dissolve completely 1 troche po 5 times d

FOR ANGULAR CHEILITIS (FUNGAL ETIOLOGY)

DRUG	NUMBER	DIRECTIONS	ABBREVIATED DIRECTIONS
Nystatin 100,000 units/g ointment	15-g tube	Sig: Apply to lesion 4 times a day until healing occurs	Sig: Apply to lesion qid until healing occurs
Nystatin 100,000 units/g and triamcinolone 0.1% ointment	15-g tube	Sig: Apply to lesion 2-3 times a day until healing occurs	Sig: Apply to lesion bid-tid until healing occurs

FOR MILD-TO-MODERATE LICHEN PLANUS, PEMPHIGUS VULGARIS, OR MUCOUS MEMBRANE PEMPHIGOID

DRUG	NUMBER	DIRECTIONS	ABBREVIATED DIRECTIONS
Fluocinonide gel 0.05%	15 g	Sig: Apply with cotton swab to affected areas twice daily	Sig: Apply c̄ cotton swab bid

FOR MILD ALLERGIC REACTIONS

DRUG	NUMBER	DIRECTIONS	ABBREVIATED DIRECTIONS
Diphenhydramine HCl 50 mg	30	Sig: 1 capsule every 6 hours as needed	Sig: 1 cap po q 6 h prn

FOR HERPETIC INFECTIONS

DRUG	NUMBER	DIRECTIONS	ABBREVIATED DIRECTIONS
Penciclovir 1% cream	2-g tube	Sig: Apply to affected area every 2 hours while awake	Sig: Apply q 2 h while awake
Valacyclovir 500 mg	8	Sig: 4 caplets every 12 hours for 1 day. Initiate dose within 2 hours of symptoms for best response.	Sig: 4 tabs po q 12 h for 1 day.

PRESCRIPTION ABBREVIATIONS

ABBREVIATION	TERM
ā	before
ac	before meals
bid	2 times a day
c̄, c	with
cap	capsule
d	day
gtt	drops
h	hour
hs, HS, hor som	at bedtime
non rep, nr, NR	do not repeat
pc	after eating
po	by mouth
prn	as needed
qh	each hour
qid	4 times a day
s̄, sine	without
sig	write on the label
ss, ss	one-half
stat	immediately
tab	tablet, caplet
tid	3 times a day

Drugs That May Cause Photosensitivity

B. Ellen Byrne, D.D.S., Ph.D.

Photosensitivity reactions may be caused by systemic or topical drugs, perfumes, cosmetics, or sunscreens. Even brief exposures to sunlight in warm or cold weather can cause intense cutaneous reactions in patients with drug-induced photosensitivity. Individual sensitivity varies widely.

The list below is not comprehensive and shows only representative brands of each generic. When in doubt, always check the specific product labeling.

SUGGESTED READING

Allen JE. Drug-induced photosensitivity. *Clin Pharm.* 1993;12:580-587.

Anderson PO, Knoben JE, Troutman WG. *Handbook of Clinical Drug Data* 1997-1998. 8th ed. New York: McGraw-Hill Professional Publishing; 1999.

Drugs that may cause photosensitivity. *Pharmacist's Letter* PHARM-FaxBACK document no. 120617. Available from: Pharmacist's Letter, 3120 W. March Lane., P.O. Box 8190, Stockton, CA 95208; or www.pharmacistsletter.com.

Moore DE. Drug-induced cutaneous photosensitivity: incidence, mechanism, prevention and management. *Drug Saf.* 2002;25:345-372.

Physicians' Desk Reference®. 63rd ed. Montvale, NJ: Physicians' Desk Reference Inc; 2009.

DRUGS THAT MAY CAUSE PHOTOSENSITIVITY

Generic	Brand
Acamprosate	Campral
Acetazolamide	Diamox
Acitretin	Soriatane
Acyclovir	Zovirax
Alendronate	Fosamax
Aliskiren/ hydrochlorothiazide	Tekturna HCT
Alitretinoin	Panretin
Almotriptan	Axert
Amiloride/ hydrochlorothiazide	
Aminolevulinic acid	Levulan Kerastick
Amiodarone	Cordarone, Pacerone
Amitriptyline	
Amitriptyline/ chlordiazepoxide	Limbitrol
Amitriptyline/ perphenazine	
Amlodipine/ atorvastatin	Caduet
Amoxapine	
Amphetamine aspartate/ amphetamine sulfate/ dextroamphetamine saccharate/ dextroamphetamine sulfate	Adderall XR
Anagrelide	Agrylin
Aripiprazole	Abilify
Atazanavir	Reyataz
Atenolol/ chlorthalidone	Tenoretic
Atorvastatin	Lipitor
Atovaquone/ proguanil	Malarone
Azithromycin	Zithromax

DRUGS THAT MAY CAUSE PHOTOSENSITIVITY

Generic	Brand
Benazepril	Lotensin
Benazepril/ hydrochlorothiazide	Lotensin HCT
Bendroflumethiazide/ nadolol	Corzide
Bexarotene	Targretin
Bismuth/ metronidazole/ tetracycline	Helidac
Bismuth subcitrate potassium/ metronidazole/ tetracycline	Pylera
Bisoprolol/ hydrochlorothiazide	Ziac
Brompheniramine/ dextromethorphan/ phenylephrine	Alacol DM
Brompheniramine/ dextromethorphan/ pseudoephedrine	
Bupropion	Wellbutrin, Wellbutrin SR, Wellbutrin XL, Zyban
Candesartan/ hydrochlorothiazide	Atacand HCT
Capecitabine	Xeloda
Captopril	Capoten
Captopril/ hydrochlorothiazide	Capozide
Carbamazepine	Carbatrol, Equetro, Tegretol, Tegretol-XR
Carvedilol	Coreg
Carvedilol phosphate	Coreg CR
Celecoxib	Celebrex
Cetirizine	Zyrtec
Cetirizine/ pseudoephedrine	Zyrtec-D
Cevimeline	Evoxac
Chlorhexidine gluconate	Hibistat
Chloroquine	Aralen
Chlorothiazide	Diuril
Chlorpheniramine/ phenylephrine	Rynatan
Chlorpromazine	
Chlorpropamide	
Chlorthalidone	Thalitone
Cidofovir	Vistide
Ciprofloxacin	Cipro, Cipro XR
Citalopram	Celexa
Clemastine	Tavist
Clindamycin phosphate	Clindagel
Clozapine	Clozaril, Fazaclo
Coagulation Factor IX (recombinant)	BeneFIX
Cromolyn sodium	Gastrocrom
Cyclobenzaprine	Flexeril
Cyproheptadine	
Dacarbazine	DTIC-Dome
Dantrolene	Dantrium
Demeclocycline	Declomycin
Desipramine	Norpramin
Diclofenac potassium	Cataflam
Diclofenac sodium	Voltaren
Diclofenac sodium/ misoprostol	Arthrotec
Diflunisal	
Dihydroergotamine	D.H.E. 45
Diltiazem	Cardizem, Tiazac
Diphenhydramine	Benadryl
Divalproex	Depakote
Doxepin	Sinequan
Doxycycline hyclate	Doryx, Periostat, Vibra-Tabs, Vibramycin
Doxycycline monohydrate	Monodox
Duloxetine	Cymbalta
Enalapril	Vasotec
Enalapril/ hydrochlorothiazide	Vaseretic
Enalaprilat (injection)	
Epirubicin	Ellence
Eprosartan mesylate/ hydrochlorothiazide	Teveten HCT
Erythromycin/ sulfisoxazole	
Escitalopram oxalate	Lexapro
Esomeprazole	Nexium
Estazolam	
Estradiol	Gynodiol, Estrogel
Eszopiclone	Lunesta
Ethionamide	
Etodolac	
Felbamate	Felbatol
Fenofibrate	Lofibra, Tricor, Triglide
Floxuridine	
Flucytosine	Ancobon
Fluorouracil	Efudex
Fluoxetine	Prozac, Sarafem
Fluoxetine/olanzapine	Symbyax
Fluphenazine	Prolixin
Flutamide	
Fluvastatin	Lescol, Lescol XL
Fluvoxamine	Luvox, Luvox CR
Fosinopril	Monopril
Fosphenytoin	Cerebyx
Furosemide	Lasix
Gabapentin	Neurontin
Gemfibrozil	Lopid
Gemifloxacin mesylate	Factive
Gentamicin	
Glatiramer acetate	Copaxone
Glimepiride	Amaryl
Glimepiride/ pioglitazone hydrochloride	Duetact
Glimepiride/ rosiglitazone maleate	Avandaryl
Glipizide	Glucotrol
Glyburide	DiaBeta, Glynase, Micronase

DRUGS THAT MAY CAUSE PHOTOSENSITIVITY

Generic	Brand
Glyburide/ metformin HCl	Glucovance
Griseofulvin	Grifulvin, Gris-PEG
Haloperidol	Haldol
Hexachlorophene	pHisoHex
Hydralazine/ hydrochlorothiazide	Hydra-zide
Hydrochlorothiazide	Microzide
Hydrochlorothiazide/ fosinopril	Monopril HCT
Hydrochlorothiazide/ irbesartan	Avalide
Hydrochlorothiazide/ lisinopril	Prinzide, Zestoretic
Hydrochlorothiazide/ methyldopa	
Hydroclorothiazide/ metoprolol tartrate	Lopressor HCT
Hydrochlorothiazide/ moexipril	Uniretic
Hydrochlorothiazide/ spironolactone	Aldactazide
Hydrochlorothiazide/ telmisartan	Micardis HCT
Hydrochlorothiazide/ triamterene	Dyazide, Maxzide
Hydrochlorothiazide/ valsartan	Diovan HCT
Hydroxocobalamin	Cyanokit Antidote
Hydroxychloroquine	Plaquenil
Hypericum perforatum	St. John's wort
Ibuprofen	Motrin
Imatinib Mesylate	Gleevec
Imipramine	Tofranil
Imiquimod	Aldara
Indapamide	
Interferon alfa-2b, recombinant	Intron A
Interferon alfa-n3 (human leukocyte derived)	Alferon-N
Interferon beta-1a	Avonex
Interferon beta-1b	Betaseron
Isocarboxazid	Marplan
Isoniazid/ pyrazinamide/ rifampin	Rifater
Isotretinoin	Accutane, Amnesteem
Itraconazole	Sporanox
Ketoprofen	
Lamotrigine	Lamictal
Leuprolide acetate	Lupron, Lupron Depot
Levamisole	Levamisole
Levofloxacin	Levaquin
Levofloxacin/ 5% dextrose	Levaquin Injection
Lisinopril	Prinivil, Zestril
Lomefloxacin	Maxaquin
Loratadine	Claritin
Loratadine/ pseudoephedrine	Claritin-D
Losartan	Cozaar
Losartan/ hydrochlorothiazide	Hyzaar
Lovastatin	Altoprev, Mevacor
Lovastatin/niacin	Advicor
Maprotiline	
Mefenamic acid	Ponstel
Meloxicam	Mobic
Mesalamine	Pentasa
Methazolamide	
Methotrexate	Trexall
Methoxsalen	Oxsoralen, Uvadex, 8-MOP
Methyclothiazide	Enduron
Metolazone	Mykrox, Zaroxolyn
Metoprolol succinate	Toprol-XL
Metoprolol tartrate	Lopressor
Minocycline	Dynacin, Minocin, Solodyn
Mirtazapine	Remeron
Moexipril	Univasc
Moxifloxacin	Avelox
Nabilone	Cesamet
Nabumetone	Relafen
Nalidixic acid	
Naproxen	Naprosyn, EC-Naprosyn
Naproxen sodium	Anaprox, Anaprox DS, Naprelan
Naratriptan	Amerge
Nefazodone	
Nifedipine	Adalat CC, Procardia
Nisoldipine	Sular
Norfloxacin	Noroxin
Nortriptyline	Pamelor
Ofloxacin	Floxin
Olanzapine	Zyprexa
Olmesartan medoxomil/ hydrochlorothiazide	Benicar HCT
Olsalazine	Dipentum
Omeprazole/ sodium bicarbonate	Zegerid
Oxaprozin	Daypro
Oxcarbazepine	Trileptal
Oxycodone	Roxicodone
Panitumumab	Vectibix
Pantoprazole	Protonix
Paroxetine hydrochloride	Paxil
Paroxetine mesylate	Pexeva
Pentosan polysulfate	Elmiron
Pentostatin	Nipent
Perphenazine	
Pilocarpine	Salagen
Piroxicam	Feldene
Polymyxin B sulfate/ trimethopim sulfate	Polytrim
Polythiazide	
Porfimer sodium	Photofrin
Pramipexole dihydrochloride	Mirapex
Pravastatin	Pravachol

DRUGS THAT MAY CAUSE PHOTOSENSITIVITY

Generic	Brand	Generic	Brand	Generic	Brand
Pregabalin	Lyrica	Selegiline	Eldepryl, Emsam	Tigecycline	Tygacil
Prochlorperazine	Compro	Sertraline	Zoloft	Tolazamide	
Promethazine	Phenergan	Sibutramine	Meridia	Tolbutamide	
Protriptyline	Vivactil	Sildenafil	Viagra	Topiramate	Topamax
Pyrimethamine/ sulfadoxine	Fansidar	Simvastatin	Zocor	Tretinoin	Avita, Retin-A
Pyrazinamide		Simvastatin/ ezetimibe	Vytorin	Triamcinolone acetonide	Azmacort Inhalation
Quetiapine	Seroquel	Sirolimus	Rapamune	Triamterene	Dyrenium
Quinapril	Accupril	Somatropin	Serostim	Trifluoperazine	
Quinapril/ hydrochlorothiazide	Accuretic	Sotalol	Betapace, Betapace AF	Trimipramine	Surmontil
Quinidine gluconate		Sulfamethoxazole/ trimethoprim	Bactrim, Septra	Valacyclovir	Valtrex
Quinidine sulfate		Sulfasalazine	Azulfidine	Valproate	Depacon
Quinine sulfate		Sulfisoxazole acetyl	Gantrisin Pediatric	Valproic acid	Depakene
Rabeprazole sodium	Aciphex	Sulindac	Clinoril	Vardenafil	Levitra
Ramipril	Altace	Sumatriptan	Imitrex	Varenicline tartrate	Chantix
Rasagiline mesylate	Azilect	Tacrolimus	Prograf, Protopic	Venlafaxine	Effexor, Effexor XR
Riluzole	Rilutek	Tazarotene	Tazorac	Verteporfin	Visudyne
Risperidone	Risperdal, Risperdal Consta	Tetracycline	Sumycin	Vinblastine	
Ritonavir	Norvir	Thalidomide	Thalomid	Voriconazole	Vfend
Rizatriptan	Maxalt, Maxalt-MLT	Thioridazine hydrochloride		Zalcitabine	Hivid
Ropinirole	Requip	Thiothixene	Navane	Zaleplon	Sonata
Rosuvastatin	Crestor	Tiagabine	Gabitril	Ziprasidone	Geodon
Ruta graveolens	Rue			Zolmitriptan	Zomig
Saquinavir mesylate	Invirase			Zolpidem	Ambien, Ambien CR

General Anesthetics

Inhalation and general anesthetics are used to induce and maintain general anesthesia.

Despite dentists' decreasing need to rely on general anesthesia, its use may be indicated for patients who:

- Are extremely anxious or fearful.
- Are mentally or physically challenged, or both.
- Are too young to cooperate with the dentist.
- Fail to respond to local anesthesia.
- Are undergoing stressful, traumatic procedures.

Selected agents have also been approved for use in providing sedation and analgesia for specific procedures that do not require general anesthesia. General anesthetics have a narrow margin of safety, and their administration must be individualized (titrated) according to the desired depth of anesthesia, the concomitant use of other medications, and the patient's physical condition, age, size, and body temperature.

The tables on the following pages provide dosing information and clinically significant drug interactions for general anesthetics.

PRESCRIBING INFORMATION FOR GENERAL ANESTHETICS

NAME	FORM/ STRENGTH	DOSAGE	WARNINGS/PRECAUTIONS & CONTRAINDICATIONS	ADVERSE EFFECTS†
Desflurane (Suprane)	**Liq:** 240mL	***Adults:*** Individualize dose. **MAC Values: 70 yrs:** 5.2% with oxygen 100% or 1.7% with 60% N_2O. **45 yrs:** 6% with oxygen 100% or 2.8% with 60% N_2O. **25 yrs:** 7.3% with oxygen 100% or 4% with 60% N_2O. **With Fentanyl or Midazolam: 31-65 yrs: No Fentanyl:** 6.3%. **With 3mcg/kg Fentanyl:** 3.1%. **With 6mcg/kg Fentanyl:** 2.3%. **No Midazolam:** 5.9%. **With Midazolam 25mcg/kg:** 4.9%. **With Midazolam 50mcg/kg:** 4.9%. **18-30 yrs: No Fentanyl:** 6.4%. **With Fentanyl 3mcg/kg:** 3.5%. **With Fentanyl 6mcg/kg:** 3%. **No Midazolam:** 6.9%. ***Pediatrics:*** Individualize dose. **MAC Values: 7 yrs:** 8.1% with oxygen 100%. **4 yrs:** 8.6% with oxygen 100%. **3 yrs:** 6.4% with 60% N_2O. **2 yrs:** 9.1% with oxygen 100%. **9 months:** 10% with oxygen 100% or 7.5% with 60% N_2O. **10 weeks:** 9.4% with oxygen 100%. **2 weeks:** 9.2% with oxygen 100%.	**W/P:** Rare increases in serum K^+ levels have resulted in cardiac arrhythmias and death in pediatric patients during post-op period. Not recommended for induction of general anesthesia via mask in infants or children. Dose-dependent decreases in BP. Concentrations >1 MAC may increase HR. Maintain normal hemodynamics with CAD; not for use as sole agent for anesthetic induction where increases in HR or BP are undesirable. Can react with dessicated CO_2 absorbents to produce CO and result in elevated carboxyhemoglobin. May cause sensitivity hepatitis in patients who have been sensitized by previous exposure to halogenated anesthetics. May trigger malignant hyperthermia. Dose-dependent increase in CSF pressure when administered to patients with intracranial space occupying lesions; administer at 0.8 MAC or less in conjunction with a barbiturate induction and hyperventilation. **Contra:** Known or suspected susceptibility to malignant hyperthermia. **P/N:** Category B, caution in nursing.	**Cough,** breath-holding, apnea, **laryngospasm,** oxyhemoglobin desaturation, **increased secretions, pharyngitis,** N/V, headache, bradycardia, HTN, nodal arrhythmia, tachycardia, conjunctivitis.
Etomidate (Amidate)	**Inj:** 2mg/mL	***Adults:*** **Range:** 0.2-0.6mg/kg IV. **Usual:** 0.3mg/kg IV, over 30 to 60 sec. ***Pediatrics:*** **>10 yrs: Range:** 0.2-0.6mg/kg IV. **Usual:** 0.3mg/kg IV, over 30 to 60 sec.	**W/P:** Not for prolonged infusion. Reduction of plasma cortisol and aldosterone concentrations have occurred; consider exogenous replacement during severely stressful conditions. **P/N:** Category C, caution in nursing.	Transient venous pain, transient skeletal muscle movements (myoclonus), hyper/hypoventilation, apnea of short duration, HTN, hypotension, tachycardia, bradycardia, N/V.
Isoflurane (Forane)	**Liq:** 100mL, 250mL	***Adults:*** **Induction:** 1.5-3%. **Maint:** 1-2.5% with concomitant N_2O or an additional 0.5-1% may be required when used with oxygen alone.	**W/P:** Hypotension and respiratory depression increase as anesthesia is deepened. Increased blood loss comparable to that seen with halothane reported in patients undergoing abortions. May cause a reversible rise in CSF pressure. May cause sensitivity hepatitis in patients sensitized by previous exposure to halogenated anesthetics. Use of inhaled anesthetics has been associated with rare increases in serum K^+ levels that have resulted in cardiac arrhythmias and death in pediatric patients during postoperative period. May trigger malignant hyperthermia in susceptible patients. Maintenance of normal hemodynamics is important to avoid myocardial ischemia in patients with coronary artery disease. Can react with dessicated CO_2 absorbents to produce CO, which may result in elevated levels of carboxyhemoglobin. **Contra:** Genetic susceptibility to malignant hyperthermia. **P/N:** Category C, caution in nursing.	Respiratory depression, hypotension, arrhythmias, shivering, N/V, ileus, transient elevations in WBC, perioperative hyperkalemia, post-op hepatic dysfunction and hepatitis, hepatic failure, hepatic necrosis.

†Bold entries denote special dental considerations.
BB = black box warning; **W/P** = warnings/precautions; **Contra** = contraindications; **P/N** = pregnancy category rating and nursing considerations.

PRESCRIBING INFORMATION FOR GENERAL ANESTHETICS *(cont.)*

NAME	FORM/ STRENGTH	DOSAGE	WARNINGS/PRECAUTIONS & CONTRAINDICATIONS	ADVERSE EFFECTS†
Ketamine HCl (Ketalar)	**Inj:** 10mg/mL, 50mg/mL, 100mg/mL	***Adults:*** **Initial: IV:** 1-4.5mg/kg (0.5-2 mg/lb). **Alternate: IV:** 1-2mg/kg at a rate of 0.5mg/kg/min. May administer with 2-5mg doses of diazepam over 60 sec. **IM:** 6.5-13 mg/kg (3-6mg/lb). **Maint:** Adjust according to anesthetic needs. May increase in increments of 1/2 to full induction dose.	**W/P:** Monitor cardiac function with HTN or cardiac decompensation. Post-op confusional states may occur during recovery. Emergence reactions reported; incidence may be reduced if verbal and tactile stimulation is minimized during recovery period; does not preclude monitoring of vital signs. Respiratory depression may occur with overdosage or too rapid a rate of administration; maintain airway and respiration. Do not use alone in pharynx, larynx, or bronchial tree procedures. Caution in chronic alcoholics and acutely intoxicated patients. May increase CSF pressure; use with extreme caution with preanesthetic cerebrospinal fluid pressure. In surgical procedures involving visceral pain, supplement with agent that obtunds visceral pain. **Contra:** Patients in whom a significant elevation in blood pressure would constitute a serious hazard. **P/N:** Not recommended during pregnancy, safety in nursing not known.	N/V, anorexia, elevated BP and pulse, hypotension, bradycardia, arrhythmia, respiratory depression, airway obstruction, diplopia, nystagmus, slight elevation of IOP, enhanced skeletal muscle tone, anaphylaxis.
Methohexital Sodium (Brevital Sodium)	**Inj:** 500mg, 2.5g	***Adults:*** Individualize dose. **IV: Induction: Usual:** 1-1.5mg/kg IV of 1% sol at 1mL/5 sec. **Range:** 50-120mg IV or more (average: 70mg). **Maint: Intermittent:** 20-40mg IV (2 to 4mL of 1% sol) q 4-7 min. **Continuous Drip:** 0.2% sol at 3mL/min (1 drop/sec). ***Pediatrics:*** **≥1 month:** Individualize dose. **IM: Induction: Usual:** 6.6-10mg/kg IM of 5% sol. **PR: Usual:** 25mg/kg rectally of 1% sol.	**BB:** Use only in hospital or ambulatory care settings that provide for continuous monitoring of respiratory and cardiac function. Ensure immediate availability of resuscitative drugs and age-/size-appropriate equipment for bag/valve/mask ventilation and intubation and personnel trained in their use and skilled in airway management. For deeply sedated patients, a designated individual other than the practitioner performing the procedure should be present to continuously monitor the patient. **W/P:** Caution apnea/hypoventilation, laryngospasm during induction. Cardiorespiratory arrest may occur. Seizures may be elicited with previous history of convulsive activity. Prolonged administration may result in cumulative effects. If extravasation is noted during injection, d/c until situation is remedied. All routes of administration associated with hiccups, coughing, and/or muscle twitching, which may also impair pulmonary ventilation. Following induction, temporary hypotension and tachycardia may occur. Caution in severe hepatic dysfunction, severe cardiovascular instability, shock-like condition, asthma, COPD, severe HTN or hypotension, MI, CHF, severe anemia, status asthmaticus, extreme obesity, debilitated patients or those with impaired function of respiratory, circulatory, renal, hepatic, or endocrine system. Unintended intra-arterial injection may produce platelet aggregates and thrombosis at site of injection. **Contra:** Patients with latent or manifest porphyria. **P/N:** Category B, caution in nursing.	Circulatory depression, thrombophlebitis, hypotension, tachycardia, respiratory depression, cardiopulmonary arrest, **laryngospasm,** skeletal muscle hypersensitivity (twitching), injury to nerves adjacent to injection site, seizures, delirium, restlessness, nausea, erythema, anaphylaxis.

†Bold entries denote special dental considerations.
BB = black box warning; **W/P** = warnings/precautions; **Contra** = contraindications; **P/N** = pregnancy category rating and nursing considerations.

NAME	FORM/ STRENGTH	DOSAGE	WARNINGS/PRECAUTIONS & CONTRAINDICATIONS	ADVERSE EFFECTS†
Propofol (Diprivan)	**Inj:** 10mg/mL	***Adults:* General Anesthesia: <55 yrs:** 40mg IV q 10 sec until induction onset (2-2.5mg/kg). **Maint:** 100-200µg/kg/min IV (6-12mg/kg/hr) or 20-50mg intermittently by IV bolus prn. **Elderly/ Debilitated/ASA-PS III & IV:** 20mg IV q 10 sec until induction onset (1-1.5mg/kg). **Maint:** 50-100µg/kg/min IV (3-6mg/kg/hr). **Cardiac Anesthesia:** 20mg IV q 10 sec until induction onset (0.5-1.5mg/kg). **Maint:** 100-150µg/kg/min IV with secondary opioid or 50-100µg/kg/min IV with primary opioid. **Neurosurgical Patients:** 20mg IV q 10 sec until induction onset (1-2mg/kg). **Maint:** 100-200µg/kg/min IV (6-12 mg/kg/hr). **MAC Sedation: <55 yrs:** 100-150µg/kg/min (6-9mg/kg/hr) IV infusion or 0.5mg/kg slow IV injection over 3-5 min followed immediately by maintenance infusion. **Maint:** 25-75µg/kg/min (1.5-4.5mg/kg/hr) IV infusion or 10-20mg incremental IV boluses. **Elderly/Debilitated/ASA-PS III & IV:** Use doses similar to healthy adults. Avoid rapid boluses. **Maint:** 80% of the usual adult dose. **ICU Sedation: Initial:** 5µg/kg/min (0.3mg/kg/hr) IV infusion for 5 min. Increase 5-10µg/kg/min (0.3-0.6mg/kg/hr) IV over 5-10 min. **Maint:** 5-50µg/kg/min IV (0.3-3mg/kg/hr) or higher may be required. ***Pediatrics:* 3-16 yrs: General Anesthesia:** 2.5-3.5mg/kg IV over 20-30 sec. **Maint: 2 months-16 yrs:** 125-300µg/kg/min IV (7.5-18mg/kg/hr). Following first half hour of maintenance, if clinical signs of light anesthesia are not present, infusion rate should be decreased.	**W/P:** Avoid rapid bolus administration in elderly, debilitated, or ASA-PS III/IV patients. Monitor oxygen saturation and for signs of significant hypotension, bradycardia, cardiovascular depression, apnea or airway obstruction. Avoid abrupt d/c. Caution with hyperlipoproteinemia, diabetic hyperlipemia, pancreatitis, epilepsy. Rare reports of anaphylaxis, post-op unconsciousness with possible increase in muscle tone, pulmonary edema, perioperative myoclonia, post-op pancreatitis, venous sequelae. Reports of bradycardia, asystole, and rarely, cardiac arrest. Use for adult and pediatric ICU sedation has been associated with propofol infusion syndrome, a constellation of metabolic derangements and organ system failures. Reports in which failure to use aseptic techniques with handling has resulted in microbial contamination and fever, infection, sepsis, other life-threatening illnesses, and death. Minimize transient local pain by using larger veins of forearm or antecubital fossa and/or prior lidocaine injection. May elevate serum TG. Do not infuse for >5 days without drug holiday to replace zinc losses; consider supplemental zinc with chronic use in those predisposed to zinc deficiency. In renal impairment, perform baseline urinalysis/urinary sediment, then monitor on alternate days during sedation. (Neurosurgical Anesthesia) Use infusion or slow bolus to avoid significant hypotension and decreases in cerebral perfusion pressure. (Cardiac Anesthesia) Use slower rates of administration in premedicated and geriatric patients, patients with recent fluid shifts or those hemodynamically unstable. Correct fluid deficits prior to use. **Contra:** Patients with allergy to eggs, egg products, soybeans, or soy products. **P/N:** Category B, not for use in nursing.	Bradycardia, arrhythmia, hypotension, HTN, tachycardia nodal, decreased cardiac output, CNS movement, injection site burning/stinging/pain, hyperlipemia, apnea, rash, pruritus, respiratory acidosis during weaning.
Sevoflurane (Ultane)	**Liq:** 250mL	***Adults:*** Individualize dose. **MAC Values: 80 yrs:** 1.4% sevoflurane in oxygen or 0.7% sevoflurane in 65% N_2O/35% oxygen. **60 yrs:** 1.7% sevoflurane in oxygen or 0.9% sevoflurane in 65% N_2O/35% oxygen. **40 yrs:** 2.1% sevoflurane in oxygen or 1.1% sevoflurane in 65% N_2O/35% oxygen. **25 yrs:** 2.6% sevoflurane in oxygen or 1.4% sevoflurane in 65% N_2O/35% oxygen. ***Pediatrics:*** Individualize dose. **MAC Values: 3-12 yrs:** 2.5% sevoflurane in oxygen. **6 months-<3 yrs:** 2.8% sevoflurane in oxygen or 2% sevoflurane in 65% N_2O/35% oxygen. **1-<6 months:** 3% sevoflurane in oxygen. **0-1 month:** 3.3% sevoflurane in oxygen.	**W/P:** Potential for renal injury. May be associated with glycosuria and proteinuria when used for long procedures at low flow rates. May cause malignant hyperthermia. Use has been associated with rare increases in serum K^+ levels that have resulted in cardiac arrhythmias and death in pediatric patients during post-op period. May decrease BP. Rare cases of seizures have been reported. Transient changes in post-op LFTs and very rare cases of post-op hepatic dysfunction or hepatitis with or without jaundice reported. Concomitant use of desiccated CO_2 absorbents, specifically those containing KOH, may result in rare cases of extreme heat, smoke, and/or spontaneous fire in anesthesia breathing circuit; replace CO_2 absorbent routinely. **Contra:** Known or suspected susceptibility to malignant hyperthermia. **P/N:** Category B, caution in nursing.	Bradycardia, hypotension, agitation, **laryngospasm,** airway obstruction, breath holding, **cough,** tachycardia, shivering, somnolence, dizziness, **increased salivation,** N/V.

PRESCRIBING INFORMATION FOR GENERAL ANESTHETICS *(cont.)*

NAME	FORM/ STRENGTH	DOSAGE	WARNINGS/PRECAUTIONS & CONTRAINDICATIONS	ADVERSE EFFECTS†
Thiopental Sodium (Pentothal)	**Inj:** 20mg/mL, 25mg/mL	***Adults:*** Individualize dose. **IV: Test Dose:** 25-75mg. **Anesthesia:** 50-75mg at 20-40 sec intervals. Once anesthesia is established, additional injections of 25-50mg may be given whenever patient moves. **Induction in Balanced Anesthesia: Initial:** 3-4mg/kg. **Convulsive States:** Following anesthesia, give 75-125mg as soon as possible after convulsion begins. Convulsions following use of local anesthetic may require 125-250mg over 10 minute period. **Neurosurgical Patients With Increased Intracranial Pressure:** Intermittent bolus of 1.5-3.5mg/kg. **Psychiatric Disorders:** After test dose, infuse at 100mg/min with patient counting backwards from 100; d/c shortly after counting becomes confused but before actual sleep is produced.	**W/P:** Avoid extravasation or intra-arterial injection. May be habit forming. If used in conditions involving relative contraindications, reduce dosage and administer slowly. Caution with advanced cardiac disease, increased ICP, ophthalmoplegia plus, asthma, myasthenia gravis, and endocrine insufficiency (pituitary, thyroid, adrenal, pancreas). **Contra:** (Absolute) Absence of suitable veins for IV administration, variegate porphyria (eg, South African) or acute intermittent porphyria. (Relative) Severe cardiovascular disease, hypotension, shock, conditions in which the hypnotic effect may be prolonged or potentiated (eg, excessive premedication, Addison's disease, hepatic/renal dysfunction, myxedema, increased blood urea, severe anemia, asthma, and myasthenia gravis), and status asthmaticus. **P/N:** Category C, caution in nursing.	Respiratory/ myocardial depression, cardiac arrhythmias, prolonged somnolence and recovery, sneezing, **cough,** bronchospasm, **laryngospasm,** shivering, anaphylactic/anaphylactoid reactions.

†Bold entries denote special dental considerations.
BB = black box warning; **W/P** = warnings/precautions; **Contra** = contraindications; **P/N** = pregnancy category rating and nursing considerations.

DRUG INTERACTIONS FOR GENERAL ANESTHETICS

Desflurane (Suprane)	
Benzodiazepines	Decreased minimum alveolar concentration (MAC) with benzodiazepines.
Neuromuscular blockers	May decrease the required dose of neuromuscular blocking agents during maintenance anesthesia.
Opioids	Decreased MAC with opioids.
Isoflurane (Forane)	
Muscle relaxants	May potentiate the muscle relaxant effect of all muscle relaxants, most notably nondepolarizing muscle relaxants.
Nitrous oxide	Decreased MAC of isoflurane.
Ketamine HCl (Ketalar)	
Barbiturates	Prolonged recovery time may occur with concurrent use of barbiturates and/or narcotics.
Opioids	Prolonged recovery time may occur with concurrent use of barbiturates and/or opioids.
Methohexital Sodium (Brevital Sodium)	
Anticoagulants	May influence the metabolism of other concomitantly used drugs, such as anticoagulants.
Barbiturates	Prior chronic administration of barbiturates may reduce the effectiveness of methohexital.
Corticosteroids	May influence the metabolism of other concomitantly used drugs, such as corticosteroids.
Ethyl alcohol	May influence the metabolism of other concomitantly used drugs, such as ethyl alcohol. Additive CNS effects may occur with concomitant use of other CNS depressants including ethyl alcohol and propylene glycol.
Halothane	May influence the metabolism of other concomitantly used drugs, such as halothane.
Phenytoin	May influence the metabolism of other concomitantly used drugs, such as phenytoin. Prior chronic administration of phenytoin may reduce the effectiveness of methohexital.
Propylene glycol	May influence the metabolism of solutions containing propylene glycol. Additive CNS effects may occur with concomitant use of other CNS depressants including ethyl alcohol and propylene glycol.

DRUG INTERACTIONS FOR GENERAL ANESTHETICS *(cont.)*

Propofol (Diprivan)	
Fentanyl	May increase the anesthetic or sedative effects of propofol and may also result in more pronounced decreases in systolic, diastolic, and mean arterial pressures and cardiac output. Concomitant use with fentanyl may cause serious bradycardia in pediatric patients.
Inhalation agents	Increased anesthetic or sedative and cardiorespiratory effects of propofol can be expected with concurrent administration of potent inhalational agents (eg, isoflurane, sevoflurane)
Opioids	Concomitant use with opioids (eg, morphine, meperidine, fentanyl) may increase the anesthetic or sedative effects of propofol and may also result in more pronounced decreases in systolic, diastolic, and mean arterial pressures and cardiac output.
Sedatives/opioids	Concomitant use with combinations of opioids and sedatives (eg, benzodiazepines, barbiturates, chloral hydrate, droperidol) may increase the anesthetic or sedative effects of propofol and may also result in more pronounced decreases in systolic, diastolic, and mean arterial pressures and cardiac output.
Sevoflurane (Ultane)	
Benzodiazepines	May decrease MAC of sevoflurane when concomitantly used with opioids.
Muscle relaxants	May increase both the intensity and duration of neuromuscular blockade induced by nondepolarizing muscle relaxants.
Nitrous oxide	Decreased MAC of sevoflurane.
Opioids	May decrease MAC of sevoflurane when concomitantly used with benzodiazepines.
Thiopental Sodium (Pentothal)	
Aminophylline	May cause thiopental antagonism.
Diazoxide	Hypotension may occur.
Midazolam	Synergism may occur.
Opioid analgesics	May cause decreased antinociceptive action.
Probenecid	May prolong the action of thiopental.

Therapeutics in Renal and Hepatic Disease

The dosage of many drugs that are normally cleared by the kidneys or liver must be adjusted in patients with renal or liver disease. If such adjustments are not made, drug accumulation and toxicity are likely to occur. The goal of therapy in a patient with renal impairment is to achieve unbound drug serum concentrations similar to those that have been associated with optimal response in patients with normal renal function. In renal disease, creatinine serves as an endogenous marker to predict the clearance of renally eliminated drugs (abbreviated in clinical tests as CrCl). Drug dosage adjustments for hepatically eliminated drugs in patients with liver disease or dysfunction are difficult to predict due to the complexity of hepatic metabolism. Unfortunately, there are no reliable endogenous markers to accurately predict a drug's hepatic clearance in patients with liver dysfunction. Because of this, unnecessary and potentially hepatotoxic medications are best avoided.

The following table lists drugs that often require dosage adjustments in patients with renal or hepatic impairment. For specific dosing information, refer to the index for page numbers of the prescribing tables where a drug may be found, or see the manufacturer's labeling.

DRUGS REQUIRING DOSAGE ADJUSTMENTS DUE TO RENAL OR HEPATIC DYSFUNCTION

GENERIC NAME (BRAND NAME)		
Abacavir/Lamivudine (Epzicom)	Allopurinol (Aloprim, Zyloprim)	Amoxicillin (Amoxil, Trimox)
Abacavir/Lamivudine/Zidovudine (Trizivir)	Almotriptan (Axert)	Amoxicillin/Clarithromycin/Lansoprazole (Prevpac)
Acarbose (Precose)	Alprazolam (Niravam, Xanax, Xanax XR)	Amoxicillin/Clavulanate (Augmentin, Augmentin ES-600)
Acebutolol (Sectral)	Amantadine (Symmetrel)	Amphotericin B (Abelcet, Ambisome, Amphotec, Fungizone)
Acetohydroxamic Acid (Lithostat)	Amifostine (Ethyol)	Ampicillin/Sulbactam (Unasyn)
Acyclovir (Zovirax)	Amikacin (Amikin)	Amprenavir
Adefovir Dipivoxil (Hepsera)	Aminophylline	Anagrelide (Agrylin)
Alendronate (Fosamax)	Amlodipine (Norvasc)	Apomorphine (Apokyn)
Alendronate/Cholecalciferol (Fosamax Plus D)	Amlodipine/Atorvastatin (Caduet)	Argatroban
Alfuzosin (Uroxatral)	Amlodipine/Benazepril (Lotrel)	
	Amobarbital (Amytal)	

DRUGS REQUIRING DOSAGE ADJUSTMENTS DUE TO RENAL OR HEPATIC DYSFUNCTION

GENERIC NAME (BRAND NAME) *(Cont.)*

Armodafinil (Nuvigil)
Arsenic Trioxide (Trisenox)
Aspirin (Bayer Aspirin, Ecotrin)
Atazanavir (Reyataz)
Atenolol (Tenormin)
Atenolol/Chlorthalidone (Tenoretic)
Atomoxetine (Strattera)
Atovaquone/Proguanil (Malarone)
Atropine/Hyoscyamine/Phenobarbital/Scopolamine (Donnatal)
Azacitidine (Vidaza)
Azathioprine (Azasan, Imuran)
Aztreonam (Azactam)
Baclofen (Kemstro)
Benazepril (Lotensin)
Benazepril/HCTZ (Lotensin HCT)
Betaxolol
Bisoprolol (Zebeta)
Bisoprolol/HCTZ (Ziac)
Bivalirudin (Angiomax)
Bupivacaine (Marcaine, Sensorcaine)
Bupivacaine/Epinephrine (Marcaine w/ Epinephrine, Sensorcaine w/ Epinephrine)
Buprenorphine (Subutex)
Buprenorphine/Naloxone (Suboxone)
Bupropion (Aplenzin, Wellbutrin SR, Wellbutrin XL, Zyban)
Butabarbital (Butisol)
Butorphanol (Stadol)
Candesartan (Atacand)
Candesartan/HCTZ (Atacand HCT)
Capecitabine (Xeloda)
Capreomycin (Capastat)
Captopril (Capoten)
Captopril/HCTZ (Capozide)
Carbamazepine (Carbatrol, Equetro, Tegretol, Tegretol XR)
Carboplatin (Paraplatin)
Carteolol
Caspofungin (Cancidas)
Cefadroxil
Cefazolin
Cefdinir (Omnicef)
Cefditoren Pivoxil (Spectracef)
Cefepime (Maxipime)
Cefixime (Suprax)
Cefoperazone (Cefobid)
Cefotaxime (Claforan)
Cefotetan
Cefoxitin (Mefoxin)
Cefpodoxime Proxetil (Vantin)
Ceftazidime (Fortaz, Tazicef)
Ceftibuten (Cedax)
Ceftizoxime
Ceftriaxone (Rocephin)
Cefuroxime (Ceftin, Zinacef)
Celecoxib (Celebrex)
Cetirizine (Zyrtec)
Cetirizine/Pseudoephedrine (Zyrtec-D)
Chloroprocaine
Chlorpropamide (Diabinese)
Choline Magnesium Trisalicylate (Trilisate)
Cidofovir (Vistide)
Cimetidine (Tagamet)
Ciprofloxacin (Cipro)
Cisplatin (Platinol-AQ)
Citalopram (Celexa)
Cladribine (Leustatin)
Clarithromycin (Biaxin, Biaxin-XL)
Clonidine (Catapres, Catapres-TTS)
Colchicine
Colchicine/Probenecid
Cromolyn (Intal)
Cyclobenzaprine (Amrix, Flexeril)
Cyclosporine (Gengraf, Neoral, Restasis, Sandimmune, Seromycin)
Dacarbazine (DTIC-Dome)
Dalfopristin/Quinupristin (Synercid)
Dalteparin (Fragmin)
Dantrolene (Dantrium)
Daptomycin (Cubicin)
Darifenacin (Enablex)
Daunorubicin (Cerubidine)
Daunorubicin Citrate Liposome (DaunoXome)
Decitabine (Dacogen)
Demeclocycline (Declomycin)
Desloratadine (Clarinex, Clarinex RediTabs, Clarinex Syrup)
Desloratadine/Pseudoephedrine (Clarinex D)
Desvenlafaxine (Pristiq)
Dexrazoxane (Totec, Zinecard)
Didanosine (Videx, Videx EC)
Digoxin (Lanoxin)
Dipyridamole/ASA (Aggrenox)
Disopyramide (Norpace)
Divalproex (Depakote)
Docetaxel (Taxotere)
Dofetilide (Tikosyn)
Doripenem (Doribax)
Doxorubicin (Doxil)
Duloxetine (Cymbalta)

DRUGS REQUIRING DOSAGE ADJUSTMENTS DUE TO RENAL OR HEPATIC DYSFUNCTION

GENERIC NAME (BRAND NAME) *(Cont.)*

Dyphylline (Lufyllin)
Efavirenz/Emtricitabine/Tenofovir Disoproxil (Atripla)
Eletriptan (Relpax)
Emtricitabine (Emtriva)
Emtricitabine/Tenofovir Disoproxil (Truvada)
Enalapril (Vasotec)
Enalapril/Felodipine (Lexxel)
Enalapril/HCTZ (Vaseretic)
Enalaprilat (Vasotec IV)
Enoxaparin (Lovenox)
Entecavir (Baraclude)
Epirubicin (Ellence)
Eplerenone (Inspra)
Eprosartan (Teveten)
Eprosartan/HCTZ (Teveten HCT)
Eptifibatide (Integrilin)
Ertapenem (Invanz)
Escitalopram (Lexapro)
Esomeprazole (Nexium)
Eszopiclone (Lunesta)
Ethambutol (Myambutol)
Etoposide (Etopophos)
Exenatide (Byetta)
Ezetimibe/Simvastatin (Vytorin)
Famciclovir (Famvir)
Famotidine (Pepcid)
Felbamate (Felbatol)
Felodipine (Plendil)
Fenofibrate (Antara, Lofibra, Tricor, Triglide)
Fexofenadine (Allegra)
Fexofenadine/Pseudoephedrine (Allegra-D)
Flecainide Acetate (Tambocor)
Fluconazole (Diflucan)
Flucytosine (Ancobon)
Fludarabine (Fludara)
Fluoxetine (Prozac, Sarafem)
Fluoxetine/Olanzapine (Symbyax)
Flurbiprofen (Ansaid)
Flutamide
Fluvastatin (Lescol, Lescol XL)
Fluvoxamine (Luvox)
Fondaparinux (Arixtra)
Fosamprenavir (Lexiva)
Foscarnet (Foscavir)
Fosinopril (Monopril)
Fosinopril/HCTZ (Monopril HCT)
Fosphenytoin (Cerebyx)
Gabapentin (Neurontin)
Galantamine (Razadyne)
Gallium (Ganite)
Ganciclovir (Cytovene)
Gemfibrozil (Lopid)
Gemifloxacin (Factive)
Gentamicin
Glimepiride (Amaryl)
Glipizide (Glucotrol, Glucotrol XL)
Glipizide/Metformin (Metaglip)
Glyburide (DiaBeta, Glynase PresTab, Micronase)
Glyburide/Metformin (Glucovance)
Hydroxyurea (Hydrea)
Ibandronate (Boniva)
Ibuprofen (Advil, Caldolor, Cap-Profen, IBU-Tab, Motrin, Profen)
Idarubicin (Idamycin PFS)
Imatinib (Gleevec)
Imipenem/Cilastatin (Primaxin IV)
Immune Globulin Intravenous, Human (Sandoglobulin I.V.)
Indinavir (Crixivan)
Insulin Detemir, rDNA (Levemir)
Interferon beta-1a (Rebif)
Irbesartan/HCTZ (Avalide)
Ixabepilone (Ixempra)
Ketoprofen
Ketorolac Tromethamine (Toradol)
Lamivudine (Epivir)
Lamivudine/Zidovudine (Combivir)
Lamotrigine (Lamictal, Lamictal CD)
Lansoprazole (Prevacid, Prevacid I.V., Prevacid SoluTab)
Lansoprazole/Naproxen (Prevacid NapraPAC)
Leflunomide (Arava)
Lepirudin (Refludan)
Letrozole (Femara)
Levetiracetam (Keppra)
Levocetirizine (Xyzal)
Levofloxacin (Levaquin)
Lisinopril (Prinivil, Zestril)
Lisinopril/HCTZ (Prinzide, Zestoretic)
Lomefloxacin (Maxaquin)
Loratadine (Claritin)
Loratadine/Pseudoephedrine (Claritin-D)
Losartan (Cozaar)
Losartan/HCTZ (Hyzaar)
Lovastatin (Altoprev, Mevacor)
Lovastatin/Niacin (Advicor)
Lymphocyte Immune Globulin, Anti-thymocyte Globulin (equine) (Atgam)
Maraviroc (Selzentry)
Melphalan (Alkeran)

DRUGS REQUIRING DOSAGE ADJUSTMENTS DUE TO RENAL OR HEPATIC DYSFUNCTION

GENERIC NAME (BRAND NAME) *(Cont.)*

Memantine (Namenda)
Meperidine (Demerol)
Meperidine/Promethazine
Mephobarbital (Mebaral)
Mercaptopurine (Purinethol)
Meropenem (Merrem)
Metformin (Fortamet, Glucophage, Glucophage XR, Glumetza, Riomet)
Methyldopa
Methyldopate
Methylnaltrexone (Relistor)
Metoclopramide (Reglan)
Metolazone (Zaroxolyn)
Metronidazole (Flagyl, Flagyl ER)
Mexiletine
Midodrine (ProAmatine)
Miglitol (Glyset)
Milrinone (Primacor)
Minocycline (Arestin, Dynacin, Minocin, Solodyn)
Minoxidil
Modafinil (Provigil)
Moexipril (Univasc)
Morphine (Astramorph-PF, Avinza, Depodur, Infumorph, Kadian, MS-Contin, Oramorph-SR, Roxanol)
Mycophenolate (CellCept, Myfortic)
Nadolol (Corgard)
Nadolol/Bendroflumethiazide (Corzide)
Naloxone
Naratriptan (Amerge)
Nebivolol (Bystolic)
Nefazodone
Nevirapine (Viramune)
Niacin (Niacor)
Niacin/Simvastatin (Simcor)
Nicardipine (Cardene, Cardene SR)
Nilotinib (Tasigna)
Nimodipine
Nisoldipine (Sular)
Nitrofurantoin (Furadantin)
Nitrofurantoin, Macrocrystals (Macrobid, Macrodantin)
Nizatidine (Axid)
Norethindrone Acetate (Aygestin)
Norfloxacin (Noroxin)
Octreotide (Sandostatin LAR)
Ofloxacin (Floxin,Floxin IV)
Olmesartan (Benicar)
Olmesartan/HCTZ (Benicar HCT)
Ondansetron (Zofran)
Oseltamivir (Tamiflu)
Oxaprozin (Daypro)
Oxcarbazepine (Trileptal)
Oxymorphone (Opana, Opana ER)
Paliperidone (Invega)
Pamidronate (Aredia)
Paroxetine (Paxil, Paxil CR, Pexeva)
Peginterferon alfa-2a (Pegasys)
Pemetrexed (Alimta)
Penicillamine (Cuprimine, Depen)
Penicillin G (Pfizerpen)
Pentobarbital (Nembutal)
Pentostatin (Nipent)
Perindopril (Aceon)
Phenobarbital
Pioglitazone (Actos)
Pioglitazone/Glimepiride (Duetact)
Pioglitazone/Metformin (Actoplus Met)
Piperacillin
Piperacillin/Tazobactam (Zosyn)
Pramipexole (Mirapex)
Pravastatin (Pravachol)
Prazosin (Minipress)
Prazosin/Polythiazide (Minizide)
Pregabalin (Lyrica)
Probenecid
Probenecid/Colchicine
Procainamide
Propafenone (Rythmol, Rythmol SR)
Propofol (Diprivan)
Propoxyphene (Darvon)
Propoxyphene/Caffeine/ASA
Propoxyphene Napsylate (Darvon-N)
Propoxyphene/Acetaminophen (Darocet-N, DarvocetA500)
Quetiapine (Seroquel, Seroquel-XR)
Quinapril (Accupril)
Quinapril/HCTZ (Accuretic, Quinaretic)
Quinidine
Ramelteon (Rozerem)
Ramipril (Altace)
Ranitidine (Zantac)
Ranolazine (Ranexa)
Rasagiline (Azilect)
Repaglinide (Prandin)
Repaglinide/Metformin (Prandimet)
Ribavirin (Copegus, Rebetol)
Rifabutin (Mycobutin)
Rimantadine (Flumadine)

DRUGS REQUIRING DOSAGE ADJUSTMENTS DUE TO RENAL OR HEPATIC DYSFUNCTION

GENERIC NAME (BRAND NAME) *(Cont.)*

Risedronate (Actonel)
Risedronate/Calcium (Actonel with Calcium)
Risperidone (Risperdal, Risperdal Consta, Risperdal M-Tab)
Rosiglitazone (Avandia)
Rosiglitazone/Glimepiride (Avandaryl)
Rosiglitazone/Metformin (Avandamet)
Rosuvastatin (Crestor)
Secobarbital (Seconal Sodium)
Sertraline (Zoloft)
Sibutramine (Meridia)
Sildenafil (Revatio, Viagra)
Simvastatin (Zocor)
Sirolimus (Rapamune)
Sitagliptin (Januvia)
Sitagliptin/Metformin (Janumet)
Sodium Oxybate (Xyrem)
Solifenacin (VESIcare)
Sotalol (Betapace AF)
Stavudine (Zerit)
Streptozocin (Zanosar)
Sumatriptan (Imitrex)
Sumatriptan/Naproxen (Treximet)
Tacrine (Cognex)
Tacrolimus (Prograf)
Tadalafil (Cialis)
Telbivudine (Tyzeka)
Telithromycin (Ketek)
Telmisartan (Micardis)
Telmisartan/HCTZ (Micardis HCT)
Teniposide (Vumon)
Tetracycline (Sumycin)
Theophylline (Theo-24, Theochron, Theolair, Uniphyl)
Ticarcillin/Clavulanate (Timentin)
Ticlopidine (Ticlid)
Tigecycline (Tygacil)
Tinidazole (Tindamax)
Tipranavir (Aptivus)
Tirofiban (Aggrastat)
Tobramycin (TOBI)
Tocainide
Tolazamide
Tolbutamide
Tolterodine (Detrol, Detrol LA)
Topiramate (Topamax)
Topotecan (Hycamtin)
Torsemide (Demadex)
Tramadol (Ultram, Ultram ER)
Tramadol/APAP (Ultracet)
Trandolapril (Mavik)
Trandolapril/Verapamil (Tarka)
Trimethoprim/Sulfamethoxazole (Bactrim, Bactrim DS, Septra, Septra DS, Sulfatrim Pediatric)
Trospium (Sanctura)
Valacyclovir (Valtrex)
Valganciclovir (Valcyte)
Valproate (Depacon, Depakene)
Valsartan (Diovan)
Valsartan/HCTZ (Diovan HCT)
Vancomycin (Vancocin)
Vardenafil (Levitra)
Varenicline (Chantix)
Venlafaxine (Effexor, Effexor XR)
Verapamil (Calan, Calan SR, Covera-HS, Verelan, Verelan PM)
Vincristine
Vinorelbine (Navelbine)
Voriconazole (Vfend)
Warfarin (Coumadin, Jantoven)
Zaleplon (Sonata)
Zidovudine (Retrovir)
Zileuton (Zyflo CR)
Zoledronic Acid (Reclast, Zometa)
Zolmitriptan (Zomig, Zomig Nasal Spray, Zomig-ZMT)
Zolpidem (Ambien, Ambien CR)
Zonisamide (Zonegran)

Updated Recommendations for Managing the Care of Patients Receiving Oral Bisphosphonate Therapy

An advisory statement from the American Dental Association Council on Scientific Affairs

Beatrice J. Edwards, MD, FACP; John W. Hellstine, DDs, MS; Peter L. Jacobsen, PhD, DDs; Steven Kaltman, DMD, MD; Angelo Mariotti, DDS, PhD; Cesar A. Migliorati, DDS, MS, PhD; for the American Dental Association Council on Scientific Affairs Expert Panel on Bisphosphonate-Associated Osteonecrosis of the Jaw

Authors' note: This advisory statement was developed as an educational tool on the basis of our opinion after a review of the literature. Because of a paucity of clinical data regarding the management of the dental care of patients receiving oral bisphosphonate therapy, these recommendations are based primarily on expert opinion and are not a product of a systematic review. These recommendations are intended as a resource for dentists to complement their own professional judgment, data obtained from the dental and medical literature and information from the patient's treating physician, and they should be balanced with the practitioner's professional judgment and the individual patient's preferences and needs.

Abstract: Background and Overview. In 2005, the American Dental Association (ADA) Council on Scientific Affairs convened an expert panel to develop clinical recommendations for dentists treating patients who are receiving oral bisphosphonate therapy. The *Journal of the American Dental Association* published the resulting report in 2006. This 2008 advisory statement is the first of projected periodic updates of the 2006 clinical recommendations.

Conclusion. This 2008 advisory statement concludes, on the basis of a review of the current literature, that for patients receiving bisphosphonate therapy, the risk of developing bisphosphonate-associated osteonecrosis (BON) of the jaw apparently remains low.

Dr. Edwards is an associate professor, Department of Medicine and Orthopaedic Surgery, Feinberg School of Medicine, Northwestern University, Chicago; Dr. Hellstein is a clinical professor, Department of Oral Pathology, Radiology and Medicine, University of Iowa, Iowa City; Dr. Jacobsen is an adjunct professor, Department of Pathology and Medicine, Arthur A. Dugoni School of Dentistry, University of the Pacific, San Francisco; Dr. Kaltman is the chairman, Department of Oral Surgery, College of Dental Medicine, Nova Southeastern University, Fort Lauderdale, Fla; Dr. Mariotti is a professor and the chair, Division of Periodontology, College of Dentistry, The Ohio State University, Columbus; Dr. Migliorati is a professor, Department of Diagnostic Sciences—Oral Medicine, College of Dental Medicine, Nova Southeastern University, Fort Lauderdale, Fla.

Address reprint requests to the American Dental Association Council on Scientific Affairs, 211 E. Chicago Ave., Chicago, Ill 60611.

Edwards BJ, Hellstine JW, Jacobsen PL, et al. *JADA*. 2008;139(12):1674-1677. Copyright © 2008 American Dental Association. All rights reserved. Reprinted by permission.

It also newly concludes that current screening and diagnostic tests are unreliable for predicting a patient's risk of developing the condition. This statement updates the 2006 recommendations regarding general dentistry, management of periodontal diseases, implant placement and maintenance, oral and maxillofacial surgery, endodontics, restorative dentistry and prosthodontics, and orthodontics.

Key Words. Bisphosphonate-associated osteonecrosis; osteoporosis; osteonecrosis. *JADA. 2008;139(12):1674-1677.*

The incidence of bisphosphonate-associated osteonecrosis (BON) of the jaw and its concomitant risk factors are not well known. As a result, dentists understandably are concerned about how to appropriately manage the care of patients receiving oral bisphosphonate therapy. The information presented here is a summary of the panel's new report, which updates the 2006 recommendations.[1] (The full report can be accessed at *www.ada.org/prof/resources/topics/topics_osteonecrosis_bisphosphonate_report.pdf.*) [2] On the basis of a review of the current literature, the panel members reiterate their conclusion from the 2006 report: that the risk of developing this condition is low for patients who are receiving oral bisphosphonate therapy. The panel newly concludes that screening tests used for the purpose of determining a patient's risk of developing BON are unreliable.

On the basis of the current literature and of the cases reported so far, the panel concludes that a patient's risk of developing BON of the jaws as a result of oral bisphosphonate therapy is minute as compared with the risk associated with intravenous bisphosphonate therapy in patients with cancer. Accordingly, the majority of reported cases of BON of the jaws have occurred in patients receiving the drugs intravenously for cancer therapy. There are no studies that adequately address the incidence of BON. Studies have estimated that BON occurs in about 20 percent of patients receiving bisphosphonates intravenously for cancer therapy (after extended use of zoledronate) and in between zero and 0.04 percent of patients taking these drugs orally.[3-10] Although total U.S. prescriptions for oral bisphosphonates in 2006 exceeded 30 million,[11] fewer than 10 percent of BON cases are associated with patients taking orally administered bisphosphonate drugs.[3,12]

The small risk of developing BON as a result of receiving oral bisphosphonate therapy must be weighed against the significant health benefits associated with the use of these drugs. Osteoporosis is a major cause of morbidity, functional dependence and institutionalization in older Americans. In 2004, the U.S. surgeon general published a report titled Bone Health and Osteoporosis that highlighted the public health imperative to address osteoporosis and prevent its health-related consequences.[13] Each year, this bone disease accounts for 1.5 million new fractures. Of these fractures, 250,000 are hip fractures that result in mortality rates exceeding 20 percent in women and 30 percent in men, recurrent hospitalizations, increased office visits and, often, the need for care at extended-treatment facilities.[13] In people who sustain hip fractures, less than 25 percent of them regain full function.[14]

All decisions with respect to use of drugs prescribed for medical conditions should be discussed with the prescribing physician. Given the risks associated with osteoporosis and the proven benefits of oral bisphosphonate therapy in treating it, the physician and patient should discuss fully any decision to alter the use of these medications.

RECOMMENDATIONS FOR MANAGEMENT OF DENTAL CARE OF PATIENTS RECEIVING ORAL BISPHOSPHONATE THERAPY

General dentistry. The expert panel makes the following recommendations for the general dental care of patients receiving oral bisphosphonate therapy:

- Routine dental treatment generally should not be modified solely because of the patient's use of oral bisphosphonates.
- All patients should receive routine dental examinations. Patients who are prescribed oral bisphosphonates and are not receiving regular dental care likely would benefit from a comprehensive oral examination before or during the early portion of their bisphosphonate therapeutic regimen.
- All patients taking the drug should be informed that:
  - oral bisphosphonate use places them at very low risk of developing BON of the jaws (the actual incidence is unknown, with estimates ranging from zero to one in 2,260 cases[3,6-10]);
  - the low risk of developing BON may be minimized but not eliminated;
  - an oral health program consisting of sound oral hygiene practices and regular dental care may be the optimal approach for lowering the risk of developing BON;
  - there is no validated diagnostic technique available to determine if patients are at increased risk of developing BON;
  - discontinuing bisphosphonate therapy may not eliminate or reduce the risk of developing BON;
  - if any problem develops in the oral cavity during oral bisphosphonate therapy, the patient should contact a dentist.

A major goal in the prevention of BON is to limit the possibility of extensive or multifocal involvement. Although there is no evidence to support a conservative clinical approach, it may be prudent to proceed conservatively in some cases, potentially allowing the practitioner to gain some insight into how a patient will heal before putting multiple quadrants at risk. On the other hand, periapical pathoses, sinus tracts, purulent periodontal pockets, severe periodontitis and active abscesses that already involve the medullary bone all may exacerbate osteonecrosis, and these areas should be treated immediately even if multiple quadrants are involved.

To the extent possible, the dentist should answer all of the patient's questions regarding bisphosphonate use and the patient's oral health. The dentist should consider documenting the discussion of risks, benefits and treatment options with the patient and obtaining the patient's written acknowledgment of that discussion and consent for the chosen course of treatment.

Management of periodontal diseases. Appropriate forms of nonsurgical therapy should be combined with the commonly recommended reevaluation at four to six weeks. If the disease fails to resolve and surgery becomes necessary, the goal of surgical treatment should be to obtain access to root surfaces. When necessary, the clinician should use modest bone-recontouring techniques. At this time, there is no evidence that periodontal procedures such as guided tissue regeneration or bone replacement grafts increase or decrease the risk of BON development or the success of implant treatment. The clinician should consider the use of such techniques judiciously on the basis of patient need. Primary soft-tissue closure after periodontal surgical procedures is desirable, when feasible.

Implant placement and maintenance. There is a paucity of data regarding the effects of implant placement in patients receiving oral bisphosphonate therapy.[15,16]

Because implant placement requires the preparation of the osteotomy site, the dentist should consider treatment options. The patient may be at increased risk of developing BON when extensive implant placement is necessary or when guided bone regeneration is required to augment a deficient alveolar ridge before implant placement.

Maintenance of implants should follow accepted mechanical and pharmaceutical methods to prevent peri-implantitis, including regular monitoring of the patient. The clinician should consider appropriate forms of nonsurgical therapy combined with a prolonged phase of initial therapy for patients with peri-implantitis. If the disease does not resolve, surgical revision of soft tissues around the implant(s) may be appropriate; when necessary, the clinician also may consider modest bone recontouring.

Oral and maxillofacial surgery. Patients undergoing invasive surgical procedures should be informed of the risk of developing BON, although that risk is small. The clinician should discuss with the patient alternative treatment plans, which include endodontics (endodontic treatment followed by removal of the clinical crown), allowing the roots to exfoliate (instead of extraction) and provision of bridges and partial dentures (instead of implant placement).

If extractions or bone surgery are necessary, the clinician should consider conservative surgical technique with primary tissue closure, when feasible. In addition, immediately before and after any surgical procedures involving bone, the patient should rinse gently with a chlorhexidine-containing rinse until the site has healed. The regimen may be extended on the basis of the patient's healing progress. Use of prophylactic antibiotics after a surgical procedure should be based on the risk of an infection and not on the patient's bisphosphonate therapy. There is no evidence that the use of antibiotics is effective in preventing BON.

Endodontics. Endodontic treatment is preferable to surgical manipulation if a tooth is salvageable. Routine endodontic technique should be used. Manipulation beyond the apex is not recommended. In some situations, depending on risk, the clinician may consider the endodontic treatment of nonrestored teeth after removal of the clinical crown, which allows passive exfoliation of the root tip. Endodontic surgical procedures should be guided by the same recommendation as is used for any oral and maxillofacial surgical procedure described above.

Restorative dentistry and prosthodontics. There is no evidence that malocclusion or masticatory forces increase the risk of developing BON. All routine restorative procedures may be conducted in a patient receiving oral bisphosphonate therapy. Prosthodontic appliances in patients should be adjusted for fit promptly to prevent ulceration and possible bone exposure.

Orthodontics. We found no published studies examining the effect of bisphosphonates on orthodontic treatment. Case reports have recounted inhibited tooth movement in patients receiving bisphosphonates.[17,18] Patients should be advised of this potential complication.

Collagen breakdown product testing and drug holidays. Recently, the use of serum levels of the collagen breakdown product C-terminal cross-linking telopeptide of Type I collagen (CTX) has been advocated as a risk predictor for development of BON.[19] Serum CTX and urinary N-telopeptide of Type I collagen (NTX) are considered markers for bone resorption. Reports suggest that dental treatment decisions should be based on the results of serum CTX/NTX level tests.[19] These recommendations are derived from clinical observations at one institution that have not been validated. It remains to be seen if these recommendations will be corroborated by well-controlled, randomized clinical trials. Therefore, while this expert panel recognizes the value of predicting and mitigating the risk of developing BON in individual patients, until objective research studies document and correlate the specificity, predictive value and reliability of such tests, we can make no recommendations.

CONCLUSION

On the basis of a review of the current literature, the expert panel concludes that the risk of developing BON of the jaw apparently remains low for patients receiving bisphosphonate therapy. Therefore, routine dental treatment generally should not be modified solely because the patient is taking oral bisphosphonates. Furthermore, given the morbidity and mortality associated with osteoporosis and the proven benefits of oral bisphosphonate therapy, patients should not alter their use of these medications without first consulting with their physicians. More research is needed to identify risk factors for developing BON, as well as screening tools to predict patients' risk.

Editor's note: To check for ADA statement updates, visit *www.ada.org/prof/resources/positions/statements/index.asp.*

Disclosure: None of the authors reported any disclosures.

1. American Dental Association Council on Scientific Affairs. Dental management of patients receiving oral bisphosphonate therapy: expert panel recommendations. *JADA*. 2006;137(8):1144-1150.
2. American Dental Association Council on Scientific Affairs. Dental management of patients receiving oral bisphosphonate therapy: expert panel recommendations—report of the Council on Scientific Affairs. "*www.ada.org/prof/resources/topics/topics_osteonecrosis_bisphosphonate_report.pdf*". Accessed Oct. 22, 2008.
3. Grbic JT, Landesberg R, Lin SQ, et al. Incidence of osteonecrosis of the jaw in women with postmenopausal osteoporosis in the Health Outcomes and Reduced Incidence With Zoledronic Acid Once Yearly Pivotal Fracture Trial. *JADA* 2008;139(1):32-40.
4. Bilezikian JP. Osteonecrosis of the jaw: do bisphosphonates pose a risk? *N Engl J Med*. 2006;355(22):2278-2281.
5. Boonyapakorn T, Schirmer I, Reichart PA, Sturm I, Massenkeil G. Bisphosphonate-induced osteonecrosis of the jaws: prospective study of 80 patients with multiple myeloma and other malignancies. *Oral Oncol*. 2008;44(9):857-869.
6. Felsenberg D, Hoffmeister B, Amling M. Bisphosphonattherapie assoziierte. *Kiefernekrosen Deutsches Arzteblatt*. 2006;46: A3078-A3080.
7. Mavrokokki T, Cheng A, Stein B, Goss A. Nature and frequency of bisphosphonate-associated osteonecrosis of the jaws in Australia. *J Oral Maxillofac Surg*. 2007;65(3):415-423.
8. Black DM, Delmas PD, Eastell R, et al.; HORIZON Pivotal Fracture Trial. Once-yearly zoledronic acid for treatment of postmenopausal osteoporosis. *N Engl J Med*. 2007;356(18):1809-1822.
9. Etminan M, Aminzadeh K, Matthew IR, Brophy JM. Use of oral bisphosphonates and the risk of aseptic osteonecrosis: a nested case control study. *J Rheumatol*. 2008;35(4):691-695.
10. Cartsos VM, Zhu S, Zavras AI. Bisphosphonate use and the risk of adverse jaw outcomes. *JADA*. 2008;139(1):23-30.
11. DrugTopics. Top 200 brand-name drugs by units in 2006. "*www.drugtopics.com/drugtopics/Pharmacy+Facts+And+Figures/Top-200-brand-name-drugs-by-units-in-2006/ArticleStandard/Article/detail/407649?contextCategoryId=7604*". Accessed Sept. 12, 2007.
12. Ruggiero SL, Mehrotra B, Rosenberg TJ, Engroff SL. Osteonecrosis of the jaws associated with the use of bisphosphonates: a review of 63 cases. *J Oral Maxillofac Surg*. 2004;62(5):527-534.
13. U.S. Department of Health & Human Services. Bone health and osteoporosis: a report of the surgeon general (2004). "*www.surgeongeneral.gov/library/bonehealth/content.html*". Accessed Oct. 2, 2008.
14. Cummings SR, Melton LJ. Epidemiology and outcomes of osteoporotic fractures. *Lancet*. 2002;359(9319):1761-1767.
15. Jeffcoat MK. Safety of oral bisphosphonates: controlled studies on alveolar bone. *Int J Oral Maxillofac Implants*. 2006;21(3):349-353.
16. Wang HL, Weber D, McCauley LK. Effect of long-term oral bisphosphonates on implant wound healing: literature review and a case report. *J Periodontol*. 2007;78(3):584-594.
17. Schwartz JE. Ask us: some drugs affect tooth movement. *Am J Orthod Dentofacial Orthop*. 2005;127(6):644.
18. Rinchuse DJ, Rinchuse DJ, Sosovicka MF, Robison JM, Pendleton R. Orthodontic treatment of patients using bisphosphonates: a report of 2 cases. *Am J Orthod Dentofacial Orthop*. 2007;131(3):321-326.
19. Marx RE, Cillo JE, Ulloa JJ. Oral bisphosphonate-induced osteonecrosis: risk factors, prediction of risk using serum CTX testing, prevention, and treatment. *J Oral Maxillofac Surg*. 2007;65(12):2397-2410.

Substance Abuse

It is important that the dentist be aware of a patient's substance abuse history. Questions included in the ADA health history form will help the dentist do this. It should be noted that the use of this information will be subject to state confidentiality law, and possibly the federal Health Insurance Portability and Accountability Act (HIPAA) privacy regulations, and also may be subject to federal, state, and local antidiscrimination laws. Information related to substance abuse treatment is subject to special federal confidentiality protection (under the U.S. Code of Federal Regulations, Title 42, Chapter 1, Part 2, Confidentiality of Alcohol and Drug Abuse Patient Records) and may not be redisclosed without express written permission of the patient.

Some patients may not reveal their history of substance abuse out of shame or fear of judgment or because they do not understand how important this information is to their dental treatment. Therefore, it is important that dentists are aware of the signs and symptoms of substance abuse. The tables on the following pages provide general information on commonly abused substances.

CONTROLLED SUBSTANCES: USES AND EFFECTS

DRUGS	CSA SCHEDULES	TRADE OR OTHER NAMES	MEDICAL USES	PHYSICAL DEPENDENCE
ANABOLIC STEROIDS				
Nandrolone (decanoate, phenpropionate)	III		Anemia, breast cancer	Unknown
Oxymetholone	III	Anadrol-50	Anemia	Unknown
Testosterone (cypionate, enanthate)	III	Depo-Testosterone, Delatestryl	Hypogonadism	Unknown
CANNABIS				
Hashish and hashish oil	I	Hash, Hash Oil	None	Unknown
Marijuana	I	Pot, Acapulco Gold, Grass, Reefer, Sinsemilla, Thai Sticks	None	Unknown
Tetrahydrocannabinol	I,II	THC, Marinol	Antinauseant	Unknown
DEPRESSANTS				
Barbiturates	II,III,IV	Fiorinal, Nembutal, Seconal, Phenobarbital, Pentobarbital	Anesthetic, anticonvulsant, sedative hypnotic, veterinary euthanasia agent	High-Moderate
Benzodiazepines	IV	Ativan, Dalmane, Diazepam, Librium, Xanax, Serax, Valium, Tranxene, Verstran, Versed, Halcion, Restoril	Antianxiety, sedative, anticonvulsant, hypnotic	Low
Chloral hydrate	IV	Noctec, Somnos, Felsules	Hypnotic	Moderate
Other depressants	I,II,III,IV	Equanil, Miltown, Noludar, Placidyl, Valmid, Methaqualone	Antianxiety, sedative, hypnotic	Moderate
HALLUCINOGENS				
Amphetamine variants	I	2, 5-DMA, STP, MDA (DOM), MDMA (Ecstasy), DOB	None	Unknown
LSD	I	Acid, Microdot	None	None
Mescaline and peyote	I	Mescal, Buttons, Cactus	None	None
Phencyclidine and analogs	I,II	PCE, PCPy, TCP, PCP, Hog, Loveboat, Angel Dust	None	Unknown
Other hallucinogens	I	Bufotenine, Ibogaine, DMT, DET, Psilocybin, Psilocyn	None	None

PSYCHOLOGICAL DEPENDENCE	TOLERANCE	DURATION (HOURS)	USUAL METHOD	POSSIBLE EFFECTS	EFFECTS OF OVERDOSE	WITHDRAWAL SYNDROME
ANABOLIC STEROIDS						
Unknown	Unknown	14-21 days	Injected	Virilization, acne, testicular atrophy, gynecomastia, aggressive behavior, edema	Unknown	Possible depression
Unknown	Unknown	24	Oral			
Unknown	Unknown	14-28 days	Injected			
CANNABIS						
Moderate	Yes	2.0-4	Smoked, oral	Euphoria, relaxed inhibitions, increased appetite, disorientation	Fatigue, paranoia, possible psychosis	Occasional reports of insomnia, hyperactivity, decreased appetite
Moderate	Yes	2.0-4	Smoked, oral			
Moderate	Yes	2.0-4	Smoked, oral			
DEPRESSANTS						
High-Moderate	Yes	1.0-16	Oral, injected	Slurred speech, disorientation, drunken behavior without odor of alcohol	Shallow respiration, clammy skin, dilated pupils, weak and rapid pulse, coma, possible death	Anxiety, insomnia, tremors, delirium, convulsions, possible death
Low	Yes	4.0-8	Oral, injected			
Moderate	Yes	5.0-8	Oral			
Moderate	Yes	4.0-8	Oral			
HALLUCINOGENS						
Unknown	Yes	Variable	Oral, injected	Illusions and hallucinations, altered perception of time and distance	Longer, more intense "trip" episodes, psychosis, possible death	Unknown
Unknown	Yes	8.0-12	Oral			
Unknown	Yes	8.0-12	Oral			
High	Yes	Days	Smoked, oral			
Unknown	Possible	Variable	Smoked, oral, injected, sniffed			

CONTROLLED SUBSTANCES: USES AND EFFECTS *(cont.)*

DRUGS	CSA SCHEDULES	TRADE OR OTHER NAMES	MEDICAL USES	PHYSICAL DEPENDENCE
NARCOTICS				
Codeine	II,III,V	Tylenol w/Codeine, Empirin w/Codeine, Robitussin A-C, Fiorinal w/Codeine	Analgesic, antitussive	Moderate
Fentanyl and analogs	I,II	Sublimaze, Alfenta, Sufenta, Duragesic	Analgesic, adjunct to anesthesia, anesthetic	High
Heroin	I	Diacetylmorphine, Horse, Smack	None in U.S., analgesic, antitussive	High
Hydrocodone	II,III	Lorcet, Tussionex, Vicodin	Analgesic, antitussive	High
Hydromorphone	II	Dilaudid	Analgesic	High
Methadone and LAAM	I,II	Dolophine, Methadose, Levoalphaacetylmethadol, Levomethadyl acetate	Analgesic, treatment of dependence	High
Morphine	II	Duramorph, MS-Contin, Roxanol, Oramorph SR	Analgesic	High
Oxycodone	II	Percodan, Percocet, Tylox, Roxicet, Roxicodone	Analgesic	High
Other narcotics	II,III,IV,V	Opium, Darvon, Talwin*, Buprenorphine, Meperidine (Pethidine), Demerol	Analgesic, antidiarrheal	High-Low
STIMULANTS				
Amphetamine/ methamphetamine	II	Desoxyn, Dexedrine, Obetrol, Ice	Attention deficit disorder, narcolepsy, weight control	Possible
Cocaine†	II	Coke, Flake, Snow, Crack	Local anesthetic	Possible
Methylphenidate	II	Ritalin	Attention deficit disorder, narcolepsy	Possible
Other stimulants	I,II,III,IV	Adipex, Didrex, Ionamin	Weight control	Possible

*Designated a narcotic under the Controlled Substances Act (CSA).
†Not designated a narcotic under the CSA.

PSYCHOLOGICAL DEPENDENCE	TOLERANCE	DURATION (HOURS)	USUAL METHOD	POSSIBLE EFFECTS	EFFECTS OF OVERDOSE	WITHDRAWAL SYNDROME
NARCOTICS						
Moderate	Yes	3.0-6	Oral, injected	Euphoria, drowsiness, respiratory depression, constricted pupils, nausea	Slow and shallow breathing, clammy skin, convulsions, coma, possible death	Watery eyes, runny nose, yawning, loss of appetite, irritability, tremors, panic, cramps, nausea, chills, sweating
High	Yes	10.0-72	Injected, transdermal patch			
High	Yes	3.0-6	Injected, sniffed, smoked			
High	Yes	3.0-6	Oral			
High	Yes	3.0-6	Oral, injected			
High	Yes	12.0-72	Oral, injected			
High	Yes	3.0-6	Oral, smoked, injected			
High	Yes	4.0-5	Oral			
High-Low	Yes	Variable	Oral, injected			
STIMULANTS						
High	Yes	2.0-4	Oral, injected, smoked	Increased alertness, excitation, euphoria, increased pulse rate and blood pressure, insomnia, loss of appetite	Agitation, increased body temperature, hallucination, convulsions, possible death	Apathy, long periods of sleep, irritability, depression, disorientation
High	Yes	1.0-2	Sniffed, smoked, injected			
High	Yes	2.0-4	Oral, injected			
High	Yes	2.0-4	Oral, injected			

SUBSTANCES OF ABUSE: DENTAL IMPLICATIONS

ABUSED SUBSTANCE	FACTS TO AID IN DIAGNOSIS	DRUGS THAT MAY INTERACT	DENTAL IMPLICATIONS
ALCOHOL			
	Patient may appear drunk or drowsy and have slurred speech. Odor of alcohol, heavy cologne, mouthwash, fruity acetone breath may be present. Patient may have difficulty maintaining position of head. Periodontal disease does not respond to therapy.	Other central nervous system (CNS) depressants (such as opioid analgesics) enhance alcohol-induced respiratory depression. Metronidazole interacts with alcohol to produce flushing, hypotension, nausea, and vomiting.	Alcohol-containing mouthrinses and liquid medications that contain high concentrations of alcohol should be avoided in dental treatment of recovering alcoholics. Recovering alcoholics with liver disease may require a lower dose of medications containing acetaminophen. Periodontal disease does not respond to therapy.
AMPHETAMINES/METHAMPHETAMINES AND DERIVATIVES (SUCH AS ECSTASY, MDMA)			
	Patient may act jittery, irritable, unable to sit still, extremely talkative, verbose, exaggerated behavior. Patient may exhibit tremors, dilated pupils, increased blood pressure and heart rate.	Intravascular injection of local anesthetics containing vasoconstrictors may enhance amphetamine-induced increase in blood pressure.	Measure blood pressure preoperatively; if high (systolic ≥180mm or diastolic ≥110mm), postpone treatment and refer to source of care. If patient is suspected of use of these drugs within 24 hrs, avoid local anesthetics containing vasoconstrictors; local anesthetics without vasoconstrictors may be used. Methamphetamine users have been reported to have high caries index; Ecstasy (MDMA, MDA, MDEA, PMA) users brux and may display wear facets and request fabrication of bite guard.
BARBITURATES AND GAMMAHYDROXYBUTYRATES (GHB, LIQUID X, HUG DRUG)			
	Patient may appear drunk or drowsy and have slurred speech. Patient may have difficulty maintaining position of head.	Other CNS depressants (such as opioid analgesics) may enhance barbiturate-induced respiratory depression.	Dose of opioids should be reduced to avoid enhanced respiratory depression.
BENZODIAZEPINES (ALPRAZOLAM [XANAX], CLONAZEPAM [KLONOPIN])			
	These CNS depressants are favorites among drug abusers.	Benzodiazepines may enhance opioid-induced respiratory depression.	Dose of opioids should be reduced to avoid enhanced respiratory depression. Xerostomia is a frequent side effect and may lead to increased caries. Although carisoprodol (Soma) is not considered a benzodiazepine and is not classified as a controlled substance by the Drug Enforcement Administration, it is often requested by the drug abuser to enhance the opioid-induced euphoria or "high."
COCAINE			
	Patient may act jittery, irritable, unable to sit still. Patient may exhibit tremors, dilated pupils, increased blood pressure and heart rate.	Intravascular injection of local anesthetics containing vasoconstrictors may enhance cocaine-induced increase in blood pressure and heart rate; cardiac arrest.	Measure blood pressure preoperatively; if high (systolic ≥180mm or diastolic ≥110mm), postpone treatment and refer to source of care. If patient is suspected of use of these drugs within 6 h, avoid local anesthetics containing vasoconstrictors; local anesthetics without vasoconstrictors may be used.
INHALANTS			
	Most, if not all, inhalants are excreted via the lungs. Patient who has abused an inhalant within a few hours will have an odor on breath.	Most inhalants are CNS depressants. Other CNS depressants (such as opioid analgesics) may enhance inhalant-induced respiratory depression.	Chronic inhalant abuse may cause liver damage, decreasing rate of inactivation of prescribed or over-the-counter drugs such as acetaminophen and thus increasing their toxicity.

ABUSED SUBSTANCE	FACTS TO AID IN DIAGNOSIS	DRUGS THAT MAY INTERACT	DENTAL IMPLICATIONS
LYSERGIC ACID DIETHYLAMIDE (LSD)			
	Patient may appear disoriented and confused. Patient may exhibit dilated pupils, increased blood pressure, and heart rate.	No confirmed interactions with dental drugs.	None of significance to dentistry.
MARIJUANA			
	Patient may appear sedated and lethargic and have bloodshot eyes. Heart rate may be increased but blood pressure will be decreased.	No confirmed interactions with dental drugs.	None of significance to dentistry.
NICOTINE			
	Patient may have history of use. Patient may exhibit staining of teeth and oral tissues, malodor characteristic of smokers.	No confirmed interactions with dental drugs.	See Appendix R, Cessation of Tobacco Use.
OPIOIDS			
	Patient may appear drowsy, lethargic, disoriented, and confused. Pupils may be constricted. Arms may exhibit scars from previous injuries or needle marks.	Other CNS depressants (such as sedatives or hypnotics) may enhance opioid-induced respiratory depression. Patients taking naltrexone, an opioid antagonist, during recovery may exhibit decreased effect of opioid analgesics.	Opioid users in recovery or actively using drugs may require increased dose of opioid analgesics to achieve analgesia. Avoid prescribing opioid-type analgesics postoperatively in patients recovering from opioid addiction. Opioid users exhibit profound xerostomia with increased craving for sweets, resulting in rampant caries.
PHENCYCLIDINE HYDROCHLORIDE (PCP, ANGEL DUST) AND KETAMINE (VITAMIN K, KETALAR, CAT TRANQUILIZER, K)			
	This anesthetic agent may program CNS depression with paradoxical CNS excitation accompanied by hallucinations.	Other CNS depressants may enhance PCP-induced respiratory depression.	None of significance to dentistry.

Note: As a general rule, patients in recovery from chemical dependency, including alcohol, should not be given any psychoactive drug, such as nitrous oxide or benzodiazepines.

Cessation of Tobacco Use

Dentists may be the first healthcare providers exposed to the signs and symptoms of oral cancer and other diseases that result from smoking or using smokeless tobacco. Signs and symptoms related to cancer may include oral sores that do not heal; lumps in the head and neck region; thickened white, red, or mixed patches on the oral mucosa (oral leukoplakia); or difficulty in chewing, swallowing, or moving the tongue or jaw. The importance of a thorough dental examination for patients who use tobacco products cannot be overemphasized. Careful extra- and intraoral examination may lead to early detection and may decrease the chance for metastases to occur. Some forms of oral malignancies are aggressive, so prompt diagnosis is critical. Beyond this, the correlation between tobacco use in a variety of forms with a variety of oral diseases and nonoral diseases that are expressed in the mouth warrants careful evaluation of patients who use tobacco products.

Helping patients quit is practical in every clinical setting and can be done by any clinician. A few moments of assistance from a clinician can be significantly more effective than self-help methods. Minimum assistance includes identifying whether patients use tobacco; advising users to stop; strengthening their interest in quitting and, for those who make a commitment to quit, equipping them with coping skills needed during the quitting process; encouraging extra-treatment social support; and providing clinical follow-up support. Nicotine patches, polacrilex gum, polacrilex lozenges, nasal sprays, and oral inhalers used alone or together with non-nicotine pharmacotherapy are to be used in combination with, not as substitutes for, support and follow-up programs. The tables on the following pages provide general usage and prescribing information for smoking cessation products.

PRESCRIBING INFORMATION FOR TOBACCO-USE CESSATION PRODUCTS

NAME	FORM/ STRENGTH	DOSAGE	WARNINGS/PRECAUTIONS & CONTRAINDICATIONS	ADVERSE EFFECTS†
CENTRALLY ACTING NON-NICOTINE AGENTS				
Bupropion SR (Zyban)	**Tab, Extended Release:** 150mg	***Adults:* ≥18 yrs: Initial:** 150mg qd for 3 days while still smoking. Set target quit date within the first 2 wks. **Usual:** 150mg bid. Separate dose intervals by at least 8 hrs. **Max:** 300mg/day. Treat for 7-12 wks; d/c at 7 wks if no progress is seen. **Renal/Hepatic Dysfunction:** Reduce dose. **Severe Hepatic Cirrhosis:** 150mg every other day.	**BB:** D/C immediately if agitation, hostility, depressed mood, or changes in thinking or behavior that are not typical for the patient are observed, or if suicidal ideation or behavior occurs. **W/P:** Dose-related risk of seizures. D/C and do not restart if seizure occurs. Extreme caution with history of seizure, cranial trauma, severe hepatic cirrhosis. Caution with recent MI, unstable heart disease, renal impairment. Agitation, insomnia, psychosis, confusion, and other neuropsychiatric phenomena reported. Allergic reactions, HTN reported. May precipitate manic episodes in bipolar disorder. **Contra:** Seizure disorder, bulimia, or anorexia nervosa; within 14 days of MAOIs, other forms of bupropion; abrupt discontinuation of alcohol or sedatives. **P/N:** Pregnancy B, not for use in nursing.	**Dry mouth**, insomnia, seizures (dose-dependent), arthralgia, dizziness, nausea, pruritus, rash, diarrhea, constipation, abnormal dreams, disturbed concentration
Varenicline (Chantix)	**Tab:** 0.5mg, 1.0mg; (Starting Pack) 1 card-0.5mg x 11 tabs, 3 cards-1.0mg x 14 tabs; (Continuing Pack) 4 cards-1.0 mg x 14 tabs	***Adults:* ≥18 yrs: Days 1-3:** 0.5mg qd. **Days 4-7:** 0.5mg bid. **Day 8-End of treatment:** 1mg bid. **Severe Renal Impairment: Initial:** 0.5mg qd. **Titrate: Max:** 0.5mg bid. **End-Stage Renal Disease: Max:** 0.5mg qd.	**BB:** D/C immediately if agitation, hostility, depressed mood, or changes in thinking or behavior that are not typical for the patient are observed, or if suicidal ideation or behavior occurs. **W/P:** Serious neuropsychiatric symptoms (eg, changes in behavior, agitation, depressed mood, suicidal ideation, suicidal behavior) reported. Physiological changes resulting from smoking cessation may alter pharmacokinetics or pharmacodynamics of some drugs (eg, theophylline, warfarin, insulin). Use caution while driving or operating machinery until the effects of varenicline are known. **P/N:** Pregnancy C, not for use in nursing.	N/V, sleep disturbance, constipation, flatulence, abdominal pain, headache, fatigue, increased appetite, abnormal dreams
NICOTINE INHALATION SYSTEM				
Nicotine inhalation system (Nicotrol Inhaler)	**Inhaler:** 10mg of nicotine [168 cartridges]	***Adults:* Initial:** Individualize dose. **Usual:** 6-16 cartridges/day. **Max:** 16 cartridges/day for 12 wks. Best effect achieved by frequent continuous puffing (20 min). Continue for 3 mos. Wean by gradual reduction of daily dose over the following 6-12 wks. Do not treat >6 mos.	**W/P:** Can be toxic and addictive. Stop smoking completely before start of therapy. May cause bronchospasm; caution with bronchospastic disease. Caution with coronary heart disease, arrhythmias, vasospastic diseases, renal/hepatic insufficiency, hyperthyroidism, pheochromocytoma, insulin-dependent diabetes, active peptic ulcers, and in elderly. Tachycardia and palpitations reported; avoid in post-MI, severe arrhythmias, severe or worsening angina. Increased risk for malignant HTN with accelerated HTN. **Contra:** Hypersensitivity or allergy to menthol. **P/N:** Category D, not for use in nursing.	**Cough,** rhinitis, sinusitis, **tooth disorders, pain in jaw** and neck, **taste alterations,** dyspepsia, nausea, diarrhea, hiccups, mouth and throat irritation, sleep disorder, dizziness, anxiety, fatigue

†Bold entries denote special dental considerations.
BB = black box warning; **W/P** = warnings/precautions; **Contra** = contraindications; **P/N** = pregnancy category rating and nursing considerations.

PRESCRIBING INFORMATION FOR TOBACCO-USE CESSATION PRODUCTS *(cont.)*

NAME	FORM/ STRENGTH	DOSAGE	WARNINGS/PRECAUTIONS & CONTRAINDICATIONS	ADVERSE EFFECTS†
NICOTINE NASAL SPRAY				
Nicotine nasal spray (Nicotrol NS)	**Spray:** 10mg/mL [10mL bottles]	***Adults:*** Stop smoking and other nicotine products completely before use. **Initial:** 2-4 sprays/hr. **Max:** 10 sprays/hr, for up to 8 wks. **Min per day:** 16 sprays/day. **Max per day:** 80 sprays/day. **Elderly:** Start at low end of the dosing range. May d/c abruptly or over 4-6 wks. Do not treat >3 mos. Do not sniff, swallow, or inhale through nose as spray is being administered; wait 2-3 min before blowing nose. Tilt head back slightly to administer.	**W/P:** Avoid with known chronic nasal disorders. Can be toxic and addictive. Stop smoking completely before start of therapy. May cause bronchospasm; caution with bronchospastic disease. Caution with coronary heart disease, arrhythmias, vasospastic diseases, renal or hepatic insufficiency, hyperthyroidism, pheochromocytoma, insulin-dependent diabetes, active peptic ulcers, and elderly. Tachycardia and palpitations reported. Increased risk for malignant HTN with accelerated HTN. **P/N:** Category D, not for use in nursing.	Runny nose, hot/peppery feeling in back of throat or nose, watery eyes, sneezing, **cough**, headache, dizziness
NICOTINE POLACRILEX GUM				
Nicotine polacrilex gum (Nicorette Original, Nicorette Mint, Nicorette Fresh Mint, Nicorette White Ice Mint, Nicorette Fruit Chill, and Nicorette Cinnamon Surge)	**Gum:** 2mg, 4mg	***Adults:*** Stop smoking and other nicotine products completely before use. **<25 Cigarettes/Day:** 2mg. **>25 Cigarettes/Day:** 4mg. Chew 1 piece for 30 minutes q1-2h for 6 wks, then 1 piece q2-4h for 3 wks, then 1 piece q4-8h for 3 wks. **Max:** 24 pieces/day for 12 wks. Do not eat/drink for 15 min before or while chewing gum. Chew until tingling feeling (nicotine release). When tingling stops, resume chewing. Do not swallow saliva when tingling is felt.	**W/P:** Do not use if continuing to smoke, chew tobacco, use snuff, nicotine patch, or other nicotine products. Caution with heart disease, recent MI, irregular heartbeat, HTN, stomach ulcers. May increase BP and HR. D/C with mouth, teeth, or jaw problems, or with symptoms of nicotine overdose (N/V, dizziness, weakness, palpitations). Use under medical supervision if <18 yrs. **P/N:** Safety in pregnancy and nursing is not known.	***Common side effects:*** **mouth, teeth, or jaw pain;** nausea; heartburn; hiccups; **teeth alterations** ***Severe side effects:*** vomiting, dizziness, weakness, sweating, irregular heartbeat, allergic reaction (redness, itchiness, hives, trouble breathing)
NICOTINE POLACRILEX LOZENGE				
Nicotine polacrilex lozenge (Commit)	**Loz:** 2mg, 4mg	***Adults:*** Stop smoking and other nicotine products completely before use. **Time to 1st Cigarette ≤30 min of Waking:** 4mg. **Time to 1st Cigarette is >30 min of Waking:** 2mg. **Weeks 1-6:** 1 loz q1-2h. **Weeks 7-9:** 1 loz q2-4h. **Weeks 10-12:** 1 loz q4-8h. **Max:** 5 loz/6 hrs or 20 loz/day. Dissolve loz in mouth for 20-30 min (minimize swallowing) moving it from one side of mouth to other. Do not chew or swallow whole. Do not eat/drink for 15 min before or during use.	**W/P:** Do not use if continuing to smoke, chew tobacco, use snuff, nicotine patch, or other nicotine products. Caution with heart disease, recent MI, irregular heartbeat, HTN, stomach ulcers, or diabetes. May increase BP and HR. D/C with mouth problems, persistent indigestion, severe sore throat, palpitations, irregular heartbeat, or with symptoms of nicotine overdose (N/V, dizziness, weakness, palpitations). Contains phenylalanine. Use 1 loz at a time. Do not continuously use one after another. Use under medical supervision if <18 yrs of age. **P/N:** Safety in pregnancy and nursing is not known.	***Common side effects:*** sore throat, **mouth problems,** heartburn ***Severe side effects:*** vomiting, dizziness, fatigue, sweating, irregular heartbeat, allergic reaction (redness, itchiness, hives, trouble breathing)
NICOTINE TRANSDERMAL SYSTEM				
Nicotine transdermal patches (Habitrol, Nicoderm CQ)	**Patch:** 7mg, 14mg, 21mg	***Adults:*** Stop smoking and other nicotine products completely. **>10 Cigarettes/day:** 21mg qd for 6 wks, then 14mg qd for 2 wks, then 7mg qd for 2 wks, then d/c. **≤10 Cigarettes/day:** 14mg qd for 6 wks, then 7mg qd for 2 wks, then d/c. Apply to clean, dry, hairless area; hold for 10 seconds and wash hands. Rotate application sites. Remove after 16 or 24 hrs; if craving for cigarettes upon waking up, wear patch for 24 hrs. If vivid dreams occur, remove before sleep. Do not wear >1 patch at a time. Do not cut patch in half. Do not use same patch >24 hrs.	**W/P:** Avoid with serious arrhythmias, severe or worsening angina, accelerated HTN, and immediately post-MI. Tachycardia, palpitations reported. D/C with irregular heartbeat, palpitations, symptoms of nicotine overdose (eg, N/V, dizziness, weakness, rapid heartbeat), skin redness or swelling, or rash >4 days. Avoid creams or lotions at application site. **P/N:** Safety in pregnancy and nursing is not known.	***Common side effects:*** vivid dreams or sleep disturbances, headache, nausea, upset stomach, and dizziness ***Severe side effects:*** skin redness, irregular heartbeats or palpitations, vomiting, fatigue, rapid heartbeat

†Bold entries denote special dental considerations.
BB = black box warning; **W/P** = warnings/precautions; **Contra** = contraindications; **P/N** = pregnancy category rating and nursing considerations.

DRUG INTERACTIONS FOR TOBACCO-USE CESSATION PRODUCTS

CENTRALLY ACTING NON-NICOTINE AGENT

Bupropion SR (Zyban)	
Alcohol	Excessive use with or abrupt discontinuation of alcohol increases the risk of seizures; minimize or avoid use of alcohol.
Amantadine	Caution; use low initial dose and gradually titrate bupropion.
Anoretics	Increased risk of seizures with concomitant use.
Antiarrhythmics, Class 1C	Caution with concomitant use; use low initial dose and gradually titrate concomitant Class 1C antiarrhythmic.
Antidepressants	Extreme caution with concomitant use.
Antidiabetic agents, oral	Increased risk of seizures with concomitant use.
Antipsychotics	Extreme caution with concomitant use.
Benzodiazepines	Excessive use with or abrupt discontinuation of benzodiazepines increases the risk of seizures.
β-Blockers	Caution with concomitant use; use low initial dose and gradually titrate concomitant β-blocker.
Bupropion-containing drugs	Avoid concomitant use with other drugs containing bupropion.
Carbamazepine	Concomitant use may induce the metabolism of bupropion.
Cimetidine	Concomitant use may inhibit the metabolism of bupropion.
Cocaine	Increased risk of seizures in patients addicted to cocaine.
Cyclophosphamide	Caution with concomitant use.
CYP2B6 substrates or inhibitors	Caution with concomitant use.
CYP2D6 substrates	Caution with concomitant use; use low initial dose and gradually titrate concomitant drug.
Insulin	Increased risk of seizures with concomitant use.
Levodopa	Caution with concomitant use; use low initial dose and gradually titrate buproprion.
MAO inhibitors	Concomitant use is contraindicated; at least 14 days should elapse between stopping an MAOI and starting bupropion.
Nicotine transdermal system	Monitor for signs and symptoms of hypertension.
Opioids	Increased risk of seizures in patients addicted to opioids.
Orphenadrine	Caution with concomitant use.
Phenobarbital	Concomitant use may induce the metabolism of bupropion.
Phenytoin	Concomitant use may induce the metabolism of bupropion.
Sedatives	Excessive use with or abrupt discontinuation of sedatives increases the risk of seizures.
Seizure threshold, drugs lowering	Extreme caution with drugs lowering seizure threshold.
SSRIs	Caution with concomitant use; use low initial dose and gradually titrate concomitant SSRI.

DRUG INTERACTIONS FOR TOBACCO-USE CESSATION PRODUCTS *(cont.)*

CENTRALLY ACTING NON-NICOTINE AGENT *(cont.)*

Bupropion SR (Zyban) *(cont.)*	
Steroids, systemic	Extreme caution with systemic corticosteroids.
Stimulants	Increased risk of seizures in patients addicted to stimulants or who are using OTC stimulants.
TCAs	Caution with concomitant use; use low initial dose and gradually titrate concomitant TCA.
Theophylline	Extreme caution with theophylline.
Varenicline tartrate (Chantix)	
Cimetidine	Concomitant use reduces the renal clearance of varenicline.
Nicotine replacement therapy (NRT)	Concomitant use may lead to an increased amount of adverse effects (eg, headache, N/V).

NICOTINE-CONTAINING PRODUCTS

Nicotine (Commit, Habitrol, Nicoderm CQ, Nicorette, Nicotrol Inhaler, Nicotrol Nasal Spray)	
Acetaminophen	May require dosage reduction of APAP following smoking cessation.
Adrenergic antagonists	May require dosage reduction of adrenergic antagonists (eg, prazosin) following smoking cessation.
Antiasthmatic agents	Concomitant use may require dosage adjustment of antiasthmatic agents.
Antidepressants	Concomitant use may require dosage adjustment of antidepressants (eg, TCAs).
β-Blockers	May require dosage reduction of β-blockers (eg, propranolol) following smoking cessation.
Caffeine	May require reduction of caffeine following smoking cessation.
Coffee	Concomitant use reduces the effects of nicotine.
Insulin	Concomitant use may require dosage adjustment of insulin.
Nicotine	Avoid concomitant use with other products containing nicotine (eg, cigarettes, chewing tobacco).
Oxazepam	May require dosage reduction of oxazepam following smoking cessation.
Pentazocine	May require dosage reduction of pentazocine following smoking cessation.
Theophylline	May require dosage adjustment of theophylline following smoking cessation.

Index

In this index, dental indications are in boldface type. Drug information found in tables is indicated by "t" after the page numbers; drugs are listed by both generic and brand names. Products that have the ADA Seal of Acceptance are indicated with a star (★).

A

E

F

H

J

K

L

M

Q

R

U

V

W

X